HERNIA

FOURTH EDITION

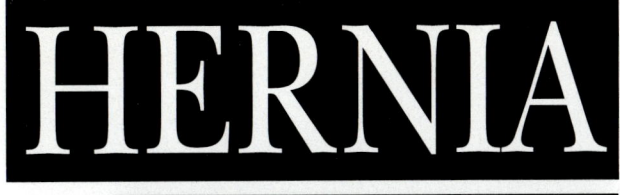

HERNIA

EDITED BY

LLOYD M. NYHUS, MD, Dres.h.c.

Warren H. Cole Professor and Head Emeritus
Department of Surgery
University of Illinois College of Medicine at Chicago
Surgeon in Chief Emeritus
University of Illinois Hospital
Chicago, Illinois

ROBERT E. CONDON, MD

Ausman Foundation Professor and Chairman
Department of Surgery
Medical College of Wisconsin
Surgeon in Chief
Froedtert Memorial Lutheran Hospital
Milwaukee, Wisconsin

FOREWORD BY

KEITH A. KELLY, MD

WITH 75 CONTRIBUTORS

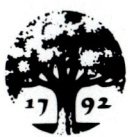

J. B. LIPPINCOTT COMPANY
PHILADELPHIA

Acquisitions Editor: Lisa McAllister
Sponsoring Editor: Paula Callaghan
Project Editor: Jody E. Gould
Indexer: Betty Herr Hallinger
Senior Design Coordinator: Kathy Kelley-Luedtke
Cover Designer: Larry Pezzato
Production Manager: Caren Erlichman
Senior Production Coordinator: Kevin P. Johnson
Compositor: Compset Inc.
Printer/Binder: Walsworth Publishing Company

Fourth Edition

6   5   4   3   2   1

Library of Congress Cataloging-in-Publication Data

Hernia / edited by Lloyd M. Nyhus, Robert E. Condon; with 75
  contributors; foreword by Keith Kelly. — 4th ed.
       p.   cm.
    Includes bibliographical references and index.
    ISBN 0-397-51286-4
    1. Hernia.   I. Nyhus, Lloyd M. (Lloyd Milton).
  II. Condon, Robert E. (Robert Edward).
    [DNLM: 1. Hernia.   WI 950 H558 1995]
  RD621.H47   1995
  617.5'59—dc20
  DNLM/DLC
  for Library of Congress   94-21056
                                                            CIP

♾ This paper meets the requirements of ANSI/NISO Z39.48–1992
(permanence of paper).

The authors and publisher have exerted every effort to ensure that drug
selection and dosage set forth in this text are in accord with current
recommendations and practice at the time of publication. However, in
view of ongoing research, changes in government regulations, and the
constant flow of information relating to drug therapy and drug
reactions, the reader is urged to check the package insert for each drug
for any change in indications and dosage and for added warnings and
precautions. This is particularly important when the recommended
agent is a new or infrequently employed drug.

Contributors

Barry Altman, MD
Associate Professor of Clinical Surgery
New York Medical College
Valhalla, New York
Director, Department of Surgery
White Plains Hospital
White Plains, New York

Parviz K. Amid, MD
Harbor-UCLA Research and Education Institute
Cedars-Sinai Medical Center
Los Angeles, California

Ricardo G. Annibali, MD
Department of Surgery One
Valduce Hospital
Como, Italy

David A. Appel, MD
Resident of General Surgery
Medical College of Wisconsin
Milwaukee, Wisconsin

Robert Bendavid, MD
Shouldice Hospital
Thornhill, Ontario, Canada

Jack Marshall Bergstein, MD
Assistant Professor of Surgery
Section of Trauma and Emergency Surgery
Medical College of Wisconsin
Milwaukee, Wisconsin

Stanley D. Berliner, MD
Associate Professor of Clinical Surgery
Albert Einstein School of Medicine
Bronx, New York
Attending Surgeon, North Shore University Hospital
Cornell University Medical College
Lake Success, New York

Sidney Black, MD
Clinical Professor Emeritus of Surgery
University of Illinois College of Medicine at Chicago
Adjunct Professor of Cell Biology and Anatomy
Head of Surgical and Clinical Anatomy Review Course
Finch University of Health Sciences
The Chicago Medical School
North Chicago, Illinois

Robert A. Brigham, MD
Clinical Associate Professor of Surgery
Uniformed Services University of the Health Sciences
Bethesda, Maryland
Attending Vascular Surgeon, The Reading Hospital and
*   Medical Center*
West Reading, Pennsylvania

James A. Bulen, MD
Clinical Assistant Professor of Surgery
University of California at San Diego
Attending Surgeon, Palomar Medical Center
Director, Hernia Center of North County
Escondido, California

Timothy G. Canty, MD
Clinical Assistant Professor of Surgery
University of California at San Diego
Senior Surgeon, Children's Hospital
San Diego, California

Robert E. Condon, MD
Ausman Foundation Professor and Chairman
Department of Surgery
Medical College of Wisconsin
Surgeon in Chief, Froedtert Memorial Lutheran Hospital
Milwaukee, Wisconsin

v

James R. DeBord, MD
Clinical Associate Professor of Surgery
University of Illinois College of Medicine at Peoria
Peoria, Illinois

Michael J. Demeure, MD
Assistant Professor, Departments of Surgery and of Cellular
*   Biology and Anatomy*
Medical College of Wisconsin
Staff Surgeon, Froedtert Memorial Lutheran Hospital,
*   John L. Doyne Hospital, and Columbia Hospital*
Milwaukee, Wisconsin

H. Brendan Devlin, MD, FRCS
Consultant Surgeon
North Tees General Hospital
Stockton-on-Tees, Cleveland
Lecturer in Clinical Surgery
University of Newcastle-upon-Tyne
Director, Clinical Epidemiology and Audit Department
Royal College of Surgeons of England
London, United Kingdom

Philip E. Donahue, MD
Professor of Surgery
University of Illinois College of Medicine at Chicago
Chairman, Division of General Surgery
Cook County Hospital
Chicago, Illinois

Mosha Dudai, MD
Head, Department of Surgery
Bikur Cholim Hospital
Jerusalem, Israel

Melvin E. Ehrhardt, MD, JD
Clinical Associate Professor
University of Illinois College of Medicine at Urbana-
*   Champaign*
Mohomet, Illinois
Staff Physician, BroMenn Healthcare
Normal, Illinois

Edward L. Felix, MD
Director of Education
The Center for Hernia Repair
Fresno, California

John J. Fildes, MD
Assistant Professor of Surgery
University of Illinois College of Medicine at Chicago
Division Chief
Trauma Education and Research
Attending Surgeon, Cook County Trauma Unit
Chicago, Illinois

Raymond Fish, MD, PhD
Clinical Assistant Professor of Surgery
Adjunct Professor of Bioengineering, and Electrical and
*   Computer Engineering*
University of Illinois College of Medicine at Urbana
Urbana, Illinois

Eric W. Fonkalsrud, MD
Professor and Chief of Pediatric Surgery
UCLA Medical Center
Los Angeles, California

W. Peter Geis, MD
Formerly, Clinical Professor of Surgery
University of Illinois College of Medicine at Chicago
Director, Minimally Invasive Surgical Training Institute of
*   Baltimore*
Chief, Minimally Invasive Surgery
St. Joseph Hospital
Towson, Maryland

Arthur I. Gilbert, MD
Associate Professor of Surgery
University of Miami School of Medicine
Miami, Florida

Stephen W. Gray, PhD
Professor Emeritus of Anatomy
Emory University School of Medicine
Atlanta, Georgia

A. Gerson Greenburg, MD
Professor of Surgery
Brown University School of Medicine
Surgeon-in-Chief, The Miriam Hospital
Providence, Rhode Island

Charles A. Griffith, MD
Clinical Professor of Surgery
University of Washington School of Medicine
Seattle, Washington

Jay L. Grosfeld, MD
Lafayette F. Page Professor and Chairman
Department of Surgery
Indiana University School of Medicine
Surgeon-in-Chief, James Whitcomb Riley Hospital for
*   Children*
Indianapolis, Indiana

Frank M. Guttman, MD, FRCS(C)
Professor of Surgery
McGill University Faculty of Medicine
Director of General Surgery
Montreal, Quebec, Canada

Arnold K. Henry, MD[†]
Emeritus Professor of Clinical Surgery
Faculty of Medicine
Cairo, Egypt
Emeritus Professor of Anatomy
Royal College of Surgeons in Ireland
Dublin, Ireland

Ronald A. Hinder, MD, PhD
Harry E. Stuckenhoff Professor of Medicine
Creighton University School of Medicine
Omaha, Nebraska

George T. Hodakowski, MD
Chief Resident in Surgery
University of Chicago Hospital
Chicago, Illinois

Yves Janin, MD
Department of Surgery
Long Island Jewish Medical Center
New Hyde Park, New York

C. Everett Koop, MD, ScD
McInherny Professor of Surgery
Dartmouth Medical School
Distinguished Scholar
Cornell University Medical College
Professor of Pediatric Surgery
University of Pennsylvania School of Medicine
Former Surgeon-in-Chief, Children's Hospital
Philadelphia, Pennsylvania
Former U.S. Surgeon General

Matthias Kux, MD
Professor of Surgery
University of Vienna Medical Center
Head, Department of Surgery
St. Joseph Hospital
Vienna, Austria

Jean-Martin Laberge, MD, FRCS(C)
Associate Professor of Surgery
McGill University Faculty of Medicine
Pediatric Surgery Program Director
Montreal Children's Hospital
Montreal, Quebec, Canada

Ernest W. Lampe, MD[†]
Clinical Professor of Anatomy and Surgery
Cornell University Medical College
New York, New York

Franck Lazorthes, MD
Professor of Digestive Surgery
Toulouse, France

Irving L. Lichtenstein, MD
Formerly, Assistant Clinical Professor of Surgery
University of California at Los Angeles
School of Medicine
Emeritus, Lichtenstein Hernia Institute
Emeritus, Cedars-Sinai Medical Center
Los Angeles, California

Edward E. Mason, MD, PhD
Professor Emeritus of Surgery
The University of Iowa College of Medicine
Department of Surgery
University of Iowa Hospitals and Clinics
Iowa City, Iowa

Sam Maywood, MD
Director of Anesthesia and Pain Management
Point Loma Surgical Center
San Diego, California

Janet L. Meller, MD
Assistant Professor of Surgery
University of Illinois College of Medicine at Chicago
Chief of Pediatric Surgery
Cook County Hospital
Chicago, Illinois

Erik Nilsson, MD
Associate Professor of Surgery
University of Linköping
Consultant Surgeon
Motala Hospital
Motala, Sweden

[†]Deceased

Lloyd M. Nyhus, MD, Dres.h.c.
Warren H. Cole Professor and Head Emeritus
Department of Surgery
University of Illinois College of Medicine at Chicago
Surgeon-in-Chief Emeritus
University of Illinois Hospital
Chicago, Illinois

José Felix Patiño, MD
Honorary Professor of Surgery
Universidad Nacional de Colombia
Centro Medico de las Andes
Fundacion Santa Fe de Bogotá
Bogotá, Columbia
Visiting Professor of Surgery
Yale University School of Medicine
New Haven, Connecticut

Russell K. Pearl, MD
Associate Professor of Surgery
University of Illinois College of Medicine at Chicago
Attending Surgeon, Division of Colon and Rectal Surgery
Cook County Hospital
Chicago, Illinois

Galen Perdikis, MD
Resident, Department of Surgery
Creighton University School of Medicine
Omaha, Nebraska

Alejandra Perez-Tamayo, MD
Assistant Professor of Surgery
University of Illinois College of Medicine at Chicago
Senior Attending Surgeon, Mercy Hospital
Chicago, Illinois

Jayant Radhakrishnan, MD
Professor of Surgery and Urology
University of Illinois College of Medicine at Chicago
Chief of Pediatric Surgery and Pediatric Urology
University of Illinois Hospital
Chicago, Illinois

Raymond C. Read, MD, FRCS
Professor of Surgery
University of Arkansas for Medical Sciences
Chief, Surgical Service
John L. McClellan Memorial Veterans Hospital
Little Rock, Arkansas

Alan W. Robbins, MD
The Hernia Center
Freehold, New Jersey

Arnold P. Robin, MD
Clinical Assistant Professor of Surgery
University of Illinois College of Medicine at Chicago
Chicago, Illinois
Attending Surgeon, Northwest Community Hospital
Arlington Heights, Illinois
Holy Family Hospital
Des Plaines, Illinois

Richard W. Rosenquist, MD
Assistant Professor of Anesthesiology
University of Illinois College of Medicine at Chicago
Director, Pain Control Center
University of Illinois Hospital and Clinic
Chicago, Illinois

Ira M. Rutkow, MD, MPH, DrPH
The Hernia Center
Freehold, New Jersey

Robb H. Rutledge, MD
Clinical Professor of Surgery
University of Texas Health Science Center at Dallas
Attending Surgeon, Harris Methodist Fort Worth Hospital
Fort Worth, Texas

Eric B. Rypins, MD
Professor of Surgery
University of Illinois College of Medicine at Chicago
Chief, Division of General Surgery
University of Illinois Hospital
Chicago, Illinois

Thomas M. Schlueter, MD
Formerly, Associate Professor of Surgery
Northwestern Ohio Universities
College of Medicine
Medical Director, Summa Health Systems
Akron, Ohio

Alex G. Shulman, MD
Attending Surgeon, Cedars-Sinai Medical Center
Los Angeles, California

David L. Sigalet, MD, PhD, FRCS(C)
Assistant Professor of Surgery
University of Alberta
Edmonton, Alberta, Canada

John E. Skandalakis, MD, PhD
Chris Carlos Distinguished Professor Emeritus
Director of the Centers for Surgical Anatomy and
  Technique
Emory University School of Medicine
Clinical Professor of Surgery
Medical College of Georgia
Senior Attending Surgeon, Piedmont Hospital
Atlanta, Georgia

Lee J. Skandalakis, MD
Clinical Associate Professor of Surgical Anatomy and
  Technique
Clinical Associate Professor of Surgery
Emory University School of Medicine
Attending Surgeon, Piedmont Hospital
Atlanta, Georgia

Panagiotis N. Skandalakis, MD
Clinical Associate Professor of Surgical Anatomy and
  Technique
Emory University School of Medicine
Atlanta, Georgia
Director of Second Department of Surgery
General Hospital
Asklepios-Athens, Greece

Frederick A. Slezak, MD
Professor of Surgery
Northwestern Ohio Universities
College of Medicine
Attending Surgeon, Akron City Hospital
Akron, Ohio

Sam G.G. Smedberg, MD, PhD
Consultant Surgeon, Helsingborg Hospital
Helsingborg, Sweden

Leif Spangen, MD
Associate Professor
Karolinska Institute
Consultant Surgeon, General Hospital
Stockholm, Sweden

James R. Starling, MD
Professor of Surgery
Medical College of Wisconsin
Milwaukee, Wisconsin

Alex M. Stone, MD
Clinical Professor of Surgery
Albert Einstein College of Medicine
Bronx, New York
Attending Surgeon, Long Island Jewish Medical Center
New Hyde Park, New York

René E. Stoppa, MD
Centre Hospitalier Univerisitaire
Amiens, France

Gordon L. Telford, MD
Professor of Surgery
Medical College of Wisconsin
Milwaukee, Wisconsin

William A. Tito, MD
Assistant Professor of Surgery
University of Illinois College of Medicine at Chicago
Senior Attending Surgeon, Mercy Hospital
Chicago, Illinois

Joseph M. Vitello, MD
Assistant Professor of Surgery
University of Illinois College of Medicine at Chicago
Senior Attending Surgeon, Mercy Hospital
Chicago, Illinois

Alonzo P. Walker, MD
Associate Professor of Surgery
Medical College of Wisconsin
Milwaukee, Wisconsin

George E. Wantz, MD
Clinical Professor of Surgery
Cornell University Medical College
Attending Surgeon, The New York Hospital–Cornell
  Medical Center
New York, New York

Alon P. Winnie, MD
Professor of Anesthesiology
University of Illinois College of Medicine at Chicago
Chairman, Department of Anesthesiology
Cook County Hospital
Chicago, Illinois

Leslie Wise, MD
Professor of Surgery
Albert Einstein College of Medicine
Professor of Surgery
Cornell University Medical College
Chairman, Department of Surgery
New York Methodist Hospital
Senior Attending Surgeon, Long Island Jewish Medical
  Center
New Hyde Park, New York

Foreword

This book addresses a topic that remains today, as it has been for centuries, of fundamental importance to surgeons. Hernia repair is still one of the most commonly performed operations and one of the first operations taught to young surgeons during their training. On finishing training, most surgeons continue to perform hernia repairs frequently and satisfactorily. Yet most surgeons could perform them better and need a greater understanding of the anatomy, the pathology, and the principles of repair on which a successful outcome is based. Moreover, although the principles must be mastered, herniorrhaphy continues to evolve as it has done since publication of the first edition of *Hernia* 30 years ago, and since publication of each subsequent edition. In fact, the pace of change has quickened recently with the advent of laparoscopic approaches, the quest for cost-effective, quality-assured, outpatient procedures, and the evolving new applications of biomaterials to the field. Hence, these circumstances warrant a new edition of *Hernia.*

The reader will find that this book covers all these new approaches and yet retains the important fundamentals for which earlier editions were well recognized: the history, the pertinent anatomy, the pathology, the pathophysiology, and the modern standard repairs. To accomplish this task, the editors have assembled a superb cast of experts. The contributing authors have written their chapters carefully and well. The illustrations that supplement the text are superb, making *Hernia* a text and atlas rolled into one. Whether the reader wants to review a standard inguinal herniorrhaphy or find the approach to an unusual abdominal or pelvic hernia, all of the needed information is here. The reader will also appreciate the helpful, newer sections on laparoscopic repair, biomaterials, and the medicolegal implications of the operations. Each chapter ends with the informative comments of the editors and other experts, who breathe life and personality into the book. The reader should pay attention to these Special Comments. Finally, the more scholarly herniotomist who wants to investigate certain topics further will find the annotated bibliography at the end of the book especially helpful.

The reader will appreciate the clear writing in *Hernia,* perhaps imparted to the work initially by the editors' senior mentor, Henry H. Harkins, but now expanded well beyond the initial effort by the current editors and authors. I predict that most readers will be pulling the book off the shelf frequently and reading it on a regular basis, as I will be doing.

Keith A. Kelly, MD
Professor of Surgery
Mayo Medical School
Chairman, Department of Surgery
Mayo Clinic
Scottsdale, Arizona

Preface

It has been 31 years since publication of the first edition of *Hernia.* While there have been many changes in the approaches to the large variety of hernial problems, operative techniques have remained the same and continue to be used regularly by their adherents. For example, the Bassini and Cooper ligament repairs of inguinal hernias remain popular with practicing general surgeons. The Shouldice, Stoppa, and Lichtenstein methods occupy an important niche in the surgeon's armamentarium.

One great area of change has been in materials used in hernial repairs. Suture materials such as silk and cotton are now used infrequently, and prosthetic materials of various types (usually nonabsorbable monofilament) have become popular. The use of prosthetic mesh to buttress ventral incisional or inguinal hernia repairs (particularly recurrent hernias) has become acceptable. A wave of enthusiasm for the use of laparoscopy in approaching many hernial problems, both primary and secondary, is sweeping the surgical world.

We are pleased to include in this volume discussion of many other aspects of hernial work. Chapters from the previous editions have been updated, and new chapters abound. This monograph is comprehensive and up-to-date. We hope the information it imparts will help surgeons throughout the world treat their patients more effectively.

We particularly thank Dr. Keith Kelly for his Foreword. Dr. Kelly was our coworker in the halcyon days under the supervision of Dr. Henry N. Harkins in the Department of Surgery of the University of Washington, Seattle, during the early 1960s. It is exciting to be publishing together again after an interval of 31 years.

We express our appreciation to Lisa McAllister, Paula Callaghan, and Jody Gould, of the Medical Books Division of J.B. Lippincott Company, for their continuing, patient support and counsel, and to C.J. Allen and June Svec of Chicago and Barbara Boyle of Milwaukee, who were of great support in our editorial offices.

Lloyd M. Nyhus, MD
Robert E. Condon, MD

Contents

HERNIA

Overview of Groin Hernia

Part One

Hernia, Fourth Edition, edited
by Lloyd M. Nyhus and Robert E. Condon.
J.B. Lippincott Company, Philadelphia © 1995.

Chapter 1

A History of the Treatment of Hernia

José Felix Patiño

Since the dawn of surgical history, hernias have been a subject of interest, and their treatment has evolved through distinct stages.[10,54,57] The history of hernia is the history of surgery.

In the past two editions of this textbook, erudite reviews were presented of the history of hernia and its treatment. Read[57] and others[3,10,51,52,54] also have dealt with this topic, which has fascinated surgeons of all latitudes through the years of recorded medical history. In an excellent historical treatise by Zimmerman and Veith,[67] the operation for hernia surges as a paramount indicator of the progress of surgical technique.

On November 17, 1892, William S. Halsted of The Johns Hopkins School of Medicine read his classic paper, "The Cure of Inguinal Hernia in the Male,"[23] at the Annual Meeting of the Medico-Chirurgical Faculty of Maryland in Easton, Maryland. The paper begins as follows:

> *Shuh said, "If no other field were offered to the surgeon for his activity than herniotomy, it would be worth while to become a surgeon and to devote an entire life to this service." Quite as well, certainly, might this be said of operations for the radical cure of hernia. There is, perhaps, no operation which, by the profession at large, would be more appreciated than a perfectly safe . . . cure for rupture.*

No other entity permits the study of the origin and evolution of surgical theory and technique as does inguinal hernia. The described details of the operation constitute a superb parameter of the scientific knowledge of anatomy and the quality of the art and science of surgery as it existed and was practiced in the different ages.

In reviewing the historical evolution in chronologic sequence, I highlight the milestones in the development of the surgical therapy of hernia through quotations from the original texts by the surgeon authors to underlay the importance of the major contributions.

ANCIENT TIMES

The *Edwin Smith Surgical Papyrus,* the oldest scientific text that deals with surgery, written during the Egyptian Old Kingdom (3000–2500 BC) and copied in the ensuing centuries (the extant copy dates from circa 1700 BC), has no reference to hernia.

The earliest recorded reference to hernias appears in the *Egyptian Papyrus of Ebers* (circa 1552 BC). According to the monumental illustrated history of medicine by Lyons and Petrucelli,[31] this papyrus contains observations on hernias: "When you judge a swelling on the surface of a belly . . . what comes out . . . caused by coughing."

GRAECO-ROMAN MEDICINE

The foundations of Western civilization, culture, and science lie in the philosophical tradition of the Ionian nature philosophers and the intellectual splendor of classical Greece.

Hippocrates (460–377 BC), "the father of medicine," and Aristotle (384–324 BC), "the philosopher," the first real theoretic and physical scientist, had the greatest influence on the development of scientific medicine, a discipline that attained distinction in Alexandria in the Hellenistic Era (310–250 BC).

Amazingly, the *Corpus Hippocraticum,*[25] the collected writings—more than 70 books—by Hippocrates and his followers, only mentions hernia in passing, although the surgical writings contain detailed anatomic descriptions and indicate refined surgical techniques. The book, *On the Surgery,* contains superb descriptions of the operating room, the people that intervene, the lighting, the instruments, the positioning of the patient, and the techniques of bandaging and dressing. Yet hernia, an easily diagnosed disease entity, is only cited in the Hippocratic text in the section on the effect of different kinds of water: "The children are specially liable to rupture (hernia) and the men to varicose veins and ulcers of the legs."[25] As stated by Zimmerman and Veith,[67] the omission of hernia and of bladder stone (a specific injunction against cutting for bladder stone is made in the "Oath") in the Hippocratic texts is puzzling and may be due to the loss of the original texts.

A great medical school flourished in the legendary Museum (from *mouseion*, sanctuary dedicated to the muses) of Alexandria, the Egyptian city founded by Alexander the Great (356–323 BC). The Museum of Alexandria was the home of the largest library of antiquity, and surgery was performed there with a high level of sophistication following the Hippocratic precepts. The outstanding medical figures in Alexandria were Herophilus of Chalcedon (circa 300 BC), recognized as the founder of anatomy, and Erasistratus of Keos (circa 330–250 BC), known as the father of physiology—both acknowledged as accomplished surgeons who practiced the ligature of vessels for hemostasis in operations for hernia, lithotomy, plastic repairs, and tracheotomy, reputedly under anesthesia induced by the administration of the juice of mandragora.[67] The practice of surgery in Alexandria during the Hellenistic Era was much more rational than the barbaric practices that prevailed in Europe in the Middle Ages and early Renaissance.

The Roman culture spans from the first century BC to about AD 500. In the first century BC and the first century AD, the Roman encyclopedists flourished, among them Aulus Cornelius Celsus (?–AD 50) and Gaius Plinius Secundus (Pliny the Elder, AD 23–79), the most famous Roman authors on medicine who were nonphysicians. Celsus, who transmitted in his writings much of what we know of Alexandrian surgery, was a disciple of Asclepiades of Prusa, the Bithynian physician who practiced in Rome. The works of Asclepiades are lost, but he and his texts are referred to by Celsus, Galen, Oribasius, and many others.[28]

As an ardent follower of Hippocrates, Celsus was the first to introduce Greek and Alexandrian medicine to Rome, for which he has been called the *Latin Hippocrates;* he is also known as the *Cicero of Medicine* for his fine literary style.[35] His *De Medicina*,[12] together with the *Corpus Hippocraticum* and the works of Galen (AD 131–201), constitute the greatest legacy of Graeco-Roman medicine.

Among Celsus' descriptions of surgical procedures is that of the operation for the treatment of hernia, preceded by a review of the anatomy and clinical presentation of "those lesions which are apt to arise in the genital parts around the testicles . . . the nature of the said region must be briefly described first."

Celsus' detailed description of the hernia operation constitutes a magnificent record of fine surgery in the Alexandrian tradition, performed with hemostasis by ligature of the vessels and careful efforts to preserve the testicle:

> When these lesions have been recognized their treatment must be discussed. . . . I shall now speak of those cases demanding the knife. . . . Now the laying open is to be done boldly, until the outer tunic, that of the scrotum itself, is cut through, and the middle tunic reached. When an incision has been made, an opening presents leading deeper. Into this the index finger of the left hand is introduced, in order that by separation of the intervening little membranes the hernial sac may be freed . . . many blood vessels are met with; the smaller ones can be summarily divided; but larger ones, to avoid dangerous bleeding, must be first be tied with rather long flax thread . . . lower down, however, not all is to be removed: for at the base of the testicle there is intimate conexion with the inner tunic, where excision is not possible without extreme danger . . . the testicle having been thus cleared is to be gently returned through the incision along with the veins and arteries and its cord. . . .

Heliodorus lived in the Graeco-Roman period at the beginning of the second century AD; he practiced as physician and surgeon during the reign of Trajan (98–117 AD). Referring to the radical cure of hernia, Leonardo[28] brings forth the following quotation: "We ligature the larger vessels, but as for the smaller ones we catch them with hooks and twist them many times, thus closing their mouths."

According to Read,[57] the concept of rupture comes from Galen of Pergamum (129–199 AD), the most prominent physician of the Graeco-Roman period. Galen traveled extensively and visited Alexandria, where the tradition of the surgical teachings and research by Herophilus and Erasistratus persisted, with "personal inspection" (ie, *autopsia*, human autopsy) as a major component of instruction. In Pergamum and in Rome, Galen was surgeon to the gladiators; he wrote extensively on surgical matters, with important observations on local pathology. Galen thought that herniation was produced by rupture of the peritoneum and overstretching of the overlying fascia and muscles. He recommended operation, which consisted of the ligature of the sac and cord with amputation of the testicle, something that represented a regression after the Alexandrian practice of preserving the testicle.

THE MIDDLE AGES

The notable technical advances of Alexandrian and Graeco-Roman surgery were largely lost during the Dark Ages, the Age of Faith and Scholasticism, the period spanning from AD 476 (fall of the Roman Empire) to the 15th century (Renaissance). Scientific and cultured idiom was Latin. The first universities were founded in Europe in the 12th and 13th centuries, and in them the formal teaching of medicine was started. Surgery was not a learned trade, being only concerned with fractures and the crude treatment of wounds of war; compared with what was practiced in Alexandria during the Hellenistic period, surgery in the Middle Ages, as performed by barbers, cutters, and incisors—people usually ignorant and often illiterate—was characterized by primitivism and regressive trends. Hemostasis was not done through ligature of vessels but rather by the dreadful cautery, and the use of any type of anesthesia was absent.

Paul of Aegina (Paulus Aegineta, seventh century AD)[1] was an important physician encyclopedist of the Byzantine period, which followed the downfall of the Roman Empire in the fifth century AD. His work, which includes one book totally dedicated to surgery—intended as a compendium of Greek and Roman medicine—became an important source for Arabic medicine in the ensuing centuries. His meticulous and accurate description of the operation for hernia, however, also constitutes a regression from the classical surgeons of Alexandria and the Roman Celsus since it includes the routine sacrifice of the testicle.

Albucasis, Abul Qasim al-Zahrawi, the great Moorish surgeon who lived between the years AD 1013 (some authors place the date of his birth in the year 936) and 1106, produced the first rational, complete and illustrated treatise, *On Surgery and Instruments*,[2] in which he described many original operative procedures and instruments of his own design. This great book, whose "purpose was to revive the art of surgery as taught by the "the Ancients," the content of which term ranges from Hippocrates to Paulus Aegineta, whose lifetimes were separated by some eleven hundred years," was translated into Latin by Gerard of Cremona and published in Toledo, Spain, in the second half of the 12th century under the title *Liber Alsaharavi de Cirurgia*; it then appeared in Venice together with Guy de Chauliac's *Cyrurgia Parva* in 1497.

With Pliny's *Historia Naturalis*, Albucasis' *On Surgery and Instruments* was among the first medical books printed in Venice in the second half of the 15th century, just several years after Gutenberg's Bible (1454). Albucasis' treatise had enormous influence on European surgeons in the ensuing centuries. Albucasis was probably born in a royal city near Cordova, Spain, where he practiced and taught. Cordova was a center of learning and culture, with a large library and several hospitals.

In the 1973 beautiful bilingual edition (Arabic and English texts) of Albucasis' text by Spink and Lewis and the Wellcome Institute of the History of Medicine,[2] one can read a detailed description of ruptures:

> On the cauterization of hernia.
> *When a rupture occurs in the groin, and part of the intestine and omentum comes down into the scrotum, being the onset of the disease, forbid the patient to take food for one day and have him use laxatives to empty the bowel. Then let him lie on his back in front of you and bid him hold his breath till the intestine or omentum comes out; then put it back with your finger. Then below the hernia over the pubic bone, mark a semicircle whose extremities point upward. Then heat a cautery of this type (illustration). When it it is white hot and emits sparks then return the intestine or omentum into his abdominal cavity, and have an assistant put his hand over the place to prevent the exit of the intestine. You should first have parted his legs and put a pillow under him; let another assistant sit on his legs and another on his chest, holding his hands. Then apply the cautery to the mark, keeping the cautery upright, and hold it till it reaches the bone. . . . You must take the greatest care that the intestine does not come out while you are cauterizing, lest you burn it and it result in death or grave injury to the patient. (pp 134–136)*
> On the treatment of intestinal hernia.
> *This hernia is due to a split occurring in the membrane stretched from the hypogastrium over the belly in the region of the groin. Through this opening the bowel descends upon one of the testes; this opening is due to the membrane's splitting or stretching. And these two kinds occur from a number of causes: from a blow or jumping or shouting, or lifting a heavy weight, or a similar cause . . . it is a slow and chronic development and does not happen on a sudden. . . . The treatment of the varieties of this disease with the knife is dangerous; so be cautious of rushing at it. . . . The incision should be sufficiently large to allow the testicle to be drawn out. Then dissect away the tissues that lie beneath the skin of the scrotum so that the hard tunica albuginea be exposed all round. . . . Feel with your finger that there be no part of the intestine that has got twisted within the tough white membrane; and should you find any push it back into the abdomen. Then take a needle with a stout tenfold thread and enter the end of the membrane which lies beneath the skin of the testicles alongside the rupture; then cut the end of the loop thread to make four sutures and arrange one over the other in the form of a cross; and with these ligate the membrane of which we have spoken with a strong ligature on each side; then twist the ends of the thread and tie them with a strong knot to prevent anything from reaching the nutrient vessels of the testicles, lest an abscess occur thereby; and make also another ligature outside the first one, rather less than two fingers' breadth from it; and after making these two ligatures leave a finger's breadth of the membrane that is beneath the skin of the testicles and cut the rest way round, and with it remove the testis.*
> On the treatment of the rupture that occurs in the groin.
> *Sometimes there occurs a rupture in the groin . . . no part of the intestine descends into the scrotum. It arises from a stretching of the membrane (i.e. the peritoneum) in the*

groin. . . . Its treatment by the cautery is as I have already described. Sometimes also is treated with the knife in this manner: . . . make an incision three fingers wide, transversally across the swelling of the rupture which projects. Then perforate the subcutaneous tissues so as to expose the white membrane (i.e. the deep fascia) that lies under the skin alongside the rupture. Take a probe and place it upon the projecting part of the fascia and push it back into the depths of the abdomen. Then sew together the two swollen portions of the membrane over the end of the probe and suture the one to the other. . . . On no account make the incision into the fascia nor touch the testis nor anything else, as I taught on the subject of treating the intestinal hernia. (p 448)

Albucasis also writes on the umbilical hernia, the "protruding navel," and describes the operation after a differential diagnosis to exclude other causes of protrusion.

The medical school at Salerno, in southern Italy, is recognized as "the first stirring in the reawakening of medicine in Western Europe"; "the flowering of the civitas Hippocratica, as Salerno came to be known," which started in the 9th century but expanded greatly in the 12th century, was due to its lay organization and to the wise rules that introduced the first system of examination for doctors, including surgeons, and the first regulations concerning medical education and licensure for practice. Salernitian surgery, including the operation for hernia, was highly developed and produced important surgical texts that had profound influence on surgical practice over the ensuing two centuries.[67]

William of Salicet (circa 1210–1277) represents an innovator in surgery. Regarding hernia, in his *Cyrurgia*, translated into French by Paul Pifteau in 1898,[53] he writes: "And if you were to be assured of this manner of opening, then permit the testicle to redescend to its place, and do not dream in any fashion of extirpating it, as do some stupid and ignorant doctors who know nothing. . . ." He is the first author since Celsus, in the first century BC, to reject mutilation of the testicle as an essential part of the operation for the cure of hernia.[67]

THE RENAISSANCE

The outstanding medical figure of the Renaissance Era (15th–mid-17th centuries) is Ambroise Paré (1510–1590; Fig. 1-1), who studied anatomy and surgery at the Hôtel Dieu of Paris and who is largely responsible, with John Hunter (1728–1793), for the development of modern surgery. One of Paré's greatest contributions was the ligature of vessels, which supplanted the method of hemostasis by the use of hot oil or cautery.

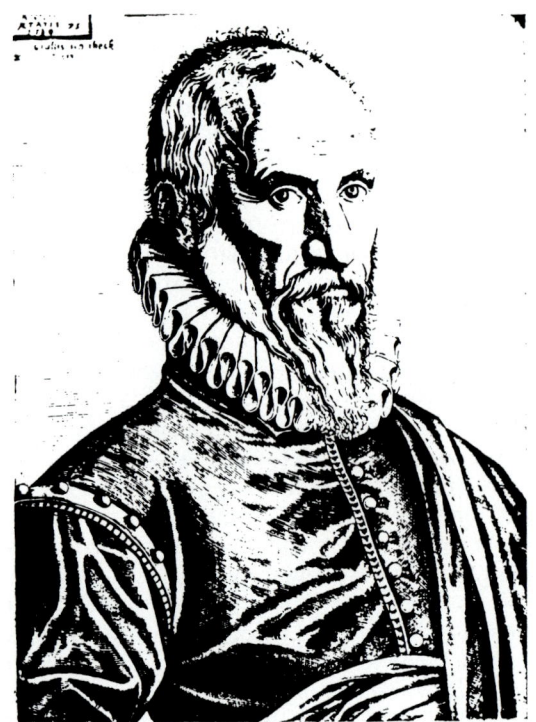

Figure 1-1. Ambroise Paré (1510–1590) at age 75. Illustration is from an engraving by Horbeck in the British Museum and is reproduced in *Selections from the Works of Ambroise Paré: With a Short Biography and Explanatory and Biographical Notes* by Dorothea Waley Singer (New York, William Wood & Co, 1824). The book is in the personal library of J.F. Patiño.

Paré elevated the surgeon's profession from an ill-reputed handicraft to a respected art. An entire chapter on hernias appears in Paré's *The Apologie and Treatise:*[50]

Of hernia. Of the tumors of the groins and codds, called Herniae, that is rupture.

The ancient Phisitions have made many kinds of Ruptures, yet indeed there are only three to be called by that name, that is, the Intestinalis, *or that of the guts, the* Zirbalis, *or that of the kall, and that which is mixed of them both. . . . And we must cure it by Chirurgery after this manner following . . . then presently make an incision in the upper part of the codde, not touching the substance of the guts. . . . We must put it into place of the incision, and put it under the production of the* Peritoneum *being cut together with the codde, all the length of the production; that so with a sharp knife we may divide the process of the* Peritoneum, *according to that cavity separated from the guts there contained. . . . When you have made an indifferent incision, the guts must be gently put up into the belly with your fingers, and then so much of the cut* Peritoneum *must be sowed up, as shall seem sufficient, that by that passage made more straight, nothing may fall into the Codde, after it is cicatrized.*

When the rupture cannot be cured as described, "by reason of the great solution of the continuity of the relaxt, or broken *Peritoneum*," Paré advises the use of the Golden Ligature, or the Punctus Aureus, the golden thread or golden tie. He gives a detailed description of the technique and illustrates the instruments, including a "croked needle, having an eye not farre from the point, through which you may put the golden wyre." Well known are Paré's illustrations of diverse trusses for the control of hernias (Fig. 1-2). He severely condemned the itinerant herniotomists who produced castration.[28]

Pierre Franco (circa 1500–1565), a provincial French surgeon, has been placed as a middleman between a barber-surgeon and an itinerant cutter. Because of his devotion to elevate the status of operative surgery and his important innovations, he also is considered by some as the premier surgeon of the 16th century. Franco was deeply interested in the surgical treatment of hernia. His *Traité des Hernies* was published by E. Nicaise in Lyon in 1561. With its detailed descriptions of the radical operation, which included

an original technique that left unharmed the spermatic vessels and testis as well as an operation for strangulated hernia, this treatise is a major surgical contribution to surgery.

Kaspar Stromayr was a cutter, or incisor, of hernia in Germany in the 16th century. His *Practica Copiosa*,[63a] a beautifully and profusely illustrated German manuscript, dated July 4, 1559, deals principally with hernia and establishes, for the first time, the distinction between indirect and direct hernias (Fig. 1-3). Removal of the testis was sanctioned in operations for hernias of the indirect type but not for the other forms.

THE POST-RENAISSANCE ERA

Antonio Scarpa (1752–1832), author of the *Treatise on Hernias*, which was published in an English translation by Wishart in Edinburgh in 1814, studied at the University of Padua, where his mentor was the renowned pathologist Giovanni Battista Morgagni. In his trea-

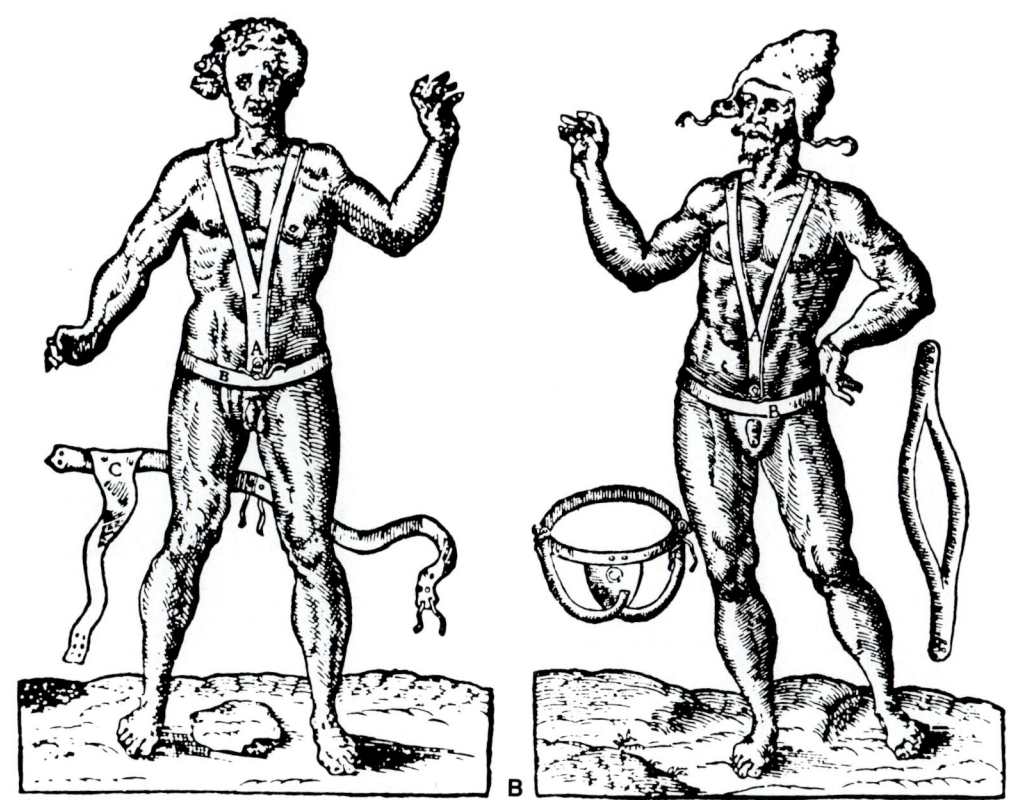

A   **B**

Figure 1-2.   (*A* and *B*) Trusses illustrated in the chapter on "Herniae, That is, Ruptures," in *Apologie and Treatise of Ambroise Paré: Containing the Voyages Made into Divers Places With Many of His Writings Upon Surgery.* From a 1951 edition of the book, in the personal library of J.F. Patiño, a gift of Professor Gustaf E. Linskog, Yale University, Christmas of 1957.

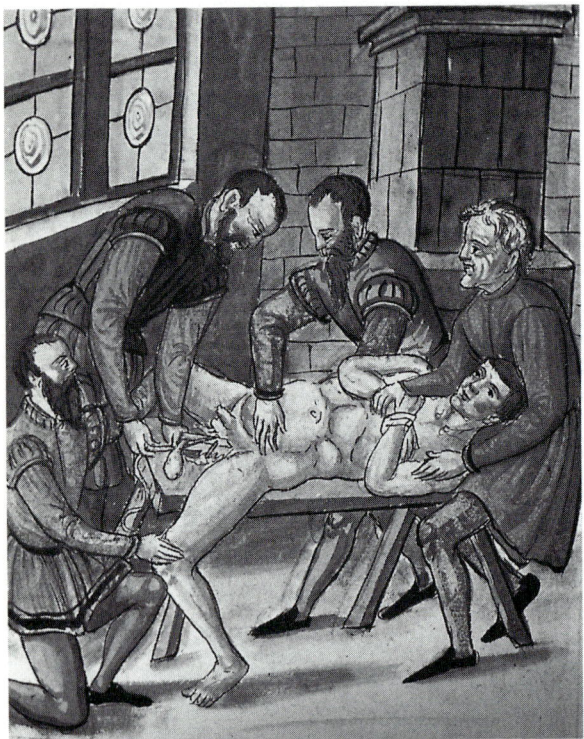

Figure 1-3. Operation for hernia, as illustrated in *Practica Copiosa* by Kaspar Stromayr, written in 1559. The author himself may have been the illustrator. According to A.G. Carmichel and R.M. Ratzan, the manuscript was not discovered until 1909. This illustration appears in their book *Medicine: A Treasury of Art and Literature* (New York, Hugh Lauter Levin Associates, 1991).

tise, Scarpa described accurately, based on autopsy studies, the sliding hernia.

The most distinguished pupil of John Hunter was Astley Paston Cooper of Norfolk (1768–1841), whose great interests resided in the study of hernia, the breast, and arterial surgery. Enormous were his contributions to anatomy and physiology. In his *Treatise on Hernia*, published in London in 1804 and 1807, and in *The Anatomy and Surgical Treatment of Abdominal Hernia*, published in Philadelphia in 1844, Cooper described for the first time the superior pubic ligament, which now bears his name, and the transversalis fascia, with full recognition of its role in the pathogenesis of hernias:

> When the lower portions of the internal oblique and transversalis muscles are raised from their subjacent attachments, a layer of fascia is found to be interposed between them and the peritoneum, through which the spermatic vessels emerge from the abdomen. This fascia, which I have ventured to name fascia transversalis, varies in density, being strong

and unyielding towards the ilium, but weak and more cellular towards the pubes.

August Gottlieb Richter (1742–1812), professor of surgery at the University of Göttingen in 1776, was the founder of the first German surgical journal (1782–1804) and was highly influential in establishing scientific surgery in Germany. His work on hernia, *Abhandlung von der Brüchen* (1777–1779), was considered the best treatise of his time.[28]

THE 19TH AND 20TH CENTURIES

Edoardo Bassini (1844–1924; Fig. 1-4) of Pavia revolutionized the treatment of inguinal hernia by the introduction of a technique designed "to restore those conditions in the area of the hernial orifice which exist under normal circumstances."[9] Read[58] published a historical review of Bassini's pioneer work at the occasion of the centenary of his landmark contribution to inguinal herniorrhaphy.

Bassini's interest in hernia surgery dates back to 1883; he had tried the different methods of correction, which resulted in a high incidence of early failure and the futile need to wear a truss after the operation with the hope of preventing recurrence. He thought that this was due to the inadequacy of a mere ligature of the sac without reconstructing the inguinal canal. Bassini's initial report to the Italian Society of

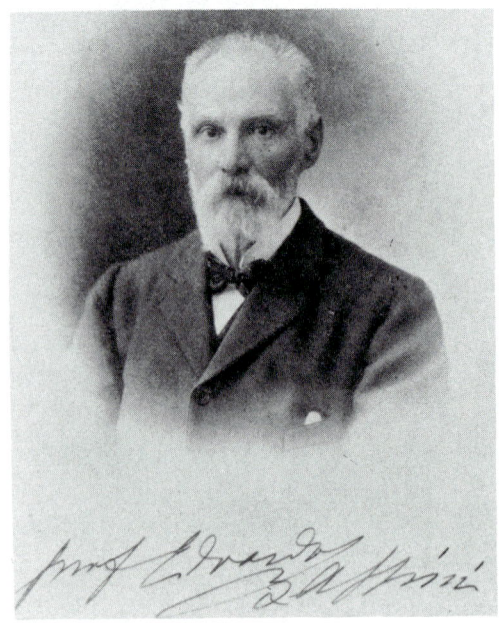

Figure 1-4. Edoardo Bassini (1844–1924). (Courtesy of the National Library of Medicine, Bethesda, MD)

Surgery at Genoa in 1887,[5] which included 38 patients, was followed later in the same year by a presentation to the Italian Medical Association at Pavia,[6] which included 72 operations, and in 1888 to the Italian Surgical Society at Naples[7] on 102 repairs. In 1889, Bassini published his celebrated monograph, which contains beautiful illustrations.[8] His paper published in Germany in 1890,[9] and later translated into Italian, made Bassini's work widely recognized.

Zimmerman and Veith[67] stated that, after Bassini's initial reports on 262 cases, with detailed illustrations, "Overnight, hernial surgery of classical antiquity gave way to that of today, and little that is basic has been added despite the myriads of alleged modifications and improvements. . . . The role of Bassini as the creator of modern hernial surgery stands unchallenged."

The Bassini repair consists of the high ligation and resection of the sac followed by the reconstruction of the floor (or posterior wall) of the inguinal canal using the conjoined tendon (internal oblique, transversus abdominis) and the transversalis fascia (fascia verticalis Cooperi), a triple layer that is sutured to the shelving border of Poupart ligament, with the cord covered by the sutured aponeurosis of the external oblique.[8]

Many modifications have been introduced to the Bassini repair, and it is performed differently by the surgeons of the world. Wantz[65] published an excellent article, which contains the full color illustrations that appear in Attilio Catterina's book published in Bologna in 1932.[11] The Shouldice repair is nothing more than a modern revival of the original Bassini procedure.[22,58]

In the United States, Marcy[33,34] (1837–1924), a North American disciple of Lister, Halsted[23] (1852–1922), of The Johns Hopkins School of Medicine, and Ferguson,[17] of the Chicago College of Physicians and Surgeons (predecessor to the University of Illinois College of Medicine) published techniques similar to the Bassini repair. Summers reviewed in 1946 the classic herniorrhaphies of Bassini, Halsted, Andrews,[4] and Ferguson.[64]

The matter of the priority in the development of these techniques has been argued over the years. Read[56] refers to Watson, who "in his textbook of 1924 stated that Bassini 'adopted' the operation of Marcy (1837–1924), the Boston surgeon, anatomist and philanthropist, a contemporary of Halsted, described at the International Surgical Congress in London in 1881." Watson continues: ". . . his epoch making technique . . . revolutionized the treatment of hernia and eclipsed the countless methods that had been used with more or less questionable results up to that time." Watson relates: "Marcy told me once that while he was

reading his paper he saw Bassini in the audience. He was listening intently, an expression of understanding about him that seemed to change to pleasant conjecture." Marcy himself stated in his book on hernia in 1892:[34] ". . . my own operation described some years previously was practically the same as that designated the Bassini."

Read[56] cites other authors who claim Marcy's priority but concludes that, as stated by Halsted, "Bassini was first," and that "Marcy never accepted Bassini's priority and labored with the help of friends to alter the history of this event, but to no avail."

Marcy was the first to indicate the importance of the high ligation of the hernial sac and closure of the dilated inguinal ring as essential steps in the repair of an inguinal hernia and the first to describe a transabdominal approach. His two landmark publications date back to 1887 and 1892.[33,34]

An "intra-abdominal method of removing inguinal and femoral hernia" was reported by LaRoque[27] in 1932. He described the advantages of the approach: accurate diagnosis, easy dissection, minimal trauma to the cord, and the safe resection of diseased bowel.

William S. Halsted (1852–1922) is the towering figure of modern surgery, and many have discussed the matter of the priority in the design and practice of the operation for the cure of inguinal hernia. The collected *Surgical Papers*[23] of William Stewart Halsted include the papers on the radical cure of inguinal hernia, first presented on November 4, 1889, and ending with "An additional note on the operation for inguinal hernia," dated August 26, 1922. In this note, Halsted refers to the work of Bassini:

> My first cases were reported at a meeting of The Johns Hopkins Hospital Medical Society, November 4, 1889, and were published in the Johns Hopkins Hospital Bulletin for January, 1890. Hence Bassini's brochure anticipated my first report by at least a month or two. Whether my first operation was performed before the appearance of Bassini's pamphlet in Italian I cannot say, for the precise date of the pamphlet is not given. In any event I had not heard of Bassini's operation until his German article appeared—possibly about one year after my first operation; neither was I or any American or German, so far as I know, aware of Bassini's first report until the appearance of the second. Bassini unquestionably has the priority. Our operations differed in several respects, but in the essential features were the same.

In the same note,[23] Halsted gives credit to Harvey Cushing, who first performed herniorrhaphies under local anesthesia.

The 1903 paper by Halsted on hernia published in the Johns Hopkins Hospital Bulletin has the famed Max Brödel's magnificent drawings, and in the text,

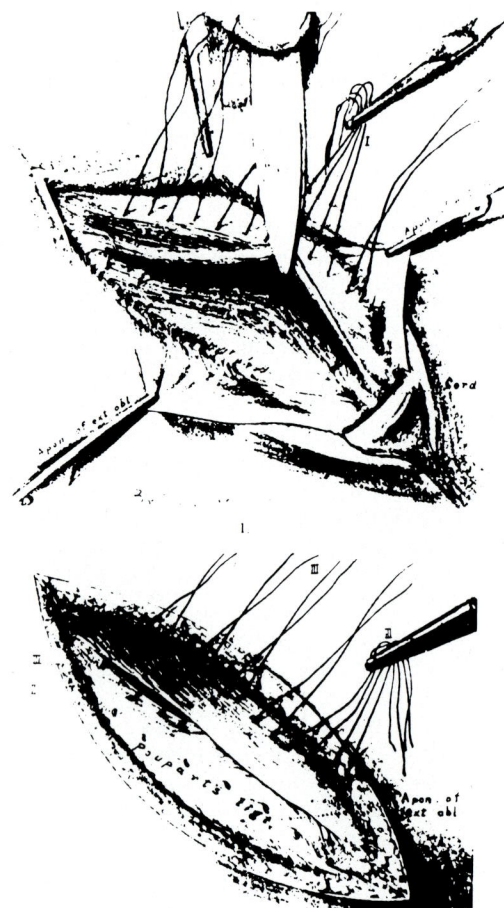

Figure 1-5. Max Brödel's drawings of the Halsted operation for the cure of hernia (plate XXII, 1 and 2). "The lower flap of the cremaster muscle and its fascia is drawn up under the mobilized internal oblique muscle and held in this position by very fine silk stitches. . . . The internal oblique muscle, mobilized, and possibly further released by incising the anterior sheath of the rectus muscle, is stitched (the conjoined tendon also) to Poupart's ligament in the Bassini-Halsted manner." (Halsted WS. The cure of the more difficult as well as the simpler inguinal ruptures. Johns Hopkins Hosp Bull 1903;14:208–214)

Halsted refers to the increasing use of rubber gloves by Bloodgood, his resident. Rubber gloves were introduced by Halsted in 1890. In this paper, Halsted first reported the modern relaxing incision over the rectus fascia (Fig. 1-5).

A widely accepted procedure is the Cooper ligament repair. The technique was described in 1898 by Georg Lotheissen[30] (1868–1935) in Vienna, but was popularized by Chester McVay (1911–1987) after his landmark article,[39] with Anson as coauthor, published in 1949. In 1958 and 1974, McVay presented the basic anatomic concept of the repair using the Cooper ligament.[36,38]

CONTEMPORARY TIMES

The basic principles of hernia repair were laid down in the late 19th century. Since then, important modifications have been added to the classic Bassini repair, and for some of the favored new procedures, local anesthesia can be advantageously used.

Local anesthesia for the repair of hernias was reported by Harvey Cushing[15,16] at the turn of the century. He used block anesthesia produced by cocaine infiltration, a method that Halsted had been largely responsible for introducing.[19] Two major techniques that have proved to be effective are usually done under local anesthesia: the Canadian Shouldice repair and the tension-free prosthetic hernioplasty.

According to Wantz,[66] the so-called Canadian repair was developed in the 1950s by Shouldice, Obney, and Ryan, but it was first described in the surgical literature in the late 1960s.[41,61] Typically, the procedure is performed under local anesthesia, and it has caused a renewed interest in local anesthesia.

The concept of the tension-free repair was introduced by Lichtenstein and colleagues[29] in 1989, who reported 1000 consecutive prosthetic hernioplasties followed for 1 to over 5 years without recurrences. The prosthetic hernioplasty consists of the reconstruction of the floor of the inguinal canal by means of a synthetic mesh.

Condon[14] described the anterior iliopubic tract repair using the traditional anterior approach through the inguinal canal, a method that evolved from the use of the iliopubic tract in operations done by the preperitoneal, or posterior, approach.

In the third edition of this book,[45] Nyhus commented: "I am convinced that all recurrent groin hernias must be approached posteriorly and the fascial repair buttressed by prosthetic material." The preperitoneal approach has been well described by Nyhus[42,44,46,48,49] and is the preferred technique for many surgeons in the treatment of all recurrent and complicated hernias.

According to Nyhus,[42,44] apparently it was Thomas Annandale of Edinburgh who first presented the concept of the preperitoneal approach in 1876; Annandale did not perform a fascial repair. Meade[40] traces it back to 1743. Bates,[9a] of Seattle, advanced the preperitoneal approach concept. Cheatle,[13] in 1920, perhaps under the influence of earlier English procedures,[57] described an operation for the radical cure of inguinal and femoral hernias through a median abdominal section, without entering the peritoneal cavity. In 1921, Cheatle reported on the use of the Pfannenstiel incision, but advised against the use of this approach for direct hernias.[57] According to Read,[57] the preperitoneal approach laid dormant until rediscovered by Henry[24] in 1936; in 1942, Jennings and

Anson[26] revived it in the United Sates. Read[55] and McVay[37] are among the authors who have reported on this approach, but it was Nyhus and associates[44] who established it firmly as a sound operation based on detailed anatomical and clinical studies:

> *My associates and I were perplexed about the failure of the method to flourish. In 1955 we began a clinical investigation in a deliberate attempt to explore the potential of the approach and to provide a large clinical group in which a long-term follow-up study could be accomplished and reported. During the ensuing years our technique for the repair of indirect and direct inguinal and femoral hernias evolved.*

In several publications,[42–49] Nyhus and associates confirmed their conviction about the merits of this approach, especially when dealing with major herniations, recurrent hernias, and femoral hernias. The detailed description of the technique, which involves repair through the preperitoneal approach, has appeared in the former editions of this textbook as well as in a recent monograph.[47] In the 1959 paper,[49] Nyhus and colleagues used for the first time a synthetic mesh (Ivalon) to buttress the posterior wall repair.

The preperitoneal approach has been favored by French surgeons,[59,62,63] who report excellent results with the implantation of Dacron and Mersilene prostheses. The military surgeons Rignault of France[59] and Rosenthal and Walters[60] of the United States also recommend it together with the use of prosthesis. Malangoni and Condon[32] recommend the preperitoneal approach for incarcerated and strangulated hernias.

The studies by Nyhus and associates and the reported results since 1959 have made this approach the preferred one for many contemporary surgeons. Our group in Bogotá prefers the use of the preperitoneal approach and repair, and because of Nyhus' leadership and pioneer work, we have proposed that it be known as the *Nyhus operation*.[51,52]

The dramatic surge of laparoscopic surgery has led to the use of the new technology for the performance of a variety of operations, including the repair of inguinal hernias. In the early 1980s, Ger[20,21] reported on a transabdominal approach for hernia repair, on the performance of a repair with staples applied under laparoscopic guidance, and on experimental studies in animals. Recent reports, such as those of Filipi and colleagues[18] of Creighton University (Omaha), describe well the attractive technique, which so far has not convincingly demonstrated superiority over the conventional extraperitoneal operations, especially over the important and effective preperitoneal approach. Laparoscopic herniorrhaphy

is still considered a procedure in the developmental stage.

REFERENCES

1. Aegineta P. Paulus Aegineta on surgery: The seven books of Paulus Aegineta. Translated from the Greek by Francis Adams with a Commentary embracing a complete view of the knowledge possessed by the Greeks, Romans, and Arabians on all subjects connected with medicine and surgery. London, Printed for the Sydenheim Society. (Special edition by The Classics of Surgery Library. Birmingham, Alabama, 1985.)
2. Albucasis. On surgery and instruments. A definitive edition of the Arabic text with English translation and commentary by MS Spink and GL Lewis. London, The Wellcome Institute of the History of Medicine, and Oxford, The University Press, 1973.
3. Andrade Perez E. Desarrollo histórico de la herniorrafia inguinal. Rev Colomb Cirugía 1988;3:182.
4. Andrews EW. Major and minor technique of Bassini's operation, as performed by himself. Medical Record 1899;56:622.
5. Bassini E. Sulla cura radicale dell'ernia inguinale. Arch Soc Ital Chir 1887;4:380.
6. Bassini E. Nuovo metodo per la cura radicale dell'ernia inguinale. Atti Congr Med Ital 1887;2:179.
7. Bassini E. Sopra 100 casi di cura radicale dell'ernia inguinale operata col metodo dell'autore. Arch ed Atti Soc Ital Chir 1888;5:315.
8. Bassini E. Nuovo metodo per la cura radicale dell'ernia inguinale. Padua, Prosperini, 1889.
9. Bassini E. Über die Behandlung des Leistenbruches. Arch fr klinische Chirurgie 1890;40:441.
9a. Bates UC. New operation for the cure of indirect inguinal hernia. JAMA 1913;60:2032.
10. Bendavid R. New techniques in hernia repairs. World J Surg 1989;13:522.
11. Catterina A. L'Operazione di Bassini per la cura radicale dell' ernia inguinale. Bologna, L Cappelli, 1932.
12. Celsus. De Medicina. With an English translation by WG Spencer. Cambridge, Harvard University Press, 1938.
13. Cheatle GL. An operation for the radical cure of inguinal and femoral hernia. Br Med J 1920;2:68.
14. Condon RE. Anterior iliopubic tract repair. In: Nyhus LM, Condon RE, eds. Hernia, ed 3. Philadelphia, JB Lippincott, 1989:153.
15. Cushing H. Cocaine anesthesia in the treatment of certain cases of hernia and in operations for thyroid tumors. Johns Hopkins Hosp Bull 1898;9:192.
16. Cushing H. The employment of local anesthesia in the radical cure of certain cases of hernia, with a note upon the nervous anatomy of the inguinal region. Ann Surg 1900;31:1.

17. Ferguson AH. Oblique inguinal hernia: typical operation for its cure. JAMA 1899;33:6.

18. Filipi CJ, Fitzgibbons RJ, Salerno GM, Hart RO. Laparoscopic herniorrhaphy. Surg Clin North Am 1992;72:1109.

19. Fulton JF. Harvey Cushing: a biography. Springfield, IL: Charles C Thomas, 1946:141.

20. Ger R. The management of certain abdominal hernias by intra-abdominal closure of the sac. Ann R Coll Surg 1982;64:342.

21. Ger R, Monroe K, Duvivier R, Mishrick A. Management of indirect inguinal hernias by laparoscopic closure of the neck of the sac. Am J Surg 1990;159:371.

22. Glassow F. The surgical repair of the inguinal and femoral hernias. Can Med J 1973;108:308.

23. Halsted WS. Surgical papers by William Stewart Halsted: the operative treatment of inguinal hernia, vol 1. Baltimore, Johns Hopkins Press, 1924 (Special edition by The Classics of Surgery Library. Birmingham, Alabama, 1984).

24. Henry AK. Operation for femoral hernia by a midline extraperitoneal approach: with a preliminary note on the use of this route for reducible inguinal hernia. Lancet 1936;1:531.

25. Hippocratic Writings. Edited with an introduction by GER Lloyd. Translated by J Chadwick and WN Mann. New York, Penguin Books, 1983.

26. Jennings WK, Anson BJ. A new method for repair of indirect inguinal hernia considered in reference to parietal anatomy. Surg Gynecol Obstet 1942; 74:697.

27. LaRoque GP. The intra-abdominal method of removing inguinal and femoral hernia. Arch Surg 1932;24:189.

28. Leonardo RA. History of surgery. New York, Froben Press, 1943.

29. Lichtenstein IL, Shulman AG, Amid PK, Montllor MM. The tension-free hernioplasty. Am J Surg 1989;157:188.

30. Lotheissen G. Radikaloperation der Schekelhernien. Zentralbl Chir 1898;25:548.

31. Lyons AS, Petrucelli RJ II. Medicine: an illustrated history. New York, Harry N Abrams Publishers, 1987.

32. Malangoni MA, Condon RE. Preperitoneal repair of acute incarcerated and estrangulated hernias of the groin. Surg Gynecol Obstet 1986;162:65.

33. Marcy HO. The cure of hernia. JAMA 1887;8:589.

34. Marcy HO. Hernia. New York, Appleton, 1892.

35. Marti-Ibáñez F. A pictorial history of medicine. London, Spring Books, 1962:86.

36. McVay CB. Inguinal and femoral hernioplasty: The evaluation of a basic concept. Ann Surg 1958;148:499.

37. McVay CB. Preperitoneal hernioplasty. Surg Gynecol Obstet 1966;123:349.

38. McVay CB. The anatomical basis for inguinal and femoral hernioplasty. Surg Gynecol Obstet 1974; 139:931.

39. McVay C, Anson BJ. Inguinal and femoral hernioplasty. Surg Gynecol Obstet 1949;88:473.

40. Meade RH. The history of the abdominal approach to hernia repair. Surgery 1965;57:908.

41. Moran RM, Blick M, Collura M. Double layer of transversalis fascia for repair of inguinal hernia. Surgery 1968;63:423.

42. Nyhus LM. The preperitoneal approach and iliopubic tract repair of inguinal hernia. In: Nyhus LM, Condon RE, eds. Hernia, ed 2. Philadelphia, JB Lippincott, 1978.

43. Nyhus LM. The recurrent groin hernia: Therapeutic solutions. World J Surg 1989;13:541.

44. Nyhus LM. The preperitoneal approach and iliopubic tract repair of inguinal hernia. In: Nyhus LM, Condon RE, eds. Hernia, ed 3. Philadelphia, JB Lippincott, 1989.

45. Nyhus LM. Editor's comment. In: Nyhus LM, Condon RE, eds. Hernia, ed 3. Philadelphia, JB Lippincott, 1989:153.

46. Nyhus LM, Condon RE, Harkins HN. Clinical experiences with preperitoneal hernial repair for all types of hernia of the groin. Am J Surg 1960; 100:234.

47. Nyhus LM, Klein MS, Rogers FB. Inguinal hernia. Curr Probl Surg XXVIII 1991;6:403.

48. Nyhus LM, Pollak R, Bombeck CT, Donahue PE. The preperitoneal approach and prosthetic buttress repair for recurrent hernia: the evolution of a technique. Ann Surg 1988;208:733.

49. Nyhus LM, Stevenson JK, Listerud MB, Harkins HN. Preperitoneal herniorrhaphy: a preliminary report in fifty patients. West J Surg Obstet Gynecol 1959;67:48.

50. Paré A. The apologie and treatise: containing the voyages made into divers places with many of his writings upon surgery. Edited with an introduction by G Keynes. London, Falcon Educational Books, 1951.

51. Patiño JF. Operación de Nyhus: hernioplastia preperitoneal. Trib Médica (Bogotá) 1992;86:62.

52. Patiño JF, García-Herreros LG, Zundel N, et al. Hernioplastia preperitoneal con prótesis. Rev Colomb Cirugía 1992;7:74.

53. Pifteau P. Chirurgie de Guillaume de Salicet. Toulouse, Imprimerie Saint-Cyprien, 1898.

54. Premuda L. The history of inguinal herniorrhaphy. Int Surg 1986;71:141.

55. Read RC. Preperitoneal exposure of inguinal herniation. Am J Surg 1968;116:653.

56. Read RC. Marcy's priority in the development of inguinal herniorrhaphy. Surgery 1980;88:682.

57. Read RC. The development of inguinal herniorrhaphy. Surg Clin North Am 1984;64:185.

58. Read RC. The centenary of Bassini's contribution to inguinal herniorrhaphy. Am J Surg 1987; 153:324.

59. Rignault DP. Properitoneal prosthetic inguinal hernioplasty through a Pfannenstiel approach. Surg Gynecol Obstet 1986;163:465.

60. Rosenthal D, Walters MJ. Preperitoneal synthetic mesh placement for recurrent hernias of the groin. Surg Gynecol Obstet 1986;163:285.
61. Shearburn EW, Myers RN. Shouldice repair for inguinal hernia. Surgery 1969;66:450.
62. Stoppa RE. The treatment of complicated groin and incisional hernias. World J Surg 1989;13:545.
63. Stoppa RE, Rives JL, Warlaumont CR, et al. The use of Dacron in the repair of hernias of the groin. Surg Clin North Am 1984;64:269.
63a. Stromayr, K. Die Handschrift des Schmitt-und Augenarztes. Lindau in Bodensee, July 4, 1659. Reprinted, Idra-Verlagsanstalt Gmbh, Berlin, 1925.
64. Summers JE. Classical herniorrhaphies of Bassini, Halsted and Ferguson. Am J Surg 1947;73:87.
65. Wantz GE. The operation of Bassini as described by Attilio Catterina. Surg Gynecol Obstet 1989;168:67.
66. Wantz GE. The Canadian repair of inguinal hernia. In: Nyhus LM, Condon RE, eds. Hernia, ed 3. Philadelphia, JB Lippincott, 1989.
67. Zimmerman LM, Veith I. Great ideas in the history of surgery. Baltimore, Williams & Wilkins, 1961.

Editor's Comment

The distinguished surgeon-historian José Felix Patiño has given us a detailed, precise review of the history of hernia studies from the ancients to the present. I particularly am pleased that he was willing to undertake this task. Patiño preceded me as the President of the International Society of Surgery (1989–1991), thus giving us the opportunity to work together for the furtherance of the Society and to discuss in-depth the many facets of the subject of hernia.

Olch and Harkins, in the first edition of *Hernia* (1964), gave an interesting interpretation of events after Bassini. I paraphrase portions of their historical presentation. William S. Halsted (1852–1922) developed an operation similar to Bassini's for the treatment of inguinal hernias. Halsted at this time was Professor of Surgery at The Johns Hopkins School of Medicine. The major difference between the Bassini procedure and the Halsted operation was the transposition of the cord to a position above the external oblique aponeurosis. Minor technical differences included the ligation of superfluous veins about the cord to reduce its size and the sectioning of fibers of the internal oblique muscle and sometimes the transversus abdominis muscle to permit more lateral displacement of the internal ring. This procedure, commonly referred to as the *Halsted I procedure* (to differentiate it from the procedure later adopted by Halsted in which the cord was not transposed, the

Halsted II procedure), was first mentioned in a brief communication to The Johns Hopkins Medical Society in 1889 and published in *The Bulletin of the Johns Hopkins Hospital* ("The Radical Cure of Hernia," 1889;1:12). The first detailed description of the procedure was published in a paper, "The Radical Cure of Inguinal Hernia in the Male" (Bull Johns Hopkins Hosp 1893;4:17). The Halsted II procedure is mentioned in Halsted's article entitled "The Cure of the More Difficult as Well as the Simpler Inguinal Ruptures" (Bull Johns Hopkins Hosp 1903;14:208).

Ravitch (Surgery 1986;100:59), in a Sherlock Holmes–type article, attempted to prove that Halsted himself had an inguinal hernia treated with a truss. Fortunately, Halsted appears to have had an umbilical hernia, so his name cannot be besmirched by association with the word *truss*.

Also incorporated in the Halsted II procedure was the imbrication of the flaps of the aponeurosis of the external oblique muscle in performing the closure. This principle of imbrication was first adopted and stressed by E. Wyllys Andrews (1856–1927) of Chicago, Professor of Surgery at the Northwestern University Medical School (Chicago Med Rec 1895;9:67). The Halsted II procedure is also known as the *Ferguson-Andrews operation* because of the two major surgical techniques involved: leaving the cord in its normal anatomic position, as proposed by Ferguson, and imbrication of the external oblique aponeurosis, as stressed by Andrews. The closure of multiple layers espoused by the Shouldice Clinic of Toronto is this imbrication technique in extensia.

The next landmark in inguinal hernia surgery was the use of the iliopectineal ligament (the Cooper ligament, ligamentum pubicum superius) to anchor the medial parietal wall in the repair. This ligament was first used by Georg Lotheissen (1868–1935) of Vienna in 1898 at the suggestion of Narath when he found the inguinal ligament destroyed in a patient with recurrent hernia. He successfully substituted the iliopectineal ligament and repeated the procedure in a series of 12 patients (Zentralbl Chir 1898;25:548). This innovation was ignored until it was revived by Seelig and Tuholske (Surg Gynecol Obstet 1914;18:55). The publications of Chester B. McVay and Barry J. Anson (Surg Gynecol Obstet 1942;74:746; 1949;88:473) led to widespread use of this technique. The contributions of McVay to the repair were so great that it was named the *McVay repair* by Henry Harkins (Surgery 1942;12:364), and this eponym has been widely adopted.

Annandale (Edinburgh Med J 1876;21:1087) is often quoted in the literature as being the first to use the Cooper ligament in hernial repair. As Koontz showed in his excellent historical analysis of the de-

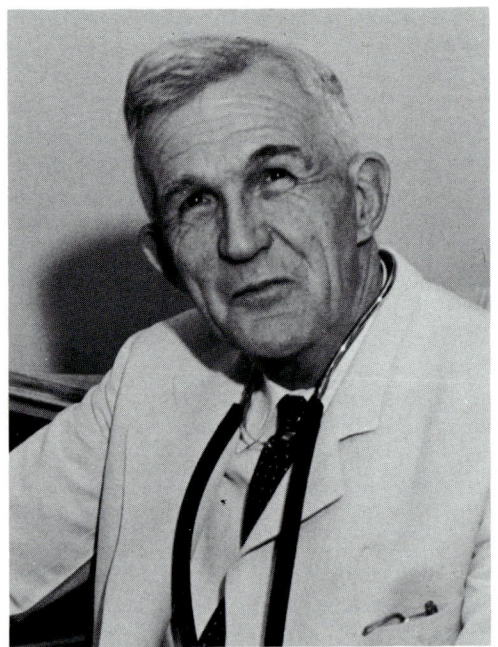

Figure 1-6. Paul W. Harrison (1883–1962).

velopment of the surgical treatment of femoral hernia (Surgery 1963;53:551), this is an example of requoting without consulting the original reference. Actually, Annandale used neither the Cooper nor the Poupart ligament in his somewhat esoteric repair of a combined direct–indirect inguinal hernia.

The recognition of the importance of the posterior inguinal wall as it relates to both the cause and the treatment of hernia is credited to many authors. One of the strongest presentations in favor of the transversalis fascia as a key factor in the anatomy of hernia was by Harrison (Arch Surg 1920;4:680). Paul W. Harrison (1883–1962; Fig. 1-6) worked for more than 40 years as a missionary doctor to the people of the Persian Gulf and Saudi Arabia. His early training in the Hunterian laboratory of Harvey Cushing is reflected in the list of other original investigations that were undertaken literally on the sands of the desert: (1) his successful fixation of a femoral fracture with an intramedullary nail of "teak" wood; (2) his early success with the original treatment of aneurysm by cellophane fibrosis; and (3) his development of the concept and clinical trial in 1948 of an aortic Venturi valve in the treatment of ascites.

Another ligament, the iliopubic tract, is important to the full understanding of hernial repair (see Chap. 8). Depicted by Hesselbach (*Neueste anatomisch-pathologische Untersuchungen über den Ursprung und das Fortschreiten der Leisten und Schenkelbrüche*, Würzburg, Baumgärtner, 1814) and described by Thomson later

during the same century, its use advocated in the anterior approach by Clark and Hashimoto (Surg Gynecol Obstet 1946;82:480) and by Griffith (Surg Clin North Am 1959;39:531). The importance of the iliopubic tract in the preperitoneal approach to repair has been emphasized by Nyhus and associates (see Chaps. 7 through 9).

Several good historical articles on hernia are:

Carlson RI. The historical development of the surgical treatment of inguinal hernia. Surgery 1956;39:1031.
Ravitch MM. The great Boston hernia controversy concerning the permanent cure of reducible hernia or rupture. Bull NY Acad Med 1969;45:767.
Rutkow IM. A selective history of groin herniorrhaphy in the 20th century. Surg Clin North Am 1993;73:395.

Dr. Henry N. Harkins (Fig. 1-7) was a coeditor of the first edition of *Hernia*. The study of hernia held his interest for almost three decades. It is appropriate to comment briefly on his life.

Henry N. Harkins was born in Missoula, Montana, on July 13, 1905. In 1912, the family moved to Chicago, where his father, William Draper Harkins, became the Andrew MacLeish Distinguished Service Professor of Physical Chemistry at the University of Chicago. After graduation from the University of Chicago in 1925 with a major in Chemistry and a minor in Mathematics, he entered Rush Medical College in 1924, was graduated in 1930, and received his MD

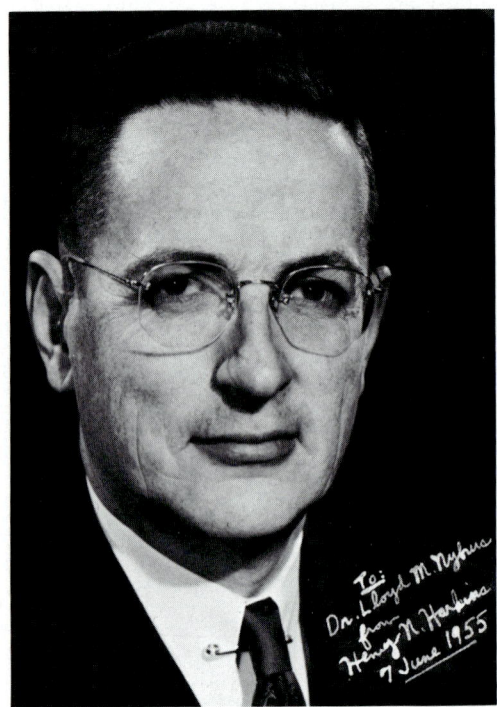

Figure 1-7. Henry N. Harkins (1905–1967).

degree after a 2-year rotating internship at Presbyterian Hospital. During this active developmental period in Dr. Harkins's life, he also received an MS degree in Chemistry in 1926 and a PhD degree in Medicine in 1928, both from the University of Chicago.

Dr. Harkins's surgical residency (1931–1936) was spent at the University of Chicago Clinics under the guidance of Dr. Dallas Phemister.

Dr. Harkins spent 4 years as an associate surgeon at the Henry Ford Hospital in Detroit. At Henry Ford, he first became interested in the surgical treatment of varicose veins and hernia, interests that resulted in many original contributions to the medical literature.

In 1943, Dr. Harkins returned to full academic pursuits at The Johns Hopkins University School of Medicine. His relatively short association (1943–1947) with Alfred Blalock made a deep impression on Dr. Harkins. In subsequent years, he combined the best of two schools of surgical thought as a guide to the practice of surgery—the Phemister school and the Halsted-Blalock school.

In 1947, Dr. Harkins accepted the position of Chairman of the Department of Surgery at the University of Washington School of Medicine in Seattle. Under his leadership, the department became recognized as one of the finest in the world. In subsequent years, Dr. Harkins's students occupied chairs of surgery at 10 universities: Robert E. Condon, the Medical College of Wisconsin; Keith A. Kelly, Mayo Medical School; Robert W. Barnes, the University of Arkansas; J. Roland Folse, Southern Illinois University; the late John E. Jesseph, Indiana University; Ryoichi Tsuchiya, Nagasaki University, Japan; Jean E. Murat, the University of Tours; Hitoshi Mohri, Yamaguchi University Teruaki Aoki, Jikei University; and Lloyd M. Nyhus, the University of Illinois.

In 1993, the Henry N. Harkins Chair of Surgery was established at the University of Washington, Seattle, to honor this surgical educator in perpetuity.

L.M.N.

Hernia, Fourth Edition, edited
by Lloyd M. Nyhus and Robert E. Condon.
J.B. Lippincott Company, Philadelphia © 1995.

Chapter 2

The Anatomy of the Inguinal Region and Its Relation to Groin Hernia

Robert E. Condon

No disease of the human body, belonging to the province of the surgeon, requires in its treatment a better combination of accurate, anatomical knowledge with surgical skill than Hernia in all its varieties.

> Sir Astley Paston Cooper, 1804

The high cure rate today, however, owes more to the exploitation of the surgical anatomy of the groin than upon any one medical or therapeutic advance.

> J.H. Talbot, 1961

Actually, however, it is frequently impossible to reconcile the structure of a region, as observed in dissection, with the conventional descriptions of the particular area.

> C.B. McVay, 1974

The identification of the iliopubic tract and assessment of its strength should be a regular feature of inguinal dissections during hernia repair.

> A.M. Gilroy et al, 1992

The groin is that portion of the anterior abdominal wall below the level of the anterior superior iliac spines. Nine of ten patients referred for surgical repair of a hernia have one of the common varieties of groin hernias: an oblique or indirect inguinal hernia, a direct inguinal hernia, or a femoral hernia.

Repair of a primary, uncomplicated hernia in a thin, reasonably muscular patient may not present much difficulty, but in obese patients, in patients with a sliding hernia, or in those who have considerable distortion or scarring of the structures of the groin after previous attempts at cure, a sound and secure hernial repair may present a distinct technical challenge. It is a surgical truism that the operator who is well versed in surgical anatomy will not flounder, no matter what distortion or variation presents itself. The converse is equally true, and the importance of a thorough understanding of this regional anatomy is self-evident.

A three-dimensional mental conception of structural relations must be acquired if one is to understand groin anatomy and the fundamental features of a groin hernial repair. Detailed descriptions and illustrations help; indeed, they are indispensable. However, in the final analysis, the required three-dimensional structural understanding is obtainable only by repeated personal dissections.

The autopsy room provides a readily available source of unfixed material similar in color and texture to the tissues seen in the operating room. Groin dissections can be carried out repeatedly in the autopsy room with a minimum of trouble, and every surgeon should take the opportunity thus presented to review surgical anatomy.

The anatomy of the inguinal region is misunderstood by some surgeons at all levels of seniority. This should not be so, for the surgical anatomy of the groin is relatively straightforward. One of the sources of misunderstanding and difficulty stems from a lack of appreciation of the full spectrum of variation in normal anatomic structure. There is a multiplicity of small structures in the groin that are variable in form and extent or are inconstantly present. Surgical teaching, on the other hand, often leaves the impression that the anatomy of this region is fixed and unvarying and places far too much emphasis on descriptions of minor structures that are of no great importance in understanding the pathogenesis of groin hernias or the principles involved in their surgical repair.

A second factor, leading to misunderstanding by both anatomists and surgeons about the relative strength of connective tissue structures of the groin, was the introduction of embalming. Embalming was primarily a public health measure but also served to free anatomists from the necessity of dissecting cadavers before putrefaction occurred. Unfortunately, the embalming process brings about coagulation of protein within connective tissue, resulting in a change both in appearance and in apparent strength. A layer of connective tissue, such as the transversalis fascia, which in life is thin, transparent, and of little intrinsic strength, is transformed by embalming into an opaque sheet that appears capable of holding sutures. Thus, dissectors working only with embalmed material develop a distorted view of connective tissue that leads, in turn, to erroneous recommendations about the technical aspects of surgical repair of a groin hernia.

A third important source of error stems from the limitations of anatomic illustrations. In a drawing, the anatomy necessarily is depicted on a flat surface, inevitably leading to some distortion of relations. This technical problem is inherent in any drawing and cannot be overcome except by stereoscopic photography. What can be overcome is the perpetuation of illustrations that are erroneous or contain deliberate obscurities.

Then there is the problem of nomenclature. Here, the surgical literature is particularly culpable. The terms *fascia* and *aponeurosis* frequently are used loosely in an interchangeable manner. A strict definition of these terms is required.

An *aponeurosis*, in the context of structures in the groin, is the flat, dense, white tendon of insertion of one of the three flat muscles of the lateral abdominal wall: external oblique, internal oblique, and transversus abdominis. These aponeuroses all come together in the midportion of the muscular lower abdominal wall to form the anterior sheath of the rectus abdominis muscle. Further, they have more or less extensive insertions into bone at the body and superior ramus of the pubis. An aponeurosis, being a tendon, is composed of strong collagenous tissue. The individual fiber bundles within the flat tendon can easily be seen.

A *fascia*, on the other hand, is a condensation of connective tissue into a definable, homogeneous layer. Fascia may vary from a diaphanous layer of no intrinsic strength to a more easily discerned and thicker lamina. Such tissues invest or cover the muscular and aponeurotic layers of the groin, but they lack the organization and intrinsic tensile strength of an aponeurosis. The designation *ligament* is applied to a wide variety of structures whose strength may vary from dense aponeurosis (eg, inguinal ligament) to delicate areolar tissue (eg, interfoveolar ligament).

Comment needs to be made regarding the several nearly identical terms that have the stem *trans-* in common. Transversus abdominis muscle, transversus abdominis aponeurosis, and transversalis fascia are all distinct structures. *Transversus abdominis muscle* is the deepest of the three flat muscles of the lateral abdominal wall. *Transversus abdominis aponeurosis* is the flat tendon of insertion of that muscle. *Transversalis fascia* is the investing fascia of the transversus abdominis muscle and its continuation, the transversus abdominis aponeurosis. Transversalis fascia in particular, although strictly defined in an anatomic sense, is loosely used by many surgeons to designate any one or all of this group of structures. This is an important point to keep in mind when reviewing the surgical literature because a great deal of emphasis has been placed on transversalis fascia and its role in hernial repair. Transversalis fascia is of varying density and often is thin, even transparent. It possesses little intrinsic strength and, by itself, is a worthless material as far as the construction of a sound hernial repair is concerned. Suture of tendinous aponeuroses and ligaments, anatomically strong structures that can hold sutures, is the key to a sound groin hernial repair.

INDIVIDUAL ANATOMIC STRUCTURES IN THE GROIN

The illustrations and descriptive text are based on 187 personal dissections of *fresh* bodies free of groin disease. In general, the descriptions of the anatomy conform to those given in standard anatomy texts. The descriptive approach is largely didactic and is primarily an anatomic one. The surgical applications of the anatomy are mentioned but not described in any detail. To help the reader keep his or her bearings, all descriptions are those of the right groin, that is, the right half of the lower abdominal wall, in a man.

I make no apologies for those points in which my descriptions herein differ from those of standard texts because the material presented is based on the human anatomy personally observed in the unfixed cadaver. So that the reader is warned, the points of difference with classic descriptions are as follows:

1. The relation of the lacunar ligament to the femoral canal—the lacunar ligament is not the *normal* medial margin of the femoral canal
2. The interparietal fasciae—a convenient and surgically practical grouping of the minor muscular investing fasciae
3. The participation of the pectineus muscle and fascia in the posterior wall or floor of the femoral canal
4. The reinforcement of the margins of the deep inguinal ring by the transversus abdominis aponeurotic arch and the iliopubic tract

Table 2-1.   Anatomic Nomenclature of Certain Structures in the Groin*

Terms Used in This Chapter	Nomina Anatomica†	Alternative Designations and Eponyms
Skeleton, Skin, Subcutaneous Tissues		
Pubis, body	Corpus ossis pubis	
Symphysis	Facies symphysialis	
Tubercle	Tuberculum pubicum	Pubic spine
Superior ramus	Ramus superior ossis pubis	
Pectineal line	Pecten ossis pubis	Pubic pecten, pectinate line
Ischiopubic ramus	Ramus inferior ossis pubis	
Iliopubic eminence	Eminentia iliopubica	Iliopectineal eminence
Ilium, crest	Crista iliaca	
Anterior superior spine	Spina iliaca anterior superior	
Subcutaneous fat	Tela subcutanea	Camper fascia, panniculus adiposus, fatty layer of the superficial fascia
Scarpa fascia		Membranous layer of superficial fascia
Musculoaponeurotic Structures		
External oblique muscle	M. obliquus externus abdominis	
Aponeurosis	Apon. obliquus externus abdominis	Descending oblique aponeurosis
Innominate fascia		Gallaudet fascia, deep abdominal fascia, outer investing fascia, external oblique fascia
Intercrural fibers	Fibrae intercrurales	
Inguinal ligament	Lig. inguinale	Poupart ligament, superficial crural arch, superficial femoral arch, iliopubic anterior ligament
Lacunar ligament	Lig. lacunare	Gimbernat ligament
Reflected inguinal ligament	Lig. inguinale reflexum	Reflex inguinal ligament, triangular ligament, Colles ligament
Superficial inguinal ring	Anulus inguinalis superficialis	External inguinal ring, subcutaneous inguinal ring
Medial crus	Crus mediale	Superior crus, internal crus
Lateral crus	Crus laterale	Inferior crus, external crus
Internal oblique muscle aponeurosis	M. obliquus internus abdominis	
Cremaster muscle	M. cremaster	
Cremasteric fascia		Cooper fascia
Transversus abdominis muscle aponeurosis	M. transversus abdominis	
Falx inguinalis (conjoined tendon)	Falx inguinalis (tendo conjunctivus)	
Transversalis fascia	Fascia transversalis	
Iliopubic tract		Deep crural arch, deep femoral arch, anterior femoral sheath, Thomson ligament, interfoveolar ligament (part), iliopubic intermediate ligament
Interfoveolar ligament	Lig. interfoveolare	Hesselbach ligament
Henle ligament		
Deep inguinal ring	Anulus inguinalis profundus	Internal inguinal ring
Transversalis fascial sling		
Superior crus		
Inferior crus		
Cooper ligament	Lig. pectineale	Superior pubic ligament, iliopubic posterior ligament
Iliopectineal arch		Iliopectineal ligament, iliopsoas fascia
Rectus abdominis muscle	M. rectus abdominis	
Rectus tendon		
Rectus sheath	Vagina m. recti abdominis	
Anterior rectus sheath	Lamina anterior	
Posterior rectus sheath	Lamina posterior	
Semicircular line	Linea arcuata	
Semilunar line	Linea semilunaris	Arcuate line, line of Douglas

(continued)

Table 2-1. *(Continued)*

Terms Used in This Chapter	Nomina Anatomica†	Alternative Designations and Eponyms
Linea alba	Linea alba	
Adminiculum	Adminiculum linea albae	
Inguinal canal	Canalis inguinalis	
External spermatic fascia		
Internal spermatic fascia		Infundibuloform fascia
Femoral sheath		Crural sheath
Canal	Canalis femoralis	
Ring	Anulus femoralis	
Septum	Septum femorale	

*With the exceptions noted in this table, the terminology throughout these descriptions is an anglicized version of the *Nomina Anatomica*.
†*Nomina Anatomica,* as revised at the 11th International Congress (Mexico City), 1980.

5. The relation between the iliopubic tract and the femoral canal—the recurring portion of the insertion of the iliopubic tract is the *normal* medial margin of the femoral canal
6. The frequent presence of a lymph node at the internal aspect of the deep inguinal ring

The nomenclature used in this chapter is generally an Anglicized version of the *Nomina Anatomica;* eponymic designations have been used for a few structures, especially when such terms are those most commonly used in conversation among surgeons. Table 2-1 lists the nomenclature used here to designate the more important groin structures as well as, for reference, the comparable terminology of the *Nomina Anatomica,* plus a number of alternative and eponymic designations that have been applied in the literature to the same structures. Terms that describe relative position have been limited to the meanings set out in Table 2-2.

The illustrations are largely derived from photographs of original dissections. The initial plan was to include several photographs, but it soon became obvious that each photograph would require an accompanying drawing for clarity. In the interests of economy of space, then, many of the photographs have been omitted. The illustrations are presented so as to display most advantageously the structure under discussion; some views are oriented from the skin inward, others from the peritoneal cavity outward.

Abdominal Wall

The lower abdominal wall is composed, in a broad sense, of several strata or layers placed one on the other from the peritoneum outward to the skin in a manner similar to the multiple layers of an onion. The muscle layers in the region of the groin all have an attachment to bone or adjacent strong fascial structures along a line from the symphysis and body of the pubis to the anterior superior iliac spine. The skin and peritoneum, and their adjacent fatty and fascial layers, both superficial and deep, are continuous with the similar tissues of adjacent areas. These continuities are outlined in Table 2-3.

Pelvic Skeleton

The pelvic bones form an anchor for the muscles and aponeuroses of the groin. Figure 2-1 shows the prominent skeletal landmarks, and Figure 2-2 indicates the areas in which the regional muscles and strong musculoaponeurotic and ligamentous structures of the groin are attached to bone. These drawings should be reviewed before the reader proceeds further.

Note that the pelvis is interposed in the axial skeleton in an angled position. The angle of tilt is about 60 degrees with regard to the shaft of the femur or the vertebral column. The superior aperture of the

Table 2-2. Terms That Describe Relative Position

Medial–lateral	Toward the midline–toward the flank
Superior–inferior, above–below	Toward the head–toward the feet
Anterior–posterior	Toward the surface of the abdomen–toward the back and vertebral column
External–internal, outward–inward, superficial–deep	Nearer the skin–nearer the peritoneum and abdominal viscera

Table 2-3. Tissue Continuities in the Groin

Abdomen and Pelvis	Spermatic Cord and Scrotum	Thigh
Skin	Skin	Skin
Superficial subcutaneous fat (Camper fascia)	Dartos (minor component)	Subcutaneous fat
Scarpa fascia	Dartos (major component)	Cribriform fascia
Innominate fascia	External spermatic fascia	Fascia lata
External oblique aponeurosis		
Superficial interparietal fascia		
Internal oblique muscle and aponeurosis	Cremasteric muscle and fascia	
Deep interparietal fascia		
Transversus abdominis muscle and aponeurosis		
Transversalis fascia	Internal spermatic fascia	Anterior and medial walls of femoral sheath
Preperitoneal tissues, including ductus deferens, vessels, nerves	Tunica vaginalis communis; ductus deferens, vessels, nerves	
Peritoneum	Tunica vaginalis testis	

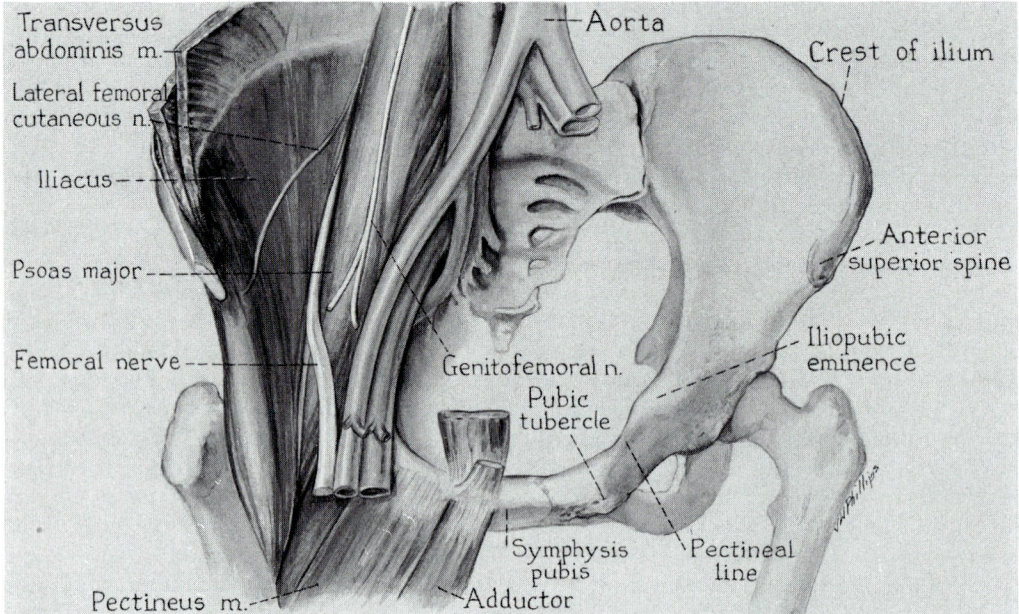

Figure 2-1. (*Left body half*) The pelvic skeleton illustrating the important bony landmarks. (*Right body half*) The muscles, vessels, and nerves that are immediately adjacent to the groin. The oblique plane of the inguinal ligament in the lateral third of the groin is also shown. The iliopectineal arch (not shown) is a fascial band continuous with the investing fascia overlying the iliacus and psoas muscles. It attaches to the pelvic skeleton at the anterosuperior spine and at the iliopubic eminence. The common trunk of origin of the inferior epigastric and deep circumflex iliac vessels from the external iliac shown here is unusual. More commonly, these branches originate separately from the artery and join the vein separately and at a somewhat more proximal level.

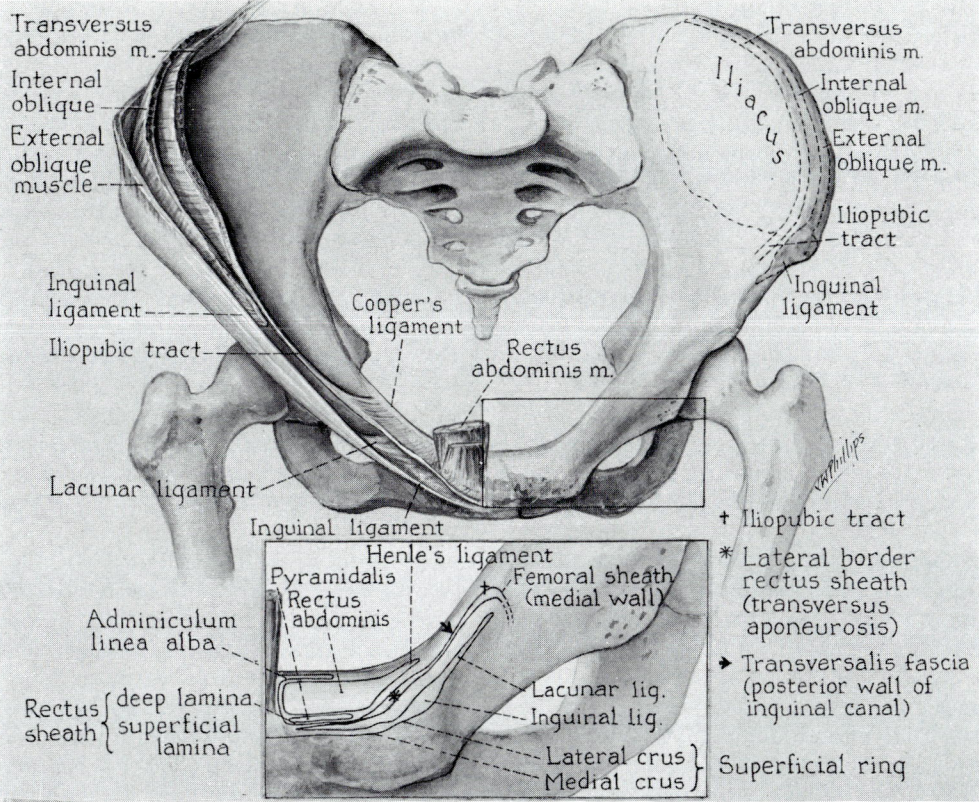

Figure 2-2. (*Left body half*) The skeletal origins of the three flat muscles are indicated in the main figure. The origins of the internal oblique and transversus abdominis muscles are not only from the crest of the ilium but also partly from iliacus fascia and the iliopectineal arch (not shown). The complex insertions of the muscle layers of the groin into the body and superior ramus of the pubis are depicted in the inset. (*Right body half*) The inferior portions of each of the three muscles of the groin have been preserved in this dissection to illustrate the relations between these layers. The drawing shows the relation between the femoral sheath and canal (removed) and the insertions of the iliopubic tract and lacunar ligament. The internal oblique muscle arches above the spermatic cord and across the groin to insert into the deep lamina of the rectus sheath.

pelvis thus opens anteriorly as well as superiorly. Because of this obliquity of the pelvis, the plane of attachment of the muscular layers of the lower abdominal wall, when viewed in parasagittal section, is not vertical, but directed obliquely outward and upward from their attachment to the pelvic skeleton.

The shape of the pelvis differs by gender. In women, the pelvis is broad and relatively flat; in men, it is more funnel-shaped, steep and narrow. As a consequence, the distance between the superior ramus of the pubis and the transversus abdominis arch is typically much less in women than in men, thus accounting for the virtual absence of direct inguinal hernia among women. Similarly, gender-based differences in the shape of the pelvis influence the occurrence of femoral hernia. The broader flat female pel-

vis is associated with a wider aperture of the femoral canal, thus permitting the more frequent occurrence of this variety of hernia in women compared with men.

Figure 2-1 shows the muscles of the pelvis and thigh that are immediately adjacent to the groin, together with the external iliofemoral vessels. This is the base on which the muscular anatomy of the groin has been constructed. These structures come into an intimate relation with the layers of the anterior abdominal wall in the inguinal region, and their spatial orientation and position need to be understood.

The anatomic layers that compose the groin are next considered seriatim, beginning at the skin and continuing progressively, insofar as possible, inward to the peritoneum.

Skin and Subcutaneous Tissues

Several landmarks are either palpable or easily visible (Fig. 2-3). The anterior superior iliac spine is found subcutaneously at the lateral aspect of the groin and is easily identified even in stout people. The body of the pubic bone can be palpated in the midline, and its upper margin is easily felt even in obese people. Also, the pubic tubercle is usually palpable at the lateral margin of the body of the pubis. It is located just above the origin of the adductor longus muscle, which can be brought into prominence by abduction of the hip.

At the lateral margin of each rectus abdominis muscle is a depression, the semilunar line, particularly marked in muscular people, that curves obliquely outward and upward from the lateral aspect of the body of the pubis to a point at about the level of the anterior superior iliac spine, after which it turns more vertically. Sometimes, it is not appreciated that the border of the rectus abdominis muscle in the region of the groin is not vertical, but more or less oblique, and that at the level of the waist the rectus abdominis muscle may occupy one third to one half of the width of the anterior abdominal wall.

In infants and obese older people, there is a prominent transverse fold in the inguinal region that demarcates the lower border of the thickest part of the abdominal panniculus.

The position of the inguinal ligament is often marked by a slight furrow just above the skin crease at the bend of the thigh. The course of the inguinal ligament between the pubic tubercle and the anterior superior iliac spine is not straight, but slightly curved, with the convexity toward the feet.

The course of the inferior epigastric vessels, which are located deep to the transversalis fascia, can be outlined by a line connecting the medial aspect of the deep inguinal ring with a point on the lateral border of the rectus abdominis muscle halfway between the pubis and the level of the umbilicus.

The skin tension lines in the groin are transverse, although they tend to curve obliquely upward laterally. Incisions should be made in the lines of skin tension (Langer lines) because this produces a wound that heals more kindly and with a better cosmetic result. Adequate flaps of skin and subcutaneous tissue always can be mobilized to allow exposure of all the groin structures through a transverse incision placed in the lines of skin tension.

Subcutaneous Fat

This layer contains the bulk of fat in the lower abdominal wall. Its thickness varies with the obesity of the person (see Fig. 2-3). The fat lobules tend to be large, and in obese people, this tissue may be further divided irregularly into several layers by thin laminae of areolar tissue. This fatty layer is continuous with the subcutaneous fat of the adjacent abdominal wall and with the corresponding layers of the thigh and perineum.

The superficial epigastric vein frequently is visible in the midportion of the groin, pursuing a more or less vertical course upward in the subcutaneous tis-

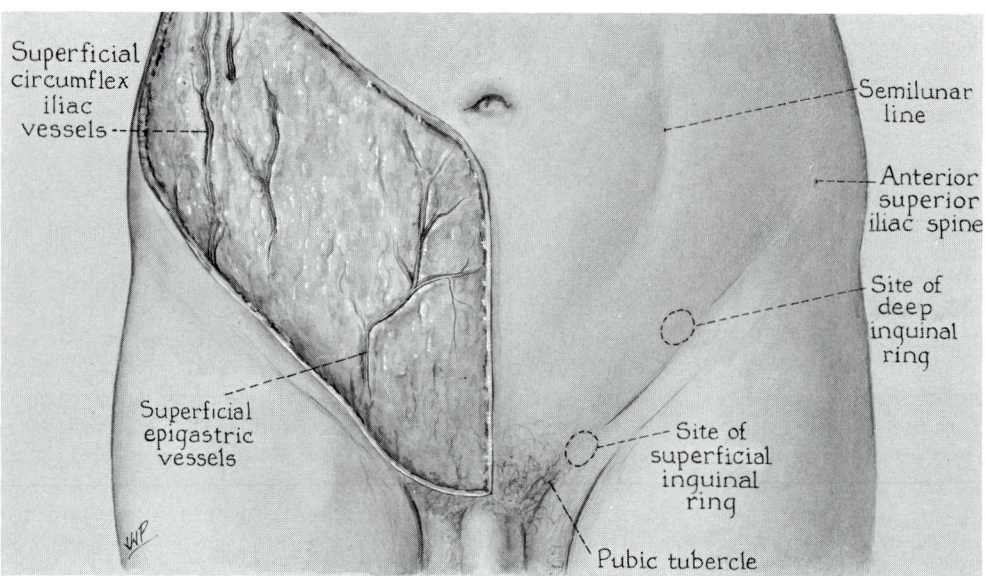

Figure 2-3.   (*Left body half*) Superficial landmarks in the groin. (*Right body half*) Dissection of the subcutaneous tissues of the groin to the level of Scarpa fascia.

sues. It is accompanied by the superficial epigastric artery. Branches of the superficial circumflex iliac vessels are present laterally near the iliac crest. At the neck of the scrotum, just inferior to the pubic tubercle, the superficial external pudendal vessels are found crossing from their origin in the region of the fossa ovalis to be distributed to the penis and scrotum.

Scarpa Fascia

Scarpa fascia is a more or less dense, homogeneous, membranous sheet of areolar tissue that forms a definite lamina in the depths of the subcutaneous tissues and usually is most prominent in the region of the groin (Fig. 2-4). It may be mistaken for the external oblique aponeurosis by the surgical novice, but it can be differentiated by the absence of the parallel collagenous fibers characteristic of an aponeurosis and by the fact that grasping Scarpa fascia and moving it back and forth causes the skin to move with this layer, whereas a similar maneuver of grasping the aponeurosis does not result in skin movement because skin is not attached to the external oblique aponeurosis.

Scarpa fascia becomes thinner superiorly and then loses its identity in the subcutaneous tissues of the flank and abdomen above the level of the umbilicus. Medially, it is attached to the linea alba in the midline, descends onto the dorsum of the penis, forming the fundiform and suspensory ligaments and the superficial fascia of that organ, and continues over the scrotum as the dartos tunic. Scarpa fascia is attached laterally to the crest of the ilium. Inferiorly, it passes over the inguinal ligament into the thigh.

In the region of the external inguinal ring, Scarpa fascia has a firm attachment to the pubis lateral to the spermatic cord and just above the origin of the abductor longus muscle; the fusion to bone is continued posteriorly along the ischiopubic ramus and into the perineum, where this layer is called *Colles fascia*. Between the pubic tubercle and the adjacent pubic bone, Scarpa fascia has no inferior attachment; the opening thus made, the abdominoscrotal passage, serves to transmit the spermatic cord.

Deep to the membranous layer of Scarpa fascia, a further collection of subcutaneous fat may be found. This layer is always much thinner and the lobules much smaller than those of the more superficial panniculus. This deep fatty layer may be entirely absent in people who are asthenic.

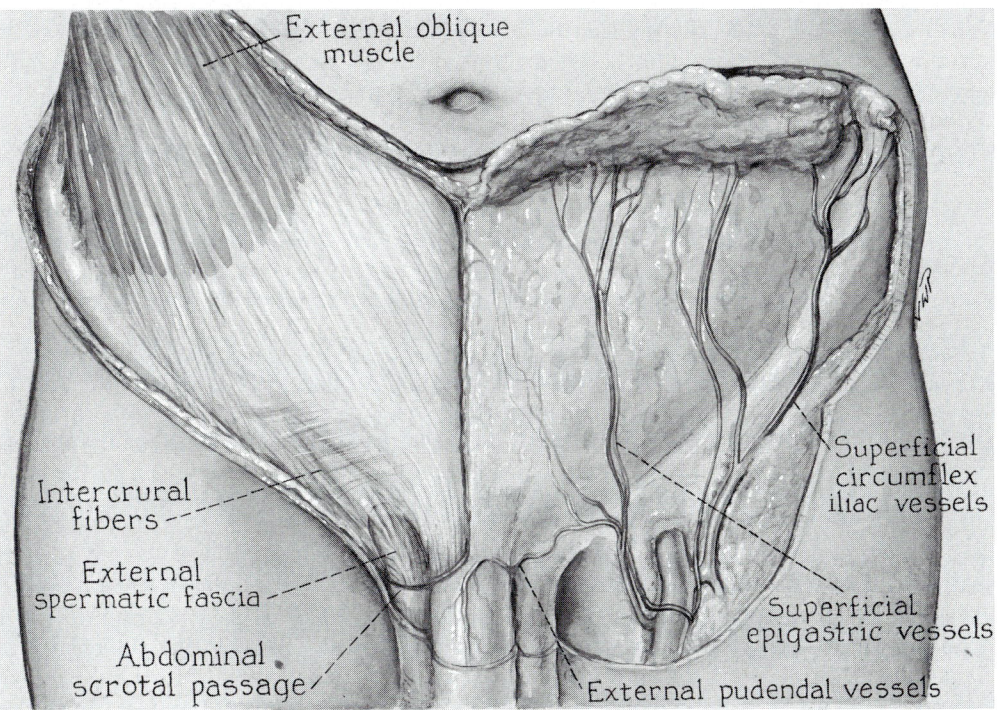

Figure 2-4. (*Left body half*) Deeper dissection of the subcutaneous tissues. The more superficial layer of fat (Camper fascia) and the membranous layer (Scarpa fascia) have been elevated to show the course of the superficial blood vessels. (*Right body half*) The subcutaneous tissues have been excised, revealing the external oblique muscle and aponeurosis covered by the innominate fascia. At the upper border of the dissection, the external oblique muscle is depicted as extending more medially than is usually the case (see Fig. 2-6).

In an occasional patient, there is no definite membrane that can be designated as Scarpa fascia; in such patients, usually obese adults, this membranous layer becomes so infiltrated and broken up by fat that its identification as a separate structure is impossible.

Abdominoscrotal Passage and Superficial Inguinal Ring

The abdominoscrotal passage, a normal opening in Scarpa fascia, is found overlying the inferolateral aspect of the pubic tubercle. This oval opening easily admits an examining finger to follow the spermatic cord up to the position of the superficial inguinal ring. The superficial ring is located immediately superolateral to the pubic tubercle. The spermatic cord, identified by palpation as it emerges from the superficial ring, can be traced to its entry into the neck of the scrotum; the ductus deferens can be felt distinctly as a firm structure on the posterior aspect of the spermatic cord.

Unless the superficial inguinal ring has been dilated by the passage of an indirect inguinal hernia, an examining finger usually cannot enter the superficial inguinal ring or the inguinal canal. Surgical teaching commonly, and mistakenly, indicates that an examining finger can be inserted into the canal; such teaching only perpetuates an error in this regard.

The deep inguinal ring is located midway between the anterior superior iliac spine and the pubic tubercle, about an inch above the skin crease between thigh and abdomen. The course of the inguinal canal is obliquely downward from the deep to the superficial ring.

Innominate Fascia

The external oblique aponeurosis is covered externally by a well-defined layer of investing fascia, the innominate fascia, which separates it from the overlying subcutaneous tissues (see Fig. 2-4). It is particularly adherent, being fixed to the aponeurosis and the much thinner posterior investing layer of external oblique fascia by small fascial bands that interdigitate between the tendinous fibers of the external oblique aponeurosis.

The innominate fascia covers the inguinal ligament and the thickened lower margin of the external oblique aponeurosis. Together with the inguinal ligament, it is firmly attached to bone at the anterior superior iliac spine and in the region of the pubic tubercle. Between these two bony attachments, the midportion of the inguinal ligament has a free lower border; the innominate fascia binds this free border to the tissues of the thigh, giving rise to the gently inferiorly curving line of the inguinal ligament as it

crosses the groin. At the superficial ring, the innominate fascia, together with the delicate posterior investing fascia of the external oblique, which here fuses with the innominate fascia, gives rise to a tubular prolongation, the external spermatic fascia (see Fig. 2-4), which is the final investment of the spermatic cord and testis just deep to the dartos tunic.

Intercrural Fibers

The intercrural fibers are present only in the lower portion of the innominate fascia in the region just above and lateral to the superficial inguinal ring (see Fig. 2-4). These aponeurotic fibers take their origin from the lateral half of the inguinal ligament and sweep medially across the triangular gap in the aponeurosis toward the midline. They are an integral part of the innominate fascia and are directed transversely or slightly obliquely upward, crossing the main fibers of the underlying external oblique aponeurosis at an acute angle. The intercrural fibers are irregularly spaced and show a great deal of variability in number and density. They serve to limit or close the apex of the triangular opening in the lower external oblique aponeurosis and bind together the aponeurotic margins of the superficial ring; thus, they resist the spreading of this aperture in instances of inguinal hernia.

External Oblique Aponeurosis

The external oblique aponeurosis is the most superficial of the three flat musculoaponeurotic (muscle and aponeurosis) layers that make up the anterolateral wall of the abdomen (Figs. 2-5 and 2-6). Imagine a curved line drawn between the anterior superior iliac spine and the midpoint of the anterior costal margin (Fig. 2-7). Lateral to this line, the external oblique layer is muscular; medial to this line, the external oblique layer usually is entirely aponeurotic. Therefore, in the region of the groin, there is no external oblique muscle, only aponeurosis. The aponeurosis is directed obliquely downward, continuing the lines of the muscular fasciculi.

Medially, the tendinous fibers of the external oblique aponeurosis pass anterior to the rectus abdominis muscle, forming the superficial layer of the rectus sheath, and then fuse with the aponeuroses of the underlying internal oblique and transversus abdominis muscles.

Inferiorly, the aponeurosis has a further insertion into the body of the pubis and the pubic tubercle and in this area presents a triangular opening through which the spermatic cord passes. This triangular apo-

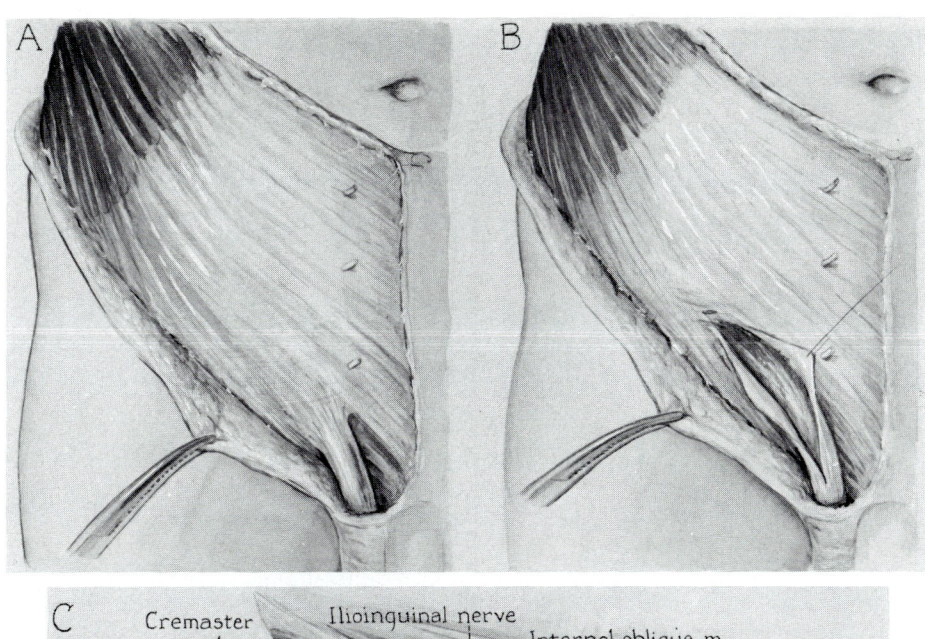

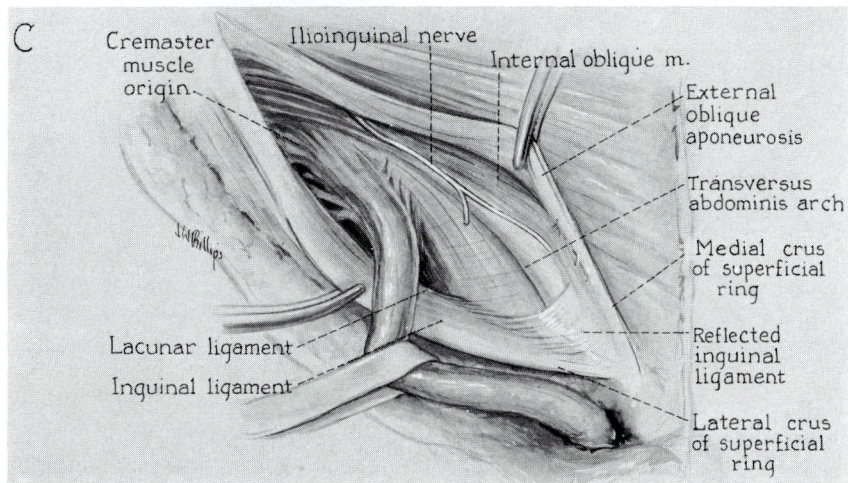

Figure 2-5. Dissection of the inguinal canal. (*A*) The intact external oblique lamina is depicted. (*B*) The external spermatic fascia and innominate fascia have been incised through the superficial inguinal ring. (*C*) The external oblique aponeurosis has been opened widely and the spermatic cord mobilized by transecting many of its areolar (cremasteric fascia) attachments to the walls of the inguinal canal.

neurotic gap is converted into the oval superficial inguinal ring principally by the overlying investing innominate fascia, with a minor contribution by the intrinsic investing fascia from the deep surface of the external oblique aponeurosis.

Inguinal Ligament

The inguinal ligament is not an isolated structure; it is the lower, thickened portion of, and is continuous with, the external oblique aponeurosis (see Figs. 2-2 and 2-5). As the fibers of the external oblique aponeu-

rosis approach the border between groin and thigh, they roll posteriorly under the next medially adjacent fibers. In parasagittal section through its lateral third, the plane of the inguinal ligament and adjacent external oblique aponeurosis is directed obliquely outward and upward (see Fig. 2-1). The inguinal ligament is thick in this region, and the fibers within it attach to the anterior superior iliac spine and to the adjacent fascia of the iliopectineal arch. The middle third of the inguinal ligament is less thick, tending to be broader, and has a free lower border. The fibers of the external oblique aponeurosis that form the inguinal ligament in this area are turning or rolling in an arc-

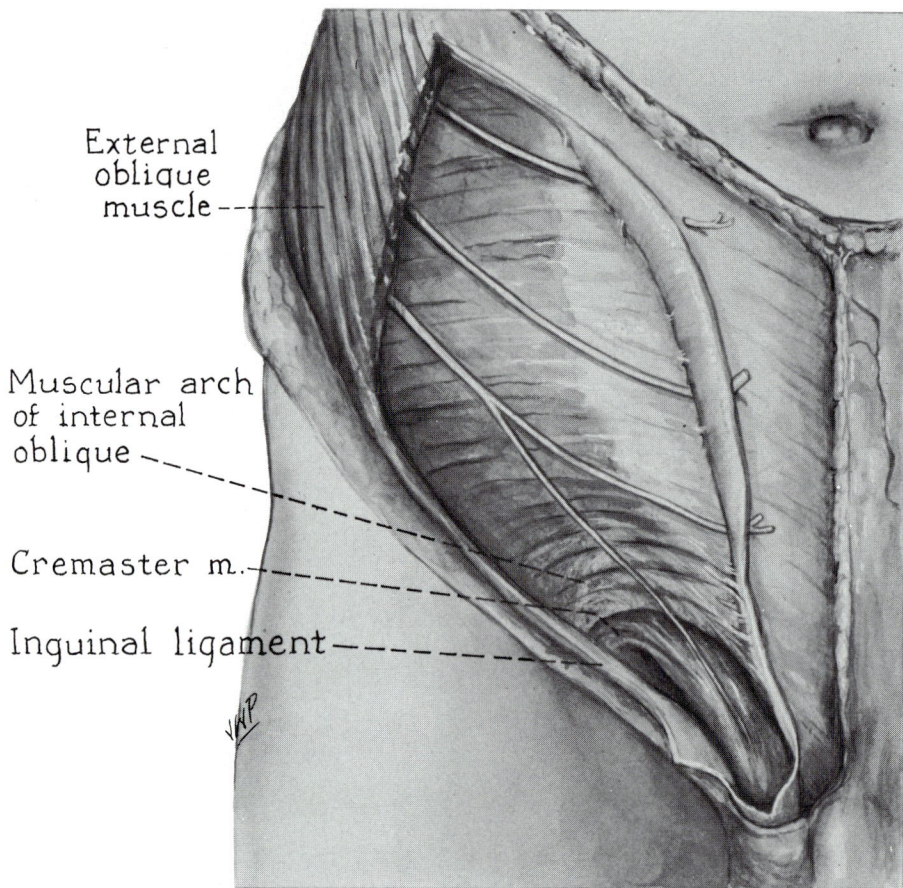

External
oblique
muscle ---

Muscular arch
of internal
oblique -

Cremaster m.-

Inguinal ligament ---

Figure 2-6. Deeper dissection of the groin (continued from Fig. 2-4, *left side*) to show the internal oblique muscle layer. The spermatic cord has been left in situ.

ing medial course across the femoral sheath to an eventual insertion into the pectineal line. This midportion of the inguinal ligament is not attached to the underlying femoral sheath and can be easily separated from it by blunt dissection.

The medial third of the inguinal ligament tends to be broad and less thick. It has rolled so that in a parasagittal section the plane of the inguinal ligament near the pubic tubercle is nearly horizontal (see Figs. 2-2 and 2-5). The fibers of the inguinal ligament in this region are firmly attached to the medial third of the superior ramus of the pubis along the pectineal line and at the pubic tubercle.

The effect of the rotation of the inguinal ligament from an oblique to a horizontal plane is to present a rounded surface toward the thigh and a hollow surface toward the inguinal canal, which acts as a supporting shelf ("the shelving border") for the spermatic cord. The gentle inferior curve toward the thigh that the inguinal ligament presents in its course between

the anterior superior iliac spine and the pubic tubercle is brought about by the attachment of its superficial investing fascia, the innominate fascia, to the fascia of the thigh.

The structure of the inguinal ligament is constant, particularly in regard to its attachment to the pubis. Important structural variations were noted in only 3 of 185 dissections. These were additional aponeurotic slips from the inguinal ligament that were attached, in common with the innominate fascia, to fascia in the thigh.

Lacunar Ligament
The lacunar ligament is merely the thinner, most inferior and lateral part of the insertion of the inguinal ligament (see Figs. 2-2 and 2-5). The separation usually is an arbitrary one and of no surgical importance. The lacunar (inguinal) ligament broadens the insertion of the parallel fibers of the inguinal ligament by

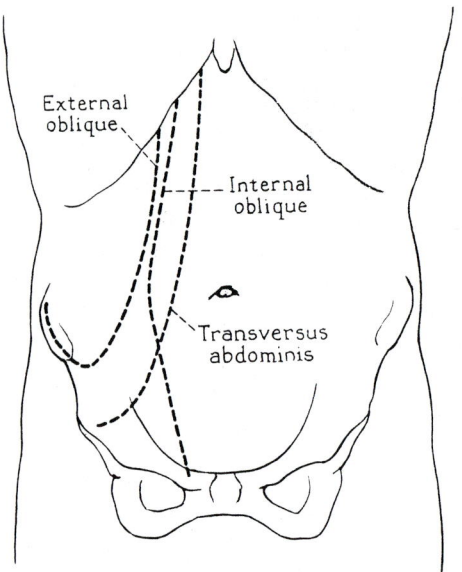

Figure 2-7. The approximate lines of transition from muscle to aponeurosis of the three flat muscles of the anterior abdominal wall. Variations of all three layers in the upper abdomen and the transversus abdominis layer in the lower abdomen are frequent.

inserting all along the pectineal line. A few fibers also may be attached to adjacent pectineus fascia.

The lacunar ligament is described in many texts as being markedly recurved and as forming the medial border of the femoral canal. The error of such statements was pointed out several years ago by McVay and Anson. The lacunar ligament, in fact, is not usually sharply recurved, and it never forms the medial border of a normal femoral canal.

In my dissections, a definitely recurved insertion of the lacunar ligament (ie, one in which the fibers of the lateral margin of the lacunar ligament recurved to their insertion through an arc of more than 45 degrees from the course of the inguinal ligament) was found in only 8 of 185 bodies. A spreading, fan-like insertion through an arc of less than 45 degrees or an insertion parallel with the inguinal ligament occurred in all other dissections.

The relation between the lacunar ligament and the femoral sheath was studied in 94 dissections with the femoral canal distended by the dissector's forefinger. In only 8 bodies did the most lateral part of the insertion of the lacunar ligament actually touch the medial border of the distended femoral canal; in 43 bodies, these two structures were separated at their attachments to pectineus fascia or the pectineal line.

Reflected Inguinal Ligament

A thin, flat group of fibers, usually tenuous in character, was noted in 70% of my dissections. The fibers were roughly triangular with a base of 2 or 3 cm along the pubic tubercle and adjacent pubic ramus in common with and at an acute angle to the attachments of the inguinal and lacunar ligaments (see Fig. 2-5). These fibers were directed upward and medially toward the linea alba. They gave an appearance of being a medial continuation of the inguinal ligament deep to the main external oblique aponeurosis and the spermatic cord, hence the designation *reflected inguinal ligament.*

This structure occupies a position on the superficial surface of the transversus abdominis aponeurosis similar to that of Henle ligament on the posterior surface of that aponeurosis. The reflected inguinal ligament has been reported to represent an insertion of decussating fibers of the external oblique aponeurosis that have crossed the linea alba from the opposite side, but I have not seen such in my dissections. The reflected inguinal ligament is of no practical importance in groin hernial repairs.

Interparietal Fasciae

The two interparietal fascial layers are so termed because of their position between the flat abdominal muscles. One is situated between the external and internal oblique layers, and the other occurs between the internal oblique and the transversus abdominis. The interparietal fasciae are formed by adjacent investing fasciae; the more superficial interparietal fascia is formed by the internal investing fascia of the external oblique muscle and the external investing fascia of the internal oblique muscle; the deeper interparietal fascia is formed by the internal investing fascia of the internal oblique muscle and the external investing fascia of the transversus abdominis muscle. The two fascial components of the two interparietal layers can be separated by careful dissection of fresh material.

These fascial layers are of interest only because they demarcate the muscle layers from one another. The deeper layer of interparietal fascia frequently is deficient in the groin, and the internal oblique muscle consequently often is intimately attached to the underlying transversus aponeurosis. Other than the fact that they serve as a landmark for the surgeon, these fasciae are of no special importance. The one exception occurs in the region of the inguinal canal, where these layers participate in the formation of the cremasteric fascia. Interparietal hernias may penetrate either of these fasciae.

Internal Oblique Muscle and Aponeurosis

The internal oblique muscle and aponeurosis are the middle one of the three flat musculoaponeurotic layers of the abdominal wall (see Fig. 2-6). Imagine a line that intersects the semilunar line near its pubic and costal ends but is somewhat more convex toward the flank so that at the level of the umbilicus, it is 1 or 2 cm lateral to the semilunar line. Lateral to this imaginary line, the internal oblique layer is muscular; medial to this line, the internal oblique becomes aponeurotic (see Fig. 2-7). The internal oblique layer, then, is mainly muscular in the inguinal region. Although this muscle is directed obliquely upward in the upper portion of the abdomen, in the region of the groin, its fibers are nearly transverse.

Sometimes, the medial bundles of the internal oblique aponeurosis interlace near the border of the rectus sheath with adjacent bundles rather than following a strictly parallel course. The main transverse direction is maintained, however, with insertion into the rectus sheath and thence into the linea alba. Occasionally, accessory muscle slips are found on the deep surface of this part of the internal oblique layer.

Throughout much of its course in the groin, the internal oblique muscle is intimately attached to the underlying fibers of the transversus abdominis aponeurosis. When the most medial part of the underlying transversus abdominis layer also is muscular (20%), the two laminae intermingle and form a functionally single muscular layer. Rarely (3%), the inferior portion of the internal oblique layer in the middle of the groin may be aponeurotic instead of muscular.

The lower muscular fasciculi of the internal oblique, arising from the iliac fascia and the iliopectineal arch near the anterior superior iliac spine, form a red muscular arch that covers the spermatic cord as it emerges from the deep inguinal ring and lies within the lateral third of the inguinal canal. As it continues medially, the lower border of this muscular arch is usually at or slightly above the level of the main aponeurotic arch of the underlying transversus abdominis layer.

The aponeurotic continuation of these lower bundles of the internal oblique usually is directed transversely to the linea alba or slightly more inferiorly to insert with the deep lamina of the rectus sheath into the body of the pubis. Only rarely (3%) do the lower fibers of the internal oblique aponeurosis turn more sharply downward to join similar fibers from the subjacent transversus aponeurosis and insert directly into the pubic tubercle and superior ramus of the pubis, thereby forming a true *conjoined tendon*.

Transversus Abdominis Muscle and Aponeurosis

The transversus abdominis muscle and aponeurosis are the innermost of the three flat abdominal muscle layers. From a clinical standpoint, this layer is the most important with regard to the pathogenesis and repair of groin hernias (Figs. 2-8 and 2-9). The relative muscular and aponeurotic extent of this layer can be ascertained by imagining a line drawn from the position of the deep inguinal ring in the middle of the groin upward to the costoxiphoid angle. Lateral to this line, the transversus layer is mainly muscular; medial to this line, the transversus layer is usually aponeurotic (see Fig. 2-7).

Variations in relative muscular and aponeurotic composition in this layer are more frequent than in the more superficial musculoaponeurotic layers, and in 20% of my dissections, the transversus abdominis muscle extended medially to near the border of the rectus sheath. Frequently, the more inferior bundles of the transversus abdominis layer in the area above and lateral to the deep inguinal ring consist of mixed muscular and aponeurotic tissues, the muscle fibers being more superficial and the aponeurotic fibers being found on the deep surface.

The most inferomedial portion of the transversus abdominis lamina, that part forming the posterior wall of the inguinal canal, becomes discontinuous. The aponeurotic fibers separate from one another, the intervening spaces being filled only by transversalis fascia. The lower border of the continuous portion of the transversus abdominis layer forms a clearly visible curved line, the *transversus abdominis arch*, which is noted most easily when this musculoaponeurotic layer is viewed from its deep or posterior aspect through the transversalis fascia (see Fig. 2-9). The transversus abdominis arch forms an important landmark for the surgeon because it is the superior border of the lateral part of most direct inguinal hernial defects. The fibers that form this arch have their muscular origin laterally from the iliopectineal arch, from which they curve upward and medially, crossing the spermatic cord structures. Aponeurotic reinforcement of this lower border of the transversus abdominis serves to limit and define the superior margin of the deep inguinal ring.

The transversus abdominis arch, having crossed over the spermatic cord at the deep ring, then curves gently downward across the groin (see Fig. 2-9). In 60% of bodies, this arching line was at least 0.5 cm but less than 2 cm above the superior ramus of the pubis, the measurement being made at a point halfway between the lateral edge of the rectus tendon and the medial edge of the femoral canal. In 17% of bod-

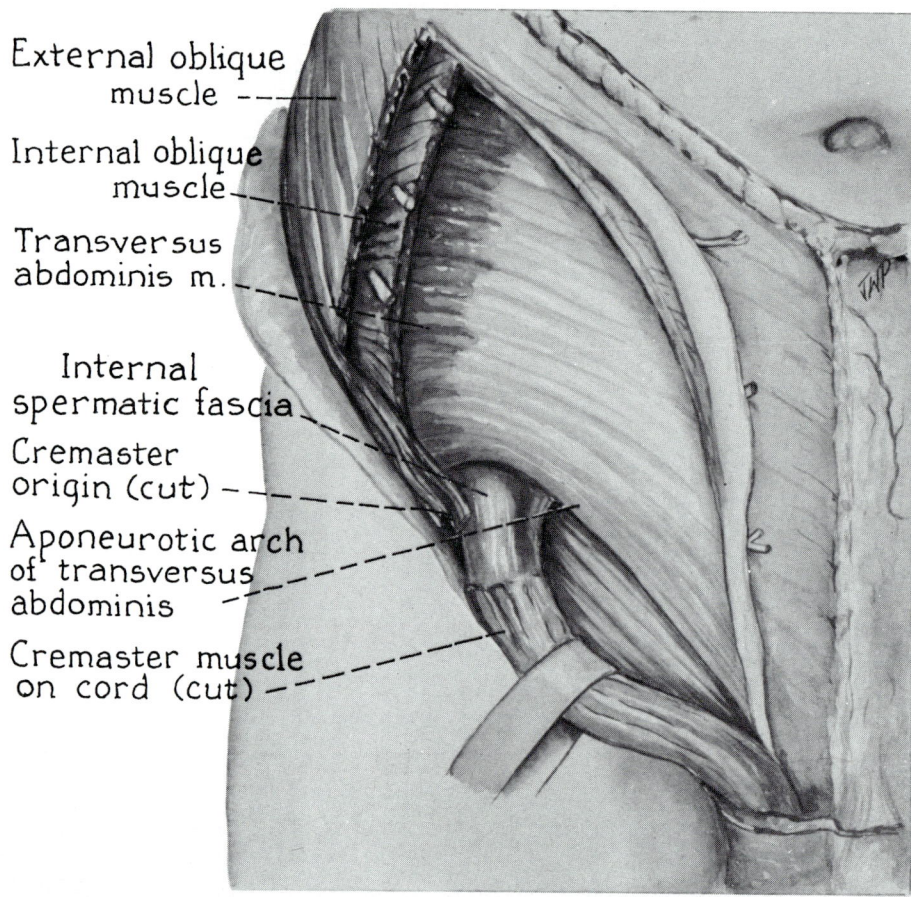

External oblique
muscle

Internal oblique
muscle

Transversus
abdominis m.

Internal
spermatic fascia

Cremaster
origin (cut)

Aponeurotic arch
of transversus
abdominis

Cremaster muscle
on cord (cut)

Figure 2-8. Dissection to show the deepest of the three muscle layers of the groin. The spermatic cord has been mobilized to show the arching muscular and aponeurotic lower margin of the transversus abdominis (the transversus abdominis arch). Inferior to this arch, the posterior wall of the inguinal canal is formed by transversalis fascia.

ies, the arch of the transversus abdominis aponeurosis was within 0.5 cm of the pubis, and in 23% of bodies, it was high in the groin, more than 2 cm above the pubic bone. In most bodies (75%), the intersection of the transversus abdominis arch with the rectus sheath occurred 0.5 cm or more above the pubic bone. In 14%, the intersection was within 0.5 cm of the pubis. In 11% of my dissections, the arching line, which represents the lower border of the main portion of the transversus abdominis aponeurosis, inserted into the superior pubic ramus lateral to the rectus tendon.

The number of aponeurotic fibers in the discontinuous lower portion of the transversus abdominis lamina varies a great deal. In some bodies, the tendinous fibers are relatively numerous; in others, they are scarce. At the most inferior aspect of this portion of the transversus abdominis layer, there is a stronger collection of aponeurotic fibers, the iliopubic tract. Because the discontinuous portion of the transversus

abdominis lamina forms the posterior wall of the inguinal canal in a typical body, and because this is the area through which direct inguinal herniation occurs, it seems likely that the extent of the discontinuous area and the number and strength of aponeurotic fibers in it are major influences in the development of a direct inguinal hernia.

Falx Inguinalis and Conjoined Tendon

In a few bodies, the continuous aponeurotic fasciculi in the lower portion of the transversus abdominis layer are not directed more or less transversely to insert into the rectus sheath, but turn more sharply downward to insert into the superior pubic ramus for a variable distance lateral to the rectus tendon. This variety of lateral insertion of the transversus abdominis aponeurosis was found in 11% of my dissections.

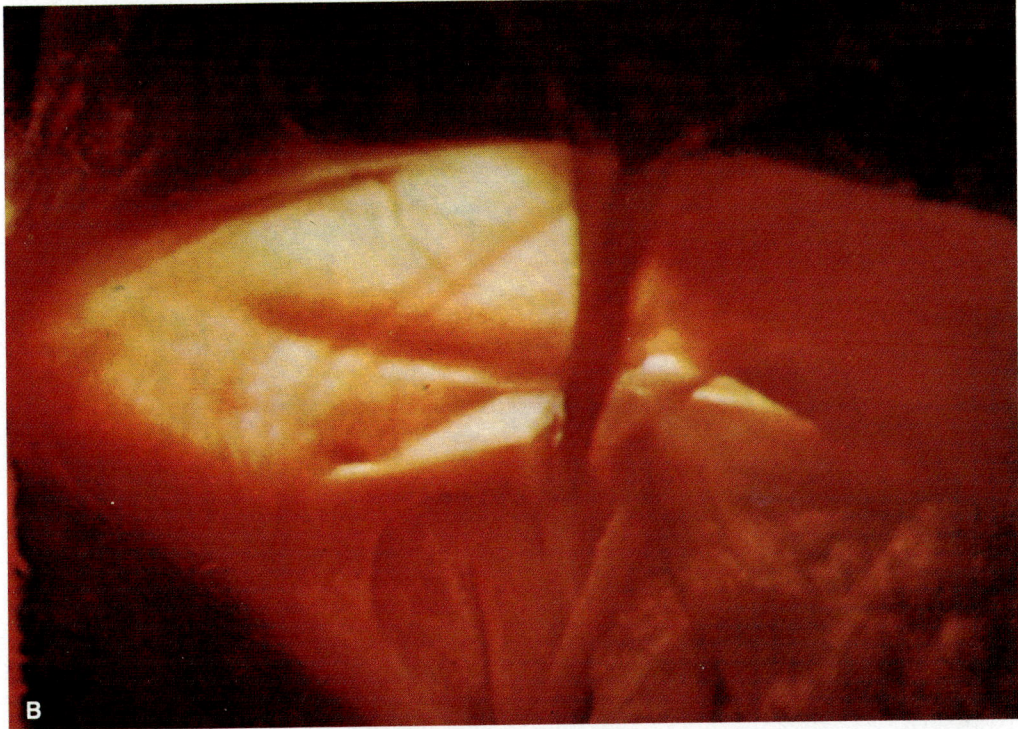

Figure 2-9. (*A*) The line drawing identifies the important structures in the transversus layer of the groin that are shown in color in Figure 2-9*B* (scale, 1:1). (*B*) This photograph was taken on completion of a dissection that removed all tissues in the groin, both superficial and deep to the transversus abdominis muscle and aponeurosis, and their associated structures. The camera was placed within the pelvis, "looking" from within, outward, and the transversus abdominis structures were delineated by transillumination. The area included in the photo is about 6 cm².

In all but one of these bodies, this portion of the transversus aponeurosis was dense, especially in the area just alongside the rectus tendon, and it is then known as the *falx inguinalis.*

The falx inguinalis has an intimate relation with the rectus sheath, as might be expected, because both are formed just above the level of the pubis by the transversus abdominis aponeurosis. Sometimes, it is difficult to see a distinction among transversus abdominis, rectus sheath, and falx inguinalis when they are viewed from the anterior aspect of the groin. The falx consists of that dense inserting portion of the transversus aponeurosis lateral to the tendon and muscular belly of the rectus abdominis. This distinction can be seen more clearly when these structures are viewed from the posterior side. The falx inguinalis, especially when it is not extensively developed, may appear to be merely a slightly expanded lateral border of the rectus sheath.

As pointed out earlier, the falx inguinalis is usually formed by fibers from the transversus abdominis

aponeurosis alone (7%). Less often (3%), the fibers of the transversus abdominis aponeurosis are joined in this area by fibers from the internal oblique aponeurosis to form a true *conjoined tendon.* The rarity of an anatomic conjunction of these two layers needs special emphasis. An insertion of dense fibers of only the transversus aponeurosis into the pubis lateral to the rectus tendon is more common (falx inguinalis); such an insertion of the internal oblique is unusual. The term *conjoined tendon* is so frequently used loosely to designate any aponeurotic insertion in this area that it provides a distinct possibility of misleading the careful dissector. However, the distinction between falx inguinalis and conjoined tendon is one of anatomic nicety and admittedly of little practical importance in the operating room provided that the distinction is understood. What the surgeon visualizes as "conjoined tendon" usually is composed of fibers of the transversus aponeurosis only and rarely is formed by a conjunction of fibers of both the transversus and internal oblique layers.

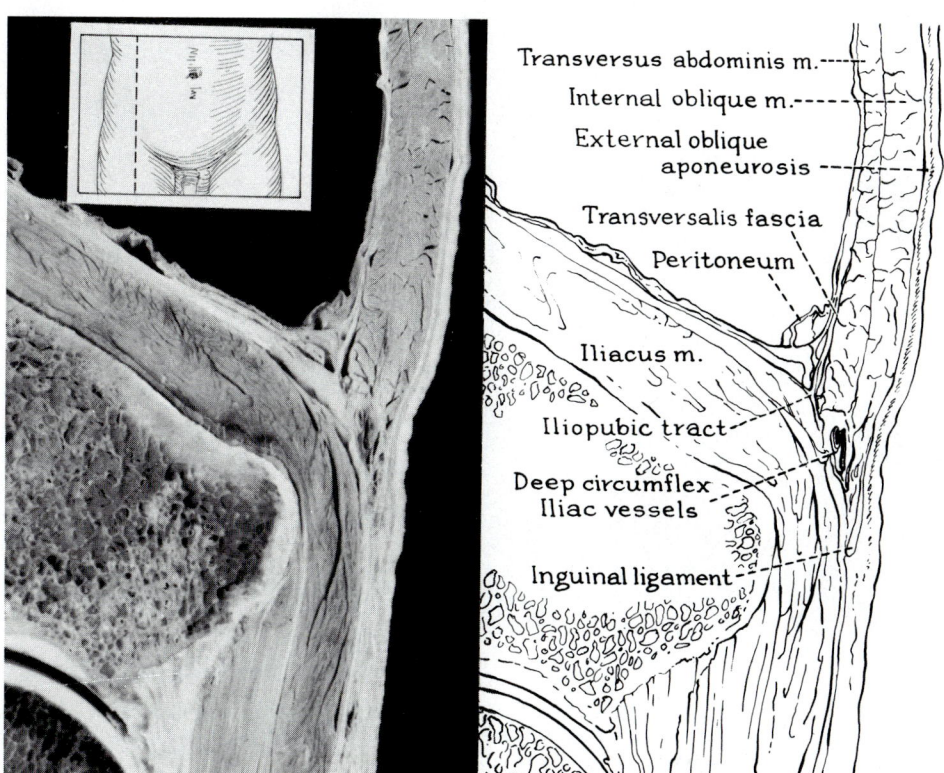

Figure 2-10. A parasagittal section of the right groin through the iliacus muscle just lateral to the femoral sheath, viewed from its lateral aspect. An embalmed cadaver was frozen, and then a parasagittal slice of tissue was cut, laid flat on its medial surface, and photographed under water. The relations of the layers of the anterior abdominal wall in the lateral portion of the groin are well shown. Note particularly the relative positions of the inguinal ligament (superficial musculoaponeurotic lamina) and the iliopubic tract (deep musculoaponeurotic lamina).

Iliopubic Tract

The iliopubic tract is a small, entirely aponeurotic band within the transversus abdominis lamina that bridges across the external iliofemoral vessels from the iliopectineal arch to the superior ramus of the pubis (Figs. 2-10 and 2-11; see Fig. 2-9). If the transversus abdominis muscle and aponeurosis are considered together with the investing transversalis fascia as a single layer, the iliopubic tract forms the most inferior margin in the groin of that deepest musculoaponeurotic lamina. Like the inguinal ligament, which has a similar relation to the external oblique aponeurosis, the iliopubic tract is firmly anchored at both ends. Unlike the inguinal ligament, the iliopubic tract shows more variation in density. It may form a strong band, or it may be represented by relatively few fibers.

Laterally, the iliopubic tract is attached to the iliopectineal arch and the iliopsoas fascia overlying the iliacus and psoas muscles. Through this fascia, the iliopubic tract gains attachment to bone at the anterior superior iliac spine and along the adjacent inner lip of the iliac crest in common with the origin of the transversus abdominis muscle. In this lateral area of the groin, the fibers of the iliopubic tract are overlapped by the inguinal ligament, which lies immediately superficial to it.

The iliopubic tract is directed medially, becoming separated from the inguinal ligament. It presents beneath the deep inguinal ring, forming the lower aponeurotic border of that aperture, and then crosses the external iliofemoral vessels, forming the line about which the transversalis fascia is reflected into the leg to form the femoral sheath. In this area, the iliopubic tract reinforces and defines the anterior margin of the femoral sheath. It is intimately connected to the transversalis fascia, forming the anterior femoral sheath, and cannot be separated from it by blunt dissection (Fig. 2-12).

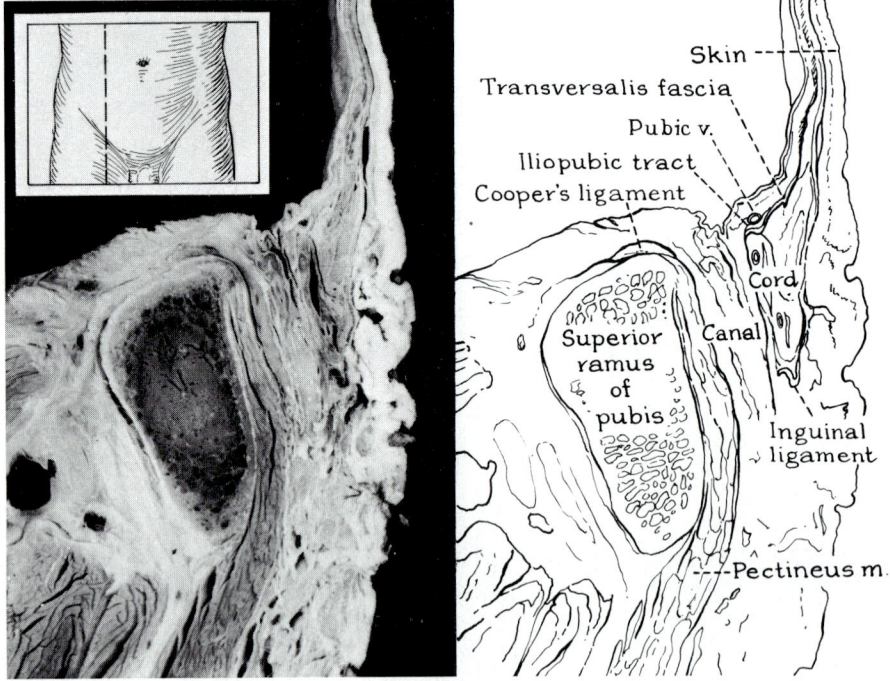

Figure 2-11. A parasagittal section of the right groin through the middle of the femoral canal, viewed from its lateral aspect. This section was cut from the same specimen as shown in Figure 2-10. Although some distortion has occurred secondary to introduction of embalming solution into the right femoral artery, the separation of the superficial and deep musculoaponeurotic layers in the midportion of the groin is well illustrated. The spermatic cord contained within the inguinal canal intervenes between the superficial layer (anterior wall of inguinal canal, inguinal and lacunar ligaments, external oblique aponeurosis) and the deep layer (posterior wall of inguinal canal, iliopubic tract, transversalis fascia, transversus abdominis aponeurosis). Note that the posterior wall or "floor" of the inguinal canal is actually posterosuperior in relation to the spermatic cord, whereas the aspect of the inguinal canal designated as the inferior wall is actually posterior in relation to the spermatic cord.

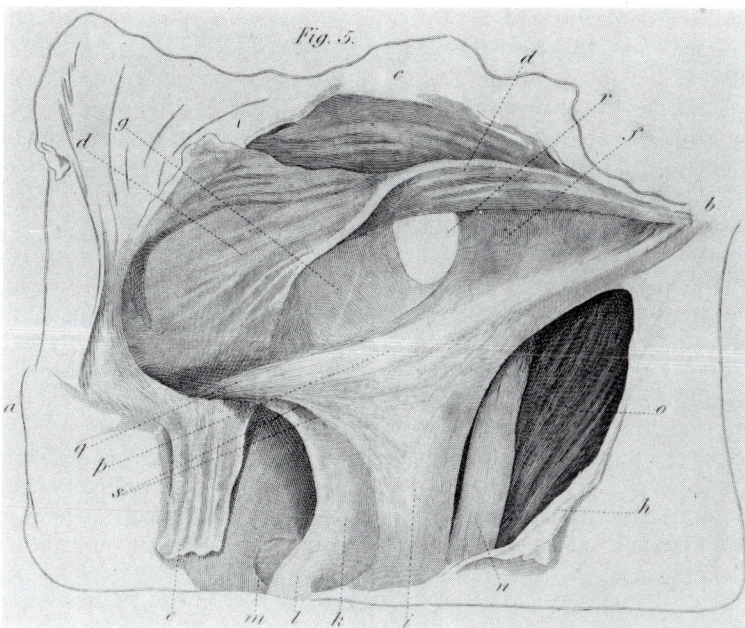

Figure 2-12.   An external view of a dissection of the left groin by Sir Astley Paston Cooper. The inguinal ligament has been transected (e) and the transversus abdominus arch elevated (d) to show the continuities of the transversalis fascia and the anterior femoral sheath. The deep inguinal ring is located at r; the transversalis fascia is depicted as a bilaminar structure (f, g). This apparent bilaminar nature of the transversalis fascia is brought about by the redundancy of the transversalis fascia as it forms the transversalis fascia sling; a dissection similar to Cooper's is produced if the transversalis fascia is dissected from its attachment to the spermatic cord, the cord excised, and the redundant transversalis fascia smoothed into flat surfaces. The iliopubic tract (p; deep crural arch) is located at the upper margin of the femoral sheath, crossing from the anterosuperior iliac spine (b) and iliacus fascia, laterally, to the superior ramus of the pubic, medially. (Fig. 5 of Plate XII from Cooper AP. The anatomy and surgical treatment of abdominal hernia, ed 2. London, Longman & Co, 1827)

The iliopubic tract then curves posteriorly and inferiorly around the femoral canal; its fibers fan out to be attached to the pectineal line along the superior ramus of the pubis. The few most inferior and then lateral fibers of the iliopubic tract turn downward most sharply to attach to pectineus fascia. This portion of the iliopubic tract forms the recurved medial fascial margin of the femoral canal in the normal groin (see Figs. 2-2, 2-9, and 2-11). It is the iliopubic tract, therefore, that defines the medial border of the normal femoral canal, *not* the lacunar ligament as is usually described. The lateral inserting margin of the lacunar ligament is not so sharply recurved as is that of the iliopubic tract, and the lacunar ligament, in relation to the iliopubic tract, lies both superficially and medially. The lacunar ligament comes into contact with the medial wall of the femoral canal only when the canal is enlarged, as in femoral hernia.

The iliopubic tract was identified in 98% of my dissections. In the few bodies in which the iliopubic tract was absent as a separate and distinct structure, the main portion of the transversus abdominis aponeurosis had an extremely wide insertion into the superior pubic ramus, extending across the posterior wall of the inguinal canal to the medial border of the femoral ring. In 22% of my dissections, the iliopubic tract was diminished in strength, as judged by gross appearance and resistance to displacement; in 28%, it was above average in density and formed a strong aponeurotic band. My observations concerning the anatomic structure and disposition of the iliopubic tract have been independently confirmed by Gilroy and associates.

The iliopubic tract frequently has been confused with the more obvious and denser inguinal ligament, which lies immediately adjacent and superficially to it.

In many textbooks of anatomy, a drawing of an internal view of the groin is presented in which the iliopubic tract is labeled "inguinal ligament." It should be obvious that in such an internal view of the groin, the inguinal ligament cannot be seen because the transversalis fascia, the transversus abdominis aponeurosis, and the spermatic cord within the inguinal canal intervene between the viewer and the inguinal ligament.

The inguinal ligament and the iliopubic tract are separate entities and belong to different musculoaponeurotic layers of the groin, a fact that readily may be ascertained by dissection of an unfixed body. The inguinal ligament is part of the external oblique layer of the groin; the iliopubic tract is part of the transversus abdominis layer. The separation or distinction of the iliopubic tract from the inguinal ligament is one of more than anatomic nicety. The mislabeling of the iliopubic tract as the inguinal ligament has been one of the principal sources of confusion in understanding anatomic relations in the groin. In addition, the iliopubic tract is of practical importance to the surgeon because, when well developed, it can and should be used in groin hernial repairs.

Transversalis Fascia

The transversus abdominis muscle and aponeurosis are covered internally by a well-defined layer of investing fascia, the transversalis fascia, which separates the muscular abdominal wall from the underlying preperitoneal fat (Fig. 2-13; see Figs. 2-10 and 2-11). There also is an investing fascia on the external surface of the transversus abdominis lamina that I have grouped with the interparietal fasciae.

The transversalis fascia is merely a portion of the continuous layer of endoabdominal fascia that com-

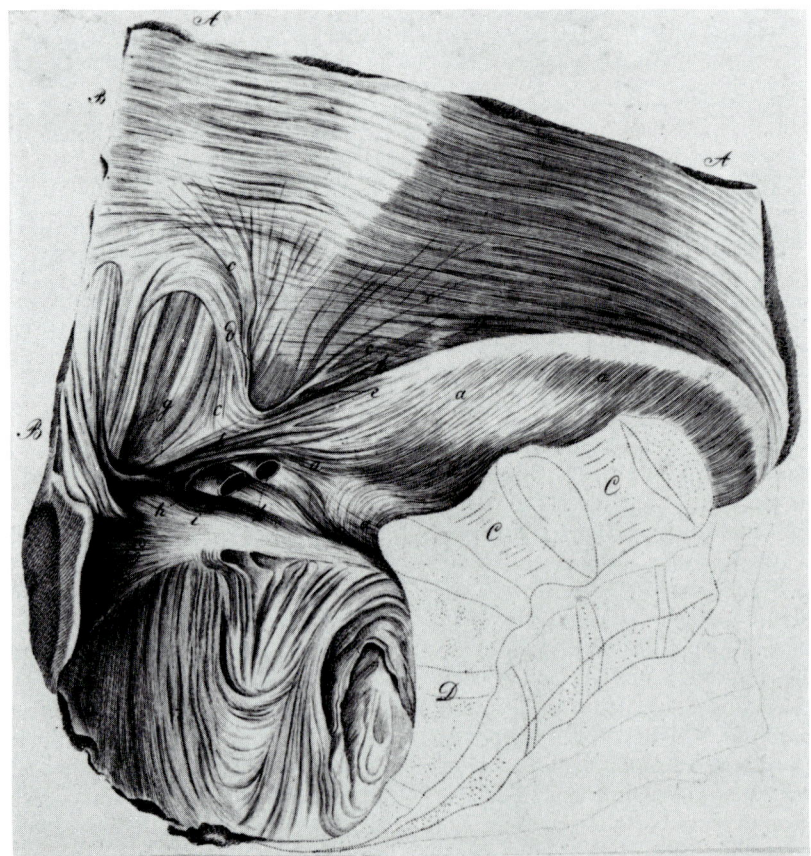

Figure 2-13. An internal view of a dissection of the right groin by Professor Hesselbach. The transversalis fascia sling (c, c) about the deep inguinal ring (d) and the iliopubic tract (b) with its recurving insertion at the medial margin of the femoral ring (h) are well shown. (Plate III from Hesselbach FC. Neueste Anatomish-pathologische Untersuchungen über den Ursprung und das Fortschreiten der Leisten- und Schenkelbrüche. Würzburg, Stahel)

pletely encloses the abdominal cavity. In various areas, the endoabdominal fascia is given particular regional designations derived from the overlying muscles, in this instance, the transversus abdominis muscle. The transversalis fascia, therefore, is immediately continuous with the lumbar, iliac, psoas, and obturator fasciae. It continues medially as the rectus fascia, forming a posterior covering of the lower part of the rectus muscle, to join the transversalis fascia of the opposite side.

The transversalis fascia is adherent over the muscular and aponeurotic extent of the transversus abdominis layer, being fixed by small fascial slips that interdigitate between the musculoaponeurotic fasciculi and anchor the transversalis fascia to the deeper layer of interparietal fascia that lies on the superficial surface of the transversus abdominis muscle and aponeurosis.

In an embalmed cadaver, the transversalis fascia is a matted opaque sheet, an appearance that can be misleading. In the living person, it is, for the most part, a thin, sometimes diaphanous, transparent membrane of little intrinsic strength. In the groin, the transversalis fascia tends to be a little thicker and therefore a little stronger than it is elsewhere in the abdominal cavity, but in the normal groin, it is still a weak fascia in absolute terms. In only 20% of my dissections was the transversalis fascia judged to be of sufficient strength unsupported to retain sutures.

The structure of the lower portion of the transversalis fascia, that part between the transversus abdominis arch superiorly and Cooper ligament and the iliopubic tract inferiorly, is of considerable interest (see Figs. 2-8 and 2-9). This is the critical weak area in which inguinal hernias are found. The transversus abdominis arch forms a relatively resistant aponeurotic superior margin in this area that begins laterally at the iliopectineal arch and is directed medially above the deep inguinal ring and across the groin to insert into the rectus sheath or the pubic bone. Similarly, the iliopubic tract and the Cooper ligament together form a resistant inferior margin in this area that begins laterally at the iliopectineal arch and is directed medially below the deep inguinal ring and across the external iliofemoral vessels to and along the superior ramus of the pubis. Between these aponeurotic margins, the continuity of the transversus abdominis layer of the groin is maintained chiefly by transversalis fascia.

The deep inguinal ring occupies the lateral half of the area between the transversus abdominis arch above and the iliopubic tract below. At the deep inguinal ring, the transversalis fascia is thrown into a fold about the spermatic cord structures, forming the *transversalis fascial sling,* and is also continued about the spermatic cord into the inguinal canal, forming the *internal spermatic fascia.* Within the transversalis

fascia along the medial aspect of the deep inguinal ring, there is a variable amount of aponeurotic reinforcement, the *interfoveolar ligament,* most of which is really periadventitial tissue of the inferior epigastric vessels.

The medial half of this area of the transversalis fascia forms the posterior wall, or "floor," of the inguinal canal. It is a relatively weak area with regard to resistance to herniation. The transversalis fascia in this area is slightly thickened by apposition to its external surface of the deeper layer of interparietal fascia. Reinforcement is also provided by the variable number of aponeurotic fibers that bridge the gap between the transversus abdominis arch above and the Cooper ligament and iliopubic tract below. These reinforcing fibers are usually directed obliquely from above downward and medially and tend to be parallel. Occasionally, additional reinforcement is provided by aponeurotic fibers directed from below obliquely upward and medially, resulting in a mesh-like arrangement. The strength of this part of the groin is directly proportional to the number of aponeurotic fibers it contains; this is the area at which disruption occurs in primary direct inguinal hernia.

Transversalis Fascial Sling

At the deep inguinal ring, there is a tubular projection of transversalis fascia, the internal spermatic fascia, that extends outward in a blunt funnel-like manner to cover the ductus deferens and the spermatic vessels. The blunt funnel is not perfectly conical, however. It is skewed; the axis of the funnel is less oblique than the axis of the ductus and vessels through the deep inguinal ring. There is therefore a relative redundancy of transversalis fascia on the medial side of the deep ring. This fascial redundancy forms a fold, shaped much like a monk's hood, that supports the spermatic cord structures as they traverse the deep inguinal ring. This is the transversalis fascial sling (see Figs. 2-9 and 2-13). The genesis of the sling can perhaps be appreciated by referring to Figure 2-14. The transversalis fascial sling in outline is somewhat like the letter V, with the open end pointing laterally and superiorly; the gradually diverging ends or arms of this sling are called the *crura.* The *superior crus* is the longer, having an extensive attachment above the deep ring through the interdigitating fascial slips that lace together the investing fasciae on the two surfaces of the transversus abdominis muscle. The shorter *inferior crus* runs parallel with and slightly above the iliopubic tract (see Figs. 2-9 and 2-13).

The transversalis fascial sling and its crura provide the basis for the shutter mechanism that is thought to operate at the deep inguinal ring. According to this hypothesis, the transversus abdominis muscle contracts during coughing or similar activity that

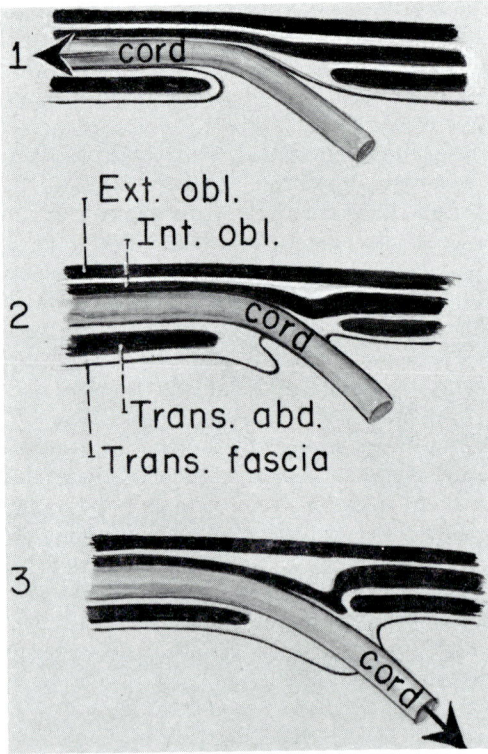

Figure 2-14. A schematic representation of the relations of the transversalis fascia and the spermatic cord. The drawing represents a transverse section made through the right groin at the level of the deep inguinal ring. The transversalis fascia is relatively redundant at the deep ring. Traction on the cord toward the scrotum (1) pulls the cone of transversalis fascia through the deep ring; it is this continuity of fascia that forms the internal spermatic fascia. Traction on the cord toward the preperitoneal space (3) completely reverses the position of the cone of transversalis fascia. When the cord is in mid-position between these extremes (2), the redundancy of the transversalis fascia forms a double layer, looping about the medial side of the cord just internal to the deep inguinal ring; this is the transversalis fascial sling.

raises intraabdominal pressure, the crura of the transversalis fascial sling are drawn closer together, and both of the crura are drawn laterally, this motion being transmitted from the contracting transversus abdominis muscle to its investing transversalis fascia. The approximation of the crura of the sling partially closes the internal inguinal ring, while the lateral sliding motion of the sling flattens the cord structures against the abdominal wall, increasing the obliquity of their course of exit. The deep inguinal ring tends to close during the maximum of increase in intraabdominal pressure, in much the same manner as the momentary action of a camera shutter, providing additional protection to this vulnerable area from forces that may lead to the development of a hernia.

Although the sling-shutter mechanism is an attractive hypothesis, note that evidence that such a mechanism actually functions in this area is incomplete. At the other extreme of opinion, some surgeons are convinced that all indirect inguinal hernias are congenital and that sudden increases in intraabdominal pressure are of primary etiologic importance in direct inguinal hernias but are not really important in the indirect variety.

In any event, the transversalis fascial sling and its crura, while forming an interesting feature of normal groin structure, are not of great importance in the repair of an indirect hernia. The essential technical feature of this repair is the approximation by suture, about the cord structures, of the transversus abdominis arch, above, to the iliopubic tract, below. The investing transversalis fascia usually is included in the sutures, but this is not essential for successful repair.

Interfoveolar Ligament

The interfoveolar ligament is usually described as a vertical band that lies at the medial aspect of the deep inguinal ring and follows the course of the inferior epigastric vessels. Its fibers are often depicted as having an extensive bony attachment along the pectineal line of the superior pubic ramus, then coming closer together to form the crescentic medial margin of the deep inguinal ring, then spreading fanwise superiorly within the transversus abdominis aponeurosis. In outline, this ligament, as depicted in some standard anatomy texts, resembles a tied sheaf of wheat. It occasionally may contain a slip of muscle. The presence of such a ligament as that described is rare; the presence of muscle within the ligament is rarer still (see Figs. 2-9 and 2-13).

The inferior deep epigastric vessels, which lie free, anatomically, in the preperitoneal space surrounded by adventitia, are located immediately subjacent to the supposed course of the interfoveolar ligament. In an embalmed body, the adventitia of the inferior epigastric vessels may appear to be attached to transversalis fascia, and perhaps this deceptive appearance accounts for the frequent overemphasis in anatomy texts regarding both the presence and the nature of the interfoveolar ligament.

If the dissection is carried out on a fresh cadaver, the structure of the interfoveolar ligament is readily apparent. Some fascial reinforcement, albeit minor, of the medial margin of the deep ring was noted in 80% of my dissections. These interfoveolar fibers have a limited distribution, being attached immediately inferiorly to the iliopubic tract and immediately superiorly to the transversus abdominis arch. Often, the fibrous reinforcement in this area was so tenuous as hardly to warrant a description separate from that of the transversus abdominis aponeurosis and the transversalis fascia. A more extensive distribution of fibrous tissue, approximating a classic interfoveolar ligament, was noted in only 14% of my dissections, and a vertical slip of muscle was noted in this area in only one body.

Cooper Ligament

Cooper ligament is remarkably constant in form and extent and represents the strongly reinforced periosteum of the superior ramus of the pubis (Fig. 2-15; see Figs. 2-9 and 2-11). On the superior and internal aspect of the superior pubic ramus, covering and immediately internal to the pectineal line, the periosteum is supplemented by a considerable quantity of dense fibrous tissue so that it usually becomes 2 mm or even 3 mm thick; less often, it is thicker, approaching 0.5 cm (6%). It is never significantly diminished. The fibers are adherent to and directed parallel with the superior ramus of the pubis. This fibrous reinforcement gradually fades away near the midline on the internal surface of the body of the pubis. Laterally, it continues posteriorly along the brim of the true pelvis, becoming progressively thinner, until it can no longer be distinguished from the periosteum of the ilium.

Cooper ligament is covered by endoabdominal fascia that is intimately attached to it and is continuous above Cooper ligament with the transversalis fascia. It is this attachment of endoabdominal fascia to Cooper ligament that provides the "insertion" of transversalis fascia into the superior ramus of the pubis. The medial half of Cooper ligament is in intimate relation with the insertions of the transversus abdominis aponeurosis and the iliopubic tract into the pectineal line. Beginning at the medial margin of the femoral canal, the bony brim of the true pelvis begins to curve more sharply posteriorly, carrying Cooper ligament with it so that laterally there is progressive divergence between Cooper ligament and the structures of the deep layer of the abdominal wall (transversalis fascia, iliopubic tract, and transversus aponeurosis). This separation exposes pectineus fascia and muscle in the floor of the femoral canal.

Cooper ligament is particularly important in the surgical correction of femoral hernias and large direct inguinal hernias because it forms a solid anchor along the inferior or posterior aspect of these hernial defects through which sutures may be placed with confidence that they will hold.

Iliopectineal Arch

The iliac fascia, covering the iliacus muscle as it leaves the pelvis for the thigh, is thickened to form a fascial arch running from the anterior superior iliac spine medially and posteriorly to the iliopubic eminence (see Figs. 2-1 and 2-10). This arch forms a sort of common meeting place for the fascial structures of the lateral groin. It acts as the insertion of fibers of the external oblique aponeurosis and the inguinal ligament, the origin of the cremaster muscle and a portion of the origin of the internal oblique and transversus abdominis muscles, the lateral attachment of the iliopubic tract, and it forms the most proximal part of the lateral wall of the femoral sheath.

Rectus Abdominis Muscle and Sheath

The rectus abdominis muscle is the paired, long, flat muscle that arises from the body of the pubis and spans the entire anterior abdomen to insert into the xiphoid and adjacent costal cartilages. The origin of the rectus tendon is constant, occupying the superior and posterior aspects of the body of the pubis from the midline to the pubic tubercle. In only 3 of 187 dissections was an attachment of rectus tendon proper found lateral to the pubic tubercle.

A thin, lateral expansion of the investing fascia of the rectus tendon, inserting along the superior ramus of the pubis, was noted in 46% of my dissections. This expansion, or *Henle ligament,* is placed behind and

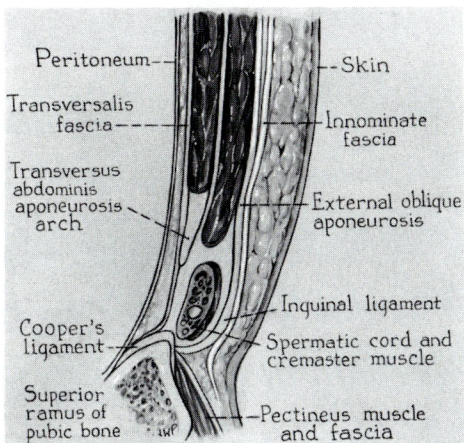

Figure 2-15. A parasagittal schematic representation of the musculoaponeurotic relations in the middle of the right inguinal canal, viewed from the lateral aspect of the section. The closer approximation, by their common insertion into the pectineal line of the pubis, of the superficial (external oblique, inguinal ligament) layer to the deep (transversus abdominis, transversalis fascia) musculoaponeurotic layer in the medial portion of the groin is shown.

reinforces the lowest and most medial part of the transversalis fascia and transversus abdominis aponeurosis in the area just lateral to the rectus tendon (see Figs. 2-2 and 2-9). Henle ligament varies a great deal in density, less so in extent. When present, it is represented in one third of instances by only a few frail fibers. More typically, it is a moderately dense structure that adheres to the transversalis fascia and the transversus abdominis aponeurosis and extends for 1 to 2 cm along the superior pubic ramus lateral to the rectus tendon. In 15 of 185 dissections, Henle ligament was prominent and formed a separate layer that extended 2 to 3 cm along Cooper ligament.

The *pyramidalis muscle* is a small, triangular muscle on the anterior surface of the rectus abdominis. It arises from the body of the pubis just anterior to the rectus tendon but deep to all layers of the rectus sheath. Its fibers are directed upward and medially to insert into the linea alba. The pyramidalis is of no surgical importance; interest lies chiefly in its great variations. It is entirely absent in about 20% of patients and minuscule in a further 20%. When well developed, it is found to overlap the rectus for about one third of the distance from pubis to umbilicus. Rarely does the pyramidalis muscle reach more than halfway to the umbilicus.

The rectus abdominis sheath is formed by fusion of the aponeuroses of the three flat muscles of the lateral abdominal wall. In the region of the groin, all three aponeuroses pass anterior to the belly of the rectus abdominis muscle. The two deeper aponeuroses—transversus abdominis and internal oblique—fuse into a single layer at the lateral border of the rectus muscle. The external oblique aponeurosis, however, remains separate for a variable distance. The line of fusion of the external oblique aponeurosis with the deeper aponeuroses forms a sigmoid-shaped curve, beginning near the lateral border of the sheath at the level of the umbilicus, but approaching nearly to the midline at the pubis. The anterior rectus sheath, then, is a partially bilaminar structure in the lower half of the abdomen.

The fused aponeuroses interdigitate in the midline, forming the dense linea alba. Most of the aponeurotic fibers terminate here. Just above the symphysis pubis, however, a portion of the aponeurotic fibers are said to be continued through the linea alba, appearing on the posterior surface of the opposite rectus tendon as a triangular expansion, the adminiculum lineae albae, to provide a broader insertion for the rectus sheath. I did not see such structures in any of my dissections.

The posterior rectus sheath is absent in the lower part of the abdomen, but somewhat more superiorly, fibers of the transversus abdominis aponeurosis begin to pass posterior to the belly of the muscle and are subsequently reinforced by a contribution from the internal oblique aponeurosis. The transition by the transversus abdominis from an anterior to a posterior position forms the lower border of the posterior rectus sheath, the semicircular line, at a point about midway between the pubis and the umbilicus (see Fig. 2-9). The transition of the transversus abdominis and internal oblique aponeuroses frequently does not occur at the same level, and there may be partial and interrupted transitions of either aponeurosis. As a consequence, several semicircular lines may be found.

The lateral margin of the rectus sheath just above the body of the pubis is sometimes reinforced by fibers of the transversus abdominis aponeurosis that turn downward alongside the rectus tendon. When the lateral extent of this portion of the rectus sheath is less than 0.5 cm beyond the border of the rectus muscle and tendon, no separate designation seems warranted. However, in 11% of my dissections, the transversus aponeurosis had a more extensive insertion clearly lateral to the rectus sheath and tendon; such a wide insertion of the transversus abdominis aponeurosis has been designated the *falx inguinalis*. Note that the falx inguinalis in most instances is composed only of fibers of the transversus abdominis aponeurosis so that this is not a conjoined tendon.

Preperitoneal Space*

The preperitoneal space is the space limited internally by the peritoneum and externally, in the groin, by the transversalis fascia. Its lateral and posterior margins are indefinite because it is continuous with the rest of the extraperitoneal and retroperitoneal tissues. It is filled with more or less fat subdivided into coarse lobules and sheets by areolar tissue. The preperitoneal space serves to transmit the blood vessels, lymphatics, and nerves to and from the leg, and the ductus deferens and vessels of the spermatic cord to and from the scrotum. The amount of fat contained in this space is a reflection of the relative obesity of the person. In an average body, fat is relatively abundant about the iliac vessels and in the iliac fossa.

---

*Preperitoneal is a hybrid from the Latin (pre-) and Greek (peritoneum). Some object to it as etymologically illegitimate and recommend the form *properitoneal*. Those who raise such an objection, however, do not object to *retroperitoneal*, which also is an etymologic hybrid (*retro-*, L.; *peritoneal*, Gr.). I prefer *preperitoneal* because it clearly conveys the intended meaning and has wide clinical acceptance. Further, *preperitoneal* is accepted by the *O.E.D.*, which should satisfy even the most abstemious etymologist.

Blood Vessels

The *external iliac artery* runs along the medial side of the psoas major muscle from which it is separated by the iliac fascia. It enters the femoral sheath by passing under the iliopubic tract and then passes beyond the level of the inguinal ligament to enter the leg as the common femoral artery. It supplies small arterial twigs to the adjacent lymph nodes and may send some small branches to the psoas major. Two major branches, the inferior epigastric and deep circumflex iliac arteries, are usually given off from the distal 2 cm of the external iliac artery, the inferior epigastric usually arising slightly proximal to the deep circumflex branch; occasionally, these branches spring from a common trunk, and not infrequently, their origin is located 1 cm or more within the femoral sheath. The *external iliac vein* accompanies the external iliac artery, lying medially and somewhat posteriorly.

The *inferior epigastric artery* gives off two small branches near its origin, the external spermatic (cremasteric) artery and the pubic branch. The main inferior epigastric artery runs vertically upward in the preperitoneal space to enter and ramify within the rectus abdominis muscle, forming collateral connections with the superior epigastric artery. The *inferior epigastric vein* is usually double, a channel lying on each side of the artery. The two channels unite as they approach the femoral sheath and then join the external iliac vein. The venous junction is usually within the preperitoneal space and 1 cm or more proximal to the origin of the artery. The inferior epigastric artery and vein are contained within the preperitoneal space throughout their course in the groin. Therefore, they are deep or internal to the transversalis fascia, not superficial to it, and these vessels have no intimate connection with the musculoaponeurotic abdominal wall in the groin. The branches of the inferior epigastric vessels usually do not pierce the transversalis fascia until they have crossed the lateral border of the rectus abdominis muscle. Between the iliac vessels and the border of the rectus muscle, the inferior epigastric vessels lie free in the preperitoneal space and have no intimate anatomic connection with the transversalis fascia; this fact is not enough appreciated.

The *deep circumflex iliac artery and vein* also arise from the distal external iliac system but quickly pierce the transversalis fascia and so occupy a position outside the preperitoneal space. They proceed laterally along the iliopectineal arch. Near the anterior superior iliac spine, their ascending branches further pierce the transversus abdominis muscle layer so that the ascending terminal branches of the deep circumflex iliac vessels lie between the transversus abdominis and internal oblique muscles and slightly medial to the iliac crest.

The *external spermatic artery*, originating from the inferior epigastric as it runs upward along the medial aspect of the deep inguinal ring, perforates the transversalis fascia to join the spermatic cord structures just outside the deep ring.

The *pubic branch* is a tiny arterial vessel that originates from the proximal centimeter of the inferior epigastric artery. It runs inferiorly, lying on the iliopubic tract and following the curve of the medial margin of the femoral ring. It crosses Cooper ligament, giving off a branch (arteria corona mortis) that courses medially on the surface of Cooper ligament. The main pubic branch continues its vertical course downward to join the obturator artery. These small arterial vessels are accompanied by relatively much larger veins. The presence of these vessels, particularly the pubic veins, constitutes a distinct hazard of hemorrhage during the conduct of direct inguinal and femoral hernial repairs. This area should always be dissected cleanly and demonstrated clearly during such repairs. These vessels usually may be ligated with impunity.

In 24% of a group of 185 groin dissections, the pubic branch was found to be relatively large, 2 or 3 mm in diameter. In such instances, the pubic branch is called the *accessory obturator artery*. In two of these dissections, this branch was the only arterial vessel that passed through the obturator foramen.

Nerves

The motor and sensory innervation of the skin and musculoaponeurotic layers of the groin is primarily supplied by the ilioinguinal and the iliohypogastric nerves. These nerves are derived from the 1st lumbar nerve but may also receive branches from the 12th thoracic nerve. The spermatic cord and testis are supplied by the spermatic plexus, which contains sympathetic and sensory fibers that enter the spinal cord through the posterior roots of the 10th, 11th, and 12th thoracic and 1st lumbar nerves. The pubic bone and its periosteum are innervated by the 2nd and 3rd lumbar nerves. The genitofemoral nerve, arising from the 1st and 2nd lumbar nerves, supplies the cremaster muscle, the skin of the scrotum, and the adjacent thigh.

The *ilioinguinal* and *iliohypogastric nerves* are formed from the lumbar plexus just outside the L1-L2 intervertebral foramina and proceed laterally and inferiorly through the psoas muscle and then across the quadratus lumborum muscle, lying just beneath the parietal peritoneum. In the flank, at a point above the middle of the iliac crest, these nerves pierce the transversus abdominis muscle and then lie between the transversus abdominis and the internal oblique muscles. Just medial and superior to the anterior iliac spine, the nerves traverse the internal oblique and come to lie beneath the aponeurosis of the external oblique muscle.

The iliohypogastric nerve divides into its iliac and hypogastric branches just after piercing the transversus abdominis muscle. The iliac branch supplies the anterior gluteal area. The hypogastric branch continues forward and downward, frequently anastomosing with the 12th thoracic (subcostal) nerve. Motor branches supply the abdominal muscles along its course. Sometimes, the hypogastric nerve gives off, beneath the internal oblique muscle, an inguinal branch that joins the ilioinguinal nerve and passes into the inguinal canal. After piercing the internal oblique muscle, the hypogastric nerve continues its medial course across the semilunar line and then divides into cutaneous branches that pierce the superficial lamina of the rectus sheath to supply the skin of the suprapubic area.

The ilioinguinal nerve follows a similar course through the layers of the abdominal wall, coming to lie on the surface of the internal oblique muscle and beneath the aponeurosis of the external oblique about 2 cm medial to the anterior superior iliac spine. The ilioinguinal nerve (together with the inguinal branch of the hypogastric nerve, when this exists) traverses the inguinal canal anterior to the spermatic cord. At the superficial inguinal ring, the ilioinguinal nerve divides into branches that supply the skin of the pubic region and the upper part of the scrotum or labia majora in the female. Along its course, the nerve gives off motor branches to the abdominal muscles.

The *genitofemoral nerve* arising from the 2nd and 3rd lumbar nerves through the lumbar plexus pursues a course obliquely downward through the substance of the psoas major muscle. It emerges on the anteromedial surface of the psoas muscle and follows the psoas muscle across the preperitoneal space to the region of the deep inguinal ring. The genitofemoral nerve usually divides into its genital and femoral branches near the deep ring, but the division may occur anywhere along its course. The genital branch, from the 1st lumbar nerve, perforates the iliopubic tract lateral to the deep inguinal ring to enter the inguinal canal and join the spermatic cord, passing medially on the posterior aspect of the spermatic cord to emerge through the superficial inguinal ring. The genital branch supplies sensory innervation to the scrotum and adjacent medial aspect of the thigh and supplies motor nerves to the cremaster muscle. The femoral branch (sometimes multiple) continues to follow the psoas muscle. It may continue to lie beneath the fascia of the psoas or it may pierce, in turn, the iliopsoas and transversalis fasciae and pass under the inguinal ligament to enter the leg. Rarely, the femoral branch may accompany the femoral artery, but its usual course is outside the femoral sheath. The terminal filaments pierce the fascia lata to be distributed to the skin of the proximal anterior thigh.

Lateral to the course of the femoral branch of the genitofemoral nerve, the femoral and lateral femoral cutaneous nerves are found under the iliac fascia. These nerves have no branches in the preperitoneal space that supply structures of the groin. They enter the thigh in a manner similar to that of the femoral branch of the genitofemoral nerve.

Lymphatics

The lymph channels in the groin follow the course of the main blood vessels. The inguinal nodes that drain the proximal thigh and perineum are, in turn, drained by the nodes within the femoral canal and thence to the chain of lymphatics surrounding the external iliac vessels. The major external iliac lymph chain is located on the medial side of the external iliac vein. However, a lymph node of the external iliac group is frequently found on the anterolateral aspect of the external iliac artery just internal to the deep inguinal ring. When enlarged, this node proves to be an annoyance during repair of indirect inguinal hernias.

The lymphatic channels from the testis and spermatic cord follow the testicular vessels and drain into the paraaortic nodes. Although this forms the main lymphatic drainage route, sometimes lymph channels can be demonstrated that drain directly into the node found at the deep inguinal ring and then course laterally and posteriorly around the external iliac artery and vein to join the main iliac chain of nodes.

Ductus Deferens

The excretory duct of the testis follows a course with the spermatic cord inward through the deep inguinal ring, where it turns sharply posteriorly and toward the midline, separating from the other components of the cord. The ductus deferens crosses the external iliac vessels about 3 cm proximal to the iliopubic eminence and enters the true pelvis. It continues a posterior and downward course along the lateral wall of the pelvis and then turns forward to the base of the bladder.

Peritoneum

The parietal peritoneum in the region of the groin is continuous with the remainder of the peritoneum lining the entire abdominal cavity. Near the pubis, the peritoneum is held away from the muscular layers of the abdominal wall by the urachus, a band of fibrous tissue that extends from the apex of the bladder to the umbilicus, the intervening space being filled by loose areolar tissue and fat, and termed the *prevesical space* (of Retzius). The elevation of the peritoneum in the midline by the urachus forms the median umbilical fold.

Laterally, the peritoneum follows the general curve of the pelvis but, in the immediate region of the groin, is separated from the abdominal wall by the fat and other tissues that occupy the preperitoneal space. Because it is separated in the groin from the transversalis fascia, the peritoneum is a relatively unsupported membrane and cannot be sutured under tension. In excising a hernial sac, therefore, some judgment must be exercised so that all redundant peritoneum is removed but enough remains to allow closure without undue tension.

In the absence of a hernia, the peritoneum presents no features of unusual interest. In the embalmed cadaver, in contrast, the peritoneum lateral to the midline is frequently elevated or ridged by the obliterated umbilical vessels that form the lateral umbilical fold and by the inferior epigastric vessels that form the inguinal or epigastric fold. Between these ridges, the groin is regionally divided into the supravesical fossa and the medial and lateral inguinal fossae. None of these lateral folds or fossae is obvious when an unfixed body is dissected. They are rarely noted during intraabdominal operations and are of no surgical importance in regard to either the causation or the repair of groin hernias.

Femoral Sheath

The femoral (crural) sheath is a fibrous tubular prolongation downward into the leg of the transversalis (endoabdominal) fascia that lines the abdominal cavity (see Figs. 2-11 and 2-12). Contained within the femoral sheath are the femoral vessels and the femoral canal. The femoral sheath is shaped like a skewed and truncated tetrahedron. The pelvic ostium is relatively wide and occupies an oblique plane, whereas the narrow lower end of the sheath terminates about 4 cm below the inguinal crease by fusing in a transverse plane with the adventitia of the femoral vessels.

The fascial continuities and relations of the femoral sheath are somewhat complex. Anteriorly and medially, the walls of the sheath are relatively longer and are continuous with the transversalis fascia that turns over the iliopubic tract to project into the leg. The short lateral wall and the lateral third of the posterior wall are continuations of the endoabdominal fascia covering the iliacus and psoas muscles. The medial portion of the posterior wall is formed by the pectineus fascia, which is continuous with the endoabdominal fascia that covers the internal periosteum of the superior ramus of the pubis.

The anterior and medial margins of the ostium of the femoral sheath are formed by the iliopubic tract to which the transversalis fascia is firmly attached and over which it is reflected into the leg. As it progresses into the leg, the anterior wall of the femoral sheath next comes into relation with the spermatic cord. About a centimeter distal to the pelvic ostium, the anterior wall of the femoral sheath is crossed by the inguinal ligament. The inguinal ligament, in contrast to the densely adherent iliopubic tract, can usually be bluntly dissected free from the underlying femoral sheath. The lowest fibers of the inguinal ligament, the lacunar ligament, curve gently posteriorly on the medial aspect of the femoral sheath to their insertion into the pectineus fascia. These fibers are not intimately approximated to the medial wall of the femoral canal, as is usually described in texts, but are slightly separated from the medial wall of the sheath. Near its inferior end, the anteromedial wall of the femoral sheath is perforated by the inguinal lymphatics.

The posterior margin of the ostium of the femoral sheath is formed by the superior ramus of the pubis. The pectineus muscle, which originates from almost the entire length of the superior ramus of the pubis, underlies the greater portion of the posterior wall of the femoral sheath, occupying the medial two thirds at the upper end of the sheath and the entire posterior aspect of its distal portion. For a short distance in the upper portion of the femoral sheath, the psoas muscle and tendon are in relation to the posterior wall. The fasciae that cover these two muscles, pectineus and psoas, form the posterior fibrous wall of the femoral sheath.

The lateral margin of the femoral sheath is supported by the main mass of the iliacus muscle and demarcated by the iliopectineal arch. The lateral wall, which is nearly vertical in orientation, is formed by the iliacus fascia. The femoral nerve lies external to the femoral sheath on the surface of the psoas and iliacus muscles. A few terminal fibers of the femoral nerve may pierce the lateral wall of the sheath in the thigh.

In summary, the fibrous walls of the femoral sheath are formed anteriorly and medially from transversalis fascia, posteriorly from pectineus and psoas fascia, and laterally from iliacus fascia. The pelvic ostium consists of a relatively fixed rim of bone and connective tissue: anteriorly and medially, the iliopubic tract; posteriorly, the superior pubic ramus; and laterally, the iliopectineal arch.

The femoral sheath is subdivided into three compartments by vertical fascial partitions that stretch between its anterior and posterior walls. The lateral compartment contains the femoral artery and the intermediate compartment, the femoral vein. The medial compartment is the smallest of the three and constitutes the femoral canal.

Femoral Canal

A half-moon, somewhat thick through its middle, approximates the cross-sectional outline of the femoral canal. The internal mouth of the femoral canal, the femoral ring, is composed of fixed tissue. Anteriorly and medially, the femoral ring consists of the iliopubic tract and its recurving insertion into the pectineal line and pectineus fascia. Laterally, the medial septum strung between the anterior and posterior walls of the femoral sheath is found, supported by the femoral vessels. Posteriorly, the ring is completed by the pectineus fascia and the superior ramus of the pubis.

The femoral canal is about 2 cm in length. It normally contains only areolar tissue and lymphatic channels and nodes that drain the overlying inguinal lymph nodes. A large node (Rosenmüller node to the Germans; Cloquet node to the French) is usually present at the upper end of the femoral canal. Sometimes, the areolar tissue within the femoral canal is found to form a thin sheet, the femoral septum, partially closing the upper end of the femoral canal. This septum is extremely weak and no barrier to the development of a femoral hernia.

Inguinal Canal and Spermatic Cord

The inguinal canal has been frequently mentioned, and the individual structures that participate in its formation have been described. However, a short review, including a sketch of the processes of testicular descent and the formation of the spermatic cord, is warranted.

Inguinal Canal

The inguinal canal, after the descent of the testis into the scrotum, remains as a triangular cleft, potential rather than actual, between the two main musculo-aponeurotic layers of the abdominal wall—the superficial external oblique layer and the deep transversus abdominis layer. The inguinal canal begins at the lateral margin of the deep inguinal ring and ends at the medial margin of the superficial inguinal ring, averaging in an adult about 4 cm in length. Through the canal, the spermatic cord travels from a preperitoneal to a subcutaneous position (see Figs. 2-11 and 2-15).

The *anterior wall* of the inguinal canal contains within its medial third the superficial inguinal ring; the remainder of the anterior wall is formed by the external oblique aponeurosis and, in particular, the inguinal ligament. At the lateral end of the inguinal canal, the muscular bundles of the lower part of the internal oblique arch over the cord, going from a position anterior to the cord to one above it, and are briefly in relation to the anterior wall.

The *inferior wall* of the inguinal canal is composed of those tissues that lie in an oblique plane inferior and posterior to the cord. The inferior wall, the base of the triangular cleft, is supported by the superior ramus of the pubis. Its medial third is formed by the horizontally rotating or "shelving" insertion of the inguinal ligament. The middle of the floor of the inguinal canal is formed by the pectineus muscle and fascia and by the insertion of the lacunar ligament. The lateral third of the inferior wall is formed by the anterior and medial walls of the femoral sheath and the iliopubic tract.

The *posterior wall* of the inguinal canal is formed by the deep layer of the groin, the transversus abdominis aponeurosis and its associated structures. The posterior wall is often referred to as the "floor" of the inguinal canal when the description is oriented to the supine position of a patient on an operating table. Anatomically, the posterior wall lies in an oblique plane posterosuperior to the spermatic cord. The deep inguinal ring occupies the lateral third of the posterior wall. The medial two thirds of the posterior wall is buttressed medially by the lateral edge of the rectus sheath or by the falx inguinalis; at the margin of the femoral canal, it is buttressed by the iliopubic tract; more superiorly, it is composed of the transversus abdominis arch and the strong transversus abdominis aponeurosis.

Between these supporting ligamentous structures, the main portion of the posterior wall of the inguinal canal usually is formed by the discontinuous portion of the transversus abdominis aponeurosis and the transversalis fascia. This is the weak area in which rupture of fascial and aponeurotic continuity first occurs in direct inguinal hernias, permitting a direct hernial sac to enter the inguinal canal and occupy a position posterior, or deep, to the spermatic cord.

The posterior inguinal wall in the region of direct herniation often is referred to as *Hesselbach triangle;* its *classic boundaries* are familiar to all: (1) the rectus sheath, (2) the inferior epigastric vessels, and (3) the inguinal ligament. It has become increasingly obvious to me that these boundaries need to be redefined so that all structures lie in association with the anatomic posterior inguinal wall. The *anatomic boundaries* of Hesselbach triangle should be (1) the rectus sheath and falx inguinalis, (2) the inferior epigastric vessels, and (3) Cooper ligament.

Superficial Inguinal Ring

The superficial inguinal ring provides a passage for the structures of the spermatic cord from the interparietal inguinal canal to the subcutaneous neck of the scrotum. The superficial inguinal ring is formed by a divergence of the fibers of the lower part of the external oblique aponeurosis immediately above and lateral to the pubic tubercle, forming a triangular aperture (see Figs. 2-4 and 2-5). The base of this triangle is at the pubic tubercle, the apex being directed obliquely upward and laterally for a variable distance. The diverging aponeurotic fibers constitute the pillars or crura of the superficial ring. The *medial crus* is flat and broad. It is merely that part of the external oblique aponeurosis next to the opening and possesses no special features. The fibers of the medial crus are attached to the body of the pubis anterior to the rectus tendon in continuity with the main insertion of the external oblique aponeurosis. The *lateral crus* is narrower. It also is formed by the external oblique aponeurosis, which here is immediately adjacent to the medial end of the inguinal ligament. The lateral crus is attached to the pubic tubercle in continuity with the attachment of the inguinal ligament.

The lateral half of the triangular aponeurotic cleft in the external oblique aponeurosis frequently is bridged by the scattered bundles of the transversely directed *intercrural fibers* contained within the investing innominate fascia. The intercrural fibers reinforce the lateral portion of the aponeurotic opening and bind the two crura together.

The closure of the triangular gap in the external oblique aponeurosis and its conversion into an oval ring are accomplished by the investing fasciae, particularly the *innominate fascia*. The innominate fascia is joined by the thinner investing fascia from the deep surface of the external oblique aponeurosis to bridge the gap between the aponeurotic crura and so maintain the uninterrupted continuity of the external oblique layer and prevent entry into the inguinal canal of fluid or pus that may come to occupy the space beneath Scarpa fascia.

At the level of the pubic tubercle, as the spermatic cord structures leave the inguinal canal to become subcutaneous in position, the innominate fascia is prolonged from all margins of the ring to form a funnel-like projection of fascia about the spermatic cord. This tube of fascia quickly becomes closely apposed to the cord and forms its final intrinsic fascial covering, the *external spermatic fascia*. It is this continuity of flat investing fascia onto the round spermatic cord that finally converts the triangular cleft in the external oblique aponeurosis into the oval superficial inguinal ring.

The ilioinguinal nerve also passes through the superficial ring, although it may occasionally pierce the aponeurosis just above and join the cord just external to the ring. The superficial ring measures about 1.5 by 2.5 cm and is readily felt by invaginating the scrotum over the tip of the examining finger, palpating the pubic tubercle, and then directing the thrust superiorly and laterally, where the finger engages the

opening but usually does not actually pass into the inguinal canal.

Deep Inguinal Ring

The structure of the deep inguinal ring bears some resemblance to that of the superficial ring in that it possesses aponeurotic tissues at its margins and is closed by investing fascia. However, the aponeurotic margins are not nearly so strong as those of the superficial ring, and they are deficient on the medial side of the ring. There also is a much wider range of significant structural variation at the deep ring. The deep inguinal ring provides a passage for the ductus deferens, the spermatic vessels, the smaller vessels that supply the ductus and the cremaster muscle from their positions in the preperitoneal space through the transversus abdominis layer of the groin to the interparietal inguinal canal, where they are bound together as the spermatic cord. The internal ring cannot be palpated externally in people with normal anatomy, but its approximate location can be determined as being halfway between the pubic tubercle and the anterior superior iliac spine. Pressure over this area with the thumb while the patient strains often helps to differentiate a small indirect from a direct hernia because this maneuver prevents extrusion of an indirect hernial mass.

The deep inguinal ring is formed basically by aponeurotic fibers of the transversus abdominis layer. The inferior border of the ring is usually entirely aponeurotic, being formed by the iliopubic tract. These fibers begin laterally from the iliopectineal arch and the adjacent iliacus fascia in common with the origin of the lower bundles of the transversus abdominis muscle and aponeurosis. They are directed medially, passing just below the deep ring, and then turn inferiorly and posteriorly to insert into the pectineal line.

The superior aponeurotic border of the deep inguinal ring is formed by the transversus abdominis arch. These bundles originate from the iliopectineal arch and adjacent iliacus fascia in common with the lateral attachments of the iliopubic tract. At its origin, the transversus abdominis arch is usually mainly muscular, but some aponeurotic fibers are present. These bundles are directed upward and medially, crossing just above the deep inguinal ring and becoming progressively more aponeurotic and less muscular. After passing above the deep ring, the transversus abdominis arch turns downward to its insertion. The lateral edge of this insertion may be found anywhere along the superior ramus and body of the pubis between the medial wall of the femoral canal and the midline.

Therefore, the aponeurotic gap between the transversus abdominis arch and the iliopubic tract is crescentic in outline. The length and width of the crescent are subject to considerable variation, depending on the course and point of insertion of the transversus abdominis arch. The closure of the crescentic aponeurotic gap in the transversus abdominis layer is accomplished by the investing transversalis fascia, which is thicker here than elsewhere in the groin.

The deep inguinal ring is located in the lateral portion of the crescentic gap. The medial portion of the crescent is the posterior wall of the inguinal canal. It is obvious that there is no firm medial aponeurotic margin of the deep inguinal ring. What, then, prevents progressive medial enlargement of the ring and resulting indirect inguinal hernia in every instance?

One factor is the reinforcement of the transversalis fascia by the more or less vertically oriented aponeurotic fibers scattered within it as it forms the main portion of the posterior inguinal wall. In addition, the presence of the interfoveolar ligament in the few instances in which it is well developed adds reinforcement. The most important element that provides structural resistance to medial displacement of the cord at the deep ring is the transversalis fascial sling. The crura of the sling converge at the medial side of the spermatic cord, thus converting the potential long crescent into an aperture that, in outline, approximates a blunt teardrop and has a transverse dimension of about 2 cm. However, all these reinforcing elements are not able to provide a solid aponeurotic rim of tissue at the medial margin of the deep ring. Therefore, this area normally shows more mobility than the other margins of the deep inguinal ring.

Testicular Descent

At an early stage in intrauterine life, an outpouching develops on each side of the groin, forming the genital swellings that later develop into the scrotum in males. The testis develops from the genital ridge located retroperitoneally in proximity to the primitive kidney at the level of the lumbar segments. At about the 2nd month of gestation, the testis becomes suspended by a peritoneal mesentery, the mesorchium. Two folds extend from this mesentery: one above, containing the spermatic vessels, and one below, transmitting the gubernaculum testis. The gubernaculum connects the testis with the developing genital swelling in the groin. It actually traverses the full thickness of the lower abdominal wall to attach to the tissues of the developing scrotum. This passage through the musculoaponeurotic layers of the lower abdominal wall marks the site of the future inguinal canal and the deep and superficial inguinal rings. At this stage of development, the two inguinal rings are superimposed, and the inguinal canal, therefore, is directed straight inferiorly and anteriorly.

Differential growth of the muscle layers in the groin, simultaneous with the early descent of the tes-

tis, subsequently leads to a change in direction of the passage of the gubernaculum through the abdominal wall. The transversus abdominis layer develops in relation to the other musculoaponeurotic layers in such a way that the site of the deep inguinal ring moves progressively more laterally as compared with the relatively fixed position of the superficial inguinal ring. As a consequence, the gubernaculum, marking the site of the future inguinal canal, comes to pass through the musculoaponeurotic layers of the groin in a more and more oblique direction.

At about the 6th month of fetal development, the testis has come to lie in the region of the deep inguinal ring. Over the ensuing 2 or 3 months, the testis moves through the abdominal wall, carrying with it the ductus deferens and its arteries, veins, nerves, and lymphatics, together with a variable small amount of areolar tissue.

The fundamental process involved in the descent of the testis remains a mystery. Despite a great deal of investigation and theorizing, the factors that control the unique migration of the gonad from its original position at the lower pole of the kidney to its position in the scrotum are simply not known. It is fairly certain that the gubernaculum does not physically pull the testis into the scrotum; as a matter of fact, peritoneal evagination to form the processus vaginalis actually precedes the descent of the testis into the scrotum.

During the descent, successive tubular projections of transversalis fascia (internal spermatic fascia), interparietal fasciae and internal oblique muscle (cremasteric fascia and muscle), and innominate fascia (external spermatic fascia) are applied as coverings of the testis and spermatic cord. This addition of investing tubes of fascia about the testis and spermatic cord is aided by the continuing differential growth of the various muscular layers of the abdominal wall that results, in turn, in a continuing relative lateral displacement of the deep inguinal ring.

After the testis has reached the scrotum, the peritoneal processus vaginalis normally atrophies except in two areas. The first exception is the most distal portion of the processus vaginalis, which remains patent and becomes the tunica vaginalis of the testis. The second exception is the small, most proximal portion of the processus vaginalis near the deep inguinal ring. In males, this portion may be open at birth, slowly reducing in caliber and finally closing during the first year of extrauterine life. If the patent proximal portion of the processus vaginalis is large or fails to close completely, an indirect hernia of the congenital variety may ensue.

Testicular descent and closure of the processus vaginalis proceed more slowly on the right side than on the left; as a consequence, the incidence of congenital indirect inguinal hernia is higher on the right side than on the left. More rarely, the closure of the processus vaginalis may fail more extensively, leading to a complete, or scrotal, indirect hernia, which is noted at birth or shortly thereafter. Failure of closure of distal or middle portions of the processus vaginalis with obliteration proceeding normally in the vicinity of the internal ring leads to formation of a hydrocele of the testis or the cord.

Spermatic Cord

The spermatic cord begins in the preperitoneal space with the confluence in the region of the deep inguinal ring of the testicular artery and vein and the ductus deferens.

The *testicular artery* is a branch of the aorta and supplies the testis. The cord contains two other arterial branches, both small. The first supplies the ductus deferens and is derived from the umbilical artery. The second supplies the cremaster and is usually a branch of the inferior epigastric artery. The venous drainage from the testis begins as a network of a dozen or more vessels, the *pampiniform plexus*, which are said to ascend the cord in three groups: one about the internal spermatic artery, one about the ductus deferens, and a third group located posteriorly that runs alone. It is usually difficult to see the triple grouping. The venous vessels of the cord tend to segregate in this manner, but it certainly is not often a clearcut separation. As they near the deep inguinal ring, the venous channels gradually reduce to one or two vessels, which then enter the preperitoneal space and follow the testicular artery upward. On the right side, these veins drain directly into the inferior vena cava and on the left side, into the left renal vein.

As the ductus deferens and vessels pass through the deep inguinal ring, they receive a tubular projection of transversalis fascia from all the margins of the deep ring. This is the *internal spermatic fascia,* which quickly becomes closely adherent to the cord structures about a centimeter along the cord external to the deep inguinal ring. In people with normal anatomy, the internal spermatic fascia cannot subsequently be easily distinguished as a layer separate from the adventitia and fat surrounding the ductus and vessels. In other words, there is usually no separate and distinct fascial stratum that constitutes the internal spermatic fascia in the distal portion of the normal and unembalmed spermatic cord, but it is true that when the spermatic cord is dissected in an embalmed cadaver, the internal spermatic fascia can be distinguished more readily and often can be followed for a considerable distance along the cord. Even here,

however, one rarely is able to separate this stratum all the way into the scrotum.

In indirect inguinal hernias, a definite internal spermatic fascial layer always is found internal to the cremasteric muscle and fascia and external to the peritoneal sac. It is possible that in instances of hernia, the connective tissues responded to the presence of the hernial mass by producing a thicker encapsulating layer. As a result of this hypertrophy, the internal spermatic fascia may become easier to see and easier to handle and dissect.

As the cord emerges through the deep inguinal ring to enter the inguinal canal, it passes under the lower edge of the internal oblique muscle and its investing fascia. A slip of this muscle and fascia is applied to the anterior aspect of the cord, forming the cremaster muscle and fascia.

The *cremaster muscle* has its origin from the medial half of the iliopectineal arch a centimeter or so lateral to the lateral margin of the deep inguinal ring. Often, it also has a few fibers that originate from the internal surface of the immediately adjacent portion of the inguinal ligament. The cremaster muscle origin is continuous with the origin of the internal oblique; the cremaster represents the lowest few bundles of the internal oblique muscle. In some instances, a contribution of fibers from the transversus abdominis muscle also is included in the cremaster, but usually the cremaster muscle is derived entirely from the internal oblique layer.

The cremaster muscle fibers, initially applied only to the anterior surface of the spermatic cord, spread out around the cord in its course through the inguinal canal so that, at the level of the superficial inguinal ring, cremaster muscle fibers are found scattered over the anterior two thirds of the circumference of the cord. This muscular encirclement then continues so that, by the time the spermatic cord enters the neck of the scrotum, cremaster muscle fibers are found on all surfaces of the cord. In the process of spreading around the cord, the individual muscle fibers become separated. The interval between muscle fibers is filled by the cremasteric fascia. In addition, the individual muscle fibers do not maintain a parallel course, but become irregularly intertwined to form a net-like arrangement. In the scrotum, these fibers lose their muscular quality, and in the usual situation, the cremasteric layer as it envelops the testis is entirely fascial.

The *cremasteric fascia* is formed by contributions from both layers of the interparietal fasciae. The superficial layer of the interparietal fascia, lying on the external surface of the internal oblique and cremaster muscle, is projected with the muscle onto the spermatic cord. All along its course in the inguinal canal, the cord receives further contributions from the interparietal fasciae investing the immediately adjacent muscle layers. These fascial contributions are noted as the areolar attachments of the cord to both anterior and posterior walls of the inguinal canal; this areolar tissue fills all the space within the inguinal canal not occupied by the cord structures per se.

A prominent attachment of the cremasteric fascia to the pubic tubercle frequently is found to lie between the bony attachments of the crura of the superficial inguinal ring. Some authors hold that this attachment in reality is the insertion of the cremaster muscle; in their view, the cremaster muscle fibers are continued down the cord, around the testis, and back again along the cord to this insertion. I have not been able to visualize such a continuity in my dissections and prefer to view this "insertion" into the public tubercle, when it occurs, merely as a secondary attachment of the cremasteric fascia. The cremaster muscle and fascia, taken together, form the second or intermediate completely enveloping fascial layer about the spermatic cord.

The cord exits from the medial end of the inguinal canal by passing through the anterior wall of the inguinal canal at the superficial inguinal ring. In a manner similar to the situation at the deep ring, nothing is added to the structure of the cord from the external oblique aponeurosis itself, but immediately the emerging cord receives a tubular contribution from the investing fascia of the external oblique, the innominate fascia. This covering derived from the innominate fascia forms the third and most superficial of the fascial coats of the cord, the *external spermatic fascia*. At this point, the structure of the spermatic cord is complete, and it enters the neck of the scrotum.

PATHOGENESIS OF GROIN HERNIAS AND PRINCIPLES OF THEIR REPAIR

Laminar Organization of the Groin: Division Into Superficial and Deep Groups of Structures

In the midportion of the groin, in the area in which groin hernias originate, there are three layers of muscle and aponeurosis—external oblique, internal oblique, and transversus abdominis. Each of the layers originates posteriorly from ribs, the lumbodorsal fascia, and the iliac crest. They curve around the flank and across the groin, becoming aponeurotic or tendinous, and fuse together anteriorly to form the rectus sheath.

Although there are three muscle layers anatomically, from a practical point of view there are only two: the external oblique, or *superficial layer,* and the transversus abdominis and internal oblique, taken together as the *deep layer.* The transversus abdominis and internal oblique are grouped together because in the groin they have a common direction and, for the most part, they function as a single layer. In the lower abdomen, the internal oblique and transversus abdominis are often not readily separable. As one spreads the muscle bundles apart during a "muscle-splitting" operative approach in the lower abdomen, the plane of separation between the internal oblique and transversus abdominis is often not obvious. In the groin, this lack of clearcut separation is almost constant.

Of the two laminae that compose the deep musculoaponeurotic layer of the groin, the transversus abdominis is by far the more important because it is more aponeurotic or tendinous in quality in the area in which hernias are found, whereas the internal oblique is soft and muscular. An understanding of the fascial structure and relations of the deep musculoaponeurotic layer is of the most fundamental importance as far as the subject of groin hernias is concerned.

If one were to push a pin from the skin into the abdominal cavity at a point in the middle of the groin, the point of the pin would encounter in succession:

1. The *skin*
2. The *subcutaneous tissues*—mostly fat, divided into a superficial layer, Camper fascia, and a deeper membranous layer, Scarpa fascia
3. The *innominate fascia,* containing the intercrural fibers and continuous with the external spermatic fascia at the superficial inguinal ring
4. The *external oblique aponeurosis* and the structures continuous with it—the inguinal ligament, the lacunar ligament, and the reflected inguinal ligament
5. The *spermatic cord,* within the inguinal canal
6. The *transversus abdominis aponeurosis,* which is continuous with the transversus abdominis muscle and ultimately associated with the internal oblique muscle
7. The *transversalis fascia* and the structures associated with it—iliopubic tract, Cooper ligament, Henle ligament, transversalis fascial sling, and deep inguinal ring
8. The *preperitoneal tissues*—mostly fat, but also containing the iliac vessels and their branches, the internal spermatic vessels, the nerves to the leg and the spermatic cord, the ductus deferens, and the regional lymphatics
9. The *peritoneum*

If one follows the course of the pin in a little less detail, one notes that it traverses in succession *skin—fat—fascia—aponeurosis—(spermatic cord)—aponeurosis—fascia—fat—peritoneum.*

The abdominal wall in the groin region can be thought of as being composed of two groups of structures—a superficial group and a deep group—that are mirror images of each other. The reflecting point is formed by the spermatic cord in the inguinal canal. Both superficial and deep to the spermatic cord is a layer composed of muscle and aponeurosis, next in succession is a layer of fascia, then one of fat, and finally the skin or peritoneum (see Figs. 2-10, 2-11, and 2-15). Although perhaps too great a simplification of the anatomy, this is a useful conceptual segregation because it emphasizes the division of groin anatomy into the deep structures, which are important in the pathogenesis and surgical repair of groin hernias, and the superficial structures, which are of no importance in the pathogenesis of hernia and of little or no importance in the conduct of repair.

This arbitrary anatomic division may be helpful, too, in understanding the structure of the inguinal canal and the terminology used in its description. The inguinal canal constitutes a cleft between the two major musculoaponeurotic layers of the groin. The anterior wall is formed by the superficial musculoaponeurotic and fascial layers (external oblique aponeurosis and innominate fascia). The posterior wall is formed by the deep musculoaponeurotic and fascial layers (transversus abdominis aponeurosis and transversalis fascia).

Fundamental Defect in Groin Hernias

What structures have ruptured in the patient who presents with a groin hernia? A direct inguinal hernia begins as a yielding of the transversus abdominis aponeurosis *and* the transversalis fascia in the weak area of the posterior inguinal wall. An indirect inguinal hernia begins with a small peritoneal sac at the deep inguinal ring, but for it to grow, there must be a yielding or relaxation of the transversalis fascia and transversus abdominis aponeurosis about the deep inguinal ring. A femoral hernia begins with an enlarged femoral ring, which is composed of tissues within the transversalis fascia–transversus abdominis layer of the groin.

The herniating intestine in each of these types of common groin hernia is covered by a sac of peritoneum. In inguinal hernias, the protruding mass is often similarly covered by a sac of attenuated transversalis fascia. In each of the varieties of groin hernia, the hernial mass escapes the abdominal cavity through the disrupted transversus abdominis layer

and then merely expands the overlying more superficial layers, producing the hernial bulge noted by the patient. To confirm this statement, one need only remember that in repairing a groin hernia, the superficial musculoaponeurotic layer, the external oblique aponeurosis, is intact and needs to be incised to expose the site of the hernial protrusion.

In less common instances of massive scrotal hernia, the external oblique fibers may be spread apart from each other secondary to the pressure against them from within. This secondary involvement of the superficial musculoaponeurotic layer occurs relatively late in the clinical development of the hernia. *The fundamental rupture, relaxation, or discontinuity in musculoaponeurotic structure in groin hernias occurs in the deeply placed transversus abdominis–transversalis fascial layer of the groin.*

An understanding of structural failure of the deep musculoaponeurotic layer as the basic defect in the genesis of inguinal hernia is of the utmost importance. The problem presented to the surgeon in terms of hernial repair is more readily apparent after this understanding of the pathogenesis of inguinal hernias has been acquired. What needs to be accomplished is *restoration of musculoaponeurotic continuity in the deep (transversus abdominis) layer of the groin,* and what is done to the more superficial layers is of relatively less importance.

It used to be held that a wide or lax superficial inguinal ring predisposed the patient to development of an inguinal hernia. Nothing could be further from the truth. The size and strength of the external ring—or indeed of any component of the external oblique layer of the abdominal wall—have little to do with the cause of hernia. The plication or partial closure of the external ring with so-called insurance stitches, however, lingers in the practice of many surgeons. This maneuver, while it rarely accomplishes any harm and may be necessary on occasion as a practical matter, is absolutely unnecessary from an anatomic standpoint.

Imbrication, darning, and other attempts at reinforcement of the external oblique aponeurosis are also unnecessary and do not have any fundamental influence on the strength of the repair or the liability to recurrence. However, strong differences of opinion over such matters are not warranted. Such accessory procedures are usually innocuous and do not add much to the risk of herniorrhaphy from the point of view of the patient. Similarly, I am not disposed to quarrel with surgeons who continue to use a Bassini type of groin hernial repair. After all, the Bassini herniorrhaphy has corrected many thousands of inguinal hernias. I do not perform such repairs, however, believing them to be anatomically irrational and associated with a higher theoretic liability to recurrence. Herniorrhaphy based on repair of the deep musculoaponeurotic layer (transversus abdominis aponeurosis *and* transversalis fascia) is my preference.

Indirect Inguinal Hernia

The important factors in the cause of indirect inguinal hernias are the presence of a protruding peritoneal sac at the deep inguinal ring and the structural variations of the transversalis fascia and transversus abdominis aponeurosis that determine the size of the deep ring and the strength of its margins.

The peritoneal sac in indirect inguinal hernias almost always protrudes through the deep inguinal ring laterally and somewhat superior to the spermatic cord structures, appearing, therefore, anterior to the spermatic cord in the inguinal canal. The reason for this configuration is obvious if one remembers the spatial relations existing during fetal growth and development. The testis, initially a retroperitoneal structure, descends through the deep inguinal ring posterior and slightly medial to the peritoneal processus vaginalis. The continuing lateral shift of the deep inguinal ring, resulting from growth of the transversus abdominis muscle layer, then tends to shift the plastic processus vaginalis further to the lateral side of the ductus deferens and testicular vessels.

This area superior and lateral to the cord between the diverging arms of the transversalis fascial sling is relatively less well protected, the overlying transversus abdominis arch usually being muscular at this point, and the tendency for herniation here is accentuated by the oblique course of the spermatic cord structures through the internal ring. In contrast, the medial aspect of the internal ring is relatively protected by the convergence of the transversalis fascial sling fibers and the slight reinforcement provided by the interfoveolar ligament. In addition, the course of the cord structures, particularly the ductus deferens, in turning over the medial margin of the ring also tends to discourage herniation here.

In indirect hernias when the mass is large and the condition of long standing, the defect also involves the posterior wall of the inguinal canal. The hernia tends to take a more and more direct course through the abdominal wall until the enlarged deep inguinal ring gradually comes to lie beneath or behind the superficial inguinal ring.

In repair of indirect inguinal hernias in all patients other than infants with the smallest hernias, attention must be paid to reinforcing the lateral area of the internal ring by suture approximation of fascial structures. This always must be done if recurrences are to be prevented. The importance of this step often is not fully appreciated. Fascial reapproximation by suture also must be accomplished on the medial side of the internal ring. But it is the need for lateral reinforcement *in every instance* that is not widely understood.

The placement of sutures lateral to the internal ring requires that the cremaster muscle at its origin be dissected up and reflected sufficiently to expose the lateral side of the ring or that the hernial defect be approached posteriorly from the preperitoneal side. In repair of either type, the sutures must include aponeurotic fibers on each margin as well as the transversalis fascia.

Direct Inguinal Hernia

The important causative factors in direct inguinal hernia are the relative strength of the posterior inguinal wall in the weak area within Hesselbach triangle and the presence of general physical factors that tend to increase abdominal straining, such as prostatic hypertrophy, chronic cough, and constipation.

The relative strength or weakness of the posterior inguinal wall—and therefore the liability of a person to have a direct inguinal hernia develop—depends on a number of factors, all of which show a great deal of variation. The main arch of the transversus abdominis may cross the groin relatively high above the superior ramus of the pubis, making the weak area relatively extensive and liable to herniation, or it may cross the groin relatively close to the bone, thereby reinforcing the posterior wall of the inguinal canal.

The insertion of the transversus abdominis arch into the pubis may be limited to an area adjacent to the rectus tendon, or it may extend laterally along the superior ramus of the pubis for 2 or 3 cm. Similarly, the iliopubic tract may be a strong or a relatively tenuous aponeurotic band, and its insertion into the pectineal line may be extensive or may be limited to a few millimeters just medial to the margin of the femoral ring.

The transversalis fascia of the posterior inguinal wall, amid the transversus abdominis arch, the lateral border of the rectus sheath, and the iliopubic tract, may thus occupy either a relatively wide or a narrow area. In addition, the number of reinforcing aponeurotic fibers contained in the fascia comprising the posterior wall of the inguinal canal varies considerably. All these structural variants are independent of one another so that a wide spectrum of structural relations is possible.

In people in whom a combination of factors produces a relatively extensive fascial posterior inguinal wall in which the amount of aponeurotic reinforcement of the potentially weak area is scant, thereby making it weak in fact, a direct inguinal hernia is a distinct possibility. If such a structural predisposition is combined with a condition that causes repetitive abdominal straining, a direct inguinal hernia is a distinct probability.

After the initial protrusion of peritoneum and transversalis fascia, which begins in the area of greatest weakness in the posterior inguinal wall, a direct inguinal hernia continues to enlarge until the resistance met along a particular margin is greater than the forces impelling the growth of the hernial mass. In direct hernias, the mass usually is limited in its growth medially by the lateral border of the rectus sheath or by the falx inguinalis, supported by the rectus tendon and Henle's ligament. Inferiorly, growth is quickly resisted by the iliopubic tract, the superior ramus of the pubis, and Cooper ligament. Laterally, growth of the direct hernial defect is limited by the structures that surround the deep inguinal ring. Direct inguinal hernias accomplish most of their initial enlargement in a superior direction, continuing to enlarge by splaying out the lowest fibers of the transversus abdominis aponeurosis until the resistance of the transversus abdominis arch becomes sufficient to halt the hernial enlargement.

Repair of a direct hernial defect is most directly accomplished by approximating the aponeurotic borders of the defect. The sutures include transversalis fascia but *must* include transversus abdominis aponeurosis superiorly and Cooper ligament or iliopubic tract inferiorly, if permanent cure of the hernia is to be expected.

Femoral Hernia

The size and shape of the femoral ring determine liability to the development of a femoral hernia. Increased intraabdominal pressure may also play a causative role in the development of this variety of groin hernia. The only important variations in the configuration of the femoral ring are those of the iliopubic tract that constitute its anterior and medial margins. The posterior margin of the ring is the superior pubic ramus, which shows no important variations. The lateral margin of the femoral ring, the femoral vein and its adjacent septum, does show some variations in size from one person to another, but these variations are of comparatively minor degree. *It is the variations of the iliopubic tract that ultimately are of prime importance in the causation of femoral herniation.*

The insertion of the iliopubic tract usually occupies a distance of about 1 to 2 cm along the pectinate line in the midportion of the superior pubic ramus. The insertion may be shifted somewhat medially, however, or the iliopubic tract may be small, resulting in a relatively broad femoral ring; or the recurving portion of the iliopubic tract, which usually turns

sharply downward along the medial margin of the femoral canal, may take a gentler curve, again resulting in a relatively broad femoral ring. In such situations, a femoral hernia is more likely to develop.

Moreover, there appears to be an inverse relation between liability to direct inguinal hernia and liability to femoral hernia. The person with an extensive weak area of posterior inguinal wall, and consequently an increased liability to direct herniation, necessarily has a smaller femoral ring and canal and, therefore, is less liable to have a femoral hernia develop. Conversely, the person with an enlarged femoral ring and an increased liability to femoral herniation has a less extensive posterior inguinal wall and, consequently, has less chance of having a direct inguinal hernia.

Note that the structural relations at the femoral ring have a direct bearing on the frequency of incarceration and strangulation in femoral hernia. Even when the femoral ring is enlarged and broad enough to permit the herniation of a peritoneal sac, the structures composing the femoral ring yield but little, compared with the relatively expandable tissues overlying the more distal femoral canal. As a result, the distal part of the peritoneal sac may enlarge readily within the femoral canal, bulging anteriorly in the upper thigh, whereas the neck of the sac is angled and held rigidly between the pubic bone and the iliopubic tract. A small amount of edema in the tissues that have herniated beyond this rigid femoral ring rapidly produces incarceration. Strangulation soon follows if this pathologic process continues. An incarcerated femoral hernia may be easily released and reduced by incision of the recurving insertion of the iliopubic tract at the medial margin of the femoral canal.

Repair of a femoral hernia requires approximation of the aponeurotic margins of the enlarged femoral canal, thereby obliterating it. The sutures should be placed through the iliopubic tract superiorly and through Cooper ligament and pectineus fascia inferiorly.

METHOD FOR DEMONSTRATING THE SURGICAL ANATOMY OF THE GROIN IN THE AUTOPSY ROOM

The unfixed cadavers available in the autopsy room provide an ideal source of material for any limited study of regional anatomy. The marked advantages of such anatomic material to the surgeon cannot be overemphasized. The relatively large number of bodies available for study enables one to perform many dissections and to gain an appreciation of the variety and variability of structural relations in the normal groin. Because the bodies are not embalmed, the tissue densities approximate those of the living, and a dissection of the groin region can be done rapidly because most of the fascial planes can be easily separated by blunt dissection.

First secure the cooperation and permission of the pathologist. Reassure the pathologist that the dissection, conducted as outlined below, does not produce any additional external defect and does not harm the vessels that subsequently must be used to embalm the body. Also reassure the pathologist that after the initial few dissections, the time required for a complete study of the anatomy of the groin in a particular specimen should not exceed 30 or 40 minutes. Study only male bodies with normal groin structures; those with a history of a previous hernial repair or other groin operation should be avoided.

Request notification from the pathologist as to when an autopsy begins and the probable time that it will be completed. This generally provides 1 or 2 hours in which to rearrange schedules so that a timely appearance in the autopsy room may be effected. Try to arrive in the autopsy room just after the major viscera have been excised so that the groin dissection can be conducted during the time that the pathologist is examining the individual organs and cutting tissue blocks. In this way, you do not delay the final closure of the body and its availability to the mortician. Ask the pathologist to leave the testis in situ so as not to disrupt the inguinal canal, to cut the ductus deferens close to the bladder, and also to leave in place as much as possible of the lateral abdominal and pelvic peritoneum when excising the pelvic viscera. You need a minimum of instruments: knife, curved dissecting scissors, toothed tissue forceps, and a few hemostats.

The ultimate objective of this method of groin dissection is to demonstrate the anatomy of the transversus abdominis and transversalis fascial layer of the abdominal wall because this is the important layer with regard to hernial repair. All specimens are dissected so that the deep inguinal ring, the femoral sheath and canal, and the intact posterior wall of the inguinal canal can be studied in situ and by *transillumination*. Only in this way can one come to understand the fundamental pathogenesis of groin hernias and the essential anatomic features of their repair.

The body usually has been opened for the postmortem examination through a standard shoulder-to-pubis Y incision. Begin your dissection by reflecting the skin and subcutaneous fat from the right side as a full-thickness layer. Start dissecting deep to the subcutaneous fat and superficially to the rectus sheath at the midline and mobilize the skin and subcutaneous fat from the entire abdomen, lower chest, and upper thigh. You may have to extend the vertical limb of the autopsy incision to the base of the penis and transect the attachments of Scarpa fascia to the pubic bone.

Carry the mobilization of skin and fat as far laterally as possible, and then fold skin on itself to rest externally to the iliac crest, exposing the muscular layers of the groin.

Study the external surface of the external oblique aponeurosis, which is covered by the innominate fascia. Note the points of emergence of the cutaneous sensory branches of the subcostal, iliohypogastric, and ilioinguinal nerves. Later in the dissection, trace these nerves proximally on the surface of the internal oblique muscle. Note the size and form of the triangular gap in the external oblique aponeurosis, the presence of any intercrural fibers, the continuity of innominate fascia over this gap as the intercrural fascia, and its prolongation over the cord as the external spermatic fascia. Note that the superficial inguinal ring is formed by the action of the innominate fascia, which converts the triangular aponeurotic gap into the oval ring.

Now reach down into the neck of the scrotum, and with a finger bluntly mobilize the distal spermatic cord. By traction and further blunt dissection, mobilize the testis out of the scrotum, and sharply transect the attachments of the inferior pole of the testis to the dartos tunic. Be careful not to cut a "buttonhole" in the scrotum. Next, sharply transect the spermatic cord at the neck of the scrotum and give the testis to the pathologist for examination. Place the stump of the spermatic cord on traction toward the scrotum and visualize again the tubular prolongation of the innominate fascia from all the margins of the superficial ring to form the external spermatic fascia.

Pick up the external spermatic fascia with a forceps, and open the superficial ring by sharply incising through this fascia in a line parallel with the spermatic cord. Then carry the line of incision laterally through the apex of the triangular gap in the external oblique aponeurosis and continue to split the external oblique layer right to its muscular origin from the iliac crest. Grasp the upper leaf of the external oblique aponeurosis, and bluntly mobilize it from the underlying internal oblique muscle, using a finger or the back of the knife handle. After noting the line on which the external oblique aponeurosis joins the underlying internal oblique and transversus abdominis aponeuroses to form the rectus sheath, excise this portion of the external oblique layer, leaving a small rim of tissue, by cutting vertically along the rectus sheath and then transversely to the iliac crest.

Mobilize the inferior leaf of the external oblique aponeurosis, again using blunt dissection. To provide better visualization, it may be convenient also to transect this lower leaf near the iliac crest down to the level of the anterior superior iliac spine. This portion of the external oblique aponeurosis, consisting mostly of the inguinal ligament, forms the anterior wall of

the inguinal canal. Bluntly mobilize the spermatic cord out of the inguinal canal. Note in the course of this dissection the numerous areolar contributions to the cremasteric fascial layer from both the anterior and posterior walls of the inguinal canal.

Grasp the upper border of the inguinal ligament in the midportion of the inguinal canal, and pull it down against the thigh. It is now possible to see the insertion of the inguinal and lacunar ligaments into the superior ramus of the pubis and the pubic tubercle. Note that the fibers of these ligaments are, for the most part, parallel to each other with a gentle curve across the groin. Also note the relation of the insertion of the inguinal and lacunar ligaments to the medial border of the femoral sheath and canal.

Having identified the inguinal and lacunar ligaments and the medial border of the femoral sheath, insert the point of the knife or scissors under the inguinal ligament anterior to the femoral sheath and cut superiorly, transecting the inguinal ligament. This maneuver relieves all tension on these structures and allows full exploration of their mode of insertion into the pubis. Grasp the cut edge of the medial fragment of the inguinal ligament and replace it in about its normal position. In this way, you can appreciate the fact that the inguinal ligament rolls on itself as it proceeds to its insertion near the pubic bone. Next, grasp the cut edge of the lateral fragment of the inguinal ligament, and by applying upward traction, strip it free from the anterior femoral sheath back to its firm lateral attachments to the iliacus fascia and the anterior superior iliac spine.

You can now see the fibers of the iliopubic tract, which run parallel with those of the inguinal ligament but in a deeper plane, crossing the anterior femoral sheath. These fibers may be traced laterally to their attachment to the iliacus fascia in common with the fibers of the inguinal ligament. The iliopubic tract, which represents the inferior limit of the transversus abdominis layer, is seen better from the internal aspect of the groin later in the dissection.

Replace the spermatic cord in more or less its normal position in the inguinal canal, and note the origin of the cremaster muscle. The cremaster fibers arise from the fascia overlying the iliacus muscle, from the iliopubic tract, and from the adjacent inguinal ligament and are applied to the anterior surface of the spermatic cord just after it emerges from the deep ring. These muscle fibers represent the lowest muscular bundles of the internal oblique layer.

The internal oblique layer in the groin is usually muscular, and its lower border arches over the spermatic cord and across the posterior wall of the inguinal canal. By gently inserting either a finger or the back of the knife handle under this muscular arch, one can usually elevate it slightly, demonstrating its intimate association with the underlying transversus abdominis aponeurosis.

Note the course of the ilioinguinal and iliohypogastric nerves on the surface of the muscle, and study the distribution of the main portion of the internal oblique muscle and aponeurosis. Note particularly that in the usual situation, the internal oblique layer and its aponeurotic continuation contribute entirely to the rectus sheath, having no pubic insertion lateral to the pubic tubercle.

Bluntly mobilize the cremaster muscle bundles by inserting the knife handle from below upward and deep to these bundles at the point where they leave the main abdominal wall and join the spermatic cord. Be careful not to injure the underlying structures of the transversus abdominis and transversalis fascial layer. After mobilizing the cremaster bundles, carefully transect them with the scissors from below upward. Distal traction on the spermatic cord now demonstrates the short projecting funnel of transversalis fascia coming through the deep ring to join the spermatic cord and to form the internal spermatic fascia.

Now direct your attention to the internal aspect of the groin. Transect the full thickness of the muscular abdominal wall at the level of the umbilicus, carrying the line of transection from the midline out into the flank. Rotate the full thickness of the lower abdominal wall as a triangular flap down against the tissues of the thigh and hold them there with a Kocher clamp.

Note the general distribution of the peritoneum in the region of the groin, carefully identifying for future preservation the major blood vessels and the ductus deferens. Strip away the peritoneum, using blunt technique. As the internal dissection proceeds, the preperitoneal fat and lymphoid tissue can be most conveniently removed by scraping them gently away from the blood vessels and the fascia covering the transversus abdominis and iliacus muscles, using the back of the knife handle.

Note the junction of the ductus deferens and the testicular vessels in the region of the deep inguinal ring to form the spermatic cord. The superior and inferior crura of the transversalis fascial sling at the deep inguinal ring now can be seen. Bring the sling into prominence by placing medial traction on the spermatic cord structures. The formation of the sling and of the funnel of transversalis fascia that forms the internal spermatic fascia can be appreciated when you pull the cord structures back and forth through the deep inguinal ring and note the movements of the transversalis fascia.

Dissect up the inferior epigastric vessels from the preperitoneal tissues, and note that they do not become covered by transversalis fascia until they are near the border of the rectus abdominis muscle.

Sometimes, the origin of the inferior epigastric vessels is within the femoral sheath. Look for the pubic or accessory obturator vein, which usually is a branch of the inferior epigastric vessels and is found along the medial margin of the femoral ring. It has a small branch running along Cooper ligament. Note also the constant presence of a tiny pubic arterial branch and the occasional presence of an accessory obturator artery.

After studying the distribution of these vessels, ligate and transect the inferior epigastric vessels close to the iliac artery and vein, and again at the semilunar line, and discard them. Similarly, mobilize the pubic or accessory obturator vessels and transect them at the obturator foramen, and discard these vessels also. Turn the ductus deferens and the testicular vessels laterally in the pelvis so they lie on the iliacus muscle. The distribution of the transversalis fascia and the transversus abdominis aponeurosis now can be readily studied.

The transversalis fascia is everywhere adherent to the transversus abdominis aponeurosis and cannot easily be separated from it. Review the anatomy of the deep inguinal ring, paying particular attention to the structure of the transversalis fascial sling. Look for fibers of the interfoveolar ligament at the medial margin of the ring. Identify the semilunar lines on the posterior aspect of the rectus muscle. Note the insertion of the rectus tendon and the extent of the lateral expansion of this tendon, known as *Henle ligament.*

Identify the main arch of the transversus abdominis aponeurosis as it crosses the posterior inguinal wall, and note its relation to the rectus tendon and to the superior pubic ramus. Cooper ligament is the thick collagenous band along the superior pubic ramus.

Remove the lymphoid tissue from the femoral canal. Insert a fingertip just into the femoral canal, and palpate anteriorly. This maneuver most easily identifies the fibers of the iliopubic tract. The iliopubic tract is a firm band along the anterior and medial margins of the femoral canal. Trace it medially to its recurving insertion into the superior pubic ramus and laterally beneath the deep inguinal ring to its attachments to the iliacus fascia and the iliac crest.

At this point, study the structures associated with the femoral sheath and canal. The pectineus muscle forms the floor of the femoral canal as viewed from the internal aspect of the groin. The lateral wall of the canal is formed by the internal septum and the femoral vein. The recurving insertion of the iliopubic tract, covered by transversalis fascia, defines the medial margin of the normal femoral ring. The relation between the medial wall of the femoral canal and the lacunar ligament can be ascertained by inserting a finger deeper into the femoral canal and distending it

while viewing the insertion of the lacunar ligament from the external aspect of the groin.

The transversus abdominis layer has now been cleaned both externally and internally and should be studied by transillumination. Place a gooseneck or similar lamp over the external aspect of the groin and view these structures from their internal aspect, elevating the full-thickness muscular flap of the lower abdominal wall with one hand.

You can now see clearly that the main portion of the transversus abdominis aponeurosis has a definite lower arching border. To view these relations most clearly, it is best to retract the spermatic cord out of the inguinal canal and hold it out of the way by clamping it to the internal oblique muscle well above the deep inguinal ring. Note that the insertion of the main arch of the transversus abdominis aponeurosis usually is in close association with the junction of the rectus tendon and the superior pubic ramus. Occasionally, however, the insertion may spread laterally along the superior ramus of the pubis, forming a falx inguinalis.

Note the insertion into the pubic ramus of the fibers of the iliopubic tract. Between the iliopubic tract and the insertion of the main portion of the transversus abdominis aponeurosis, the posterior wall of the inguinal canal is mainly filled by transversalis fascia, in which there are scattered aponeurotic fibers. This is the weak area in which direct herniation occurs. A direct hernia may be simulated when a fingertip is thrust through the fascia of the posterior inguinal wall, thus nearly duplicating the fundamental fascial defect in direct inguinal hernia. With a finger inserted in the defect thus created, note that the superior margin of a direct hernial defect is formed by the transversus abdominis aponeurosis, whereas the inferior margin is formed by the iliopubic tract and Cooper ligament. This makes obvious the essential requirement in surgical repair of such a defect—the suture reapproximation of the transversus abdominis aponeurosis to Cooper ligament and the iliopubic tract.

Similarly, the fascial defect in indirect inguinal hernias can be simulated with a fingertip placed superiorly and laterally to the spermatic cord within the sling at the deep inguinal ring and thrust outward along the course of the spermatic cord and inguinal canal. This maneuver demonstrates that the upper margin of an indirect hernial defect is formed by the superior crus of the transversalis fascial sling and the adjacent transversus abdominis aponeurosis, and the inferior border is formed by the inferior crus of the sling and the iliopubic tract. The requirements for repair are suture approximation of these two borders.

With a finger inserted in the artificially created indirect hernial defect, tension applied medially duplicates the process by which the indirect inguinal

hernia enlarges and finally breaks down all the posterior inguinal wall. In such hernias, the essential requirement of surgical repair is more extensive approximation, on the superior aspect of the defect, of the transversus abdominis aponeurosis and its investing transversalis fascia to the iliopubic tract and Cooper ligament on the inferior aspect of the defect.

The course of a femoral hernia can be duplicated by insertion of a finger into the femoral canal. Palpation distally with a fingertip shows that the tissues in the upper thigh are relatively more expandable than those at the femoral ring. It is these fixed tissues at the neck of the sac that lead to incarceration and strangulation of femoral hernias. Palpation of the femoral ring also demonstrates the fascial margins that require reapproximation in femoral hernial repair. The upper margin is the iliopubic tract; the lower margin is the Cooper ligament and the adjacent pectineus fascia.

It is instructive at this point to take the scissors and transect the remainder of the abdominal muscular aponeurotic wall at a level 2 or 3 cm above the superior pubic ramus. Begin medially along the border of the rectus abdominis tendon and sheath, and carry the line of transection just above the deep inguinal ring. The important relations of the insertions of the anterior and posterior walls of the inguinal canal to each other and to the femoral sheath and internal ring now can be perceived most easily.

After completing the dissections, make certain of the ligatures on the stumps of the inferior epigastric vessels. The abdominal muscle and skin flaps may then be returned toward their former position, and the body is ready to be closed in the usual manner.

It cannot be emphasized too strongly that multiple dissections and demonstrations of the regional surgical anatomy of the groin are the surest path to secure understanding of the anatomy of the structures in this area. Repeated dissections should be made so that the surgeon may become thoroughly familiar with the usual anatomy and with all the common variants.

BIBLIOGRAPHY

No effort has been made to include all pertinent literature (a truly formidable task!), nor has any attempt been made to include all publications on which historical priorities are based. Rather, this is a short list of monographs and articles that are of value to the surgeon because of their excellence of description or illustration.

This chapter represents a synthesis of my original observations combined with those portions of the anatomic studies listed below that could be confirmed by personal dissection. The important contributions of these workers have been freely included without specific credit being given in the body of the text, and it is hoped that their citation here will partially remedy this omission.

Anson BJ, Morgan EH, McVay CB. Surgical anatomy of the inguinal region based upon a study of 500 body-halves. Surg Gynecol Obstet 1960;111:707.

Bassett DL. A stereoscopic atlas of human anatomy: the abdomen. Portland, OR, Sawyer's, 1960.

Clark JH, Hashimoto EI. Utilization of Henle's ligament, iliopubic tract, aponeurosis transversus abdominis and Cooper ligament in inguinal herniorrhaphy. Surg Gynecol Obstet 1946;82:480.

Condon RE. Surgical anatomy of the transversus abdominis and transversalis fascia. Ann Surg 1971;173:1.

Cooper AP. The anatomy and surgical treatment of abdominal hernia, ed 2. Rev. by CA Key. Philadelphia, Lea & Blanchard, 1844:17–58.

Donald DC. The value derived from utilizing the component parts of the transversalis fascia and Cooper ligament in the repair of large indirect and direct inguinal hernia: a group of cases. Surgery 1948;24:662.

Gilroy AM, Marks SC Jr, Lei Q, Page DW. Anatomical characteristics of the iliopubic tract: implications for the repair of inguinal hernias. Clin Anat 1992;5:255.

Gray SW, Skandalakis JE. Atlas of surgical anatomy for general surgeons. Baltimore, Williams & Wilkins, 1985.

Lytle WJ. The internal inguinal ring. Br J Surg 1945;32:441.

McVay CB. Hernia: the pathologic anatomy of the more common hernias and their anatomic repair. Springfield, IL., Charles C Thomas, 1954.

McVay CB. The anatomic basis for inguinal and femoral hernioplasty. Surg Gynecol Obstet 1974;139:931.

McVay CB, Anson BJ. Aponeurotic and fascial continuities in the abdomen, pelvis, and thigh. Anat Rec 1940;76:213.

McVay CB, Savage LE. Etiology of femoral hernia. Ann Surg 1961;154:25.

Tobin CE, Benjamin JA, Wells JC. Continuity of the fasciae lining the abdomen, pelvis and spermatic cord. Surg Gynecol Obstet 1946;83:575.

Special Comment

The Transversalis Fascia
Ernest W. Lampe

The transversalis fascia is a membranous layer that lines the abdominal cavity like a bag. Its outer aspect is in contact with the muscles, aponeuroses, and bones that bound the abdominal cavity. Its inner aspect is in contact with the preperitoneal or extraperitoneal layer of areolar tissue, which may or may not contain fat.

Superiorly, the transversalis fascia is fused intimately with the diaphragm, where some refer to it needlessly as the *diaphragmatic fascia*. The right and left medial arcuate ligaments or medial lumbocostal arches are band-like thickenings of the transversalis fascia that extend from the tips of the right and left transverse processes of the 1st lumbar vertebra and across the psoas muscles to become attached to the disk between the 1st and 2nd lumbar vertebrae and adjacent tendinous parts of the crura of the diaphragm. The right and left lateral arcuate ligaments or lateral lumbocostal arches are also band-like thickenings of the transversalis fascia that extend from the tips of the transverse processes of the 1st lumbar vertebra and across their respective quadratus lumborum muscles to become attached near the tips of the 12th ribs. These band-like ligaments perform a dual function: they serve as sites of origin of adjacent parts of the diaphragm, and they form the upper border of the anterior layer of lumbodorsal fascia.

Posteriorly and centrally, the transversalis fascia is pressed up against the bodies of the lower three or four lumbar vertebrae and the anterior aspects of the sacrum and coccyx. This means that it is posterior to the kidneys, adrenal glands, stomach, duodenum, and pancreas.

Posteriorly and laterally, this fascia fuses intimately with a thin layer of fascia (epimysium?) covering the psoas and quadratus lumborum muscles. On the psoas muscles, it is frequently referred to as the *psoas fascia*, which continues with the psoas muscle deep to the inguinal ligament and down to the lesser trochanter of the femur for insertion. Everyone recalls the clinical reason for remembering this: In lumbar Pott disease or any other suppurative process, deep to the so-called psoas fascia the pus may gravitate under the inguinal ligament into the upper lateral part of the femoral triangle and down to the lesser trochanter of the femur.

Continuing laterally from the psoas fascia portion the transversalis fascia fuses with the fascia (epimysium?) covering the anterior aspect of the quadratus lumborum muscles to form the anterior layer of the so-called lumbodorsal fascia, which extends from the 12th rib to about the posterior third of the crest of the ilium.

Anteriorly, the transversalis fascia is fused with the posterior sheath of the rectus abdominis muscles down to the semicircular fold of Douglas. From this level, the transversalis fascia continues downward and is in intimate contact not only with the posterior aspects of the lower portions of the rectus muscles but also with about the upper half of the body of each pubic bone. At about the midpoint of the posterior aspect of the body of each pubic bone, the transversalis fascia becomes again a noticeably white, thick-

ened, band-like structure that extends posteriorly across the upper third of the obturator internus muscle to the spine of the ischium. It is commonly referred to as the *white line* or *arcus tendineus* (Fig. 2-16, label 10).

Laterally and anterolaterally, the transversalis fascia extends from the lateral borders of the quadratus lumborum muscles to the lateral borders of the rectus muscles. En route, it is in intimate contact with the posterior aponeurotic portion of the transverse ab-

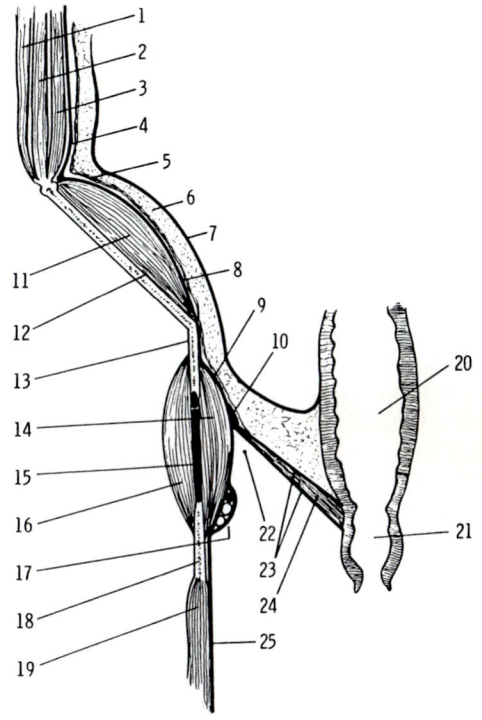

Figure 2-16. Transversalis fascia in lateral and lower parts of abdominal cavity. (1) External oblique muscle and its superficial and deep fasciae. (2) Internal oblique muscle and its fasciae. (3) Transversus abdominis muscle and fasciae. (4) Transversalis fascia. Note that the muscles above and the transversalis fascia are attached to the crest of ilium. (5) Condensation of the fibrous stroma of the preperitoneal or subserous fat layer into a (6) membrane-like layer—mistaken by some as the transversalis fascia. The same membrane-like condensation of fibrous stroma occurs in the subcutaneous fat layer and is known as the Scarpa fascia. (7) Peritoneum. (8) Iliac fascia. (9) Obturator fascia, intraabdominal portion. (10) Arcus tendineus or "white line" extends from the back of the pubic bone to the spine of the ischium. (11) Iliacus muscle. (12) Iliac fossa. (13) Superior iliopubic ramus. (14) Obturator internus muscle. (15) Obturator membrane. (16) Obturator externus muscle. (17) Alcock canal containing pudendal nerve, internal pudendal artery, and vein. (18) Inferior puboischial ramus. (19) Muscles on medial aspect of the thigh. (20) Rectum. (21) Anal canal. (22) Ischiorectal fossa. (23) Superior and inferior pelvic diaphragmatic fasciae. (24) Levator ani muscle. (25) Fascia lata on medial aspect of thigh.

dominis muscles, then with the muscular parts, and finally with their anterior aponeuroses.

The iliac fascia is that part of the transversalis fascia that covers the iliacus muscles found in the iliac fossae (see Fig. 2-16, label 8). This portion of the fascia is adherent at the iliac crests and the brim of the true pelvis. It continues downward to the arcus tendineus as the intraabdominal part of the obturator fascia, which covers the upper half of the obturator internus and coccygeus muscles (see Fig. 2-16, label 9). Recall that the arcus tendineus, or white line, is a white, band-like thickening of this part of the transversalis fascia that extends from the ischial spine to a point at about the middle of the posterior aspect of the body of the pubic bone (see Fig. 2-16, label 10). It serves as a line of origin for portions of the levator ani and coccygeus muscles (see Fig. 2-16, label 24) and marks the site where the obturator fascia splits to form a thin membranous covering for the superior and inferior surfaces of these two muscles. They are commonly referred to as the *superior* and *inferior pelvic diaphragmatic fasciae* (see Fig. 2-16, label 23). Observe how the lower half of the obturator fascia (extraabdominal portion) and the inferior pelvic diaphragmatic fascia help to serve, respectively, as the lateral and the medial boundaries of the ischiorectal fossa (see Fig. 2-16, label 22). Also note how the extraabdominal part of the obturator fascia helps to form the Alcock canal (see Fig. 2-16, label 17) and, after gaining attachment to the inferior puboischial rami, becomes continuous with the deep fascia on the medial aspect of the thigh (see Fig. 2-16, label 25).

In the inguinal region, posterior to about the lateral third of the inguinal ligament, the transversalis fascia on the posterior aspect of the anterior abdominal wall meets the iliopsoas portion of the fascia to form a band-like thickening called the *iliopectineal ligament*. Portions of the cremaster muscle and the lowermost parts of the internal oblique and transversus abdominis muscles originate from it. The lateral part of the inguinal ligament is intimately attached to the iliopectineal ligament and the adjacent part of the fascia lata.

From the medial part of the iliopectineal ligament, the thickened lower border of the transversalis fascia continues medially over the femoral vessels as the iliopubic tract. At the operating table, with a preperitoneal exposure, one can easily palpate the taut inguinal ligament anterior and slightly inferior to the iliopubic tract (Fig. 2-17, labels 14 and 18) and by tugging with a thumb forceps on the tract, one can clearly demonstrate how its medial end fans out to gain attachment to the Cooper ligament. Then, by elevating the tract slightly, immediately over the femoral vessels, one can see how the transversalis fascia is carried

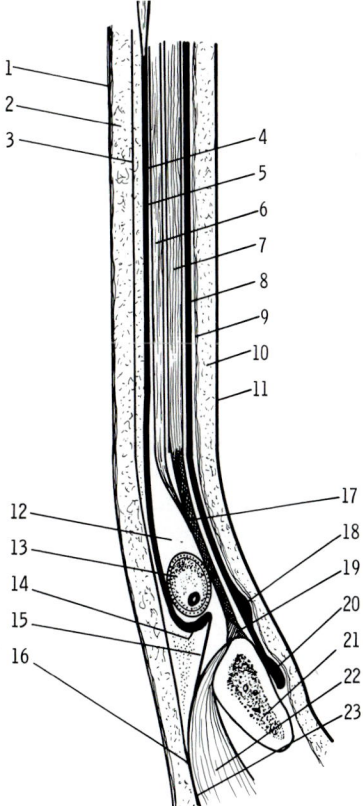

Figure 2-17.   Cross section of a strong posterior canal wall. (1) Skin. (2) Camper fascia, the soft fatty component of the superficial fascia. (3) Scarpa fascia, a membranous condensation of the fibrous stroma of the superficial fatty layer. (4, 5) Aponeurosis of the external oblique muscle and its intimately fused fasciae. (6) Internal oblique muscle and fasciae. (7) Transversus abdominis muscle and fasciae. (8) Transversalis fascia. (9) Membrane-like condensation of fibrous stroma of preperitoneal fatty or fascial layer. Mistakenly interpreted by some as the transversalis fascial layer. (10) Preperitoneal fascia or fatty layer. (11) Peritoneum. (12) Inguinal canal. (13) Spermatic cord. (14) Shelving border of the inguinal ligament. (15) Continuation of the fasciae of the external oblique aponeurosis down to the fascia lata (16). (17) Aponeurosis of transversus abdominis and its fasciae here form a strong posterior canal wall. The lowermost arching fibers of the internal oblique are low and just anterior to 17. Ideal for obtaining the shutter or sphincter action. (18) Iliopubic tract, a thickening of the lower part of the transversalis fascia, which is usually intimately adherent to the aponeurosis of the transversus abdominis. (19) Cooper ligament. (20) Arcus tendineus or "white line," which here is the lowest part of the transversalis fascia and extends from the back of the pubic bone to the spine of the ischium. (21) Superior ramus of the pubic bone. (22) Pectineus muscle. (23) Pectineal part of the fascia lata.

distal as the femoral sheath. This maneuver also demonstrates how much easier and safer it is to place the so-called transition sutures of McVay by the preperitoneal exposure than by the external approach for repairing a hernia.

Remember that the aponeurosis of the transversus abdominis muscle gains insertion into a variable length of the Cooper ligament—anywhere from the pubic tubercle to the edge of the femoral vein—and that the transversalis fascia is intimately adherent to it (Fig. 2-18*L*, label 4, and *R*, label 5).

That portion of the transversalis fascia in the Hesselbach triangle varies from a membrane that is strong to one that is thin and weak.

The ideally strong posterior inguinal canal wall is shown schematically in Figures 2-17 and 2-18*R*. Here, the arching part of the internal oblique muscle or its aponeurosis extends down as low as the pubic tubercle for its insertion, enabling the muscle to exert its shutter or sphincter action when it contracts (see Fig. 2-18*R*, label 4). Also note that the aponeurosis of the transversus abdominis muscle and its superficial and deep fasciae, including the adherent transversalis fascia, form a good strong posterior wall for the canal (see Fig. 2-17 and Fig. 2-18*R*, labels 4, 8, and 17). Anson and colleagues,[1] in their review of 500 body halves, found the strong combination in about 26% of the bodies. In about 8% of bodies, they found the unhappy combination of structures shown schematically in Figures 2-18 and 2-19. Note that the arching fibers

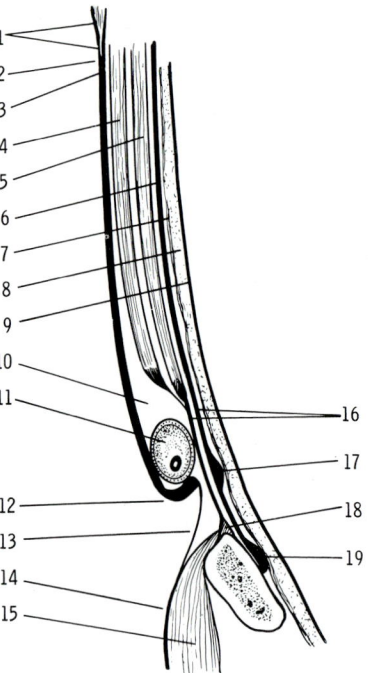

Figure 2-19. Cross section of a weak posterior canal wall. (1, 2) External oblique muscle and its superficial and deep fasciae. (3) External oblique aponeurosis. (4) Internal oblique muscle and fasciae. (5) Transversus abdominis muscle and its fasciae. (6) Transversalis fascia. (7) Membrane-like condensation of the fibrous stroma of the preperitoneal fatty layer. Mistaken by some as the transversalis fascia. (8) Preperitoneal fascia. (9) Peritoneum. (10) Inguinal canal. (11) Spermatic cord. (12) Shelving border of the inguinal ligament. (13) Fasciae of the external oblique muscle fusing with fascia lata (14). It is this attachment that prevents the lifting up or upward bowing of the inguinal ligament. (15) Pectineus muscle. (16) Fasciae of the transversus abdominis muscle are fused with one another and the transversalis fascia (6) to form a weak posterior inguinal canal wall. Note that the lowermost fibers of the internal oblique muscle are too high to be able to exert the shutter or sphincter action and that no part of the aponeurosis of the transversus abdominis reaches the Cooper ligament to help form a strong posterior canal wall. (17) Iliopubic tract, a thickening of the medial half of the transversalis fascia behind the inguinal ligament. (18) Cooper ligament. (19) Arcus tendineus or "white line," a thickened band of transversalis fascia that extends from back of pubic bone to spine of ischium.

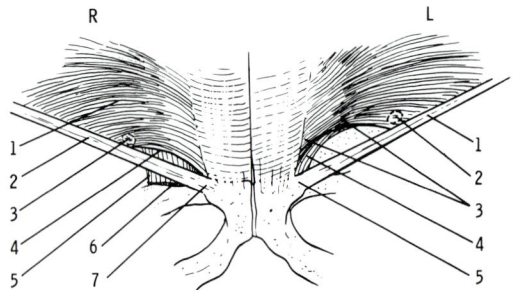

Figure 2-18. (*R*) Ideal disposition of lowermost fibers of internal oblique and transversus abdominis muscles for strong posterior canal wall. (1) Internal oblique muscle. (2) Inguinal ligament. (3) Internal inguinal ring. (4) Lowermost arching fibers of the internal oblique muscle, extending to the pubic tubercle (7) for insertion—ideal for obtaining the protective shutter or sphincter action. (5) Aponeurosis of transversus abdominis muscle and fascia attached along full length of Cooper ligament (6), adding strength to the posterior inguinal canal wall. (6) Cooper ligament. (7) Pubic tubercle. (*L*) Nonideal disposition of lowermost fibers of internal oblique and transversus abdominis muscles results in weak posterior inguinal canal wall. Compare with Figure 2-19. (1) Inguinal ligament. (2) Internal inguinal ring. (3) Lowermost arching fibers of internal oblique muscle inserting high above pubic tubercle (5), making it impossible to obtain shutter or sphincter action. (4) Lowermost fibers of transversus abdominis aponeurosis insert into pubic tubercle. They do not extend along Cooper ligament as on opposite side (5, 6) and, therefore, offer little support to the posterior wall of inguinal canal. The dotted space inferior to lowermost fibers represents fasciae of transversus abdominis muscle back to back with transversalis fascia. (See Fig. 2-19, label 16.)

of the internal oblique muscle have their insertion well above the pubic tubercle (see Fig. 2-18*L*, label 3), making the protective shutter or sphincter action on exertion impossible. Also note that the aponeurosis of the transversus abdominis muscle apparently does not extend laterally along the Cooper ligament for its insertion (see Fig. 2-18*R*, label 4), leaving nothing but the superficial and deep fasciae of the transversus abdominis aponeurosis back to back and fused with a thin, unsubstantial transversalis fascia (see Fig. 2-19, label 16). This clearly is not a strong posterior wall for the inguinal canal. Anson and colleagues[1] believed that this weak combination of structures might have accounted for most of the recurrences of direct hernias (about 9%) after the repair of indirect inguinal hernias. Thus, it can be seen that the lower the arching fibers of the internal oblique, and the stronger the aponeurosis of the transversus abdominis, and the farther it extends laterally along the Cooper ligament for its insertion, the less is the likelihood for a direct hernia to form. A thickened transversalis fascia in the Hesselbach triangle helps but does not count as much as the other two factors.

REFERENCE

1. Anson BJ, Morgan EH, McVay CB. Surgical anatomy of the inguinal region based upon a study of 500 body-halves. Surg Gynecol Obstet 1960;111:707.

Editor's Comment (First Edition)

The undersigned will never forget a hot June 1960 afternoon spent with Drs. Harkins and Condon on the 15th floor of Cornell Hospital. The three Westerners soon forgot the heat (not an easy thing for a Westerner to do) as Dr. Lampe led us through myriads of beautiful blackboard drawings of groin anatomy. We were honored to spend a few short hours attempting to grasp some of this teacher's insight into groin anatomy. *Teacher* is stressed because Lampe has taught innumerable students surgical anatomy at that venerable institution.

The reader will enjoy comparing these concepts with those presented by Dr. Condon. It must be stated that the drawings in Dr. Lampe's *Special Comment* are very schematic. In Figure 2-17, the transversalis fascia appears to be fully as strong as the external oblique aponeurosis, which it is not.

With the help of source material such as this, the elusive (in some observers' minds) iliopubic tract will become a well-recognized and appreciated entity.

L.M.N.

Editor's Comment (Second Edition)

Dr. Lampe, who died on October 19, 1966, trained many young surgeons in surgical anatomy. His contributions to surgical education at Cornell and in the New York region are outstanding. His *Special Comment* in the first edition of *Hernia,* concerning the transversalis fascia, is included here as a tribute to Dr. Lampe by the Editors.

W.J. Lytle has recently pointed out to me that the special relation between the inguinal ligament and Cooper ligament contained in Figure 2-17 is inexact—the inguinal ligament should lie at or below the level of Cooper ligament. Mr. Lytle is right, and I am sure that Dr. Lampe would have agreed with him were he with us to participate in discussion. Dr. Lampe, throughout his productive professional lifetime, taught many a surgeon to be a better anatomist. He will be missed not only by his former students but also by the students of the current generation, who will not have the benefit of his counsel and teaching.

R.E.C.

Editor's Comment

Yes, Condon and I continue to highlight the work of Lampe by reprinting his *Special Comment*, which stems from our meeting in 1960. A master surgeon-anatomist, we forever are indebted to him for his clear delineation of the anatomy of the lower abdominal wall.

Careful attention should be given to the Condon review of the nerves innervating the groin area. Early results of laparoscopic hernia operations have suggested damage to the neural connections traversing the lower abdominal wall. The blind placement of staples lateral to the internal abdominal ring to attach the prosthetic mesh has caused severe pain in the distribution of the ilioinguinal, iliohypogastric, femoral, and genitofemoral nerves. I hope that this serious complication can be prevented as we review the neural anatomy and learn new and better ways to apply laparoscopic skills.

L.M.N.

Special Comment

The Transversalis and Preperitoneal Fasciae—A Reevaluation
Raymond C. Read

No disease of the human body belonging to the province of the surgeon requires in its treatment a better combination of accurate anatomical knowledge with surgical skill than hernia in all its varieties.

Cooper, 1804

Harrison[12] in 1922 stressed the importance of the fascia transversalis in the pathology and repair of inguinal herniation. Recently, Condon[8] affirmed this fact, "The fundamental rupture, relation or disconti-

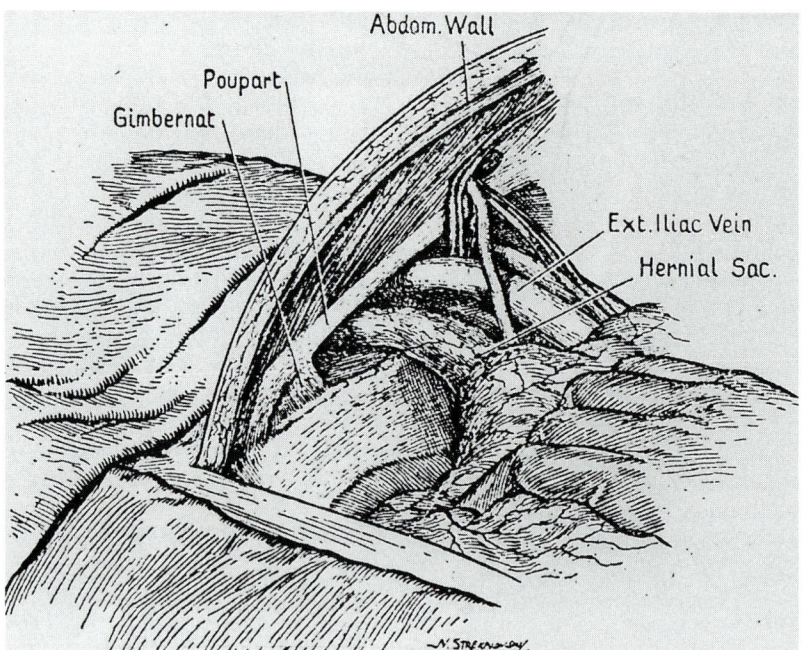

Figure 2-20.   Preperitoneal approach through the linea alba. Note that exposure is internal to the inferior epigastric vessels retracted with the rectus abdominis. (Henry AK. Operation for femoral hernia by a midline extraperitoneal approach. Lancet 1936;1:531)

nuity in the musculo-aponeurotic structure in cases of groin hernia occurs in the deeply placed transversus abdominis-transversalis fascial layer." Henry[13] in 1936 not only rediscovered the preperitoneal approach to the groin reported by Cheatle[6] but also was able to make an important contribution to our understanding of surgical anatomy. Henry pointed out that division of the infraumbilical linea alba allowed the rectus muscles to be divaricated with their blood supply, the inferior epigastric vessels. Dissection of the underlying extraperitoneal space loosened the vas deferens and spermatic vessels and any peritoneal protrusion that could be ligated high at its origin from the general peritoneal cavity (Fig. 2-20). He emphasized that this should be performed at the wider "true neck," which in indirect herniation is some distance from the "false neck" at the internal abdominal ring in the transversalis fascia (Fig. 2-21). Failure to appreciate this distinction results in the retention of a protrusion, which can later expand into a recurrence. Support for his contention was provided by Postlethwaite[21] in 1971 when he reported over half of 300 recurrences that followed repair of inguinal herniation were "indirect with the sac descending within the cord in the manner of a primary indirect hernia."

Lytle[16] in 1945 cast more light on this area by describing two layers to the posterior wall of the inguinal canal—the superficial transversalis muscle lamina and

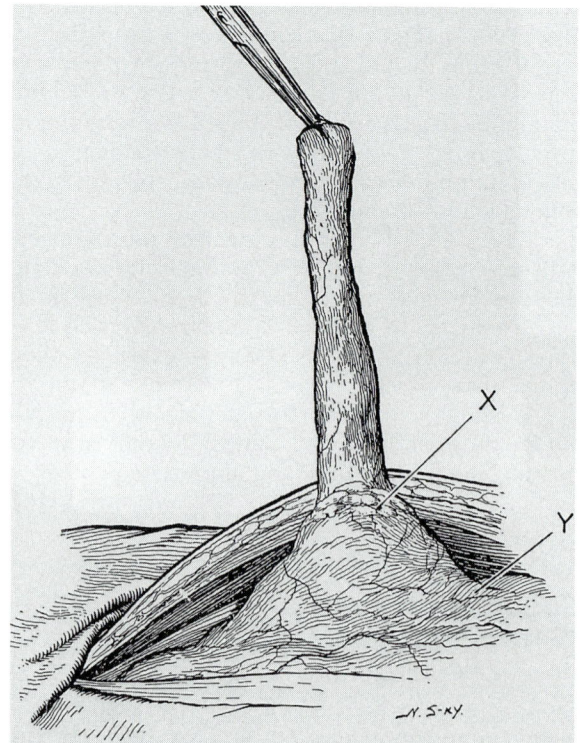

Figure 2-21.   False (X) and true (Y) necks of the processus vaginalis. (Henry AK. Operation for femoral hernia by a midline extraperitoneal approach. Lancet 1936;1:531)

a deeper layer, the transversalis fascia. Each had an internal ring (actually, Lytle termed them *internal* and *middle*). He said the inferior epigastric could pierce the transversalis fascia and lie on a more superficial plane (between the two transverse laminae). This is illustrated in Figure 2-22. The superficial transversalis muscle layer in the floor of the canal Lytle reported as being "the continuation downward of the transversalis [sic, transversus] muscle and its aponeurosis. It is the stouter of the two posterior laminae forming the floor of the inguinal canal. It is formed by the blending of the muscle fasciae lining its superficial and deep surfaces." He stated, "over the edge of the middle ring (the opening in the transversalis muscle layer through which the cord emerges) at a point below and medial to the internal ring (which it encircles like a collar) emerge the cremasteric vessels together with the genital branch of the genitofemoral nerve." It would appear that Lytle's more superficial "middle ring" is what most surgical anatomists refer to as the *internal abdominal ring,* whereas his deeper internal ring is novel. He says that this opening in the transversalis fascia is bounded medially by the Hesselbach ligament and inferiorly by the Thomson (iliopubic) tract. "The transversalis fascia joins with the superficial layer in forming the anterior wall of the femoral sheath."

This concept of two internal abdominal rings was confirmed and expanded in 1975 by Fowler,[10] a pediatric surgeon from Melbourne, Australia. He considered Lytle's deeper internal ring to be in the preperitoneal fascia, a condensation of the extraperitoneal layer similar to Scarpa fascia in the subcutaneous layer (but here an outer lamina, not inner). This lamina, thicker and stronger in the groin, had been depicted by Lampe.[15] Fowler called the deeper ring the *secondary* internal ring. The inferior epigastric vasculature ran in the plane between the transversalis and preperitoneal fascial rings. He agreed with Lytle that there was considerable individual variation in the strength of these layers and the amount of fat interspersed. He reported that fairly tough pre-

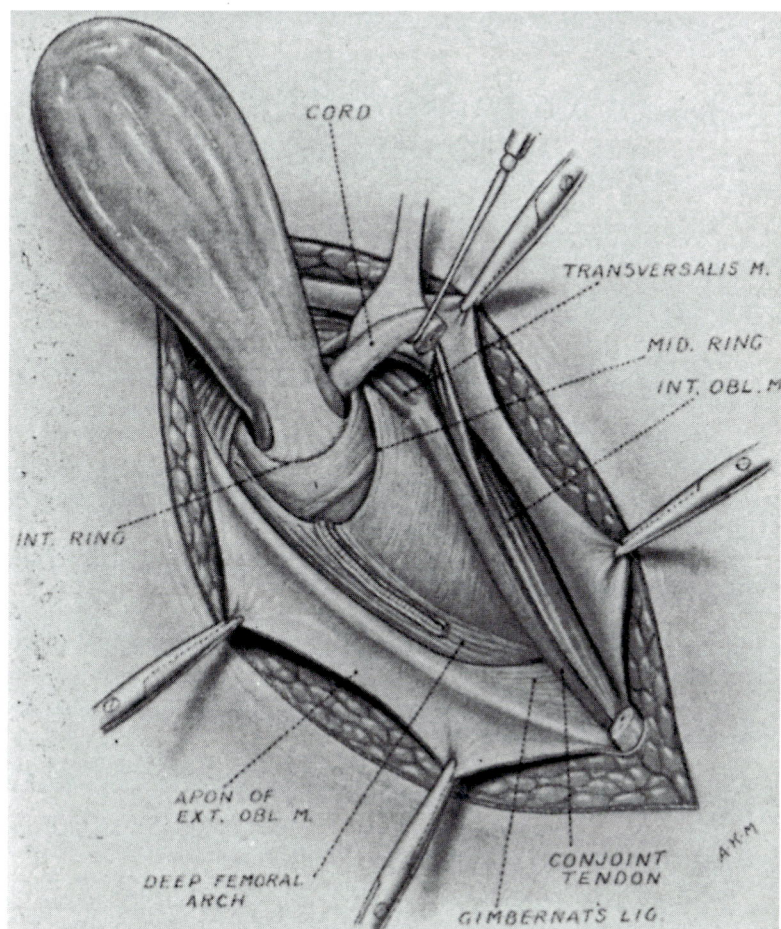

Figure 2-22. Floor of the inguinal canal, illustrating two internal rings with epigastric vessels running on the posterior lamina transversalis fascia. (Lytle WJ. The internal inguinal ring. Br J Surg 1945;32:441, by permission of the publisher, Blackwell Scientific Publications)

peritoneal fascial fibers surrounded the spermatic vessels, the vas deferens, and any patent processus vaginalis as they came together to constitute the spermatic cord, forming a secondary deeper internal ring. "They have to be deliberately disrupted to fully expose a hernial sac opening up a fissile plane or little "cave" of loose areolar tissue leading to the retroperitoneal plane . . . through which the vas and spermatic vessels course." This cavity he encountered is presumably the interparietoperitoneal space of Bogros[4] and Hureau.[14] Fowler went further: "Recognition of the secondary internal ring identifies the true neck of the sac and avoids the pitfall of leaving a residual funnel. . . . The vas deferens angles acutely around the medial lip of this deeper ring, which has to be divided during orchidolysis." Stoppa,[27] in his "parietalization" of the cord, performs this maneuver.

My interest[22,23] in preperitoneal herniorrhaphy was stimulated by Nyhus, Condon, and Harkins.[20] They, at the behest of Bruce,[5] had adopted McEvedy's[17] (Fig. 2-23) unilateral approach to the in-

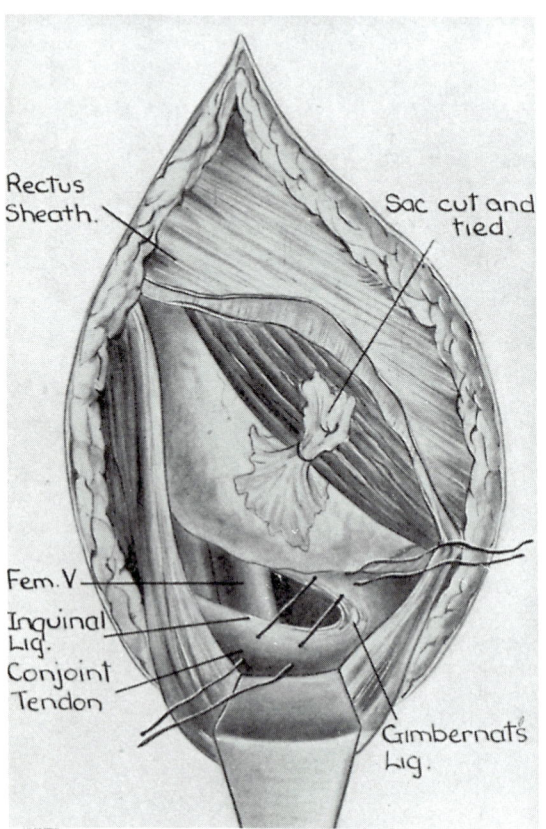

Figure 2-23. McEvedy rectus sheath unilateral approach to the preperitoneal space in 1950, modified soon thereafter to a transverse incision. (McEvedy PG. Femoral hernia. Ann R Coll Surg Engl 1950;7:484)

fraumbilical preperitoneal space through the rectus sheath with medial rather than lateral displacement of the muscle. I reported in the late 1960s[22] that, consonant with Lampe's observation, there was a definite layer internal to the epigastric vasculature separating the transversus-transversalis layer from the peritoneum. However, I also found that this preperitoneal fascia fused with the transversalis at the internal ring, where the former gave rise to most of the internal spermatic fascia lining the contents of the spermatic cord. This structure is supposed to arise from the transversalis layer. It was only after the preperitoneal fascia had been divided with retraction of the inferior epigastric vessels that the fissile fatty extraperitoneal space could be entered. Thus, whereas the Cheatle-Henry incision divides both layers of the transversalis fascia at the linea alba and brings one down immediately into the preperitoneal space, McEvedy's unilateral incision in the rectus sheath does not. The posterior lamina supporting the inferior epigastric vessels still has to be disrupted.

More recently, performing preperitoneal prosthetic placement from the groin for large hernias, I found that, after a transversalis fascial layer in the floor of the inguinal canal had been divided, the inferior epigastric vessels with their pubic, circumflex, cremasteric, accessory obturator, and rectusial branches encased in fat were displayed[2] (Fig. 2-24) lying on a separate translucent but tough layer overlying extraperitoneal fat.[24] This suggested it was a preperitoneal fibrous membrane. However, this layer attached to the pubic or iliopectineal ligament of Cooper, the linea alba, and the linea semicircularis. Again, it was only after this second layer was disrupted, avoiding injury to the epigastric vasculature lying on it, that the finger could be passed freely outside the preperitoneal fat down into the pelvis, medially to the space of Retzius, laterally to the space of Bogros and the iliopsoas fascia, retroperitoneally over the iliac vessels, and anteriorly up under the lineae semilunaris and semicircularis. The vas deferens and spermatic vessels could then be dissected separately and parietalized onto the iliopsoas fascia. A "jockstrap" angle-iron polypropylene (Marlex) prosthesis, 12 × 16 centimeters, could then be easily underlapped deep to the inferior epigastric vessels in the fissile preperitoneal space of Bogros using Stoppa's principles (enthusiastically supported by Bendavid[3] and Gilbert[11]) of essentially sutureless fixation. My experience led to the conclusion, in agreement with Lytle but different from Fowler, that this extra layer was not a condensation of the preperitoneal fat, but a second plate of transversalis fascia enclosing with its more superficial layer a fatty vascular envelope for the blood supply to the anterior abdominal wall. Thus, this vasculature does not course in the

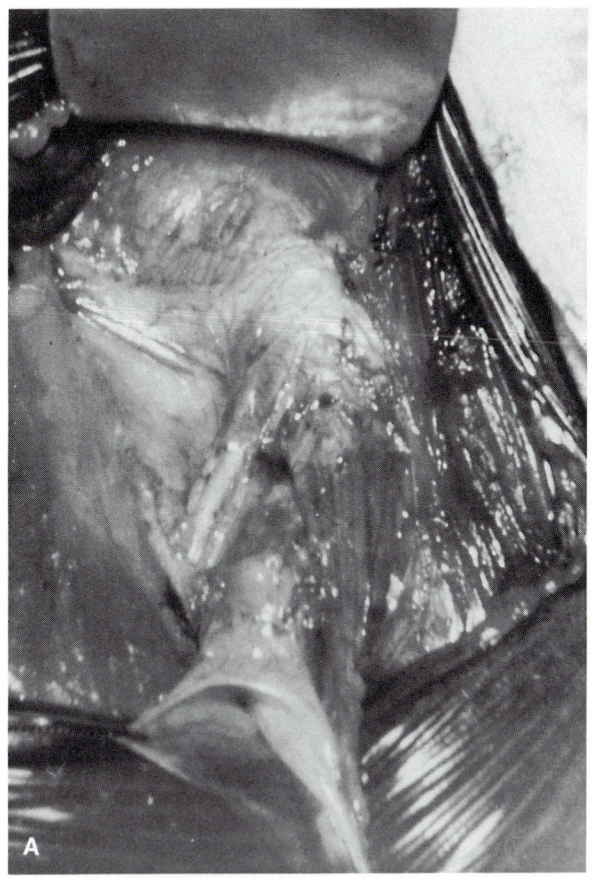

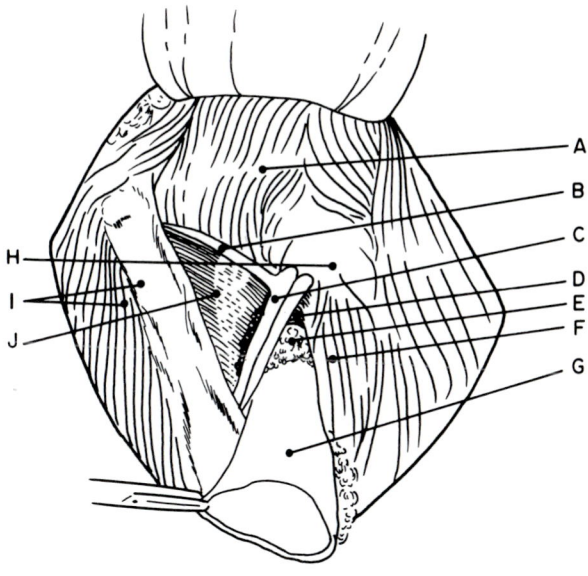

Figure 2-24. (*A*) Photograph taken during the repair of a right indirect inguinal herniation through a modified McEvedy (transverse) rectus sheath incision. (*B*) Drawing made from (*A*). (A) Retracted anterior rectus sheath. (B) Pubic vein. (C) Inferior epigastric artery and vein with fat. (D) Secondary internal ring. (E) Preperitoneal fat in the space of Bogros. (F) Spermatic blood vessels beneath the posterior lamina transversalis fascia. (G) Hernia sac. (H) Internal abdominal ring. (I) Rectus muscle and tendon. (J) Posterior lamina transversalis fascia.

preperitoneal (parietoperitoneal) space of Bogros, as indicated by Bendavid,[2] but external to it, separated by the deepest fascia, the posterior lamina of transversalis.

Interestingly, a detailed examination[24] of the original description of the transversalis fascia by Astley Cooper[9] documents two layers of this structure, that is, "the fascia transversalis may be divided into two portions, the one being placed a little before the other. . . . The inner portion is thinner than the former; . . . it rises to the tendon of the transversalis muscle on the inner side of the spermatic cord and is firmly attached to the linea semilunaris. It appears that the internal ring is not a circumscribed aperture like the external abdominal ring but is formed by the separation of two portions." Cooper was upset when the posterior lamina was denied by Scarpa,[26] "From below the umbilicus to the pubis the rectus muscle has

no aponeurotic sheath and lies immediately upon the peritoneum." This prejudice against a bilaminar nature continued. Anson and McVay, writing in 1938, state, "the medially placed tendinous plate is, in almost all descriptions, correctly termed aponeurosis, but curiously enough the inferior continuation of the same structure is called a fascia, more specifically, 'transversalis fascia.' That the two are merely areas of the same layer is self-evident." Nevertheless, an important supporter of Cooper was MacKay, who in 1889 stated, "What we have been taught to call the 'preperitoneal membrane' lying between the rectus muscles with their investing fascia and the peritoneum is a part of the transversalis fascia."

Therefore, with MacKay and Lytle's support, I believe that the preperitoneal fascia of Lampe is actually Cooper's long ignored posterior lamina of transversalis fascia. This distinction is important not only academically but practically because the proper location for the placement of preperitoneal prostheses, taking advantage of the anatomic parietoperitoneal spaces,[8] cannot be reached unless one is internal to both transversalis fascial laminae and to the inferior epigastric vessels (Fig. 2-25). We must become cognizant of both internal abdominal rings and the inner inguinal canal between. High ligation requires disruption of this fibrous funnel to prevent retention within the inner inguinal canal and eventually recurrence of peritoneal (or extraperitoneal fatty) protrusions. Deviation of the inferior epigastric vessels almost to the pubis by large indirect herniation is explained by the fact that these blood vessels pierce the posterior lamina of transversalis fascia soon after their origin from the external iliac vessels and run in between the transversalis laminae of the anterior abdominal wall, coursing medially to the inner inguinal fibrous canal. They are held there by Hesselbach ligament and are deviated by the inner, interstitial component of large hernial sacs.

In conclusion, an earlier statement by Condon needs to be revised in the light of the evidence cited above. Condon had said that the inferior epigastric vessels:

> . . . are contained within the preperitoneal space throughout their course in the groin. Therefore, they are deep or internal to the transversalis fascia, not superficial to it, and these vessels have no intimate connection with the musculoaponeurotic abdominal wall in the groin. . . . Between the iliac vessels and the border of the rectus muscle, the inferior epigastric vessels lie free in the preperitoneal space and have no intimate anatomical connection with the transversalis fascia; this fact is not enough appreciated.[8]

The recent introduction of laparoscopic approaches[1] to preperitoneal herniorrhaphy underscores Hureau's[14] comment: "Too often has it been said that all has been described in anatomy! Nothing is further from the truth. No sooner than a new surgical technique appears . . . than our science appears suddenly deficient." Or, perhaps more to the point, is his countryman, Andre Gide's, well-known sally: "Everything has been said before, but since nobody listens, we have to keep going back and begin all over again."

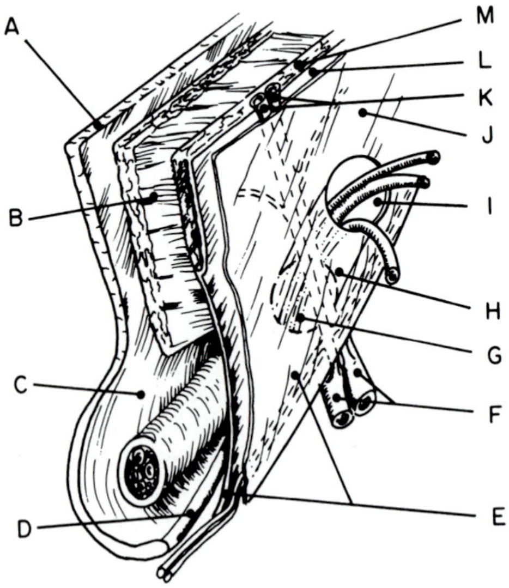

Figure 2-25. Nyhus' classical parasagittal diagram of the right midinguinal region illustrating the muscular aponeurotic laminae separated into anterior and posterior walls. The posterior lamina of the transversalis fascia has been added, with the inferior epigastric vessels coursing through the abdominal wall medially to the inner inguinal canal. (A) External oblique muscle. (B) Internal oblique muscle. (C) Inguinal canal. (D) Poupart ligament. (E) Iliopubic tract. (F) External iliac artery and vein. (G) Internal abdominal ring. (H) Inner inguinal canal. (I) Secondary internal ring. (J) Transversalis fascia (posterior lamina). (K) Inferior epigastric artery and vein. (L) Transversalis fascia (anterior lamina). (M) Transversus abdominis muscle.

REFERENCES

1. Arregui ME, Navarrete JL. Laparoscopic repair of inguinal hernias with mesh. In: Rosin D, ed. Minimal access general surgery. Oxford, Radcliffe Medical Press, 1994:96–121.
2. Bendavid R. The space of Bogros and the deep inguinal venous circulation. Surg Gynecol Obstet 1992;174:355.
3. Bendavid R. New techniques in hernia repair. World J Surg 1989;13:522.
4. Bogros AJ. Essai sur l'anatomie chirurgicale de la région iliaque et description d'un nouveau procédé pour faire la ligature des artères épigastrique et iliaque externe. Th. Paris 1823, no. 153. A Paris, de l'imprimerie de Didot le Jeune, imprimeur de la Faculté de médicine, rue des Maçons, Sorbonne no. 13.
5. Bruce J. Discussion of Nyhus LM, Stevenson JK, Listeraud MB, Harkins HN. Preperitoneal herniorrhaphy: a preliminary report in fifty patients. West J Surg Obstet Gynecol 1959;67:48.
6. Cheatle GL. An operation for the radical cure of inguinal and femoral hernia. Br Med J 1920;2:68.
7. Cleland J, MacKay JY, Young RB. The relations of the aponeurosis of the transversalis and internal oblique muscles to the deep epigastric artery and to the inguinal canal. In: Memoirs and memoranda in anatomy, vol 1. London, Williams & Norgate, 1889:142.
8. Condon RE. The anatomy of the inguinal region and its relationship to groin hernia. In: Nyhus LM, Condon RE, eds. Hernia, ed 3. Philadelphia, JB Lippincott, 1989:18.

9. Cooper AP. The anatomy and surgical treatment of inguinal and congenital hernia. London, Longman, 1804.
10. Fowler R. The applied surgical anatomy of the peritoneal fascia of the groin and the "secondary" internal inguinal ring. Aust N Z J Surg 1975;45:8.
11. Gilbert AJ. Inguinal hernia repair: biomaterials and sutureless repair. Perspect Gen Surg 1991;2:113.
12. Harrison PW. Inguinal hernia: a study of the principles involved in surgical treatment. Arch Surg 1922;4:680.
13. Henry AK. Operation for femoral hernia by a midline extraperitoneal approach: with a preliminary note on the use of this route for reducible inguinal hernia. Lancet 1936;1:531.
14. Hureau J. The space of Bogros and the interparietoperitoneal spaces. In: Bendavid R, ed. Prostheses in abdominal wall hernias. Austin, RG Landes Medical Publishers, in press.
15. Lampe EW. Experiences with preperitoneal hernioplasty. In: Nyhus LM, Harkins HN, eds. Hernia. Philadelphia, JB Lippincott, 1964:295.
16. Lytle WJ. The internal inguinal ring. Br J Surg 1945;32:441.
17. McEvedy PG. Femoral hernia. Ann R Coll Surg Engl 1950;7:484.
18. McVay CB, Read RC, Ravitch MM. Inguinal hernia. Curr Probl Surg 1967;Oct:17.
19. Nyhus LM. The preperitoneal approach and iliopubic tract repair of inguinal hernia. In: Nyhus LM, Condon RE, eds. Hernia, ed 3. Philadelphia, JB Lippincott, 1989:154.
20. Nyhus LM, Condon RE, Harkins HN. Clinical experiences with preperitoneal hernial repair for all types of hernia of the groin. Am J Surg 1960;100:234.
21. Postlethwaite RW. Causes of recurrence after inguinal herniorrhaphy. Surgery 1971;69:772.
22. Read RC. Pre-extraperitoneal approach to inguinofemoral herniorrhaphy. Am J Surg 1967;114:672.
23. Read RC. Preperitoneal exposure of inguinal herniation. Am J Surg 1968;116:653.
24. Read RC, Barone GW, Hauer-Jensen M, Yoder GG. Properitoneal prosthetic placement through the groin: the anterior (Mahorner-Goss, Rives-Stoppa) approach. Surg Clin North Am 1993;73:545.
25. Read RC. Cooper's posterior lamina of transversalis fascia. Surg Gynecol Obstet 1992;174:426.
26. Scarpa A. A treatise on hernia. Translated by John Henry Wishart. Edinburgh, Longman, Hurst, Rees, 1814.
27. Stoppa RE. The treatment of complicated groin and incisional hernias. World J Surg 1989;13:545.

Editor's Comment

There certainly are multiple layers of connective tissue in patients, particularly obvious in those who are obese, between the transversus abdominis muscle and the peritoneum. The transversalis fascia was originally described by Astley Paston Cooper in 1804. In that work, Cooper defined the transversalis fascia as "it lines the posterior part of that muscle (the transversus abdominis)." Cooper also recognized that there were other fascial layers between the peritoneum and the transversus abdominis muscle, but he did not designate these layers as transversalis fascia. That error entered in later editions of his text, primarily in those editions edited by Key.

Perhaps the best discussion of the issues concerning the transversalis fascia is contained in a paper by one of my teachers, Professor Charles E. Tobin (Surg Gynecol Obstet 1946;83:575). Tobin points out the many contradictory definitions regarding transversalis fascia contained in anatomic and surgical texts. He groups these various definitions of transversalis fascia as: (1) the investing fascia on the inner surface of the transversus abdominis muscle, (2) all the tissue between that investing fascia and the retroperitoneal tissues, and (3) all the tissues between the transversus abdominis muscle and the peritoneum. Modern anatomists are agreed that the first of these definitions is the correct one. Read, however, appears to prefer the third definition.

The limited definition of transversalis fascia as the membrane lining the internal surface of the transversus abdominis muscle is preferable because it has historical priority. It is also simple and straightforward, thereby reducing the possibilities of confusion when one surgeon attempts to communicate with another about groin anatomy. If one accepts the strict definition of transversalis fascia, then what should we call the other multiple (there may be as many as 21!) fascial layers in the preperitoneal space? I think calling them preperitoneal, properitoneal, or retroperitoneal fascia would serve. I cannot get overly excited about this issue because these thin, filmy fascial layers have no practical importance in the repair of a groin hernia. They are of no practical value because they lack sufficient strength.

I recognize that there is some practical value in understanding or in knowing about the presence of these multiple fascial layers, particularly as surgeons begin to approach hernias from the peritoneal or preperitoneal side. Annibali (see the following Special Comment) also alludes to the confusion that can result when a laparoscopic approach is made from the peritoneum through these multiple layers of tissue gauze to the true hernial orifice in the transversus abdominis muscle layer. But, in our zeal to prevent amateur herniotomists from getting lost in the preperitoneal space, we should not confuse matters further by mislabeling everything in sight as *transversalis fascia*.

R.E.C.

Special Comment

Surgical Anatomy of the Inguinal Region and Lower Abdominal Wall From the Laparoscopic Perspective
Ricardo G. Annibali

Introducing his popular handbook of operative surgery on the repair of hernias, Ravitch[14] stated in 1969 that "operations for the cure of hernia would seem to be established and well known beyond the possible need for further discussion and demonstration." In fact, at that time, the only real variable in the field of hernia surgery was the type of repair preferred. In reality, after more than two decades, the last word on the surgical treatment of groin hernias has not been written yet. The recent introduction of laparoscopic surgery has challenged the surgeon with a totally new perspective of the problem hernia, both in anatomy and technique. Through the laparoscope, a hernia is no longer viewed as the *protrusion,* but rather as the *extrusion,* of a viscus from the abdominal cavity.

The study of anatomy of the groin and inguinal canal has always presented a challenge to medical students, residents in surgery, and practitioners alike. Although the anatomy of the inguinal region is obviously unvaried, a different approach to its study is required before performing laparoscopic repairs. Most anatomy and surgery textbooks describe the critical layers in sequence as a dissection or operation would proceed from the superficial to the deep layers, giving little consideration to the internal view of the abdominal wall. This is probably why, already in 1945, Lytle[9] wrote that "the operating surgeon knows little of the posterior wall of the inguinal canal, so well is it hidden from his view." To become familiar with laparoscopic hernia repair, it may be appropriate to reverse this approach and begin the study from the deepest layers, which are the working field for the laparoscopic surgeon. The unusual perspective offered by the videocamera reveals some particular anatomic structures that are relevant to laparoscopic hernia repair. They are briefly outlined here.

PERITONEUM

In the anatomy section, Dr. Condon remarks that the umbilical fossae are rarely noted during intraabdominal operations and are of no surgical importance in regard to either the etiology or the repair of groin hernias. Since the development of laparoscopic techniques for hernia repair, however, increased attention has been paid to the internal aspect of the abdominal wall, and a consistent relation between inguinal her-

niation and the umbilical fossae has been routinely observed. In addition, the peritoneal fossae delimited by the umbilical ligaments are an important landmark used by the laparoscopic surgeon for orientation during hernia repairs (Figs. 2-26 and 2-27). Note that there is some confusion about the correct terminology applied to the umbilical folds. The more contemporary terminology followed by *Nomina Anatomica* defines as *median umbilical ligament* the peritoneal fold uplifted by the remnant of the embryonic urachus, as *medial umbilical ligament* the fold covering the obliterated distal portion of the umbilical artery, and as *lateral umbilical ligament* the fold around the inferior epigastric vessels. Some authors, however, refer to the fold outlined by the umbilical artery as the *lateral umbilical ligament,* while the fold associated with the inferior epigastric vessels has been called *plica epigastrica.*[18,20]

PREPERITONEAL SPACE

Transversalis Fascia

Traditionally, the transversalis fascia has been viewed as the anterior border of the preperitoneal space. However, as pointed out by Read,[15] the original description by Sir Astley Cooper suggests that the transversalis fascia is composed of an outer (or anterior) and an inner (or posterior) lamina. According to this assumption, the anterior layer would cover the internal aspect of the transversus muscle aponeurosis; it would insert inferiorly to Cooper ligament and medially envelop the rectus muscle. The posterior layer, on the other hand, would be attached superiorly to the linea semicircularis of Douglas, medially to the linea alba, and inferiorly to the superior ramus of pubis. The inferior epigastric vessels would not lie freely inside the preperitoneal space, but would instead be contained within the two layers of the transversalis fascia. The existence of a posterior layer of the transversalis fascia has been confirmed by Cleland and colleagues,[4] but disputed by McVay and Anson.[1] Other authors have recognized a *preperitoneal membrane.*[19] Others, again, have identified the preperitoneal membrane with the posterior layer of the transversalis fascia.[7–9] More recently, Arregui and colleagues[1] described a thin fascial layer superficial to the peritoneum, observed almost constantly during 187 laparoscopic hernia repairs in 145 patients. The magnification obtained with the videocamera allows a better identification of this fascia, which is somehow difficult to isolate in the embalmed cadaver. This layer, identified by Arregui as the Cooper posterior transversalis fascia, divides the preperitoneal space

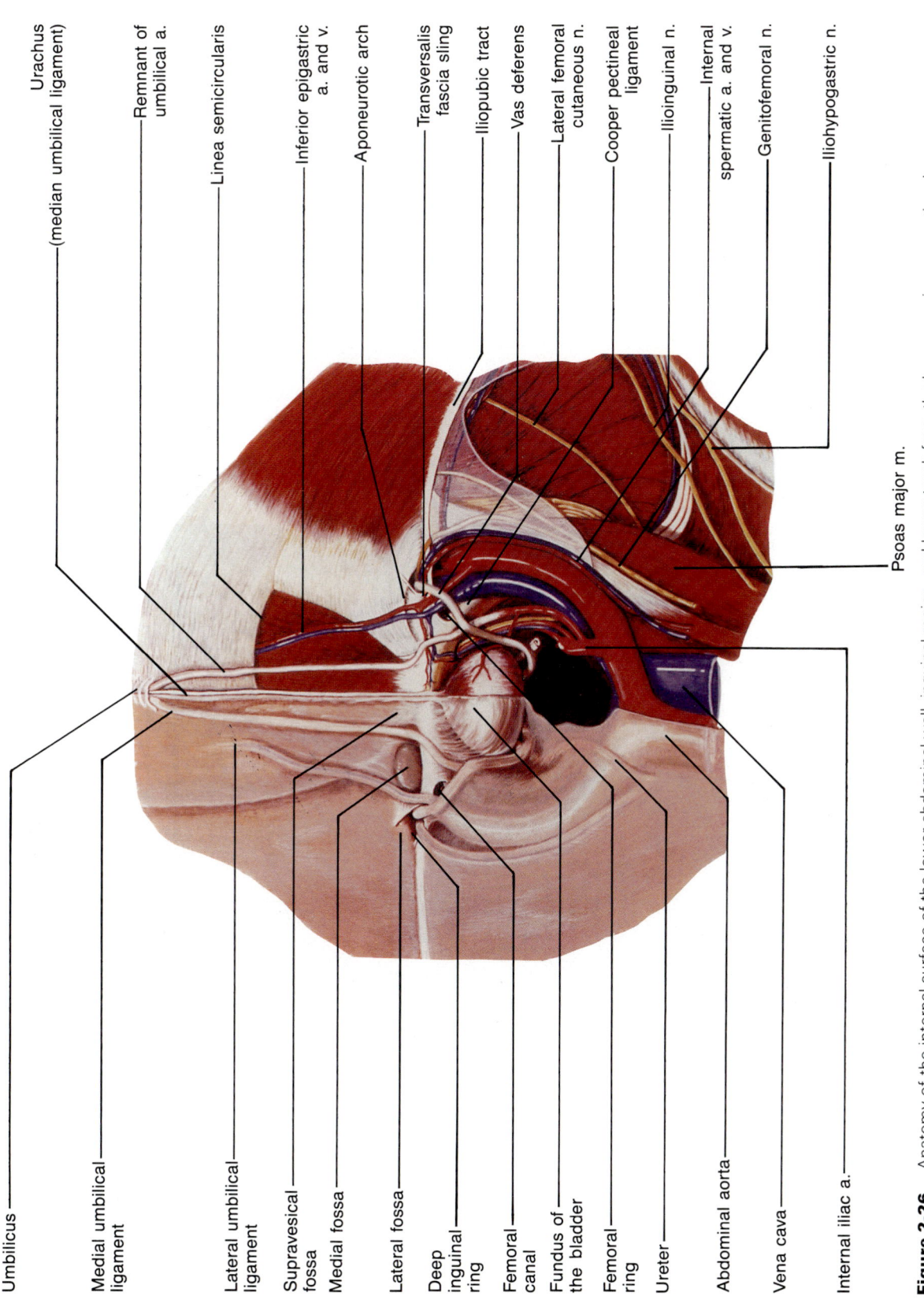

Umbilicus

Urachus (median umbilical ligament)

Remnant of umbilical a.

Linea semicircularis

Inferior epigastric a. and v.

Aponeurotic arch

Transversalis fascia sling

Iliopubic tract

Vas deferens

Lateral femoral cutaneous n.

Cooper pectineal ligament

Ilioinguinal n.

Internal spermatic a. and v.

Genitofemoral n.

Iliohypogastric n.

Psoas major m.

Medial umbilical ligament

Lateral umbilical ligament

Supravesical fossa

Medial fossa

Lateral fossa

Deep inguinal ring

Femoral canal

Fundus of the bladder

Femoral ring

Ureter

Abdominal aorta

Vena cava

Internal iliac a.

Figure 2-26. Anatomy of the internal surface of the lower abdominal wall, inguinal region, and lower trunk from the laparoscopic perspective. In the right half of the picture, the peritoneum has been removed to show the anatomic structures contained within the preperitoneal space. (Adapted from Annibali RG, Fitzgibbons R Jr, Filipi C, Litke B, Salerno G. Laparoscopic hernia repair. In: Green FL, Ponsky JL, Nealon WH, eds. Endoscopic surgery. Philadelphia, WB Saunders, 1994)

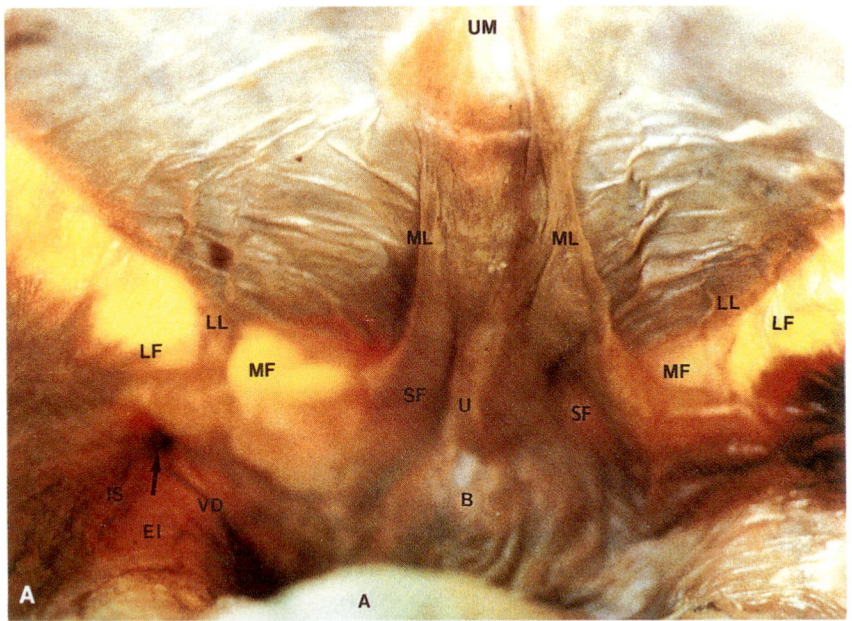

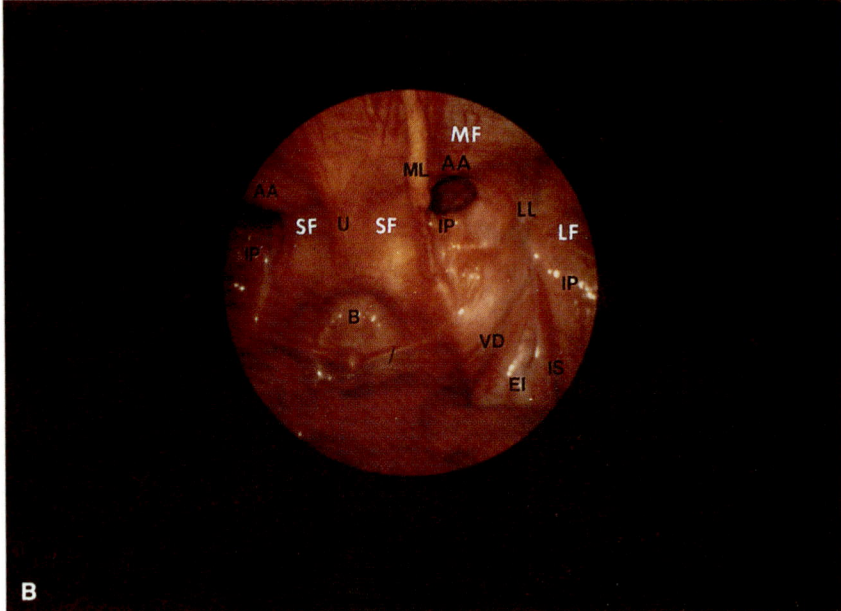

Figure 2-27. (A) The peritoneal fossae, demonstrated with transillumination of the lower anterior abdominal wall. (B) Peritoneal folds and fossae as they are seen at laparoscopy. A direct hernia is visible bilaterally and appears as a circular defect included between the aponeurotic arch of the transversus abdominis muscle superiorly and the iliopubic tract inferiorly. A, abdominal aorta; AA, aponeurotic arch of the transversus abdominis muscle; B, fundus of the bladder; EI, external iliac vessels; IP, iliopubic tract; IS, internal spermatic (testicular) vessels; LF, lateral fossa; LL, lateral umbilical ligament (inferior epigastric vessels); MF, medial fossa; ML, medial umbilical ligament; SF, supravesical fossa; U, median umbilical ligament; UM, umbilicus; VD, vas deferens. The arrow in (A) indicates the deep inguinal ring. (Annibali RG, Fitzgibbons R Jr, Filipi C, Litke B, Salerno G. Laparosopic hernia repair. In: Green FL, Ponsky JL, Nealon WH, eds. Endoscopic surgery. Philadelphia, WB Saunders, 1994)

into two different compartments, and its opening is required to enter the preperitoneal space (of Bogros) proper. According to this model, the space between the peritoneum and the posterior layer of the transversalis fascia would contain a small amount of adipose and areolar tissue, the remnant of the umbilical artery, and the inferior epigastric vessels that produce the two peritoneal folds on either side of the midline. Arregui also supports the hypothesis that, at the level of the internal inguinal ring, the posterior layer of the transversalis fascia is intimately fused with the peritoneum and provides the conical sheath that is visible laparoscopically around the vas deferens and the internal spermatic vessels. It then continues distally, following the spermatic cord, to form the inner layer of the internal spermatic fascia. During laparoscopic repair of an indirect hernia, this fascial covering must be entered to clear the sac from the other structures of the cord to reduce, ligate, and transect the hernial sac. Finally, the plane between the peritoneum and the posterior layer of the transversalis fascia may be mistakenly entered during either a laparoscopic transabdominal preperitoneal procedure or a totally extraperitoneal repair. This could lead to injury to the bladder if the dissection is carried medial to the medial umbilical ligament.

Inguinal (Hesselbach) Triangle

According to the original description, the boundaries of the inguinal triangle were described as the inferior epigastric vessels superolaterally, the rectus sheath medially, and Cooper ligament inferiorly.[10,16] These borders have been subsequently modified with the substitution of the inguinal ligament for Cooper ligament, to allow an easier identification of the area by surgeons who use the traditional anterior approach for herniorrhaphy. For the laparoscopic procedure, however, it may be more appropriate to return to Hesselbach's original description because the inguinal ligament is not visible laparoscopically. Alternatively, if we want to refer to the inguinal triangle as the area where only direct hernias develop (thus excluding the femoral ring, which is the outlet for femoral hernias), we might set the iliopubic tract as its inferior border (Fig. 2-28).

Vessels and Nerves

A precise knowledge of the vascular and neurologic structures included in the preperitoneal and retroperitoneal space of the lower trunk is essential for the laparoscopic surgeon intending to perform a preperitoneal hernia repair. In fact, the major risks involved

with this procedure are linked to possible damages to vessels and nerves located deeply within the preperitoneal space, most of which are not even encountered during the conventional anterior approach. The *vascular structures* may be easily damaged, mostly during dissection of the preperitoneal space, often resulting in the formation of a serious hematoma. In 1991, Spaw and colleagues[17] introduced the term "triangle of doom" to designate the area between the vas deferens medially and spermatic vessels laterally (Fig. 2-29). Its importance is related to the fact that the external iliac vessels lie in its floor, usually hidden by the peritoneum and the transversalis fascia, and may be damaged with serious consequences. It is also recommended that care be taken not to injure the *inferior epigastric vessels;* however, care has to be paid also to some minor vascular structures, whose importance should not be underestimated (Fig. 2-30A; see Figs. 2-26, 2-28, and 2-29A). The *anastomotic pubic branches* originate from the inferior epigastric vessels and run to the obturator foramen, where they join the obturator vessels. The artery gives rise to the *anterior pubic branch,* accompanied by the iliopubic vein, where it crosses the superior ramus of the pubis. The whole anastomotic ring is sometimes called *corona mortis* ("the crown of death") because of the bleeding that occurs if it is injured while dissecting or applying staples to Cooper ligament. The risk linked to a potential damage is even higher when the obturator artery originates from the inferior epigastric or external iliac, as observed in about 30% of subjects.[5,11-13] In these cases, the obturator artery usually appears as a considerably large branch, and an obturator artery from the hypogastric artery is missing. The *deep circumflex iliac artery* and *vein* are also important. They originate from the external iliac vessels, cross laterally over the femoral sheath, run between the iliopubic tract and the iliopectineal arch, pierce the transversalis fascia, and finally, end in the space between the transversus abdominis and the internal oblique muscles. Here, they complete an anastomotic circle by joining the *iliolumbar* and *superior gluteal vessels* (see Fig. 2-28). Staples applied below the iliopubic tract may injure these vessels (see Fig. 2-28). A familiarity with the veins that form the deep venous circulation of the preperitoneal space is also important for all surgeons interested in placing prosthetic materials inside the preperitoneal space for hernia repair because damage of these structures during preperitoneal dissection is easy and usually leads to hematoma formation (see Fig. 2-27). The *iliopubic vein* courses deeply to the iliopubic tract and accompanies the anterior pubic branch when this is present. It either empties directly into the inferior epigastric vein or joins the venous anastomotic pubic branch to form a common trunk that drains into the inferior epigastric vein. An-

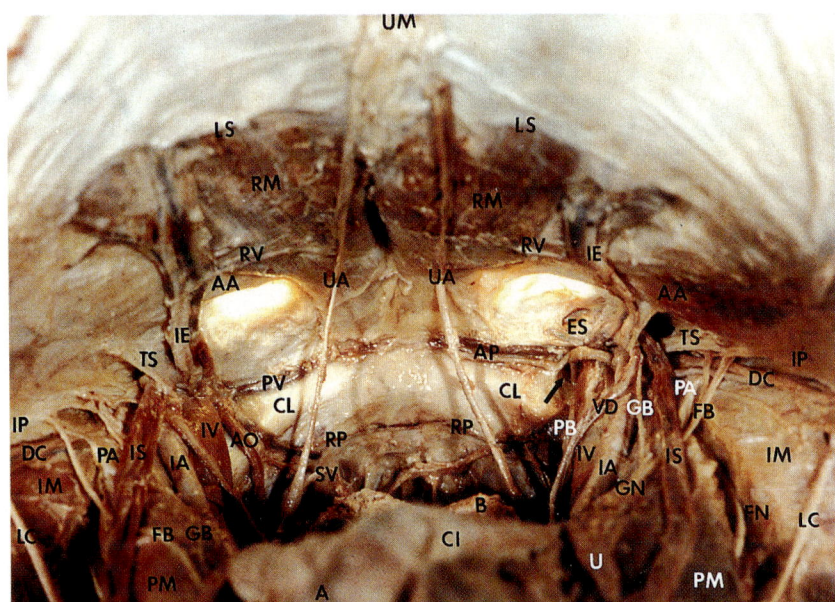

Figure 2-28. The internal surface of the lower anterior abdominal wall prepared in a cadaver to demonstrate the structures contained in the preperitoneal space. The weak areas inside the inguinal triangles through which direct herniations occur, and included between the aponeurotic arch of the transversus abdominis muscle superiorly and the Cooper pectineal ligament inferiorly, are better demonstrated here by transillumination of the lower anterior abdominal wall. A, aorta; AA, aponeurotic arch of the transversus abdominis muscle; AO, anomalous obturator artery; AP, anterior pubic branch and iliopubic vein; B, bladder; CI, common iliac artery; CL, Cooper ligament; DC, deep circumflex iliac vessels; ES, external spermatic vessels; FB, femoral branch of the genitofemoral nerve; FN, femoral nerve; GB, genital branch of the genitofemoral nerve; GN, genitofemoral nerve; IA, external iliac artery; IE, inferior epigastric vessels; IM, iliacus muscle; IP, iliopubic tract; IS, internal spermatic vessels; IV, external iliac vein; LC, lateral femoral cutaneous nerve; LS, linea semicircularis (of Douglas); PA, iliopectineal arch; PB, anastomotic pubic branch; PM, psoas major muscle; PV, iliopubic vein; RM, rectus abdominis muscle; RP, retropubic vein; RV, rectusial vein; SV, superior vesical arteries; TS, transversalis fascia sling; U, ureter; UA, umbilical arteries; UM, umbilicus; VD, vas deferens. The arrow indicates the femoral ring. (Annibali RG, Fitzgibbons R Jr, Filipi C, Litke B, Salerno G. Laparoscopic hernia repair. In: Green FL, Ponsky JL, Nealon WH, eds. Endoscopic surgery. Philadelphia, WB Saunders, 1994)

other tributary of the inferior epigastric vein, the *rectusial vein*, runs along, or is embedded within, the lower lateral fibers of the rectus muscle. According to Bendavid,[3] who first gave a name to this vessel, it consistently forms a venous anastomotic ring by joining the iliopubic vein above the pubic crest. Occasionally, it is possible to demonstrate this connection in cadaver dissections; however, the venous anastomoses are better identified at the operating table, rather than in the anatomy laboratory, because the small veins are often collapsed and empty in the cadaver, but darkened in color and engorged in the patient undergoing surgical treatment. Finally, a small collateral branch of the anastomotic pubic vein is commonly observed on the lower posterior aspect of the pubic ramus, beneath the Cooper pectineal ligament, and has been called the *retropubic vein*.

Important *neurologic sequelae* due to improper placement of staples for mesh fixation have been reported after the introduction of laparoscopic hernia repair. Preliminary results of a multicentered clinical trial considering 816 repairs in 636 patients, promoted by our group at Creighton University,[6] revealed that nerve injury causing transient or permanent pain is by far the most frequently observed local complication after laparoscopic hernia repair (Table 2-4). The resulting pain is due mostly to the improper placement of staples along the course of the major nerves responsible for the innervation of the lower abdominal wall, the inguinal and genital region, the thigh and the leg. The reason for the frequent damage to the nerves is due partly to an inadequate knowledge of their anatomy and probably also to a misconception of the notion of the "triangle of

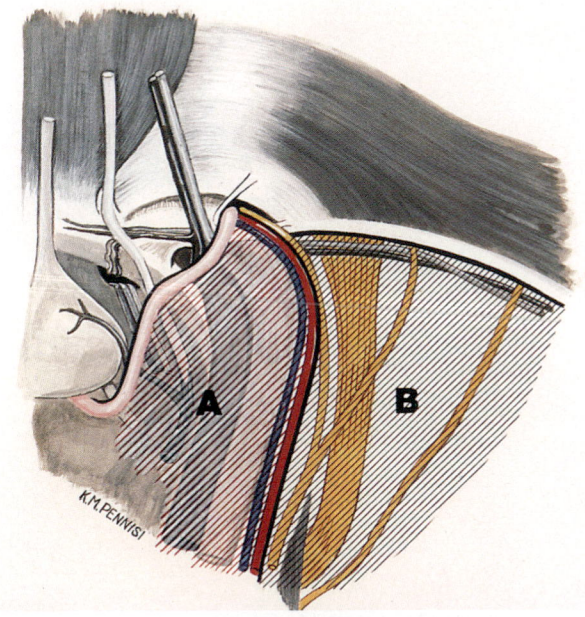

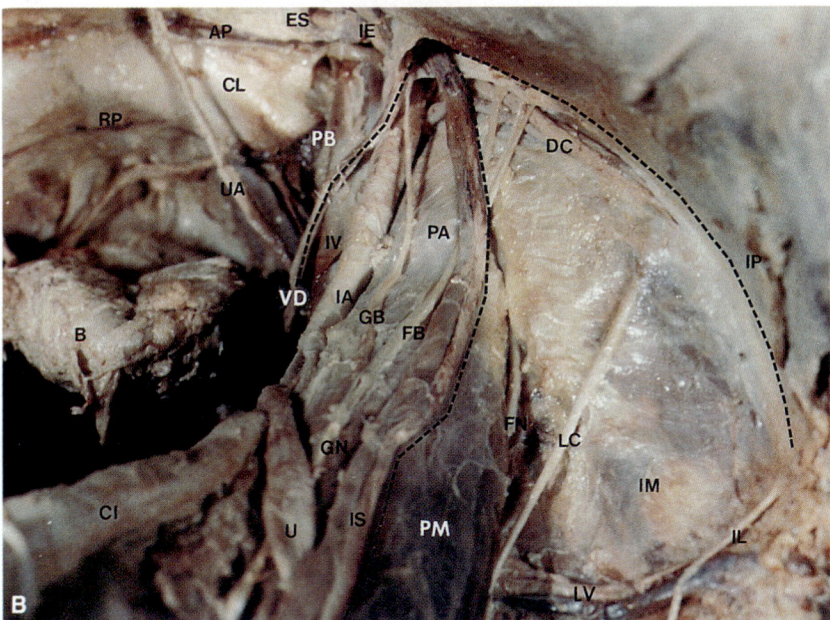

Figure 2-29. (*A*) The area known as "triangle of doom" (A) is included between the vas deferens medially and the internal spermatic vessels laterally. The "triangle of pain" (B) is bordered superolaterally by the iliopubic tract. (*B*) Cadaver preparation (*right side*) that shows the structures included within the "triangle of doom" (medial triangle) and the "triangle of pain" (lateral triangle). AP, anterior pubic branch and iliopubic vein; B, bladder (reflected posteriorly); CI, common iliac artery; CL, Cooper pectineal ligament; DC, deep circumflex iliac vessels; ES, external spermatic (cremasteric) vessels; FB, femoral branch of the genitofemoral nerve; FN, femoral nerve; GB, genital branch of the genitofemoral nerve; GN, genitofemoral nerve; IA, external iliac artery; IE, inferior epigastric vessels; IL, ilioinguinal nerve; IM, iliac muscle; IP, iliopubic tract; IS, internal spermatic vessels; IV, external iliac vein; LC, lateral femoral cutaneous nerve; LV, iliolumbar vessels; PA, iliopectineal arch; PB, anastomotic pubic branch; PM, psoas major muscle; RP, retropubic vein; U, ureter; UA, umbilical artery; VD, vas deferens. (Annibali RG, Fitzgibbons R Jr, Filipi C, Litke B, Salerno G. Laparoscopic hernia repair. In: Green FL, Ponsky JL, Nealon WH, eds. Endoscopic surgery. Philadelphia, WB Saunders, 1994)

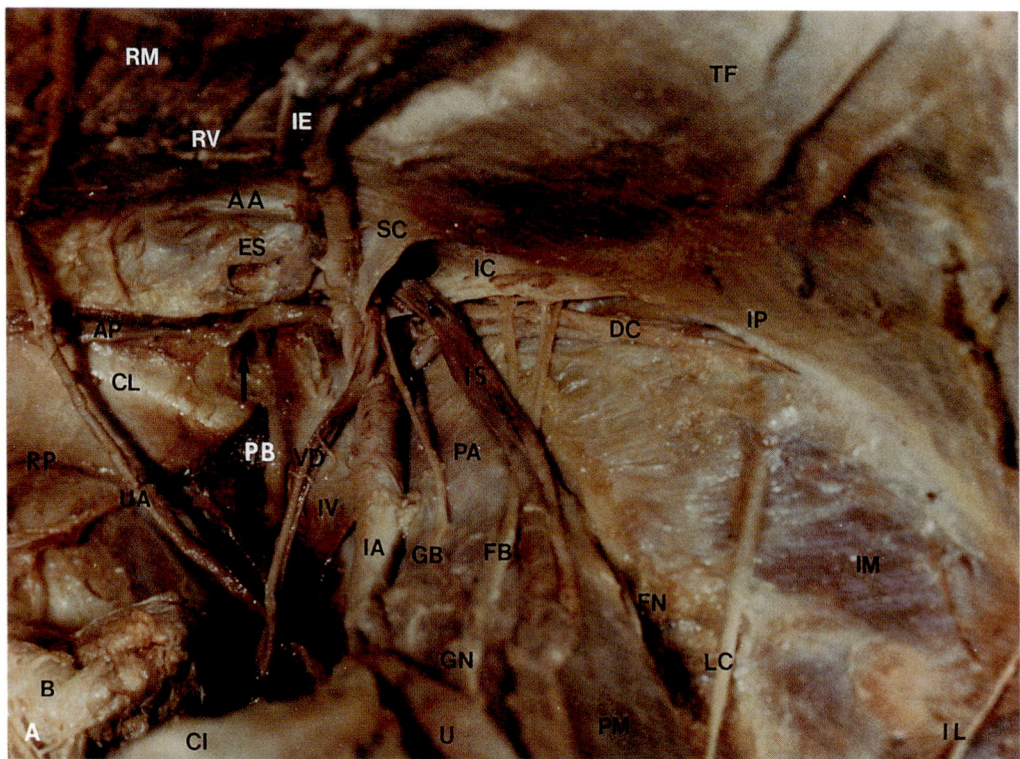

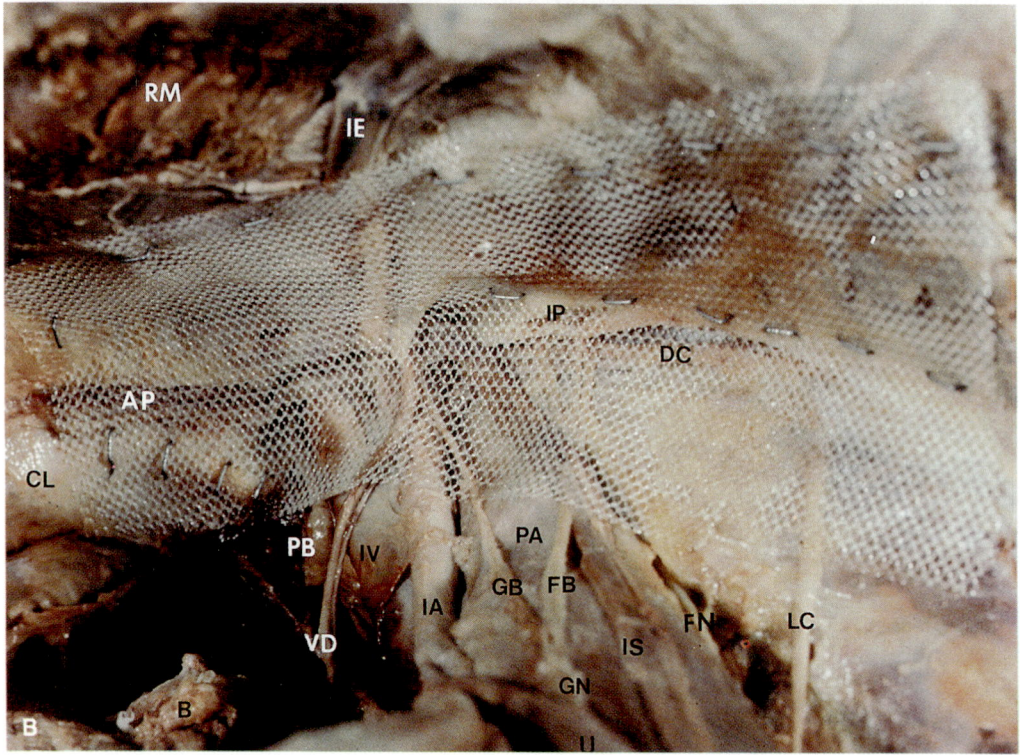

Table 2-4. Local Complications of Laparoscopic Hernia Repair: Preliminary Results of a Multicenter Trial

Complication*	No. (%)
Transient cord or testicular pain	8 (0.98)
Persistent cord or testicular pain	4 (0.49)
Transient groin pain	51 (6.25)
Persistent groin pain	15 (1.84)
Transient thigh pain	26 (3.18)
Persistent groin pain	8 (0.98)
Hematoma	18 (2.20)
Seroma requiring aspiration	12 (1.47)
Seroma with spontaneous resolution	26 (3.19)
Prosthesis infection	1 (0.12)
Orchitis, epididymitis	5 (0.61)

*Transient pain, pain that lasts less than 2 months; persistent pain, pain that lasts more than 2 months. (Courtesy of R. J. Fitzgibbons, Jr., M.D. Creighton University, Sch. of Med., Omaha, NB)

doom." As mentioned earlier, this term refers to the area between the vas deferens medially and spermatic vessels laterally and includes the external iliac vessels. To avoid injury to these important structures, it is strongly recommended that suturing or stapling be done only *medial to the vas deferens* or *lateral to the spermatic vessels*[17] (see Fig. 2-29). This statement might have lead to the false belief that all major dangers involved in laparoscopic herniorrhaphy are located only in that triangular area and consequently to a false sense of confidence when placing staples needed to hold the prosthetic mesh in place. Actually, the borders of the dangerous area should be extended. In fact, lateral to the spermatic vessels and immediately below (or, in some instances, directly through) the fibers of the iliopubic tract are the genital and femoral branches of the genitofemoral nerve, the femoral nerve, and the lateral femoral cutaneous nerve (see Figs. 2-29 and 2-30A). Consequently, staples placed caudally to the iliopubic tract and laterally to the in-

ternal spermatic vessels can result in transient or permanent neuralgias involving one or more of the previously mentioned nerves or branches (see Fig. 2-30B).

The *genital branch of the genitofemoral nerve* is not encountered commonly in the area in which staples are applied. It may be damaged, however, by the maneuvers used to reduce the sac of an indirect hernia. The *femoral branch of the genitofemoral nerve* and the *lateral femoral cutaneous nerve* lie on the anterior surface of the psoas and iliacus muscles respectively, along the course where staples are usually applied to tack the inferior border and the outer corner of the mesh. Because they are more superficial, they are also more exposed to a possible injury (see Fig. 2-30B). The femoral branch provides sensory innervation to the anteromedial surface of the upper thigh, while the area innervated by the lateral femoral cutaneous nerve extends from the greater trocanter to the midcalf level; this is where pain develops if the corresponding trunks are damaged. The *femoral nerve* is medial, usually hidden in the groove between the iliacus and psoas muscles. It is considered to be less vulnerable because of its deeper position, but may nevertheless be injured by staples placed to tack the mesh inferomedially, close to the iliopectineal arch. Possible sensory (usually pain in the anteromedial region of the thigh) or functional consequences (inability to extend the leg, quadriceps atrophy) may occur as a result of its damage. Pain in the groin or lower abdomen is noted if the *ilioinguinal* or the *iliohypogastric nerve* is injured, whereas pain along the cord and scrotum occurs if the genital branch of the genitofemoral nerve is damaged. Injury of the iliohypogastric and ilioinguinal nerves, however, occurs much less frequently during laparoscopic hernia repair than with conventional anterior herniorrhaphy because these nerves lie in a plane superficial to the preperitoneal space. At times, however, they can be compromised when sta-

◄Figure 2-30. (A) Photograph of a cadaver preparation (*right side*) showing the inguinal area at level of the preperitoneal space, after removal of the peritoneum and preperitoneal adipose tissue (the uracus has been resected and the bladder retracted posteriorly.) (B) Mesh correctly positioned and tacked with staples to cover the three weak areas corresponding to the deep inguinal ring, the inguinal triangle, and the femoral ring. Note that the staples have been placed above the iliopubic tract. AA, aponeurotic arch of the transversus abdominis muscle; AP, anterior pubic branch and accompanying iliopubic vein; B, bladder (reflected posteriorly); CI, common iliac artery; CL, Cooper pectineal ligament; DC, deep circumflex iliac vessels; ES, external spermatic vessels; FB, femoral branch of the genitofemoral nerve; FN, femoral nerve; GB, genital branch of the genitofemoral nerve; GN, genitofemoral nerve; IA, external iliac artery; IC, inferior crus of the transversalis fascia sling; IE, inferior epigastric vessels; IL, ilioinguinal nerve; IM, iliac muscle; IP, iliopubic tract; IS, internal spermatic vessels; IV, external iliac vein; LC, lateral femoral cutaneous nerve; PA, iliopectineal arch; PB, anastomotic pubic branch; PM, psoas major muscle; RM, rectus abdominis muscle; RP, retropubic vein; RV, rectusial vein; SC, superior crus of the transversalis fascia sling; TF, transversalis fascia; U, ureter; UA, umbilical artery; VD, vas deferens. The arrow in (A) points to the femoral ring. (Annibali RG, Fitzgibbons R JR, Filipi C, Litke B, Salerno G. Laparoscopic hernia repair. In: Green FL, Ponsky JL, Nealon WH, eds. Endoscopic surgery. Philadelphia, WB Saunders, 1994)

ples are placed deeply, especially if a vigorous bimanual technique is used.

In conclusion, it appears appropriate to introduce another dangerous zone in addition to the triangle of doom, where important nerves are found that need to be preserved intact. This second triangular area, the *triangle of pain,* is bordered by the internal spermatic vessels inferomedially and the iliopubic tract superolaterally and lies lateral and next to the triangle of doom (see Fig. 2-29). Prevention of injury to the nerves, but also to the external iliac and deep circumflex iliac vessels, is obtained by simply applying staples only above and parallel to the iliopubic tract when tacking the prosthetic patch lateral to the vas deferens and the internal inguinal ring (see Fig. 2-30B). Medial to the vas deferens, staples for the inferior border of the mesh should be applied on the Cooper pectineal ligament only because damage to the terminal portion of the external iliac vein before it passes below the iliopubic tract may occur if the staples are placed too close to the transversalis fascia sling (see Fig. 2-30).

REFERENCES

1. Anson BJ, McVay CB. Inguinal hernia. I. The anatomy of the region. Surg Gynecol Obstet 1938;66:186.
2. Arregui ME, Navarrete J, Davis CJ, Castro D, Nagan RF. Laparoscopic inguinal herniorrhaphy: techniques and controversies. Surg Clin North Am 1993; 73(3).
3. Bendavid R. The space of Bogros and the deep inguinal venous circulation. Surg Gynecol Obstet 1992;174:355.
4. Cleland J, Mackay JY, Young BJ. The relations of the aponeurosis of the transversalis and internal oblique muscles to the deep epigastric artery and to the inguinal canal. In: Memoirs and memoranda in anatomy. London, Williams & Norgate, 1889.
5. Edwards EA, Malone PD, MacArthur JD. Operative anatomy of abdomen and pelvis. Philadelphia, Lea & Febiger, 1975.
6. Fitzgibbons RJ Jr. Personal communication at the annual SAGES meeting. Phoenix, April 1993.
7. Fowler R. The applied surgical anatomy of the peritoneal fascia of the groin and the "secondary" internal inguinal ring. Aust N Z J Surg 1975;45:8.
8. Lampe EW. Experiences with preperitoneal hernioplasty. In: Nyhus LM, Condon RE, eds. Hernia, ed 3. Philadelphia, JB Lippincott, 1978.
9. Lytle W. The internal inguinal ring. Br J Surg 1945;32:441.
10. Nyhus LM, Klein MS, Rogers FB. Inguinal hernia. Curr Probl Surg 1991;6:401.
11. Pfitzer W. Über die Ursprungverhöltnisse der arteria oburatorie. Anat Anz 1889;4:504.
12. Pick JW, Anson BJ, Ashley FL. The origin of the obturator artery: study of 640 body halves. Am J Anat 1942;70:317.
13. Poynter C. Congenital anomalies of the arteries and veins of the human body with bibliography. University Studies 1922;22:33.
14. Ravitch MM. Repair of hernias. Chicago, Year Book Medical Publishers, 1969.
15. Read RC. Cooper's posterior lamina of transversalis fascia. Surg Gynecol Obstet 1992;174:426.
16. Skandalakis J, Colborn G, Gray S, Skandalakis L, Pemberton L. The surgical anatomy of the inguinal area: part I. Contemp Surg 1991;38(1):20.
17. Spaw AT, Ennis BW, Spaw LP. Laparoscopic hernia repair: the anatomic basis. J Laparoendosc Surg 1991;1(5):269.
18. Thorek P. Anatomy surgery. Philadelphia, JB Lippincott, 1962.
19. Tobin CE, Benjamin CA, Wells JC. Continuity of the fasciae lining the abdomen, pelvis and spermatic cord. Surg Gynecol Obstet 1946;83:575.
20. Zimmermann L, Anson B. Anatomy and surgery of hernia. Baltimore, Williams & Wilkins, 1967.

Hernia, Fourth Edition, edited
by Lloyd M. Nyhus and Robert E. Condon.
J.B. Lippincott Company, Philadelphia © 1995.

Chapter 3

Theoretic Aspects of Hernia

Philip E. Donahue

No matter how many hernial repairs an experienced surgeon has performed, an individual patient can still provide seemingly endless variations on the common theme. This is true with respect to the patient's symptoms, the particular tissue relations in and around the hernia, and the course after repair. Most patients have an uneventful repair of the hernia and promptly return to work. An unfortunate few are plagued by a complication of the procedure or by a recurrence of the hernia after the original repair. Hernial repair is still considered a major surgical event that demands both technical awareness and skill in performance.

The word *hernia,* a Latin term that means rupture of a portion of a structure, is apt indeed. The connotation of the abdominal wall as the site of opposing physical forces that eventually resolve according to mechanical principles by the appearance of a hernia is both accurate and productive. It is accurate because the mechanical factors are considered the dominant explanation for the emergence of hernias and productive because any repair performed without regard to these mechanical factors is at an increased risk of failure.

GROIN HERNIA

The illuminating work of Condon[8] defined several aspects of the anatomy of the groin, the area in which most hernias occur. The precise definitions of the terms *fascia* and *aponeurosis* are important in this context, as is the precise definition of a *ligament*. A *fascia* is a condensation of connective tissue into a definable, homogeneous layer, which may vary from a thin layer to an easily observed, stout structure. An *aponeurosis* is a tendinous insertion of a major muscle that is composed of strong individual collagenous fiber bundles. *Ligament* is applied to any definable tissue that bands two or more structures, whether bony or visceral, and may refer to structures of either areolar or aponeurotic consistency.

When referring to groin hernias, one must be careful not to confuse *transversus abdominis aponeurosis* and *transversalis fascia.* The latter term is incorrectly applied at times to the transversalis abdominis muscle and the transversus abdominis aponeurosis. Transversalis fascia by itself varies in density and possesses little intrinsic strength. It usually represents the first anatomic boundary to visceral structures as they herniate through the abdominal wall, but by itself it cannot form the basis for groin hernial repairs. Instead, all herniated structures must first be restored to their anatomic position behind and deep to the transversalis fascia, and the repair of the hernial defect must be performed by suturing neighboring tendinous aponeuroses and ligaments that can hold sutures properly (see Chap. 2).

Anatomy of the Groin

The repairs of all common groin hernias are designed to eliminate permanently defects in the abdominal wall by means of sutures placed into the solid structures that line the defect.

The aponeurosis of the external oblique muscle inserts at the pubic tubercle and has a flattened medial portion that is recurved beneath the floor of the inguinal canal. The relation of the inguinal ligament to the fascia of the transversus abdominis muscle is that of contiguous, separate structures. The lacunar ligament, a structure that extends from the posterior border of the inguinal ligament to the pectineal fascia, is separate and superficial to the iliopubic tract. One must be aware of this relation because the rationale for modern hernial repair involves the reconstruction of separate layers of the abdominal wall, with an attempt to preserve the shutter mechanism effected by the different layers of the abdominal wall. This shutter mechanism consists of structures that move simultaneously in different planes and is analogous to the shutter on a camera: the planes of motion occur within the internal oblique and transversus layers of the abdominal wall.[24] Conventional herniorrhaphy does not result in a functional shutter mechanism unless the principles of anatomic repair of hernia are followed: the dynamic components of the shutter are compression of the potential hernial defect by traction on the superior and inferior crus of the internal inguinal ring. This contraction of the transversus muscle results in narrowing of the internal ring and lateral traction on the spermatic cord.

The shutter mechanism thus affords continuous protection for the two most vulnerable areas of the groin—the area in which direct hernias exit through the Hesselbach triangle and the inguinal canal, through which "oblique" herniation, beginning at the internal inguinal ring, occurs.

Congenital Factors in the Genesis of Groin Hernia

Of factors associated with herniation in the groin, congenital ones probably are the most important. Both the anatomic and the clinical laboratories have provided supportive data for this concept. The anatomic data were the first to be recorded and show that discrete structural abnormalities are present in most areas of hernia occurrence.[2]

The inguinal area, for example, is the site of indirect inguinal hernias (oblique hernias) that occur through an unobliterated processus vaginalis and of direct hernias that occur through the weak area (the Hesselbach triangle) between the pubic ramus and the musculofascial components of the lower abdominal wall.

The peak incidence of hernia is during infancy, when about half of boys have a patent vaginal process. Therefore, the predisposing factor in the development of common indirect inguinal hernias is anatomic configuration. Equally important causes that cannot be easily described are related to the wear and tear of living, such as repetitive local trauma, degenerative changes associated with increased abdominal pressure, and altered collagen synthesis in middle age.[1,30] For example, autopsy studies show that up to 20% of people have had a patent processus vaginalis for a lifetime without any clinical appearance of hernia.[19] In this context, the similar incidence of contralateral patency of the processus vaginalis in patients who have had an inguinal hernia discovered or repaired forces one to admit that patency of the processus vaginalis alone does not necessarily lead to inguinal herniation.[23] Similarly, Gullmo and colleagues[15] observed that 5% of young women who had incidental herniography after hysterosalpingography had open processus vaginalis without clinical hernias. These diverticula of Nuck were asymptomatic.

Several studies shed further light on the role of the age of the infant as a particular risk factor for the presence of inguinal hernia. For example, in children who weighed less than 1500 g at birth, a total of 18.9% developed an inguinal hernia within 1 to 3 years of birth, compared with an incidence of hernia in 10.3% of those who weighed less than 2000 g; these numbers, however, represent those with clinical hernia, as opposed to those with a patent processus vaginalis.[10] When systematic exploration of the contralateral groin is carried out during operations for inguinal hernia, the number of patients with patent processus vaginalis is related to the age of the infant; one recent study in Nigerian children showed a wide range of patency in children of various age groups, including 39% in those younger than 1 year old, 22% at 2 years, and 17% beyond 2 years of age. By 5 years of age, the exploration was negative.[12] These studies are of interest in showing that the data from the clinical laboratory do not always mirror those from the postmortem investigation and for showing the effect of age and development on clinical observations. The exploration of the contralateral groin is not recommended, despite the high incidence of abnormal findings, for several reasons, not the least of which is a risk of injury to the spermatic cord. As mentioned later (see Iatrogenic Factors: Previous Operations), there is substantial evidence that the processus vaginalis remains open or potentially open in (probably) most patients, based on the high rate of inguinal herniation in patients with ascites or chronic intraabdominal fluid collections.

Other congenital factors that affect the presence of groin hernia are those that result in abnormalities of the inguinal canal, such as exstrophy of the urinary bladder, which results in lack of obliquity of the canal due to pubic bone diastasis. Husmann and colleagues,[20] in a series of 134 cases of bladder exstrophy, found that 56% of the boys and 15% of the girls developed hernia in a 10-year interval. Many of the children required emergent repair of these hernias owing to incarceration, leading the authors to reinforce the importance of careful examination and primary repair when possible.

Direct inguinal hernias, which occur between the pubic ramus and the arching border of the transversus abdominis muscle, medial to the deep inferior epigastric vessels, are also associated with both congenital and environmental factors. For example, patients who possess a transversus abdominis aponeurosis with a high, arching lower border are at risk for the development of this hernia. Congenital factors, however, do not explain the increased incidence of direct inguinal hernias in advanced age groups or the tendency of elderly patients to have attenuated fascial structures.

HERNIAS OF THE ABDOMINAL WALL

The anterior abdominal wall also has anatomic abnormalities that appear to be antecedents to the appearance of hernias. The most common of these abnormalities are umbilical hernias, which occur where the umbilical ring has failed to obliterate the opening of the allantoic duct and which are ordinarily prevented by growth of the contiguous fascia of the linea alba. It is clear why this site is prone to development of hernia, but as was noted for inguinal hernias, there is often no clear explanation as to why some people have hernias but most of those at risk do not. Some people are known to be at risk for the development of umbilical hernias in later years. These include patients with massive ascites or those with induced ascites, such as those undergoing chronic ambulatory peritoneal dialysis, and patients with abnormal or defective collagen synthesis secondary to nutritional deficiencies or aging.

The next most common hernias of the anterior abdominal wall occur in the linea alba, usually above but occasionally below the umbilicus. These are usually small, often multiple, and typically contain preperitoneal fat. Some of these hernias are deceptive and may be apparent only as a pinpoint convexity overlying the standing patient's linea alba. If the results of the physical examination are normal but the patient's complaint is persistent, surgical exploration may be necessary to provide a definite diagnosis. The most plausible explanation for these hernias is provided by anatomic studies of the linea alba. This structure is a complex network of the three musculoaponeurotic components of the rectus sheath[4] and varies considerably in its inherent strength. There are at least three recognizable patterns of decussation of these fibers in the midline, all of which may be aggravated by marked distention of the abdominal wall. In addition, there are discrete areas midway between the xiphoid and umbilicus that are subjected to repetitive stresses by phrenic aponeurotic bands that insert into the midline fascia. Perhaps the latter structures eventually weaken the midline fascia and, therefore, help to explain the location of most hernias in this area.[4]

Another group of hernias that deserves consideration in the context of predisposing anatomic factors consists of those hernias that develop in the lateral edge of the rectus abdominis aponeurosis. This area is known as the *spigelian fascia* (named after the Flemish anatomist Adriaan van der Spieghel, who described it in the 1600s) and is the site of hernias that are usually below the umbilicus and may be multiple. Variations in the anatomic structure of the spigelian fascia are either congenital or acquired, as discussed earlier, and lead to the appearance of these hernias, which are often subtle and often present a diagnostic challenge.[33] Most of the confusion results from the fact that these are usually intramural hernias, covered by the external oblique muscle, and are therefore not as obvious as hernias that traverse the entire abdominal wall.

This emphasis on congenital factors is not meant to imply that sudden stresses, such as abdominal trauma or industrial accidents, or chronic processes, such as multiparity, may not play a role in the sudden appearance of hernia in a patient previously without symptoms. The latter factors are thought to be provocateurs only in the presence of "fertile ground"— the weak or attenuated transversus–transversalis layer.

BIOLOGIC FACTORS IN THE GENESIS OF HERNIATION

Renewed interest in the biochemical and structural aspects of herniology followed the description of some of the molecular and cellular elements of the protective fascia and collagenous tissues that normally prevent the formation of hernias.

Collagen, the major constituent of the various aponeuroses and fascial structures of the body, has been studied intensively. Like all other tissues in the body, it is in a state of dynamic equilibrium. There appears to be a constant synthesis of collagen, which is matched by a parallel and constant rate of degradation. When they studied the transversalis fascia medial to the contralateral internal inguinal ring in patients with unilateral hernias, Peacock and Madden[28] compared rates of collagen synthesis and collagenolysis in both inguinal areas and found that the rates of both processes were markedly increased. These findings were thought to support the concept that an abnormality of local collagen metabolism might be a factor in the eventual appearance of a hernia.[27] Further support for the abnormal collagen view is provided by studies of hydroxyproline (the major amino acid constituent of collagen) content in the rectus muscle aponeurosis of patients with and without groin hernias. There was a frank decrease in the hydroxyproline level in patients with groin hernias, and these decreased amounts did not relate to age or muscle mass. Fibroblasts cultured from the anterior rectus sheath of these patients proliferated poorly, incorporating labeled precursors at a much lower rate than did control specimens. In addition, the ultrastructure of rectus sheath collagen from other patients with direct hernias was found to contain irregular microfibrils, supporting the concept of both a structural and a biochemical abnormality in adult patients in whom hernias develop.[29]

Collagen metabolism is a natural focal point for investigations of wound strength and wound healing, and modern techniques provide unique ways to define collagen strength. For example, it is known that extracellular matrix molecules, such as the collagens, are affected by superoxide anions.[26] Superoxide radicals, which are produced in a variety of physiologic and pathologic conditions, appear to cleave collagen into small molecules and could conceivably cause damaging effects in the structure of abdominal and groin fascial structures. It is even conceivable that some of the deleterious effects of inflammation in wound healing are due to mechanisms of this type; for example, a report[31] showed that experimental collagen synthesis was a function of the status of endogenous tumor necrosis factor-α (TNF-α) activity.

Although these factors are of great interest, it is obvious that wound healing is a multifactorial process and that many factors exert their effects simultaneously. One ingenious study[17] looked at the amount of collagen deposition in standardized wounds in patients with abdominal operations as a function of the amount of fluid resuscitation given perioperatively. When postoperative fluid resuscitation was provided on the basis of subcutaneous oxygen tension, there was a resulting increase in collagen deposition, as reflected by hydroxyproline accumulation in polytetrafluoroethylene tubes inserted subcutaneously; these patients received more fluid perioperatively than those patients in whom fluid therapy was guided by clinical criteria.

The debate about the relative effects of TNF-α or other lymphokines, therefore, is not entirely theoretic as it relates to collagen metabolism in healing incisions. Studies that evaluated many potential factors in the evolution of recurrent hernia have evaluated a possible role of infection; this is logical because some clinicians have considered wound infection as a definite risk factor for subsequent hernia development. Hesselink and colleagues[18] were not able to show a role for wound infection as a specific risk factor for the development of recurrent ventral hernia; further, obesity, diabetes mellitus, and a site in the lower midline were not found to be specific risk factors for recurrence. The only factor in this study that had a direct correlation with the risk of recurrent hernia was the size of the hernia, with those smaller than 4 cm at significantly less risk of recurrence. Because the rate of recurrence was so high in both groups (25% versus 41%), the authors were supportive of changes in technique, such as the routine use of prosthetic mesh insertion.

Another study[6] came to the same conclusion relative to the risk of infection but observed a lower incidence of recurrence (4.2%) than cited earlier. These authors were able to exclude the presence of specific wound infection subtypes (clean, clean-contaminated, and dirty) as specific risks for subsequent ventral hernia.

Malnutrition

The specific effects of malnutrition on the evolution of hernias of the groin or abdominal wall are as yet undefined. Many people with adult-onset hernias and malnutrition are encountered in the surgical clinics of large public hospitals. For many years, I have been suspicious of a possible correlation between malnutrition and hernia and believe that the question should be carefully studied. If the collagenous structures that gird the abdominal wall are vital, constantly experiencing remolding and resynthesis, then there is a balance between synthesis and destruction of these supporting structures. Most people live an entire lifetime without hernias, but the question remains, Why do so many adults have hernias of the groin and abdominal wall structures?

One of the first insights into the problem was provided on the sailing ships whose crews suffered scurvy. In addition to bleeding gums, periosteal pain, and weakness, these sailors were reported to have hernias or ruptures of healed scars. Later, a specific effect of vitamin C on collagen maturation was described, allowing a reasonable explanation of the observed effects.

Another condition that provides insight into the nature of acquired hernias is lathyrism, a disease that results from ingestion of the flowering sweet pea. The active agent β-aminoproprionitrile prevents the maturation of collagen and is capable of causing groin hernias in young rats and mice.[9] Groin hernias developed in rats less than 1 month old who were given sweet pea seeds in their diet, in contrast to older rats in whom hernias did not develop when the rats were fed a similar diet. This disease process is interesting in the current context because it illustrates how environmental factors affect the natural balance between collagen synthesis and lysis, eventually leading to the appearance of herniation. We may eventually be able to discern similar defects in patients who are malnourished who appear to have excessive numbers of hernias and more than their share of recurrent hernias after primary repair.

Lathyrism is still a major problem in some parts of the world, but the effects of the neurotoxic amino acid β-N-oxalylamino-1-alanine acid do not present as disorders of collagen metabolism in humans; instead, a syndrome of neurotoxicity is observed. The syndrome, which was described in Ethiopia,[16] developed after a period of heavy consumption of the grass pea for over 2 months, with a prevalence rate of 0.1 to 7.5 cases per 1000.

If patients in these areas were to undergo tests of dermal collagen content as related to tensile strength, there would no doubt be substantial decreases in these measures of skin strength compared with a normal population. A study[11] in rats with or without lathyrism revealed precisely these differences, using the resistance of the skin to both high and low rates of tension-loading.

The relation of hernial wound healing to overall nutritional status must be viewed in a multifactorial context. That is, the hernia wound per se exists in a patient who may or may not have latent vitamin or mineral deficiencies, altered immunity or resistance to infection, or underlying systemic disease. In addition, such patients may have an impaired ability to generate the proteinaceous constituents of collagen and the various components of a repaired healed defect.

Patients with Laennec cirrhosis who have ascites illustrate how people predisposed to hernias eventually have clinical hernias when undergoing stress, specifically a hydrostatic pressure challenge. Groin and umbilical hernias may be a particular challenge in these patients if the overlying skin is affected. For example, skin overlying large umbilical hernias is frequently traumatized. In the worst instances, the resulting small ulcerations become infected, leading to further erosion of the subcutaneous tissues overlying the hernial sac, which is distended by ascitic fluid pressure. The critical management of patients with cirrhosis and ascites is conservative, and usually the ascites can be controlled with diuretics and salt restriction. One caveat is in order with respect to the peritoneovenous shunt: Resist the urge to insert the shunt (for ascites control) simultaneously with repair of the hernia, to avoid contamination of the shunt. The suggested alternative in these situations is first to manage aggressively the cirrhosis and ascites, and then, if medical management has reduced the amount of ascitic fluid, to electively repair the hernia. On the contrary, if the ulcerated skin has been progressively eroded, resulting in an ascitic fluid leak, the hernia alone should be repaired using standard surgical practices, and the question of peritoneovenous shunt should be deferred until at least 2 to 3 weeks have passed and residual peritoneal contamination has been excluded by diagnostic paracentesis.

Environmental Toxins

The recent description of altered levels of circulating enzymes in patients with emphysema adds another dimension to the question. In a provocatively entitled presentation, Cannon and Read[5] discussed metastatic emphysema, a mechanism for acquiring inguinal herniation. These authors measured serum elastolytic and antiproteolytic activity in cigarette smokers and nonsmokers. They found that the smokers had the potentially undesirable combination of increases in proteolytic activity and reductions in α_1-antitrypsin, the major naturally occurring circulating antiprotease. This combination could set the stage for the evolution of a hernia by affecting the synthesis–degradation equilibrium of groin collagen and could be a pathologic sequence initiated by excessive smoking.

The smoking habit cannot always be implicated as a factor in the elevated levels of certain enzymes found in patients with hernia. When Lehnert and Wadouh[23a] evaluated the incidence of inguinal hernia in patients with aortic aneurysm and aortic occlusive disease, those with aneurysm were found to have a 41% incidence of hernia versus an incidence of less than 19% in those with aortic occlusive disease. In addition, almost as many patients with aneurysm had a recent hernia repair. The incidence of smoking in both groups was similar, suggesting that the smoking per se did not explain all the increased risk observed in the patients with aneurysm; the authors ascribed the observed changes to differences in elastase levels in the two groups of patients.

Athletics

People who perform repeated strenuous physical activities offer another example of hernias produced by a combination of predisposed anatomy and situational stress. One illustrative series was reported by Gullmo and associates,[15] who used herniography to define the cause of obscure groin pain in a group of young athletes. The patients were able to describe a number of unusual hernias, including obturator hernias and incipient hernial defects at the internal ring, which could not be diagnosed by other means. The young athletes were examined because many of them had severe pain that prevented their usual activity, yet they had an unremarkable initial examination. The abnormal herniograms were helpful because they led to surgical cures. All surgeons should be aware of the technique of herniography and its potential for helping to establish the correct diagnosis in difficult situations.

Iatrogenic Factors: Previous Operations

A body of evidence suggests that appendectomy may predispose to the later appearance of ipsilateral oblique (indirect) inguinal hernia. The presumptive mechanism is that damage to the innervation of the muscular constrictors of the internal ring shutter mechanism during appendectomy allows later herniation of abdominal contents through a patent processus vaginalis. Insights from patients support this premise; for example, laparoscopic views of the internal ring soon after acute appendicitis demonstrated poor to absent contraction of the internal ring during coughing or straining.[34] The possibility of a temporary neuropraxia related to surgical trauma must be kept in mind in this specific situation, but there is other evidence to support the thesis. There is statistical correlation between the presence of appendicitis and the later evolution of ipsilateral hernias, as shown by Arnbjornsson,[3] who described a threefold greater incidence of right inguinal hernia in men who had a previous appendectomy compared with right inguinal hernia in men without a previous operation.

The role of previous appendectomy, however, as a particular risk factor for the evolution of inguinal hernia is by no means established. One study, for example, investigated the incidence of right groin hernia in patients with previous appendectomy (n = 42) to that of right groin hernia in patients without previous operation. In a group of 583 hernia patients, the incidence of right-sided hernia (male or female) was similar in those with or without previous operation.[25]

During surgical exposure of the common femoral artery and the distal external iliac artery, the inguinal ligament and the musculoaponeurotic borders of the internal ring must be divided. Groin hernias occur in patients undergoing such a procedure occasionally in the first few months after the operation, suggesting a definite relation to the first operation. The most plausible explanation for these hernias is that closure of the abdominal wall was done without attention to the principles of primary herniorrhaphy. Reconstruction of the specific layers of the abdominal wall, including the internal ring, after any surgical transection of the internal inguinal ring is extremely important. Patients with a patent processus vaginalis are most susceptible to this complication, but anyone can have this problem. For example, some patients with severe groin pain after vascular access have no discrete hernial sac, but instead have a lax internal ring, which allows preperitoneal fat to herniate. These patients do extremely well with surgical closure of the ring by the principles mentioned previously, whether an anterior or posterior approach is used. The internal ring is first exposed, its borders widely dissected, and during vascular access or after indirect hernial sac excision, a repair of the abdominal wall results in a snug internal ring. An anatomic reconstruction of the specific layers of the abdominal wall must be done if recurrent hernias at the internal ring are to be avoided.

Growing evidence indicates that the increased hydrostatic intraabdominal pressure associated with chronic ambulatory peritoneal dialysis frequently results in a hernia.[13] The reported incidence varies between 1% and 30%, with most of the hernias occurring in the groin and umbilicus and occasionally in the exit site, diaphragm, or spigelian areas. Because the groin is the most frequent site, there is an obvious chance that congenital factors have set the stage for the appearance of a hernia. However, because renal failure per se has a deleterious effect on collagen metabolism, there is a possibility that a multifactorial pathogenesis is operating.[7,21,32] The problems of patients with chronic ambulatory peritoneal dialysis are thus similar to those of patients with advanced cirrhosis and ascites. These problems involve a high risk for the evolution of hernial defects caused by increased abdominal pressure and aggravated by nutritional or metabolic factors that result in poor wound healing and defective or suboptimal collagen synthesis.

Hernias that appear at the site of large latex rubber drain tracts are infrequent and are caused by the enthusiastic creation of a drainage tract by the surgeon. Some surgeons believe that a two-finger aperture is required for optimal drain function and that any drainage tract of smaller dimension is both ineffectual and imprudent. This belief is erroneous and likely to cause iatrogenic hernias. Furthermore, there is good evidence that most drains after common surgical procedures are unnecessary and that most postoperative drains are therapeutic only for the surgeon. There are certainly situations, however, that do necessitate generous drainage, but these are usually best handled by suction drains rather than multiple latex rubber drains and do not require extremely large openings.

One group of patients appears to be at specific risk for subsequent hernia, analogously to patients with large drain tracts. Patients undergoing laparoscopic surgery often have multiple large ports inserted through the abdominal wall, in sizes ranging from 5 to 40 mm. There have already been numerous anecdotal reports of hernias occurring at trocar sites, but many surgeons remain unaware of the potential size of the problem. The recent report of Kadar and colleagues[22] is of great interest in this regard because it shows a difference in hernia rate between 10- and 12-mm ports (0.23% versus 3.1%). The need for careful attempts to close the anterior fascia are warranted, although this maneuver cannot guarantee that hernia will not develop. Because of the sheer number of laparoscopic procedures being performed nationally and worldwide, there will definitely be future reports about this topic.

Finally, there are occasional instances in which surgeons elect to perform open drainage of part or all of the peritoneal or retroperitoneal surfaces. The situation most commonly treated by this means is hemorrhagic or necrotizing pancreatitis. When open drainage is used, it is done with full awareness that hernias of the abdominal wall are made; the repair of these hernias should be planned for at a later date. I endorse this approach, especially in patients with pancreatic and peripancreatic necrosis. Although there is serious doubt as to whether mortalities are lowered by open packing, it seems apparent that postoperative and perioperative care immediately is simplified because the question of a recurrent abscess is usually eliminated by the ability to inspect directly the sources of possible recurrence.

DIAGNOSIS OF HERNIAS

Physical Examination

Physical examination remains the most important part of diagnosis of all types of hernia. The usual complaint that brings the patient to the physician's attention is a persistent or intermittent bulge or persistent or intermittent pain. The pain associated with simple hernias depends on the contiguous structures, which are either compressed or irritated by the hernia. The pain is usually localized, sharp, aggravated by changes in position or by straining, and relieved by cessation of the physical activity that precipitated it. When a hernia contains incarcerated or strangulated structures, the pain becomes persistent and is often associated with systemic signs or symptoms, such as elevated temperature, tachycardia, vomiting, and abdominal distention. Because of the variability in the manner of hernias in the respective typical areas, a region-by-region approach allows elucidation of specific pitfalls, differential diagnosis, and common errors in diagnosis.

Some groin hernias are extremely difficult to diagnose, and others are apparent. The standard maneuvers to diagnose a groin hernia are based on digital palpation of the floor of the inguinal canal. The patient should initially stand while visual inspection of the groin is conducted. The physician examines the external genitalia to check for any localized swellings along the spermatic cord on either side or for abnormalities in the testis or the scrotal contents. In a female patient, there may be palpable swelling on the side of the patient's complaints. In either instance, ipsilateral abnormalities require definite explanation,

and the inference that a hernia is present becomes tenable.

Three prerequisites are recommended for a complete examination of the floor of the inguinal canal. The first is palpation of the fascial border or external inguinal ring after the scrotal skin is invaginated along the axis of the inguinal canal. The second is digital palpation of the floor of the canal and the overlying spermatic cord. The third is examination of the internal ring. The examiner performs the last by palpating the area of the ring and then withdrawing the examining finger 1 cm while the patient strains for 5 to 10 seconds to increase intraabdominal pressure. The patient is then asked to give a gentle cough. A positive response is a palpable tap against the fingertip, made as the distended hernial sac transmits the cough-induced increase in pressure. Alternatively, a gurgle of peritoneal fluid may pass beneath the examining finger. At times, the positive response is a reproduction of the patient's pain; the latter situation demands careful interpretation to exclude other possibilities.

If the patient has had a previous inguinal hernial repair, the same principles of examination are followed. On the occasions when the patient complains of pain during the examination, the differential diagnosis must include ilioinguinal nerve entrapment or neuroma of a branch of the nerve severed previously. Occasionally, the patient complains of a typical pain syndrome, but the physical examination is normal. I usually then recommend a waiting period, during which I examine the patient at monthly intervals. During this time, there is an opportunity to study the colon and rectum and the genitourinary tract. In such patients, there is often a place for surgical exploration of the groin even when the examiner has no absolute evidence that a hernia exists. The patient must have realistic expectations of results after surgical intervention, however, and be informed that whereas most patients do well after an operation, some have persistent postoperative discomfort.

One must be extremely cautious in recommending operations in the absence of absolute evidence that a hernia exists. However, in my own clinic there have been occasional patients, usually one every year or two (0.1%–0.3% of groin hernias), who report a typical pain syndrome but have no definite hernia. After several normal examinations, the patient comes in with an ultimatum from his or her employer to return to work immediately or face the loss of his or her job and accrued benefits. Often, a previous examiner has considered malingering or a latent personality disorder more likely than an occult hernia. Following the principles described, I always found a definite explanation for the complaint when a localized groin or epigastric area of tenderness was present; either a small indirect hernia or a patulous internal ring was the explanation for the pain.

Herniography

The only diagnostic test worth consideration is peritoneography (herniography), which relies on intraperitoneal injection of contrast medium. If one has an interested radiologist, the use of this test has great theoretic appeal. After using it sporadically for several years, however, I do not believe that it can serve as a definitive test unless it is performed frequently by a team of enthusiasts. The problem is that the test is needed so infrequently that decisions are based mainly on traditional clinical concepts; decisions cannot be based on the vague results of a contrast examination.

Specific Hernias

Femoral Hernias

Femoral hernias are often a challenge and usually present as a subtle mass lesion in the inguinal crease, somewhat medial to the femoral artery. It is extremely important that examiners realize that the mass lesion may be small (1 cm or less in diameter) and that in obese people or patients with an edematous overlying skin, the hernia may be clinically occult. At such times, the general condition of the patient serves as a guide for the specific management plan. Patients who have unexplained, acute-onset local pain or signs of disease, who also have systemic signs or symptoms consistent with an incarcerated hernia, should have prompt surgical exploration. The prudent surgeon must attempt to identify patients at risk before the 6 to 24 hours required before ischemic segments of intestine suffer irreversible changes.

Epigastric and Ventral Hernias

Epigastric and ventral hernias are usually noticed as small convexities situated along the ventral midline and are frequently asymptomatic. Occasionally, an epigastric hernia can be associated with severe pain similar to that described for groin hernia. One of my most vivid memories concerns a 20-year-old man who was incapacitated from gainful employment by lower abdominal pain and unable to work; his young family was threatened with dissolution because of associated economic factors. After several normal examinations elsewhere, he appeared for another opinion. Because his story and complaints of deep tenderness were consistent, I explored his linea alba in the lower midline

and found a 1-cm hernia in the ventral midline. This patient's findings reinforce the concept that persistent complaints usually have a cause, which must be established; ultrasonography may provide a definite explanation for the pain.

Often, congenital ventral hernias are asymptomatic and discovered incidentally. Most occur above the umbilicus, and there are often multiple hernial defects. The contents of tiny ventral hernias are usually small collections of preperitoneal fat, but they should always be approached with caution lest an intestinal injury occur.

Ventral hernias are usually apparent when the patient is standing and are accentuated by having the patient strain. If the area of the bulge is palpated, the fascial edge of the hernial defect can be felt unless there is an incarceration or cellulitis.

At times, a patient with ventral hernias after previous midline operations may be examined more efficiently in the supine position, in which subcutaneous fat is less apparent and the firm fascial border of the hernial defect more obvious. A midline hernia is usually obvious unless there is an incarcerated component, in which case it is sometimes difficult to separate the boundary of the inflammatory reaction from the hernia and its contents. Also, it is important to recognize that the obvious hernia may be presenting because another intraabdominal problem has made the hernia more obvious. One example of this phenomenon was a 40-year-old man who presented with an incarcerated umbilical hernia; he had unsuspected malignant ascitic fluid and diffuse peritoneal carcinomatosis. There have been several similar instances in which occult peritonitis has caused the patient's abdomen to become distended, and the examining physician has been misled to ascribe the illness to the hernia.

Spigelian Hernias

Spigelian hernias can be subtle and must be considered in the differential diagnosis of any painful crisis in which the pain is located along the spigelian line, that is, along the outer border of the rectus muscle. The typical spigelian hernia is interparietal and therefore does not penetrate all layers of the abdominal wall. Instead, the defect in the transversalis fascia and the lateral border of the aponeurosis of the rectus muscle is bounded anteriorly by the external oblique muscle, resulting in a hernia that can be difficult to detect. The key to diagnosis is a high index of suspicion in any person with either persistent or intermittent focal pain in the typical location or evidence of local tenderness (or the suspicion of a mass) overlying the spigelian line. For many years, these classic findings were the only evidence that could be used in making a diagnosis of a spigelian hernia. There is no question that complaints of pain often herald the appearance of a hernia, and the physical examination is the most important first step in arriving at the diagnosis.

The use of ultrasonography has forced a reevaluation of the traditional views of spigelian hernia. Spangen[33] reported that B-mode scans were useful in discovering spigelian hernias in a relatively large number of patients. My associates and I also have had some success with ultrasonic diagnosis of spigelian hernias and believe that it is a useful adjunct in the diagnosis of unexplained abdominal wall pain. For most surgeons, the sine qua non of accepting a patient for herniorrhaphy is the demonstration of the hernia in question by methodic physical examination. On the one hand, when no hernia is palpable, there is always concern that the wrong diagnosis has been made and that the operation will not help the patient in question. On the other hand, it is a fact that most spigelian hernias seen before the advent of ultrasonic diagnosis were discovered intraoperatively in patients with strangulation obstruction of a portion of small intestine. I use ultrasonography selectively in patients with persistent pain and in whom I cannot feel a mass or a specific hernial defect. The advantage of using this diagnostic modality is that some patients with a painful hernia, obvious or occult, who may be reluctant to undergo surgical exploration without concrete evidence, can be counseled that they have a good chance for elimination of the presenting complaints. However, if they have a clinical syndrome of pain at or near the spigelian line without a definable hernia, they may still be candidates for surgical exploration of the target area because they may suffer from a spigelian stretch syndrome. They should be aware that surgical exploration and suture reinforcement of attenuated fascia in the area of the spigelian fascia may relieve their symptoms but that the relief of painful symptoms is less predictable in this setting.

Herniography is an alternative technique that has been described as attractive by its proponents. I have used the technique of Gullmo,[14] which consists of paracentesis and injection of 50 to 60 mL of diatrizoate meglumine (Renografin) after instillation of diluted lidocaine into the peritoneal cavity. The procedure has great potential for the discovery and definition of unusual hernias, but patients who are undergoing the procedure need careful reassurance and preparation. The technique is not successfully applied by a casual approach. A committed radiologist is vital to the success of the study. Gullmo's definitive article describes and illustrates some of the best examples of unusual hernias that any surgeon is likely to encounter.[14]

Pitfalls

Many of the problematic areas for the diagnosis of inguinal hernia are listed in Table 3-1. Any structure in and around the inguinal canal can give rise to signs or symptoms consistent with or easily mistaken for a groin hernia. Most of these problems are apparent to the experienced clinician, but in occasional patients, the findings can only be correctly interpreted at the operating table.

The conditions that must be carefully sought are those that cause low-grade peritonitis or a gradual increase in both the size of the abdomen and the hydrostatic pressure acting against the abdominal wall. For example, patients with cirrhosis and those undergoing chronic ambulatory peritoneal dialysis notice a gradual appearance of hernias in the usual areas. However, it may not be appreciated that infection or metabolic crises aggravate the hydrostatic pressure relations within the abdomen, leading to protrusion (pseudoincarceration of elements of the hernia). If deterioration of the patient's condition and ileus supervene, the hernia may appear to be strangulated when in fact it is not.

Another common clinical condition, small intestinal obstruction, masquerades as an incarcerated inguinal hernia at times. The differential diagnosis of this condition may include strangulated inguinal her-

Table 3-1. Differential Diagnosis of Hernia

Direct or indirect inguinal hernia
Femoral hernia
Lipomas of the cord
Epididymitis
Torsion of the testis
Urinary tract infection
Prostatitis
Abscess or inflammation of inguinal nodes: tuberculosis, psoas abscess, bubo
Pseudoaneurysm of femoral artery
Abscess or hematoma associated with vascular graft
Inflammatory retroperitoneal phlegmon (pancreatitis)
Appendicitis
Meckel diverticulitis
Intestinal obstruction
Peritonitis
Thrombophlebitis
Ascitic fluid accumulation
Cellulitis of groin
Sebaceous cyst
Hidradenitis of inguinal apocrine glands
Stitch reaction (suture abscess)
Perirectal abscess
Urethral extravasation

nia, either direct, indirect, or femoral, including the Richter hernia; strangulated or incarcerated obturator hernia; or the variety of conditions that cause a typical small intestinal obstruction. The virtue of caution in assessing such patients is that a complete set of diagnostic tests is performed and the correct surgical approaches are undertaken. A transverse incision or preperitoneal incision often provides the greatest latitude when the diagnosis is unclear.

REFERENCES

1. Andrews E. A method of herniotomy utilizing only white fascia. Ann Surg 1924;80:225.
2. Anson BJ, Morgan EH, McVay CB. Surgical anatomy of the inguinal region based upon a study of 500 body-halves. Surg Gynecol Obstet 1960;111:707.
3. Arnbjornsson E. Development of right inguinal hernia after appendectomy. Am J Surg 1982;143:174.
4. Askar O. Surgical anatomy of the aponeurotic expansions of the anterior abdominal wall. Ann R Coll Surg Engl 1977;59:313.
5. Cannon DJ, Read RC. Metastatic emphysema: a mechanism for acquiring inguinal herniation. Ann Surg 1981;194:270.
6. Carlson MA, Ludwig KA, Condon RE. Ventral hernia and other complications of 1077 midline wounds. Proc West Surg Assoc 1993;101:25.
7. Colin JF, Elliot P, Ellis H. The effect of uraemia upon wound healing: an experimental study. Br J Surg 1979;66:793.
8. Condon RE. Surgical anatomy of the transversus abdominis and transversalis fascia. Ann Surg 1971; 173:1.
9. Conner WT, Peacock EE Jr. Some studies on the etiology of inguinal hernia. Am J Surg 1973;126:732.
10. Darlow BA, Dawson KP, Mogridge N. Inguinal hernia and low birthweight. N Z Med J 1987;100:492.
11. Dombi GW, Haut RC, Sullivan WG. Correlation of high-speed tensile strength with collagen content in control and lathyritic rat skin. J Surg Res 1993; 54:21.
12. Duvie SO. The incidence of contralateral patent processus vaginalis in unilateral inguinal hernia in Nigerian children. Trop Geogr Med 1984;36:371.
13. Engeset J, Youngson GG. Ambulatory peritoneal dialysis and hernia complications. Surg Clin North Am 1984;64:386.
14. Gullmo A. Herniography: the diagnosis of hernia in the groin and incompetence of the pouch of Douglas and pelvic floor. Acta Radiol Scand 1981;(Suppl 361):1.
15. Gullmo A, Broome A, Smedberg S. Herniography. Surg Clin North Am 1984;64:229.
16. Haimanot RT, Kidane Y, Wuhib E, et al. The epidemiology of lathyrism in North and Central Ethiopia. Ethiop Med J 1993;31:15.
17. Hartmann M, Jonsson K, Zederfeldt B. Effect of tissue perfusion and oxygenation on accumulation of collagen in healing wounds: randomized study in patients after major abdominal operations. Eur J Surg 1992;158:521.
18. Hesselink VJ, Juijendijk RW, de Wilt JH, Heide R, Jeekel J. An evaluation of risk factors in incisional hernia recurrence. Surg Gynecol Obstet 1993;176: 228.
19. Hughson W. The persistent or preformed sac in relation to oblique inguinal hernia. Surg Gynecol Obstet 1925;41:610.
20. Husmann DA, McLorie GA, Churchill BM, Ein SH. Inguinal pathology and its association with classical bladder exstrophy. J Pediatr Surg 1990;25:332.
21. Jorkasky D, Goldfarb S. Abdominal wall hernia complicating chronic ambulatory peritoneal dialysis. Am J Nephrol 1982;2:323.
22. Kadar N, Reich H, Liu CY, Manko GF, Gimpelson R. Incisional hernias after major laparoscopic gynecologic procedures. Am J Obstet Gynecol 1993;168: 1493.
23. Keith A. On the origin and nature of hernia. Br J Surg 1924;11:455.
23a. Lehnert B, Wadouh F. High coincidence of inguinal hernias and abdominal aortic aneurysms. Ann Vasc Surg 1992;6:134.
24. Lytle WJ. Internal inguinal ring. Br J Surg 1945; 32:441.
25. Malazgirt Z, Ozen N, Ozkan K. Effect of appendicectomy on development of right inguinal hernia. Eur J Surg 1992;158:43.
26. Monboisse JC, Borel JP. Oxidative damage to collagen. Experientia Suppl 1992;62:323.
27. Peacock EE Jr. Biology of hernia. In: Nyhus LM, Condon RE, eds. Hernia, ed 2. Philadelphia, JB Lippincott, 1978:79.
28. Peacock EE Jr, Madden JW. Studies on the biology and treatment of recurrent inguinal hernia: II. Morphological changes. Ann Surg 1974;179:567.
29. Read RC. Attenuation of rectus sheath in inguinal herniation. Am J Surg 1970;120:610.
30. Read RC. The development of inguinal herniorrhaphy. Surg Clin North Am 1984;64:185.
31. Regan MC, Kirk SJ, Hurson M, Sodeyama M, Wasserkrug HL, Barbul A. Tumor necrosis factor-alpha inhibits in vivo collagen synthesis. Surgery 1993; 113:173.
32. Robinson RR, Leapman SB, Wetherington GM, Hamburger RJ, Finebery NS, Filo RS. Surgical considerations of continuous ambulatory peritoneal dialysis. Surgery 1984;96:723.
33. Spangen L. Spigelian hernia. Surg Clin North Am 1984;64:351.
34. Tobin GR, Clark DS, Peacock EE Jr. A neuromuscular basis for development of indirect inguinal hernia. Arch Surg 1976;11:464.
35. Van Asseldonk JP, Schroder CH, Severijnen RS, de Jong MC, Monnens LA. Infectious and surgical complications of continuous ambulatory peritoneal dialysis. Eur J Pediatr 1992;151:377.

Special Comment

Audit of Groin Hernia Repair

Erik Nilsson

Pragmatically, *audit* may be defined as a systematic evaluation with the ultimate aim of identifying possibilities of improvements and implementing appropriate changes. The key questions of audit have been formulated as follows:[4] What do we do? Do we do what we think we do? What should we do? Are we doing what we should be doing? How can we improve what we do? Have we improved?

During the last decade, the audit concept has stimulated development in many areas of health care, including surgery.[13,18,20] In hernia surgery, it is of particular importance for several reasons. Herniorrhaphy is the most common operation performed on adults in general surgery.[19] Hernia specialists report recurrence rates lower than 2% after primary inguinal hernia repair,[23] whereas figures from nonspecialist centers vary from 5% to 20%.[8,10] The renewed interest in cost-effectiveness and the introduction of a new technology, laparoscopic surgery, underlines the importance of audit in hernia surgery. Using data from two reports that described hernia surgery in nonspecialist hospitals,[10,16] implications and possible beneficial effects of audit are discussed next.

WHAT DO WE DO?

To address this question, all groin hernia repairs on patients older than 15 years of age were recorded in eight Swedish hospitals according to a common protocol during 1992.[16] The total catchment area covered by this survey was 7.61×10^5 inhabitants, and the main findings were:

- An over-all operation rate of 254 per 10^5 inhabitants per year. The range among the hospitals was 147 to 478 operations per 10^5 inhabitants per year.
- A reoperation rate of 17% (323 of all 1936 operations were for recurrences). The range among hospitals was 10% to 21%.
- The Bassini and Shouldice methods were used in 29% and 25% of the repairs, respectively, and laparoscopy was used in 5% (88 operations, 72 of which were done during the latter half of 1992). In 26% of all operations, polyglycolic acid (Dexon) and polyglactin 910 (Vicryl) sutures were used.
- Thirty percent of all operations were done within the frame of day surgery. The range among hospitals was 0% to 59%.

WHAT SHOULD WE DO?

Operation Rate

The operation rate is a manifestation of both demand and availability of resources. In countries where access to elective hernia surgery is good, as in the United States, Australia, and Norway, operation rates are of the same size of order as observed in the Swedish survey.[15] The rationing of hernia surgery has been questioned.[23] Hence, selection of subjects who may benefit from hernia surgery, although of critical importance for the individual patient, is not a major issue for audit.

Reoperation Rate

The reoperation rate should be distinguished from the recurrence rate. The reoperation rate in hernia surgery may be considered an indicator of past failures. It does not give information about when (or where) recurrent hernias primarily were treated nor about previously operated patients who do not return with their recurrences. The recurrence rate refers to a cohort of patients who were reinvestigated at a given time after surgery, and it requires knowledge of the definition of recurrence used, the method of control, and the completeness of follow-up to make comparisons with other series meaningful. Unless drastic changes occur in hernia treatment after the initial treatment, a correlation between reoperation rate and recurrence rate is to be expected. Hence, a reoperation rate of 17% is a matter of great concern. The aim of the eight participating hospitals should be to reduce this figure by a factor of 5% or 10% within a limited number of years.

Method of Repair

Only one fourth of our operations were performed using the Shouldice technique, the only method that, in experienced hands, has produced worldwide recurrence rates of about 1%.[2,3,5,7,9] In one randomized controlled study,[17] the Shouldice technique proved superior to the conventional modification of the Bassini repair employed in 29% of operations in the survey. Another randomized controlled trial emphasized that supervision of junior surgeons for more than six operations during the Shouldice learning period is required to achieve excellent results.[11] The increasing, although still infrequent, use of laparoscopic hernia repair is worth considering. The possible but unproven advantages of laparoscopy in hernia surgery may be less postoperative discomfort and shorter time off work. For statistical reasons, however, recurrence rates after laparoscopic hernia surgery may never claim superiority over results obtained by experts using the Shouldice or mesh techniques.[21] Laparoscopy has its own learning curve in hernia surgery. It transforms an operation for primary inguinal hernia that can be safely done with conventional methods under local anesthesia into a procedure that requires general anesthesia, associated with potential anesthesiologic and intraabdominal hazards. In one fourth of all procedures in this survey, polyglycolic acid or polyglactin 910 sutures were used. These sutures have variable retention of tensile strength in vivo (half of their strength may be lost in 15 days[6]), and their use in hernia repair is incompatible with early return to work, because wound healing may restore only 40% of normal tissue integrity after 2 months.[12]

Day Surgery

The great variation in day surgery rates (0%–59%) observed among the eight hospitals in the survey indicates that hospital stay for hernia patients is determined by organizational rather than clinical issues. The same conclusion was reached by the Audit Commission in its 1990[1] survey on day surgery in England and Wales. In addition, Medicare, the US federal program that reimburses hospitals and physicians for medical care of the elderly, in 1989 disallowed reimbursement for patients over the age of 65 years undergoing elective inguinal herniorrhaphy as inpatients.

ARE WE DOING WHAT WE SHOULD BE DOING?

Discrepancies between hernia surgery as practiced in our eight hospitals and objectives achieved in centers with a special interest in this field have been revealed. The aim for nonspecialists should be to approach the clinical outcomes reached by experts cost-effectively, with acceptability and satisfaction for their patients.

HOW CAN WE IMPROVE WHAT WE DO?

Improvements in outcome and cost-effectiveness outside specialist hernia centers may require changes in organization and education. It is mandatory to have an ongoing recording of outcome after hernia repair

that is compatible with busy clinical work. In the evaluation of groin hernia surgery, a clear terminology must be adopted. The limitations of reoperation rate and the prerequisites of recurrence rate were stated earlier.

The importance of method of control and definition of recurrence was analyzed in one study.[10] The two definitions used were: (1) an expansile cough impulse[22] or, synonymously, a bulge that protrudes during abdominal straining; and (2) a weakness of the operation area necessitating a further operation or the provision of a truss.[14] Five years after hernia surgery, letters were sent to 137 patients who were between 15 and 80 years of age at operation that asked about pain or a lump in the operated groin, with an invitation to clinical follow-up. Ninety-two percent of these patients answered the letter, and 88% came for follow-up examination (120 patients, representing 124 hernias). In the follow-up examinations (Table 3-2), recurrence was defined as "the presence of a clearly palpable bulge during abdominal straining." Thirteen patients answered that they felt a lump in the operated groin; nine of these patients had a recurrence. Among the 111 patients who answered that no lump was evident, 6 had recurrences. The predictive values of positive and negative answers were 69% and 95%, respectively. When recurrence was classified as "a weakness of the operation area necessitating a further operation or the provision of a truss," 5 recurrences were found among the 13 patients with positive answers, and 1 recurrence was found among the 111 patients with negative answers. The predictive values for positive and negative answers under these conditions were 38% and 99%, respectively. These two figures have important clinical implications. Examination of the 13 patients whose questionnaire answers aroused suspicion of recurrence revealed that 5 of the 6 patients with previously unknown recurrences were considered to benefit from a further operation.

Thirteen of the 137 patients with 142 hernias had been reoperated before follow-up, which placed the recurrence rate at 9%. When the recurrence rate was based on the definition, "already reoperated or in need of a reoperation or a truss," and only patients with positive questionnaire answers were reinvestigated, a recurrence rate of 14% was reached. Widening the definition to "previous reoperation or a bulge during abdominal straining" added another recurrence to this group of patients and resulted in the same recurrence rate. Inclusion of all patients who were followed and use of the definition "reoperated or in need of a reoperation or a truss" again led to a recurrence rate of 14%. When the wider definition was applied to these patients, the recurrence rate was 19%. It is unlikely that all patients who did not attend

Table 3-2. Questionnaire Answers and Results of Clinical Examination of 120 Patients*

Questionnaire Answer	Recurrence	No Recurrence	Total
Positive (lump)	True positive (TP) = 9	False positive (FP) = 4	13
Negative (no lump)	False positive (FN) = 6	True negative (TN) = 105	111
TOTAL	15	109	124

Sensitivity: $\dfrac{\text{TP}}{\text{TP} + \text{FN}} = \dfrac{9}{9 + 6} = 60\%$

Specificity: $\dfrac{\text{TN}}{\text{TN} + \text{FP}} = \dfrac{105}{105 + 4} = 96\%$

Predictive value, positive answer: $\dfrac{\text{TP}}{\text{TP} + \text{FP}} = \dfrac{9}{9 + 4} = 69\%$

Predictive value, negative answer: $\dfrac{\text{TN}}{\text{TN} + \text{FN}} = \dfrac{105}{105 + 6} = 95\%$

*Four patients had operations on both sides, and one patient was reoperated on, owing to recurrence in 1984. Hence, validation of questionnaire is based upon 124 operations. (Kald A, Nilsson E. Quality assessment in hernia surgery. Quality Assurance in Health Care 1991;3:205–210, with kind permission from Elsevier Science Ltd, The Boulevard, Langford Lane, Kidlington OX5 1GB, UK.)

follow-up examination had a recurrence. If this were true, however, the recurrence rate would reach 29%. These data are summarized in Table 3-3.

It is obvious that whatever definition and method of control is chosen, the ultimate aim for outcome after hernia repair in the hospital must be to reduce the recurrence rate by a factor of 10.

After completion of this study, the following changes were carried through in hernia treatment at the hospital:

1. The Shouldice technique has been introduced as the routine method for primary groin hernias.

Table 3-3. Recurrence Rate in Relation to Type of Follow-up and Definition of Recurrence

Type of Follow-up	Definition of Recurrence	Recurrence Rate 5 Years After Operation	
		No.	%
No follow-up	Reoperation (or truss) necessary	13/142	9
Questionnaire, clinical examination of patients who answered "lump"	" "	17/125	14
" "	Bulge during straining or previous reoperation	18/125	14
Clinical examination offered to all patients	Reoperation (or truss) necessary	18/125	14
" "	Bulge during straining or previous reoperation	25/125*	19
" "	Bulge during straining or previous reoperation, assuming positive findings in patients not attending follow-up	25 + 16/142	29

*Type and number of hernias with number of recurrences in brackets: medial 30 (9), lateral 69 (8), combined 5 (2), femoral 2 (0), recurrent 19 (5). (Kald A, Nilsson E. Quality assessment in hernia surgery. Quality Assurance in Health Care 1991;3:205–210, with kind permission from Elsevier Science Ltd, The Boulevard, Langford Lane, Kidlington OX5 1GB, UK.)

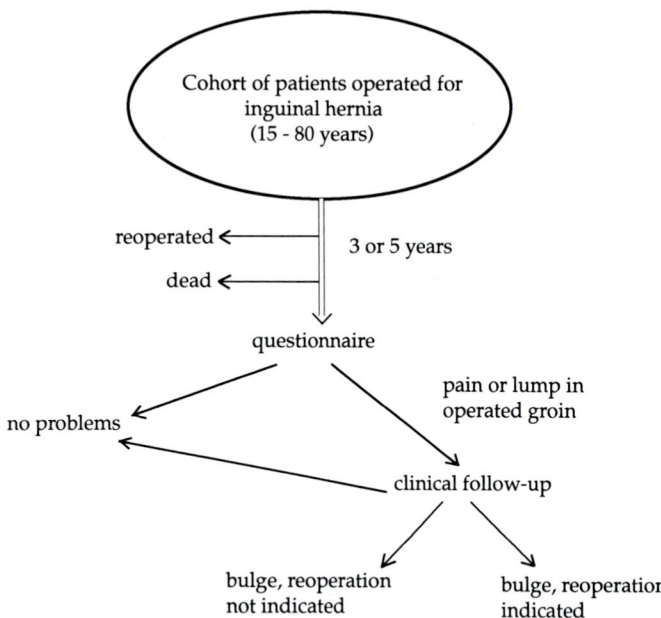

Figure 3-1. Audit scheme based on questionnaire, selective follow-up, and the definition of recurrence as having undergone reoperation or in need of a further operation.

2. Nonabsorbable sutures are used exclusively.
3. A prospective, computerized recording of all hernia operations has started, forming the basis for questionnaire follow-up and, in appropriate cases, clinical examination.

An audit scheme based on questionnaire, selective follow-up, and the definition of recurrence as "reoperated or in need of a further operation" is shown in Figure 3-1. Once established within a department, all steps to the clinical follow-up may be executed by secretaries. Surgeons, optimally independent observers, have to perform examinations of the minority of patients whose questionnaire answers may indicate signs of recurrence.

In summary, I have tried to illustrate that audit of hernia surgery based on comparisons between hospitals as well as questionnaire and selective follow-up may provide means of reducing the gap in recurrence rates between specialist and nonspecialist units.

REFERENCES

1. Audit Commission. A short cut to better services: day surgery in England and Wales. London: HMSO, 1990.
2. Barwell NJ. Recurrence and early activity after groin hernia repair. Lancet 1981;2:985.
3. Berliner SD. An approach to groin hernia. Surg Clin North Am 1984;64:197.
4. Bhopal RS, Thomson R. A form to help learn and teach about assessing medical audit papers. In: Smith R, ed. Audit in action. London: Br Med J, 1992.
5. Cubertafond P, Gainant A. Traitement des hernies de l'aine par kélorraphie type Shouldice: analyse d'une série de 403 opérés. Chirurgie 1989;115:133.
6. Devlin HB. Management of abdominal hernias. London, Butterworths, 1988:48.
7. Devlin HB, Gillen PHA, Waxman BP, MacNay RA. Short stay surgery for inguinal hernia: experience of the Shouldice operation, 1970–1982. Br J Surg 1986;73:123.
8. Deysine M, Soroff HS. Must we specialize herniorrhaphy for better results? Am J Surg 1990;160:239.
9. Glassow F. Inguinal hernia repair using local anaesthesia. Ann R Coll Surg Engl 1984;66:382.
10. Kald A, Nilsson E. Quality assessment in hernia surgery. Quality Assurance in Health Care 1991;3:205.
11. Kingsnorth AN, Gray MR, Nott DM. Prospective randomized trial comparing the Shouldice technique and plication darn for inguinal hernia. Br J Surg 1992;79:1068.
12. Lichtenstein IL, Shore JM. Exploding the myths of hernia repair. Am J Surg 1976;132:307.
13. Lyons C, Gumpert R. Medical audit data: counting is not enough. In: Smith R, ed. Audit in action. BMJ, 1900;300:1563.
14. Marsden AJ. The results of inguinal hernia repairs: a problem of assessment. Lancet 1959;1:461.
15. McPherson K. Why do variations occur? In: Anderson TF, Mooney G, eds. The challenge of medical practice variations. London, MacMillan, 1990.
16. Nilsson E, Anderberg B, Bragmark M, et al. Hernia surgery in a defined population: improvements possible in outcome and cost-effectiveness. J Ambulatory Surgery 1993;1:150.

17. Paul A, Troidl H, Rixen D, Williams J. Leistenbruch-operationen nach Shouldice oder Bassini. Ergebnisse einer kontrollierten randomisierten Studie. Manuscript. 1993.
18. Pollock A, Evans M. Surgical audit. London, Butterworths, 1993.
19. Quill DS, Devlin HB, Plant JA, Denham KR, McNay RA, Morris D. Surgical operation rates: a twelve year experience in Stockton-on-Tees. Ann R Coll Surg Engl 1983;65:248.
20. Royal College of Surgeons of England. Guidelines to clinical audit in surgical practice. London, RCS, 1989.
21. Shulman AG, Amid PK, Lichtenstein IL. The safety of mesh repair for primary inguinal hernias: results of 3019 operations from five diverse surgical sources. Am Surg 1992;58:255.
22. Shuttleworth KED, Davies WH. Treatment of inguinal herniae. Lancet 1960;1:126.
23. Williams M, Frankel S, Nanchahal K, Coast J, Donovan J. Hernia repair. London, NHS Management Executive, 1993:77–86.

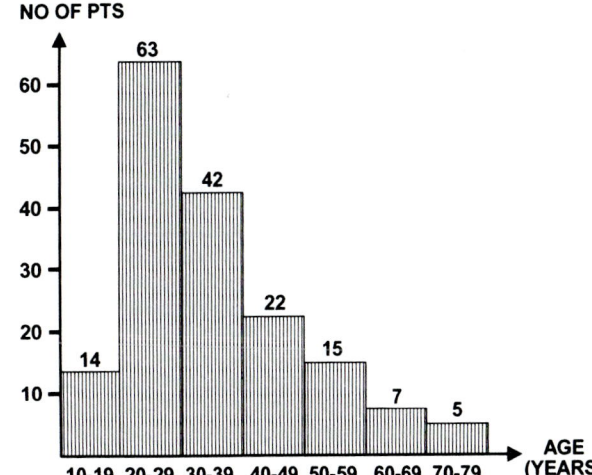

Figure 3-2. Age distribution of 180 patients with a history and clinical findings that prompted exploration for suspected occult inguinal hernia.

Special Comment

Nonpalpable Inguinal Hernia in Women
Leif Spangen

A nonpalpable hernia as the possible cause of inguinal pain in women is often overseen. On review of the literature, one is struck by how few reports there are on this type of hernia.[4,7,10,12] I believe, however, that symptomatic, nonpalpable (incipient, occult) inguinal hernia is relatively common in women but seldom diagnosed.

MATERIAL

To obtain more information on history, diagnosis, and operative findings, we carried out a follow-up study of 168 patients judged preoperatively to have non-palpable inguinal hernia. The patients had not undergone previous inguinal hernia repair on the involved side, and there was absence of detectable impulse while coughing. The study took place over a 12-year period. Most of the patients were 20 to 50 years of age (Fig. 3-2). The most important diagnostic and surgical findings are presented in Tables 3-4 through 3-6. In most instances, a woman with a nonpalpable indirect inguinal hernia reports dull inguinal pain aggravated by physical exertion. About three fourths of the patients notice intermittent neuralgic-type pain during periods of accentuated symptoms, and in almost two thirds, there is pinprick hyperalgesia of the skin corresponding to the distribution of the ilioinguinal

nerve. The patient always experiences a distinct point tenderness on palpation over the deep inguinal ring during a Valsalva maneuver, and the pressure reproduces or increases her current pain. In all patients studied, the deep inguinal ring was abnormally wide (2.5 cm or more).

DISCUSSION

In men, the external inguinal ring usually permits insertion of a finger in the inguinal canal by inversion of the scrotal skin whereby even minor hernias can be diagnosed. The skin of the labium majus cannot be inverted in the same way, and the external inguinal ring in women is usually so narrow that a palpating

Table 3-4. Preoperative Symptoms in 172 Cases of Occult Inguinal Hernias

Symptom	No.
Type of inguinal pain:	
Dull, drawing pain	170
Neuralgic pain only	2
Combined dull and neuralgic pain	126
Pain radiating from the groin to the ipsilateral:	
Thigh	96
Flank	61
Hypogastrium	28
Pain accentuated by:	
Physical exertion	161
Menstruation	18
Mental stress	3

Table 3-5. Clinical Findings in 172 Cases
of Occult Inguinal Hernia

Finding	No.
Tenderness corresponding to the deep inguinal ring upon palpation during Valsalva maneuver	172
Hyperalgesia of the skin corresponding to the distribution of the ilioinguinal nerve	109

finger cannot reach the inguinal canal. Inguinal hernias in women are therefore often diagnosed after a prolonged symptomatic period.

During a Valsalva maneuver, the posterior wall of the inguinal canal is partly protected by a shutter mechanism, and the deep inguinal ring is normally closed by a closure or sphincter mechanism. (Fig. 3-3). In women, the insertion of the internal oblique and transversus abdominis muscles into the rectus sheath is located more distally than in men, and the insertion in the Cooper ligament is broader. Hesselbach triangle is thus narrower, and the transversalis fascia and transversus abdominis muscle are usually better developed and stronger in women than in men. All these factors contribute to make women less susceptible to direct inguinal hernia.[1,9] Because the round ligament is a structure of less diameter than the spermatic cord, the internal ring is correspondingly narrower in women. This creates a more effective closure mechanism and reduces the risk of acquired indirect inguinal hernia. The oblique path taken by the round ligament through the abdominal wall laminae indirectly serves to protect against herniation. As the transversus abdominis muscle contracts, the obliquity of exit of the round ligament through the deep ring increases, and an additional protection of the opening against the onset of a hernia is obtained. To understand the patient's symptoms, it is also important to be familiar with the topographic anatomy of the ilioinguinal nerve. This nerve runs from the retroperitoneal space and penetrates the abdominal wall cra-

Table 3-6. Findings at Operation in 180 Inguinal Explorations (in 168 Patients) for Suspected Occult Inguinal Hernia

Finding	No.
Indirect inguinal hernia consisting of:	
Hernial sac	119
Preperitoneal fat only	51
Sliding hernia	1
Combined indirect and direct hernia	1
Direct inguinal hernia	0
Femoral hernia only	1
Normal operation findings	7

nially and somewhat laterally to the deep inguinal ring. The nerve passes the transversus abdominis and internal oblique muscles stepwise. The entrapment point is therefore located in the area where the nerve passes these two muscles. The deep inguinal ring in our patients with nonpalpable inguinal hernia was always wider than normal. During a Valsalva maneuver, the contraction of the muscles of the abdominal wall reduces the width of the deep inguinal ring without closing it completely (see Fig. 3-3). The dull pain is likely to be caused by stimulation of the pain fibers present in large numbers in both the preperitoneal fat and the parietal peritoneum when these structures are forced out through the deep inguinal ring. The pain is aggravated on palpation because the hernia is pressed against the hernial ring, which during a Valsalva maneuver is well defined and firm. The cause of the neuralgic-like pain is uncertain, but a direct mechanical influence of the hernia on the ilioinguinal nerve is unlikely. We consider the following explanation more probable. The dull inguinal hernia pain causes a local reflex increase of tone in the internal oblique and transversus abdominis muscles. As the nerve passes between the fibers of these muscles, it may be subject to mechanical pressure, thereby giving rise to neuralgic pain (entrapment neuropathy). The fact that the increase in tone is only intermittent would explain why the neuralgic-like pain and the pinprick hyperalgesia occur simultaneously. The fact that the hyperalgesia, on the other hand, can sometimes be demonstrated several days or weeks after the neuralgic pain may be interpreted as an indication that the pressure can cause neuropraxia.

Herniography has been found to be a sensitive and reliable diagnostic aid capable of demonstrating nonpalpable hernial sacs in the groin. The use of herniography in adults with unexplained groin pain has been advocated by Gullmo. Note, however, that in about one third of nonpalpable inguinal hernias in women, the hernia consists entirely of preperitoneal fat (see Table 3-6). Preperitoneal lipomas represent a variety of indirect inguinal herniation. Characteristically, the lipoma is found within the cremasteric sheath. Herniography is not capable of demonstrating lipoma of the round ligament or cord, but appears to be more sensitive than surgical exploration in demonstrating small hernial sacs.[3,6,11] Thus, if the history and clinical findings in a woman suggest the presence of a hernia, exploration should be considered despite a normal herniogram in the patient with no other explanation of groin pain.

Laparoscopy has been reported and recommended as a possible diagnostic modality in patients with groin pain.[8] If laparoscopy is performed on the indication of obscure groin and lower abdominal pain, the lower abdominal wall should be carefully in-

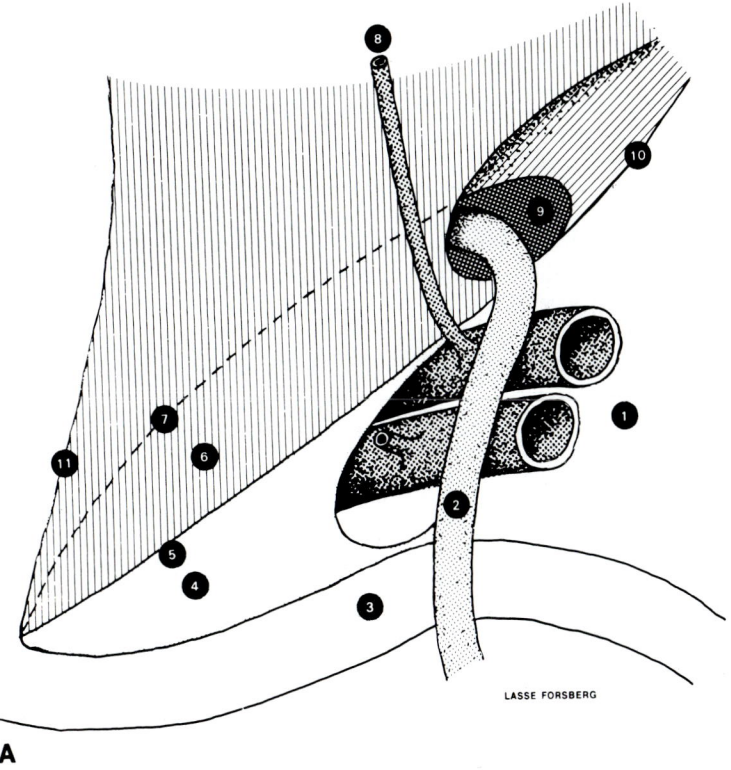

A

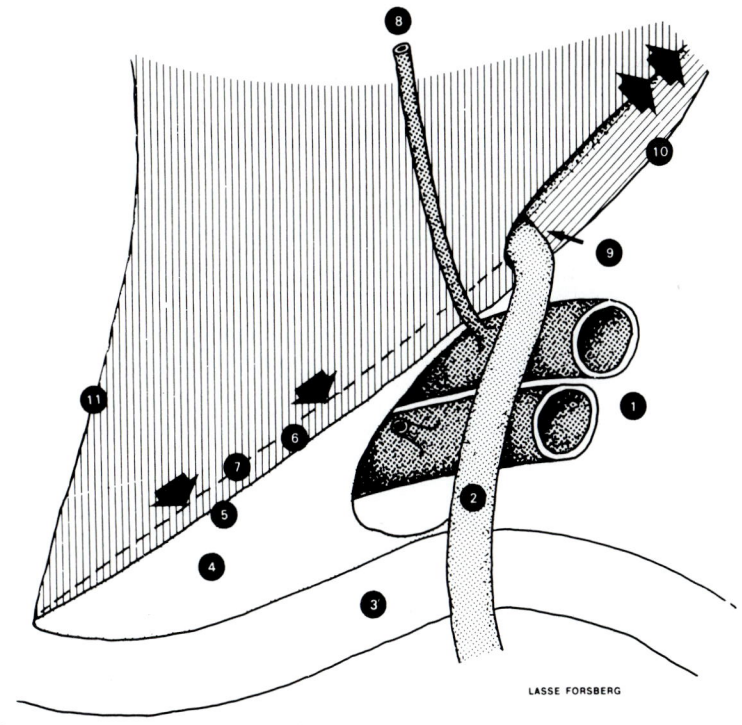

B

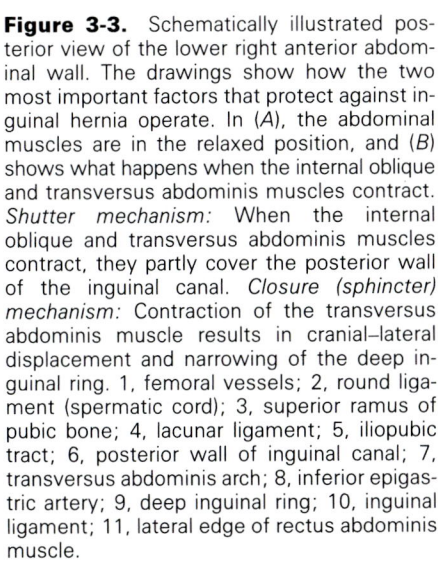

Figure 3-3. Schematically illustrated posterior view of the lower right anterior abdominal wall. The drawings show how the two most important factors that protect against inguinal hernia operate. In (A), the abdominal muscles are in the relaxed position, and (B) shows what happens when the internal oblique and transversus abdominis muscles contract. *Shutter mechanism:* When the internal oblique and transversus abdominis muscles contract, they partly cover the posterior wall of the inguinal canal. *Closure (sphincter) mechanism:* Contraction of the transversus abdominis muscle results in cranial–lateral displacement and narrowing of the deep inguinal ring. 1, femoral vessels; 2, round ligament (spermatic cord); 3, superior ramus of pubic bone; 4, lacunar ligament; 5, iliopubic tract; 6, posterior wall of inguinal canal; 7, transversus abdominis arch; 8, inferior epigastric artery; 9, deep inguinal ring; 10, inguinal ligament; 11, lateral edge of rectus abdominis muscle.

spected to discover existing hernias. There is need for a simpler method than laparoscopy in the diagnosis of inguinal hernia.

Ultrasonography has been used but does not appear to be reliable in the diagnosis of nonpalpable inguinal hernia.[2]

In conclusion, nonpalpable indirect inguinal hernia in the female patient may be the cause of persistent groin and lower abdominal pain. This hernia is clinically recognizable on the basis of intermittency, character, and location of the pain and typical findings on examination. Herniography is of great help in the investigation of these patients. However, inguinal pain is a common symptom with multifactorial causes. The patient should therefore be thoroughly investigated for other possible or concomitant causes of pain before the decision is made to carry out an inguinal exploration.

REFERENCES

1. Condon RE. Surgical anatomy of the transversus abdominis and transversalis fascia. Ann Surg 1971; 173(1):1.
2. Deitch EA, Soncrant MC. Ultrasonic diagnosis of surgical disease of the inguinal-femoral region. Surg Gynecol Obstet 1981;152:319.
3. Ekberg O, Blomqvist P, Olsson S. Positive contrast herniography in adult patient with obscure groin pain. Surgery 1981;89:532.
4. Fodor PB, Webb WA. Indirect inguinal hernia in the female with no palpable sac. South Med J 1971;64:15.
5. Gullmo A. Herniography. Acta Chir Scand 1980; 132(Suppl):361.
6. Hall C, Hall PN, Wingate JP, Neoptolemos JP. Evaluation of herniography in the diagnosis of an occult abdominal wall hernia in symptomatic adults. Br J Surg 1990;77:902.
7. Herrington JK. Occult inguinal hernia in the female. Ann Surg 1975;181:481.
8. Hunt RB, Camer SJ. Laparoscopy in the diagnosis of occult inguinal hernia. Am J Obstet Gynecol 1982; 142:924.
9. Ponka JL. The hernia problem in the female. In: Ponka JL. Hernias of the abdominal wall. Philadelphia, WB Saunders, 1980:82–90.
10. Roos H, Smedberg S. Symptomatic non-palpable inguinal hernias. Postgrad Gen Surg 1992;4(2):131.
11. Smedberg SGG, Broomé AEA, Elmér O, Gullmo A. Herniography in the diagnosis of obscure groin pain. Acta Chir Scand 1985;151:663.
12. Spangen L, Andersson R, Ohlsson L. Non-palpable inguinal hernia in the female. Am Surg 1988; 54(9):574.

Clinical Aspects of Groin Hernia

Part Two

Hernia, Fourth Edition, edited
by Lloyd M. Nyhus and Robert E. Condon.
J.B. Lippincott Company, Philadelphia © 1995.

Chapter 4

Groin Hernia in Infants and Children

Jay L. Grosfeld

Inguinal hernia is common in infants and children. Repair of congenital inguinal hernia is the most frequently performed operation in the pediatric age group. Advances in pediatric anesthesia, ambulatory care, neonatal intensive care, and certain aspects of operative technique have revised some of the early considerations regarding patient management and the correct timing of repair. This chapter reviews the embryology and clinical presentation of inguinal hernia in children and provides an update of the contemporary aspects of managing this common pediatric condition.

HISTORICAL BACKGROUND

A historical survey regarding the treatment of inguinal hernia by Olch and Harkins[57] refers to Ambroise Paré, who was the first to advocate the repair of hernia in children. Percival Pott is given credit for the first description, in 1756, of congenital inguinal hernia. In 1877, Czerny (Vienna) and Banks (England) recommended ligation of the hernial sac through the external inguinal ring. In 1881, Lucas-Championniere described incising the external oblique aponeurosis for adequate exposure of the internal ring and high ligation of the hernial sac. In 1899, Ferguson[17] first described leaving the spermatic cord undisturbed during the repair. Turner,[75] MacLennon,[51] and Russell[69] all reaffirmed that cure required only simple high ligation of the sac. Gertrude Herzfeld[35] initiated outpatient surgery for pediatric inguinal hernia in 1938 in Edinburgh, Scotland. In 1941, William E. Ladd and Robert E. Gross[45] of Boston recommended early hernial repair. Willis Potts and colleagues[59] in Chicago were also strong advocates of early repair and, in addition, condemned the use of a truss as a method of treatment. Both Gross and Potts documented a high rate of bilaterality. Duckett,[14] however, was the first to introduce contralateral inguinal exploration. This was followed by a number of reports by Rothenberg and Barnett,[65] Clausen and associates,[7] Gilbert and Clatworthy,[21] Lynn and Johnson,[50] and Sparkman,[73] who all enthu-

siastically recommended bilateral exploration. During the past two decades, the development of sophisticated neonatal intensive care has resulted in a high survival of premature infants and introduced a new, relatively large group of patients requiring hernia repair.[23,27] These infants also required the development of a new fund of knowledge regarding both anesthesia and clinical patient care management skills.

EMBRYOLOGY OF HERNIA AND HYDROCELE

An adequate understanding of congenital indirect inguinal hernia requires some insight into its embryology. The occurrence of a hernia is related to events involved with the descent of the testes and the processus vaginalis. During the third month of gestation, the testis begins its descent from a retroperitoneal location, following the course of the gubernaculum testis. The gubernaculum testis is a mesenchymal fold that develops from the caudal end of the mesonephros and is attached to the caudal portion of the developing gonad.[46] The mesonephros is extended in a cranial direction by the development of the vertebral column, separating the kidney and testis. The superior portion of the testicular blood supply is involved with the cranial migration of the kidney and renal vessels from which the spermatic vessels arise. In boys, the wolffian duct persists and develops into the vas deferens and epididymis, whereas the müllerian structures (paramesonephric tissues) regress. In girls, the mesonephros regresses, and there is minimal development of a gubernaculum. The müllerian structures fuse to form the upper third of the vagina, the uterus, and the fallopian tubes. The gonads (ovaries) usually remain within the pelvis in a position caudal to the fallopian tubes. Because the gubernaculum in girls is relatively unimportant, there is little stimulus for penetration of the processus vaginalis into the groin. The inguinal canal is narrow, and a shallow diverticulum of peritoneum may persist; this is called the *canal of Nuck* and is similar to the processus vaginalis in boys. It usually disappears by the seventh or eighth intrauterine month, but it may persist and remain open and extend into the labia majora (the female homologue of the scrotum). The wolffian structures regress with the exception of the round ligament, which enters the canal and is the female homologue of the vas deferens.

In boys, the gubernaculum grows and passes through the internal inguinal ring, widening the inguinal canal. A diverticulum of peritoneum, the processus vaginalis, follows the gubernaculum and testis through the internal ring into the inguinal canal, usually at the seventh intrauterine month. The gubernaculum extends down to the scrotum, leading the testis to its final destination. This process is probably related to hormonal stimulation and adequate end-organ receptors. Evidence exists that testicular descent can be prevented by division of the genitofemoral nerve, which innervates the cremasteric muscle.[16] This suggests that an abnormality of the genitofemoral nerve may also play a role in incomplete gonadal descent and subsequent hernia occurrence. The fate of the associated peritoneal diverticulum (the processus vaginalis) is variable. In most children (90%), the processus involutes by obliteration, leaving a remnant attached to the testis, the tunica vaginalis. In a consid-

erable number of children, however, persistent patency of all or part of the processus vaginalis may result in the development of a variety of inguinal anomalies (Fig. 4-1). Complete patency from the internal ring to the scrotum results in a diverticular scrotal hernia. Obliteration of the processus distally and persistent patency in the proximal portion result in the usual inguinal hernia.

Hydroceles (water sacs) are also the result of incomplete obliteration of the processus vaginalis. These include the isolated hydrocele of the tunica vaginalis, which is the most common, with proximal obliteration; hydrocele of the spermatic cord in boys or canal of Nuck in girls with distal and proximal obliteration; and communicating hydroceles, which are indirect inguinal hernias with a small neck at the internal ring, communicating with the peritoneal cavity. In some instances, when the proximal end is obliterated, the hydrocele can be large and extend into the retroperitoneum (abdominoscrotal hydrocele).[15] In other instances, both a proximal indirect inguinal hernia and a separate hydrocele of the tunica vaginalis that do not communicate may coexist. The rate of persistent patency of the processus vaginalis is high in

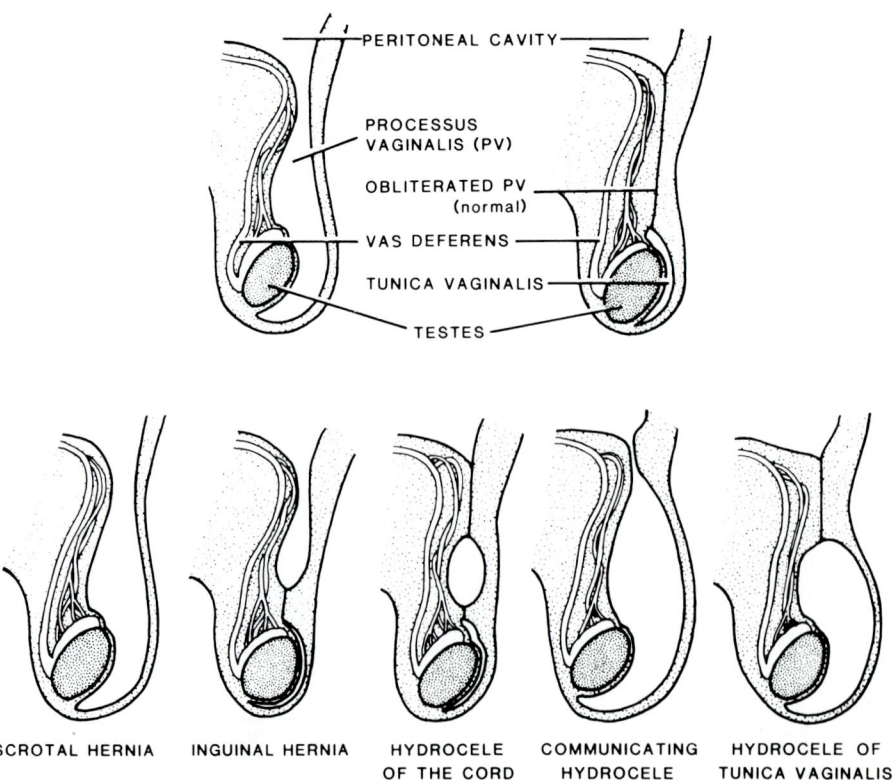

Figure 4-1. (*Top*) The fetal (*left*) and normal anatomy of the inguinoscrotal area in the term infant. (*Bottom*) The various anomalies related to patency of all or part of the processus vaginalis.

instances of undescended testes, possibly because normal testicular descent may be necessary for the obliterative event to take place.

CLINICAL PRESENTATION

Although inguinal hernia can present at any age, the peak incidence is during infancy and childhood. About 3% to 5% of full-term infants may be born with a clinical inguinal hernia.[22,36] The incidence is substantially increased in premature infants, 5% to 30% of whom may present with a hernia.[34] A positive family history for congenital indirect inguinal hernia is observed in 11.5% of instances.[36] Hernia occurrence has been noted in twins;[1] however, no specific hereditary factors have been detected. About 80% to 90% of pediatric hernias occur in boys.[7,36] The processus vaginalis is patent in 90% of all newborn infants and in 40% of boys at 2 years of age.[67,71] About one third of the hernias present in the first 6 months of life. Congenital inguinal hernia presents more commonly (55%–60%) on the right side[36,67] (Fig. 4-2). About 25% of hernias occur clinically on the left side, and 15% have a bilateral presentation (Fig. 4-3). The high incidence of right-sided hernia is probably related to late descent of the right testis and delayed obliteration of the processus vaginalis.

A number of conditions are associated with an increased incidence of inguinal hernia.[64] These include prematurity, a positive family history of inguinal hernia, hydrops, meconium peritonitis, chylous ascites, abdominal wall defects,[31] exstrophy of the bladder or

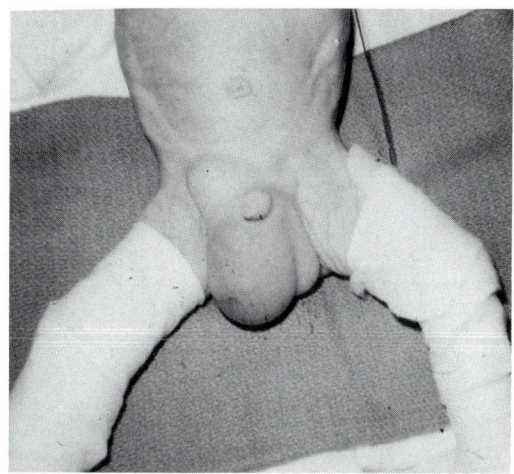

Figure 4-2.   A large right inguinal hernia extending into the scrotal sac in a premature infant weighing 3 lb. Sixty percent of clinical hernias present on the right side.

cloaca,[77] undescended testis, hypospadias, epispadias, connective tissue disorders,[11,36] and liver disease with ascites. In addition, infants with intersex problems, particularly phenotypic girls with testicular feminization syndrome, frequently have inguinal hernia.[58,61] One should pay special attention to girls with bilaterally palpable gonads in the labia majora. It is suggested that these girls should be screened with a buccal smear and appropriate genetic evaluation before their hernial repair.[77] In instances of testicular feminization syndrome, bilateral gonadectomy can be ac-

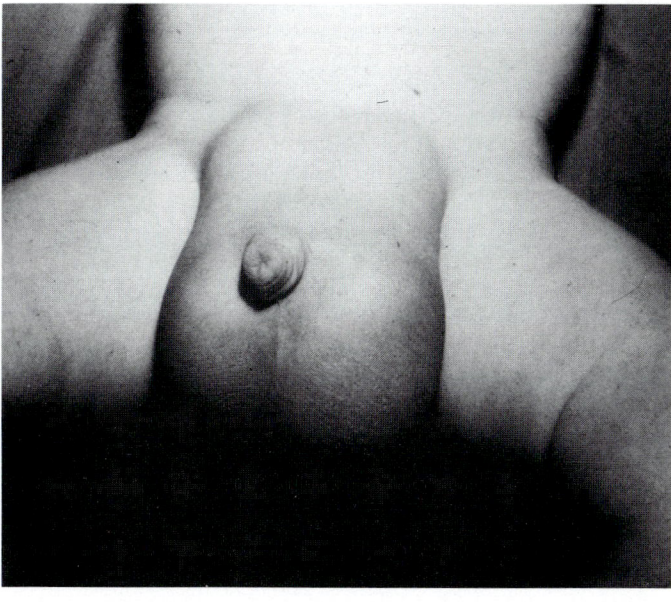

Figure 4-3.   Bilateral inguinal hernias.

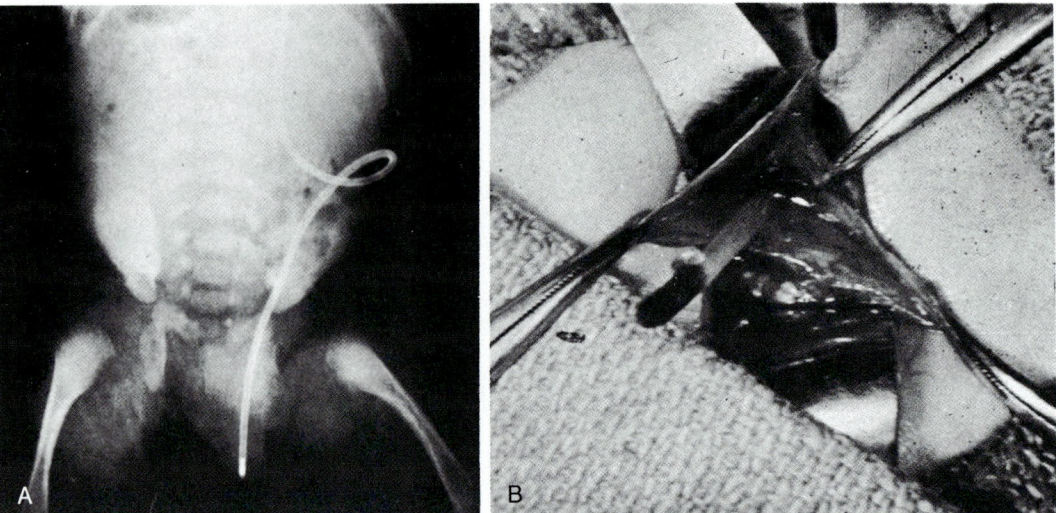

Figure 4-4. (*A*) Abdominal roentgenogram showing the presence of a ventriculoperitoneal shunt catheter in the left scrotal sac. The catheter tip migrated into the hernial sac through the internal ring. (*B*) Ventriculoperitoneal shunt catheter was found in the hernial sac at operation and was carefully returned to the peritoneal cavity before high ligation of the sac.

complished by the inguinal approach at the time of the hernial repair. A considerable increase in the incidence of inguinoscrotal anomalies in children with cystic fibrosis and their unaffected relatives has also been observed.[37,76]

Absence of the vas deferens and a small epididymis were observed in 31 of 32 boys with cystic fibrosis described by Wang and coworkers.[76] Absence of the vas deferens at the time of hernial repair or orchiopexy should suggest the possibility of mucoviscidosis. Absence of the vas deferens was also described in boys without mucoviscidosis in association with ipsilateral renal agenesis.[49]

An increased incidence of inguinal hernia also was noted after the performance of ventriculoperitoneal shunt procedures for hydrocephalus.[28] Sixteen percent of infants with hydrocephalus who were operated on in the first few months of life developed a previously unrecognized inguinal hernia (Fig. 4-4). It is theorized that the production of cerebrospinal fluid exceeds the peritoneal absorption rate, resulting in cerebrospinal fluid ascites. The ascites increases intraabdominal pressure in young infants at risk of having a patent processus vaginalis. The ventriculoperitoneal shunt changes a potential hernia (eg, a patent processus) into a clinically apparent hernia.[25,29] The same mechanism is responsible for the increased incidence of inguinal hernia in patients receiving continuous ambulatory peritoneal dialysis for renal failure[26] (Table 4-1).

PHYSICAL EXAMINATION AND MANAGEMENT

Examination of the inguinal area for a hernia may show an obvious bulge at the site of the external ring or within the scrotum (see Fig. 4-1). This bulge can often be gently reduced. The examiner may feel gas-filled viscera in the sac. The bulge may be seen only during severe straining, such as with crying or with

Table 4-1. Conditions Associated With an Increased Incidence of Inguinal Hernia*

Prematurity
Positive family history
Hydrops
Meconium peritonitis
Chylous ascites
Liver disease with ascites
Abdominal wall defects
Ambiguous genitalia
Hypospadias, epispadias
Exstrophy of bladder, cloaca
Cryptorchid testes
Cystic fibrosis
Connective tissue disorders
Ventriculoperitoneal shunt
Continuous ambulatory peritoneal dialysis
Hunter-Hurler syndrome
Mucopolysaccharidosis

*Based on patients seen at the James Whitcomb Riley Hospital for Children, Indiana University Medical Center, Indianapolis.

defecation, when increased intraabdominal pressure exists. When the infant relaxes, the mass frequently reduces spontaneously. If the infant is old enough to stand, he or she should be examined in both the supine and the erect positions. If not, the parent or a nurse can hold the infant upright so that the surgeon can closely observe the inguinoscrotal area. In instances in which the intestine descends into the scrotum, the viscera may be easily palpated in the scrotal sac.

The so-called silk sign, which may be observed by rubbing the index finger over the thickened cord structures and is caused by the presence of the sac, is suggestive, but not pathognomonic, of a hernia, and may be an unreliable finding.[21] Before an examination for an inguinal hernia, it is also essential to make sure that the testis is within the scrotal sac to avoid mistaking a retractile testis for a hernial bulge. In older children, one can palpate the external ring by digital examination upward and by asking the youngster to cough or strain to assist in the evaluation. In young infants, however, this is both difficult for the examiner and painful for the child and should be omitted. It may occasionally be difficult to demonstrate the presence of a hernial sac in some children. One may usually rely on the referring physician's observation of the hernia or more rarely on the infant's mother or father. It is desirable for at least one physician to document the presence of a hernia before a surgical repair is attempted.[24] Occasional false-positive errors have been noted, with no hernia observed at operation.[36,78] Because of the high rate of incarceration, early repair is advised for all inguinal hernias.

Communicating hydroceles frequently present with a history of a mass that changes size. The scrotal size increases during activities such as running, jumping, or crying and decreases after the child takes a nap. This is related to an exchange of fluid from the peritoneal cavity to the scrotal sac through a narrow communication at the internal ring. These are essentially inguinal hernias and require surgical repair. Hydroceles of the spermatic cord in boys or the canal of Nuck in girls are usually smaller, nontender, and slightly mobile and are located in the mid-inguinal canal or upper labia. A hydrocele of the tunica vaginalis is a soft, usually nontender, fluid-filled sac that transilluminates and envelops the testis. This type of hydrocele does not change size and may involute spontaneously in the first 6 months of life. Hydroceles that persist beyond that time are usually associated with an inguinal hernia and should be treated surgically. Congenital hydroceles should be differentiated from the acquired type more commonly seen in older children and young adults as a result of trauma, tumor, or inflammation.

The presence of an empty scrotum should alert the examining physician to a possible undescended or ectopic testis, which is associated with an inguinal hernia (or at least a patent processus) more than 90% of the time. Although routine orchiopexy is usually delayed until the child is 1 year of age, if a symptomatic inguinal hernia coexists, it should be promptly repaired and orchiopexy accomplished at the same time.

INCARCERATED HERNIA

Inguinal hernias are prone to incarcerate. *Incarceration* is defined as a hernia, usually containing viable small intestine, that is "stuck" or confined, and therefore irreducible. It is observed in 17% of right-sided hernias and 7% of left-sided hernias; the overall rate is 12%.[66] Incarceration is most common in the first 6 months of life, when more than half of instances are observed.[24,62,66] The rate of incarceration in the first few months to the first year of life is over 30%.[62,64] The incidence of incarceration is higher in girls, even though 80% to 90% of all inguinal hernias occur in boys. In addition, an emergency operation for incarceration is more frequently required in girls (21%) than in boys (17%).[66]

An incarcerated hernia usually presents as an acute, tender mass in the inguinal canal. The mass may protrude beyond the external inguinal ring or into the scrotum (Fig. 4-5). The skin over the mass may be discolored, edematous, erythematous, or blue.

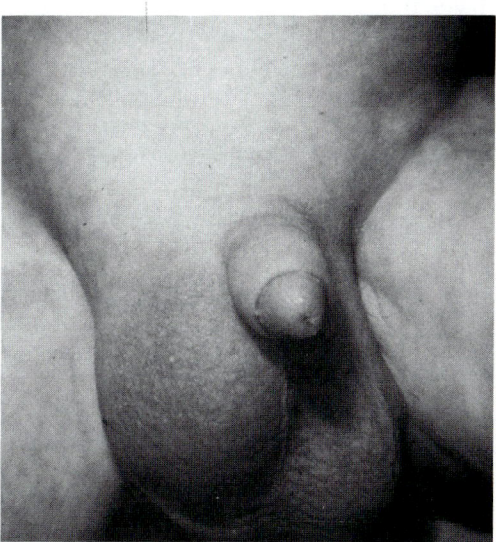

Figure 4-5. A 5-week-old boy with an incarcerated right inguinal hernia. The skin over the mass is somewhat discolored.

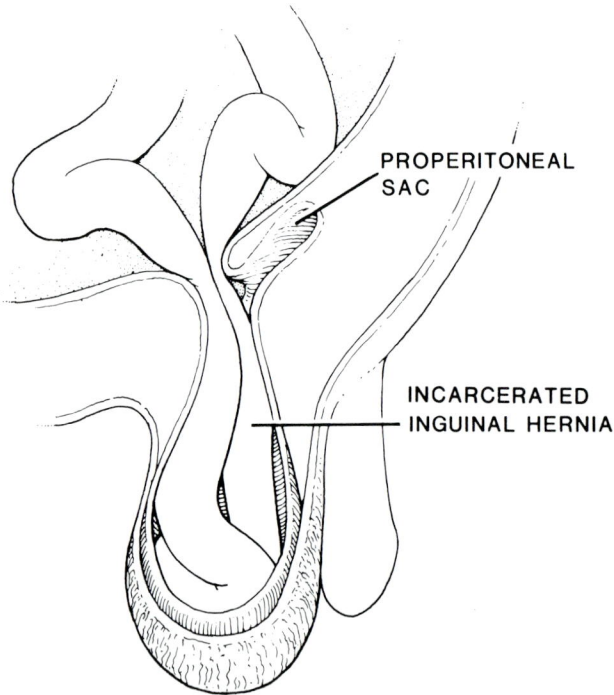

Figure 4-6. Intestine incarcerated in an indirect inguinal hernia. Incarceration usually occurs at the internal inguinal ring.

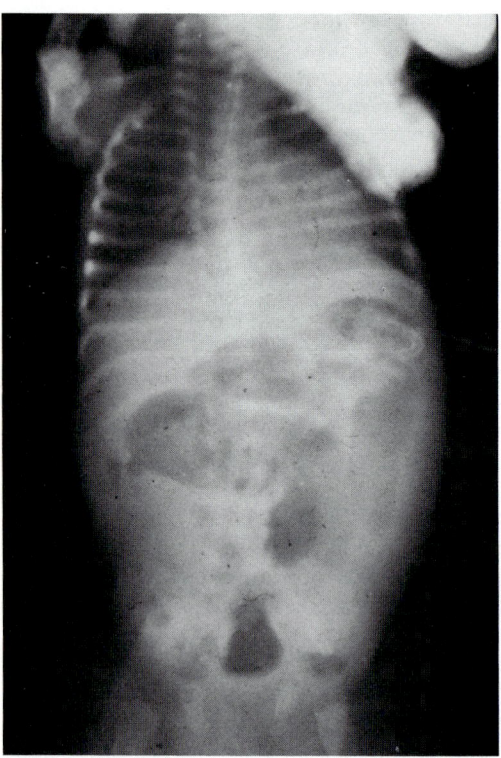

Figure 4-7. Abdominal roentgenogram of the infant in Figure 4-5. Dilated loops of small intestine are consistent with intestinal obstruction. Note the gas in the inguinal canal area.

Inability to reduce the mass may result in compromise of the blood supply (intestinal hypoxia), causing strangulation obstruction (Fig. 4-6). This is characterized by abdominal distention, bilious vomiting, failure to pass rectal gas or fecal material, tachycardia, and an obstructive small intestinal pattern on abdominal roentgenograms (Fig. 4-7). The latter findings all suggest an early operation for relief of obstruction, intestinal salvage, and hernial repair.

Fortunately, most (80%) incarcerated hernias in children can be managed by conservative measures. The diagnosis is usually achieved early in the course and the patient promptly brought to the attention of a physician. In patients with incarceration of short du-

ration and without evidence of toxicity (defined as fever, tachycardia, abdominal distention, blue discoloration over the hernia, and an obstructive pattern on abdominal roentgenogram), a conservative approach can be used. This consists of a four-point program of (1) sedation (Table 4-2); (2) placing the baby in a Trendelenburg position; (3) using a cold pack (over petrolatum gauze to prevent cold injury to the skin in the inguinoscrotal or inguinal labial region); and (4) when the baby is quiet, and when spontaneous reduction has not occurred, gentle "taxis" applied over the

Table 4-2. Sedation for Attempted Reduction of Incarcerated Hernia

Age	Medication	Dosage
0–3 mo	Pentobarbital	2–6 mg/kg/24 h IM Max. dose: 100 mg/24 h IM
3–12 mo	Secobarbital or	4–6 mg/kg/24 h
	Meperidine	1–1.5 mg/kg/dose Max. dose: 100 mg/dose IM
>1 y	Morphine sulfate	0.1–0.2 mg/kg/dose Max. dose: 15 mg/dose IM

involved hernia. This program usually allows reduction and avoids an emergency surgical procedure.

In nontoxic instances, one can usually safely delay exploration for incarcerated hernia, to allow either spontaneous reduction or gentle manipulative reduction with the aforementioned measures, for about 4 to 6 hours. Delay beyond this period of time, if the hernia remains irreducible, is unwarranted. I have not been able to successfully reduce instances of infarcted intestine. The complication rate is 18 to 20 times greater after emergency operations for incarcerated hernia than after elective procedures.[66] It is therefore worthwhile to reduce the hernia when possible (more than 75%–80% of the time) and perform an elective herniorrhaphy within 24 to 48 hours of the reduction. Recurrent incarceration occurs frequently when an operation is further delayed.

Management of Premature Infants

The development of contemporary neonatal intensive care has resulted in the survival of many seriously ill preterm and older infants, who frequently present with a symptomatic inguinal hernia. Although inguinal hernial repair is commonly performed in childhood, controversy exists concerning the appropriate timing and actual safety of hernial repair in the perinatal period. In a survey of pediatric surgeons, 30% of those surveyed were reluctant to operate on premature infants who had reducible hernias.[68] In a review of 100 consecutive inguinal hernial repairs in previously hospitalized newborn infants younger than 2 months of age, Rescorla and Grosfeld[64] documented that inguinal hernia (1) was common in preterm and other seriously ill hospitalized newborns; (2) had a high (31%) incidence of incarceration, about two times that of the general childhood population; (3) had a 9% rate of intestinal obstruction; (4) had a 2% rate of gonadal infarction; and (5) was a potentially life-threatening condition.

Early elective hernial repairs can be done safely, before discharge, in premature infants hospitalized for concurrent illness.[23,64] Premature infants who present with hernias while at home, after their discharge, should be managed in an extended observation area or as inpatients and carefully observed after anesthesia because of an increased risk of apnea and bradycardia.[27,74] Full-term infants without previous respiratory episodes can be safely treated as outpatients. If appropriate precautions are followed in the presence of qualified pediatric surgical and anesthetic expertise, early repair is associated with reduced morbidity and no mortality.[64]

The Role of Herniography

In 1967, Ducharme and colleagues[12] described the use of intraperitoneal herniography as a diagnostic aid in the detection of inguinal hernias. The procedure requires percutaneous transperitoneal injection of a contrast medium. The infant is placed in the prone position with the head of the roentgenographic examining table elevated. The contrast material is allowed to collect at the internal ring, and a simple exposure is obtained at 5 to 10 minutes.[79] Delayed roentgenograms are obtained at 45 to 60 minutes to obtain an absorption urogram as a screening measure to identify suspected renal anomalies, which occur in 1% to 2% of patients.[39,77] Proponents of inguinal herniography suggest that this technique is most useful in instances in which the hernia cannot be confirmed by a physician, for evaluation of the opposite side as an indicator for contralateral exploration, and for an assessment of cryptorchidism.[43,77] Complications have been observed in about 11% of patients.[39] These include abdominal wall hematoma, dehydration and hypovolemia, intestinal hematoma, intestinal entry, bladder entry, and false-negative examinations.[5] The use of herniography is somewhat controversial, and few pediatric surgeons (less than 2%) rely on it.[6,36] The disadvantages of herniography that have been cited include discomfort and pain from peritoneal injection, unnecessary radiation exposure, a complication rate greater than the elective operation complication rate, false-negative studies, and the added expense of the procedure. Herniography has not gained wide popularity, and Ducharme also recommended limiting the use of this procedure after some untoward complications.[13]

Intraoperative transperitoneal probing and air injection have been advocated to detect the contralateral patent processus vaginalis;[4,47,60] these techniques are seldom used, however.

My associates and I have not used herniography, probing techniques, or pneumoperitoneum in the management of our patients. Some surgeons advocate direct observation of the opposite internal ring during hernia repair by passing an endoscope through the clinically apparent hernia sac. We have no experience with this technique but would be concerned about tearing the often fragile peritoneal sac noted in small infants.

TREATMENT

The high risk for incarceration in the pediatric age group makes the presence of an inguinal hernia an indication for surgical repair. Repair should be performed soon after the diagnosis is made. Herniorrhaphy may be postponed because of concurrent infection, such as otitis media or upper respiratory tract illness; a terminal illness, such as a progressive malignant tumor; or severe prematurity. In instances of severe prematurity, repair should be accomplished just before the infant's discharge from the neonatal intensive care unit.

All full-term infants and older children without underlying illness may undergo hernial repair as outpatients. Ambulatory surgery for infants and children requires skilled pediatric anesthesia and nursing staffs, a pleasant environment, appropriately sized pediatric equipment and monitoring, and the ability to admit the infant to a pediatric inpatient facility if necessary. Outpatient hernial operations have been safe, effective, and well tolerated.[8,56] Outpatient surgical procedures also have the benefit of reducing the child's psychological trauma by avoiding hospitalization, limiting family separation, and reducing costs related to hospitalization as well as the incidence of cross-infection. A preoperative visit and tour of the outpatient facility and performance of laboratory tests before the day of the operation have been useful. Patients who require perioperative antibiotics for congenital heart defects, who are asplenic, or who have ventriculoperitoneal shunts may begin receiving their antibiotics at home 24 hours before the operation. After the operation, they should be managed postoperatively in a 12- to 23-hour extended observation area, avoiding a formal hospital admission in most cases.

OPERATIVE MANAGEMENT

On arrival in the operating room, the patient undergoes a number of steps in preparation for the procedure. Infants younger than 6 months of age have their extremities wrapped in Webril. The patient is placed on a warming pad under an overhead heater. Temperature is monitored with an axillary or skin thermal probe. Electrocardiogram, blood pressure, Doppler pulse, and an oximeter for oxygen saturation are carefully monitored. An intravenous line is started, using a percutaneously placed 24-gauge Silastic or Teflon catheter. A percutaneous arterial line is seldom indicated, except for infants with bronchopulmonary dysplasia or congenital heart disease. An endotracheal tube is inserted, and a humidified halogenated anesthetic agent is usually used. A grounding pad is applied for use of an electrocoagulator. Some authors recommend local anesthesia, caudal or spinal anesthesia in premature infants;[20,70] however, we prefer a general anesthetic.

The patient is placed in the supine position with the legs slightly spread, the knees slightly bent lat-erally, and the feet together. Skin preparation is accomplished using a gentle application of iodophor solution to the lower abdomen and inguinoscrotal (or labial) area, including the upper thighs and perineum. The field is draped with towels and linens, which includes the scrotum in the sterile field. If intestine is present within the hernial sac, in the inguinal canal, or in the scrotum, it should be reduced before the incision is made.

Incision

A short (1-inch) transverse incision is made in the lowest inguinal skin crease, always starting on the side of the obvious clinical hernia (Fig. 4-8A). Bleeding is usually minimal and can be easily controlled with a fine-tip infant electrocoagulator.

Dissection

The superficial fascia (Scarpa fascia) is incised, and the external oblique aponeurosis is identified (see Fig. 4-8B). The aponeurosis is traced laterally to identify the inguinal ligament, and the dissection is continued inferiorly to expose the exact location of the external inguinal ring. The external oblique fascia should not be opened until these anatomic landmarks are identified.

Although some surgeons advocate repair through the external ring in young infants (Mitchell Banks technique[44]), I incise the external oblique fascia to gain direct access to the internal ring. The external oblique fascia is incised in the long axis of its fibers, perpendicular to the external inguinal ring (see Fig. 4-8C). Caution must be taken to avoid injury to the ilioinguinal and genitofemoral nerves. The oblique fascia is opened through the ring to expose the cremasteric muscle and fascia, which envelop the cord structures. I avoid placing hemostats on the edges of the external oblique muscle in young infants because they may injure the delicate tissues. The cremasteric fibers are gently elevated and teased open by blunt dissection on the medial surface to expose the white, glistening, indirect inguinal hernial sac (see Fig. 4-8D).

The hernial sac is always located in an anteromedial position in relation to the cord. The sac is elevated with a hemostat and the cremasteric fibers carefully freed from the anterior and lateral aspects. The sac is retracted medially, allowing identification of the spermatic vessels and vas deferens (see Fig. 4-8E). The areolar tissue between these structures and the edge of the sac is grasped with a DeBakey forceps, and the retroperitoneal structures are gently teased

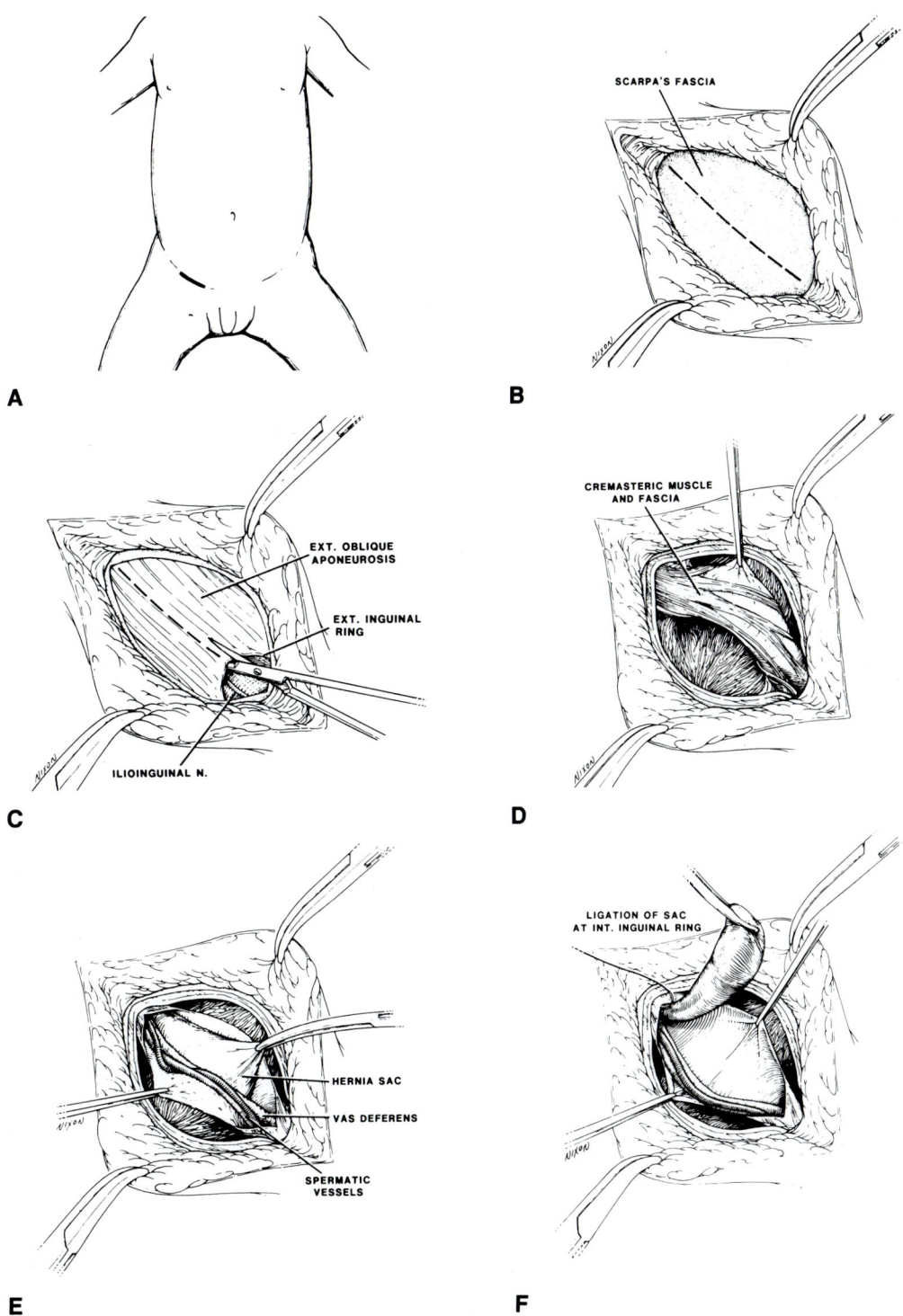

A

B SCARPA'S FASCIA

C EXT. OBLIQUE APONEUROSIS / EXT. INGUINAL RING / ILIOINGUINAL N.

D CREMASTERIC MUSCLE AND FASCIA

E HERNIA SAC / VAS DEFERENS / SPERMATIC VESSELS

F LIGATION OF SAC AT INT. INGUINAL RING

Figure 4-8. (*A*) The site of the transverse incision in the lowest inguinal crease. (*B*) Scarpa fascia is incised. (*C*) The external ring is identified, and the external oblique fascia is opened perpendicular to the ring in the long axis of its fibers. (*D*) The cremasteric muscle is teased open and the glistening hernial sac identified. (*E*) The sac is retracted medially, and the vas deferens and spermatic vessels are separated from the sac. (*F*) High ligation of the hernial sac is accomplished at the internal ring with interrupted suture ligatures.

away from the sac in a posterolateral direction. The vas itself should not be grasped directly with the forceps to avoid injury to this structure. The floor of the inguinal canal is not disturbed. If the sac is short, the end is freed, and the careful separation of the sac and spermatic structures is carried superiorly to the level of the internal inguinal ring. A small segment of retroperitoneal fat usually signals the upper limit of the dissection. If the sac is a diverticular structure that extends down to the scrotum, it may be divided once the cord structures are identified and protected from harm. The proximal end of the sac is then grasped for traction with a hemostat, and dissection is carried out up to the level of the internal ring, as noted. The base of the sac is carefully inspected and gently twisted to reduce any fluid or viscera into the abdominal cavity.

Repair

Suture ligation of the base of the sac is accomplished with two interrupted 4-0 silk suture ligatures (see Fig. 4-8F). Free ties should never be used because they may be dislodged if abdominal distention occurs. Gentle pressure is exerted on the lower abdomen to assure the operator that no leak of peritoneal fluid occurs because of an unrecognized tear at the base of the sac. The tied suture ends are cut before the sac is excised. The peritoneal stump should retract proximally through the internal ring. If the base of the sac is large, a pursestring suture may prove useful in performing the high ligation. If it is excessively large, the internal inguinal ring should be "snugged" with an interrupted 4-0 silk suture that approximates the transversalis fascia inferior to the cord structures. Closing the ring too tightly, however, may result in vascular compression of the cord and severe swelling.

If the floor of the inguinal canal is weak, two sutures from the conjoined tendon (internal oblique aponeurosis and transversalis fascia) to the iliopubic tract usually suffice in solving this problem. In instances in which the diverticular sac was previously divided (after high ligation), the distal end of the sac is simply widely incised on the anterior surface only, to avoid injury to the spermatic vessels and vas deferens. This maneuver almost always avoids annoying bleeding that may occur during attempts at extensive dissection of the testicular end of the congenital hernial sac. If, however, a noncommunicating hydrocele coexists with a proximal hernia, the hydrocele requires excision. The hydrocele sac is excised anterolaterally with great care to avoid damage to the spermatic vessels and vas deferens. A rim of the posterior wall of the hydrocele sac is left on the anteromedial surface of the testis and vital structures.

After adequate hemostasis (with an infant electrocoagulator) is ensured, the testis is returned to its normal intrascrotal position with the aid of a blunt-tipped joker elevator. The operator holds the testis in place externally by downward transscrotal traction as the joker elevator is removed from the inguinal wound. This action prevents iatrogenic entrapment of the testis in the inguinal canal.

Wound closure is accomplished in layers. The external oblique fascia is approximated with interrupted 4-0 (5-0 in infants) silk sutures to restore the inguinal anatomy. Bupivacaine is injected along the ilioinguinal and iliohypogastric nerve to reduce postoperative discomfort. A regional caudal block may also effectively reduce postoperative pain.[9] The subcutaneous fascia is closed with two or three interrupted 5-0 absorbable sutures with the knots buried. The skin edges are approximated with two interrupted 4-0 plain catgut subcuticular sutures. The skin edges are everted and sealed with a collodion dressing. The collodion protects the wound from urine, avoids the need for Steri-Strips or other tape and dressings in the diaper area, and obviates the trauma of subsequent suture or tape removal in the office or clinic at follow-up examination. No outer dressing is required. Although laparoscopic hernia repair has become a popular technique for repair of inguinal hernia in adults, there is little to no indication to use this technique in infants and young children. There may be a role for laparoscopic hernia repair in older children or adolescents with recurrent hernia in whom a preperitoneal procedure requiring mesh insertion is anticipated.

Circumcision

If a circumcision was not previously performed, and the parents desire this procedure, the excision of the foreskin should follow the hernial repair. Retraction of the foreskin and preparation should be delayed until completion of the hernial repair to avoid excessive edema of the subcoronal tissues. After a brief iodophor preparation to clean away any hidden smegma, removal of the foreskin can be carried out by either clamp or freehand technique.

Orchiopexy

In instances of hernia associated with an undescended testis, orchiopexy can be carried out at the time of the hernial repair. The hernial sac in instances of cryptorchid testis may be particularly thin and fragile. Gentle technique is essential in the separation of the sac from the cord structures. Once the diverticular hernial sac is freed up and divided, significant length of the testicular vessels and cord is obtained. High ligation of the hernial sac is accomplished by suture ligation (Fig. 4-9*A*). Further dissection is usually necessary, and division of the lateral spermatic fascia along the spermatic vessels as they pass through the internal ring into the retroperitoneal space usually frees up enough length to allow the testis to reach the scrotum. If further length is required, the epigastric vessels can be divided and the floor of the inguinal canal taken down to convert a triangular course to a straight line, which gains 1 to 2 inches in length for the spermatic vessels (see Fig. 4-9*B*). The previously unused scrotal sac is made into a pouch by digital dissection and pressure, to receive the testis. A small transscrotal incision is made and a dartos muscle pouch created (see Fig. 4-9*C*). The testis is then passed into the dartos muscle pouch and fixed with interrupted 3-0 or 4-0 Vicryl suture to prevent testicular retraction (see Fig. 4-9*D*). The scrotal skin wound is closed with interrupted 4-0 plain catgut sutures (see Fig. 4-9*E*). If the floor of the inguinal canal was taken down during the dissection, this is repaired with interrupted 3-0 or 4-0 silk sutures. This step creates a single inguinal ring at the site of the external ring and the pubic tubercle. I have not seen a recurrent hernia when this technique was used. Wound closure is accomplished in the usual manner.

Operation for Incarcerated Hernia

Patients with an incarcerated hernia, toxicity, and obvious intestinal obstruction, or who fail attempts at reduction, require an emergency operation. Physicians should be alert to search for an incarcerated hernia in children who present with signs of intestinal obstruction without a previous laparotomy scar. Careful palpation of the inguinal area may detect a mass caused by a Richter type of inguinal hernia, with a knuckle of the antimesenteric border of the intestine trapped at the internal ring, or, rarely, a Littre hernia, with a Meckel diverticulum strangulated at the internal ring. Infants and children with incarcerated hernias should be given antibiotics (ampicillin, gentamicin, or clindamycin) before operation. A nasogastric tube is inserted, and intravenous volume repletion using crystalloid solution, 20 mL/kg of 5% dextrose in lactated Ringer's solution, is initiated. Monitoring precautions and operating room preparation are similar to those previously noted. The entire abdomen is also pre-

pared with an iodophor solution in case laparotomy is required.

The operation begins through the inguinal area, and the incarcerated intestine must be carefully inspected for viability once the obstruction at the internal ring is relieved. A rapid return of pink color, sheen, peristalsis, and palpable or visible pulsations at the mesenteric border should be observed. A sterile Doppler probe or fluorescein dye may be useful. The odor and nature of the peritoneal fluid should be assessed and cultures obtained for both aerobic and anaerobic organisms. If there is any question regarding intestinal viability, a resection and anastomosis should be carried out, and hernial repair accomplished.

In certain instances, the incarcerated intestine may reduce during surgical manipulation, before the operator has an opportunity to visualize the intestine. If the peritoneal fluid is bloody, malodorous, or cloudy, a counterincision should be made and a formal laparotomy performed to more accurately assess intestinal viability (Fig. 4-10).

An operation for incarcerated hernia may be difficult because of edema, tissue friability, and the presence of the mass, which can obscure the anatomy. The gonad should be carefully inspected because it may become infarcted by vascular compression caused by the incarcerated intestine.[55] The undescended testis is more vulnerable to this complication in the presence of incarcerated intestine (Fig. 4-11).

The preperitoneal approach has been advocated by a number of surgeons as an effective method of managing incarcerated groin hernias.[40,52]

Operation for Sliding Hernia

A *sliding inguinal hernia* is defined as one in which part of the sac wall is a viscous structure. This may involve the cecum, appendix, bladder, sigmoid colon, ovaries, fallopian tubes, and rarely, uterus. These hernias must be recognized to avoid injury to the aforementioned structures. In girls, the ovary and fallopian tube are carefully dissected free and returned to the abdominal cavity before suture ligation of the base of the hernial sac. Because there are no vital structures in the inguinal canal in girls, the internal ring is closed with a figure-of-eight 4-0 silk suture to prevent any possibility of indirect inguinal hernial recurrence. The ovary and fallopian tube may be found in the sac in as many as 15% of hernias in girls. Torsion of the ovary within the sac and ovarian incarceration can also occur. Girls with an irreducible gonad should undergo prompt surgical repair.

In cecal sliding hernia, in which the appendix is in the sac, my associates and I usually attempt to re-

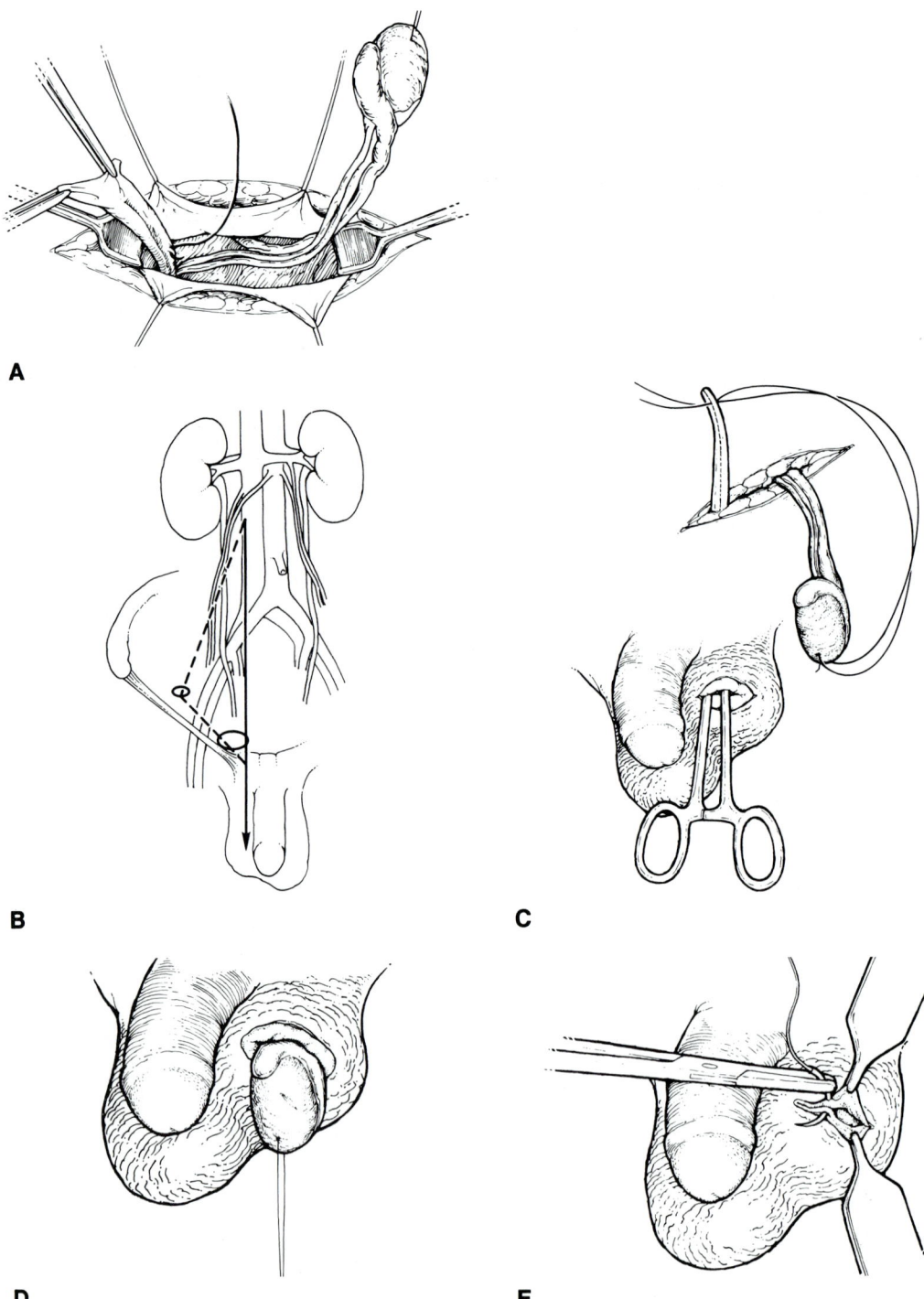

Figure 4-9. (*A*) The hernial sac has been divided and high suture ligation accomplished at the internal ring. The sac division allows significant lengthening of the cord vessels to the cryptorchid testis. (*B*) The added length one can attain by taking down the floor of the inguinal canal and converting the path of the spermatic vessels from a triangular to a straight line course to the scrotum. (*C*) A scrotal incision is placed and a dartos muscle pouch prepared. The cryptorchid testis is brought down using a traction suture. (*D*) Dartos muscle fixation is accomplished using 3-0 chromic catgut suture to prevent testicular retraction. (*E*) The scrotal skin is closed with 4-0 plain catgut, and a collodion dressing is applied.

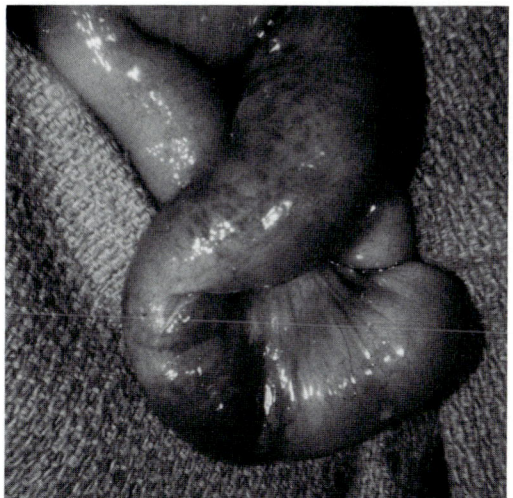

Figure 4-10. A loop of incarcerated intestine that slipped back into the peritoneal cavity before inspection. Laparotomy was performed because of the presence of cloudy, serosanguineous peritoneal fluid. Although the serosa was ecchymotic, a Doppler examination confirmed viability. The infant recovered uneventfully without the need for intestinal resection.

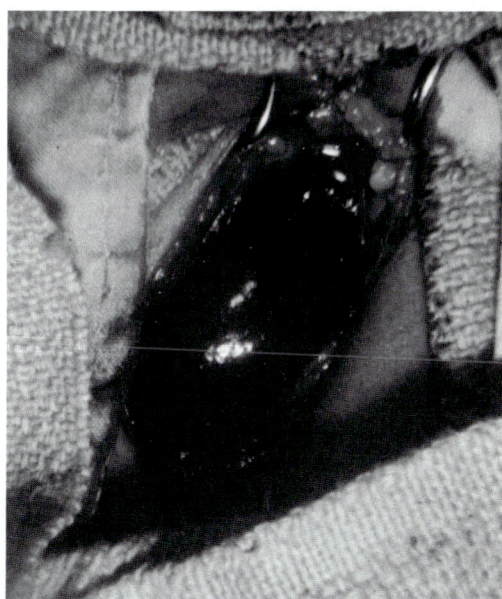

Figure 4-11. This infarcted undescended testis was noted at the time of exploration for an incarcerated inguinal hernia.

duce the appendix into the abdominal cavity rather than risk contamination by performing an inguinal appendectomy.

Contralateral Inguinal Exploration

Although there is unanimity regarding the need to perform early repair of a clinically apparent unilateral inguinal hernia, some controversy exists about the treatment of the contralateral side. Many pediatric surgeons routinely explore the opposite groin because of the great likelihood of a patent processus vaginalis, a potential hernia, being present.[36,63,67,72,73] A few surgeons repair only the clinically obvious side and simply observe the other side.

The natural history of the processus vaginalis was described by Rowe and associates in 1969.[67] In a report concerning more than 2300 hernias, they noted that in 30% of patients, the processus vaginalis disappeared within the first 2 or 3 months of life. In an additional 30%, the processus vaginalis disappeared by the time the child was 2 years of age. Of the remaining 40% of patients with patency, 20% subsequently had a clinically apparent hernia, whereas the other 20% maintained a patent processus vaginalis throughout life (documented by late necropsy) without having any clinical signs of hernia. It is difficult, however, to detect which hernia will fit into which category.

Although a clinically apparent inguinal hernia occurs more frequently on the right side, a patent processus vaginalis is more commonly found on the right side if the unilateral clinical hernia presents on the left. Furthermore, young girls with inguinal hernias more commonly have a contralateral patent processus vaginalis than do boys. The long-term patency rate for girls is 58%, whereas for boys, it is only 42%.[67] Bock and Sobye[2] noted that 47% of infants who underwent unilateral repair in the first year of life required reoperation for a second hernia on the opposite side. This rate was compared with a reoperative rate of only 11% for contralateral hernia in patients undergoing unilateral repair after they were 1 year of age. Similarly, Kiesewetter and Parenzan[41] described a 31% rate of reoperation for contralateral hernia after unilateral hernial repair in patients younger than 2 years of age. More recent reports, however, suggest a relatively lower incidence of subsequent contralateral clinical hernia when only one side is repaired.

My practice is to explore routinely the contralateral side in selected cases, particularly those infants younger than 2 years of age, girls younger than 5 years of age, and patients with a clinically apparent left inguinal hernia. Contralateral exploration is reasonable if the operator is experienced and skilled in performing inguinal hernial repairs in infants, if the anesthesiologist has considerable expertise in administering anesthesia to young infants, and if the patient has no serious underlying condition that increases the risk of an operation. An operation is always performed first on the side with the clinically obvious hernia.

Complications

Complications of inguinal hernial repair are divided into intraoperative and postoperative categories. For experienced pediatric surgeons, the complication rate should be extremely low for elective repair. Injury to the ilioinguinal nerve can usually be avoided by elevating the external oblique fascia before incision. This nerve lies in the cremasteric fascia and passes down through the external ring to give sensory innervation to the base of the penis and scrotum. If the nerve is cut, I usually do not attempt to repair it, and I avoid entrapment during closure. Placing a small silver clip on the cut end prevents neuroma formation.

Injury to the vas deferens is unusual. If divided, the vas should be repaired with interrupted 7-0 monofilament sutures. The use of a magnifying loupe or an operating microscope makes the repair more precise.

Intraoperative bleeding is also an unusual complication unless the floor of the canal is weakened and requires repair. Needle-hole injury to the epigastric vessels or the femoral vein can usually be controlled by withdrawal of the suture and direct pressure. If bleeding continues, however, exposure and direct control may be necessary.

Postoperative complications include wound infection, scrotal hematoma, postoperative hydrocele, and recurrent inguinal hernia. The wound infection rate at most major pediatric centers is low (1%–2%).[36] An increased incidence of infection may be expected in incarcerated hernias.[66] The presence of diaper rash should delay the performance of hernial repair because skin excoriation may be superficially infected, increasing the risk of infectious complications.

Unlike in adults, recurrent inguinal hernia is a relatively uncommon complication in children. Recurrence rates of less than 1% have been reported by experienced pediatric surgeons.[30,36,67] This is compared with a greater than 5% rate of indirect hernial recurrence in adults.[53] Eighty percent of recurrences in children are noted within the first postoperative year.[27] The major causes of recurrent inguinal hernia in infants and children include (1) a missed hernial sac or an unrecognized tear in the peritoneum; (2) a broken suture ligature at the neck of the sac; (3) failure to repair a large internal inguinal ring; (4) injury to the floor of the inguinal canal, resulting in the development of a direct inguinal hernia; (5) severe infec-

tion in the inguinal canal; and (6) increased intraabdominal pressure, as is noted in patients with ascites after ventriculoperitoneal shunts,[28] in children with cystic fibrosis,[32] after previous operation for incarceration,[30] and in patients with connective tissue disorders.[36] Reoperations for recurrent inguinal hernia may be a technical challenge. A preperitoneal operation may be an extremely useful surgical approach in recurrent hernia.[3,19,42]

The finding of a direct inguinal hernia at reoperation usually necessitates a more formal hernial repair by suturing the conjoined tendon to Cooper ligament. Primary direct inguinal hernias in children are relatively rare, representing 0.5% of all groin hernias.[36] Direct inguinal hernias are observed more frequently in boys than in girls and are associated with an increased rate of recurrence.[53] Femoral hernias are also unusual in the pediatric age group and are more frequently noted in girls than in boys.[18,38,48]

Postoperative hydrocele may rarely occur after high ligation of the proximal hernial sac and incomplete excision of the distal portion. To avoid this complication, I usually split the anterior surface of the distal hernial sac and partially resect the anterior and lateral aspects of the sac. The postoperative hydrocele often resolves spontaneously. Although contraindicated before hernial repair, needle aspiration may prove useful in selected instances of resistant postoperative hydrocele. Rarely, long-term persistence of the hydrocele may require a formal hydrocelectomy.

Testicular atrophy has been observed after incarcerated hernias and acute tense hydroceles in young infants. In addition, testicular atrophy has also been noted after severe postoperative scrotal swelling. Such atrophy may be related to ischemia and venous engorgement resulting from tight closure of the internal ring.

SUMMARY

Congenital inguinal hernia is common in infants and children. This anomaly is a high-risk problem caused by an increased rate of incarceration. The incidence of intestinal incarceration and strangulation is greatest in the first few months of life. Inguinal hernia in infants and children should be promptly repaired once the diagnosis has been established. Preterm infants in whom a clinical hernia develops during hospitalization for other neonatal conditions should have their hernia repaired before they are discharged from the hospital. Most full-term infants without underlying comorbid conditions can undergo safe repair on an outpatient basis. Bilateral exploration is reasonable in infants younger than 2 years of age, in girls younger than 5 years of age, and in patients presenting with a left-sided unilateral hernia. For qualified pediatric surgeons and anesthesiologists, the morbidity is low, and the mortality related to hernial repair should be zero.

REFERENCES

1. Bakwin H. Indirect inguinal hernia in twins. J Pediatr Surg 1971;6:165.
2. Bock JE, Sobye JV. Frequency of contralateral inguinal hernia in children. Acta Chir Scand 1970; 136:707.
3. Boley SJ, Kleinhaus SA. A place for the Cheatle-Henry approach in pediatric surgery. J Pediatr Surg 1966;1:394.
4. Brown RK. Hernia diagnosis by transperitoneal probing of the contralateral groin. Surg Gynecol Obstet 1964;118:123.
5. Butsch JL, Kuhn JP. Intramural hematoma of the small bowel: a possible lethal complication of herniography. Surgery 1978;83:121.
6. Clatworthy HW Jr. Routine bilateral herniorrhaphy for infants and children. In: Nyhus LN, Condon RE, eds. Hernia, ed 2. Philadelphia, JB Lippincott, 1978: 132–133.
7. Clausen EG, Jake RJ, Binkley FM. Contralateral inguinal exploration of unilateral hernia in infants and children. Surgery 1958;44:735.
8. Cloud DT, Reed WA, Ford JL, Linkner LM, Trump DS, Dorman GW. The surgicenter: a fresh concept in outpatient pediatric surgery. J Pediatr Surg 1972; 7:206.
9. Conroy JM, Othersen HB Jr, Dorman BH, Gottesman JD, Wallace CT, Brahan NH. A comparison of wound installation and caudal block for analgesia following pediatric inguinal herniorrhaphy. J Pediatr Surg 1993;28:565.
10. Cooney DR. Repair of inguinal hernia in children with ventriculoperitoneal shunts In: Grosfeld JL, ed. Current problems in pediatric surgery. Chicago, Year Book Medical Publishers, 1991:17–28.
11. Coran AG, Eraklis AH. Inguinal hernia in the Hurler-Hunter syndrome. Surgery 1967;61:302.
12. Ducharme JC, Bertrand R, Chocas R. Is it possible to diagnose inguinal hernia by x-ray? J Can Assoc Radiol 1967;18:448.
13. Ducharme JC, Guttman FM, Poljicak M. Hematoma of bowel and cellulitis of the abdominal wall complicating herniography. J Pediatr Surg 1980;15:318.
14. Duckett JW. Treatment of congenital inguinal hernia. Ann Surg 1952;135:879.
15. Erdener A, Mevsim A, Herek O. Abdominoscrotal hydrocele: case report and review of the literature. Pediatr Surg Int 1992;7:398.
16. Fallat ME, Williams WPL, Farmer PG, Hutson JM. Histologic evaluation of inguinoscrotal migration of the gubernaculum in rodents during testicular descent and its relationship to the genitofemoral nerve. Pediatr Surg Int 1992;7:271.
17. Ferguson AH. Oblique inguinal hernia. Typic [*sic*] operation for its radical cure. JAMA 1899;33:6.
18. Fonkalsrud EW, DeLorimier AA, Clatworthy HW. Femoral and direct inguinal hernias in infants and children. JAMA 1965;192:597.
19. Fowler R. Preperitoneal repair of inguinal hernias in infancy and childhood. Aust Pediatr J 1973;9:85.
20. Furman JR, Smith MD. Caudal anesthesia and intravenous sedation for repair of giant bilateral inguinal hernias in a ventilator-dependent premature infant. Anesthesiology 1990;72:573.
21. Gilbert M, Clatworthy HW Jr. Bilateral operation for inguinal hernia and hydrocele in infancy and childhood. Am J Surg 1959;97:255.
22. Gray SW, Skandalakis JE. Embryology for surgeons. Philadelphia, WB Saunders, 1972:417–422.
23. Groff D, Nagaraj HS, Pietsch JB. Inguinal hernias in premature infants operated on before discharge from the neonatal intensive care unit. Arch Surg 1985; 120:962.
24. Grosfeld JL. Management of inguinal hernia and hydrocele in infants and children. J Ind St Med Assoc 1975;68:261.
25. Grosfeld JL. Inguinal hernia and ventriculoperitoneal shunt for hydrocephalus. In: Nyhus LN, Condon RE, eds. Hernia, ed 2. Philadelphia, JB Lippincott, 1978:134–136.
26. Grosfeld JL. Current concepts in inguinal hernia in infants and children. World J Surg 1989;13:506.
27. Grosfeld JL. Inguinal hernia in the premature neonate. In: Grosfeld JL, ed. Current problems in pediatric surgery. Chicago, Year Book Medical Publishers, 1991:3–8.
28. Grosfeld JL, Cooney DR. Inguinal hernia after ventriculoperitoneal shunt for hydrocephalus. J Pediatr Surg 1974;9:311.
29. Grosfeld JL, Cooney DR, Smith J, Campbell RL. Intra-abdominal complications following ventriculoperitoneal shunt procedures. Pediatrics 1974;54:791.
30. Grosfeld JL, Minnick K, Shedd F, West KW, Rescorla FJ, Vane DW. Inguinal hernia in children: factors affecting recurrence in 62 cases. J Pediatr Surg 1991;26:283.
31. Grosfeld JL, Weber TR. Congenital abdominal wall defects: gastroschisis and omphalocele. Curr Probl Surg 1982;19:159.
32. Gross K, DeSanto A, Grosfeld JL, West KW, Eigen H. Intraabdominal complications of cystic fibrosis. J Pediatr Surg 1985;20:431.
33. Gunter JB, Watcha MF, Forestner JE, et al. Caudal epidural anesthesia in conscious premature and high risk infants. J Pediatr Surg 1991;26:9.
34. Harper RC, Carcia A, Sin C. Inguinal hernia: a common problem of premature infants weighing 1000 grams or less at birth. Pediatrics 1975;56:112.
35. Herzfeld G. Hernia in infancy. Am J Surg 1938; 39:422.

36. Holder TM, Ashcraft KW. Groin hernias and hydroceles. In: Holder TM, Ashcraft KW, eds. Pediatric surgery. Philadelphia, WB Saunders, 1980:594–608.

37. Holsclaw DS, Schwachman H. Increased incidence of inguinal hernia, hydrocele and undescended testicles in males with cystic fibrosis. Pediatrics 1971;3:442.

38. Immordino PA. Femoral hernia in infancy and childhood. J Pediatr Surg 1972;7:40.

39. Jewett TC, Kuhn J, Allan JE. Herniography in children. J Pediatr Surg 1976;11:451.

40. Jones PF, Towns GM. An abdominal extraperitoneal approach for the incarcerated inguinal hernia of infancy. Br J Surg 1983;70:719.

41. Kiesewetter WB, Parenzan L. When should hernia in the infant be treated bilaterally? JAMA 1959;171:287.

42. Kleinhaus S, Boley SJ. Recurrent inguinal hernia in children. In: Grosfeld JL, ed. Current problems in pediatric surgery. Chicago, Year Book Medical Publishers, 1991:29–35.

43. Kuhn JP. Herniography in perspective. Am J Dis Child 1977;131:1206.

44. Kurlan MZ, Web PB, Piedad OH. Inguinal herniorrhaphy by the Mitchell Banks technique. J Pediatr Surg 1972;7:427.

45. Ladd WE, Gross RE. Abdominal surgery of infancy and childhood. Philadelphia, WB Saunders, 1941:357–359.

46. Lemeh CB. A study of the development and structural relationships of the testis and gubernaculum. Surg Gynecol Obstet 1960;110:164.

47. Levy JL. Evaluation of transperitoneal probing for detection of contralateral inguinal hernia in infants. Surgery 1972;72:412.

48. Lickley HLA, Trusler GH. Femoral hernia in children. J Pediatr Surg 1966;1:338.

49. Lukash F, Zwiren CT, Andrews HG. Significance of absent vas deferens at herniorrhaphy in infants and children. J Pediatr Surg 1975;10:165.

50. Lynn HG, Johnson WW. Inguinal herniorrhaphy in children. Arch Surg 1961;83:105.

51. MacLennon A. The radical cure of inguinal hernias in children. Br J Surg 1922;9:445.

52. Malangoni MA, Condon RE. Preperitoneal repair of acute incarcerated and strangulated hernias of the groin. Surg Gynecol Obstet 1986;162:65.

53. Marsden AJ. Inguinal hernia: a 3 year review of 2000 cases. Br J Surg 1962;216:384.

54. Melone JH, Schwartz MZ, Tyson RT, et al. Outpatient inguinal herniorrhaphy in premature infants: Is it safe? J Pediatr Surg 1992;27:203.

55. Menardi F, Sauer M. Gangrene of the testis as a complication of incarcerated inguinal hernia in infancy. Z Kinderchir 1975;16:421.

56. Morse TS. Pediatric outpatient surgery. J Pediatr Surg 1972;7:283.

57. Olch PD, Harkins HN. Historical survey of the treatment of inguinal hernias. In: Nyhus LM, Harkins HN, eds. Hernia, ed 1. Philadelphia, JB Lippincott, 1964:1–13.

58. Pergament E, Heimler A, Shah P. Testicular feminization and inguinal hernia. Lancet 1973;2:740.

59. Potts WE, Riker WL, Lewis JE. The treatment of inguinal hernias in infants and children. Ann Surg 1950;132:566.

60. Powell RW. Intraoperative diagnostic pneumoperitoneum in pediatric patients with unilateral inguinal hernias: the Goldstein test. J Pediatr Surg 1985;20:418.

61. Punnett HH, Kistenmacher ML, Toro-Sola M. Testicular feminisation and inguinal hernia. Lancet 1973;2:852.

62. Puri P, Guincy EJ, O'Donnell B. Inguinal hernia in infants: the fate of the testes following incarceration. Pediatr Surg 1984;19:44.

63. Rathauser F. Historical overview of the bilateral approach to pediatric inguinal hernias. Am J Surg 1985;150:527.

64. Rescorla FJ, Grosfeld JL. Inguinal hernia repair in the perinatal period and early infancy: clinical considerations. J Pediatr Surg 1984;19:832.

65. Rothenberg RE, Barnett T. Bilateral herniotomy in infants and children. Surgery 1955;37:947.

66. Rowe MI, Clatworthy HW Jr. Incarcerated and strangulated hernias in children. Arch Surg 1970;101:136.

67. Rowe MI, Copelson LW, Clatworthy HW Jr. The patent processus vaginalis and the inguinal hernia. J Pediatr Surg 1969;4:102.

68. Rowe MI, Marchildon MG. Inguinal hernia and hydrocele in infants and children. Surg Clin North Am 1981;61:1137.

69. Russell RH. Inguinal hernia and operative procedure. Surg Gynecol Obstet 1925;41:605.

70. Sartorelli KH, Abajian JC, Kreutz JM. Improved outcome utilizing spinal anesthesia in high risk infants. J Pediatr Surg 1992;27:1.

71. Snyder WH Jr, Greaney EM Jr. Inguinal hernia. In: Benson CD, Mustard WT, Ravitch MM, Snyder WH Jr, Welch KJ, eds. Pediatric surgery. Chicago, Year Book Medical Publishers, 1962:573.

72. Solomon JR. The practice and implications of contralateral exploration in children with unilateral inguinal hernias. Aust N Z J Surg 1967;37:125.

73. Sparkman RS. Bilateral exploration in inguinal hernia in juvenile patients. Surgery 1962;51:393.

74. Steward DJ. Preterm infants are more prone to complications following minor surgery than are term infants. Anesthesiology 1982;56:304.

75. Turner P. The radical cure of inguinal hernia in children. Proc R Soc Med 1912;5:133.

76. Wang CI, Kwok S, Edelbrock H. Inguinal hernia, hydrocele and other genitourinary abnormalities in boys with cystic fibrosis and their male siblings. Am J Dis Child 1970;119:236.

77. White JJ, Haller JA. Groin hernia in infants and children. In: Nyhus LN, Condon RE, eds. Hernia, ed 2.. Philadelphia, JB Lippincott, 1978:110–121.

78. White JJ, Haller JA, Dorst JB. Congenital inguinal

hernia and inguinal herniography. Surg Clin North Am 1970;50:823.

79. White JJ, Parks LC, Haller JA. The inguinal herniogram: a radiologic aid for accurate diagnosis of inguinal hernia in infants. Surgery 1968;63:991.

Special Comment

Groin Hernia In Infants and Children
C. Everett Koop

Hernias of the groin in infants and children are different in etiology, management, and prognosis from similar hernias found in adults. Hernias in children are frequently associated with hydroceles, which are nonsecreting and exist only because they communicate with the abdominal cavity by means of the patent tunica vaginalis. Such hydroceles can fluctuate in size when there is two-way flow of peritoneal fluid, but on occasion, when flow into the hydrocele is easy but flow out is difficult, the size of the hydrocele may steadily increase. A hernia is usually called to the attention of a parent by the presence of a hydrocele, much less frequently by an actual bulge in the groin caused by protrusion of an abdominal viscus into the patent tunica vaginalis. Scrotal hernias containing bowel are rare. Cryptorchidism, or undescended testicle, is almost always accompanied by an indirect inguinal hernia, and therefore no discussion of hernias in children is complete without consideration of the diagnosis of the hernia associated with an undescended testicle. The examination of the scrotum is the place to begin.

If one side of the scrotum is larger than the other (not meaning the lower left testicle), this leads to the question of which side is abnormal. Asymmetry of the scrotum could mean that one side contains a hydrocele and is therefore larger, or it could mean that one side contains no testis and is therefore smaller. Examination of the corrugations of the skin of the scrotum may be helpful; they are narrower on the side that has never been the domicile of a testicle. The corrugations are important to examine because they are identical on both sides of the scrotum if one testicle is retracted (physiologically) rather than undescended. Eliciting a cremaster reflex is also helpful. Palpation of the scrotum is usually diagnostic. Transillumination of a suspected hydrocele can be misleading because on the rare occasion when there is bowel in a child's hernia, it too may appear translucent.

Hernias in children are either congenital or iatrogenic, usually from previous surgery during which the sac was not properly ligated or an adult-like (unnecessary) repair was done without understanding the special nature of a juvenile hernia and the needless concern about adequate repair. Simple ligation of the hernial sac as high as possible is sufficient treatment for indirect inguinal hernias in children.

HYDROCELES

A hydrocele is merely the collection of fluid in the bottom of the hernial sac. Therefore, a hydrocele may be a physiologic phenomenon if the processus vaginalis closed before birth, trapping peritoneal fluid in the scrotal portion of the patent processus vaginalis. If this is the case, the trapped fluid will be resorbed, and the hydrocele will disappear slowly but uniformly over a period of about 3 months. It is usually safe to say that a hydrocele in an infant older than 4 months of age is indicative of a hernia. Hydroceles in children are not secreting lesions.

If a hydrocele in a child older than 4 months of age visibly changes in size so that the parents notice it, such change is not caused by absorption and secretion, but can only represent fluid entering and leaving the patent processus vaginalis, which indicates an indirect inguinal hernia. A hydrocele that is first noticed as a small swelling and then on repeated examination increases in size is an indication that the fluid of the abdomen is finding its way into the processus vaginalis, but not finding its way out. Therefore, a fairly safe rule is that a hydrocele that enlarges, fluctuates in size, or is present in a child older than 4 months of age is indicative of the presence of an indirect inguinal hernia—a congenital defect.

The embryology behind all this is helpful. About 3 to 4 weeks before expected delivery, the left processus vaginalis normally closes. About 7 to 10 days later, the right processus vaginalis follows suit. Therefore, it is logical to expect that if a newborn or young infant has a visible or palpable hernia on the left side, a similar lesion on the right is likely, even if it is not seen or palpated. The contrary is not necessarily true. Obviously, in babies born prematurely or babies born with low birthweight, indirect inguinal hernias are more commonly found than in larger newborns.

Hydrocele of the spermatic cord is a cystic lesion usually not freely movable, palpable between the pubic tubercle and the internal inguinal ring. It is nothing more than encapsulated fluid in the tunica vaginalis. Such a hydrocele almost always indicates the presence of an indirect inguinal hernia and almost certainly does so in a child older than 4 months of age. Hydroceles of the tunica vaginalis in girls frequently form an encysted mass in the inguinal canal. Although they carry the traditional name of *hydroceles of the canal of Nuck,* the term really refers to hydroceles of the patent processus vaginalis.

INDIRECT INGUINAL HERNIA

It is simple to diagnose an inguinal hernia of the indirect variety if it contains abdominal viscera—usually bowel in the male, the ovary in the female. Such hernias are relatively rare. As one becomes familiar with palpation of the spermatic cord in male infants, an increased thickness of the cord is not difficult to detect. Another sign, relied on by astute diagnosticians, is the so-called silk sign or silk-glove sign, which the examiner can elicit by gently stroking the spermatic cord at right angles to its long axis with a finger. If a hernia is present, the trained finger can usually detect the slippery sensation produced by rubbing the tunica vaginalis on itself. The adult technique of examining for an inguinal hernia where the scrotum is inverted and the palpating finger feels an impulse or an enlargement of the external inguinal ring is not reliable in children. Indeed, it can be misleading; a youngster can have a large external ring and no hernia or a large hernia and no enlargement of the external ring.

OTHER HERNIAS

Congenital direct inguinal hernias are relatively rare in children. When they exist, most are iatrogenic from previous surgery on an indirect hernia where the posterior wall of the canal was damaged and not recognized or not repaired. In a patient with a history of a previous indirect inguinal herniography, with the bulge closer to the pubis and the midline than the expected line of the spermatic cord, a direct hernia is the best bet.

Femoral hernias are even more rare than direct hernias and frequently are misdiagnosed before operation. Many can be readily palpated in the femoral triangle below the inguinal ligament, but others bulge above the inguinal ligament, leading to the misdiagnosis.

Indirect inguinal hernias in girls are almost always sliding, with the viscus attached to the wall of the tunica vaginalis being the ovary. Sometimes, the blood supply is splayed out across the circumference of the tunica. Many times, the bulge in a girl's groin is an incarcerated ovary. The ovary exits through the internal ring into the patent processus vaginalis and cannot readily return. Fortunately, the blood supply is seldom damaged. Unless the ovary is necrotic, it should be replaced within the abdomen.

INCARCERATED INDIRECT INGUINAL HERNIAS

Children with incarcerated inguinal hernias usually exhibit systemic signs of early intestinal obstruction. Incarcerated hernias seldom require immediate surgical correction. Relaxation is the most essential part of reducing an incarceration. The simplest way to achieve this is to have the infant's mother rock the infant in a chair during feeding. More often than not, the incarcerated bowel slips back unnoticed into the peritoneal cavity. Surgical repair then can be undertaken at one's leisure.

Frequently, an incarcerated hernia diagnosed by a referring physician reduces itself en route to the hospital just because the child is relaxed in the jostling motion of the automobile.

Manual reduction is simple and should be learned to avoid the unnecessary emergency operation on an incarcerated hernia. First, two fingers, such as the index and thumb of one hand, are brought together at the tips and placed above the internal ring, creating a barrier above the ring to prevent the incarcerated bowel from slipping up over the abdominal wall. Second, inasmuch as the incarcerated bowel in children is usually filled with liquid and gas, the gas can be emptied by placing the thumb and forefinger of the other hand over the mass and opening and closing the two sets of fingers alternately so that the gas and liquid is pushed into the belly and the size of the bowel reduced. Usually, without further effort, the emptied bowel slides back into the abdomen.

Simplicity is the key to success in the management of hernias of the groin in infants and children. The diagnosis is simple, reduction of an incarceration when present is simple, the surgery should be kept simple, and after repair, which should not take more than a few minutes, the child can be sent home on complete activity without external sutures or bandages.

Hernia, Fourth Edition, edited
by Lloyd M. Nyhus and Robert E. Condon.
J.B. Lippincott Company, Philadelphia © 1995.

Chapter 5

The Marcy Repair of Indirect Inguinal Hernia: 1870 to the Present

Charles A. Griffith

In 1871 I first published in the *Boston Medical and Surgical Journal* two cases, operated upon by me in the previous year, in which I closed the [internal] ring with interrupted sutures of carbolized cat-gut, followed by permanent cure. So far as yet I know they were the first cases operated upon in this manner.

H.O. Marcy, 1881

HENRY ORLANDO MARCY (1837–1924)

Amherst College and Harvard Medical School; surgeon, Union Army, Civil War; student of Virchow, Paget, Wells, and Lister; unaffiliated private practitioner, Cambridge, Massachusetts; first advocate in Boston area of Lister's doctrine of antisepsis and Lister's carbolized catgut sutures; first surgeon-author to describe the "radical cure" of hernia at the internal ring; rebuffed by Bigelow and all other Boston surgeons for these methods; president of gynecologic section at 9th International Medical Congress, 1887; President of American Medical Association, 1892; reclaimed marshland from Charles River bank for construction of Massachusetts Institute of Technology; instrumental in building the Harvard Bridge, renovating the Charles River Basin, and designing Esplanade Parkway; honorary A.M. from Amherst College and L.L.D. from Wesleyan University.

Since the last edition of this book (ed 3, 1989), the herniorrhaphists have become more outspoken and frequent in citing national statistics that compare their rates of recurrent inguinal hernia with those of general surgeons. After primary inguinal repair, the recurrent rate for herniorrhaphists is 1% versus 5% for general surgeons; after repair of recurrent hernias, the same rates are 10% for herniorrhaphists versus 25% for surgeons.[2] These statistics are not confined to large, complex, and difficult hernias (as some might surmise), but include so-called simple indirect inguinal hernias as well. I first suspected that a simple indirect hernia is not so simple some 50 years ago—the era of World War II—while serving a term of duty at a large military hospital (Madigan Army). Many of the patients were young soldiers with indirect inguinal hernias, and among these patients, the numbers with indirect recurrences after operations in childhood were high. Similarly, in the 1950s at the Seattle Veterans Administration Hospital, many of

the hernias were indirect recurrences after operations done some 10 years earlier during World War II.

THE REPAIR

The Marcy repair of indirect inguinal hernia entails high ligation of the sac plus closure of the internal ring with only transversalis fascia (Fig. 5-1). This exclusive use of transversalis fascia distinguishes the Marcy repair from all other inguinal repairs that use the inguinal ligament and demands a dissection that accurately exposes, identifies, and closes the internal ring as a distinct anatomic entity. The resultant repair is the same as the preperitoneal repair described in Chapters 7 and 8. Only by using transversalis fascia with the Marcy repair and the preperitoneal techniques (or both) can general surgeons eliminate the aforementioned disparity enjoyed by herniorrhaphists regarding hernia recurrence.

CLOSING THE INTERNAL RING VERSUS REPAIRIING THE INGUINAL CANAL

Bassini and Halsted used transversalis fascia plus the more superficial inguinal ligament and musculoaponeuroses to close the internal ring for indirect hernia and the inguinal canal for direct hernia. Their techniques, however, were subsequently modified by other surgeons who had the idea of "repairing the inguinal canal," which focused attention on exactly *what* musculoaponeurosis should be sutured to the inguinal ligament and exactly *how* it should be sutured, with or without transposing the cord and with or without imbricating the external oblique aponeurosis. These details of repairing the canal gradually, and in some in-

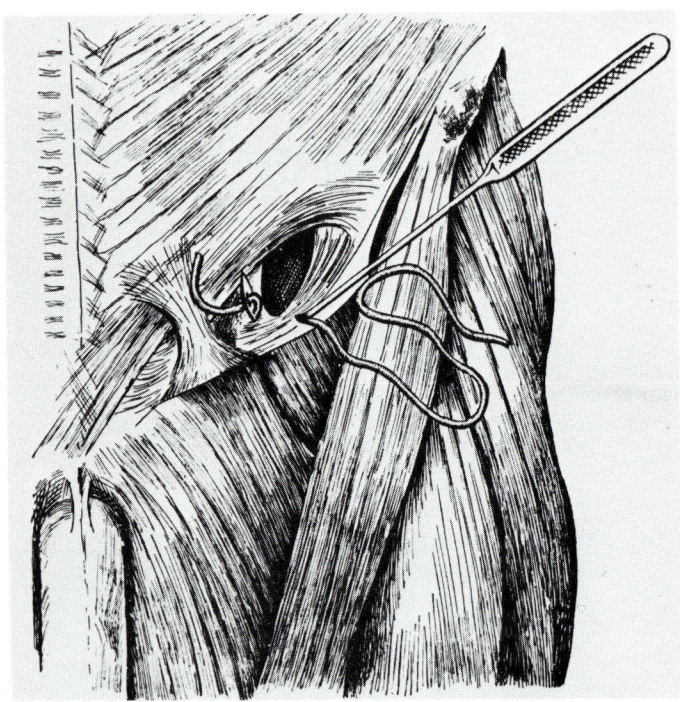

Figure 5-1. The Marcy operation. The needle passes through the transversalis fascia, "the first stitch taken for the closure of the internal ring from below upward, in order to reform the inguinal canal." In this illustration, Marcy elected to demonstrate the transversalis fascia by removing the inguinal ligament and abdominal muscles. His purpose was to prove that he closed the internal ring and not the external ring (as many of his critics claimed, and some still do). (Marcy HO. The anatomy and surgical treatment of hernia, New York, Appleton, 1892)

stances completely, detracted from the details of using transversalis fascia to close the internal ring. The result was, and still is, indirect inguinal recurrence. The recurrent sac herniates through the *unrepaired* ring and proceeds along the *repaired* canal, usually beneath whatever has been sutured to the inguinal ligament.

THE AUTHOR'S AND EDITORS' EXPERIENCE: TERMINOLOGY

During my early surgical training with a modified Bassini technique, I learned how to repair the inguinal canal but did not learn how to expose or close the internal ring. The editors of this book (Nyhus and Condon) experienced the same problem. Of equal, if not more, importance, we did not recognize this deficiency in our training until we did anatomic dissections with simultaneous exposure of the ring from above through the abdominal cavity and from below through the inguinal canal.*

---

*Although Marcy, Bassini, and Halsted removed part or all of the cremaster muscle, specific emphasis on this technical detail in the voluminous literature is rare. This lack stems from the idea of repairing the canal, which can be done easily by suturing something to the inguinal ligament without removing the cremaster muscle. Thus, many surgeons still fumble through and around the cremaster (as the editors and I once did) without getting a good look at the ring. The trouble lies in the fact that these fumblers *think* they can see the ring. I cannot, particularly in muscular young men.[4]

In my case, the late General Clinton S. Lyter, MC, UAS taught me the Marcy repair at Madigan in the 1940s but attached no name to it. The repair remained nameless to me for some 20 years until I visited Sheffield, England in the 1960s to see "Jimmy" Lytle, one of Great Britain's leaders (if not *the* leader) in the field of hernia. Lytle taught me what I know about Marcy and what he did. Lytle had much to do with the popularity of the term *Marcy repair* in Britain and emphasized two points. First, all four of Marcy's papers,[9–12] from 1871 to 1887, predate those of Bassini and Halsted. Second, scrutiny of Figure 5-1 confirms that Marcy closed the internal and not the external ring.

General Lyter's lessons in the operating room were complemented by my gross dissections in the morgue of the lower abdomen and inguinal areas above and below the internal ring. These dissections were supervised by Robert Johnson, Professor of Anatomy at the University of Washington and consultant to Madigan. Whereas the inguinal phases of the dissections revealed definite obstacles to the internal ring (eg, the cremaster muscle, the inguinal ligament, and the shelving edges of the internal oblique and the transverses abdominis muscles), I failed to appreciate the relatively clearer approach to the internal ring and entire inguinal floor from above, as did the editors in their subsequent and independent dissections of the intraabdominal and preperitoneal approaches. Thus, while I stayed with the Marcy repair, the editors wisely devised their preperitoneal techniques (see Chap. 8).

THE INTERNAL RING

To present a workable anatomic concept, highlights from Chapter 2 are summarized. The entire peritoneal cavity is encased by a continuous sheet of endoabdominal fascia. The transversalis and iliac components of endoabdominal fascia in the groin exist alone and separate from their intrinsic muscles (the transversus abdominis and iliopsoas). Transversalis fascia (the site of inguinal hernias) and iliac fascia (the site of femoral hernias) fuse to form the dense iliopubic tract. The fallacy expressed by some that the iliopubic tract does not exist stems from the fact that it lies hidden from view beneath the inguinal ligament and can be exposed only by retracting the ligament.

The Hole

As the iliopubic tract is a thickening of endoabdominal fascia, so is the internal ring a thickening of transversalis fascia. The medial thickening is the interfoveolar ligament of Hesselbach, which joins the superomedial and inferolateral crural thickenings (pillars) to form a horseshoe. Thinner transversalis fascia at the open end of the horseshoe completes the ring. In the presence of an indirect inguinal hernia, the internal ring is the hole in the abdominal wall through which the indirect sac herniates (Fig. 5-2).

Surgical Exposure

The ring may be exposed by three anatomic routes: the transabdominal, the preperitoneal, and the inguinal. Whichever route is used, repair of the ring is the same (Fig. 5-3).

REPAIR FROM ABOVE: THE TRANSABDOMINAL AND PREPERITONEAL APPROACHES

It may rarely happen to the operator, who has opened the abdomen for some other purpose, to find the complication of hernia. When the section has been made considerably large, as in the removal of a large tumor, the internal abdominal ring is within reach of the surgeon. Upon reflection, it would naturally occur to any operator that under these conditions it is better to close the internal ring, and reform the smooth internal parietal surface from within by means of suturing.

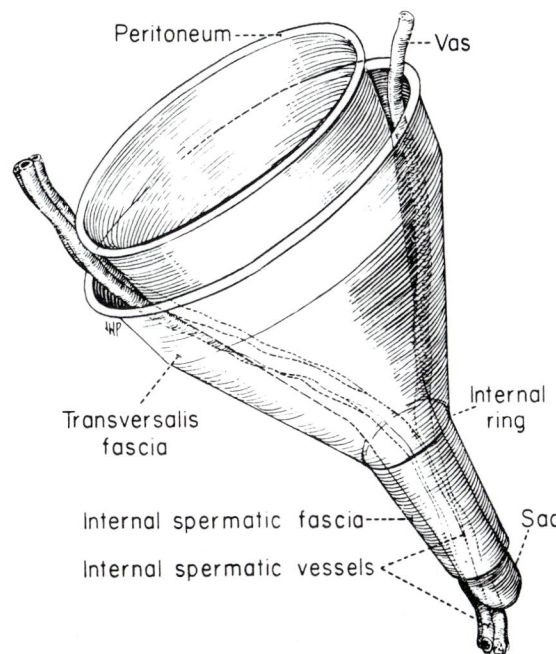

Figure 5-2.   The anatomic concept of indirect inguinal hernia. The internal spermatic vessels, vas deferens, and indirect sac leave the abdomen and enter the inguinal canal at the internal ring. At this point, the transversalis fascia funnels around the vessels, vas, and sac to form the internal ring. From the internal ring, the transversalis fascia continues as the internal spermatic fascia, which encases the vessels, vas, and sac in the inguinal canal.

My friend, Dr. N. Bozeman, of New York, easily did this at my suggestion in a case of ovariotomy more than ten years ago.—H.O. Marcy, 1892

Even now it is clearly recognized that the most efficient way to close a hernial ring is from within. If one is performing any laparotomy in the neighborhood, a few stitches in the peritoneum and fascia are far more effectual than any other herniotomy. One has the feeling he is really sewing up a hole and not going through the motions of a complicated plastic operation.—E. Andrews, 1924

Deliberate and routine removal of the hernial sac from within the peritoneal cavity was introduced by LaRoque,[5] who referred to his technique as the *intraabdominal* or *combined inguinoabdominal method.* The first phase of the LaRoque operation consists of a conventional inguinal incision and dissection of the sac out of the inguinal canal; but instead of performing high ligation by this conventional inguinal exposure, LaRoque entered the abdomen above the internal ring (Fig. 5-4). This muscle-splitting transabdominal approach to the hernial sac constitutes the second phase of the LaRoque operation.

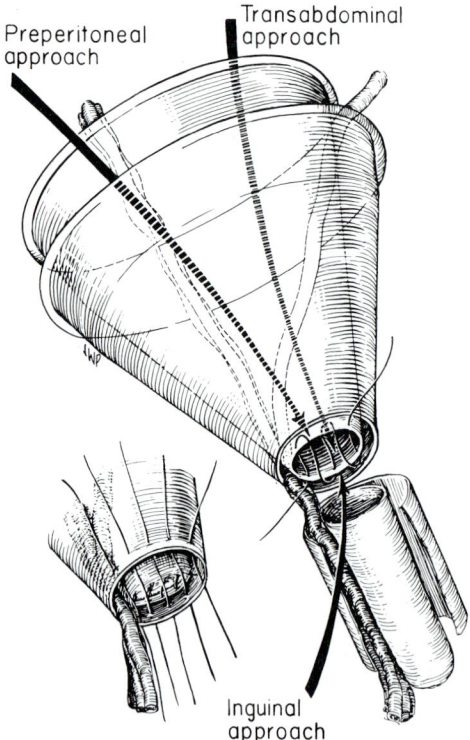

Preperitoneal approach

Transabdominal approach

Inguinal approach

Figure 5-3. The surgical concept of indirect inguinal hernia. The arrows indicate the transabdominal, the preperitoneal, and the inguinal approaches to the internal ring. In the inguinal approach, the spout of the funnel (internal spermatic fascia) is incised longitudinally to expose the sac and cord structures (vas deferens and internal spermatic vessels). The spout of the funnel is next incised circumferentially at its junction with the wide mouth of the funnel to define the internal ring as a hole in the transversalis fascia. The sac is then dissected and removed, and the peritoneum is sutured above the internal ring within the funnel of transversalis fascia. This is high ligation. The internal ring is then closed to cover the peritoneum with its normal encasement of transversalis fascia. This is a fascial repair of the internal ring, which is the normal anatomic keystone that makes the repair strong enough to prevent recurrence of the indirect hernia.

LaRoque's principal consideration in advocating the transabdominal approach was the absolute assurance of accomplishing high ligation by removing the hernial sac from within the abdomen. However, rather than closing the internal ring and peritoneum from within the abdomen, as suggested by Marcy, LaRoque returned to his inguinal dissection to "repair the inguinal canal."

The ease of entering the abdomen after starting the inguinal approach often facilitates (1) feasible intraabdominal procedures (eg, prophylactic appendectomy), (2) resection of strangulated intestine and omentum, and (3) reduction of large sliding hernias

of the cecum, sigmoid, fallopian tube, and ovary. Also, as noted in the legend to Figure 5-4, entering the preperitoneal and retroperitoneal spaces offers essentially two advantages. The first is to avoid extensive scar tissue in the inguinal canals of patients with recurrent hernias. The second is to mobilize the internal spermatic vessels in instances of cryptorchidism, particularly when not enough has been gained by freeing the vessels from the internal spermatic fascia and transplanting the internal ring medially.

REPAIR FROM BELOW: THE INGUINAL APPROACH OR MARCY OPERATION

Draw up the peritoneal pouch quite sufficient to cause its obliteration upon the inner side and sew it evenly. . . . Then cut away the redundant pouch and allow the peritoneum to drop back. . . . With the finger within the ring, to protect the peritoneum and guide the needle, I introduce it quite one half inch from the outer portion of the ring. . . . The stitches are repeated at distances of about one third of an inch, including both pillars of the ring, until the opening is securely closed—in the female completely . . . in the male, the parts are closed so as to carefully protect and secure the cord from injury.—H.O. Marcy, 1887

Thin young men are the ideal patients for demonstrating the Marcy repair. The same technique applies to infants and children with dilated internal rings. In middle-aged and older patients with larger indirect plus direct inguinal hernias, the internal ring is closed as part of a more extensive repair.

Removal of the Cremaster Muscle

The technique described below is used in men whose cremaster muscle is well developed. The procedure is usually unnecessary in infants, children, and women.

In the inguinal canal, the cremaster and internal oblique muscles are invested and bound together by a common thin fascia. One can display this fascia by grasping the cremaster at about the level of the external ring and pulling it away from the internal oblique muscle. Incising the stretched-out fascia with knife or scissors results in a clean separation of the cremaster from the internal oblique muscle.

Elevation of the cremaster now reveals that a thin sheet of fascia anchors it to the iliopubic tract, which is exposed by sharp downward retraction of the inguinal ligament. Incising this thin fascial sheet along the iliopubic tract completely mobilizes the cremaster and cord (see Fig. 5-4).

With continued retraction of the inguinal ligament, the surgeon incises the cremaster muscle lon-

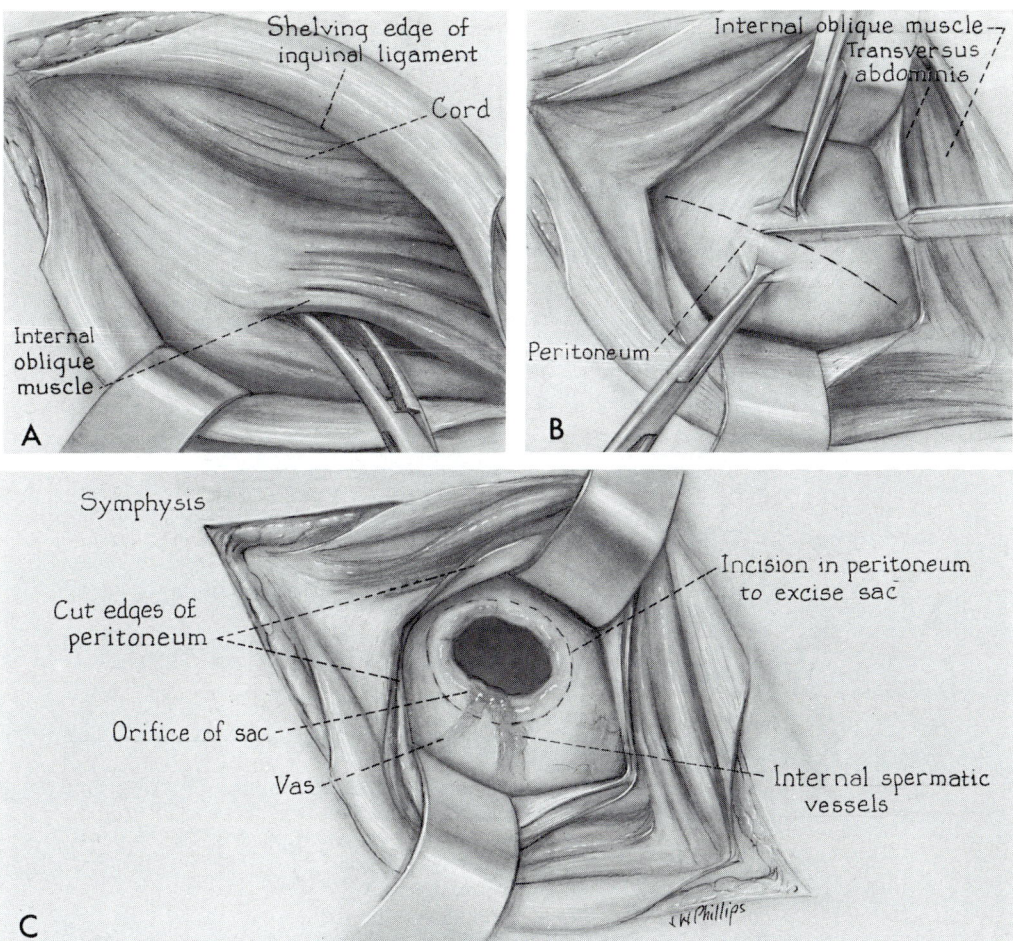

Figure 5-4.   The LaRoque operation. (*A*) The upper flap of the external oblique aponeurosis has been reflected superiorly to expose the internal oblique muscle. Forceps are splitting the internal oblique and transversus abdominis muscles (about 3 cm above the free arcuate edge of the internal oblique muscle) to expose the peritoneum above the internal ring. (*B*) The peritoneum is exposed. Dotted lines indicate the incision through the peritoneum. (*C*) Orifice of the hernial sac exposed from within the peritoneal cavity. Dotted lines indicate incision of the peritoneum around the orifice of the sac to remove the sac from the inguinal canal. Rather than incise the peritoneum, as in (*B*), the surgeon may reflect the intact peritoneum to gain access to the preperitoneal and retroperitoneal spaces.

gitudinally and dissects it from the cord in two segments—a lower and an upper flap (Fig. 5-5). The lower flap is removed by an incision separating the fascial origin of the cremaster muscle from the iliopubic tract. This incision necessarily transects the external spermatic (cremasteric) vessels, which, as described later, are useful landmarks for finding fascia to repair the internal ring. Excision of the upper flap of the cremaster from the internal oblique permits optimal retraction of the internal oblique–transversus abdominis arcuate edge for exposure of the ring superiorly.

Location of the Internal Ring

A common mistake at this stage of the operation is the separation of the sac from the cord structures by a blunt dissection (wiping with a sponge) that destroys fascial relations and landmarks. Instead, the sac and cord structures are handled as a unit that emerges through the internal ring and lies within the sheath of internal spermatic fascia. This sheath is incised longitudinally to permit dissection of the sac. Preserving the internal spermatic fascia as a sheath provides two advantages. First, tracing the sheath proximally leads

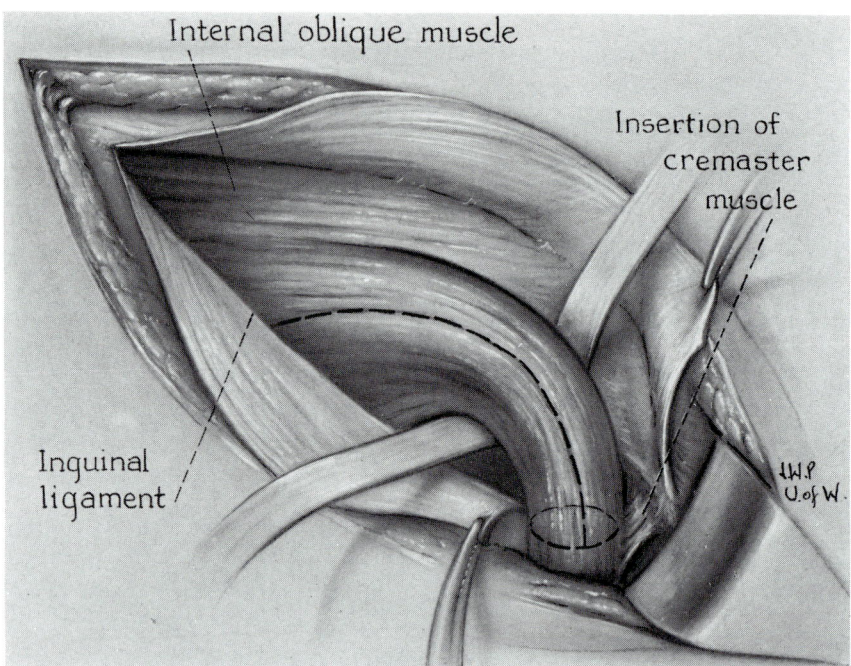

Figure 5-5. The mobilized cord. Cremasteric fibers depart from the internal oblique muscle, descend around the spermatic cord, encircle the testicle, and then ascend to insert on the pubis just below the pubic insertion of the arcuate fibers of internal oblique muscle. Thus, the so-called medial head of origin of the cremaster muscle from the pubis is actually its insertion. Dotted lines indicate proposed incisions through the cremaster muscle for its removal. The ilioinguinal and iliohypogastric nerves are not shown. (Griffith CA. Inguinal hernia: an anatomic-surgical correlation. Surg Clin North Am 1959;39:531)

directly to the transversalis fascia and internal ring. Second, incising the sheath circumferentially starts the dissection for defining the margins of the ring (Fig. 5-6).

The next common mistake is the ligation of the sac before the internal ring is separated from the peritoneum. If this mistake is made, particularly if the suture of ligation includes transversalis fascia, the ring retracts into the abdomen with the sutured peritoneum after the sac is excised. To prevent this error, the transversalis fascia must be completely separated from the peritoneum above the neck of the sac and secured within the surgical field by clamps before the sac is ligated (Fig. 5-7). During this dissection, the vas deferens and internal spermatic vessels are separated from both the peritoneum and the transversalis fascia, and occasionally from each other, above the ring. In other words, as written by Lytle:[6,8]

The chief difficulty is to find the internal ring at operations, for if the routine method of removing the sac is followed, the ring with the stump of the sac retracts back into the abdomen and disappears from view. When the hernial sac has been dissected free from the cord, the ring can, however, be brought into full view by pressing it forward with the index finger which has been passed through the neck of the opened sac. The ring edge is then easily secured in artery forceps and its medial and lateral pillars are separated from the neck of the sac and from the spermatic cord. To expose, secure and separate the ring margins in this way, is the most important step in the operation.

The Fascia Worthy of Suture

The ease or difficulty of finding transversalis fascia worthy of suture to reconstruct the internal ring depends on how much the ring has been stretched by the sac. When the neck of the sac and the ring are relatively small, strong and tough fascia is present in the immediate surgical field. In contrast, when a large sac has stretched the ring to a hole that admits two or more fingers, further dissection and retraction are required to find worthy fascia. Medially, and encasing the inferior epigastric vessels, the transversalis fascia thickens to form the ligament of Hesselbach. Traction on a clamp applied to this ligament stretches out the superomedial and inferolateral crura and facilitates their identification. Superiorly, exposure of worthy fascia (the crus) requires firm retraction of the inter-

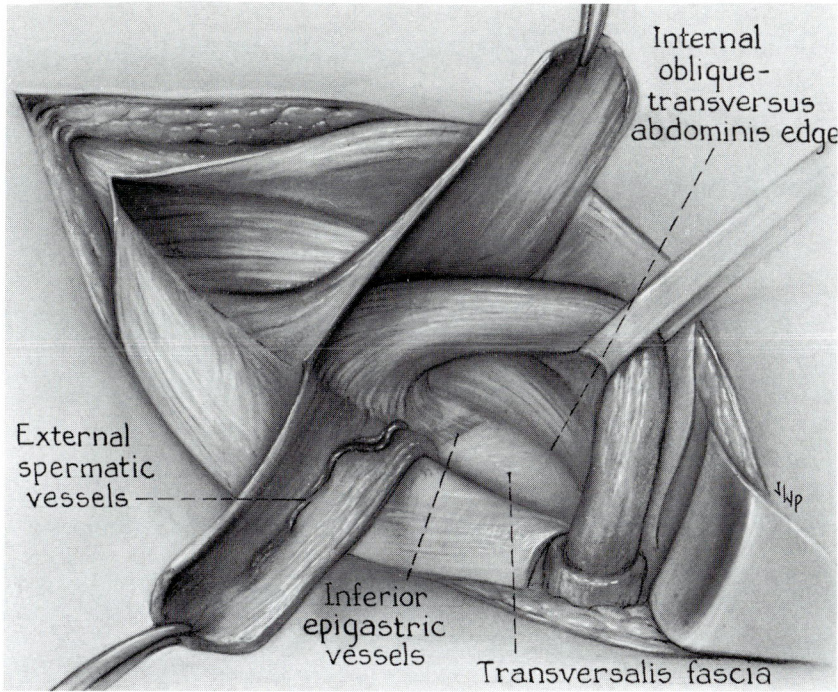

Figure 5-6. Removal of the cremaster muscle. The cremaster muscle is being removed in two segments after complete circumferential amputation distally. It has been halved by two longitudinal incisions from this point proximally, one incision on top of the cord and the other behind it. The upper half is split from the internal oblique muscle. The lower half is cut from its fascial origin, through which the external spermatic (cremasteric) vessels run to the cremaster muscle. The internal spermatic fascia remains on the cord. Note how the transversalis fascia funnels around the cord at the internal ring and continues as the internal spermatic fascia. (Griffith CA. Inguinal hernia: an anatomic-surgical correlation. Surg Clin North Am 1959;39:531)

nal oblique–transversus abdominis arcuate edge. Occasionally, the arcuate edge must be rolled upward with clamps. The superomedial crus is brought into the field and secured with a clamp. Inferiorly, the fascial origin of the cremaster muscle (containing the ligated external spermatic vessels) is continuous with the iliopubic tract, the anterior femoral sheath, and the inferolateral crus of the ring. Traction on the cremaster's fascial origin with a clamp and downward retraction of the inguinal ligament are essential for optimal exposure. The clamps on the crura and the ligament of Hesselbach are left in place to keep the internal ring within the surgical field.

High Ligation

As noted in Figure 5-3, the term *high ligation* means ligating the sac *above* the internal ring so that the ring's transversalis fascial edges may be sutured *below*

the ligated sac. Accordingly, identification of the internal ring as the anatomic landmark is a prerequisite for determining where the sac should be ligated.

The sac is opened with care to avoid entering the contents of any sliding hernia that may be present (cecum, sigmoid, fallopian tube, ovary, bladder, or bladder diverticulum). Digital exploration is done to find any associated femoral or direct inguinal hernia. If prophylactic appendectomy is an incidental objective, and the appendix cannot be exposed through the hernial sac, the abdomen may be entered (see Fig. 5-4).

The peritoneum is closed by any convenient method. I usually use a transfixion suture through the twisted neck of a narrow sac and a running suture for a sac with a wide neck. In regard to the sac of a sliding hernia, complicated techniques of creating peritoneal flaps have been devised to perform a high ligation in the conventional sense. With a proper repair of the internal ring, these techniques are no longer consid-

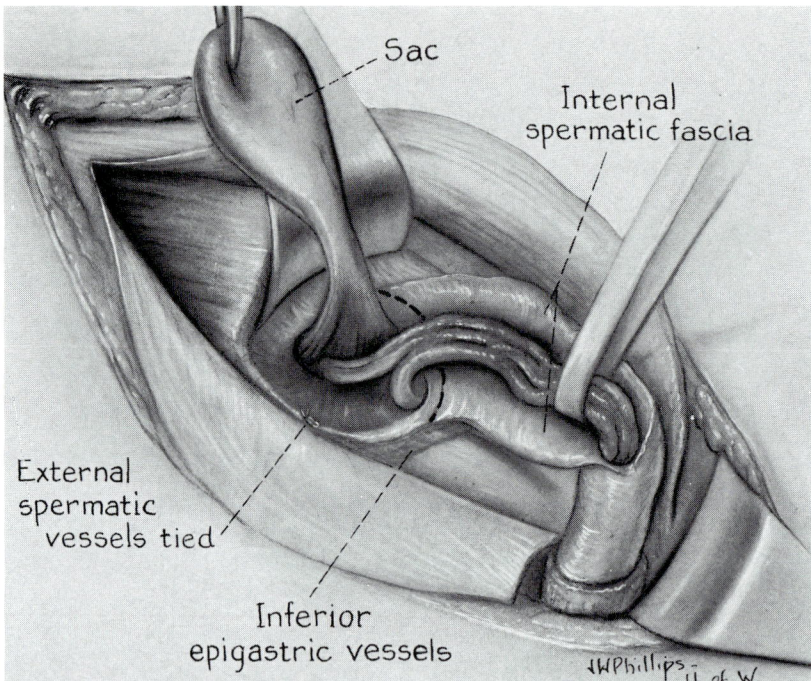

Figure 5-7. Exposure of the internal ring. The cremaster muscle has been removed. Note the tied external spermatic artery and the fascia adjacent to this artery. The internal ring is exposed by superolateral retraction of the internal oblique and transversus abdominis muscles. The internal spermatic fascia has been opened longitudinally to permit dissection of the sac and cord structures. The vas and vessels have been freed from the sheath of internal spermatic fascia and encircled with a Penrose drain. The fascia has been removed from the sac superolaterally to define this aspect of the internal ring. It is cut (as indicated by the dotted line) to define the medial margin of the internal ring. (Griffith CA. Inguinal hernia: an anatomic-surgical correlation. Surg Clin North Am 1959;39:531)

ered necessary. The sliding sac is simply reduced and kept in place by the closed ring.

Motility of the Ring

At this stage of the operation, if it is done under local anesthesia and the patient coughs on request, the surgeon may demonstrate why the transversalis fascial edges of the internal ring should not be sutured to the inguinal ligament. The sudden contraction of the transversus abdominis muscle is transmitted to its intrinsic transversalis fascia and literally jerks the internal ring out of the inguinal canal to a position beneath this muscle's arcuate edge. In addition, the patulous ring at rest is abruptly transformed into a narrow slit by the oblique pull of the transversus abdominis fibers, which are oblique in the inguinal region. Once this motility of the ring is observed, it is easy to appreciate that the transversus muscle is powerful

enough to tear its transversalis fascia through any sutures anchoring it to the inguinal ligament.†

Evaluation of the Inguinal Floor

Digital exploration through the hernial sac, as previously mentioned, does not permit direct palpation of the transversalis fascia because peritoneum and pre-

---

† These changes in the position and shape of the ring provide a valvular function that protects against hernia.[6,8] In response to the denial of this function on the basis that an indirect inguinal sac is always congenital, if such is indeed the case, the ring prevents herniation of abdominal contents into the congenital sac of the patient whose hernia is not apparent at birth but becomes apparent a few to many years after birth. With regard to preventing indirect recurrence at the time of operation, the motility and protective function of the ring are preserved by the Marcy repair and destroyed by immobilizing the ring with sutures that transfix it to the inguinal ligament.

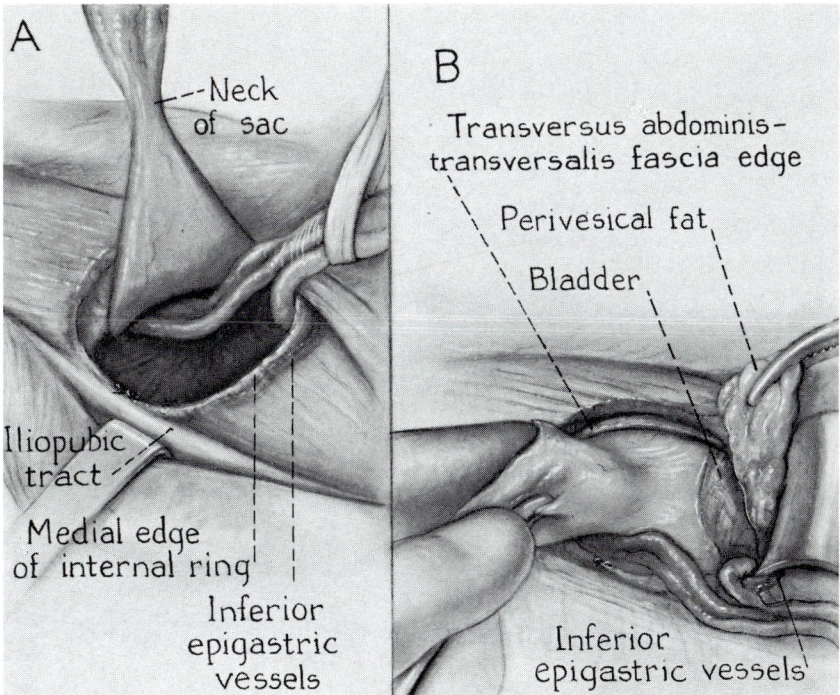

Figure 5-8. Identification of the internal ring. (*A*) The vas and vessels have been separated from the peritoneum posteriorly. The vas turns medially while the vessels continue upward. Note how the neck of the sac is freed and pulled beyond the internal ring for ligation well above the neck. The medial boundary of the internal ring is well defined after removal of the internal spermatic fascia. The iliopubic tract is exposed by downward retraction of the inguinal ligament. The iliopubic tract blends with that fascia adjacent to the ligated external spermatic artery. (*B*) The retractor inserted into the internal ring pulls the medial edge of the internal ring and inferior epigastric vessels medially. The sac is opened, and a finger inserted into the sac pulls the peritoneum out. The perivesical fat is dissected from the peritoneum to expose bladder muscle. Although this exposure of bladder is rare in children and young men, it is not rare in older men with concomitant direct inguinal hernia, particularly when the direct sac is converted into the indirect sac by the Hoguet maneuver and the "bladder" is actually a diverticulum of the bladder. (Griffith CA. Inguinal hernia: an anatomic-surgical correlation. Surg Clin North Am 1959; 39:531)

peritoneal fat are between the finger and the fascia. A more accurate method entails insertion of the finger through the internal ring into the preperitoneal space (Figs. 5-8 and 5-9).

The so-called inguinal shutter, as well as the integrity of the transversalis fascia, is evaluated. It comes into play when the internal oblique–transversus abdominis arcuate edge apposes the iliopubic tract and the inguinal ligament. By virtue of the fact that the arcuate edge varies in height, the efficiency of the shutter also varies; that is, the higher the arcuate edge, the less efficient is the shutter with less protection against direct herniation. Optimal evaluation is obtained by seeing and feeling the shutter when the patient coughs.

Closure of the Ring

The internal ring is closed with displacement of the cord structures laterally. The Marcy repair is now complete (Fig. 5-10).

Nothing can be added to this repair with the idea of preventing an *indirect* recurrence. Prevention of the development of a *direct* hernia is an entirely different matter.

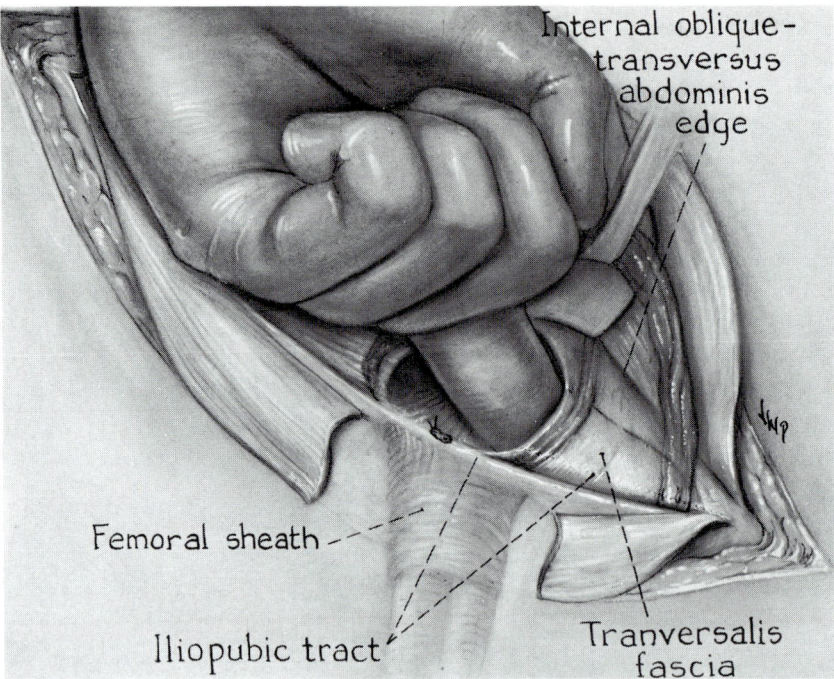

Figure 5-9. The hole in the transversalis fascia. The sac has been ligated and removed. A finger inserted through the internal ring, behind the transversalis fascia preperitoneally down to the pubic spine, palpates the inguinal floor. A section of inguinal ligament has been removed from the illustration to show the transversalis fascia composing the inguinal floor. This illustration and Figure 5-8 demonstrate that the iliopubic tract continues with that fascia adjacent to the ligated external spermatic artery. This fascia is also continuous with the femoral sheath. The stump of the external spermatic artery is therefore a landmark for the fascia composing the inferior edge of the internal ring. Superiorly, the transversalis fascia continues beneath the transversus abdominis aponeurosis. (Griffith CA. Inguinal hernia: an anatomic-surgical correlation. Surg Clin North Am 1959;39:531)

The Buttress

With but rare exception, the inguinal floor in children, young men, and all women is sound. It is also sound in some elderly men. In other middle-aged and older men, the transversalis fascia is weak and attenuated with a latent or overt direct inguinal hernia. In these men, a buttress of the inguinal floor is added to the Marcy repair.

In making the buttress, two points are noteworthy. First, we are not buttressing the internal ring and inguinal canal laterally. The repaired ring is sound, and it has its own buttress by its motility and shutter action. We can do more harm than good by securing it to something with sutures that tear out with the first cough. Second, we are buttressing the impending direct hernia over the Hesselbach triangle with sutures in the medial inguinal canal that come to lie in a plane superficial to Hesselbach fascia. The buttress ends at the medial edge of the repaired internal ring and superficial to it.

In general, the buttress is made by suturing transversalis fascia plus aponeurosis to transversalis fascia plus aponeurosis. Inferiorly and medially, the needle incorporates the iliopubic tract and the inguinal ligament. What the needle incorporates superiorly depends on the specific anatomic variation at hand. At one rare extreme, the internal oblique and transversus abdominis muscles are aponeurotic in the inguinal region, and these aponeuroses are fused to compose a conjoined tendon. At the other rare extreme, the internal oblique and transversus abdominis muscles are present as separate red muscles that do not become aponeurotic until they form the lateral border of the rectus sheath. Between these extremes, and most commonly, the transversus abdominis aponeurosis is available at variable distances from the inguinal ligament. Finding the aponeurosis and adjacent fascia occasionally requires splitting the arcuate muscular edge of the transversus abdominis muscle or rolling it upward with clamps. In any case, *the completed buttress is separate from, and superficial to, the Marcy*

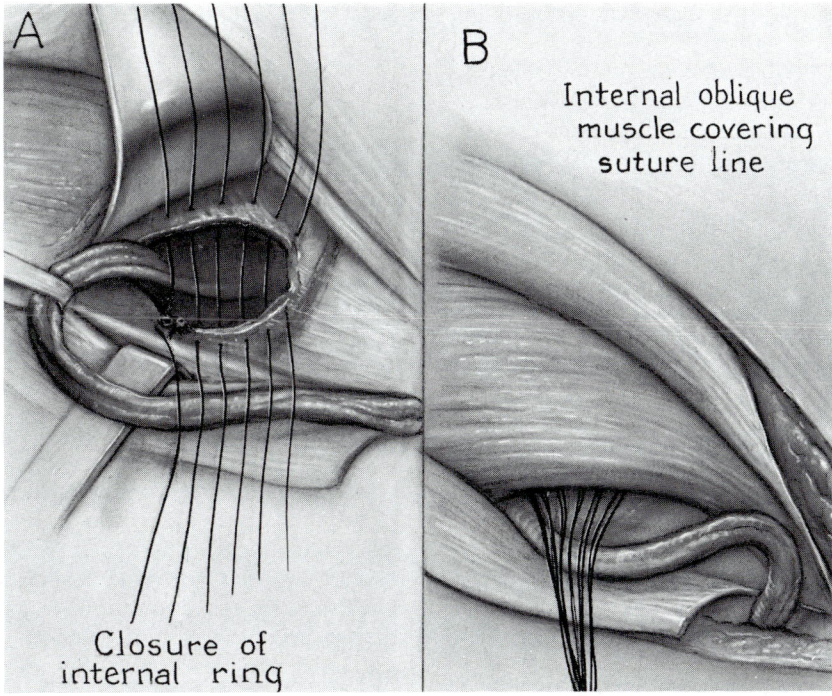

Figure 5-10. Repair of the internal ring. (*A*) Sutures are placed only through the transversalis fascia. The cord structures are displaced laterally. The reconstructed ring admits only the tip of a hemostat. This repair is made possible by removal of the cremaster muscle and retraction, as illustrated. (*B*) Retractors are removed to allow the inguinal ligament and the internal oblique and transversus abdominis muscles to assume their normal positions at rest. The internal ring is buttressed by overlying muscle. If at this stage under local anesthesia, the patient coughs at request, the sutures snap upward and laterally (displacement of the internal ring), and the arcuate fibers slam against the inguinal ligament (inguinal shutter). (Griffith CA. Inguinal hernia: an anatomic-surgical correlation. Surg Clin North Am. 1959;39:531)

repair of the internal ring so that the motility of the ring is not impaired or reduced.

SUMMARY

The cause of indirect recurrence is failure to close the patulous internal ring. This failure stems from essentially two fallacies. The first fallacy holds that all infants and children have tight internal rings and need only high ligation of the sac. When these hernias recur in adulthood, the inguinal canal and internal ring are more or less virginal. Either a low ligation was done, in which case a patulous ring was not even exposed, or a high ligation was done, but a patulous ring was not closed. Recurrence from these errors is prevented by evaluating the internal ring in all infants and children. Digital exploration through the opened sac reveals that the finger or even the thumb goes

through the ring in a few instances. When the fingertip encounters a tiny constriction, it is still best to identify the ring to exclude the occasional sac with a tight neck and a loose ring just above it.

The second and more common fallacy concerns the numerous modifications of Bassini's and Halsted's original techniques with the misconception that suturing one or more musculoaponeuroses to the inguinal ligament automatically closes the internal ring. No matter what is sutured to the inguinal (or Cooper) ligament, a recurrent sac can still herniate through an unclosed ring. Preventing recurrence from this error requires that indirect inguinal hernial repair be conceived in terms of the transversalis fascia and not the more superficial muscles and aponeuroses, as Marcy conceived in Figure 5-1 and as diagrammed in Figure 5-2. This concept removes the repair from the traditional category of simple and places it in the category of an accurate anatomic dissection that demands adequate exposure and positive identification of the internal ring.

In 40 years of private practice, neither my associates nor I have seen a recurrence after a Marcy repair. This does not mean that the recurrence rate is zero or approaches zero because, after 40 years, too many patients have been lost to follow-up for valid statistical analysis. It does mean that recurrence after a Marcy repair is rare. At up to 40 years and beyond, however, more direct bulges in patients without buttresses return.

REFERENCES

1. Andrews E. A method of herniotomy utilizing only white fascia. Ann Surg 1924;80:225.
2. Deysine M, Soroff HS. Must we specialize in herniorrhaphy for better results? Am J Surg 1990;160:239.
3. Griffith CA. Inguinal hernia: an anatomic-surgical correlation. Surg Clin North Am 1959;39:531.
4. Griffith CA. The Marcy repair revisited. Surg Clin North Am 1984;64:215.
5. LaRoque GP. The intra-abdominal method of removing inguinal and femoral hernia. Arch Surg 1932;24:189.
6. Lytle WJ. The internal inguinal ring. Br J Surg 1945;32:441.
7. Lytle WJ. A history of hernia. Med Press 1954;232:1.
8. Lytle WJ. Anatomy and function in hernia repair. Proc R Soc Med 1961;54:967.
9. Marcy HO. A new use of carbolized catgut ligatures. Boston Med Surg J 1871;85:315.
10. Marcy HO. The radical cure of hernia by the antiseptic use of the carbolized catgut ligature. Trans Am Med Assoc 1878;29:295.
11. Marcy HO. The cure of hernia by the antiseptic use of animal ligature. Trans Int Med Cong 1881;2:446.
12. Marcy HO. The cure of hernia. JAMA 1887;8:589.
13. Marcy HO. The anatomy and surgical treatment of hernia. New York, Appleton, 1892.

Editor's Comment

Dr. Griffith establishes two important points: the historic place of the Marcy repair and the reasons for its success. The initial reports of Marcy clearly antedate the reports of Bassini and Halsted regarding methods for repair of inguinal hernia. Marcy repaired small to medium indirect inguinal hernias with reconstruction of the deep inguinal ring, the entire repair being conducted within the transversus abdominis layer of the groin. The Bassini and Halsted repairs, which use the inguinal ligament, came along several years later.

There are those, myself included, who view the Bassini and Halsted repairs as setting the stage for the high recurrence rates that have plagued groin hernia repair over the last century. This is so because they cross anatomic layers in the conduct of the repair, and this then leads to unnecessary stress within the repair when the patient resumes activity. The reason for success of the Marcy repair, as clearly pointed out by Griffith, is that the repair is conducted entirely within the transversus abdominis lamina of the groin. Physical activity by the patient then does not lead to disruptive forces, but rather allows the repaired tissues within this layer to move more normally.

I differ with Dr. Griffith in his insistence that the Marcy repair uses only transversalis fascia. If one accepts the definition of transversalis fascia (see my comments that follow Chap. 2) as the thin, diaphanous, lining membrane on the internal surface of the transversus abdominis muscle and aponeurosis, then one has to accept that this is not the sort of material from which a secure groin hernia repair can be constructed. Transversalis fascia simply does not have the strength. The Marcy repair actually uses other tissues within the transversus abdominis lamina, principally aponeurotic fibers that are regularly present on the margins of the deep ring within the transversalis fascia as well as the transversus abdominis muscle. Thus, I believe that Griffith's description would be more anatomically accurate if it recognized the inclusion of these additional reinforcing fibers.

R.E.C.

Hernia, Fourth Edition, edited
by Lloyd M. Nyhus and Robert E. Condon.
J.B. Lippincott Company, Philadelphia © 1995.

Chapter 6

The Cooper Ligament Repair of Groin Hernias

Robb H. Rutledge

The Cooper ligament repair is the only anterior hernia operation that repairs all the hernias that can occur in the groin. It is a more extensive procedure than most hernia operations, but it gives excellent results for all groin hernias in adults.

HISTORICAL DEVELOPMENT

The story of the Cooper ligament repair really should begin with Sir Astley Cooper himself. In 1784, at the age of 16 years, Cooper was apprenticed to Mr. Henry Cline, the leading surgeon at St. Thomas' Hospital in London. One night, when Astley was attending one of Mr. Cline's lectures on hernias, he realized that he, himself, was the subject of that complaint. He ran home, dashed upstairs to his room, threw himself on the bed, elevated his legs on the bedpost, and waited for Mr. Cline to come home. When Mr. Cline arrived, he confirmed the diagnosis and fitted young Astley with a truss that he wore faithfully for 5 years. He apparently had no further trouble.[2]

This episode stimulated Cooper's interest in hernias. In 1804, Cooper published his classic hernia work[1] and dedicated it to Mr. Cline. In this, he demonstrated the anatomic defects of groin hernias, described the transversalis fascia, and defined the superior pubic ligament that later bore his name. Anesthesia and asepsis were unknown then, and Cooper recommended surgery only for incarceration. He did not use his own ligament in his repairs, and he treated his own hernia with a truss.

In 1892, Guiseppe Ruggi[19] was the first to use the Cooper ligament in any type of hernia surgery. He sutured the inguinal ligament down to the Cooper ligament in his femoral repairs.

In 1897, Georg Lotheissen, one of Billroth's pupils, was the first to suture the conjoined tendon to the Cooper ligament. He was operating in Innsbruck on a 45-year-old woman with a twice-recurrent inguinal hernia after previous Bassini repairs. Lotheissen found that the patient's inguinal ligament had been destroyed, so he anchored the conjoined tendon to the Cooper ligament instead. He subsequently reported success with his Cooper ligament technique for both inguinal and femoral hernias, but he did not use a relaxing incision.[8]

In 1939, Chester McVay submitted his thesis on the anatomy of the inguinal and femoral areas for his doctorate at Northwestern University. He pointed out that the normal insertion of the transversus abdominis and the transversalis fascia was on the Cooper ligament, not the inguinal ligament. From these dissections, McVay developed his technique of a Cooper ligament repair and reported this from Ann Arbor in 1942 while he was a surgical resident.[11] He was unaware of Lotheissen's work then. McVay emphasized that the Cooper ligament was the anatomically correct anchor for a posterior wall reconstruction and recommended a Cooper ligament repair for direct, large indirect, and femoral hernias. He used a relaxing incision to avoid tension. His work provided a sound anatomic basis for a Cooper ligament repair and popularized its use in America.[6,9,12]

A relaxing incision is an essential part of a Cooper ligament repair. Although Anton Wolfler did not use the Cooper ligament in his hernia surgery, he is given credit for making the first relaxing incision. In 1892, in the Festschrift for Theodor Billroth, Wolfler described making an incision in the anterior rectus sheath whenever he noted tension approximating the rectus sheath to the inguinal ligament. He did this, not primarily to relieve tension, but to gain access to the rectus muscle to transplant it to reinforce the repair.[28] Subsequently, the concept of a relaxing incision has evolved to its present purpose of reducing tension on a posterior wall reconstruction. It is difficult to credit one surgeon for this (Fig. 6-1). The contributions of Bloodgood, Fallis, Rienhoff, Tanner, and McVay have all been important.[18]

ANATOMIC BASIS FOR A COOPER LIGAMENT REPAIR

A strong posterior inguinal wall is the best protection against a groin hernia in an adult. Normally, this is provided by the insertion of the transversus abdom-

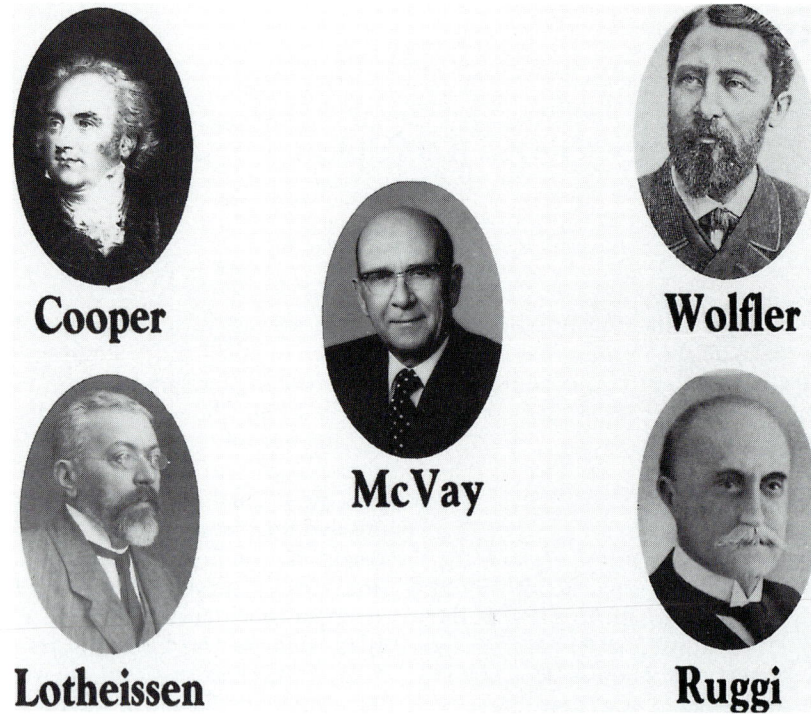

Figure 6-1. The developers of the Cooper ligament repair (Rutledge RH. Cooper's ligament repair: a 25-year experience with a single technique for all groin hernias in adults. Surgery 1988;103:1)

inis and the underlying transversalis fascia from the pubic tubercle to the medial margin of the femoral ring.

There is a wide variation in the length of the insertion of the transversus abdominis on the Cooper ligament. In about 75% of McVay's dissections, this was a long insertion with a broad aponeurotic plate, giving a strong posterior wall. These people are unlikely to develop a direct hernia. In the remaining 25%, the insertion was short, and the continuity of the posterior wall was made up only of the transversalis fascia, making the wall potentially much weaker.[10]

This weak area of the posterior wall that is protected only by the transversalis fascia has been called the *myopectineal orifice* by Fruchaud.[4] It is bounded by the rectus muscle medially, the internal oblique and transversus abdominis superiorly, the iliopsoas muscle laterally, and the Cooper ligament and pubis inferiorly. It is spanned and divided by the inguinal ligament, traversed by the spermatic cord and femoral vessels, and bridged on its inner surface by the transversalis fascia[27] (Fig. 6-2).

All groin hernias begin as a weak area in this myopectineal orifice. With a decrease in the area's aponeurotic fibers from defective collagen metabolism and a gradual attenuation from increased intraab-

dominal pressure (eg, prostatism, constipation, or chronic lung disease), a hernia can result. The transversalis fascia deteriorates and allows a peritoneal protrusion through it. Depending on the length of the insertion of the transversus abdominis on the Cooper ligament, the presence of a patent processus vaginalis, and the width of the femoral ring, the hernia could be direct, indirect, femoral or any combination of the three (Fig. 6-3).

Groin hernias are corrected either by repairing all or part of this myopectineal orifice or by substituting a prosthesis for the deteriorated transversalis fascia.

INDICATIONS FOR A COOPER LIGAMENT REPAIR

A Cooper ligament repair is indicated whenever a posterior wall reconstruction is done. Many surgeons, including McVay, chose a Cooper ligament repair only for direct, large indirect, and femoral hernias. They did not use this repair for small or medium indirect hernias because they thought that a posterior wall reconstruction was unnecessary in these cases.

Using this selective approach, McVay in 1958 reported a recurrence rate of 3.2% for abdominal ring repairs for small or medium indirect hernias, but only

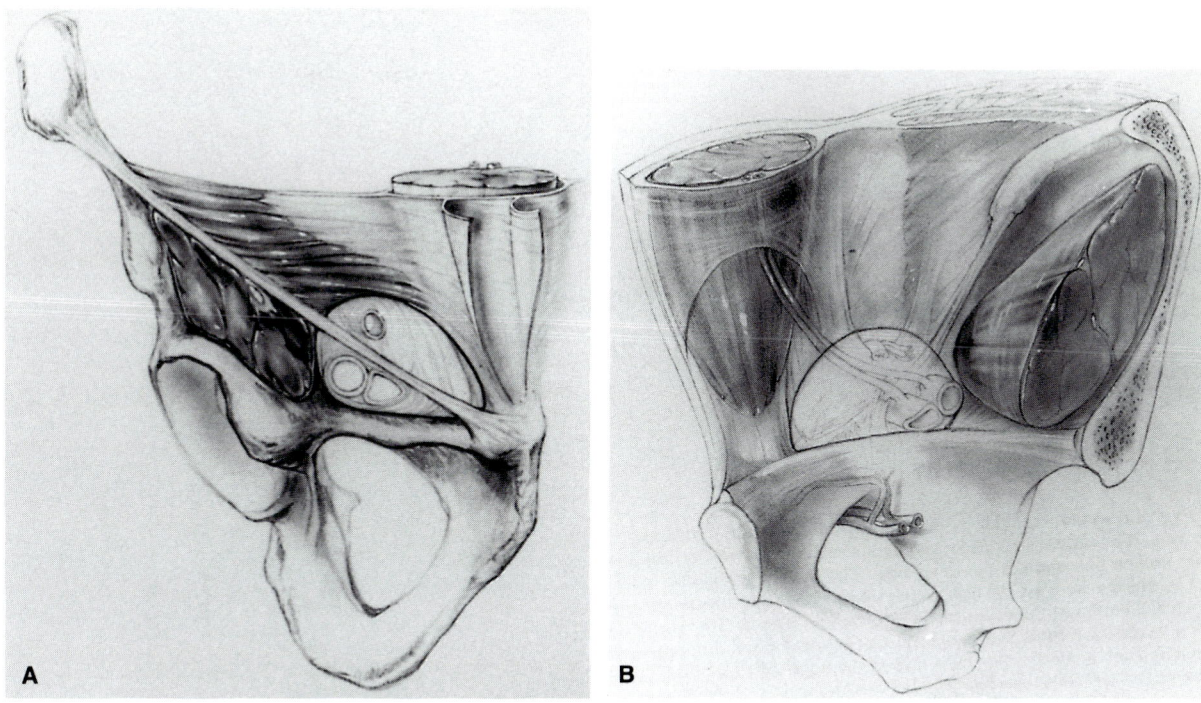

Figure 6-2. Anterior (*A*) and posterior (*B*) views of the myopectineal orifice. See text for boundaries. (Wantz GE. Atlas of hernia surgery. New York, Raven Press, 1991:4,5)

a 0.85% recurrence rate for Cooper ligament repairs for the more difficult direct, large indirect, or femoral hernias.[12] McVay's report is one of the few that has a higher recurrence rate for indirect hernias than for direct ones. A more complete repair on the small and medium indirect hernias should give better results.

My preference is to do a Cooper ligament repair on all groin hernias in adults. About 15% to 20% of patients have multiple ipsilateral defects at the original operation. Most recurrences are due to missed hernias, inadequate dissection, or subsequent further deterioration of the transversalis fascia. Recurrences

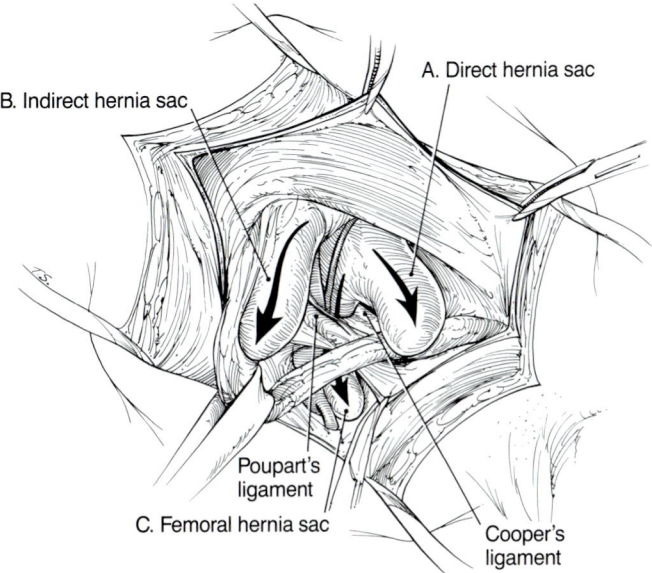

A. Direct hernia sac

B. Indirect hernia sac

Poupart's ligament

C. Femoral hernia sac

Cooper's ligament

Figure 6-3. Direct, indirect, and femoral hernias all present through the myopectineal orifice and can be repaired with one operation. (Rutledge RH. Cooper's ligament repair: a 25-year experience with a single technique for all groin hernias in adults. Surgery 1988;103:1)

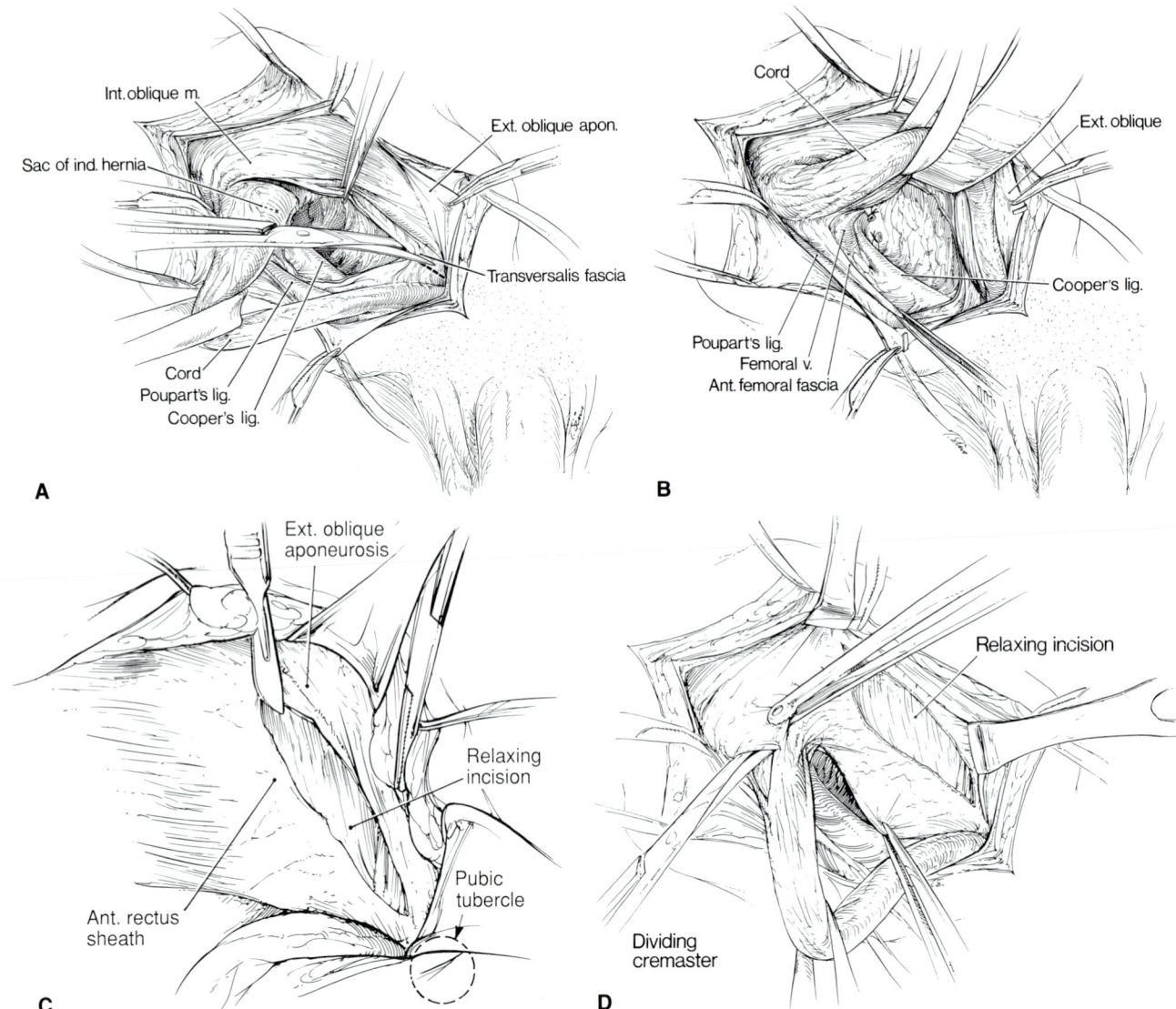

Figure 6-4. Basic steps in a Cooper ligament repair. See text for current surgical technique. (Rutledge RH. Cooper's ligament repair: a 25-year experience with a single technique for all groin hernias in adults. Surgery 1988;103:1)

should be less if all possible defects are repaired and the myopectineal orifice completely closed at the original operation. Since 1959, I have done a Cooper ligament repair on all groin hernias in adults, primary or recurrent, regardless of the presenting type.[20,21,23]

SURGICAL MANAGEMENT

Before operation, all patients are told of the use of Marlex mesh and the possible sacrifice of the ilioinguinal nerve. All male patients are told of the possible occurrence of ischemic orchitis and subsequent testicular atrophy regardless of careful technique.

General anesthesia has been used routinely. A short course of perioperative antibiotics (cefazolin) is given. A Foley catheter is placed in the bladder before operation and removed in the recovery room. My technique is described in detail next. An identical repair is done whether the hernia is primary or recurrent and direct, indirect, or femoral. More detailed remarks about recurrent hernias, bilaterality, Marlex mesh, relaxing incisions, the femoral vessels, and testicular problems follow under Special Considerations.[22,23]

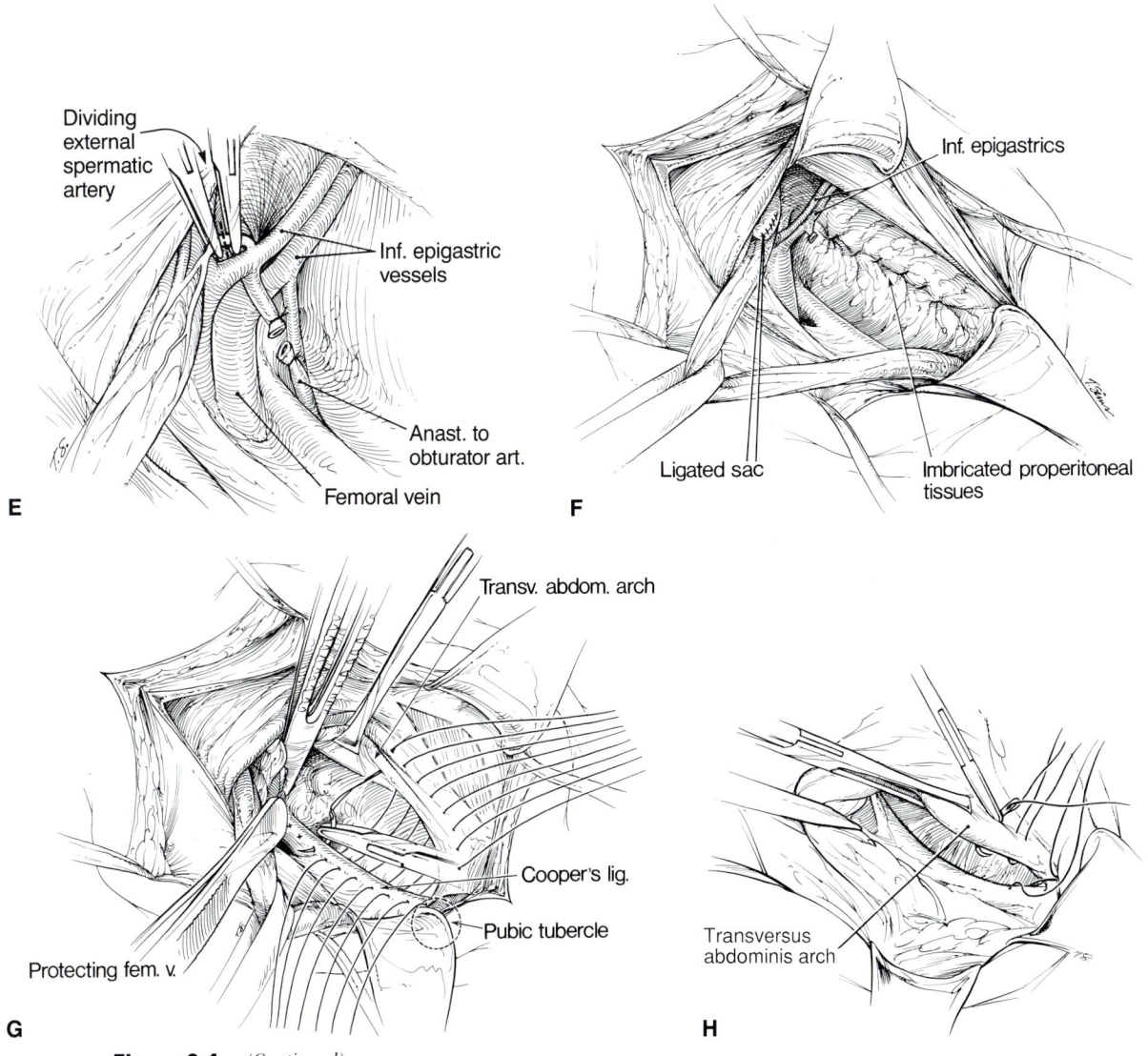

Dividing external spermatic artery

Inf. epigastric vessels

Anast. to obturator art.

Femoral vein

E

Inf. epigastrics

Ligated sac

Imbricated properitoneal tissues

F

Transv. abdom. arch

Cooper's lig.

Pubic tubercle

Protecting fem. v.

G

Transversus abdominis arch

H

Figure 6-4. *(Continued)*

Technique

A low, almost transverse incision is made. The external oblique is opened through the external ring. Small hemostatic clips mark the boundaries of the external ring as a guide for the new external ring diameter. The ilioinguinal nerve is usually preserved, but I frequently clip and divide it laterally if I think it has been injured during the surgery. The spermatic cord is mobilized in the canal but is not mobilized medial to the pubic tubercle to preserve testicular collateral circulation.

The posterior wall of the inguinal canal is incised completely, destroying the internal ring. The iliopu-bic veins are controlled, and the Cooper ligament is dissected free (Fig. 6-4A). The spermatic cord is retracted superiorly with a broad Deaver retractor, and the deeper portion of the Cooper ligament is cleared (see Fig. 6-4B).

Then, starting lateral to the femoral vessels, the anterior femoral fascia is identified and dissected free. Working medially, the anterior surface of the femoral artery and vein are seen and cleared off as the anterior femoral fascia is developed. The dissection continues medially, and the fat and lymph nodes are removed from the femoral canal. Any femoral sac is converted to an inguinal one. Finally, any vascular connections to the obturator circulation are divided and ligated so they will not be torn during the repair.

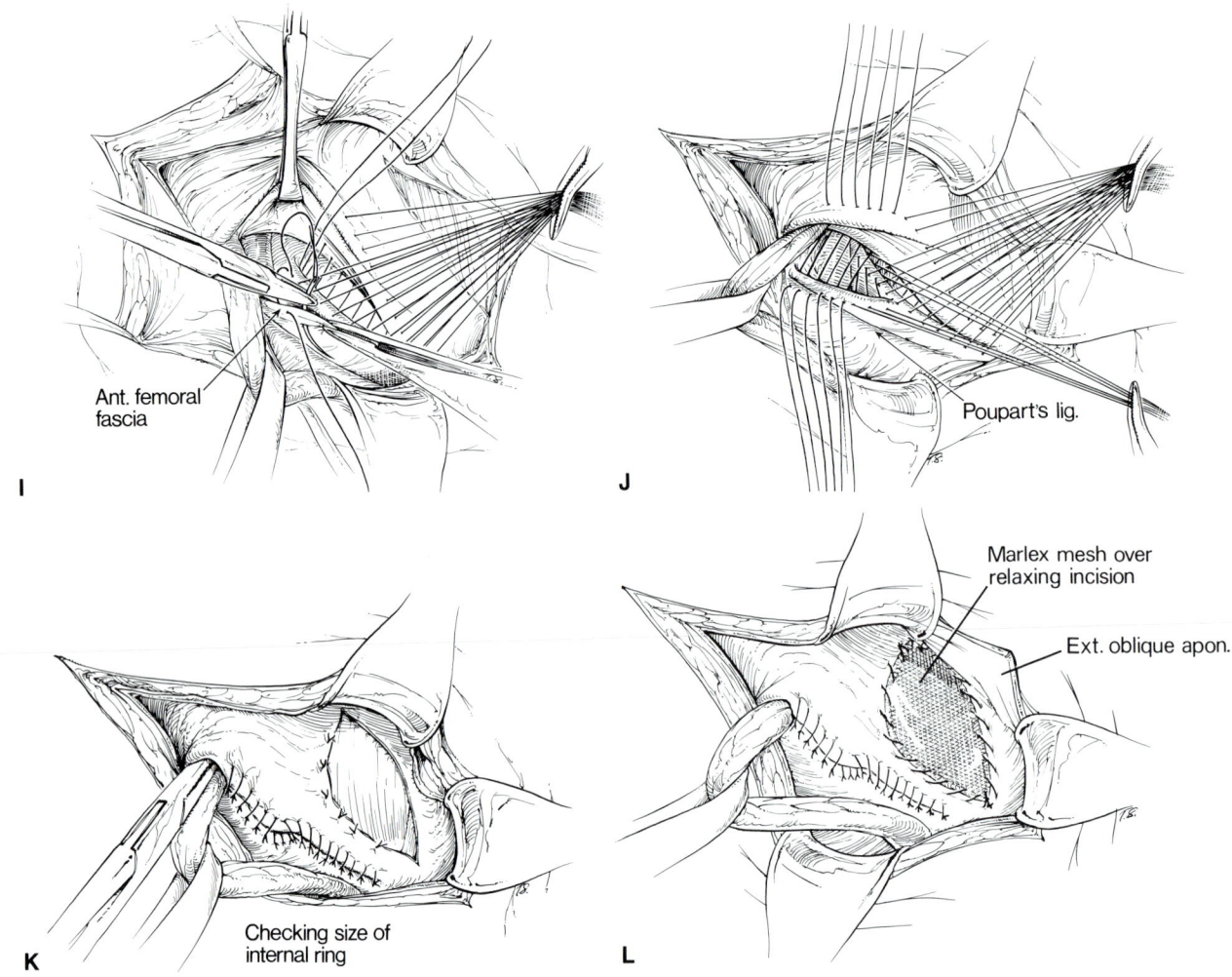

Ant. femoral
fascia

I

Poupart's lig.

J

Checking size of
internal ring

K

Marlex mesh over
relaxing incision

Ext. oblique apon.

L

Figure 6-4. *(Continued)*

After the inferior dissection is completed, the transversus abdominis arch is mobilized superiorly from the underlying preperitoneal tissues, and any attenuated transversalis fascia and internal oblique are excised. Then, a relaxing incision is made at the point of fusion of the external oblique aponeurosis and the anterior rectus sheath. This starts at the pubic tubercle and extends superiorly about 4 to 5 inches (see Fig. 6-4C).

The patient is placed in the Trendelenburg position to decrease the likelihood of intestinal injury. The spermatic cord is opened, and the cremaster fibers are divided at the internal ring (see Fig. 6-4D). Any fat or lipoma is removed from the cord. The external sper-

matic artery is divided as it comes off the inferior epigastric so the cord can be moved laterally during the repair (see Fig. 6-4E).

Indirect sacs are opened and explored to evaluate any intraabdominal pathology and to be certain that no intestine is adherent directly under the area of the repair. Small indirect sacs are removed and the peritoneum closed. Large indirect sacs are transected just distal to the internal ring. The proximal sac is freed from the cord by sharp dissection and closed. To decrease the chances of developing an ischemic orchitis, the distal sac is left in place and filleted on its anterior surface to prevent hydrocele formation. If no indirect sac is apparent, the anteromedial portion of the cord

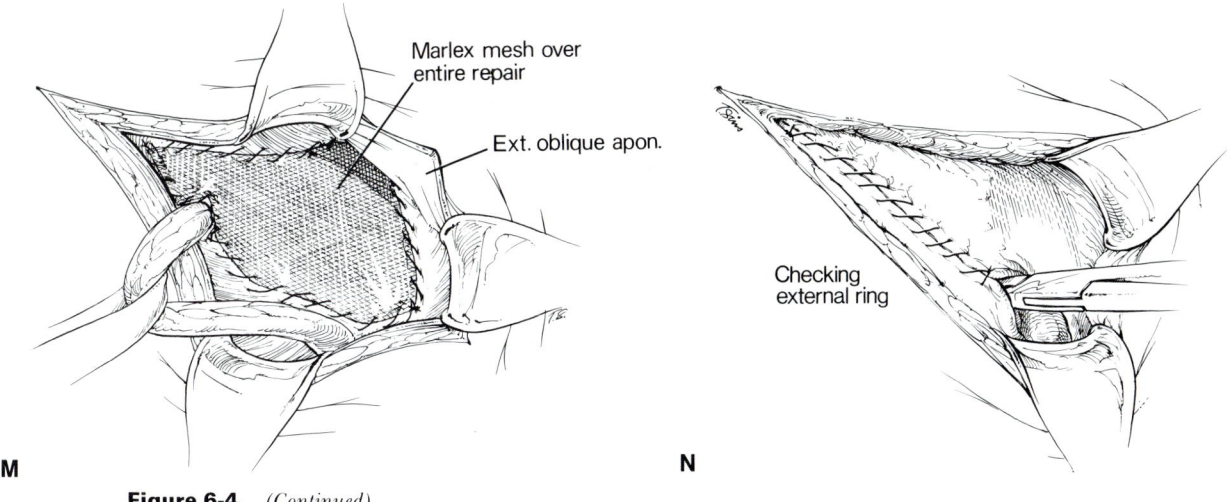

Marlex mesh over
entire repair

Ext. oblique apon.

Checking
external ring

M   **N**

Figure 6-4. *(Continued)*

is dissected superiorly to identify and ligate the small peritoneal tab that is always present to avoid overlooking an indirect sac.

Most direct sacs are inverted, but large ones are occasionally excised. Large combined direct and indirect sacs are joined by dividing the inferior epigastric vessels and closing the sacs as one defect.

Sliding hernias are reduced, either by working through the sac or by freeing the sac from the cord by sharp dissection and then reducing the whole sac into the abdomen.

The repair is begun by inverting the preperitoneal tissues with a continuous 1-0 chromic catgut suture to reduce them away from the main repair (see Fig. 6-4F). This must be done carefully to avoid injuring the underlying intestine. Then, beginning at the pubic tubercle, a layer of interrupted sutures is placed between the transversus abdominis arch and the Cooper ligament going as far laterally as the medial edge of the femoral vein (see Fig. 6-4G). An Allis clamp is used to grasp the transversus abdominis arch to be certain that good bites are placed in it, not merely in the overlying internal oblique (see Fig. 6-4H). A short thick tonsillectomy needle is used for the Cooper ligament sutures. They are more easily placed right-handed on right-sided hernias and left-handed on left-sided hernias.

The femoral canal is closed by three or four transition sutures between the Cooper ligament and the anterior femoral fascia (see Fig. 6-4I). The lateral one is placed just lateral to the last suture placed in the Cooper ligament. The medial two or three then are placed between the most lateral sutures in the Cooper ligament.

Using a larger needle, the repair is continued by placing sutures between the transversus abdominis arch and the anterior femoral fascia, continuing laterally beyond any indirect sac so the spermatic cord comes out obliquely laterally at the new internal ring. No sutures are placed lateral to the cord (see Fig. 6-4J).

This entire layer is done with 1-0 silk sutures (Siliconized—Davis and Geck). They are tied from medial to lateral and the patient is brought out of the Trendelenburg position.

The new internal ring is snug and admits only a Kelly clamp (see Fig. 6-4K). Although the relaxing incision can be secured in position with a few interrupted sutures, I prefer to fill the defect with a Marlex mesh patch held in position by a continuous 1-0 Prolene suture (see Fig. 6-4L). Occasionally, a sheet of Marlex mesh is sutured on top of this whole basic layer as an onlay graft reinforcement (see Fig. 6-4M). The cord is returned to its natural position, and the external oblique is closed over the cord with continuous 2-0 Vicryl (see Fig. 6-4N). The new external ring is loose, easily admitting a finger. The soft tissues are closed, and the skin is closed with subcuticular 4-0 Dexon sutures and Steri-Strips.

Special Considerations

Recurrent Hernias
A Cooper ligament repair from an anterior approach was done on all recurrent hernias. Beginning laterally in clean tissues, the previous repair is dismantled completely regardless of the type of recurrence.

Nearly always, the transversus abdominis arch, the Cooper ligament, and the anterior femoral fascia can be safely dissected and used for a good repair. A long relaxing incision is made, and the spermatic cord is carefully preserved. If indicated, either an inlay or on-lay prosthetic graft can be added for reinforcement.

It is popular to repair recurrent hernias through a preperitoneal approach with a prosthetic inlay graft.[13,17] Recurrent hernia repairs can be done successfully from either an anterior or posterior approach. Complete closure of the myopectineal orifice, not the particular approach, is responsible for the good results.

Bilaterality

An underlying metabolic collagen defect is found in most adult hernia patients. Forty six percent of my patients either had a bilateral repair or had a contra-lateral hernia that was repaired earlier or developed subsequently.[21] This high percentage of eventual bilaterality emphasizes two points. First, all patients who have a unilateral repair must have the opposite side carefully checked before operation. Second, a complete repair should be done at the primary operation to avoid further problems with that side.

Most bilateral hernias are repaired at the same operation through two separate incisions, leaving a broad area between them to minimize scrotal swelling. If the first repair was prolonged or difficult, the second side is postponed until that repair is clinically indicated.

Marlex Mesh

The use of prosthetic grafts in hernia surgery increases steadily. Marlex mesh is the most popular. It is good for patches and plugs, but not as satisfactory for large inlay grafts. It is widely available, easy to use, and safe.[25] Patients frequently ask for Marlex mesh and feel reassured if it is used in their repair. I use it much more than I did 10 years ago, but cannot justify this practice with statistics.

A Marlex mesh patch is used routinely to fill the relaxing incision defect. About 20% of the time, I reinforce the basic layer of the repair with a Marlex mesh onlay graft.

To minimize the chance of infection, perioperative antibiotics are used. The mesh is soaked in an antibiotic solution that is also used to irrigate the wound. The mesh is sutured in place with monofilament polypropylene (Prolene) sutures.

Relaxing Incisions

A generous relaxing incision is essential to prevent tension on the repair. This incision begins just above the pubis and extends 4 to 5 inches superiorly in the plane of fusion of the external oblique aponeurosis and the anterior rectus sheath. If there is tension while tying these sutures, the incision is lengthened superiorly. This nearly always gives enough relaxation. On the rare occasion that this is unsuccessful, I look for aberrant aponeurotic fibers lateral to the pyramidalis. Dividing these fibers provides adequate relaxation.[10]

Others have described patients in whom a Cooper ligament repair could not be performed without tension despite all the maneuvers just described. Then a piece of Marlex mesh can be placed in the preperitoneal position as an inlay graft for a new posterior wall. It is attached to the Cooper ligament and anterior femoral fascia inferiorly, to the rectus medially, and to the transversus abdominis superiorly. This has not been necessary in my practice (Fig. 6-5).

A hernia through the relaxing incision is normally prevented by the medial extension of the transversalis fascia as the rectus fascia. Occasionally, a patient has a prominence of the rectus muscle through the relaxing incision. To prevent this, I routinely fill the relaxing incision defect with a Marlex mesh patch.

Femoral Vessels

Careful technique around the femoral vessels is required. Well-trained surgeons are familiar with basic vascular techniques and should have no trouble with this. I find it easier to develop the anterior femoral fascia lateral to the femoral vessels first. Then, working medially, the anterior femoral fascia is developed, and the front surface of the femoral artery and vein are cleaned off. With the femoral vein clearly identified, the femoral canal is cleaned out. This gives excellent exposure to any tributaries to the obturator circulation. These are then divided and ligated so they will not be torn during the repair. Placement of sutures in the Cooper ligament is stopped at the medial edge of the femoral vein to prevent any venous constriction and decrease the likelihood of thrombophlebitis.

Testicular Problems

To minimize risks to the testicle, several maneuvers are important. No dissection is done medial to the pubic tubercle. The external ring is left loose. An ipsilateral hydrocele is not removed unless an orchiectomy is done. Only sharp dissection is used around the cord. Large indirect sacs are transected at the internal ring, and the distal portion is left in place. Although the external spermatic artery is routinely divided and the internal ring made snug, no sutures are placed lateral to the cord so it can move laterally without constriction. All these technical steps protect testicular circulation and decrease the chances of thrombophlebitis of the spermatic cord and ischemic orchitis.

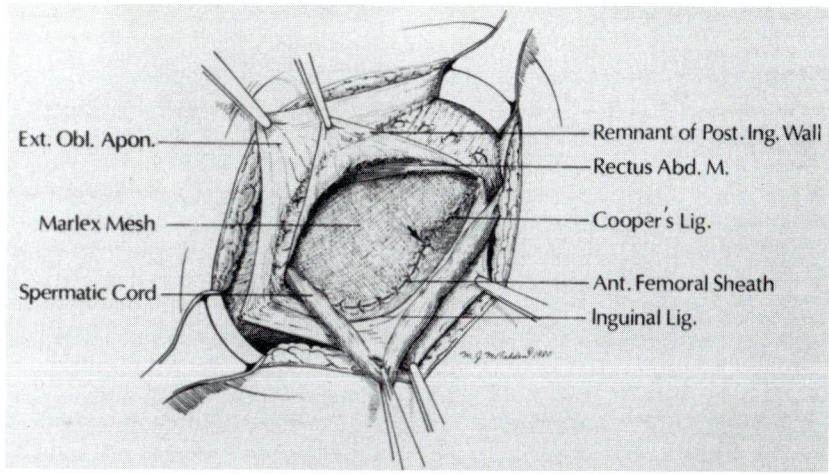

Figure 6-5. Marlex mesh inlay graft used when posterior wall is deficient for a primary Cooper ligament repair. (McVay CB. Anson and McVay surgical anatomy, ed 6. Philadelphia, WB Saunders, 1984:560)

Orchiectomy is rarely necessary in hernia surgery. It is done only with prior consent. Indications include patients with an undescended, painful, or atrophic testicle. A coexisting large ipsilateral hydrocele in an elderly patient is also an indication. Recurrent hernia patients only rarely require an orchiectomy. Nearly always, enough of the cord can be preserved to save a good testicle. A normal testicle is never removed.

RESULTS FROM A PERSONAL SERIES

My total experience from 1959 through 1992 is shown in Table 6-1. My last complete report[21] was in 1988 on 1142 Cooper ligament repairs in 942 patients done between 1959 and 1984 with a 97% follow-up. The only operative death was in a 65-year-old man with a proven myocardial infarction on the fourth postoperative day. One hundred and sixty-seven patients (202 hernia repairs) had died by the time of the follow-up. They were followed an average of 7.2 years before death, with one suspected recurrence. None of this group had an operation for a recurrence. The late death patients were not included in the statistics. Twenty-eight patients (34 hernia repairs) were lost to follow-up. The remaining 747 live patients (906 hernia repairs) were followed an average of 9 years. I personally examined 80% and talked to the remaining 20% on the telephone.[21]

There were 18 recurrences, for a 2% overall recurrence rate. Seventeen of these were indirect along the cord in a subgroup of 147 repairs done with a sub-

cutaneously transplanted cord. This method was discarded in 1972. There was one recurrence in 572 repairs with the cord in the natural position; there was no recurrence in 154 repairs in female patients; and there was no recurrence in 33 repairs in male patients with an orchiectomy. Excluding the group with the subcutaneously transplanted cord, the recurrence rate was 0.13% for 759 repairs followed an average of 7.4 years.

The only three recurrences in the 127 recurrent repairs were indirect along the cord in the subcutaneously transplanted group. There has been no recurrence in a recurrent repair using the present technique that was begun in 1972.

Although a complete follow-up has not been done since my 1988 report,[21] I continue to follow my patients closely and am aware of the results. My impression is that the recurrence rates are essentially unchanged.

Table 6-1. Cooper Ligament Repair*

Type of Repair	1351 Primary No. (%)	231 Recurrent No. (%)
Direct	482 (35)	133 (58)
Indirect	818 (61)	90 (39)
Femoral	51 (4)	8 (3)
TOTAL	1351 (100) (85% of total)	231 (100) (15% of total)

*1582 repairs conducted between 1959 and 1992.

DISCUSSION

Advantages of a Cooper Ligament Repair

The Cooper ligament repair restores normal anatomic planes and provides the best anchor for a strong posterior wall reconstruction. It closes the femoral canal and displays the femoral vessels to protect them from injury. It is the only anterior repair that closes the complete myopectineal orifice. It repairs all the hernias that can occur in the groin.

Disadvantages of a Cooper Ligament Repair

The Cooper ligament repair is a more extensive operation than most other hernia repairs. The patients have a slower convalescence and generally have more discomfort for the first 3 or 4 days after surgery. Wound irrigations with bupivacaine have not decreased this early postoperative pain. Although some patients go home the afternoon of surgery, most patients spend 1 night in the hospital. They are advised to stay home for 1 week and walk daily for exercise. More active sports are encouraged in several weeks.

Sixty percent of my patients are older than 50 years of age. Many are retired, and most of those who are working are not required to do heavy lifting. Patients with desk jobs return to work in 1 to 2 weeks, while those who must do heavy labor return in about 4 weeks. This latter figure is usually set by the company's rules, not by the type of hernia repair. Most patients have resumed all their preoperative activities by 1 month. Patient motivation is a strong factor governing the duration of the convalescence.

Tension is considered to be another disadvantage of a Cooper ligament repair. This can be avoided by a generous relaxing incision.

Vascular injuries and thromboembolic problems are cited as dangers of the Cooper ligament repair.[14,15,24] Careful technique around the femoral vessels should prevent both of these concerns. The chances of vascular injury are minimal because the vessels are seen and protected. The deep layer of the repair is stopped at the medial edge of the femoral vein to prevent venous constriction and decrease the risk of thrombophlebitis. In my series of 1582 Cooper ligament repairs, there was no vascular injury, and only two patients had pulmonary emboli that required heparin therapy. Phlebograms on each of these did not show the operative side to be the source. The femoral vessels need not be a problem if careful technique is used.

Which Hernia Repair To Use?

No standard method has been developed of reporting recurrences or complications in hernia surgery. There has never been a significant prospective randomized trial of hernia repairs in adults. Consequently, there are no data to indicate whether one particular repair is superior.

Surgeons do not agree on methods of repair. Some surgeons prefer a selective method of repair.[16] They tailor the repair to the type of hernia. Others do a direct–indirect repair on nearly all groin hernia repairs in adults.[3,5,7,26] My preference is to do a Cooper ligament repair on all adults.

Excellent results have been obtained with all these methods. The points in common appear to be a thorough dissection to avoid overlooked hernias and a complete repair of the myopectineal orifice without tension.

SUMMARY

A Cooper ligament repair provides the best anchor for a strong posterior wall reconstruction, closes the femoral canal, and repairs all the hernia defects that can occur in the groin. It requires a generous relaxing incision and careful technique around the femoral vessels. Although it is a more extensive operation than most hernia repairs, it can be done safely with minimal morbidity and a low recurrence rate. Many surgeons choose a Cooper ligament repair for direct, large indirect, and femoral hernias only. I use it for all groin hernias in adults, primary or recurrent, and have been pleased with the results.

REFERENCES

1. Cooper A. The anatomy and surgical treatment of inguinal and congenital hernia. London, JT Cox, 1804.
2. Cooper A. Lectures on the principles and practice of surgery. London, E Portwine and JT Cox, 1835.
3. Devlin HB, Gillen PHA, Waxman BP, et al. Short stay surgery for inguinal hernia; experience of the Shouldice operation. Br J Surg 1986;73:123.
4. Fruchaud H. Anatomie chirurgicale des hernies de l'aine. Paris, G Doin, 1956.
5. Glassow F. Short stay surgery (Shouldice technique) for repair of inguinal hernia. Ann R Coll Surg Engl 1976;58:133.
6. Halverson K, McVay CB. Inguinal and femoral hernioplasty: a 22-year study of the authors' methods. Arch Surg 1970;101:127.
7. Lichtenstein IL, Shulman AG, Amid GK, et al. The tension-free hernioplasty. Am J Surg 1989;157:188.

8. Lotheissen G. Zur radikaloperation der schenkelher-nien. Centralbl Chir 1898;25:548.

9. McVay CB. The anatomic basis for inguinal and femo-ral hernioplasty. Surg Gynecol Obstet 1974;139:931.

10. McVay CB. Anson and McVay: surgical anatomy, ed 6. Philadelphia, WB Saunders, 1984:556.

11. McVay CB, Anson BJ. A fundamental error in cur-rent methods of inguinal herniorrhaphy. Surg Gyne-col Obstet 1942;74:746.

12. McVay CB, Chapp JD. Inguinal and femoral hernio-plasty. Ann Surg 1958;148:499.

13. Mozingo DW, Walters MJ, Otchy DP, et al. Properi-toneal synthetic mesh repair of recurrent inguinal hernias. Surg Gynecol Obstet 1992;174:33.

14. Nissen HM. Constriction of the femoral vein follow-ing hernia repair. Acta Chir Scand 1975;141:279.

15. Normington EY, Franklin DP, Brotman SL. Constric-tion of the femoral vein after McVay inguinal hernia repair. Surgery 1992;111:343.

16. Nyhus LM, Klein MS, Rogers FB. Inguinal hernia. Curr Probl Surg 1991;28:407.

17. Nyhus LM, Pollack R, Bombeck T, et al. The preperi-toneal approach and prosthetic buttress repair for re-current hernia. Ann Surg 1988;208:733.

18. Ponka JL. The relaxing incision in hernia repair. Am J Surg 1968;115:552.

19. Ruggi G. Metado operativo meovo per la cura radi-cale dell'ernia crurale. Bull Sci Med Bologna 1892; 7(3):223.

20. Rutledge RH. Cooper's ligament repair for adult groin hernias. Surgery 1980;87:601.

21. Rutledge RH. Cooper's ligament repair: a 25-year ex-perience with a single technique for all groin hernias in adults. Surgery 1988;103:1.

22. Rutledge RH. Cooper's ligament repair. Surgical Rounds 1989;12:17.

23. Rutledge RH. The Cooper ligament repair. Surg Clin North Am 1993;73:451.

24. Shamberger RC, Ottinger LW, Malt RA. Arterial in-juries during inguinal herniorrhaphy. Ann Surg 1984; 200:83.

25. Shulman AG, Amid PK, Lichtenstein IL. The safety of mesh repair for primary inguinal hernias. Am Surg 1992;58:255.

26. Wantz GE. The Canadian repair: personal observa-tions. World J Surg 1989;13:516.

27. Wantz GE. Atlas of hernia surgery. New York, Raven Press, 1991:4.

28. Wolfler A. Zur radikaloperation des freien leisten-bruches. In: Festschrift Theodor Billroth, ed. Bei-trage Zur Chirurgie. Stuttgart, Verlag Von Ferdinand Enke, 1892:552.

TRIBUTE: CHESTER B. McVAY, 1911–1987

Chester McVay's accomplishments stand as a re-minder of the valuable contributions that an individ-ual surgeon can make in our complex society. He continued to contribute throughout his entire profes-sional career. McVay's anatomic dissections were done while he was a medical student. He completed his 9-year term as a Regent of the American College of Sur-geons 4 years before his death.

McVay was born on August 1, 1911, in Yankton, South Dakota. His high school and college education were in Yankton, and he received his Bachelor of Sci-ence degree from Yankton College in 1933. He grad-uated with honors, majoring in chemistry and biology.

In the fall of 1933, McVay entered Northwestern University Medical School in Chicago. Throughout his medical school training, he did extra research work in the anatomy department. He served as an As-sistant in Anatomy and received his Master of Science degree in 1937. Much of his work was concentrated on the anatomy of the abdominal wall. He received his Doctor of Medicine degree in 1938. In 1939, he was awarded his Doctor of Philosophy degree from the anatomy department of Northwestern University after the completion of his thesis: "Studies of the An-terior Abdominal Wall. I. The anatomy of the in-guinal and femoral regions. II. Composition of the rectus sheath."

While at Northwestern, McVay worked with the anatomist Barry Anson. They began a long-term col-laboration until Anson's death in 1974. Their publi-cations include many anatomic and surgical reports and their textbook, *Surgical Anatomy* (Philadelphia, WB Saunders, 1933).

In 1938, McVay began his surgical training at the University of Michigan in Ann Arbor. There he de-veloped his technique of Cooper ligament repair, which he reported in 1942 (Fig. 6-6).

On completion of his surgical residency, McVay entered the US Army Medical Corps in 1943 and served until 1946. He was attached to the 298th Gen-eral Hospital Division (University of Michigan) and was stationed in England, France, and Belgium. He was at Liege, Belgium, during the Battle of the Bulge.

After World War II, McVay returned home to Yankton and founded the Yankton Clinic. He did all his clinical work there. He was Chief of Surgery at the Yankton Clinic and the Sacred Heart Hospital until he retired in 1981.

McVay kept up his academic work by joining the staff of the 2-year medical school of the University of South Dakota at Vermillion, 30 miles away from Yankton. He became Associate Professor of Anatomy and Clinical Professor of Surgery there. In 1974, he was largely responsible for the change in the medical school to a 4-year school. He was made Professor and was the first chairman of the Department of Surgery. He was then elevated to Emeritus status in 1977 (Fig. 6-7).

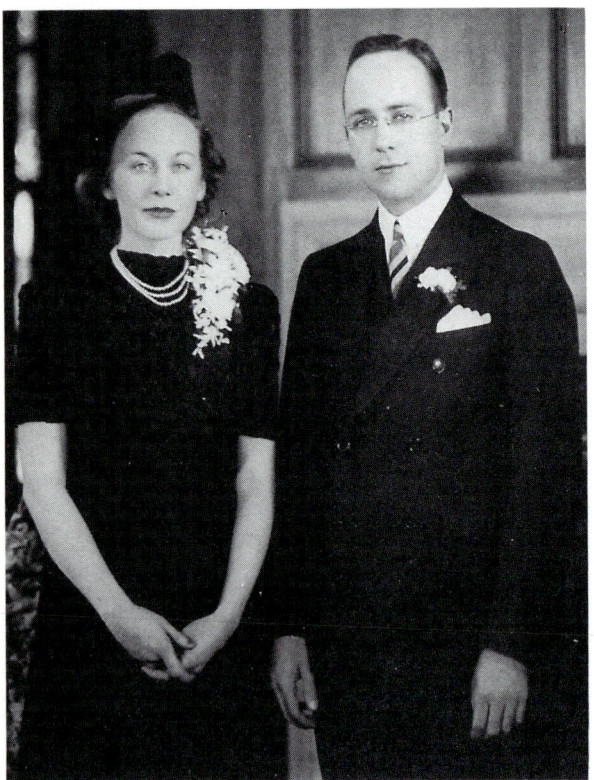

Figure 6-6. Chester McVay and June Brubacher on their wedding day in Ann Arbor in 1938.

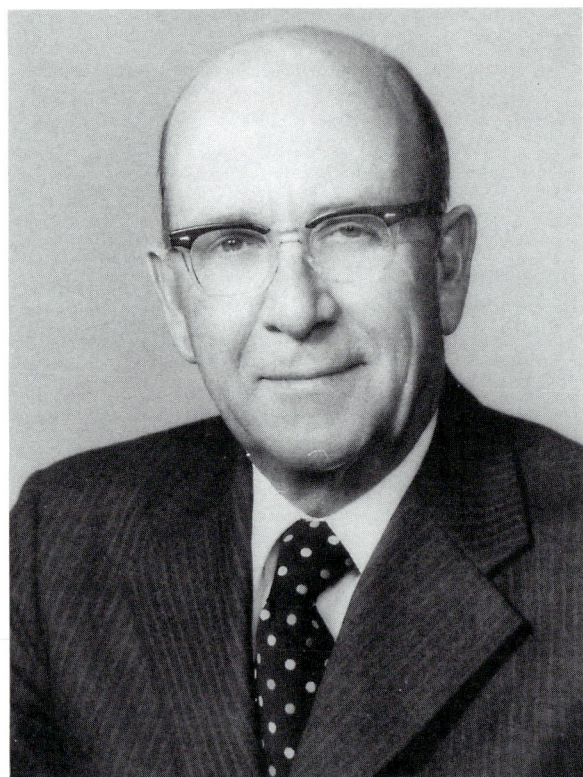

Figure 6-7. The mature surgeon in Yankton, SD.

McVay retired from active surgery in 1981 but continued his studies until his death in 1987. His wife, a daughter, and two physician sons survive.

McVay's honors include the presidencies of the Western Surgical Association, the Central Surgical Association, and the Frederick A. Coller Surgical Society. He was a second vice president of the American Surgical Association. He served 9 years as a Regent of the American College of Surgeons.

Throughout his career, McVay continued his careful clinical work and anatomic studies. He reported long-term results on his hernia patients, and continued, with Anson, to revise their textbook on surgical anatomy. His last major work was the sixth edition of that textbook, *Anson and McVay: Surgical Anatomy,* published in 1984, 10 years after Anson's death.

McVay never lost his enthusiasm for surgery or anatomy. He was a good example of that old tale: "Academic surgery is a state of mind, not a place." Chester McVay was an academic surgeon.

Editor's Comment

The presentation reports a 0.13% recurrent hernia rate for 759 repairs: an amazing result. Why then, do not we all change our various biases and follow this lead? The Cooper ligament repair does involve extensive operative dissection, similar to the Shouldice technique. Most students of the hernia problem continue to search for a way to obtain similar results using less operative trauma, that is, no-tension repairs and laparoscopic approaches. The answer is not available today, therefore, we must continue to accept that these more extensive operative repairs are the gold standard to which all other techniques must be compared.

Rutledge continues to use the term *anterior femoral fascia* (McVay anterior femoral sheath) for the iliopubic tract (see Fig. 6-4E). This tends to confuse the neophyte student of anatomy as well as those who consider themselves to be expert.

I am concerned with the use of silk and polypropylene sutures in the same wound. We found this combination of suture material to complicate the care of a wound infection and, therefore, have rigidly used only polypropylene for our hernia repairs.

Ott, Dudda, and Wenzel (McVay und Nyhus: Alternativen? Langenbecks Arch Chir, Kongressband 1993:242) pointed to the similarity of the Cooper ligament and the posterior iliopubic tract repair as described by us. I often have said that there is possibly one suture difference between the two methods, that is, at the level of the McVay-Rutledge transition suture. Their transition suture moves the plane of repair anteriorly to the iliopubic tract (anterior femoral sheath) after about five medial sutures. In contrast, with the posterior iliopubic tract repair, the anterior plane (transition) is started after only two or three medial sutures into the Cooper ligament. Thus, the distance the aponeurosis transversus abdominis must be moved posteriorly is lessened. These comparisons hold equally for the anterior iliopubic tract repair of Condon.

L.M.N.

Hernia, Fourth Edition, edited
by Lloyd M. Nyhus and Robert E. Condon.
J.B. Lippincott Company, Philadelphia © 1995.

Chapter 7

The Anterior Iliopubic Tract Repair

Robert E. Condon

The method of hernial repair described in this chapter, using the traditional anterior approach through the inguinal canal, evolved from an appreciation of groin anatomy gained by cadaver dissection and from use of the iliopubic tract in repair of groin hernias by the posterior, or preperitoneal, approach (see Chap. 8).

The iliopubic tract is the lower border of the transversus abdominis layer of muscle and aponeurosis. The hernial defect, in both indirect and direct varieties of groin hernia, is found within the transversus abdominis layer. It is within this layer that repair of the hernial defect is constructed.

Although some surgeons have expressed doubts about the existence of the iliopubic tract or its suitability for groin hernia repair, such concerns are based, for the most part, on inadequate practical experience with this method of repair. Difficulties with anatomic understanding are best resolved by a review of groin structure as outlined in Chapter 2. Judgment about the use of the iliopubic tract or, for that matter, of any aponeurotic structure for repair of a groin hernia is made by intraoperative testing of tissues as described in this chapter.

The important elements in the successful construction of a sound repair of any groin hernia are as follows:

1. Know the anatomy.
2. Identify the hernia by dissection.
3. Excise weak and redundant tissues.
4. Clear the hernial borders to strong tissue.
5. Suture the hernial defect without tension, accomplishing a primary repair.
6. If primary repair without tension cannot be accomplished, insert a prosthesis to replace missing tissue as the means of repair.

The anterior iliopubic tract repair is applicable to most inguinal hernias. In this chapter, techniques are described for repair of typical indirect and direct inguinal hernias. Repair of a complete hernia, a large indirect inguinal hernia that has destroyed the posterior wall of the inguinal canal and for which repair

combines the features of both a direct and an indirect hernia repair, also is outlined. The technique of prosthetic repair is described in Chapter 10.

The anterior iliopubic tract repair is not preferred for management of recurrent hernias previously repaired by an anterior approach or for suspected sliding hernias or femoral hernias, all of which are better and more easily managed by the posterior approach. The method should not be used for repair of small indirect hernias, such as usually are found in infants. These hernias have not greatly enlarged the deep inguinal ring, and they require only excision of the sac and perhaps one or two stitches to tighten the deep ring. The method also should not be used for repair of small diverticular direct hernias, which also are best managed by simple direct closure of the defect with two or three stitches.

REPAIR OF INDIRECT INGUINAL HERNIAS

Preparation of the Operative Field

It is not necessary to shave all the perineum bald. Shave only the area around the proposed incision that will be covered postoperatively by the dressing and adhesive tape. Wash and scrub the scrotum and upper thighs as well as the lower abdomen with an iodophor or chlorhexidine solution or soap. Do not use alcohol-based solutions for skin preparation; they cause painful scrotitis.

In draping, place a sterile towel under the scrotum and a second one over it to permit aseptic access to the scrotum if needed during the operation.

Landmarks and Incision

The deep inguinal ring, through which an indirect inguinal hernia obtrudes, is situated exactly halfway between the pubic tubercle and the anterior superior iliac spine. The incision is centered directly over the projected location of the deep inguinal ring and is made more or less transversely, following a natural skin crease or tension line (Fig. 7-1). The skin and most of the subcutaneous fat are incised in one sweep. Branches of the superficial epigastric vessels are encountered in the medial half of the incision, and branches of the superficial circumflex iliac vessels are encountered in the lateral half of the incision. Ligatures and sutures of 3-0 polyglycolic acid are used throughout the operation, except for repair of the hernia and for wound closure. The incision is completed with a knife to expose the external oblique aponeurosis with its overlying investing (innominate) fascia.

Sometimes, Scarpa fascia can be identified within the subcutaneous fat as an opaque layer. Particularly in infants and in obese adults, Scarpa fascia may appear to be so thick to the novice surgeon that it is confused with the external oblique aponeurosis. It is readily distinguished by the fact that when grasped, Scarpa fascia moves the skin and overlying subcutaneous fat with it, whereas the external oblique aponeurosis does not. Much ado has been made in the past about Scarpa fascia. For the most part, no particular attention should be paid to it. It should not be sought by dissection, and it need not be sutured during closure.

Opening the Inguinal Canal

The skin and subcutaneous fat are retracted sufficiently to expose the upper portion of the superficial inguinal ring. It is not necessary, and indeed is harmful, to clean thoroughly innominate fascia from the surface of the external oblique aponeurosis. A small nick, about 1 cm long, is made with the knife between fibers of the external oblique aponeurosis in the midportion of the main incision (Fig. 7-2) and is placed so that, if extended, it carries into or just inferior to the apex of the superficial inguinal ring.

The lower border of the small incision in the external oblique aponeurosis is picked up with a Cushing forceps, and the closed points of Metzenbaum scissors are inserted and passed gently laterally, separating both the underlying internal oblique musculature and the iliohypogastric and ilioinguinal nerves from the external oblique aponeurosis. One blade of the scissors is now inserted deep to the aponeurosis and the other maintained superficially to it; the scissors, in a slightly opened position, are pushed laterally between contiguous fibers of the external oblique aponeurosis and musculature to open the lateral aspect of the external oblique layer. Fine hemostats are applied to the edges of the external oblique aponeurosis to provide traction.

The closed scissors tip is now directed medially beneath the external oblique aponeurosis, separating the underlying nerves, the internal oblique musculature, and the spermatic cord from the overlying external oblique aponeurosis. The aponeurosis then is split down to the superficial inguinal ring.

Depending on circumstances, it may be necessary to open into the superficial inguinal ring; certainly, it is not necessary to do so on a routine basis. The objective is to provide sufficient exposure to allow mobilization of the spermatic cord and the hernial sac. If the hernia is sufficiently elongated to have escaped the superficial inguinal ring and entered the scrotum, in most instances it is necessary to open the superficial ring widely to mobilize completely the hernial sac. In less extensive hernias, it often is not necessary to open the superficial ring. A self-retaining retractor is placed deep to the external oblique lamina at either end of the incision to maintain exposure of the deeper tissues.

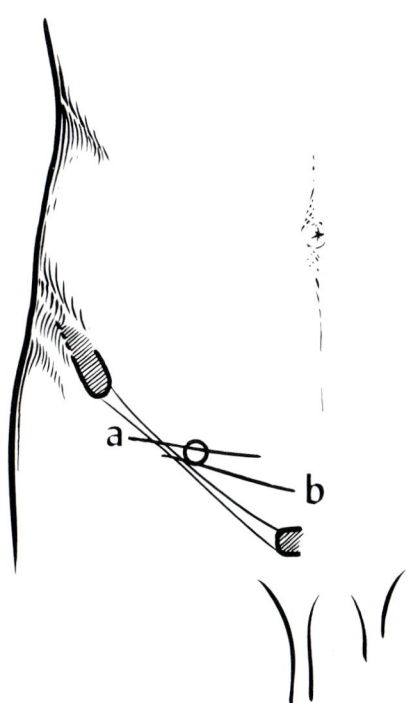

Figure 7-1. Landmarks for the skin incision in the repair of an inguinal hernia. The incision for an indirect hernia (a) is made transversely in a skin crease, centered on the location of the deep inguinal ring halfway between the pubic tubercle and the anterior superior iliac spine. The incision for a direct hernia (b) is made transversely in a skin crease, centered on the hernial bulge and placed just below the palpable superior border of the hernial defect.

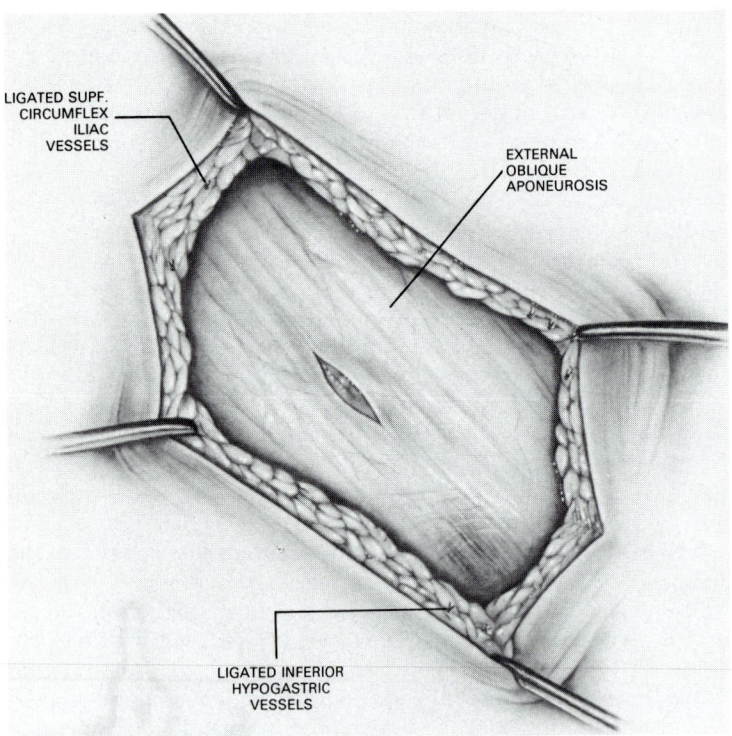

LIGATED SUPF.
CIRCUMFLEX
ILIAC
VESSELS

EXTERNAL
OBLIQUE
APONEUROSIS

LIGATED INFERIOR
HYPOGASTRIC
VESSELS

Figure 7-2. The incision has been completed through the skin and subcutaneous tissues (retracted) to expose the external oblique aponeurosis. The initial incision into the external oblique aponeurosis is made between fibers so that when it is extended, it will enter the apex of the superficial inguinal ring.

Mobilizing the Spermatic Cord

The ilioinguinal and, on occasion, the iliohypogastric nerves should be identified, widely mobilized, and gently displaced (Fig. 7-3). The spermatic cord is identified immediately subjacent to the superficial inguinal ring. The lower leaf of the external oblique aponeurosis is grasped in its midportion and retracted inferiorly. The spermatic cord is grasped gently and retracted anteriorly and superiorly. The areolar attachments of cremasteric fascia to the deep surface of the external oblique aponeurosis and the inguinal ligament are separated bluntly, the dissection continuing posteriorly until the deepest aspect ("shelving border") of the inguinal ligament has been exposed from the pubic tubercle to the deep inguinal ring.

The spermatic cord is then gently retracted inferiorly. One finds the lower border of the internal oblique muscle by identifying, just above the deep inguinal ring, the muscle bundles that are continuous from their lateral attachment to the inguinal ligament (and to the iliopubic tract, currently hidden from view) to their medial attachment to the rectus sheath or, in rare instances, the conjoined tendon. One identifies the bundles of the cremaster muscle by following them from their lateral attachment to the inguinal lig-

ament and iliopectineal arch, just medial to the attachments of the inferior oblique muscle, and noting that the cremaster fibers continue with the spermatic cord. Superior traction is made with a Cushing forceps grasping the lower border of the internal oblique muscle, and inferior traction is similarly made on the cremaster muscle, thus opening the plane between these structures. Dissection is continued in the plane between the inferior oblique and cremaster muscles on the superior aspect of the cord (see Fig. 7-3), separating the cord entirely from the posterior inguinal wall between the pubic tubercle and the medial border of the deep inguinal ring.

In many instances, as this dissection proceeds, there appears to be a small "mesentery" of cremasteric fascia on the deep aspect of the cord at the junction of the posterior inguinal wall (transversus abdominis aponeurosis and transversalis fascia) and the inguinal ligament (external oblique aponeurosis) as they attach to the superior ramus of the pubis. Once the cord is sufficiently mobilized, any mesentery should be transected and the cord encircled with a small Penrose drain. The dissection is continued on the undersurface of the cord, progressing laterally beyond the deep inguinal ring to the origin of the cremaster muscle (Fig. 7-4).

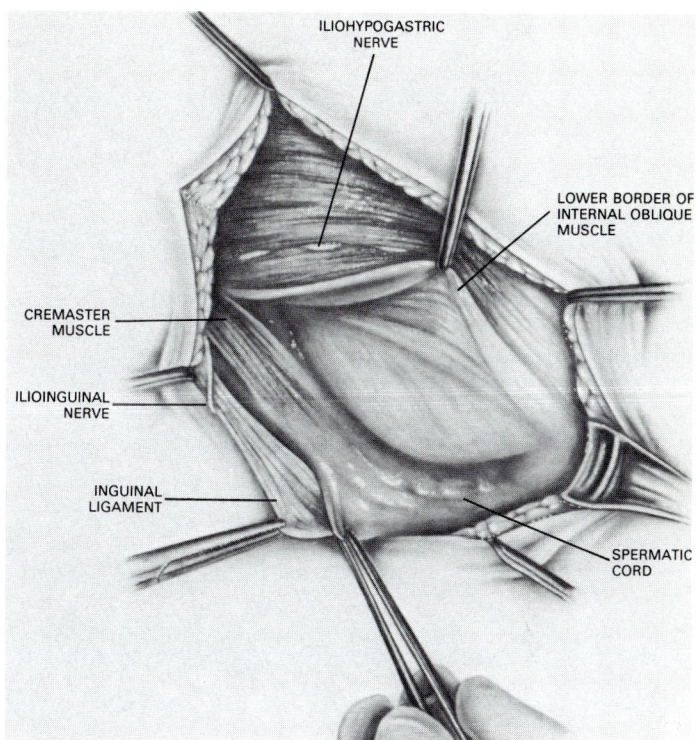

Figure 7-3. The external oblique aponeurosis has been opened and retracted, the ilioinguinal nerve has been mobilized and placed behind a hemostat, and the attachments of the spermatic cord to the inguinal ligament have been transected. The plane between the internal oblique and cremaster muscles is opened to completely mobilize the spermatic cord between the pubic tubercle and the deep inguinal ring.

Dissection of the Deep Inguinal Ring

The tip of a fine hemostat is inserted at the lateral aspect of the deep inguinal ring, bluntly from above downward, beneath the origin of the cremaster muscle but superficial to the iliopubic tract and the inguinal ligament. In many instances, the cremaster muscle lateral to the deep inguinal ring can be elevated with a small retractor to expose the lateral margin of the ring. In other instances, the cremaster muscle must be transected to provide this exposure. After the ilioinguinal nerve is carefully retracted and protected, paired hemostats are applied across the origin of the cremaster muscle, and the muscle is transected between these clamps (see Fig. 7-4). In an occasional patient, it may be necessary to divide the origin of the cremaster muscle in two bites. The proximal stump of the cremaster muscle is suture-ligated to control the cremasteric artery; a simple ligature is sufficient to manage the distal muscle stump.

Mobilization and, if needed, transection of the origin of the cremaster muscle commonly are omitted in other methods of repair of indirect inguinal hernias. But without this maneuver, it is impossible to adequately visualize the lateral aspect of the deep inguinal ring. Because nearly all recurrences that follow repair of a primary indirect hernia occur at the lateral aspect of the deep inguinal ring, it is obvious that exposure and suture-reconstruction of this aspect of the deep inguinal ring are essential steps to reduce the risk of recurrence.

Any remaining fascicular or areolar attachments of cremasteric fascia at the deep inguinal ring are transected about the entire circumference of the cord. Distal traction on the cord now makes the internal spermatic fascia (transversalis fascia) stand out. The internal spermatic fascia is transected circumferentially around the hernial sac and cord about 1 cm distal from the deep inguinal ring (see Fig. 7-4, *top*). A small arterial branch, the external spermatic artery, may perforate the iliopubic tract at the inferior aspect of the deep ring to join the spermatic cord. It may be transected and ligated.

These maneuvers expose the peritoneal hernial sac and the fascial margins of the deep inguinal ring. The fascial margins will be dissected more extensively after excision of the hernial sac. But for the present, the iliopubic tract should be identified immediately subjacent to the inguinal ligament at the inferior aspect of the deep inguinal ring. The transversus abdominis arch may be palpated after the overlying lip of internal oblique muscle is retracted at the superior aspect of the deep inguinal ring.

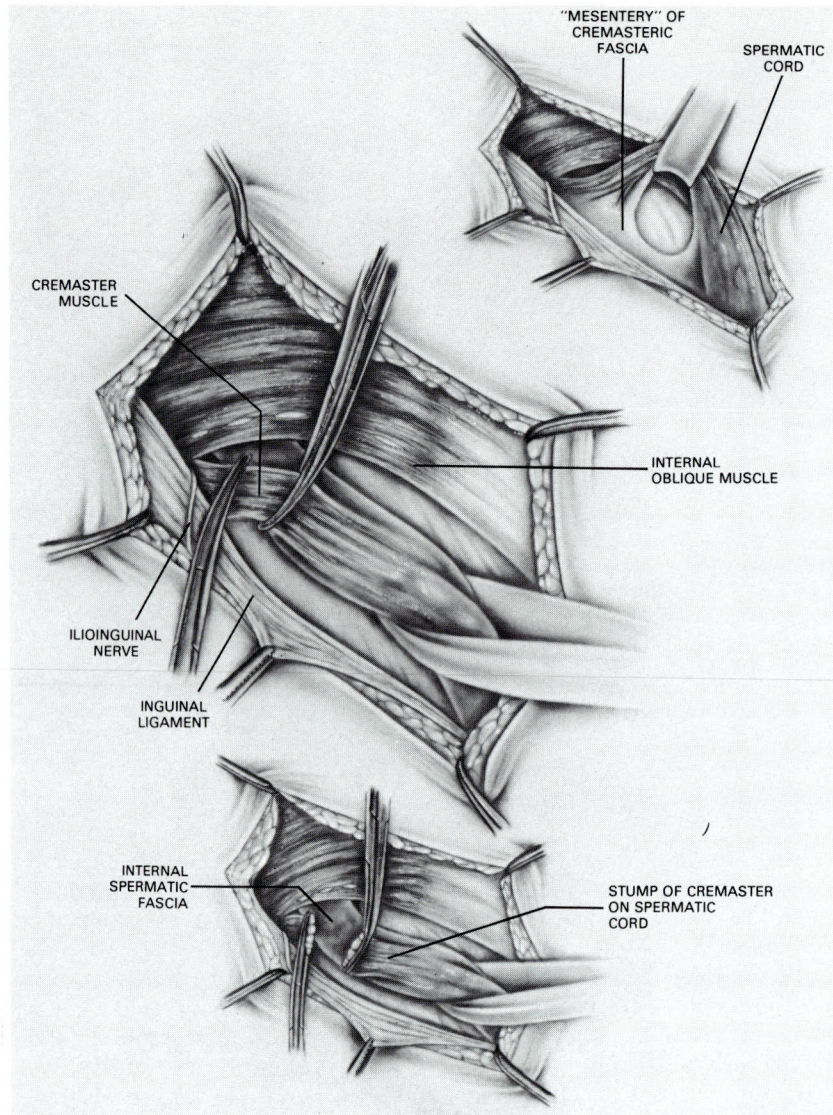

Figure 7-4. (*Top*) The spermatic cord is retracted, and the "mesentery" and all other attachments of cremasteric fascia are transected. The external spermatic artery may be encountered beneath the deep inguinal ring, perforating the iliopubic tract, and should be ligated. (*Center*) The cremaster muscle is mobilized freely near its origin and clamped. (*Bottom*) The origin of the cremaster muscle is transected between hemostats. Distal traction on the cord places the internal spermatic fascia, a protruding sleeve of transversalis fascia, under tension.

Mobilization and Excision of the Peritoneal Sac

In a primary indirect inguinal hernia, the peritoneal sac protrudes through the superior aspect of the deep inguinal ring and is found along the superior aspect of the cord. In recurrent hernias, the sac usually protrudes at the lateral aspect of the deep ring; in rare instances, the sac may be at the medial aspect of the ring between the spermatic cord and the inferior epigastric vessels.

The tissues covering the hernial sac within the cord, the cremasteric and internal spermatic fasciae, are further cleared from the sac by sharp dissection along the superior aspect of the cord for a distance of 2 to 3 cm. A small incision is made into the sac 2 to 3 cm distal to the deep inguinal ring. The forefinger of the operator's nondominant hand is inserted through the incision into the sac, directed distally; a

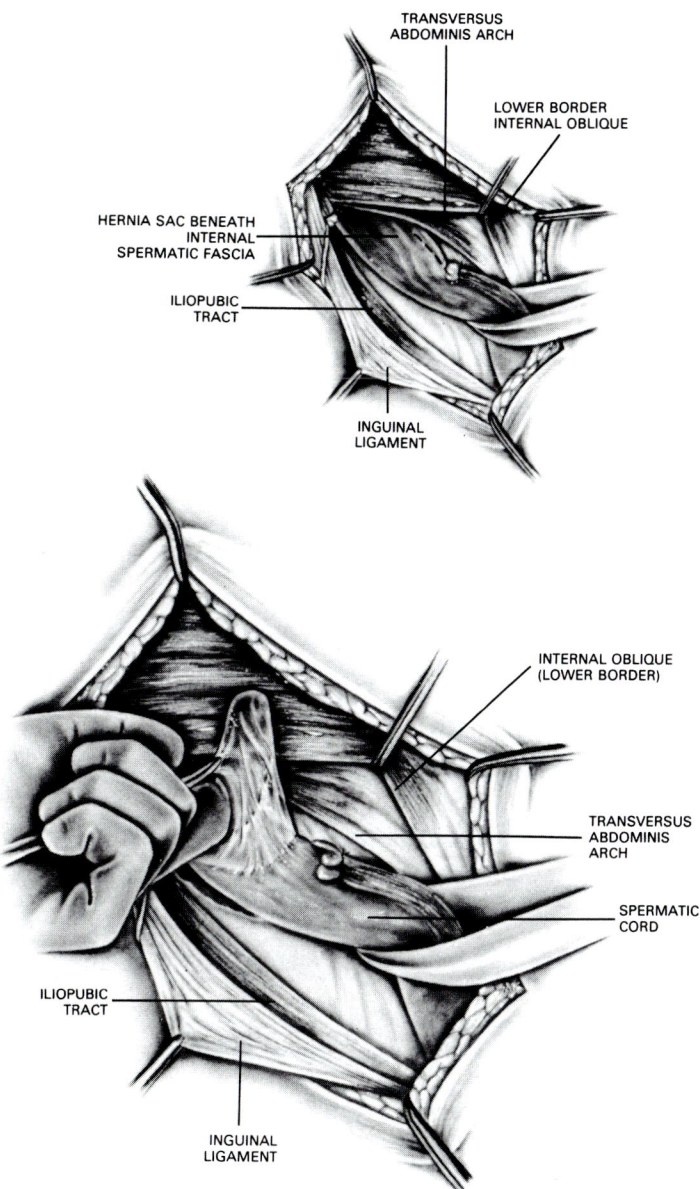

Figure 7-5. (*Top*) The internal spermatic fascia is incised and then transected circumferentially about the cord a centimeter or so from the deep inguinal ring. The peritoneal sac is next incised, indicated by the dashed line. (*Bottom*) The hernial sac is mobilized from the spermatic cord.

fine hemostat is applied to the distal apex of the sac incision and held on traction in the operator's palm to facilitate subsequent dissection (Fig. 7-5).

The cremasteric and internal spermatic fasciae overlying the peritoneal sac are cleared, chiefly by sharp dissection. Sharp dissection is emphasized because the blunt dissection used by most surgeons for these maneuvers increases the risk of injury to the vital spermatic cord structures, which are spread out on the surface of the hernial sac.

Clearing of the cremasteric and internal spermatic fasciae from the hernial sac is facilitated by maintaining traction on the sac while an assistant re-tracts the margins of the cremasteric and internal spermatic fasciae. Dissection is made in the plane between the sac and fasciae, initially clearing the superficial two thirds of the circumference of the sac.

As the initial segment is cleared, the incision in the sac is extended distally, the hemostat is replaced at the apex of the incision, the finger is thrust further distally, and the dissection is continued as before. When the most distal end of the peritoneal sac is reached, the tip of the finger within the sac is curled anteriorly, and dissection on the posterior aspect of the sac is continued back to the level of the deep inguinal ring.

Before excision and closure of the sac, a finger is inserted into the peritoneal cavity, and the areas of femoral and direct inguinal herniation are palpated to ensure the absence of a hernia in these areas. In palpating the posterior wall of the inguinal canal from its internal aspect, sufficient tension should be applied to the tissues to judge whether or not the area is liable to future direct herniation. If these tissues are weak, the hernia should be managed as described subsequently for complete indirect inguinal hernias.

The interior of the sac is inspected, with the surgeon looking for a more or less continuous ring of peritoneal thickening or scarring. This peritoneal scar identifies the level of the deep inguinal ring and the point at which initial peritoneal rupture occurred. The suture of the base of the sac that restores peritoneal continuity is placed at or above the level of this peritoneal scar.

The sac either may be twisted and its apex transfixed with a suture ligature or may be closed with an external or internal pursestring suture. The redundant peritoneal protrusion is excised. Finally, the aponeurotic margins of the deep inguinal ring are cleared of any remaining bits of fatty or areolar tissue so that the entire circumference of the deep inguinal ring is clearly delineated.

Assessment of Tissues for Repair

The margins of the deep inguinal ring are now palpated and inspected. In particular, the aponeurotic portion of the transversus abdominis arch at the superior aspect of the ring must be identified. The overlying internal oblique muscle and the superficial portions of the transversus abdominis muscle are rolled and retracted superiorly. On occasion, these tissues need to be grasped with an Allis forceps to expose the partially aponeurotic tissues on the deep surface of the transversus abdominis layer. Aponeurosis (ie, tendon) is easily identifiable medially; at the superior aspect of the deep ring, there is progressive transition to muscle. It is important to secure tissues along the superior margin of the deep inguinal ring that are sufficiently strong so that sutures will be retained.

The iliopubic tract is visible along the inferior margin of the deep inguinal ring. Its full extent can be appreciated by grasping its upper margin with a forceps or hemostat and retracting superiorly while the inguinal ligament is retracted inferiorly. The posterior margin of the inguinal ligament is easily identified by its thicker, whiter fibers. The inguinal ligament partially covers the iliopubic tract near the deep inguinal ring and is attached to the iliopubic tract by fusion of their respective thin investing fasciae. If this fusion is broken with the tip of a hemostat, the instru-

ment can be passed beneath the inguinal ligament into the leg. Such a maneuver is not recommended as a routine procedure, but it can demonstrate the anatomically distinct lower border of the inguinal ligament (external oblique lamina) and the continuity of the iliopubic tract (transversus abdominis lamina) with the femoral sheath in the leg.

Closure of the Deep Inguinal Ring

Braided 2-0 nylon suture swedged to a strong half-round taper-point needle is preferred for the repair. The cord is retracted to the lateral aspect of the deep inguinal ring. The first suture is placed through the transversus abdominis aponeurotic arch superomedially to the deep inguinal ring adjacent to the inferior epigastric vessels (Fig. 7-6, *bottom*). The overlying internal oblique muscle has to be retracted to gain exposure. The needle point is inserted from without to within the preperitoneal space and directed outward through the open deep inguinal ring.

After the needle is placed in the tissues but before it is pulled completely through, outward traction should be applied to test the ability of the tissue to hold the needle and, subsequently, the suture. As each bite of tissue is taken on each margin of the deep inguinal ring, the tissue is tested by tugging on the needle before completing its passage to ensure that the tissues encompassed are strong enough to retain the suture against moderate stress.

After placing and testing the first suture bite on the mediosuperior aspect of the deep ring and passing the needle outward through the deep inguinal ring, the surgeon passes the needle point back through the deep ring into the preperitoneal space, directing it just beneath the iliopubic tract and then distally in a flat path anterior to the femoral vein for a centimeter or more before the wrist is turned to bring the point of the needle back through the iliopubic tract and into the inguinal canal.

Occasionally, as the needle point turns back into the inguinal canal, it catches one or two fibers of the overlying inguinal ligament. Although it is unnecessary to encompass inguinal ligament within the suture, in most instances, I make no particular effort to replace the suture if a few fibers of the inguinal ligament happen to be caught within it. Indeed, in the occasional instances in which the iliopubic tract is not sufficiently strong, it may be necessary to deliberately include a portion of the overlying inguinal ligament to secure a sufficiently strong repair.

The ends of the initial suture are held by the assistant and placed on moderate traction. The second suture is placed 5 to 7 mm lateral to the first, again encompassing a tested strong bite of transversus ab-

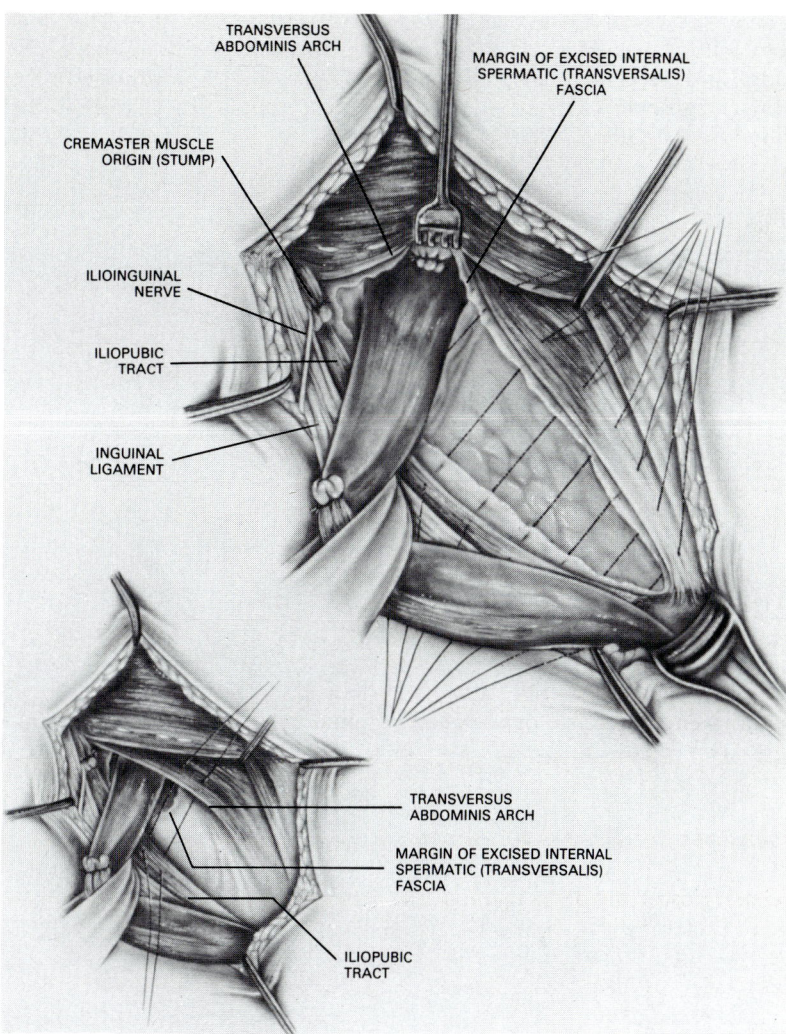

Figure 7-6. (*Top*) The repair of a complete indirect inguinal hernia in which the posterior wall of the inguinal canal is weakened or broken down requires suture reconstruction of the entire groin. The medial sutures are placed, beginning at the pubic tubercle, through the transversus abdominis arch above and the iliopubic tract below. (*Bottom*) The initial repair sutures for the typical indirect inguinal hernia are placed medially through the transversus abdominis arch above and the iliopubic tract below. For repair of this type of uncomplicated indirect inguinal hernia, only a few sutures on the medial side of the spermatic cord are needed.

dominis aponeurosis and muscle superiorly and iliopubic tract inferiorly. In passing the needle beneath the iliopubic tract, one must be aware that the deep circumflex iliac vessels are immediately subjacent; they are avoided by passing the needle tip flatly just beneath the iliopubic tract, encompassing a shallow amount of tissue in the anatomic anterior-posterior plane, but a substantial bite of tissue in the anatomic superior-inferior plane.

Sufficient additional sutures are placed, spaced 5 to 7 mm apart, to accomplish closure of the medial portion of the deep inguinal ring (see Fig. 7-6, *bottom*). The objective should be to close the tissues so that the cord exits lying immediately superiorly and just laterally to the subjacent external iliac artery.

Once all the medial sutures have been placed, they are maintained on gentle traction by the assistant, and the spermatic cord is retracted medially to

expose the lateral aspect of the deep inguinal ring. Sutures now are inserted lateral to the spermatic cord, encompassing the transversus abdominis arch above and the iliopubic tract and origin of the cremaster muscle below (Fig. 7-7). In the lateral portion of the groin, the transversus abdominis arch may be almost entirely muscular; nonetheless, it must be tested by applying traction to the inserted needle to ensure that the bite of tissue will hold the suture in place. A sufficient number of sutures, usually one to three, are used laterally to ensure closure of the deep ring about the cord. The closure should not be so tight as to cause strangulation. Leaving a gap of 0.5 cm between the cord and the nearest sutures permits the expected swelling of the cord postoperatively but does not lead to recurrence.

The sutures in the lateral aspect of the deep ring are tied after their placement. The cord is once again

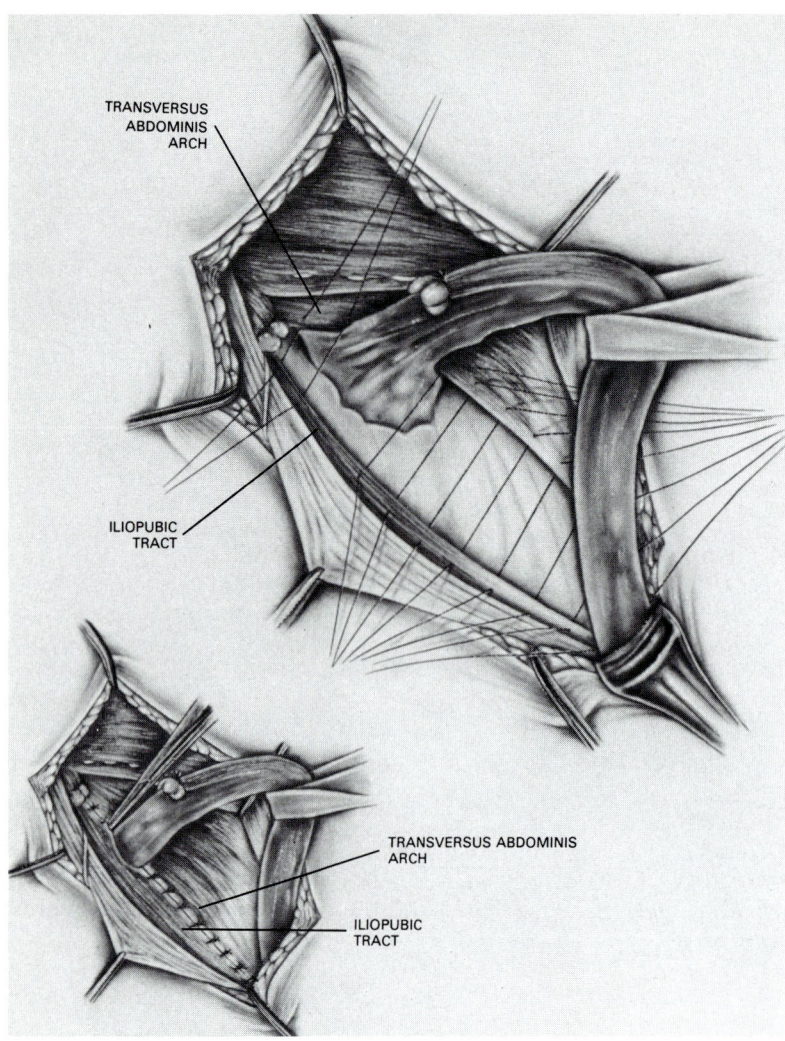

TRANSVERSUS ABDOMINIS ARCH

ILIOPUBIC TRACT

TRANSVERSUS ABDOMINIS ARCH

ILIOPUBIC TRACT

Figure 7-7. (*Top*) Sutures lateral to the cord complete reconstruction of the deep inguinal ring. These sutures encompass the transversus abdominis arch above and the cremaster origin and iliopubic tract below. (*Bottom*) The reconstruction of the deep ring should be snug but also loose enough to admit the tip of a hemostat.

retracted laterally, and the sutures in the medial portion of the deep inguinal ring are tied, beginning with the most medial suture and progressing laterally. At completion of closure of the deep inguinal ring, it should be just possible to pass the tip of a hemostat alongside the cord (see Fig. 7-7, *bottom*).

Wound Closure

The wound is irrigated with saline or saline-antibiotic solution: kanamycin, 500 mg, and bacitracin, 50,000 U in 500 mL of normal saline solution. Retractors are removed, and hemostasis is assured. The assistant grasps the testis and by gentle traction ensures its appropriate location in the scrotum. This maneuver also usually accomplishes replacement of the spermatic cord neatly within the inguinal canal.

If it has been transected, no attempt is made to reattach the cremaster muscle to its origin. The cremaster becomes adherent to tissues within the inguinal canal and, surprisingly, appears to function postoperatively in many patients.

The margins of the external oblique aponeurosis are reapproximated with interrupted or running sutures of 3-0 braided nylon. If the superficial inguinal ring has been widely dilated by passage of a scrotal hernial sac, it may be necessary to close the apical portion of the superficial ring by suture-approximation of its margins. At completion of the closure of the external oblique lamina, it should be possible to insert a fingertip, but not more, into the superficial inguinal ring alongside the spermatic cord.

The wound is again irrigated. The subcutaneous fat is not sutured. If the patient is excessively obese, the possibility of dead space is managed by placement of a few deep, locked mattress sutures.[2] The skin is closed with interrupted or running monofilament 3-0 nylon sutures, and a dressing is applied.

I do not adhere to the modern fetish of early exposure of wounds. The dressing applied in the operating room usually is left in place until suture removal, on the fifth or sixth postoperative day. If the dressing becomes stained with blood or serum, or if there is any suspicion of developing wound infection or any other reason to inspect the wound, I have no hesitation about removing the dressing—but I do not routinely pull the dressing off on the first postoperative day. Sutures are removed on the fifth or sixth postoperative day and replaced with Steri-Strips.*

REPAIR OF DIRECT INGUINAL HERNIAS

Direct hernias occur through the posterior wall of the inguinal canal, medial to the deep inguinal ring, and produce a diffuse bulge in the groin. Anatomically, direct hernias are excluded from the spermatic cord structures in the inguinal canal and thus are retained only by the overlying external spermatic fascia and the external oblique aponeurosis. The typical direct hernia does not have a constricting ring or "neck," and incarceration and strangulation are less likely complications. Of course, with the diverticular direct variety of hernia, a neck does exist. These atypical direct hernias usually appear as a recurrence after a previous repair, the hernia usually protruding through a tear made by a suture placed under tension.

Landmarks and Incision

The deep inguinal ring is situated halfway between the pubic tubercle and the anterior superior iliac spine. The direct hernial defect is situated between the deep inguinal ring and the pubic tubercle. The upper border of the hernial defect should be identified by palpation. The incision is placed just below the level of the superior margin of the direct inguinal hernial defect, centered on the hernial bulge, and is made transversely following a skin crease (see Fig. 7-1). Incisions for repair of direct hernias are located more medially than those used for repair of indirect inguinal hernias.

The incision is carried down to the underlying external oblique aponeurosis. Blood vessels, as encoun-

tered, are ligated with 3-0 polyglycolic acid suture material.

Opening the Inguinal Canal

The external oblique aponeurosis is opened, as in repair of an indirect hernia, by placing a small incision, 1 to 2 cm in length, between fibers of the aponeurosis just above the apex of the superficial inguinal ring (see Fig. 7-2). The tip of a scissors is inserted through this incision, and the underlying nerves and muscles are reflected away, after which the aponeurosis is split, first laterally and then medially, through the superficial inguinal ring. The incision should be continued through the external spermatic fascia on to the spermatic cord for a distance of 3 to 4 cm. The superior and inferior margins of the external oblique aponeurosis are grasped with hemostats and retracted, the underlying tissues being separated bluntly. Care needs to be taken throughout this dissection to protect both the iliohypogastric and the ilioinguinal nerves. Self-retaining retractors are inserted at each end of the wound to maintain exposure of the deeper tissues.

The line of division between the cremaster and internal oblique muscles is opened, as in repair of indirect hernias (see Fig. 7-3), and the intact spermatic cord is mobilized from the underlying direct hernial sac and adjacent posterior inguinal wall by sharp dissection. The cord then is encompassed by a Penrose drain and gently retracted inferiorly. Compared with repair of indirect hernias, mobilization of the cord should be more extensive medially in the region of the pubic tubercle and the superficial inguinal ring, but the area lateral to the deep inguinal ring need not be dissected.

The direct inguinal hernia now is visualized as a diffuse bulging or redundancy of tissue in the posterior wall of the inguinal canal (Fig. 7-8). A few fibers of transversus abdominis aponeurosis may be found spread widely over the surface of the hernial sac, but for the most part, the hernial sac is composed only of stretched transversalis fascia and peritoneum. The transversalis fascia often is opaque and may appear thickened and strong; the appearance is a delusion. Transversus aponeurosis, not transversalis fascia, must be used for the repair.

Management of the Hernial Sac and Dissection of the Hernia

Although it is not necessary to excise the peritoneal sac of a typical direct inguinal hernia, it is necessary to incise the transversalis fascia to gain access to the

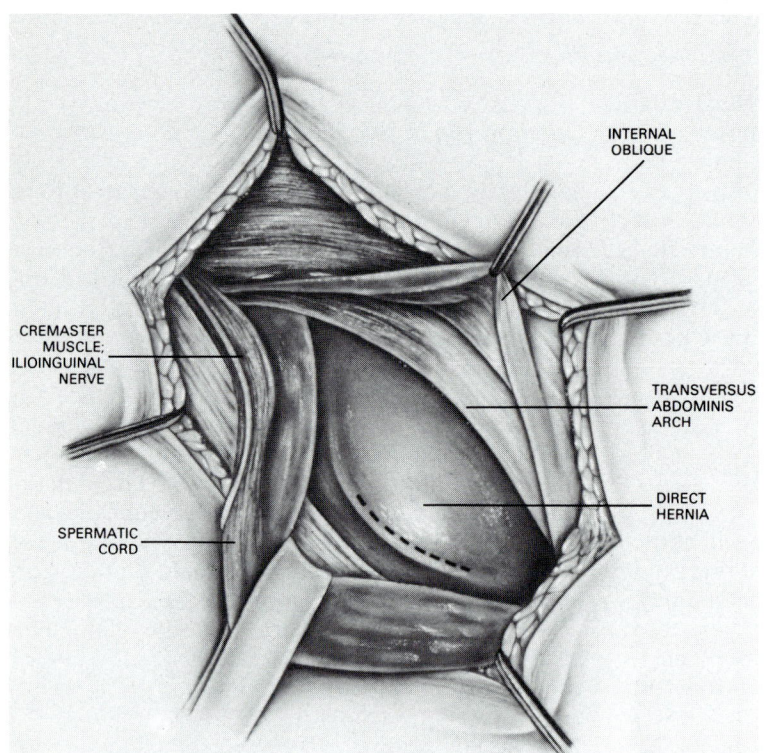

INTERNAL OBLIQUE

CREMASTER MUSCLE; ILIOINGUINAL NERVE

TRANSVERSUS ABDOMINIS ARCH

DIRECT HERNIA

SPERMATIC CORD

Figure 7-8. A direct hernia is exposed by mobilization of the spermatic cord. The hernia bulges through the posterior wall of the inguinal canal (transversalis fascia) The initial incision in the transversalis fascia is indicated by the dashed line. All redundant and weakened tissue in the posterior wall of the inguinal canal is to be excised.

preperitoneal space to facilitate identification and dissection of the fascial margins of the direct hernia. The redundant stretched-out transversalis fascia is excised. In the rare instances in which there also is a great excess of redundant peritoneum, the peritoneum may be opened and the excess excised, followed by running closure with absorbable suture.

In the typical situation, a small incision is made through the transversalis fascia (posterior wall of the inguinal canal) about 1 to 1.5 cm above the superior ramus of the pubis (see Fig. 7-8). The lower margin of the transversalis fascia is grasped with a hemostat and retracted inferiorly. Blunt dissection, with a "peanut" or similar dissector, is used to begin initial mobilization of the preperitoneal tissues from the overlying transversalis fascia. The underlying peritoneum and preperitoneal fat are pushed away from the internal aspect of the transversalis fascia all along the superior ramus of the pubis. This dissection should be carried out with care taken not to damage the arterial and venous blood vessels (corona mortis), which are found lying on or near Cooper ligament. The pubic tubercle, Cooper ligament, and adjacent portions of the iliopubic tract all should be identified and cleared.

In dissecting along the medial aspect of a direct hernial defect, one must take care not to injure the urinary bladder, which may have become incorporated in a larger direct inguinal hernia. Care also needs to be exercised to avoid entering the prevesical space or damaging the many blood vessels situated therein.

The inferior epigastric vessels are identified along the lateral margin of the direct hernial defect and gently mobilized with the preperitoneal tissues and away from the overlying transversus abdominis aponeurosis and muscle. Finally, a finger is inserted into the developing preperitoneal dissection plane and swept superiorly to identify the transversus abdominis aponeurotic arch along the superior margin of the direct hernial defect. Redundant and weakened transversalis fascia now can be excised to expose all the fascial margins about the direct hernia (Fig. 7-9).

A decision now needs to be made whether to proceed with primary suture repair, using a relaxing incision, or to proceed with reconstruction with a prosthesis because primary repair would engender too much tension. This is a matter of judgment for which there are no rules. The objective is to avoid tension in the repair. Because tissue is missing in many direct hernias, prosthetic repair is needed more frequently than in other varieties of groin hernia.

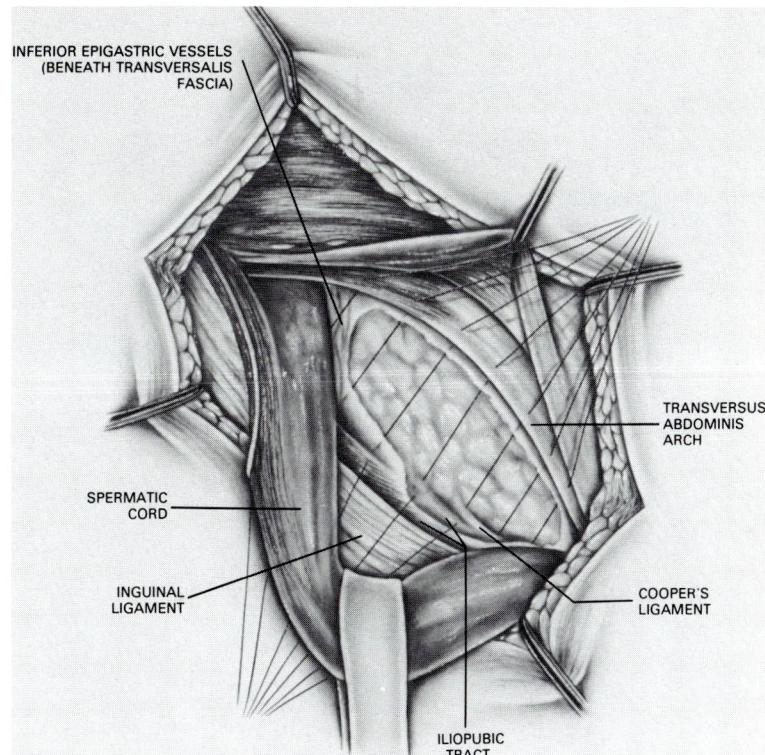

Figure 7-9. In a completed dissection of a direct inguinal hernia, the redundant transversalis fascia has been excised around all the borders of the hernia. The inferior epigastric vessels at the lateral aspect of the hernial defect have been carefully preserved. Sutures for repair of the hernia are placed, beginning at the pubic tubercle and progressing laterally, to the approximate transversus abdominis arch above and to Cooper ligament and the iliopubic tract below. Each suture is tested by traction on the needle to determine that the tissues are sufficiently strong.

Suture Closure of the Hernial Defect

Nonabsorbable 2-0 braided nylon suture swedged to a sturdy half-circle needle is used for primary repair. I prefer to place the sutures as individual interrupted sutures, although running suture technique is acceptable.

The initial suture is placed through the transversus abdominis aponeurosis immediately superior to the pubic tubercle, carried from without to within the preperitoneal space. Often, this suture also grasps a portion of rectus sheath, but the tendon of the rectus abdominis muscle should be avoided. As the needle is passed through the transversus abdominis aponeurosis, the strength of tissue encompassed is tested by placing the needle on traction.

The initial suture is extracted through the hernial defect, regrasped, passed back into the hernial defect, and carried through the periosteum and ligaments overlying the pubic tubercle, testing for solid placement as described earlier (see Fig. 7-9).

Sutures are now placed successively, about 7 to 8 mm apart, through the transversus abdominis aponeurosis arch, which forms the superior border of the direct hernial defect, and through the strong fascial structures along the inferior border of the hernial de-

fect; in turn, two or three sutures are placed through Cooper ligament and then the remainder through the iliopubic tract overlying the femoral canal. Sutures are all placed before being tied. In some patients, particularly those with a large direct hernial defect, it is not possible to tie sutures and close the hernial defect before making a relaxing incision.

Relaxing Incision

A relaxing incision is used in every primary repair of a direct hernia, excepting only the smallest diverticular direct types of hernia. A relaxing incision is essential if tension in the hernial repair, and consequent liability to recurrence, is to be avoided.

The superior flap of the external oblique aponeurosis is dissected bluntly back toward the linea alba in the area immediately above the pubic symphysis. This plane of dissection is developed superiorly and laterally to a depth of about 10 cm. In effect, this dissection mobilizes the superficial lamina of the lower one fourth of the rectus sheath (Fig. 7-10).

An incision is then made through the deep lamina of the rectus sheath to expose the underlying rectus abdominis muscle. The incision begins 2 or 3 cm

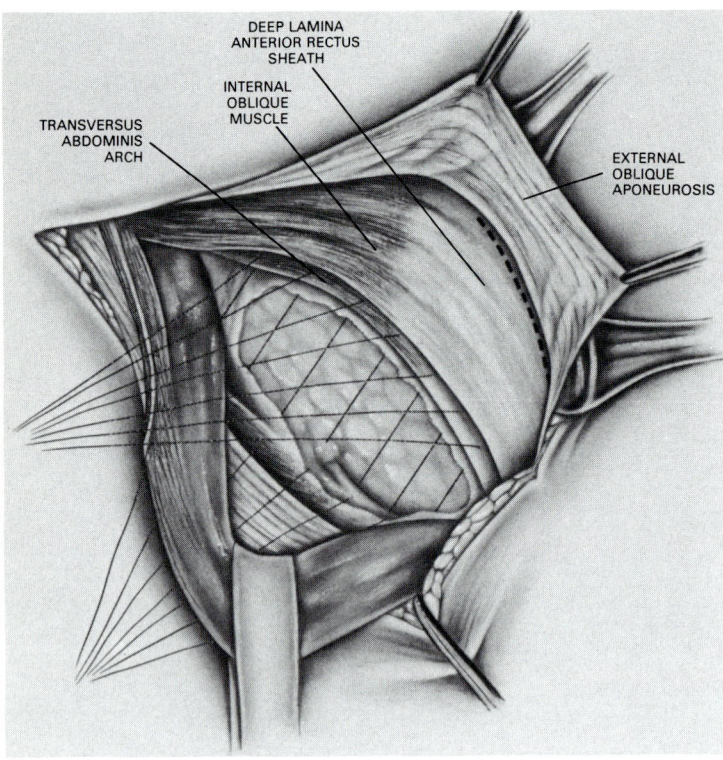

DEEP LAMINA
ANTERIOR RECTUS
SHEATH

INTERNAL
OBLIQUE
MUSCLE

TRANSVERSUS
ABDOMINIS
ARCH

EXTERNAL
OBLIQUE
APONEUROSIS

Figure 7-10. The external oblique aponeurosis (superficial lamina of the rectus sheath) has been dissected medially and superiorly to its line of fusion with the rectus sheath. The placement of a relaxing incision in the deep lamina of the rectus sheath (transversus abdominis and internal oblique aponeuroses) is indicated by the dashed line. Once the relaxing incision is made, all sutures are placed for closure of the direct hernia.

above the symphysis pubis immediately adjacent to the line of synthesis of the superficial and deep laminae. It is continued superiorly, following the line of laminar fusion, curving gently laterally to the border of the rectus sheath. Traction inferiorly on the transversus abdominis arch slides the resulting bipedicled musculoaponeurotic flap inferiorly and releases tension in the hernial repair (Fig. 7-11). If the tissue does not slide easily, its deep surface should be cleared by sharp dissection, with care taken to ligate branches of the inferior epigastric vessels.

Indications for Insertion of a Prosthesis

In many patients with a direct hernia, and particularly when repairing a recurrent direct inguinal hernia, it is found that the major condition for successful repair—closure without tension—cannot be achieved. After extensive excision of weakened tissues, the aponeurotic margins of the direct hernial defect are sufficiently far apart that they cannot be approximated, even with the help of a relaxing incision. If the repair is made under tension, recurrence is more likely to ensue. Under such circumstances, a prosthesis must be inserted to substitute for missing tissue or to rein-

force the hernial repair. If the need for a prosthesis can be identified preoperatively, it is much more convenient to approach the hernia posteriorly (preperitoneal approach) because application of the prosthesis on the deep (internal) surface of the transversus abdominis aponeurosis is much easier.

A piece of Marlex about 2 cm larger than the hernial defect in all dimensions is cut. All sutures should be placed before any are tied. I find it useful to use heavy sutures of 2-0 or 1-0 braided nylon with needles swedged to both ends. Alternatively, Marlex suture can be used, but it is stiffer, which makes handling awkward.

The initial suture is placed as a mattress suture along the inferior margin of the prosthesis in its midportion; one end of the suture is simply passed through the Marlex about 1 cm from its free border and encompassing about 1 cm of Marlex; the suture is placed so the loop is on the internal aspect of the prosthesis. The prosthesis is then stuffed through the direct hernial defect into the preperitoneal space. Each end of the suture is then passed separately through Cooper's ligament from within to without, the needles are cut off, and the suture ends are held.

Successive similar mattress sutures are placed about 1 cm apart along the remainder of the inferior

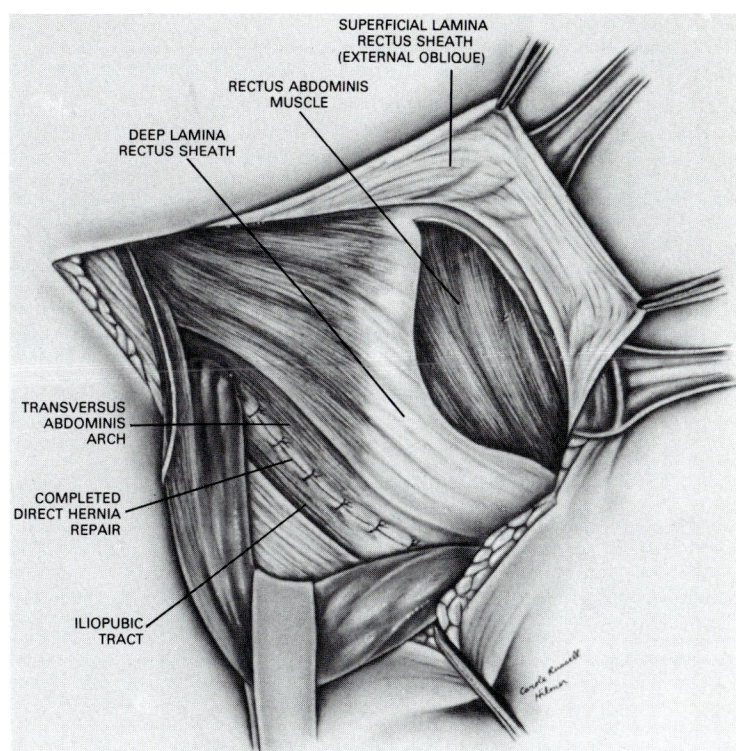

Figure 7-11. The completed direct hernial repair demonstrates that the relaxing incision allows the transversus abdominis to slide inferiorly. As the relaxing incision opens, the rectus muscle is exposed, but the overlying intact superficial lamina (external oblique aponeurosis) of the rectus sheath prevents the development of a hernia.

border, then the medial border, then the lateral border, and finally the superior border of the direct hernial defect. Sometimes, this process is tedious and awkward because of the necessity to work through the hernial defect to place the prosthesis on the deep aspect of the transversus abdominis lamina. When all sutures are placed, they are all pulled up and tied successively. No attempt is made, necessarily, to suture the borders of the hernial defect after placement of the prosthesis.

Wound Closure

The wound is irrigated with saline or antibiotic-saline solution and hemostasis assured. The external oblique aponeurosis is closed with 3-0 braided nylon interrupted sutures and the skin with 3-0 monofilament nylon continuous suture, as described for repair of indirect hernias. If a Marlex prosthesis has been placed, suction drains can be omitted (in contrast to most situations in which Marlex is used). Dressing care and suture removal are as described for indirect repair.

REPAIR OF A COMBINED OR COMPLETE HERNIA

A combined or complete hernia is an indirect inguinal hernia that has sufficiently enlarged medially that it has completely, or nearly completely, broken down the posterior wall of the inguinal canal. Repair of this hernia combines features of repair of indirect hernias of a more ordinary size with those of a direct inguinal hernia; the techniques of these repairs should be reviewed. Because the hernia is so large, it is usual to find the sac in the scrotum, and it is not uncommon to find that the scrotum is greatly enlarged and hangs pendulously at the level of mid-thigh or even below.

The skin incision is made transversely at a level just below the superior border of the hernial defect. The inguinal canal is opened by splitting the external oblique aponeurosis. The cord is mobilized and the cremaster muscle transected at its origin, as described for repair of indirect hernias. Dissection of the peritoneal sac from within the cremasteric and internal spermatic fasciae of the cord occasionally is a tedious process.

Often, when mobilization of the hernial sac has been completed, the scrotum is found inverted, and the testis is in the inguinal canal. In such instances, after excision of the peritoneal sac and its closure, the testis should be replaced within the scrotum and the normal relations of scrotum, testis, and spermatic cord restored by gentle distal traction. It is not necessary to anchor the mobilized testis by suture within the scrotum. If the sac envelops the testis as a hydrocele, that portion of the peritoneum adherent to the testis should be left in situ, hemostasis along the cut margins being achieved with a running locking stitch of absorbable suture material.

It is necessary to dissect cleanly the superior border of this large hernial defect from the pubic tubercle to the lateral aspect of the deep inguinal ring. Weakened and redundant transversalis fascia is excised during this dissection, leaving the transversus abdominis arch, which is muscular on its superficial surface and aponeurotic on its deep surface. Similarly, the lower border of the hernial defect must be cleared of areolar tissue and redundant transversalis fascia beginning at the pubic tubercle, progressing along Cooper ligament and the iliopubic tract to the lateral aspect of the deep inguinal ring. In this dissection, the external spermatic and cremasteric vessels are ligated. Care is taken to avoid injury to the inferior epigastric vessels and their branches within the preperitoneal space.

Suture repair of this large defect is begun medially at the pubic tubercle. As in closure of less extensive hernias, as the needle is passed through the tissue at the borders of the hernial defect, the strength of the tissue is tested by traction on the needle to ensure that the suture will hold. The initial suture is placed from the superficial to the deep aspect through the transversus abdominis arch about 1 cm above the pubic tubercle; the needle is regrasped and passed from within to without through the periosteum of the pubis immediately adjacent to the pubic tubercle. Sutures then are placed every 5 to 7 mm along each border until the spermatic cord lies in a position immediately superficial to the external iliac artery (see Fig. 7-6, *top*). At this point, the cord is retracted medially, and the repair is completed on the lateral aspect of the deep inguinal ring with one to three additional sutures (see Fig. 7-7).

A large relaxing incision is an essential feature of repair of an extensive hernia of this type. In an occasional instance, it may be found that, even with a relaxing incision that extends, as described for direct hernial repair, from above the symphysis pubis upward and outward to the border of the rectus sheath, some tension still remains in the midportion of the hernial repair. In such situations, the relaxing incision can be carried beyond the lateral border of the rectus sheath, transecting the transversus abdominis muscle

at a level just below the umbilicus. There is a small risk of a subsequent interstitial hernia when the relaxing incision is extended in this manner; the alternative is to insert a prosthesis. Optimal surgical judgment must apply in such instances.

Editor's Comment

Alexander Thomson (J Conn Med Prac 1836;4:137) would have been proud to see how the iliopubic tract, which he described, has become such an integral part of hernial repairs (Rheault, et al. Surg Gynecol Obstet 1965;121:601). This presentation by Robert Condon rings with authority. My approach varies slightly, but in essence, Dr. Condon and I are in agreement. This is the approach and repair for uncomplicated direct and indirect inguinal hernias (Types IIIA and IIIB; see Chap. 8). The importance given to the relaxing incision for direct and combined hernias in the Condon discussion must be highlighted.

I am now convinced that all recurrent groin hernias (Type IV) must be approached posteriorly and the fascial repair buttressed by prosthetic material. For surgeons unfamiliar with the preperitoneal approach, the anterior approach with prosthetic repair described in this chapter has merit.

L.M.N.

Special Comment

An Anterior Iliopubic Tract— Transversus Abdominis Repair Using an Inlay Graft for Selected Type III and IV Inguinal Hernias
Stanley D. Berliner

During the past decade, a biomaterial has been employed with increasing frequency in repairing groin hernias. With a personal experience of more than 6000 inguinal hernias, I have not found one operation that is applicable for all situations.

The type of repair employed is determined by the pathology encountered. For a Nyhus type I and type II hernia (see Chap. 8), a Marcy high dissection and removal of the indirect sac, combined with a transversalis fascia reinforcement about the internal ring, is sufficient. The intact posterior wall is not disturbed.

For most Nyhus type III and type IV hernias, a two-layer overlap hernioplasty is performed, which is a modification of the four-layer Shouldice technique. In about 20% of the cases, however, a major recon-

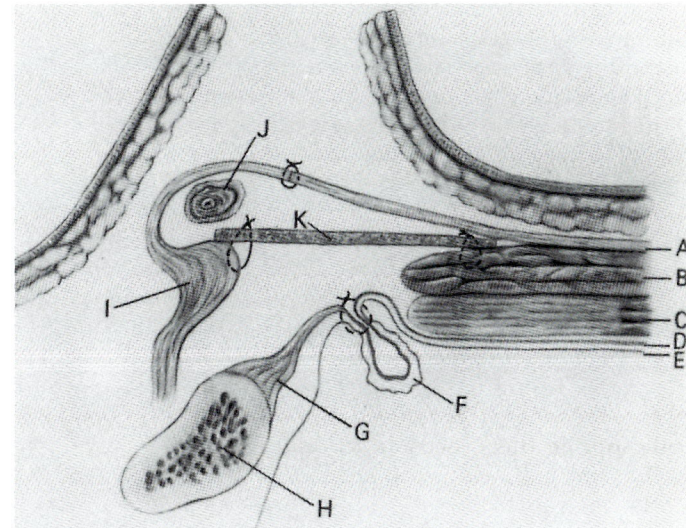

Figure 7-12. Sagittal view of the Lichtenstein on-lay graft repair. The posterior wall defect is corrected with an imbrication of the direct sac (F). The mesh patch is sutured to the inguinal ligament (I) and to the internal oblique muscle (B). This leaves a vulnerable area between the inguinal ligament and the iliopubic tract (G). A, external oblique aponeurosis; C, transversus aponeurosis; D, transversalis fascia; E, peritoneum; H, pubis; J, spermatic cord; K, mesh. (Lichtenstein IL, Shulman AG, Anid PK, Montllor MM. The tension-free hernioplasty. Am J Surg 1989;157:192.)

struction of the posterior wall and internal ring is necessary. Here, a preperitoneal graft is used to bridge the defect between the transversus arch above and the iliopubic tract below.

An onlay graft does not address the posterior wall defect (Fig. 7-12). If a major reconstruction is necessary to avoid tension, the inlay graft is physiologically, anatomically, and mechanically sound. The posterior wall is the transversus abdominis aponeurosis and its investing sheath of transversalis fascia. Its inferior margin is the iliopubic tract condensation of transversalis, not the inguinal ligament. An incision into this transversalis fascia–transversus abdominis aponeurosis posterior wall encourages fibroplasia and permits the mobile fibroblasts to envelop the biomaterial and deposit their collagen and proteoglycans.

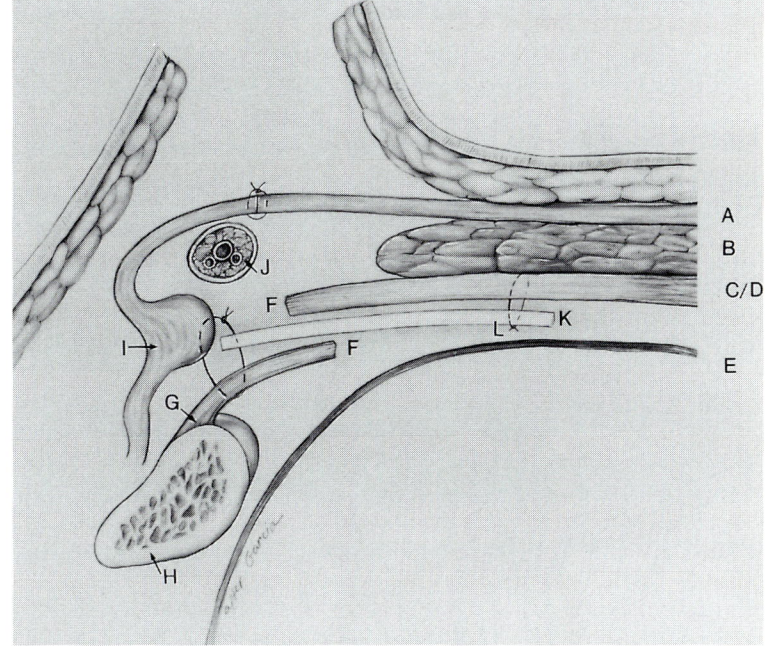

Figure 7-13. The inlay graft is sutured inferiorly to both the inguinal ligament (I) and the transversalis fascia (F) and superiorly to the white line of the transversus arch (L). Excess direct sac has been exised (F). A, external oblique aponeurosis; B, internal oblique muscle; C and D, transversalis fascia (TF) and transversus abdominis aponeurosis (TAA) posterior wall; E, peritoneum; F, incised TF and TAA posterior wall, direct sac excised; G, iliopubic tract insertion on Cooper ligament; H, pubis; J, spermatic cord; K, expanded polytetrafluoroethylene soft tissue patch. (Lichtenstein IL, Shulman AG, Anid PK, Montllor MM. The tension-free hernioplasty. Am J Surg 1989;157:192)

A flap is developed superiorly to the rectus margin, and the mesh is attached preperitoneally to the white line above and to both the incised posterior wall and the inguinal ligament below. This repairs the anatomic defect between the transversus arch and the iliopubic tract without tension and establishes a new internal ring lateral to the epigastric vessels (Fig. 7-13). Pubic tubercle failures are due to improper medial fixation of the graft. Lateral recurrences have not occurred.

Despite the fact that the inlay grafts represent cases with more extensive pathology, the results have been rewarding. In 350 operations, with a mean follow-up of 4.5 years, the failure rate is 1.1%.[1]

REFERENCES

1. Berliner SD. Clinical experience with an inlay expanded polytetrafluoroethylene soft tissue patch as an adjunct in inguinal hernia repair. Surg Gynecol Obstet 1993;176:323.
2. Hermann RE. Transabdominal repair of esophageal hiatal hernia anterior to the esophagus. Surg Gynecol Obstet 1968;127:839.

Hernia, Fourth Edition, edited
by Lloyd M. Nyhus and Robert E. Condon.
J.B. Lippincott Company, Philadelphia © 1995.

Chapter 8

The Preperitoneal Approach and Iliopubic Tract Repair of Inguinal Hernias

Lloyd M. Nyhus

There is no doubt that the first appearance of the mammal, with his unexplained need to push his testicles out of their proper home into the air, made a mess of the three layered abdominal wall that had done the reptiles well for 200 million years.

Sir Heneage Ogilvie, 1960

If hernias occur because of the failure of the transversalis fascia to withstand the pressure to which it is subjected, the natural method of operative correction would seem to be the repair and strengthening of the fascia.

P.W. Harrison, 1922

The development of the posterior approach to the groin has made it possible for surgeons to treat recurrences by using an alternative route, since in most instances the anterior approach has been used for the first procedure. This avoids scarring, limits damage to the blood supply to the cord and reduces postoperative complications from bleeding and infection.

Raymond C. Read, 1995

The purpose of this chapter is to present an evaluation of the preperitoneal (properitoneal, extraperitoneal, posterior) approach to and iliopubic tract repair of inguinal (indirect and direct) hernias. The anatomy of the groin must be thoroughly understood, and the anatomic concepts as presented by Condon (see Chap. 2) should be studied as a prerequisite to reading this section. The anatomy of the posterior inguinal wall, particularly the transversalis fascial layer and the iliopubic tract, is discussed further in this chapter as it relates to the technique of the recommended repair. The terms *properitoneal, extraperitoneal,* and *posterior approach* are synonymous with *preperitoneal* approach. Femoral hernia and its treatment by this approach are presented in Chapter 9.

HISTORY

Preperitoneal Approach

The early history of the posterior approach to groin hernias is interesting. In a report of one patient, Thomas Annandale[1] of Edinburgh in 1876 presented for the first time the concept of the preperitoneal approach. The incision used was not dissimilar to that advocated today. Annandale did not perform a fascial

repair. Lawson Tait[102,103] of Birmingham, England, in 1883 and 1891, reported the advantages of the treatment of hernia by "median abdominal section." He also recognized that, for "radical cure" to occur, "elements of the tendinous aperture must be agglutinated in order that the aperture may be effectively closed." Thus, the concept of repair of the posterior inguinal wall was presented in association with the intraperitoneal approach. There were many similar suggestions in the literature at this time.[58] The September 26, 1891, issue of the *British Medical Journal* is particularly interesting to peruse because it contains many allusions to the posterior approach, as presented to the Annual Meeting of the British Medical Association in Bournemouth, England, July 1891.

Bates[3] of Seattle should be credited with further advancing this concept. Bates repaired the defect from the posterior approach using *transversalis fascia.* The historical impact of Bates's contribution is significant. Therefore, the first two paragraphs of his paper are quoted:

This operation consists in making an incision, about two inches long, parallel with Poupart's ligament. The end of the incision should be about one inch above the usual location of the internal ring. The fascia of the external oblique muscle is divided in line of its fibers. The arching fibers of

Table 8-1. Methods of Anatomic Repair of a Defect With a Preperitoneal Approach to Hemioplasty

Author	Type of Hernia	Method of Repair
Annandale (1876)[1]	Indirect	Ligation of hernial sac
	Direct	Ligation of hernial sac
	Femoral	Obscure
Tait (1883)[102]	Groin	Obscure
Maunsell (1887)[58]	Femoral	Suture of pectineus fascia and pectineal line to Poupart ligament
Tait (1891)[103]	Indirect	Suture of fascial defect, "external column of ring to inner column"
	Femoral	Obscure
Bates (1913)[3]	Indirect	Suture of transversalis fascia of internal ring
Cheatle (1920)[8]	Indirect	Occlusion of internal ring by suture
	Femoral	Flap periosteum of pubis to Poupart ligament
Cheatle (1921)[9]	Indirect	High ligation of sac only
	Femoral	Flap periosteum of pubis to Poupart ligament
Henry (1936)[38]	Indirect	Plastic to internal ring—transversalis fascia to fascia deep surface internal oblique muscle
	Femoral	Flap of pectineus fascia to Poupart ligament
Jennings et al. (1942)[44]	Indirect	Plastic closure of internal ring—suture of transversalis fascial sling lateral to the cord
Musgrove and McCready (1949)[67]	Femoral	Suture of Poupart ligament to Cooper ligament
McEvedy, P. G. (1950)[63]	Femoral	Suture of conjoined tendon to Cooper ligament
Riba and Mehn* (1952)[87]	Indirect	Plastic closure of internal ring—suture of transversalis fascial sling
	Direct	Suture of transversalis fascia to Cooper ligament
Hull and Ganey (1953)[39]	Femoral	Suture of Poupart ligament to Cooper ligament or pectineus fascia flap technique of Henry
Mikkelsen and Berne (1954)[65]	Femoral	Suture of transversalis fascia and transversus aponeurosis to Cooper ligament
	Small indirect	Plastic repair of internal ring—transversalis fascia
	Large indirect	Similar to femoral closure
Mouzas and Diggory (1956)[66]	Femoral	Suture of conjoined tendon to Cooper ligament
McEvedy, B. V. (1958)[62]	Femoral	As described by his father in 1950
	Indirect	Suture of inguinal ligament to transversalis fascia and reinforced by conjoined tendon to Cooper ligament
	Direct	Suture of conjoined tendon to Cooper ligament
Nyhus et al. (1959)[76]	Indirect	Suture of transversalis fascial sling medial to the cord
	Direct	Suture of transversalis fascia or conjoined tendon or both to Cooper ligament
	Femoral	Suture of transversalis fascia to Cooper ligament
Nyhus et al. (1960)[72]	Indirect	Suture of transversalis fascial sling medial or lateral to the cord or both
	Direct	Suture of transversalis fascia, arch of transversus abdominis aponeurosis, or both to iliopubic tract
	Femoral	Suture of iliopubic tract to Cooper ligament
Sheehan (1961)[95]	Femoral	Suture of transversalis fascia and conjoined tendon to Cooper ligament
Smith (1962)[97]	Medial recurrent	Suture of transversalis fascia to Poupart ligament
	Lateral recurrent	Same
Estrin et al. (1963)[23]	Femoral	Suture of transversalis fascia to Cooper ligament
	Indirect	Suture of transversalis fascia to inguinal ligament
	Direct	Suture of transversalis fascia to Cooper ligament
Stoppa et al. (1972)[100]	Indirect, direct	Preperitoneal insertion of large Dacron prosthesis without fascial repair
Stoppa et al. (1984)[101]	Femoral, recurrent	Same

(continued)

Table 8-1. *(Continued)*

Author	Type of Hernia	Method of Repair
Ger 1990	Indirect	Laparoscopic closure neck of sac
Greenburg 1995 (Current)	All types plus recurrent	Similar to Nyhus (below)
Nyhus 1995 (Current)	Small indirect (type II)	Suture of transversalis fascial sling medial to the cord
	Large indirect (type IIIB)	Suture of transversalis fascia and transversus abdominis aponeurosis to iliopubic tract medial to cord. Occasionally, one or two sutures placed between transversalis fascial sling and iliopubic tract lateral to cord to ensure adequate closure of internal ring. Cord at level of femoral vessels. If massive, use components of direct repair as well. Buttress with Marlex mesh.
	Direct (type IIIA)	Suture of transversalis fascia and transversus abdominis aponeurosis to iliopubic tract.
	Femoral (type IIIC)	Suture of iliopubic tract to Cooper ligament
	Recurrent (type IV)	Repair defect, and buttress with Marlex mesh

*Performed in conjunction with retropubic prostatectomy

the internal oblique are separated and retracted. The fascia of the transversalis, together with the peritoneum, is opened. If adhesions are encountered they can be broken up by traction and blunt dissection with the finger within the sac.

The internal ring, including the neck of the sac, is caught up with an Allison [sic] tissue forceps or a hemostat and pulled up to the incision, where a purse-string suture of No. 3 plain catgut, on a needle, is passed around the circumference of the ring, engaging the fascia of the transversalis except at the junction of the inner and lower quadrant, where the vas deferens or round ligament is encountered; this is excluded externally from the ligature. Pulling up the internal ring and transversalis fascia restores them to the original position held before a hernia was produced.

Cheatle[8,9] renewed interest in the preperitoneal approach. The concept was slow to gain adherents; however, through subsequent decades, a number of advocates presented views on the subject (Table 8-1). Cheatle and later Henry[38] suggested that the approach might facilitate the technical handling of inguinal and femoral hernias. However, with few exceptions, the approach was used only for femoral hernias. There was little use of the approach for direct hernias.

My associates and I were perplexed about the failure of this method to flourish. In 1955, we began a clinical investigation in a deliberate attempt to explore the potential of the approach and to provide a large clinical group in which a long-term follow-up study could be accomplished and reported. During the ensuing years, our technique for the repair of indirect and direct inguinal and femoral hernias evolved.[72–74,76] As indicated in Table 8-1, many other

anatomic concepts and operative techniques used in conjunction with the preperitoneal approach to hernial repair were reported between 1876 and 1995.

Intraperitoneal Approach

Some confusion exists concerning the position of LaRoque[48–50] in the historical sequence under consideration. Basically, this surgeon from Richmond, Virginia, suggested that the peritoneal cavity be entered at the outset, through an incision slightly above the standard hernial incision. He then removed the hernial sac and performed a high ligation of the neck of the sac. LaRoque made no attempt to repair the posterior inguinal wall, but performed a standard anterior repair.

A number of articles were written on the intraperitoneal approach in subsequent years.[40,41,56,79,106,107]

Iliopubic Tract

The iliopubic tract was first described by Alexander Thomson[104] (frequently misspelled Thompson) in 1836.[84] Thomson recognized this important thickening in the posterior inguinal wall as an entity distinctly separate from the inguinal ligament. He wrote: "There is not one single fiber coming from the external oblique muscle. . . . We always find behind the tendinous portion of the external oblique, which forms Poupart's ligament, a strong aponeurotic bandelette, which has been, but wrongly, confused with the tendon itself."

Eugen Polya[81] also was a strong proponent of the individuality of the iliopubic tract. Polya made several interesting comments concerning this structure: "The opinions are not unanimous whether the ligament is part of the transversalis fascia, Poupart's ligament, femoral sheath or the psoas fascia. As far as I am concerned, and most of the other authors agree, this ligament constitutes a part of the transversalis fascia."

In his anatomic dissections (see Chap. 2), Condon transected or excised the inguinal ligament to visualize the iliopubic tract. Polya,[81] in 1912, recognized the importance of this technique to adequately demonstrate this structure. It was Polya who suggested that the *bandelette iliopubienne* be named the *ligamentum iliopubicum Thomsonii*. Ogilvie (personal communication, 1960), in discussing the iliopubic tract, added support to the concept of its separate origin from the Poupart ligament by stating, "There is a very obvious band that continues in the plane of Poupart's ligament backwards, but that clearly has no contribution from the external oblique aponeurosis." Finally, Fruchaud[25,26] described both in script and pictorially the iliopubic tract in the greatest detail presented in the modern medical literature.

The importance of the transversalis fascia and the internal abdominal ring in the repair of groin hernias has been recognized by many authors. The role of the iliopubic tract in these matters, however, is obscure.

Attention was focused on the iliopubic tract in the modern era of hernial repair by Clark and Hashimoto.[10] These authors demonstrated the iliopubic tract repair of the posterior inguinal wall by the anterior approach. Donald[17] used the iliopubic tract in a similar type of anterior repair. Griffith[31] should be credited with bringing many of the concepts of the anterior approach and the iliopubic tract into proper perspective.

Although my colleagues and I were unaware of the iliopubic tract as an anatomic entity at the beginning of our clinical study, the ideal exposure of the posterior inguinal wall by the preperitoneal approach allowed for early recognition of this thickening in the transversalis fascial layer as well as the recognition of the overall importance of this structure in the repair of all groin hernias.

SURGICAL ANATOMY

General and detailed concepts of groin anatomy are presented in Chapter 2. Further expansion on the subject would readily lead to the accusation of excess verbiage. There are, however, a few anatomic considerations that relate to iliopubic tract repair that must be stressed.

Laminar Structure of the Inguinal Region

The abdominal wall is composed of musculoaponeurotic layers protected externally by skin and subcutaneous fat and covered internally by preperitoneal fat and peritoneum. An anatomic hernial repair should restore the continuity and integrity of each disrupted musculoaponeurotic lamina. In uncomplicated groin hernias, only the lamina of the transversalis fascia is disrupted; other structures are merely displaced. In the repair of groin hernias, then, the essential task is the repair and restoration of the transversalis fascial lamina.

A parasagittal or vertical section through the midportion of the inguinal region (Fig. 8-1) illustrates the separation of the laminae of the abdominal wall into two groups of structures. The spermatic cord is contained between these layers within a cleft or space, the inguinal canal. The group of structures that lies anterior to the spermatic cord constitutes the anterior inguinal wall, or the superficial musculoaponeurotic lamina, and is composed of innominate fascia, the external oblique aponeurosis and its lowermost fibers, and the inguinal (Poupart) ligament. The spermatic cord exits from the medial end of the inguinal canal by passing through the anterior wall at the external inguinal ring. The structures posterior to the spermatic cord constitute the posterior inguinal wall, or the deep musculoaponeurotic lamina, and are composed of the transversalis fascia and the transversalis fascial analogues—iliopubic tract, crura and sling of the internal ring, transversus abdominis aponeurosis, proximal femoral sheath, and Cooper ligament. The spermatic cord enters the lateral end of the inguinal canal by passing through the posterior inguinal wall at the internal abdominal ring. The floor of the inguinal canal is primarily formed by the bony superior ramus of the pubis and its closely associated structures: the pectineus muscle, the pectineus fascia, and the more distal portion of the anterior femoral sheath.

Transversalis Fascia

A groin hernia results anatomically from a disruption or relaxation of the transversalis fascia. This concept is fundamental to understanding the anatomy of all groin hernial repairs. If surgical cure of the hernia is to be expected, the anatomic integrity of the transversalis fascia must be restored, no matter what tech-

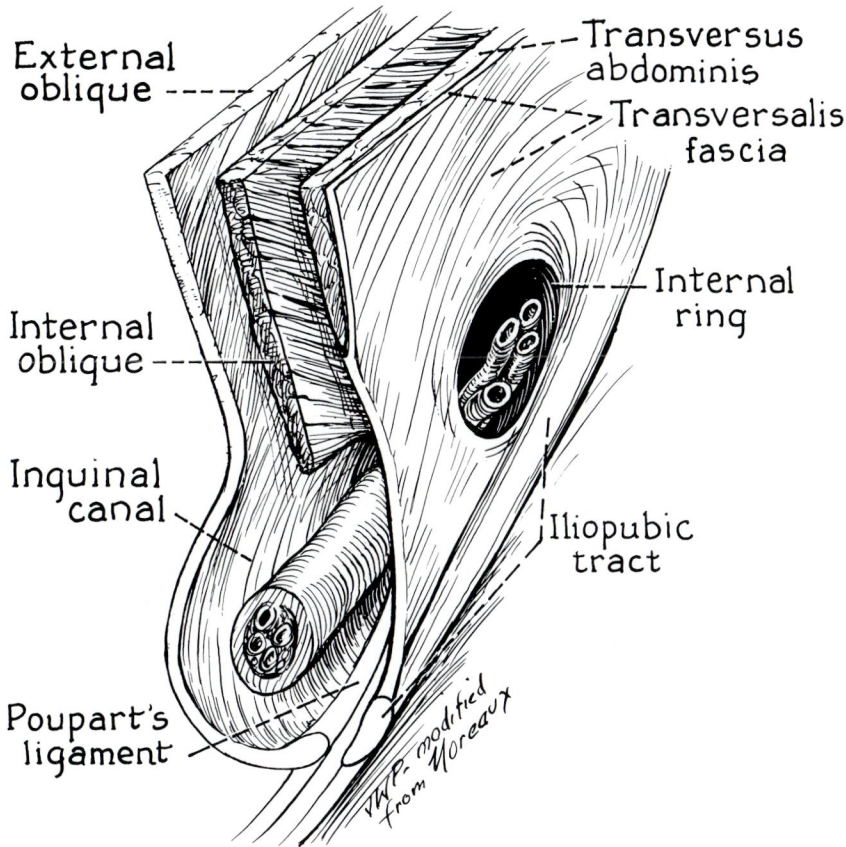

Figure 8-1. Parasagittal section through the right mid-inguinal region illustrating the separation of the musculoaponeurotic lamina into the anterior and posterior inguinal walls. All figures in this chapter are drawn on the right side.

nique of repair is used. No matter what else is done, the defect in the transversalis fascia must be repaired or a high rate of recurrence will follow. In the usual anterior approach to hernial repair, the exposure of the transversalis fascia is less than ideal. This may account, in part, for some surgeons' relatively high recurrence rates with the anterior approach.

Adherence to the principle of restoration of the anatomic integrity of the transversalis fascia in groin herniorrhaphy does not imply an unalterable commitment to use only transversalis fascia in the repair. It does imply, however, that the structures used for the repair must all lie within the transversalis lamina of the inguinal region (ie, in the posterior inguinal wall). This layer still forms the essential guide to repair because it defines the lamina within which repair should be carried out. The structures that actually are often used in the hernioplasty are a group of ligamentous and aponeurotic structures closely associated with the transversalis fascia. They are capable of retaining heavy sutures, and they provide the strength

required for the reapproximation and restoration of continuity of the transversalis fascia.

Iliopubic Tract (Ligamentum Iliopubicum Thomsonii, Bandelette Iliopubienne)

The iliopubic tract is a strong fascial band that begins laterally along the crest of the ilium and at the anterior superior iliac spine. In this area, it gives origin to the iliacus muscle and the lowermost fibers of the transversus abdominis muscle. The iliopubic tract arches over the psoas muscle and the femoral vessels; at the arch, it forms an integral part of the anterior femoral sheath. In its midportion, the iliopubic tract lies immediately subjacent to the inguinal ligament. It is, however, completely separated from the inguinal ligament, and the relation is one of proximity only. Continuing medially, the iliopubic tract inserts fanwise into the superior ramus of the pubis and into the Cooper ligament. The most inferior fibers of the ilio-

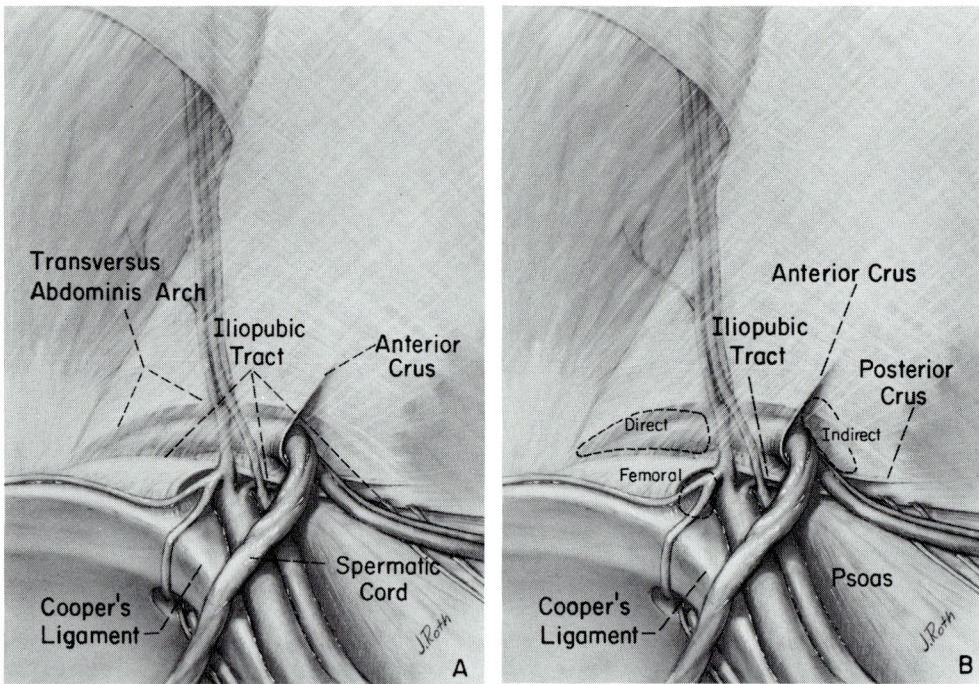

Figure 8-2. (*A*) The important anatomic structures of the posterior inguinal wall as seen from the preperitoneal approach. (*B*) The same view demonstrating sites of common groin hernias.

pubic tract—those that insert most laterally into the Cooper ligament—are sharply recurved in the normal groin. It is this recurved portion of the iliopubic tract that defines the medial border of the femoral canal, not the lacunar (Gimbernat) ligament of classic description.

The fundamental importance of the iliopubic tract is understanding the anatomy of groin hernias is appreciated when one realizes that the iliopubic tract forms one of the margins of the hernial defect in each of the common groin hernias. Direct and indirect inguinal hernial defects are limited on their posterior aspects by the fibers of the iliopubic tract; femoral hernial defects are similarly limited on their medial and anterior aspects.

Transversalis Crura and Sling of the Internal (Abdominal) Inguinal Ring

The internal ring is given an elliptic shape by the presence on its anterior and posterior aspects of a double fold of transversalis fascia that cradles and supports the spermatic cord in this region. This sling appears to be open laterally, but as is implied by the name internal abdominal *ring*, transversalis fascia can be delineated on all sides of the defect. The posterior crus or arm of this sling consists of fibers that parallel the iliopubic tract and finally fuse with it. The anterior crus is a denser band that has an extensive origin in the transversalis fascia above the internal ring. The two crura are continuous with each other on the medial aspect of the internal ring and the spermatic cord, and because they are more prominent at this level, a sling effect is given; thus, the terminology, transversalis fascial sling of the internal abdominal ring.

Conjoined Tendon—A Misrepresentation

Fusion of the aponeuroses of the internal oblique and transversus abdominis muscles to form one structure is the exception rather than the rule. This phenomenon occurs in less than 10% of dissected specimens. Thus, the term *conjoined tendon* should be discarded in favor of more specific terminology.[98]

Layers in the Hesselbach Triangle

Two layers of fascia cover the Hesselbach triangle—transversalis fascia and fibers of the transversus abdominis aponeurosis. The adherence of these tissue layers to each other is also apparent at and above the heavy curved arch of the transversus abdominis aponeurosis. Thus, these structures are not isolated, but sutured as one layer in the repair.

The anatomic structures contained within the posterior inguinal wall important to the surgeon are shown in Figure 8-2.

CLASSIFICATION OF GROIN HERNIAS

Human anatomy provides a natural system for guarding against indirect inguinal hernias (the sphincter mechanism of the internal abdominal ring) and direct inguinal hernias (the shutter mechanism of the transversus abdominis aponeurotic arch). The goal of successful operative procedures to repair these common inguinal hernias is to duplicate the natural mechanisms (ie, to close the sphincter or the shutter permanently). If suture lines are placed to approximate the posterior inguinal wall to itself (ie, transversus abdominis aponeurotic arch to iliopubic tract [shutter] and anterior transversalis fascia crus to posterior crus–iliopubic tract [sphincter]), a relatively tension-free repair results. Prosthetic mesh is not necessary for routine hernia repairs. Mesh may be useful in patients with large direct or combined direct-indirect hernias. To aid in surgical decision making, it is helpful to classify the types of inguinal hernias. Classifying hernias and matching the types of hernia with specific operations serve as a technical guide to hernia repair. This guide allows objective evaluation of treatment and verification of results.

> *Type I:* Type I hernias are indirect inguinal hernias in which the internal abdominal ring is of normal size, configuration, and structure. They usually occur in infants, children, or young adults. The boundaries are well delineated, and Hesselbach triangle is normal. An indirect hernial sac extends variably from just distal to the internal abdominal ring to the middle of the inguinal canal.
> *Type II:* Type II hernias are indirect inguinal hernias in which the internal ring is enlarged and distorted without impinging on the floor of the inguinal canal. Hesselbach triangle (floor of the canal) is normal when palpated through the opened peritoneal sac. The hernial sac is not in the scrotum, but it may occupy the entire inguinal canal.
> *Type III:* Type III hernias are of three subtypes: direct, indirect, and femoral.
> Type IIIA are direct inguinal hernias in which the protrusion does not herniate through the internal abdominal (inguinal) ring. The weakened transversalis fascia (pos-

terior inguinal wall medial to the inferior epigastric vessels) bulges outward in front of the hernial mass. All direct hernias, small or large, are type IIIA.

Type IIIB hernias are indirect inguinal hernias with a large dilated ring that has expanded medially and encroaches on the posterior inguinal wall (floor) to a greater or lesser degree. The hernial sac frequently is in the scrotum. Occasionally, the cecum on the right or the sigmoid colon on the left makes up a portion of the wall of the sac. These sliding hernias always destroy a portion of the inguinal floor. (The internal abdominal ring *may* be dilated without displacement of the inferior epigastric vessels. Direct and indirect components of the hernial sac may straddle those vessels to form a pantaloon hernia.)

Type IIIC hernias are femoral hernias, a specialized form of posterior wall defect.

> *Type IV:* Type IV hernias are recurrent hernias. They can be direct (type IVA), indirect (type IVB), femoral (type IVC), or a combination of these types (type IVD). They cause intricate management problems and carry a higher morbidity than do other hernias.[71]

THE OPERATION—PREPERITONEAL APPROACH AND THE ILIOPUBIC TRACT REPAIR

Indications

The preperitoneal approach is an ideal method for circumventing the scar tissue in operations for recurrent hernia. This technique has given a definite advantage in these patients. In addition, I have been pleased to find the posterior inguinal wall usually untouched during the previous operation or operations; therefore, that the iliopubic tract repair has been feasible in every instance.

Sliding hernia, so frequently the cause of consternation, is readily recognized and handled. All incarcerated and strangulated hernias of the groin can be released with relative ease. The constricting ring can be cut with minimal danger to vital blood vessels and nerves. If it is necessary to resect necrotic intestine, the peritoneum may be opened and the appropriate resection and anastomosis undertaken.[54] The problem of cryptorchidism is discussed later; however, the preperitoneal approach is ideally suited for correction of the defect.

As our techniques evolved, my associates and I became convinced that the approach was good for all complicated groin hernial problems. Therefore, we expanded our list of indications to include complicated hernias in adults.

Contraindications

Poor Anesthesia
The lower abdominal wall must be relaxed to facilitate visualization of the posterior inguinal wall. The operation *can* be performed successfully with only one assistant, provided good abdominal wall relaxation has been achieved, whether this be by general or regional block anesthesia.

Infants
General agreement exists that excision and high ligation of the hernial sac is a technique sufficient for the cure of ordinary hernias in infants with type I hernias. Because repair of the posterior inguinal wall is unnecessary and the hernial sac can be handled readily by the anterior approach, the posterior approach in infants appears to be superfluous. In general, I do not use the preperitoneal approach in children younger than 6 years of age.

Obesity
Extreme obesity complicates any hernial repair. It is my impression that because of the necessity of dealing with an anterior abdominal wall flap during the exposure of the posterior inguinal wall, the natural difficulties encountered in obesity are multiplied considerably by the preperitoneal approach. Many of my colleagues, however, do not agree that there is a disadvantage to the posterior approach in obese patients, and they persist in using it for all patients, lean or fat.

Direct Hernia
I do *not* consider direct hernia a contraindication to the preperitoneal approach. I must make a definitive statement in this regard because of the high recurrence rates reported after the use of this repair by several authors. It is now recognized that the judicious use of an inlay of polypropylene mesh to buttress the repair of large defects regularly gives good long-term results.[70,75]

Technique

Approach to the Preperitoneal Space
The preperitoneal space is entered through a transverse lower abdominal incision placed 3 cm above the inguinal ligament. The incision, then, is about two fingerbreadths above the symphysis pubis and slightly above the usual inguinal incision used in conventional anterior hernial repairs (Fig. 8-3).

The dissection is carried successively through the skin, subcutaneous tissue, and anterior rectus sheath. Before incision of the rectus sheath, exposure of the external inguinal ring as a basic landmark allows a more accurate estimation of the position of the internal abdominal ring. The incision through the anterior abdominal wall *must* be placed so that it is above (cephalad to) the internal abdominal ring (Fig. 8-4). The initial incision is placed over the rectus muscle (Fig. 8-5, *top*). The rectus muscle is retracted slightly toward the midline, and the transverse incision is extended laterally a few centimeters through the full thickness of the musculoaponeurotic layers formed by the external oblique aponeurosis and the internal oblique and transversus abdominis muscles (see Fig. 8-5, *bottom*).

The transversalis fascia is now exposed. It is opened transversely, special care being taken *not to enter the underlying peritoneum*. The preperitoneal space is entered (Fig. 8-6). Slight retraction of the lower margin of the incision exposes the posterior inguinal wall and the area of herniation. The general pelvic peritoneum and the preperitoneal fat are reflected

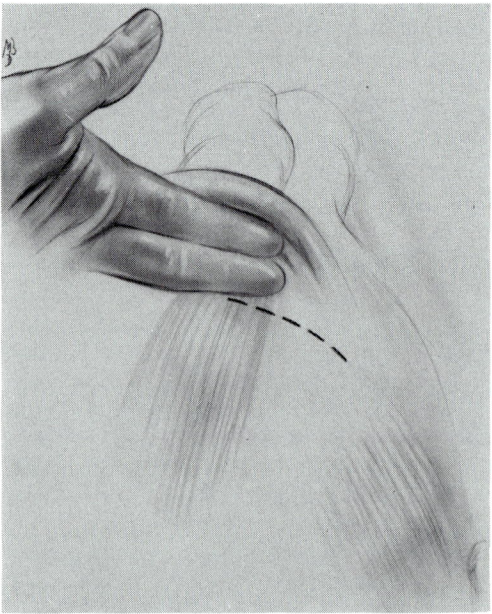

Figure 8-3. The skin incision for the preperitoneal approach is placed about two fingerbreadths above the symphysis pubis in a transverse direction. The incision may be extended into the preperitoneal space at this level, however, the maneuver depicted in Figure 8-4 prevents the incision from being placed too high or too low.

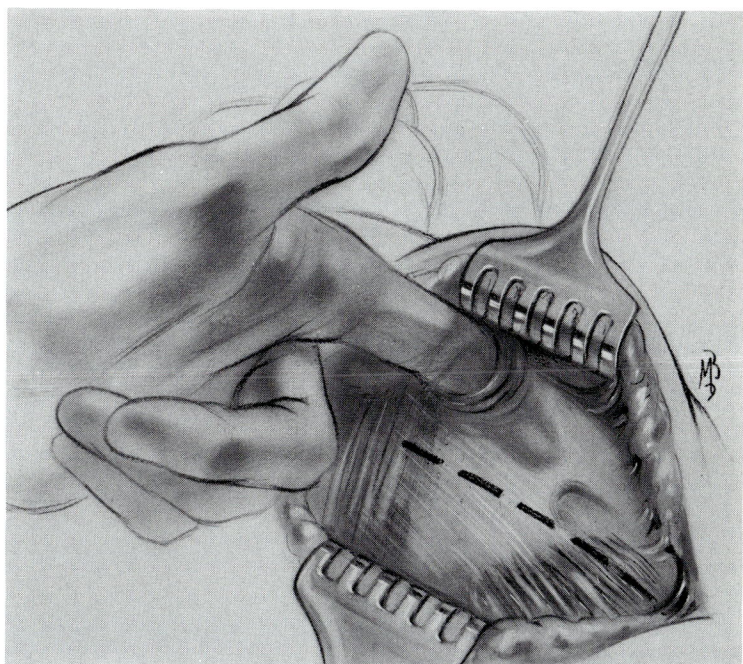

Figure 8-4. After the skin and subcutaneous tissues have been incised and the rectus sheath has been exposed, the level of the internal ring may be estimated by insertion of the left index finger into the external ring. This simple maneuver allows the surgeon to imagine the location of the internal ring, which is hidden from view. The incision in the anterior rectus fascia should be placed so that it passes just superior (cephalad) to the internal ring.

by blunt dissection, and any peritoneal projections through the posterior inguinal wall are readily visualized.

Repair of a Direct Inguinal Hernia

A direct hernial sac (type IIIA) is easily reduced by gentle traction and dissection (Fig. 8-7). As the sac is reduced, the tissues should be carefully watched. The attenuated transversalis fascia at the apex of the sac everts along with the peritoneal sac and can be noted as a prominent fold or white line. This fascia can be grasped, and the margins of the hernial defect are rapidly defined.

The usual peritoneal sac associated with a direct hernia need not be excised. If the peritoneum appears particularly redundant, however, the sac may be invaginated into a pursestring suture or excised and the peritoneum closed flush with its normal curve. The proximity of the bladder in a direct hernia must be considered when a peritoneal sac is being excised and care exercised to prevent damage to the bladder wall.

The direct hernial defect is repaired with interrupted sutures (1-0 monofilament polypropylene, the last of the five knots compressed with a stainless steel clip) to approximate the upper and lower borders of the defect. The upper border of the defect is thickened transversalis fascia and the arch of the aponeurosis of transversus abdominis muscle. The inferior margin of the direct defect is the iliopubic tract, which may be identified visually, or by palpation, or using

both methods. It is not unusual for the first and second medial sutures to be placed through both the iliopubic tract and the Cooper ligament. The more lateral sutures are placed into the iliopubic tract. If the iliopubic tract has been attenuated by the pressure of a large direct hernia, all the lower sutures may be placed in the Cooper ligament.

Repair of an Indirect Inguinal Hernia

An indirect hernial sac is reduced by traction, a pursestring suture is placed about its neck, the excess sac is excised, and the pursestring suture is tied (Fig. 8-8). An optimally high ligation is performed. Alternatively, the sac may be left in situ, the contents reduced, the neck transected, and the peritoneum closed; the distal sac is left open. Although I usually reduce and excise indirect hernial sacs, it is preferable to leave the distal sac in situ if extensive dissection is needed for its mobilization. I have not encountered hydrocele formation when the distal sac has been left in situ. Even if an occasional hydrocele formed, this would be preferable to the damage to the spermatic cord, vessels, and testis that accompanies the difficult and extensive dissection needed to remove a scarred indirect sac. This principle also applies to the conventional anterior approach to indirect inguinal hernia and is not unique to the preperitoneal approach.

After the high ligation of the neck of the hernial sac, the hernial defect is repaired. For the smaller indirect hernias (type II), a few sutures placed medial or lateral to the cord, approximating fibers of the an-

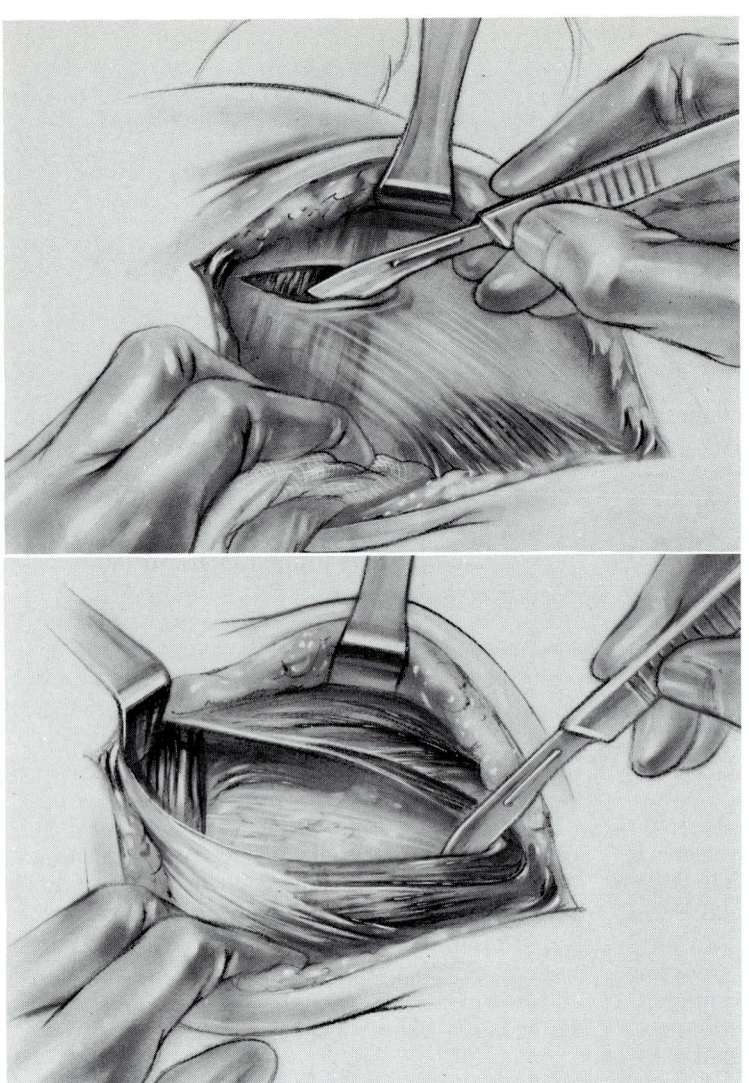

Figure 8-5. Transverse fascial incision. (*Top*) The incision begins over the mid-rectus muscle of the affected side. (*Bottom*) The surgeon enlarges the incision by separating and cutting fascia and muscle fibers of the external oblique, internal oblique, and transversus abdominis muscles. The transversalis fascia is seen in the depth of the wound. When the transversalis fascia is cut, the preperitoneal space is entered, and the proper plane of dissection is achieved.

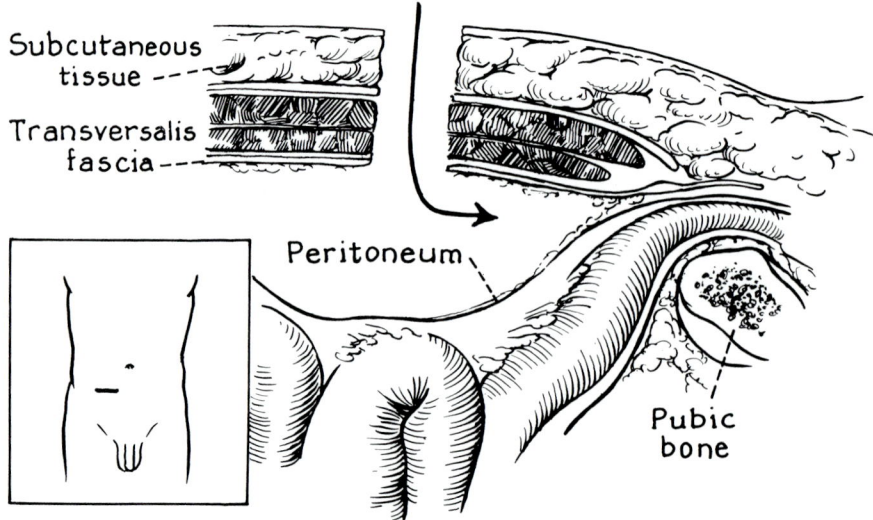

Figure 8-6. The operative approach to the preperitoneal space. It is seldom necessary to ligate and sever the inferior epigastric artery and vein.

162

terior crus of the internal ring to the posterior crus and iliopubic tract, suffice. For larger indirect hernias, the cord is first gently retracted laterally, and sutures are placed between the anterior crus of the transversalis fascial sling and the iliopubic tract medial to the cord. Sufficient sutures—one or two in the usual hernia, more with extensive defects (type IIIB)—are placed so that the internal ring and associated spermatic cord are restored to their normal anatomic position above and slightly lateral to the femoral artery. The cord is then retracted medially, and the repair of the hernial defect is continued laterally. Two or three sutures usually suffice for the lateral closure. In massive indirect hernias with associated medial displacement of the inferior epigastric vessels and destruction of the posterior inguinal wall in the area of the Hesselbach triangle, the principles of repair in both direct and indirect hernioplasty are used. The medial portion of the hernial defect is repaired as a direct hernia; the repair is continued laterally, and a new internal abdominal ring is created at the level of the femoral vessels (see Fig. 8-8*E*).

Closure of the Wound

After the hernial repair is complete, the remainder of the groin must be carefully searched for other hernias or areas of weakness. If such a "missed" hernia is not found and repaired, it may appear postoperatively as a "recurrent" hernia.

Meticulous care must be taken to secure complete hemostasis before closure of the wound. The preperitoneal space is then well irrigated with saline solution. The thin layer of transversalis fascia entered below the semicircular line of Douglas is usually not closed. The anterior sheath and lateral muscle aponeuroses are sutured in layers with interrupted medium polypropylene suture, followed by closure of the subcutaneous tissue and skin.

General Remarks

In my early experience, ligation of the inferior epigastric artery and vein was routine. As my experience has broadened, I have not found it necessary routinely to add this maneuver for adequate exposure.

If an Allis clamp is placed on the iliopubic tract at the level of the anterior femoral sheath and pulled laterally, it helps immeasurably to delineate the medial projection of the iliopubic tract. Similarly, lateral traction on an Allis clamp placed on the anterior crus of the internal abdominal ring (the clamp includes the transversalis fascia and the transversus abdominis aponeurosis) helps to delineate the superior edge of direct hernial defects as well as the superior edge of large indirect hernial defects. The fascial bands and thickening may on occasion be easier to palpate than to visualize.

The iliopubic tract should be lifted in an anterior direction when sutures are placed into it at the level of the femoral artery and vein. Unless this precaution is taken, the vessels may be traumatized.

The standard suture material used in the fascial layer of the iliopubic tract repair is 1-0 polypropylene.

Results of Treatment

Total operative morbidity, particularly late morbidity, is much lower after the posterior approach is used; there is much less atrophy of the testis and less evidence of neuropathy. In a continuing 38-year review (November 1955–November 1993) by my associates and I,[70] the operative complications, including mortality, have remained at the level reported previously.

Incidence of Recurrence

My associates' and my series[70] of 1200 primary hernial repairs gave the following results: indirect, 3% recurrence; direct, 6% recurrence. The relaxing incision was not used, nor was plastic material used to buttress these repairs.

Similar satisfactory results have been reported by others.[11,30,33,60,83] McClelland and associates[60] used a relaxing incision in every instance and also stressed the use of the Cooper ligament rather than the iliopubic tract in repair of direct hernias. I have shown that, when properly performed, the so-called Cooper ligament repair from the anterior approach may differ from my technique by as little as one or two sutures. In both techniques, the most medial sutures are placed into the combined iliopubic tract and Cooper ligament. As the repair progresses laterally, I do not continue to place sutures into the Cooper ligament; rather, at the midportion of the repair, I place posterior sutures only into the iliopubic tract. The transition suture of McVay is unnecessary. Thus, the medial and lateral sutures of these repairs are similarly placed. It probably is only the transition suture of McVay and the suture placed just before it that differentiate the two repairs.[77]

Unfortunately, excellent results have not been universally reported. There has been no problem with the posterior repair when performed for indirect primary hernias. However, representative reports of recurrence rates for direct hernias are as follows: 28%,[57] 16%,[35] 17%,[92] 21%,[27] 35%,[18] and 18%.[96] Many authors used the vertical midline approach of Cheatle and Henry without considering the finer nuances of anatomic information and operative technique available.

These reports certainly are discouraging. In one of our first papers on this subject,[72] my colleagues and I stated, "Any operative approach in inguinofemoral

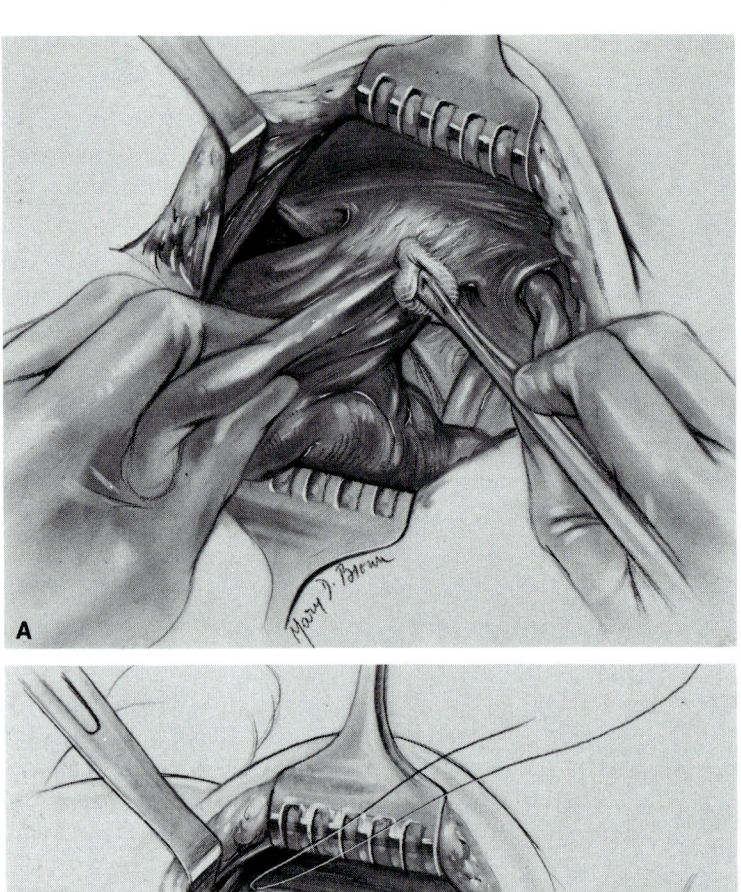

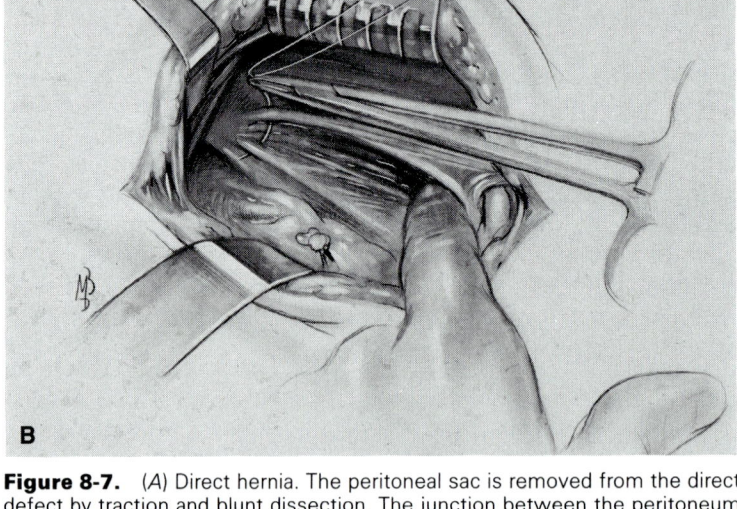

Figure 8-7. (*A*) Direct hernia. The peritoneal sac is removed from the direct defect by traction and blunt dissection. The junction between the peritoneum and the weakened transversalis fascia is usually seen as a definite fold or white line. The peritoneum in a direct hernia usually has a broad base and does not need to be excised. The redundant peritoneum may be inverted into a purse-string suture if desired. (*B*) The superior edge of this direct defect is the fused transversalis fascia–transversus abdominis aponeurosis layer. A suture is being placed into this upper edge and into the iliopubic tract below. One may delineate these structures by placing a finger into the direct defect and placing lateral traction on the tissues. (*C*) The direct defect has been closed. The transversalis fascial sling of the internal abdominal ring is tightened as a prophylactic measure.

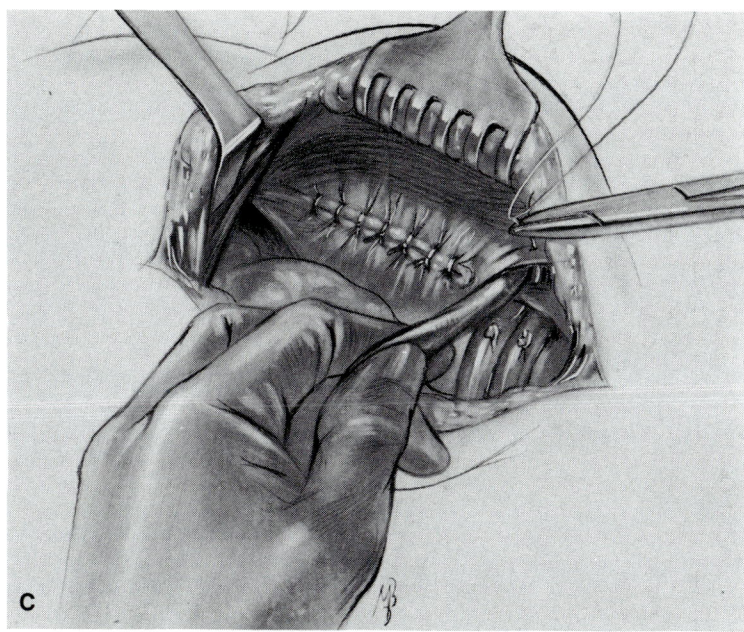

Figure 8-7. *(Continued)*

hernias, to be practical, must intrinsically allow for immediate repair of indirect, direct, or femoral hernias."

We, and others[30] (see Special Comment), showed that the posterior approach can give satisfactory results in the repair of *all* types of groin hernia. However, it is our premise that surgeons should choose the operative procedure best suited to their own abilities and to the actual type of hernia found. Thus, the posterior approach and iliopubic tract repair with or without an inlay prosthetic buttress should be a part of the selection process (Table 8-2).

Relaxing Incision
A relaxing incision of the McVay-Tanner method has never been necessary in the repair of type II or IIIC hernias, that is, for small indirect or femoral defects. We have urged that this tension-relieving maneuver be used for the repair of all type IIIA, IIIB, and IV hernias. It is in these same complex defects that we now recognize the need to support the repair by placement of the inlay prosthetic buttress. Although it appears heretic, we have not used a relaxing incision concomitant to use the buttress and have noted no change in our good results. The prosthesis acts to bolster the wall (a force against tension–distraction) in addition to its protection against intraabdominal pressure.

By careful attention to the detail of hernia types, we have been able to modify our procedure significantly. This allows for greater ease of performing the operation, without sacrificing the quality of the repair.

Use of Prosthetic Material for Recurrent Hernias
I recommend the use of prosthetic materials in primary repairs of types IIIA, IIIB, IV hernias. Recommendations for this modification, particularly for repair of direct hernias, are common.*

The technique of the preperitoneal approach and repair of a recurrent defect is not different from that previously described for the primary repair. Indeed, it may not be necessary to repair the defect after the hernial sac has been removed, according to the Stoppa principle (see Chap. 10). Having made this seemingly radical statement, I must emphasize that we do close the defects with 1-0 polypropylene monofilament suture. A 6-cm × 14-cm rectangle of polypropylene mesh is anchored posteriorly to the Cooper ligament with interrupted 1-0 polypropylene sutures (Fig. 8-9). The mesh is then tacked above the aforementioned repair with 3-0 polypropylene (Fig. 8-10). Finally, the mesh is folded cephalad to fit beneath the wound of entrance into the preperitoneal space (Fig. 8-11).

My colleagues and I have been satisfied with the preperitoneal approach and mesh buttress of the repair of recurrent hernias. We began to use the mesh buttress regularly in 1975. Our recurrence rate with the technique is less than 2%.[74,75] I believe that placing the buttress mesh posteriorly takes full advantage of

*References 2, 4–7, 12, 14, 15, 24, 28, 35, 47, 51, 78, 82, 89, 90, 101, 105.

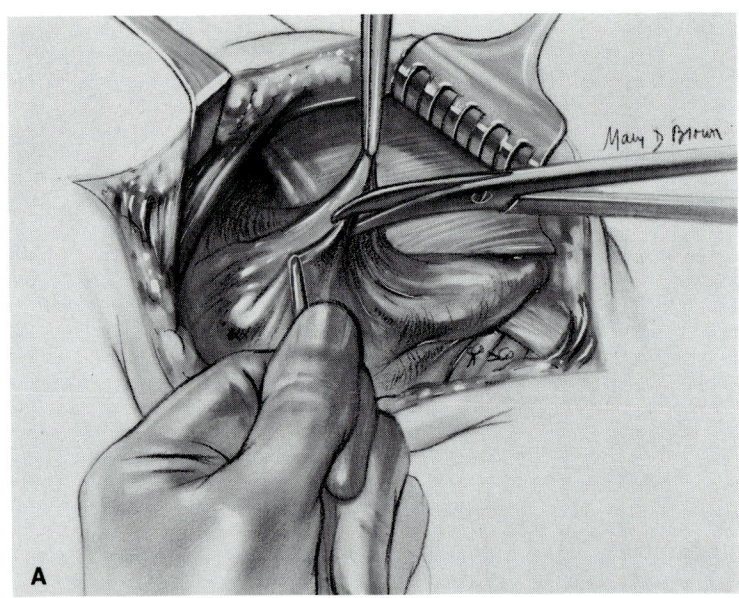

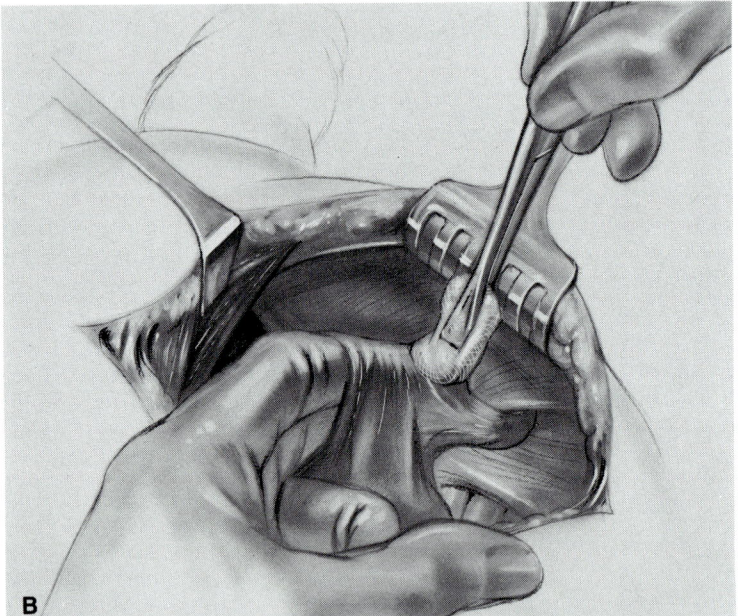

Figure 8-8. (*A*) Indirect hernia (type IIIB). After the spermatic cord and hernial sac are encompassed, the peritoneum is opened. (*B*) A finger is placed into
the indirect hernial sac, and by means of traction and blunt dissection, the sac
is removed from the inguinal canal. (*C*) Before excision of this indirect sac, the
peritoneal defect is closed with a pursestring suture. (*D*) In small indirect hernias (type II), the lateral or medial aspect of the internal abdominal ring is
closed, usually from the anterior approach. (*E*) An indirect hernia enlarges in a
medial direction. In massive (sliding) indirect hernias (type IIIB), the medial repair is similar to that of a direct hernia. The spermatic cord is placed at the level
of the femoral vessels, and a new internal abdominal ring is made by sutures
placed between the anterior crus of the sling and the posterior crus (iliopubic
tract).

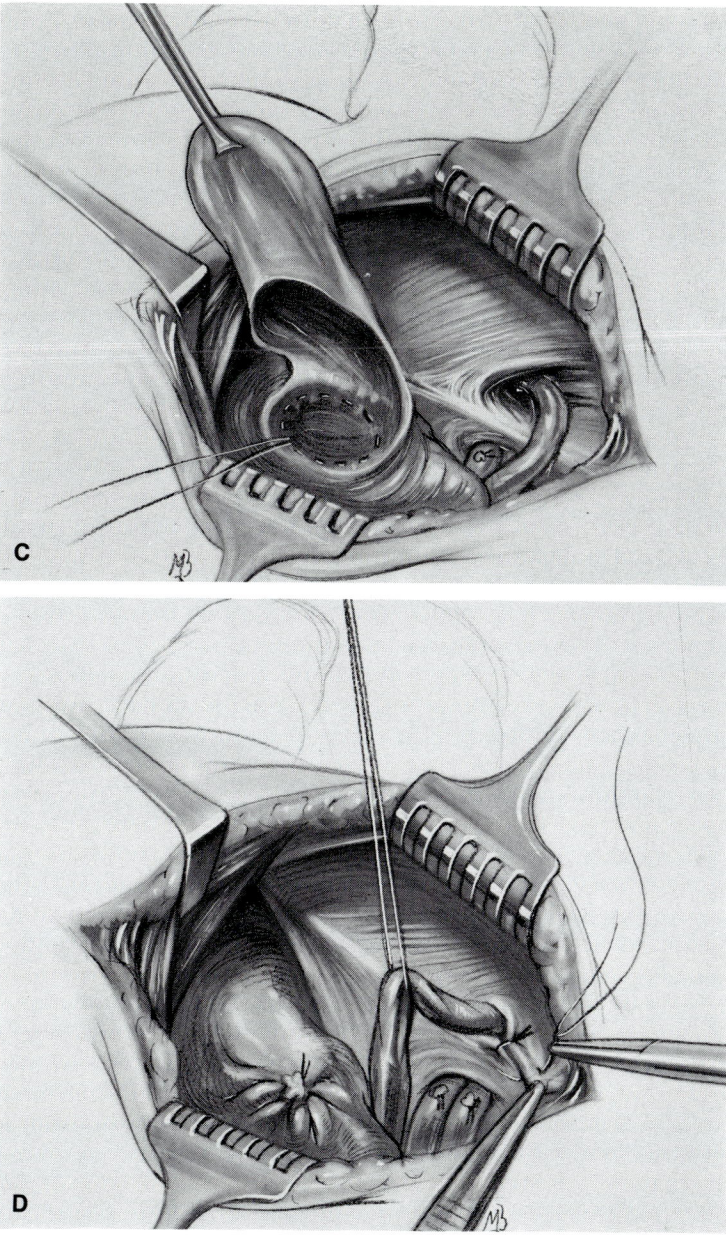

Figure 8-8. *(Continued)*

the hydrostatic principle of Pascal (see Chap. 10), unlike the use of anteriorly placed mesh, which demonstrates no advantage in either primary or secondary repairs.

McVay and Halverson,[64] Rignault,[88] Rosenthal and Walters,[93] Greenburg,[30] and Wantz (see Special Comment to Chap. 10) also are studying the posterior approach and the use of prosthetic mesh for patients with multiple recurrent hernias. It will be years before the results of this modification are known. After ap-

plication of the prosthetic buttress from the posterior approach, the surgeon has a sense of well-being. My concerns relative to the potentially increased incidence of infection or rejection of the polypropylene mesh have not been warranted to date. The worldwide experience with polypropylene mesh used in the presence of infection has been outstanding.[53] The use of the mesh in a clean wound should be most salutary. In 1959, my colleagues and I[76] reported on the use of prosthetic material (Ivalon) to buttress hernial repairs

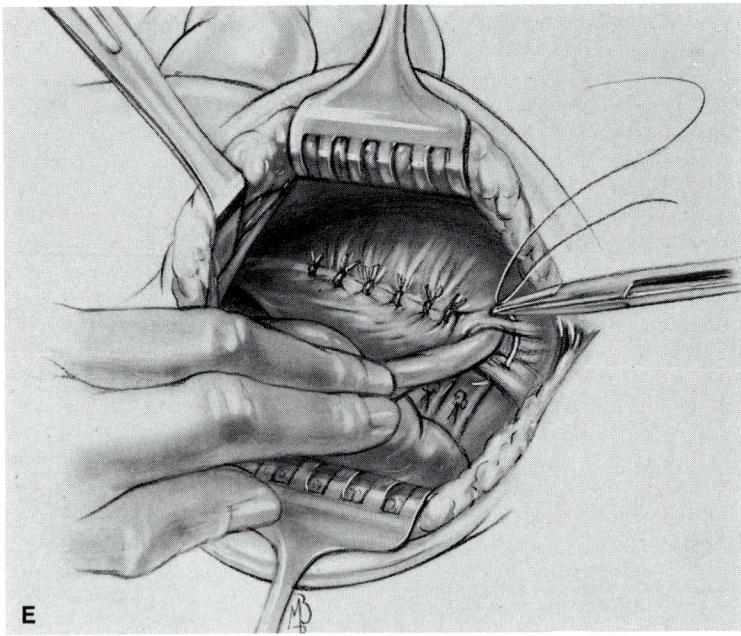

Figure 8-8. *(Continued)*

from the posterior approach. My 36 years of study of this method make me certain that recurrent groin hernias in the future in large measure will be approached preperitoneally and buttressed with prosthetic material.

Laparoscopic herniotomy (see Chap. 15) clearly is an operative method in which the posterior approach and synthetic prosthetic materials are key elements of the procedure. By the year 2000, an answer to the effectiveness of these new and innovative techniques should be available.

MISCELLANEOUS CONSIDERATIONS

Prostatectomy and the Preperitoneal Approach

McDonald and Huggins[61] stated that "simultaneous herniorrhaphy and prostatectomy are well tolerated and constitute a practical procedure." These two authors and others[16,42,55] did not use the posterior approach to repair the hernia, but used the standard

Table 8-2. Repair Individualized to Type of Hernia

Type of Hernia	Repair
Type I—Indirect with normal internal abdominal ring	High ligation of sac*; no repair
Type II—Indirect with internal abdominal ring dilated, posterior abdominal wall intact	High ligation of sac; transversalis fascia repair of internal abdominal ring (plastic repair)

Type III—Posterior wall defects
  A. Direct
  B. Large indirect
	Anterior approach—IPTR without mesh (Condon); Shouldice repair; Cooper ligament repair or
	Posterior approach—IPTR with inlay buttress of polypropylene mesh; Stoppa GPRVS with Mersilene

C. Femoral	Posterior approach—IPTR without mesh
Type IV—Recurrent	Posterior approach—IPTR with inlay buttress of polypropylene mesh

*Excision and ligation of hernial sac are performed for all indirect and femoral hernias. A direct sac is usually not opened, excised, or ligated.
GPRVS, giant prosthetic reinforcement of the visceral sac; IPTR, iliopubic tract repair.

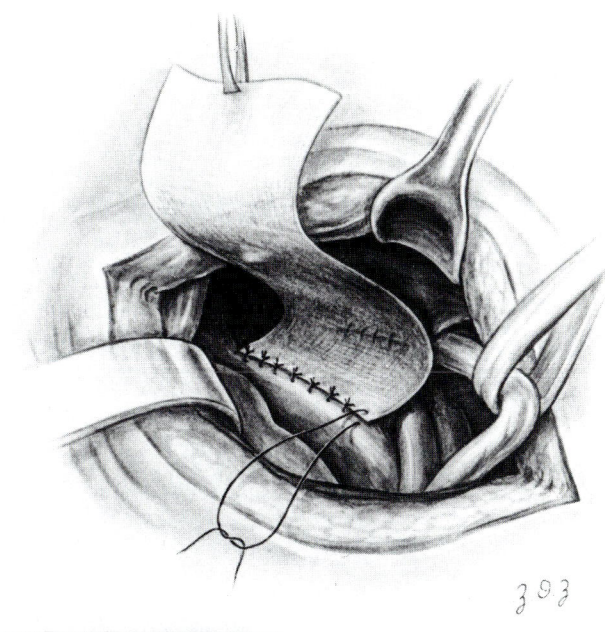

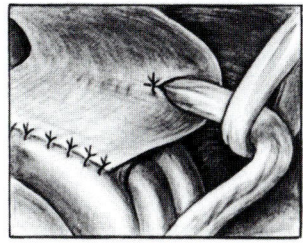

Figure 8-9. A polypropylene mesh buttress is attached posteriorly to the Cooper ligament (after repair of the recurrent defect in the wall) with 1-0 polypropylene suture material. If there is concern about closure of the internal abdominal ring (in indirect recurrences), the mesh may be folded around the spermatic cord (*inset*).

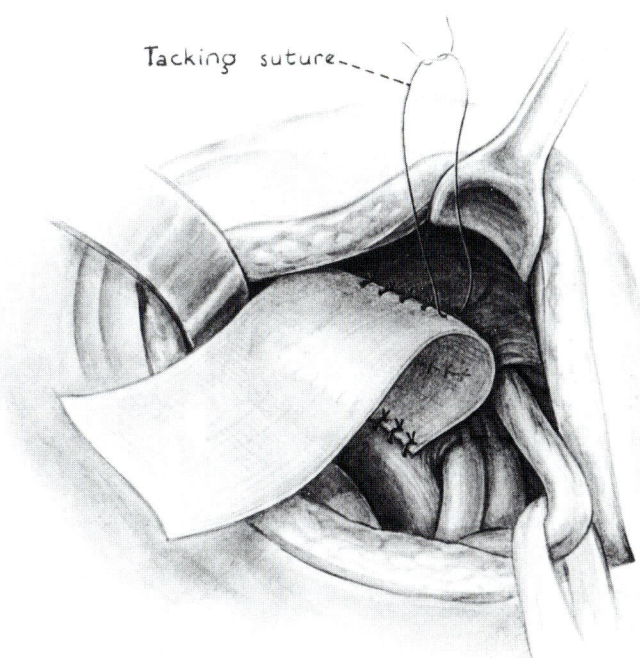

Figure 8-10. The mesh is tacked above the repair of the recurrent defect in the wall with 3-0 polypropylene suture material.

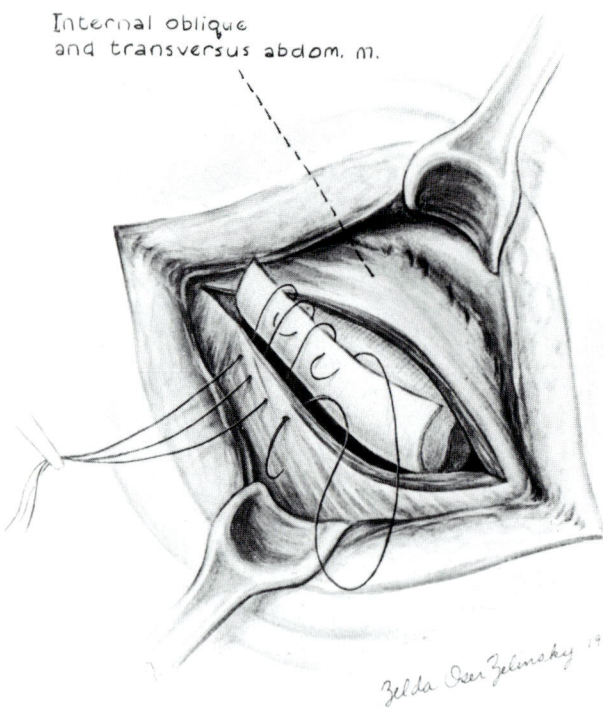

Internal oblique and transversus abdom. m.

Zelda Oser Zelinsky 1987

Figure 8-11. Sutures of 3-0 polypropylene are used to mold the mesh to the undersurface of the wound of entrance into the preperitoneal space before layered closure of the abdominal wound.

anterior repair of Bassini and Halsted in conjunction with the prostatectomy.

Riba and Mehn[86,87] should be credited with combining prostatectomy and hernial repair by the extraperitoneal approach. The potential for the development of a deep wound infection appears to be magnified by the combined extraperitoneal prostatectomy and hernial repair. Riba and colleagues[85] reported on a 10-year experience with this technique. They indicated that infections had not been associated with the hernioplasty and that the hernial repairs had been permanent. They concluded that "intrapelvic hernial repair can be combined with prostatectomy with good results and the patient is spared another operative procedure." This concept has been confirmed by Jasper[43] and by Kursh and Persky.[46] An editorial[68] gives further insight into this use of the posterior approach.

The same principle that applies to an already *extraperitoneal* operation such as a prostatectomy can also be applied to certain lower abdominal intraperitoneal operations such as an abdominoperineal resection. In such instances, if a groin hernia exists, a flap of peritoneum over the defect can be turned down. Then, the iliopubic tract repair is done and the flap

of peritoneum sutured back in place over the repair, much as one closes the peritoneal pelvic diaphragm.[34]

Radical Pelvic Operations and the Preperitoneal Approach to Hernial Repair

Schlegel and Walsh[94] performed groin hernial repairs safely and expeditiously during radical pelvic operations, using the preperitoneal approach through a median longitudinal incision. They performed 41 preperitoneal herniorrhaphies simultaneously with 343 radical retropubic prostatectomies and 26 radical cystoprostatectomies. As of the date of their report, there was no evidence of recurrent hernias, and there were no complications attributable to the hernial repairs.

Orchiopexy and the Preperitoneal Approach

It has been recognized for many years that mobilization of the spermatic artery and vas deferens, so-called skeletonization of the cord, is the most important maneuver in the treatment of an undescended testis. Unfortunately, this mobilization is usually performed in the inguinal canal, and little attention is given to increasing the length of the vas deferens and spermatic artery in the preperitoneal space. During the course of my hernioplasty study, it soon became apparent that the cord structures might easily be skeletonized in the preperitoneal space and further length obtained. On the basis of this observation, I operated, by the preperitoneal approach, on children with undescended testes. In every instance, there was an indirect inguinal hernia.

A standard preperitoneal approach is undertaken. After the hernial sac is removed, the testis—in my patients, the testis was in the mid-inguinal canal— is readily brought out through the internal abdominal inguinal ring. Meticulous dissection of the important spermatic cord structures allows sufficient mobilization for placement of the testis into the scrotum without the slightest tension. The route to the scrotum is created by gentle blunt dissection with the finger through the internal ring, inguinal canal, external ring, and scrotum. On occasion, there may be an indication to open the external ring and external oblique fascia to aid in either initial mobilization of the testis or placement of the testis into the scrotum.[52] A single stitch is placed through the skin at the apex of the scrotum into the gubernaculum testis at the completion of the procedure so that the testis does not slip backward into the inguinal canal during the first 48 hours after the operation. Sufficient tissue reaction occurs after this time for the testis to maintain an appropriate scrotal position without a stay. The transversalis fascial sling of the enlarged internal ring is closed with two or three sutures lateral to the cord. Finally, the anterior wound is closed in a standard manner.

This technique has proved to be of exceptional value. Several authors have suggested that the external inguinal canal should be approached first. If adequate cord length cannot be readily obtained, an approach to the preperitoneal space is considered.[22,37]

Vascular Operations and the Preperitoneal Approach

The preperitoneal space has been for many years subject to many invasions by surgeons, for example, lumbar sympathectomy, operations on the kidney and ureter, and retroperitoneal lymph node dissections. A successful use of the preperitoneal or extraperitoneal approach has developed in the field of vascular surgery. Rob[91] used this approach for the repair of abdominal aortic defects in more than 500 patients. He indicated that this method permits a shorter and smoother postoperative course.

Appendectomy and a Modification of the Preperitoneal Approach Incision

Interest has been revived in incidental appendectomy during repairs of groin hernia.[19,20,45] The incision for the preperitoneal approach, being slightly cephalad to that for the more standard approach, appeared ideal for accepting the challenge of the incidental appendectomy. Thus, I perform elective appendectomy during the right preperitoneal hernioplasty whenever the appendix presents itself in the wound before high ligation of the sac. I have seen no complications.

I am always displeased with the exposure of the cecal area after the gridiron incision of McBurney,[59] which appears unnecessarily traumatic. The wide exposure of the posterior inguinal wall routinely obtained by the relatively small incision used in the preperitoneal approach suggests that if the incision were modified slightly, it not only would be esthetically more satisfactory, but also would give better exposure than standard appendectomy incisions. On the basis of this observation, the incision for the preperitoneal approach was modified and used routinely for emergency appendectomies.

A 3-inch transverse skin incision is made in the right lower quadrant. The midportion of the incision should be at a point where a line drawn from the umbilicus to the anterior iliac spine crosses the lateral border of the rectus muscle. This incision passes through the skin and subcutaneous tissue. A transverse incision is made in the anterior rectus sheath over the muscle belly of the rectus at its lateral border. This transverse incision in the fasciae of the external oblique, internal oblique, and transversus abdominis muscles is extended lateral to the rectus for 2 inches. It may be necessary in the most lateral aspect of the incision to split, in line with the fibers, the internal oblique and transversus abdominis muscles. The incision as described should be below the linea semicircularis. The transversalis fascia and peritoneum remain to be incised. The rectus muscle may be mobilized medially for better exposure. A surprising degree of wound mobility is readily apparent as soon as exploration of the peritoneal cavity begins. At the conclusion of the appendectomy, the peritoneum is closed. The remainder of the abdominal wound closure is simplified by the presence of at least two excellent fascial layers. For added strength in the lateral wound, the epimysium of the transversus abdominis muscle may be sutured.

The incision as described bears close resemblance to the incisions of Elliott[21] and of Davis.[13] The technique is recommended for use in the treatment of acute appendicitis.

SUMMARY

Spivack[99] stated:

The transversalis fascia is a continuous layer which surrounds the entire abdominal cavity external to the peritoneum. It is known by different names in different regions, being at the same time one continuous layer. Thus in the anterior abdominal wall it is known as the transversalis fascia; in the upper part, where it serves as a lining for the diaphragm, it is known as the diaphragmatic fascia; in the fossa iliaca, as the iliac fascia; in front of the psoas and quadratus lumborum muscles, as the lumbar fascia; and on the pelvic floor as the pelvic fascia. This layer is very important because it is strongly elastic and, according to modern views, it prevents the formation of hernia more than any other single factor.

This chapter has shown how defects in the transversalis fascial layer of the posterior inguinal wall may be approached and repaired: that is, the *preperitoneal approach* and the *iliopubic tract repair*.

In years of study of this subject, we have learned the following:

1. The preperitoneal approach and iliopubic tract repair with inlay synthetic mesh buttress are satisfactory for type IIIA (direct), type IIIB (large indirect), type IIIC (femoral—mesh usually not necessary) and type IV (recurrent) hernias. Incarcerated or strangulated femoral and indirect hernias are ideally approached posteriorly. The Stoppa method is particularly effective in the presence of bilateral complex hernias.

2. Small indirect hernias are best treated from the anterior approach by high ligation of the sac (type I) and plastic closure of the transversalis fascia at the internal ring (type II).

3. Large indirect and direct hernias (types IIIA, IIIB, and IV—recurrent) may be treated by several other anterior approaches, for example, the techniques of Condon, Shouldice, or McVay.

REFERENCES

1. Annandale T. Case in which a reducible oblique and direct inguinal and femoral hernia existed on the same side and were successfully treated by operation. Edinburgh Med J 1876;21:1087.

2. Baader W. Preperitoneal hernioplasty with Marlex reinforcement. Presented to the Seattle Surgical Society, January 16, 1987, Seattle.

3. Bates UC. New operation for the cure of indirect inguinal hernia. JAMA 1913;60:2032.

4. Bellis CJ. Immediate unrestricted activity after inguinal herniorrhaphy: 9727 personal cases with specific reference to local anesthesia and polyester fiber mesh. Int Surg 1969;52:107.

5. Bulman JFH. The use of floss nylon in the repair of inguinal hernia, with a 2 year's followup of 70 consecutive cases. Br J Surg 1963;50:636.

6. Calne RY. Repair of bilateral hernia. Br J Surg 1967;54:917.

7. Calne RY. Repair of bilateral hernia with Mersilene mesh behind rectus abdominus [*sic*]. Arch Surg 1974;109:532.

8. Cheatle GL. An operation for the radical cure of inguinal and femoral hernia. Br Med J 1920;2:68.

9. Cheatle GL. An operation for inguinal hernia. Br Med J 1921;2:1025.

10. Clark JH, Hashimoto EI. Utilization of Henle's ligament, iliopubic tract, aponeurosis transversus abdominis and Cooper's ligament in inguinal herniorrhaphy. Surg Gynecol Obstet 1946;82:480.

11. Condon RE. Posterior repair of groin hernias. Techniques in Surgery, Ethicon, Inc., 1972.

12. Copello AJ. Technic and results of Teflon mesh repair of complicated recurrent groin hernias. Rev Surg 1968;25:95.

13. Davis GG. A transverse incision for the removal of the appendix. Ann Surg 1906;43:106.

14. Deter RL, Wilcox LE, Harris RJ. Reparacion extraperitoneal de la hernia: Reporte de doscientos casos. Memorias de la 8A. Asamblea Medica de Occidente, 1965:539.

15. Devadhar DSC. Levoplasty: a new principle in the treatment of groin hernias. Br J Surg 1968;55:411.

16. Dickey LD. Simultaneous retropubic prostatectomy and inguinal herniorrhaphy. Rocky Mt Med J 1961;58:34.

17. Donald DC. The value derived from utilizing the component parts of the transversalis fascia and Cooper's ligament in the repair of large indirect and direct inguinal hernias. Surgery 1948;24:662.

18. Dyson WL, Pierce WS. Changing concept of inguinal herniorrhaphy: experience with preperitoneal approach. Arch Surg 1965;91:971.

19. Eiseman B, Fowler WG, Robinson JM. Appendectomy during right inguinal herniorrhaphy. Ann Surg 1959;149:110.

20. Eiseman B, Robinson RM, Brown FH. Simultaneous appendectomy and herniorrhaphy without prophylactic antibiotic therapy. Surgery 1962;51:578.

21. Elliott JW. A modification of the McBurney incision for appendectomy. Boston Med Surg J 1896;135:433.

22. Estrin J. An improved technique of orchidopexy. Surg Gynecol Obstet 1963;116:379.

23. Estrin J, Lipton S, Block IR. The posterior approach to inguinal and femoral hernias. Surg Gynecol Obstet 1963;116:547.

24. Freidman EA, Meltzer RM. Collagen mesh prosthesis for repair of endopelvic fascial defects. Am J Obstet Gynecol 1970;106:430.

25. Fruchaud H. Anatomie chirurgicale des Hernies de l'Aine. Paris, Doin, 1956.

26. Fruchaud H. Le traitement chirurgical des Hernies de l'Aine chez l'Adulte. Paris, Doin, 1956.

27. Gaspar MR, Casberg MA. An appraisal of preperitoneal repair of inguinal hernia. Surg Gynecol Obstet 1971;132:207.

28. Gautier-Benoit MC, Quandalle P, Florin M, Faillon JM. Le traitement des éventrations postopératoires par plaque de Mersilène. Lille Chir 1968;23:13.

29. Ger R, Monroe K, Duvivier R, Mishrick A. Management of indirect inguinal hernias by laparoscopic closure of the neck of the sac. Am J Surg 1990;159:370.

30. Greenburg AG. Revisiting the recurrent groin hernia. Am J Surg 1987;154:35.

31. Griffith CA. Inguinal hernia: an anatomic-surgical correlation. Surg Clin North Am 1959;39:531.

32. Halverson K, McVay CB. Inguinal and femoral hernioplasty. Arch Surg 1970;101:127.

33. Harcourt KF. Henry's "heinous" herniorrhaphy. Am Surg 1978;44:465.

34. Harkins HN. Editorial comment. Rev Surg 1963;20:346.

35. Harris RJ, Deter RL, Wilcox LE. Extraperitoneal hernia repair: a report of 800 consecutive hernioplasties. Presented to the Texas Surgical Society, Fort Worth, Texas, 1971.

36. Harrison PW. Inguinal hernia: a study of the principles involved in the surgical treatment. Arch Surg 1922;4:680.

37. Hartman SW, Greaney EM Jr. Technique of orchidopexy. Surg Gynecol Obstet 1963;116:629.

38. Henry AK. Operation for femoral hernia by a midline extraperitoneal approach. Lancet 1936;1:531.

39. Hull HC, Ganey JB. The Henry approach to femoral hernia. Ann Surg 1953;137:57.

40. Jacobson P. Inguinal herniorrhaphy from the intra-abdominal perspective. Am J Surg 1946;71:797.

41. Jacobson P. Intra-abdominal approach to inguinal herniorrhaphy. Am J Surg 1950;79:557.

42. Jasper WS. Combined open prostatectomy and herniorrhaphy. J Urol 1963;89:728.

43. Jasper WS Sr. Combined open prostatectomy and herniorrhaphy. J Urol 1974;111:370.

44. Jennings WK, Anson BJ, Wright RR. A new method of repair for indirect inguinal hernia considered in reference to parietal anatomy. Surg Gynecol Obstet 1942;74:697.

45. Keeley JL, Schairer AE. Incidental appendectomy during repair of groin hernias. Surgery 1962;52:421.

46. Kursh ED, Persky L. Preperitoneal herniorrhaphy: adjunct to prostatic surgery. Urology 1975;5:322.

47. Lardennois B, Benoist M, Hibon J, Flament JB. Résultats de l'utilisation d'une étoffe en Dacron dans le traitement des grandes éventrations: a propos de 37 cas. Acta Chir Belg 1971;70:287.

48. LaRoque GP. The permanent cure of inguinal and femoral hernia: a modification of the standard operative procedures. Surg Gynecol Obstet 1919;29:507.

49. LaRoque GP. The intra-abdominal operation for femoral hernia. Ann Surg 1922;75:110.

50. LaRoque GP. The intra-abdominal method of removing inguinal and femoral hernia. Arch Surg 1932;24:189.

51. Lifschutz H, Juler GL. The inguinal darn. Arch Surg 1986;121:717.

52. Lipton S. Use of the Cheatle-Henry approach in the treatment of cryptorchidism. Surgery 1961;50:846.

53. Long WB III, Howatson A, Gill W. Marlex mesh in gas gangrene. J Trauma 1976;16:948.

54. Malangoni MA, Condon RE. Preperitoneal repair of acute incarcerated and strangulated hernias of the groin. Surg Gynecol Obstet 1986;162:65.

55. Maluf NSR, Tauber AS. Combined prostatectomy and herniorrhaphy through the Pfannenstiel incision. Urol Int 1961;11:51.

56. Mansfield RD. A new approach to the treatment of hernias of the groin. Am J Surg 1960;100:462.

57. Margoles JS, Braun RA. Preperitoneal versus classical hernioplasty. Am J Surg 1971;121:641.

58. Maunsell HW. Advantages of suprapubic laparotomy in strangulated femoral hernia. N Z Med J 1887;1:23.

59. McBurney C. The incision made in the abdominal wall in cases of appendicitis, with a description of a new method of operating. Ann Surg 1894;20:38.

60. McClelland RN, Sparkman R, eds. Selected readings in general surgery: hernia. Dallas, University of Texas Southwestern Medical School, 1975.

61. McDonald DF, Huggins C. Simultaneous prostatectomy and inguinal herniorrhaphy. Surg Gynecol Obstet 1949;89:621.

62. McEvedy BV. Inguinal hernia: the rectus sheath approach. West Afr Med J 1958;7:106.

63. McEvedy PG. Femoral hernia. Ann R Coll Surg Engl 1950;7:484.

64. McVay CB, Halverson K. Inguinal and femoral hernias. In: Beahrs O, Beart RW Jr, eds. General surgical therapy. New York, Wiley, 1981.

65. Mikkelsen WP, Berne CJ. Femoral hernioplasty: suprapubic extraperitoneal (Cheatle-Henry) approach. Surgery 1954;35:743.

66. Mouzas GL, Diggory PLC. A modification of the McEvedy repair of femoral hernia. Lancet 1956;2:1073.

67. Musgrove JE, McCready FJ. The Henry approach to femoral hernia. Surgery 1949;26:608.

68. Nyhus LM. Posterior hernial repair and prostatic operations. (Editorial) Arch Surg 1972;104:17.

69. Nyhus LM. The recurrent groin hernia: therapeutic solutions. World J Surg 1989;13:541.

70. Nyhus LM. Iliopubic tract repair of inguinal and

femoral hernia: the posterior (preperitoneal) approach. Surg Clin North Am 1993;73:487.

71. Nyhus LM. Individualization of hernia repair: a new era. Surgery 1993;114:1.

72. Nyhus LM, Condon RE, Harkins HN. Clinical experiences with preperitoneal hernial repair for all types of hernia of the groin. Am J Surg 1960; 100:234.

73. Nyhus LM, Condon RE, Harkins HN. Preperitoneal hernioplasty: a technic for the repair of all groin hernias. A brochure presented at the Scientific Exhibit, 111th Annual Meeting, A.M.A., June 1962.

74. Nyhus LM, Klein MS, Rogers FB. Inguinal hernia. Curr Probl Surg 1991;28:407.

75. Nyhus LM, Pollak R, Bombeck CT, Donahue PE. The preperitoneal approach and prosthetic buttress repair for recurrent hernia: the evolution of a technique. Ann Surg 1988;208:733.

76. Nyhus LM, Stevenson JK, Listerud MB, Harkins HN. Preperitoneal herniorrhaphy: a preliminary report in fifty patients. West J Surg 1959;67:48.

77. Ott G, Dudda W, Wenzel E. McVay und Nyhus: Alternativen? Langenbecks Arch Chir Suppl 1993: 242.

78. Petit J. Methode originale de traitement des hernies de l'aine et de leurs recidives: l'interposition sans fixation d'une prosthese en tulle de Dacron par voie indirecte. A propos de 168 observations. These pour le doctorat en medicine, January 1974.

79. Phetteplace CH. The intra-abdominal (LaRoque) approach to hernioplasty. West J Surg 1955;63:490.

80. Pollak R, Nyhus LM. Groin hernia. Curr Surg Ther 1986;2:268.

81. Polya E. Die Ursachen der Recidive nach Radicaloperation des Leistenbruches. Arch Klin Chir 1912; 99:816.

82. Read RC. Preperitoneal prosthetic inguinal herniorrhaphy without a relaxing incision. Am J Surg 1976;132:749.

83. Read RC. Basic features of abdominal wall herniation and its repair. In: Zuidema GD, Nyhus LM. Surgery of the Alimentary Tract, vol 5, ed 4. Philadelphia, WB Saunders (in press).

84. Rheault MJ, Oppenheimer J, Nyhus LM. Portrait of the anatomist Alexander Thomson. Surg Gynecol Obstet 1965;121:601.

85. Riba LW, Apfelbach GL, Uehling D. Vesicocapsular prostatectomy and elective intrapelvic hernial repair. J Urol 1963;90:75.

86. Riba LW, Mehn WH. Combined inguinal hernia repair and retropubic prostatectomy. Q Bull Northwestern Univ Med School 1951;25:62.

87. Riba LW, Mehn WH. Retropubic prostatectomy and inguinal hernia repair. J Urol 1952;67:106.

88. Rignault DP. Properitoneal prosthetic hernioplasty through a Pfannenstiel approach. Surg Gynecol Obstet 1986;163:465.

89. Rives J. Surgical treatment of the inguinal hernia with Dacron patch: principles, indications, technic and results. Int Surg 1967;47:360.

90. Rives J, Stoppa R, Fortesa L, Nicaise H. Les pièces en Dacron et leur place dans la chirurgie des hernies de l'aine. Ann Chir 1968;22:159.

91. Rob C. Extraperitoneal route for abdominal aorta work. Surg World 1962;2:5.

92. Robertson HT. Preperitoneal approach in the repair of inguinal hernias. Am J Surg 1966;112:627.

93. Rosenthal D, Walters MJ. Preperitoneal synthetic mesh placement for recurrent hernias of the groin. Surg Gynecol Obstet 1986;163:285.

94. Schlegel PN, Walsh PC. Simultaneous preperitoneal hernia repair during radical pelvic surgery. J Urol 1987;137:1180.

95. Sheehan MV. The supra-inguinal operation for femoral hernia. Proc 19th Congress Int Soc Surg, Dublin, 1961.

96. Skeie E, Borgeskov S. Praeperitoneal herniotomi. 35 Nordiske Kirurg Kongres, 1971.

97. Smith AN. A rectus-sheath extraperitoneal operation for recurrent inguinal hernia. J R Coll Surg Edinburgh 1962;7:195.

98. Sorg J, Skandalakis JE, Gray SW. The emperor's new clothes, or the myth of the conjoined tendon. Am Surg 1979;45:588.

99. Spivack JL. The surgical technic of abdominal operation. Springfield, IL, Charles C Thomas, 1946.

100. Stoppa R, Petit J, Henry X, et al. Plastie des hernies de l'aine par voie mediane sous-peritoneale: acta chirurgicales. Paris, Masson, 1972.

101. Stoppa RE, Rives JL, Warlaumont CR, et al. The use of Dacron in the repair of hernias of the groin. Surg Clin North Am 1984;64:269.

102. Tait L. Radical cure of exomphalos. Br Med J 1883;2:922.

103. Tait L. Treatment of hernia by median abdominal section. Br Med J 1891;2:685.

104. Thomson A. Cause anatomique de la hernie inguinale externe. J Conn Méd Prat 1836;4:137.

105. Van Damme J-PJ. A preperitoneal approach in the prosthetic repair of inguinal hernia. Int Surg 1985; 70:223.

106. Williams C. The advantages of the abdominal approach to inguinal hernia. Ann Surg 1938;107: 917.

107. Williams C. Repair of sliding inguinal hernia through the abdominal (LaRoque) approach. Ann Surg 1947;126:612.

Editor's Comment

Preperitoneal hernioplasty has been a subject of controversy since it was reintroduced into surgical practice by Dr. Nyhus 36 years ago. The objections, comparing the preperitoneal approach with the conventional anterior approach through the inguinal canal, revolve around two concerns: (1) the difficulty of dissection and exposure of the hernial defect and (2) the recurrence rate.

Two concepts are embodied in this chapter that directly address these issues and concern themselves with (1) the preperitoneal or posterior approach to the repair of inguinal hernias and (2) the iliopubic tract repair.

There is no question that the preperitoneal (posterior) approach is a valuable procedure for every surgeon. Anyone who has used this approach to repair a femoral hernia would agree that both the exposure and the repair are conducted more easily by the posterior approach (see Chap. 9) than by either the anterior approach through the inguinal canal or an approach below the inguinal ligament through the thigh.

Are there other situations in which a preperitoneal approach to hernia is useful? Sliding hernias are much less confusing when approached through the preperitoneal space, and their replacement within the peritoneal cavity is much more easily managed; I would recommend a posterior approach to every sliding hernia. Repair of a recurrent hernia previously repaired by the anterior (inguinal canal) approach also is conducted more easily if approached from behind.

What about the primary repair of inguinal hernias? There is general agreement that the posterior approach should not be used for a small indirect inguinal hernia. There is more controversy about the utility of a preperitoneal approach in the management of medium and larger indirect inguinal hernias. My view is that this is really a "fielder's choice" situation, but the larger the hernia becomes, the more rapidly and clearly can one delineate the anatomy by a posterior approach. The major controversy in choice of anterior versus posterior approach concerns the management of direct hernias. My own view is that large direct hernias are better repaired through a preperitoneal approach. I take this view because the relevant anatomy is more easily visualized directly when the hernia is approached through the preperitoneal space.

Turning to the issue surrounding the iliopubic tract method of hernial repair and associated recurrence rates, we must recognize two subsidiary questions: (1) Does a preperitoneal approach to hernial repair lead to a higher recurrence rate per se, and (2) is the iliopubic tract an appropriate and useful structure in the conduct of hernial repair? Note that the approach, anterior or posterior, should not influence recurrence rates if sound principles of hernial repair are applied. In any given hernia, the same structures are sutured to accomplish hernial repair, whether the approach is made anteriorly or posteriorly. Any argument that a posterior approach is responsible for a higher rate of recurrence is specious. No author who has reported high recurrence rates after repair of inguinal hernias by the preperitoneal route has both-

ered to learn the method from a knowledgeable preceptor. Self-taught surgeons unfamiliar with groin anatomy as viewed from its inner aspect who make an inadequate dissection and repair of a groin hernia should condemn themselves, not the approach.

The final comment, and perhaps the most important issue in this discussion, concerns the utility of the iliopubic tract in hernial repair. This is another "tempest-in-a-teapot" discussion, conducted among those who view hernial repair with a degree of anatomic rigidity inappropriate to the spectrum of structural variation that is found in the groin of a patient with a hernia. The major principle to be remembered in the conduct of hernial repair is that strong tissue on the border of the hernia needs to be closed without tension. Is the iliopubic tract such a strong structure on the border of groin hernias? Yes, usually in the case of both indirect and direct inguinal hernias, and always in instances of femoral hernia. Should sutures for hernial repair be anchored in the iliopubic tract? Yes, they should, provided the sutures hold—which is determined by testing each one as it is placed (see Chap. 7). Are not repairs anchored to inguinal ligament or to Cooper ligament preferable? In most circumstances, they are not preferable, but can be satisfactory; one should use whatever strong connective tissue structure is most available at the border of the hernia and not reach for another structure because of preconceived notions about hernial repair. Each hernia is unique; but each one should be repaired according to the principle of suturing together without tension whatever strong structures are present on the borders of the hernial defect. If primary repair cannot be done without inducing tension, then a prosthesis should be inserted. Any questions on the part of the reader about the iliopubic tract are best resolved by personal dissection (see Chap. 2) rather than by reading about disparate views in a textbook.

R.E.C.

Special Comment

Expanded Indications for the Posterior Hernia Repair: The High-Risk Patient
A. Gerson Greenburg

As surgeons, we are frequently asked to see patients with significant chronic single- or multiple-organ system compromise and a symptomatic groin hernia. Generally considered prohibitive surgical risks, these patients are often classified as nonoperable for elective repair. Unfortunately, an emergency surgical procedure related to an incarcerated, strangulated, or obstructing hernia is often required in this patient population. Recognizing that emergency surgery generally carries a higher risk for most procedures in any, but especially in this patient population, the possibility of an undesirable outcome is accentuated. I believe elective hernia repair in these high-risk patients is a preferable management option.

Between January 1974 and March 1993, I repaired over 650 recurrent groin hernias, 90% of which were done using the preperitoneal approach. Early in this experience, I was impressed by the exposure of the groin anatomy afforded by this procedure and decided to pursue preperitoneal repair in certain high-risk patients with an indication for hernia repair because I found it to be a safe, effective, efficient, and anatomically sound procedure.

The preperitoneal, or posterior, approach to hernia repair was not new at the time; its application to a group of high-risk patients was an expanded indication for its use.[1] Traditionally, the preperitoneal approach was reserved for recurrent inguinal hernias. With the advent of laparoscopic repair of groin hernias, this traditional wisdom is being challenged because that procedure relies on a similar anatomic approach but uses a different concept for repair. Whether the laparoscopic repair is of the same quality or associated with fewer complications is not yet clear as applied to routine herniorrhaphy in noncompromised patients. At this writing, I would be hesitant to apply the technique to any, but especially the high-risk, patient.

The preperitoneal approach usually involves virgin anatomy and affords ready access to the peritoneal cavity if needed. For these reasons, I use it for all incarcerated inguinal hernias as well as for recurrent groin hernias. Moreover, based on the information and experience obtained during the repair of over 650 recurrent groin hernias, there is a relatively high (10%–12%) incidence of multiple defects detected. These often involve an unsuspected femoral component.[2] Performed as classically described or with a few embellishments based on modern experience, the preperitoneal approach obviates any potential for overlooking associated defects.[3,4] In my opinion, the most complete exploration and repair of the groin hernia is only possible using this approach. This is precisely the kind of procedure required for the high-risk patient. Missing a repairable defect or failing to adequately repair an offending defect could contribute to a poor outcome requiring yet another operative procedure and must be avoided.

High-risk patients are usually of advanced age with significant pulmonary disease sufficient to impair gas exchange or respiratory mechanics. Significant cardiovascular disease, impaired renal function, and documented hepatic compromise also qualify a pa-

tient for this category. Some patients with major neurologic disease also fall into this group. In 1979, a group of 36 high-risk patients were reported.[1] This number now exceeds 140. The basic observations made at that time appear to remain valid. A history of multiple, symptomatic, recurrent incarcerations with difficulty reducing the hernia in the high-risk group qualifies these patients for surgical consideration. An incarcerated nonreducible hernia is a definite indication in this patient population. Of note, 30% to 40% of these are recurrent hernias. Operating time ranges from 20 to 80 minutes, with a mean of just under 1 hour.[2] Direct and femoral defects are repaired by approximation of the transversalis arch to the pubic tubercle and periosteum of the pubis (Cooper ligament) or the iliopubic tract. Internal ring defects are repaired using the transversus arch and the iliopubic tract as part of the femoral investing fascia at the level of the femoral canal.[3]

Occasionally, a medial or mid-floor direct defect is encountered that appears to be a simple hernia, a small, less than 3-cm fascial defect; this defect is amenable to a simple interrupted or running suture closure, in a vertical manner, without anchoring to the inferior ligamentous structures. This is possible using the posterior approach because no further extensive dissection is required to define the presence of multiple defects. Using the anterior approach, there would be a tendency to see the single defect and avoid disruption of the anatomy in search of other lesions.

For repair, I use interrupted 1-0 coated, braided polyester suture swedged onto a Mayo-7 needle or a running polypropylene suture of the same size with the same needle.[3] Infrequently, I employ mesh or other prosthetic material. If required, polypropylene mesh is placed with a running suture, anchoring it to the iliopubic tract or Cooper ligament. If possible, the primary defect is approximated and the repair reinforced and buttressed with mesh. In the posterior position, the mesh is without tension well below the skin. Antibiotic coverage intraoperatively and for 24 hours postoperatively is used with intraoperative placement of mesh.

In comparing operating times, in-hospital stays, recurrence rates, complications, and mortality against all other herniorrhaphy patients, the results remain favorable. For the high-risk patient, this remains a valid surgical approach. It is not just the surgical procedure that is critical for success in these cases. The concept of complete patient management is equally important. Implementation of a protocol designed to minimize the risks of surgery is essential for all but especially so in these patients. Excellent regional anesthesia is crucial to the success of this approach. Epidural anesthesia is my choice, especially for the patient with pulmonary disease. The catheter may be used postoperatively for pain control as well. For patients with cardiac disease, general anesthesia with monitoring as indicated is preferred because it affords the best opportunity for the control of physiologic variables needed to maintain tissue perfusion. The preperitoneal repair is difficult to perform under local anesthesia because of the wide field required and the direct interaction and intervention with the peritoneum. Patients with significant pulmonary impairment can be operated on using regional anesthesia with the head elevated to 30 degrees, allowing them spontaneous respiration with minimal anxiety.

I have expanded my use of the preperitoneal approach to a wider group of patients, including those having first-time repair of groin hernias. It is as effective and as easily accomplished as a standard anterior approach. My rationale has been to apply the procedure, which is known to be useful in complicated situations, to a primary surgical environment. If it works for the complicated situations, it should be equally effective as a primary procedure. In so doing, the anatomy is clarified, and familiarity is obtained. Critics of the procedure should reexamine the bases of their views and should read the older literature carefully before relegating the preperitoneal approach to obscurity. Properly performed, this is an excellent approach for the repair of *all* groin hernias.

REFERENCES

1. Greenburg AG, Saik RP, Peskin GW. Expanded indications for preperitoneal hernia repair: the high risk patient. Am J Surg 1979;138:149.
2. Greenburg AG. Revisiting the recurrent groin hernia. Am J Surg 1987;154:35.
3. Greenburg AG. Preperitoneal repair of recurrent groin hernia. Perspect Gen Surg 1991;2:43.
4. Shahinian TK, Greenburg AG. Groin hernia. In: Levine BA, Copeland EM, Howard RJ, Surgerman H, Warshaw AL, eds. Current practice of surgery, vol 3. New York, Churchill Livingstone, 1993.

Hernia, Fourth Edition, edited
by Lloyd M. Nyhus and Robert E. Condon.
J.B. Lippincott Company, Philadelphia © 1995.

Chapter 9

The Preperitoneal Approach and Iliopubic Tract Repair of Femoral Hernias

Lloyd M. Nyhus

The three approaches to the repair of a femoral hernia are: high, low, and inguinal. Expert herniotomists can obtain excellent results with their own familiar approaches. However, the preperitoneal approach (high) and the iliopubic tract repair are so simple and give such excellent results that I recommend their use to the exclusion of other operations for femoral hernia.

NORMAL ANATOMY

Confusion has reigned because of wide acceptance of the incorrect concept that the medial aspect of the femoral ring is composed of the lacunar (Gimbernat) ligament. Condon[5] and McVay[20] have given convincing evidence that the fascia in question at the femoral ring is the insertion of the posterior inguinal wall into the Cooper ligament. Semantics play an important role here. Whereas McVay[21] denied the presence of an iliopubic tract, he at the same time stated that the "medial wall of the femoral ring is not the lacunar ligament but is the lateralmost attachment of the posterior inguinal wall onto Cooper's ligament." It is my contention that the medial insertion of the iliopubic tract described by Condon in the following words, "the iliopubic tract bridges the femoral canal and then curves posteriorly and inferiorly, its fibers spreading fanwise to insert adjacent to Cooper's ligament into a broad area of the superior ramus of the pubis," is the same structure as that described by McVay. Lytle[13-15] concurred in this concept of the femoral ring; he wrote of the three-dimensional femoral ring, canal, and distal orifice. Lytle believed that the femoral orifice in the distal femoral canal is the key to the operative manipulation and repair of femoral hernias. He also believed that the Gimbernat ligament plays a prominent role in the anatomic boundaries of the femoral orifice and in the repair of the femoral hernial defect by the low operative approach. The Gimbernat ligament cannot be seen from the posterior approach to the repair of femoral hernias; thus, Lytle's

views are given only to place this anatomic structure in proper perspective—its total lack of importance to the posterior and inguinal approaches to repair and its continued importance to the low approach.

CAUSES OF FEMORAL HERNIA

The concept that a preformed (congenital) peritoneal sac is important to the development of femoral hernias is no longer believed. Keith[8] discredited this concept, which had many proponents.[26,29,32]

In my many explorations of the femoral ring (always done during the preperitoneal approach to groin hernias), I am always surprised at the presence of a relatively large defect that has no accompanying femoral hernia. This widening of the femoral ring is caused by a narrow insertion of the posterior inguinal wall onto the Cooper ligament[22] or, put in another way, a narrow insertion of the iliopubic tract onto the Cooper ligament (see Chap. 2).

The enlarged femoral ring predisposes to the development of an acquired hernia. This acquired hernia is probably caused by increased intraabdominal pressure. As an example, femoral hernia is most commonly found in multiparous women. McVay,[19] however, found that femoral hernias are three times more common in men than in nulliparous women. The mechanism, then, for development of a femoral hernia is increased intraabdominal pressure, which results in preperitoneal fat insinuating itself into the femoral ring (small or large). This bolus of fat drags along pelvic peritoneum to develop a femoral peritoneal sac. I tend to concur with Lytle[15] that a peritoneal projection just within the femoral hernial ring is of no consequence; if the peritoneal sac moves the short distance down the canal and out the femoral orifice, however, it becomes apparent and of consequence. Not only does the hernia become visible and palpable after passage through the femoral orifice, but the contents of the peritoneal sac are in a prime position for incarceration, strangulation, or both. Fortunately, the distance between the entrance and the exit of the femoral canal is short, and the constricting fascia can be released by either the low or the high operation.

Why femoral hernias develop in elderly people, particularly women, is a mystery. An attractive concept involves the muscle bulk adjacent to the distal femoral canal. Normally, the iliopsoas and pectineus muscle bundles encroach on the canal and thus act as a barrier to the development of a femoral hernia. With the natural atrophy of muscle tissue that occurs with senescence, the actual volume of muscle within the canal decreases, allowing positive intraabdominal pressure to push the peritoneum into the canal. This would explain the high rate of femoral hernia among elderly women as well as men. In women of all ages, the muscle mass is not as great as it is in men. Thus, women are predisposed to femoral hernias as the result of any condition that increases intraabdominal pressure, such as pregnancy or morbid obesity.

Because the femoral ring has its orifice in the posterior inguinal wall, it is in the same layer as the orifices of both the direct and indirect inguinal hernias. Thus, it is our tenet that the three common groin hernias should be considered together. In our classification of groin hernias (see Chap. 8), we, therefore, include femoral hernias as type IIIC. This conceptual change in thinking of the femoral hernia has simplified the classification of groin hernias, making it more workable.

DIAGNOSIS

A femoral hernia passes into the upper thigh beneath the inguinal ligament, appearing at the saphenous opening in the deep fascia. It may be difficult to determine its relation to the inguinal ligament. Confusion also may occur because an enlarged inguinal lymph node, lipoma, saphenous varix, or psoas abscess may mimic a femoral hernial enlargement in many details. Williams[31] described a venous thrill that can be elicited by palpating the upper thigh in patients with femoral hernias. The patient is placed in a supine position, and a Valsalva maneuver is performed. A narrowing (temporary stenosis) occurs at the level of the fascial walls, hernial sac, and femoral vein that produces the palpable thrill.

Sir Heneage Ogilvie[28] gave considerable insight into how we may prevent making these errors in diagnosis:

The differential diagnosis of a femoral hernia will depend on whether it is reducible or not.

The common femoral hernia is irreducible but symptomless. The sac contains nothing but a tag of adherent omentum and the outer coverings are fat laden and bulky. There is no impulse on coughing. Such a swelling is merely a rounded elastic tumour in the inner half of Scarpa's triangle that must be distinguished from an enlarged lymph gland and a lipoma, the only conditions which it resembles.

The distinctive feature of the hernia is that it has a neck, and the neck passes backwards below Poupart's ligament and medial to the femoral vessels. When the lump is moved about this deep attachment becomes obvious. A lymphatic gland lies in the plane of the superficial fascia, and in that plane it can be moved to an approximately equal extent in all directions. A single enlarged inguinal gland is in any case unusual. A lipoma is in the subcutaneous fat, and can be lifted off the deep fascia. A femoral hernia can be moved in circles within the range allowed by its "stalk," like the joystick of an aeroplane: in most cases the "stalk" can be traced to Poupart's ligament.

A reducible femoral hernia may be quite clearly a hernia, that is it is reduced by manipulation, and returns not immediately, but after coughing or straining. Reduction and reappearance are accompanied by the gurgle of intestine, and the swelling is resonant to percussion. The only difficulty in such a case is the distinction between a femoral hernia lying over the external ring and an inguinal hernia.

The distinction between femoral and inguinal hernia rests on two points; on the relation of the swelling to the pubic spine, and whether the swelling after reduction reappears above or below Poupart's ligament. An inguinal hernia that has reached the external ring overlies the pubic spine, but the spine can be felt by putting a finger below and lateral to the swelling and displacing it inwards. In femoral hernia the pubic spine can be felt only by a finger placed above and medial to the swelling. After reduction of a hernia whose nature is in doubt, a finger should be kept on the inner end of Poupart's ligament while the patient coughs. It can then be determined whether the swelling reappears from below the ligament, that is from the crural canal, or above it from the inguinal canal.

Two reducible swellings in Scarpa's triangle, saphenous varix and psoas abscess, may be mistaken for the femoral hernia by the inexperienced or over-confident. Both are reducible swellings below Poupart's ligament, but neither has the true characters of a hernia. Both appear in the erect position and disappear on recumbency, and neither has the firm rounded outline of a hernia, gives a gurgle when handled, or is resonant to percussion.

TREATMENT

As indicated, there are three operative approaches to the repair of femoral hernias: (1) low,[13,24] (2) inguinal,[7,12,19,25] and (3) high[1,4,6,9,16,17,23,27,30] (see Special Comment and Chap. 15).

Prostheses have been used for repairs of both primary and recurrent hernias. Lichtenstein[10] inserts a plug of plastic mesh. During a groin exploration below the inguinal ligament, I found myself looking at a femoral hernia from the low approach. The edges of the defect were rigid and immobile. Having removed the hernial sac and its contents from the femoral canal, I sutured a rolled-up piece of polypropylene mesh into the defect as a plug. I was satisfied with the results. Bendavid[2,3] developed a prosthesis of polypropylene mesh that looks like an umbrella, the stem or handle of which is excised, the disk remaining in the preperitoneal space as a barrier against recurrence of the femoral hernia. Stoppa places a large prosthetic mesh into the preperitoneal space (see Chap. 10). The mesh covers all potential or real groin defects as a blanket.

Techniques of femoral hernia repair that open the posterior inguinal wall for exposure and repair (the inguinal approaches of Bassini, Shouldice, McVay-Cooper, Halsted, and Andrews) rarely should be used. It is unnecessary and, therefore, unacceptable to tear down this natural fascial barrier in Hesselbach triangle for exposure; the low or high posterior approach leaves the inguinal floor intact.

The laparoscopic techniques of hernia repair use prosthetic mesh. We continue to watch the developments in this new high approach with interest. I am convinced, however, that the high or preperitoneal approach is the simplest method and that the iliopubic tract repair effectively prevents recurrence of the problem.

Surgical Technique

The approach to and exit from the preperitoneal space are fully described in Chapter 8.

A femoral hernial sac is reduced by traction (Figs. 9-1 and 9-2). If the hernia is incarcerated, one releases the sac by carefully incising the insertion of the iliopubic tract into the Cooper ligament at the medial margin of the femoral ring. The sac should then be opened for inspection of its contents (Fig. 9-3). The repair of the hernia is begun with high ligation of the sac (Fig. 9-4). The anterior margin of the hernial defect is formed by the iliopubic tract and the posterior margin by the Cooper ligament. The hernioplasty is completed by suturing these two structures together, thereby obliterating the femoral canal medial to the femoral vein (Figs. 9-5 and 9-6). In the preperitoneal approach, there is no problem in regard to visualization of the external iliofemoral vein; it is easily seen and easily protected, and the correct degree of closure of the canal medial to it without compressing it is more readily obtained. The aberrant obturator artery (corona mortis) crossing the Cooper ligament is seen and protected when present.

If the restraining fascia is distal at the femoral canal orifice (Gimbernat ligament), release can be attained from above. I can envision, however, the rare

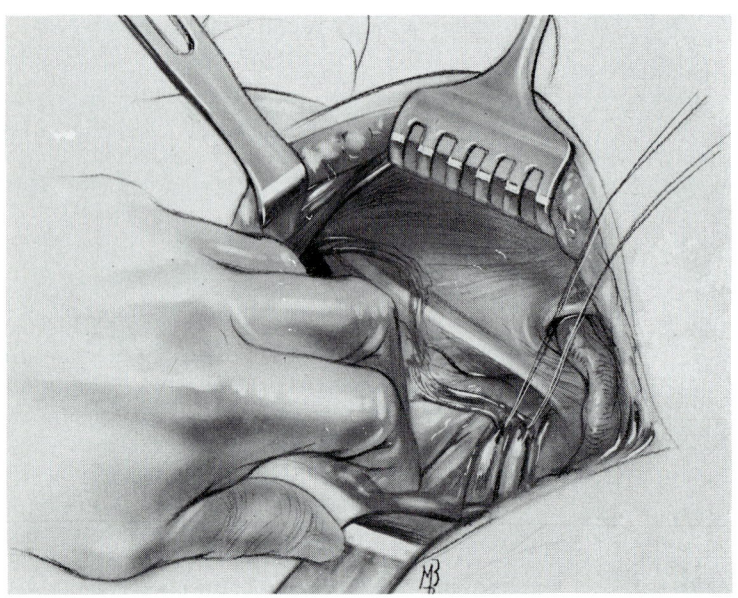

Figure 9-1. Femoral hernia. The peritoneal sac of a femoral hernia is reduced by traction and blunt dissection.

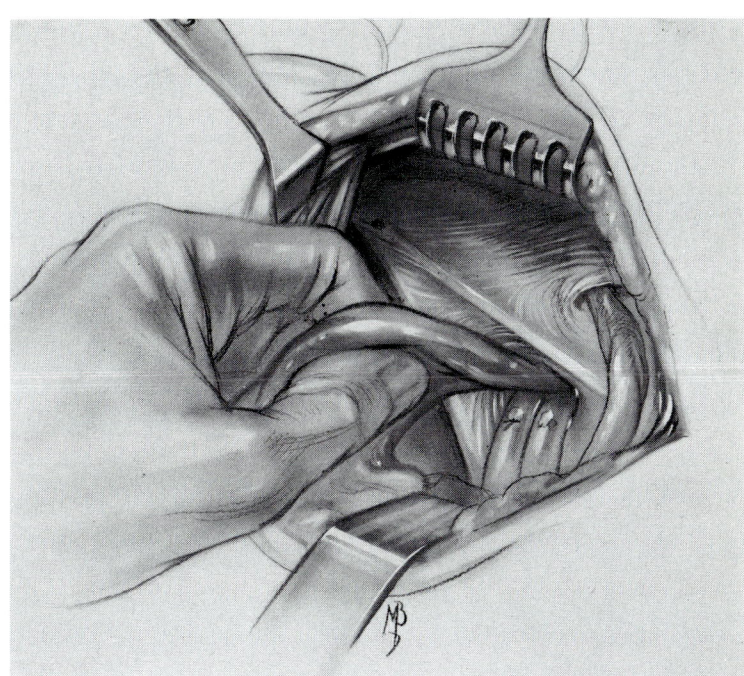

Figure 9-2. The inferior epigastric vessels have been ligated for better exposure. The hernial sac is being further reduced.

possibility of performing a counterincision in the upper thigh over the femoral hernial mass for release of this restricting fascia. I have never found this necessary. Use of relaxing incisions or of polypropylene mesh has not been necessary for the iliopubic tract repair of femoral hernias.

Incarcerated or Strangulated Femoral Hernia

Incarceration or strangulation is managed with relative ease. Transperitoneal control of the unaffected intestine at the hernial ring allows full control of the necrotic intestine and its lethal contents. After proxi-

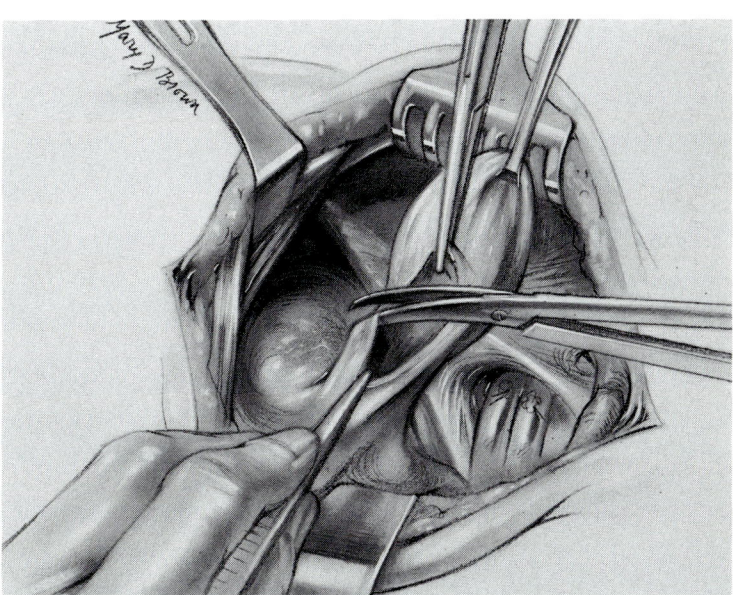

Figure 9-3. The femoral hernial sac is excised.

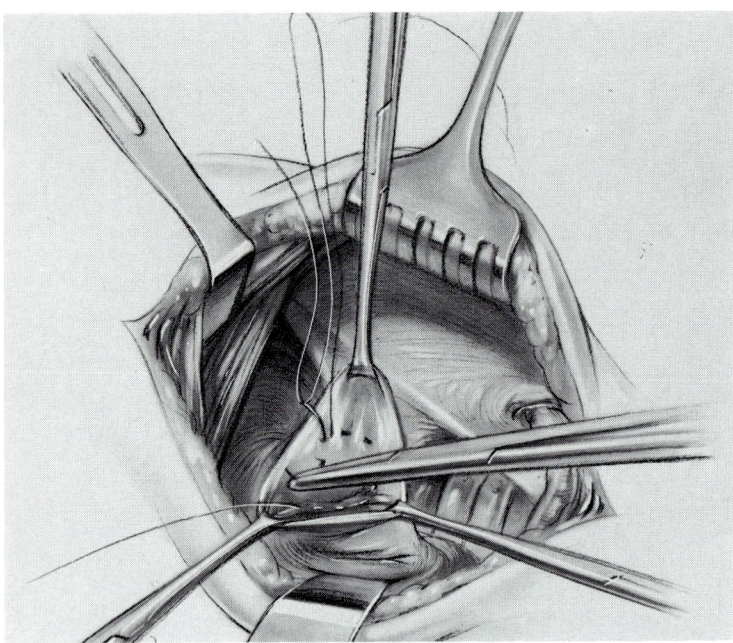

Figure 9-4. The peritoneum is closed.

mal control of the intestine is achieved through the posterior approach (and, in this instance, preperitoneal and transperitoneal exposure), release of the constricting insertion of the posterior inguinal wall into the Cooper ligament at the femoral ring, of the Gimbernat ligament at the distal femoral orifice, or of both allows for easy intestinal resection and anastomosis. The classic iliopubic tract repair follows.

Results

My recurrence rate remains at 1% or less. I have never repaired a femoral hernia that has recurred after my recommended approach and repair. These exceptional results have been confirmed by McNaught,[18] Mikkelsen and Berne,[23] Keynes and Withycombe,[9] and Ljungdahl.[11] Thus, I continue to espouse the pre-

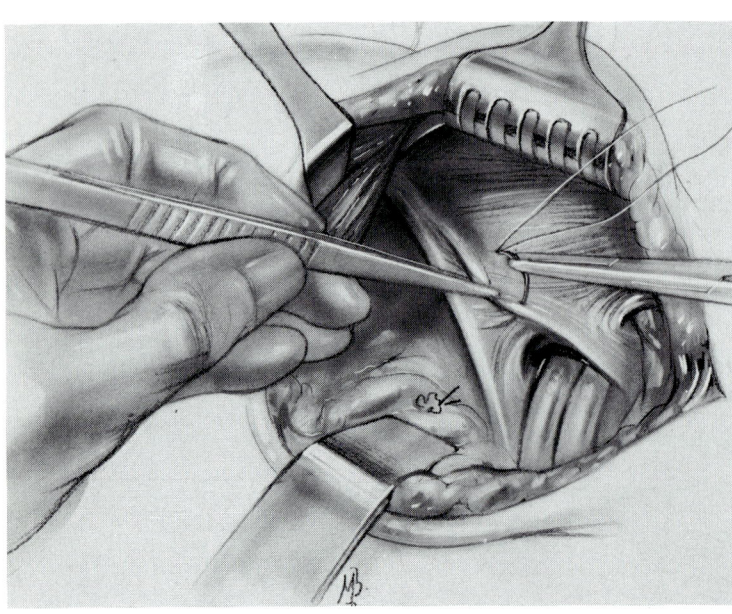

Figure 9-5. The femoral canal is narrowed by sutures placed between the iliopubic tract above and the Cooper ligament below.

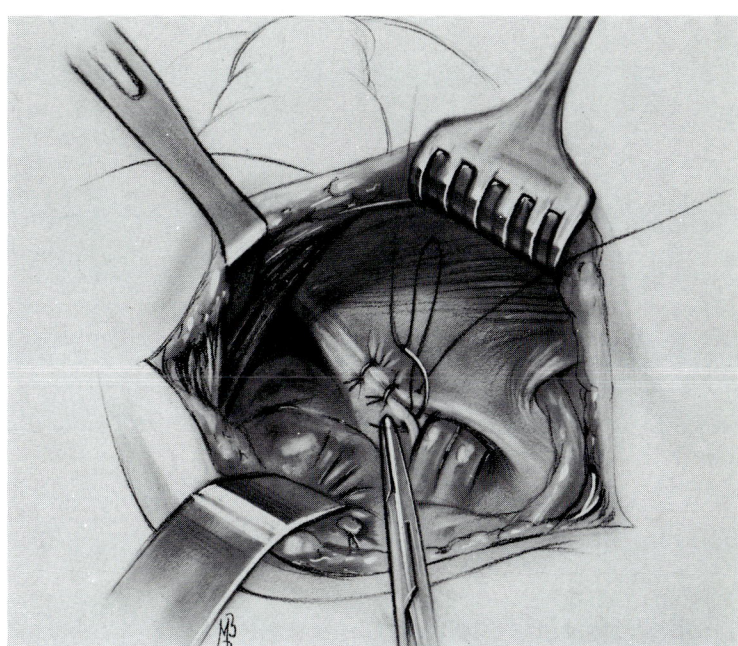

Figure 9-6. Completion of the femoral hernial repair.

peritoneal approach and iliopubic tract repair as the methods of choice for the treatment of femoral hernia.

REFERENCES

1. Annandale T. Case in which a reducible oblique and direct inguinal and femoral hernia existed on the same side and were successfully treated by operation. Edinburgh Med J 1876;21:1087.
2. Bendavid R. A femoral "umbrella" for femoral hernia repair. Surg Gynecol Obstet 1987;184:153.
3. Bendavid R. Recurrent femoral hernia treated by the insertion of a Marlex umbrella. Postgrad Gen Surg 1992;4:117.
4. Cheatle GL. An operation for the radical cure of inguinal and femoral hernia. Br Med J 1920;2:68.
5. Condon RE. Surgical anatomy of the transversus abdominis and transversalis fascia. Ann Surg 1971; 173:1.
6. Henry AK. Operation for femoral hernia by a midline extraperitoneal approach. Lancet 1936;1:531.
7. Horton MD, Florence MG. Simplified preperitoneal Marlex mesh hernia repair. Am J Surg 1993;165:595.
8. Keith A. On the origin and nature of hernia. Br J Surg 1923–1924;11:455.
9. Keynes WM, Withycombe J. Hudson's operation for femoral hernia. In: Nyhus LM, Harkins HN, eds. Hernia. Philadelphia, JB Lippincott, 1964.
10. Lichtenstein IL. Hernia repair without disability, ed. 2. St Louis, Ishiyaku EuroAmerica, 1986.
11. Ljungdahl I. Inguinal and femoral hernia: personal experience with 502 operations. Acta Chir Scand 1973;439(Suppl):7.
12. Lotheissen G. Zur Radikaloperation der Schenkelhernien. Zentralbl Chir 1898;25:548.
13. Lytle WJ. Femoral hernia. Ann R Coll Surg Engl 1957;21:244.
14. Lytle WJ. Femoral hernia. Br J Hosp Med 1970; July:17.
15. Lytle WJ. The inguinal and lacunar ligaments. J Anat 1974;118:241.
16. Maunsell HW. Advantages of suprapubic laparotomy in strangulated femoral hernia. N Z Med J 1887;1:23.
17. McEvedy PG. Femoral hernia. Ann R Coll Surg Engl 1950;7:484.
18. McNaught GHD. Femoral hernia: the rectus sheath operation of McEvedy. JR Coll Surg Edinburgh 1956;1:309.
19. McVay CB. The normal and pathologic anatomy of the transversus abdominis muscle in inguinal and femoral hernia. Surg Clin North Am 1971;51:1251.
20. McVay CB. The anatomic basis for inguinal and femoral hernioplasty. Surg Gynecol Obstet 1974; 139:931.
21. McVay CB. Cooper's ligament hernioplasty. In: Varco RL, Delaney JP, eds. Controversy in surgery. Philadelphia, WB Saunders, 1976.
22. McVay CB, Savage LE. Etiology of femoral hernia. Ann Surg 1961;154(Suppl.):25.
23. Mikkelsen WP, Berne CJ. Femoral hernioplasty: suprapubic extraperitoneal (Cheatle-Henry) approach. Surgery 1954;35:743.
24. Monro A. Femoral hernia: the lower approach. In: Nyhus LM, Harkins HN, eds. Hernia. Philadelphia, JB Lippincott, 1964.

25. Moschcowitz AV. Femoral hernia: a new operation for radical cure. NY J Med 1907;7:396.
26. Murray RW. Is the sac of a femoral hernia of congenital or acquired origin? Ann Surg 1910;52:668.
27. Nyhus LM, Donahue PE. Femoral hernia. Ann Ital Chir 1993;64:157.
28. Ogilvie H. Hernia. London, Edward Arnold, 1959.
29. Russell RH. Femoral hernia and the saccular theory. Br J Surg 1923–1924;11:148.
30. Tait L. Radical cure of exomphalos. Br Med J 1883;2:922.
31. Williams JS. Venous thrill and femoral hernia. Surg Gynecol Obstet 1966;123:1083.
32. Wood AC. Appendicular femoral hernia with a report of 100 cases. Ann Surg 1906;43:668.

Special Comment

The Extraperitoneal Approach to Femoral Hernias

Arnold K. Henry

This method of dealing with femoral hernia came into my hands by the sort of association that Rudyard Kipling, in his speech to the English Royal College (1923) on surgical advances, called, a "marriage of observation upon accident." The "accident" happened in my case to be the wholesale infestation by the flukeworm, or Bilharzia parasite, of the population of Egypt. The "observation" came with repeated opportunity; from the galaxy of lesions this parasite can produce in humans, two in the pelvis are relevant to the technique for femoral hernia: (1) juxtavesical stones in one or both ureters, and (2) a juxtavesical stricture in one or the other conduit.

These lesions may occur together or separately and are often bilateral, and because to see them I had to strip and raise the peritoneum from the pelvis, they were the sole foundation, source, and inspiration of my method.

So common were these lesions during my time in Cairo that a week seldom passed without the appearance of one or other of them in the surgical theater, and because of their frequent occurrence, bilateral extraperitoneal exposure of both ureters within the bony pelvis became a routine spectacle.

After a ritual assessment of the patient, the operation proceeds as follows: using a midline hypogastric incision through skin and fascia, the surgeon exposes the two recti muscles of the belly because the knife opens both sheaths and shows an overlap of rectus belly from right or left. Clean separation is easy to effect because the two muscles—as at a traffic round-

about—pass the navel on opposite sides. If then one prolongs the top of the midline incision to skirt the navel, one can there expose the wide umbilical parting of the muscles and follow down their cleavage to the symphysis, leaving the joint unscotched. This allows the surgeon to exploit the widest part of the potential space of Retzius, which is the part that lies to the left and right of the bladder and thus allows its expansion.

The long incision gives room for subsequent maneuvers and is not a waste of time. But because the incision reaches to the symphysis, a cautionary stitch at the close of operation is advisable: a single mattress suture in the divided sheath of rectus brings the deep faces of the aponeurosis flatly together, like two hands in prayer, and may baulk the advent of a hernia.[2]

Outside the intact peritoneum, the surgeon's hand passes down beside the bladder on either side and there detaches and lifts the still unopened sac from bladder and from the pelvic walls, exposing the structures that cling to these walls.

The juxtavesical parts of both ureters are left practically undisturbed because these parts—unlike the rest of their length—are *not* formally adherent to peritoneal membranes and, therefore, are not raised when it is lifted. Certain structures, except during inflammatory incidents, adhere normally to the sac and follow its displacement when the surgeon lifts it up; structures that are relevant are the rest of the pelvic ureter, which is not juxtavesical, and the obliterated umbilical artery. The vas in particular is firmly adherent to the peritoneum, so firmly that when the sac has been lifted to its upper limit, the cord-like loop of the vas warns the surgeon to stop by pressing almost painfully on his or her wrist.

Now it happens that this stripping of the bony pelvic wall affords a commanding view from above of all the anatomy one could wish to see or use in any operation for femoral hernia, each part displayed with the satisfying clarity of a diagram. I should have been blind if I had missed this amazing windfall.

There are seven structures. These include (1) the Poupart ligament; (2) the Gimbernat or the lacunar ligament; (3) the posterior pillar of the superficial ring, or ligament of Colles, whose fibers lose their identity under their modern alias *reflected fibers* (actually, they are contralateral fibers that decussate in the linea alba with their opposite fellows and hence are often stronger in right-handed people at the *left* superficial inguinal ring than at the right[1]); (4) the fascia over the pectineus; (5) the conjoint tendon; (6) the ligament of Henle that continues the edge of the sheath of the rectus abdominis muscle in a lateral direction; and (7) the adminiculum (the so-called *prop* of the linea alba).

The *Poupart ligament* is too familiar to require more than a note. R. Atkinson Stoney, of Dublin, long insisted on the importance of its hinder edge as a prominent landmark. This white band stands up clearly from the main ligament, and I learned long since from Stoney to mark it with an easily recognized atraumatic forceps at the start of an operation for inguinal hernia so that it is ready for recognition at the close, where it may be less evident. The same maneuver is equally valuable in operations for femoral hernia.

I have found this ligamentous edge described under the name of *Thomson's iliopubic band* in volume I of Paturet's fine Taité d'Anatomie Humaine.[4]

The Poupart ligament has bony medial attachments not merely to the *tip* of the pubic spine, or tubercle, but also to its base on the pubic ramus. Thus, as Paturet states, the Gimbernat ligament is absent at birth, but as "the Poupart" and the ramus separate during growth, these *basal* fibers form a web uniting the two, which bridges the gap, or lacuna, and forms the lacunar ligament (Gimbernat), just as happens when one separates two fingers, leaving a web with a sharp free edge lying between—an edge that in the Gimbernat ligament is the favorite site for strangulation.

Fibers from the seven sources listed earlier form a thick incrustation covering the pectineal crest of the pubis, a covering now called the *pectineal ligament of Astley Cooper.* The threefold trend of the direction of these fibers gives the ligament great strength and prevents sutures placed in it from tearing out.

I find it hard to approve the longitudinal section of the Cooper ligament that has been advocated to allow its foremost half to relax sufficiently to bend forward and reach the hinder edge of the Poupart ligament without tension in case the two fail to approximate easily because it would be difficult to split the Cooper ligament usefully without reaching periosteum. It is perhaps worth noting that oozing points have been recorded at the base of a split Cooper ligament,[3] and these, conceivably, may serve as foci for the troublesome neuroses that are the plague of pubic bones.

Although the twofold ureteral occasion of stone and stricture was part of the daily surgery of Kasr el Aini Hospital, femoral hernia (in marked contrast with the inguinal kind) was a thing most rare and could always be counted on as a sure draw for a packed audience in the operating theater.

During my last year in Cairo, the double rarity of a girl with manifest bilateral femoral hernias entered my surgical unit. This gave me the long-awaited opportunity to use the knowledge I had gained from exposing both ureters extraperitoneally in the pelvis.

But for admission of that patient, the femoral method might have lapsed.

Apart from certain obvious benefits of the method, for example, a single incision, whether midline as I described or a Pfannenstiel, each allowing the possible discovery of an early unsuspected femoral hernia contralateral to the obvious one, the dominating view from above favors easy recognition and an easy means of noting the percentage of incidence of prevascular, external, and other varieties of femoral hernia, whose positions matter more to the surgeon than the feat of recalling their multiple eponyms. Meanwhile, the favorable view of the Gimbernat ligament from above cancels the danger from abnormal obturator arteries.

Mr. Nigel Kinnear, President of the Royal College of Surgeons of Ireland, who has used the extraperitoneal method for femoral hernia since its inception in 1936, sent me the following comment:

> It is possible and profitable always [*emphasis mine*] to open the general peritoneal cavity and explore the whole abdomen through a midline approach. By doing so a totally unsuspected intestinal carcinoma was found on one occasion. On another occasion it was seen that the cause of an acute intestinal obstruction was a carcinoma of the caecum and not a co-existing, irreducible, femoral hernia.

Kinnear reminded us, too, that appendectomy can often be combined with an operation for femoral hernia. It would indeed be difficult to find a formula at once more acceptable and less dogmatic than Kinnear's "It is possible and profitable always. . . ."

Kinnear thus converted the purely extraperitoneal method for femoral hernia into a combined operation—intraperitoneal and extraperitoneal. The intraperitoneal part is mainly for exploration, when our fingers may grasp the hernial organ, whether intestine or omentum, and follow it downward.

PELVIC HERNIA

The pelvic nature of a hernia may thus appear and its variety be established. The extraperitoneal part of the combined operation lays bare the pelvic wall and allows one to confirm the pelvic nature of the hernia, to see and close its site of escape, and to attempt a radical cure.

A further advantage in the precise location of three of the more common pelvic hernias springs from the fact that each of them follows the course of a major branch of the internal iliac artery—obturator, gluteal, and sciatic. The origin of these three vessels lies close to that of the obliterated hypogastric artery, and when a surgeon mobilizes its fibrous part and draws gently on that tough leash, the branches of the posterior division of the parent internal iliac artery stand up in clear relief. They show through the layer of thin tissue that binds them closely to the deep face of the pelvic wall and the muscles that partly clothe it.

Numerous ways are recommended for curing femoral hernia—metal staples, nailing down the Poupart ligament to the pubis, or with a free bony block removed from the head of the femur.

Aird's summary is admirable: "These operative extravaganzas are not followed by recurrence; neither is simple ligation of the sac, supplemented by two or three sutures inserted between 'Poupart's' and pectineal fascia."

INGUINAL HERNIA

An attempt to enlist the extraperitoneal method for work on inguinal hernia was met on three occasions with the rebuff of rapid recurrence in two patients within 10 days of their operations. The speed of this event surprised me because I believed that I had found the presence of something associated with an inguinal hernia that might help in preventing, or at worst retarding, such a mischance. I had noticed on the deep aspect of the peritoneum, proximal to the neck of the inguinal sac, a thickening in the deep layer of peritoneum, sometimes appearing as a milky circle about a hand's breadth in diameter that, when the sac was pulled downward, seemed to mark an entrance to a second, wider neck that lay at the mouth of a funnel, which I thought of as awaiting a further hernial consignment. I determined at the time that I would close this funnel at the milky ring with a pursestring suture after I had dealt with the ordinary sac. But I found that this closure of the funnel's mouth failed to influence the rate of recurrence.

I am aware of no confirmation of the presence of these thickenings, which I described in an article in 1936, though they were then clear enough.

I have long relinquished the extraperitoneal approach for inguinal hernia as discouraging and unsatisfactory, but I have come to believe that it may be usefully adapted in dealing with the large but much rarer group of pelvic hernias, whose variety and inaccessibility still present problems.

In conclusion, I have no long list to place in evidence for statistical use. As I said in 1936, my method was based on a single patient, but at the same time on some 11 years of clinical observation, during which it was possible to obtain the know-how that exposed not merely the juxtavesical ureters, but also the impressive windfall of structures concerned with femoral hernia.

REFERENCES

1. Charpy, Poirier. Fascicle I, ed 2, vol II. 1901:488.
2. Henry AK. Extensile exposure, ed 2. Baltimore, Williams & Wilkins, 1963:160–165.
3. Mouzas GL, Diggory P. Modification of McEvedy repair of femoral hernia. Lancet 1956;2:1073.
4. Paturet. Taité d'Anatomie Humaine, vol I. 1938.

Editor's Comment

One of the high points in the preparation of the first edition of *Hernia* was the receipt of this comment from Professor Henry (Fig. 9-7). Dr. Harkins and I first met him on the balcony of the Convention Hall in Copenhagen on the occasion of the XVI Congress of the International Society of Surgery in 1955. He was most gracious, and we could sense an enthusiasm for learning unusual for his advanced years.

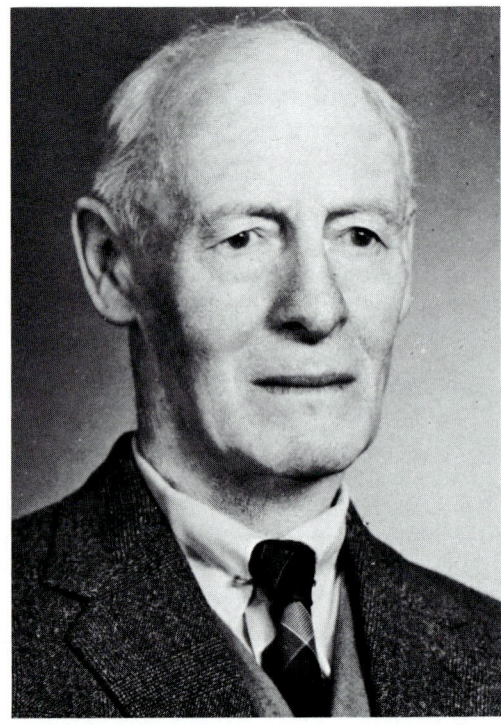

Figure 9-7. Arnold K. Henry (1886–1962).

Professor Henry died soon after writing this comment. In a letter to me postmarked February 20, 1961, he made the following observation:

My recent illness has kept me away from the Royal College of Surgeons of Ireland and from the chance of studying your interesting suggestions. I am sure that, like you, I should long since have abandoned the vertical incision. I feel that the effort provoked by the relatively cramped view of in- *guinal components obtained with the vertical approach may have caused a terminal laxity of sutures, that might have favoured recurrence of an inguinal protrusion. N. Kinnear suggested that possibility to me.*

Professor Henry was a great man. His contributions to the fields of surgery and anatomy are classics.
L.M.N.

Hernia, Fourth Edition, edited
by Lloyd M. Nyhus and Robert E. Condon.
J.B. Lippincott Company, Philadelphia © 1995.

Chapter 10

The Preperitoneal Approach and Prosthetic Repair of Groin Hernias

René E. Stoppa

Since the publication of the third edition of this text, the use of prosthetic materials has gained an extensive spread in groin hernia surgery, when adding all the methods actually proposed. These include classic patches, plugs, giant prostheses, and, still being appraised, laparoscopic attempts at repair (at times exclusively using mesh). Diverse principles have been put forward regarding the use of prosthetic materials, including tension-free or suture-free repairs and large wrapping of the visceral sac.

In this chapter, I present my method combining a midline preperitoneal approach and the placement of a very large bilateral piece of polyester (Dacron) mesh in the retroparietal cleavage spaces. This can be regarded as the maximal extension of hernia prosthetic repair and as an almost absolute weapon against recurrences, on the condition that the original technique, which we have improved, is performed.

I do not propose this operation as a panacea but rather as a worthwhile method for the treatment of difficult cases. As many others, I believe that hernias are polymorphous lesions that require surgeons to understand and learn several well-assessed techniques kept up in the surgical arms conservatory that has been impressively produced by the successive editions of this text.

PROSTHESES

We have reached an era in which we must deal with recurrence-preventing operations, not only with respect to the patient's benefit and surgeon's pride, but also considering justifiable economic concerns caused by the great number of hernias operated on. In the name of efficacy, there is no doubt that the reinforcement or replacement of the transversalis fascia by a synthetic mesh arrived in the nick of time for rendering possible the repair of irremediably damaged inguinal walls.

Anatomic Purposes

Good anatomic knowledge is a basic principle for improving operations for hernia. Fruchaud[15,16] proposed a possible unification of groin hernias: whatever their superficial emergence (inguinal or femoral), they pass through the inguinal wall across the musculopectineal opening (Fig. 10-1). The size of this hole varies according to the structure of the inguinal muscular triangle, shown in the work of Condon and Nyhus[13,14] and Gaston,[17] and the variations of the "inguinal angles" of Radojevic[35] and Barbin (cited in Panou de Faymoreau[32]), or the "pubic height" of Ami[2] (Fig. 10-2).

Within the weak area of the musculopectineal opening, the transversalis fascia (the inguinal portion of the endoabdominal fascia)[3,4,25,26] and its analogues represent the only (and often poorly) resistant layer— the intraabdominal, pressure-tight layer—of the wall. This is the best depth for inguinal repairs, in which the wall must be sutured without tension or reinforced. I believe that perfect and permanent tightness of the deep inguinal layer is easily ensured by a piece of synthetic mesh.

Behind the transversalis fascia is a wide cleavable cellular space that spreads to the two sides of the infraumbilical midline—the retrofascial preperitoneal and prevesical spaces—which widely overspread the spaces of Retzius and Bogros. With Odimba,[30] we have made precise measurements of its shape, dimensions, and variations by dissection and radioanatomic study. Thus, we have been able to show the practicing surgeon the shape and size of the retrofascial space, a natural site for large prostheses replacing or reinforcing the transversalis fascia (Fig. 10-3), and at the same time a fine route for placing them.

An interesting anatomic detail related to a key gesture in our prosthetic repair is the retroparietal anatomic disposition of the elements that constitute the spermatic cord.[50,57] Every surgeon has observed that, of the two pedicles that pass through the musculopec-

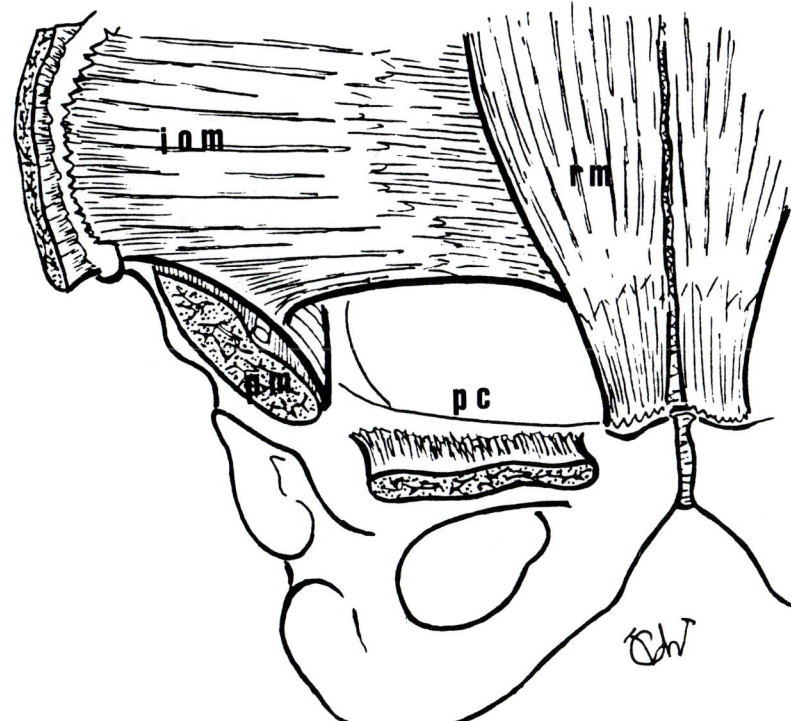

Figure 10-1. Schematic drawing of Fruchaud musculopectineal hole limited by a regional solid frame and limited by the rectus muscle (rm), its medial pilar; the psoas muscle (pm), its lateral pilar; the internal oblique muscle arch (iom), its superior limit; and the pectineal crest (pc), its inferior bony margin. (Adapted from Nyhus LM, Baker RJ, eds. Mastery of surgery, ed 2, vol 2. Boston, Little, Brown, 1992:1616)

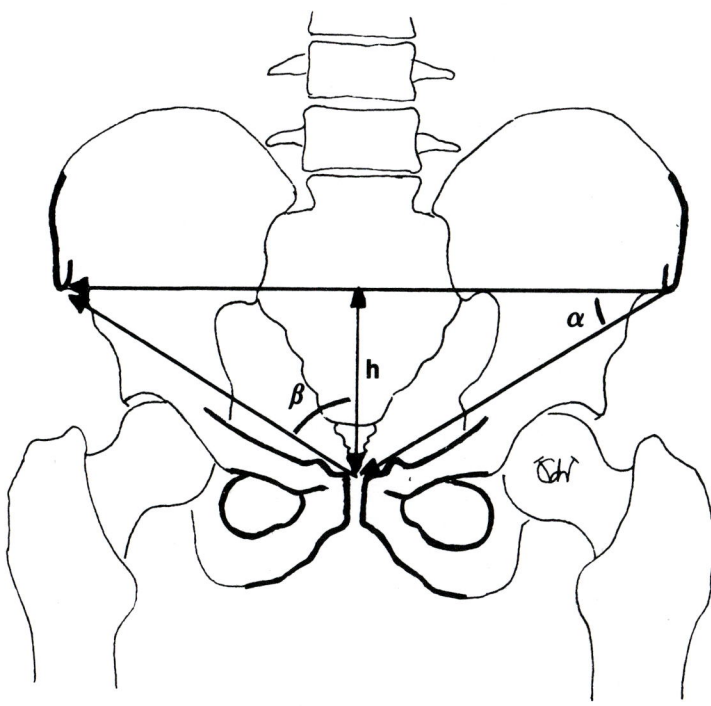

Figure 10-2. Schematic representation of the angles of Radojevic (α) and Barbin (β) and the pubic height of Ami (h), which are related to the dimensions of the musculopectineal opening described by Fruchaud.

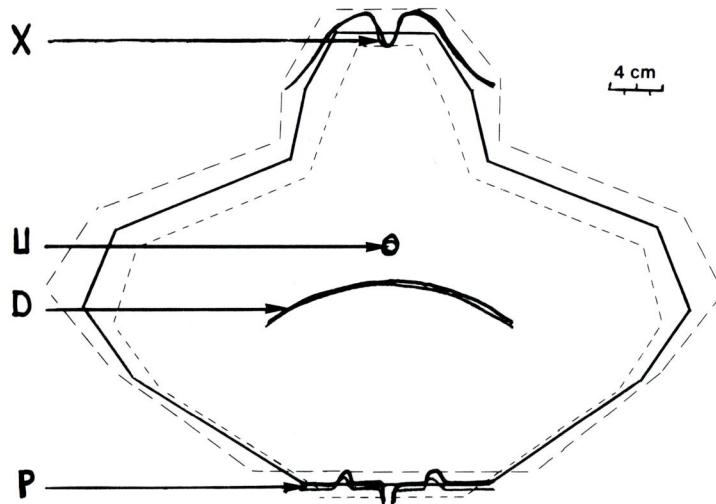

Figure 10-3. Schematic plane projection on the abdominal wall of the preperitoneal prevesical retrofascial space after anatomic and roentgenographic measurements. The continuous line represents the median size and shape of this cleavable space. The outer dashed line represents the maximal dimensions, and the inner dashed line represents the minimal size. D, Douglas linea arcuata; P, pubis; U, umbilicus; X, xiphoid appendix.

tineal opening, the iliofemoral vascular pedicle is a parietal element, whereas the spermatic pedicle traverses the inguinal retroparietal cellular space when the preperitoneal cleavage has been performed. The elements of the cord can be separated from the peritoneum and parietalized when a preperitoneal prosthesis is placed. There are three advantages to this technique: (1) The transverse enlargement of the zigzag course of the cord is transferred several centimeters more laterally. (2) Consequently, the inguinal passage is better protected against a dangerous sudden increase in intraabdominal pressure. (3) The need to cut the mesh for passage of the spermatic cord is eliminated; the prosthesis can be easily placed in a retroparietal and retrofunicular location (Fig. 10-4).

On the whole, one must remember the conditions naturally favorable to the possible use of prostheses: (1) the frequent propensity to weakness of the inguinal structures that sustain the tight layer of the wall, the transversalis fascia itself being of variable strength, and (2) the existence of a retroparietal, easily cleavable wide space, a natural site for insertion of large prostheses.

Pathologic Purposes

In the field of prosthetic repairs by the preperitoneal approach, we restrict ourselves to discussing the respective efficiency of the two main methods of treatment of groin hernias—herniorrhaphy and prosthesis insertion. If herniorrhaphies, elective by nature, call for a precise study of hernial orifices, prosthetic repair accommodates itself to Fruchaud's singular concept: that all groin hernias, inguinal or femoral, pass through the musculopectineal opening. From this point of view, there are two types of groin hernias: *congenital* hernias, caused by persistence of the peritoneovaginal channel, which are easily repaired by herniorrhaphy, and *weakness* hernias, always resulting from the failure of the transversalis fascia. The latter type may necessitate the use of a prosthesis when an irremediable loss of substance exists in the inguinal musculofascial layer (Fig. 10-5). In addition to congenital abnormalities of the transversalis fascia and the internal oblique muscle arch, one hears more and more of a probable biologic insufficiency of the groin, a sort of "fascial diathesis" predisposing mostly to direct hernias,[32,33,36,37,59–61] a weakening by aging of the aponeurotic structures, or diverse progressive deficiencies of scars.[7,8]

Hernial lesions are diverse and call for diverse methods of repair. For the most benign lesions, a simple technique may be sufficient, if the herniorrhaphy provides a permanently strong scar that overlaps viable structures, creating "living" collagen with no tension and correct oxygenation.[7,8] This type of repair would be ideal if surgical scars did not grow old.[20,21] But such is not the case, and recurrences develop.

For the severest lesions of the inguinal structures and mostly for multiply recurring hernias (those with the Poupart or Cooper ligament and transversalis fascia destroyed), prosthetic repair is a preferable solution. Herniorrhaphy is nearly always appropriate for congenital hernias. Prosthetic repair of the transversalis fascia is logical for weakness hernias caused by deterioration of the inguinal musculofascial layer.

The best reason for the use of prostheses is their efficacy. They solve instantly and definitively the mechanical problem created by the deficiency of the impervious layer of the abdominal wall in hernias caused by weakness because they reinforce the endoabdominal fascia or replace it. They are also a definitive so-

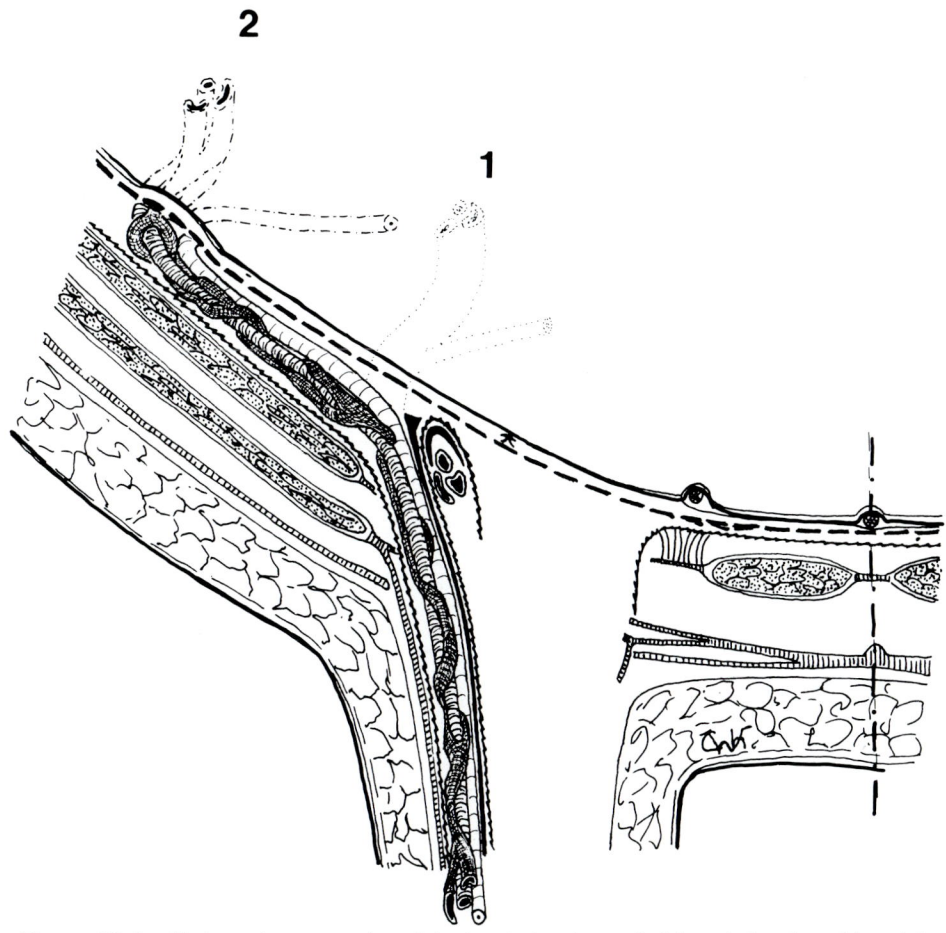

Figure 10-4.   Horizontal cross section of the inguinal region and of the relative disposition of the cord after "parietalization" of its constituting elements. Note the deeper lateral position of the cord so that its zigzag course is enlarged transversally before (1) and after (2) parietalization.

lution against scar aging, which provokes deterioration of a herniorrhaphy. This scar deterioration does not happen with prosthetic repair. The result of a prosthetic repair is quickly and definitively secured. These advantages, however, are counterbalanced by some possible complications. The worst of these complications used to be sepsis, but sepsis is no longer a high risk.

PURPOSE OF THE PREPERITONEAL APPROACH

Because the more damaged inguinal layer is the deeper one, in groin hernia, the abdominal preperitoneal approach is most logical. Among the abdominal or posterior approaches, the preperitoneal approach offers the richest well-known resources (see Chap. 8). Since 1965, Rives, in France, has emphasized the approach.[40,47,48] Since 1969, I have used the preperitoneal subumbilical approach.[51,52] The advantages of the approach are facility of separation of the retrofascial cellular space, direct access to the posterior inguinal structures, clear understanding of hernial lesions, and good exposure of the musculopectineal opening. The movements in placing a prosthesis are easily carried out. This is most noticeable when one repairs multirecurrent hernias, which proceed from normal anatomy (of the midline) toward abnormal anatomy (of the hernial lesions)—there is no additional deterioration of the already weakened inguinal structures. Familiarity with this approach and with prostheses encourages us to distinguish no longer between the different types of groin hernias (inguinal or femoral). The main interest in this approach is the ability to place a large piece of synthetic mesh behind the weak inguinal area for tightening the wall, whatever the damage to its structural layers, at the same time widely wrapping the visceral sac—rendering it inextensible—so that herniation can no

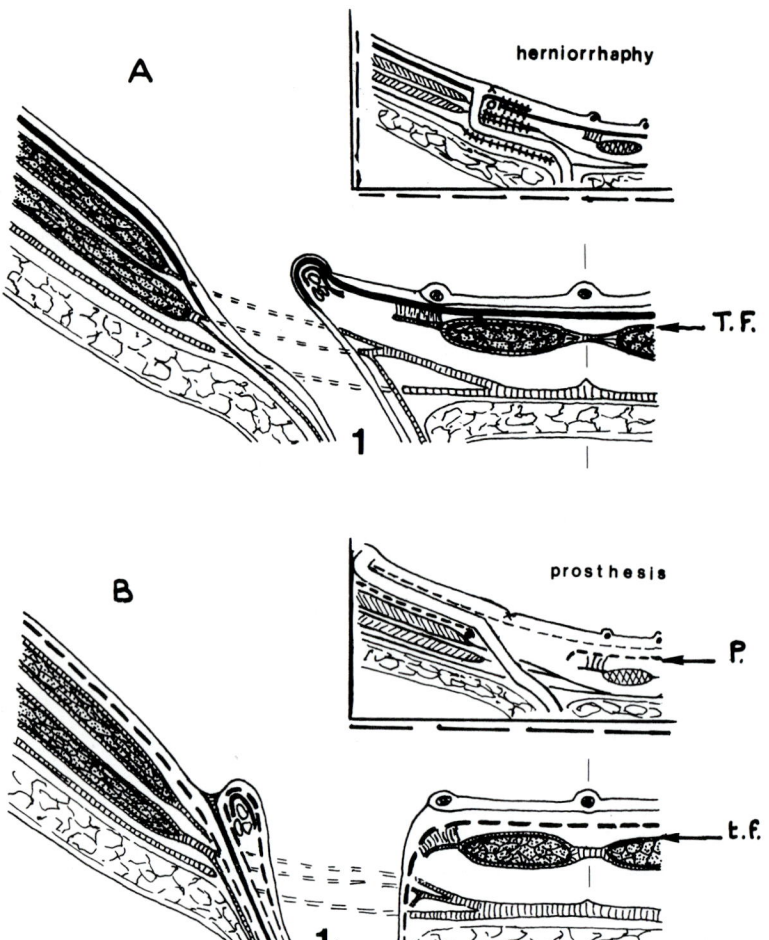

Figure 10-5. Schematic horizontal cross sections of the inguinal region, showing a congenital indirect inguinal hernia (*A*) and one caused by direct weakness (*B*). The insets show the methods of treatment: herniorrhaphy (*A*) and prosthetic repair (*B*). 1, 1b, hernial sacs; T.F., strong transversalis fascia; t.f., weakened transversalis fascia; P., prosthesis.

more occur. The preperitoneal approach is perfectly convenient for even the most difficult hernial repairs, such as those of multirecurrent, prevascular, sliding, enormous, and bilateral hernias.

When one avoids the superficial inguinal nerves in the preperitoneal approach, the number of testicular atrophies and painful sequelae is decreased.[11,12] In the same way, this technique preserves the mechanisms that protect the inguinal region from the effects of intraabdominal pressure (Keith's inguinal shutter, Lytle's Hesselbach ligament sling, Ogilvie's cord lifting).

The median preperitoneal approach may induce the risk of incisional hernia, and I respond to this risk by using large bilateral pieces of prosthetic material, which tighten the weak inguinal areas of both sides and at the same time protect the subumbilical midline closure. I have had limited experience with Nyhus's suprainguinal incision[28] because I prefer to use the retroparietal large bilateral prosthesis, which cannot be placed by this approach. Nyhus's approach has the advantage of not damaging the median raphe, but in

my experience, it does not secure the repair from the risk of eventration after wound suppuration. Some French surgeons, following Rignault and coworkers,[38,39] have used a Pfannenstiel incision, but opening and closing the wall are time-consuming, the risk of damaging superficial nerves is present, and I believe that there is only a cosmetic advantage to this transverse incision.

One must distinguish between the preperitoneal approach and prosthetic repair of inguinal hernias by the direct approach, which is used in France.[40–48] As in all inguinal approaches, this procedure requires dissection of the spermatic cord, inguinal layers, and hernial sac; this dissection may be difficult in recurrent hernias. The square prosthesis used is small (6–8 cm²) and must be carefully sewn laterally to the iliac fascia, with care taken to avoid the crural nerve; to the femoral vessel sheath, with care to avoid the femoral vein; and to the medial and superior edges of the musculopectineal hole. The prosthetic mesh is cut to let the cord through, which creates a risk of recurrence through the gap in the patch. This technique is more difficult than insertion of the large bilateral prosthesis by the preperitoneal approach and must be used only by experienced surgeons. I do know that Rives and associates have been successful, and I have some personal experience with the technique,[50,53,56] with less consistent results than with the use of our large bilateral prosthesis.

Do not confuse the preperitoneal approach with the transperitoneal route, another posterior approach, suggested by Laroque in 1929 and scarcely used until it became the preferred route for laparoscopic repair of groin hernia. This route, which allows creation of a pneumoperitoneum under general anesthesia as well as exposure to the risks of postoperative adhesions, cannot be presented as an advantage of laparoscopic procedures for hernia repair.

In conclusion, I use the preperitoneal approach—well known in the United States for elective repair of hernial orifices—for the placement of large pieces of mesh that reinforce or replace the damaged transversalis fascia. Prosthetic repair by this method is easier than by the inguinal approach. I prefer the median approach over others because it allows the surgeon to approach both sides at once, quickly and with good exposure, and to insert large bilateral pieces of Dacron mesh. Wantz proposed the unilateral giant prosthetic repair, which is the same as our bilateral procedure, but cut in half; the preperitoneal space is reached by a transverse incision extending from the midline laterally for 8 to 9 cm, made 2 to 3 cm below the level of the anterior superior iliac spines.

HOW TO USE PROSTHESES

Choosing a Good Prosthesis

Good prostheses replace or reinforce the tight inguinal layer (the transversalis fascia) and are a fundamental modern therapeutic option. Classic research and clinical experience[1,5,22,23,34,38,41,44,49,50,56] have produced well-known data, which are not reproduced here. A good prosthetic material must provoke a moderate inflammatory reaction and have strong fibroblastic activity. Mesh must be preferred because of its good biologic tolerance of septic conditions and its fast invasion by the connective tissue.

I routinely have used Dacron mesh, advocated in France by Rives and associates,[40–48] for 25 years. Our experiments with Petit[34] showed the good biologic tolerance of Dacron mesh, and Arnaud and colleagues[5] stressed the quality of the fibroblastic-to-inflammatory cell ratio. Marlex or Prolene mesh and Rhodergon 8000 can be used, but they are less supple than Dacron and less convenient for groin hernia repair by giant prostheses as assessed by Wantz.[65] Other materials, such as Vicryl mesh (low absorbency), offer only a temporary buttress, and Silastic sheets (impervious) and Rhodergon velours (joining a sheet of Silastic and synthetic velvet) should never be used because they are badly tolerated by the body.

Important Principles of Prosthesis Use

I conceive the prosthetic repair of groin hernias, like that of eventrations, as the placement of synthetic nonabsorbable mesh between the deeper inguinal layer and the visceral sac in the retroparietal cleavable space described earlier. In so doing, I do not place a simple patch, but make a large interposition of prosthetic mesh able to hold face to face with the neighboring layers and to support instantly and permanently the inguinal wall. For this purpose, the prosthesis must extend broadly beyond the weak inguinal area in all directions (Fig. 10-6) so that when the peritoneal sac is replaced, the prosthesis is pressed by intraabdominal pressure against the inner face of the abdominal wall and quickly attached by the development of the connective tissue through the mesh. By this method, the surgeon uses the force that has created the hernia—the intraabdominal pressure—to obtain a radical cure.

I and my colleagues have demonstrated that in accordance with Pascal's hydrostatic principle, abdominal pressure procures a stability that exempts the surgeon from fixation of the prosthesis, provided it is large. Gosset[19] wrote that the prosthesis was like "a gaiter between the inner tube and the tire," and Van Damme[58] compared the tactic with "plugging a leak in a bathtub." The central principle of our method is: the larger the prosthesis, the more efficient is the repair. In our conception, there are two possible types of operations that use Dacron mesh as a piece of artificial endoabdominal fascia placed by the preperitoneal approach—the unilateral patch, which needs to be fixed carefully because of its small size, and the large bilateral prosthesis, widely wrapping the visceral sac, which needs no suture because it holds instantly and definitively with the intraperitoneal pressure.

TECHNICAL ASPECTS OF PROSTHETIC REPAIR

Preoperative Preparation

Operations for extremely large hernias necessitate respiratory preparations and on occasion the use of the progressive pneumoperitoneum, as suggested by

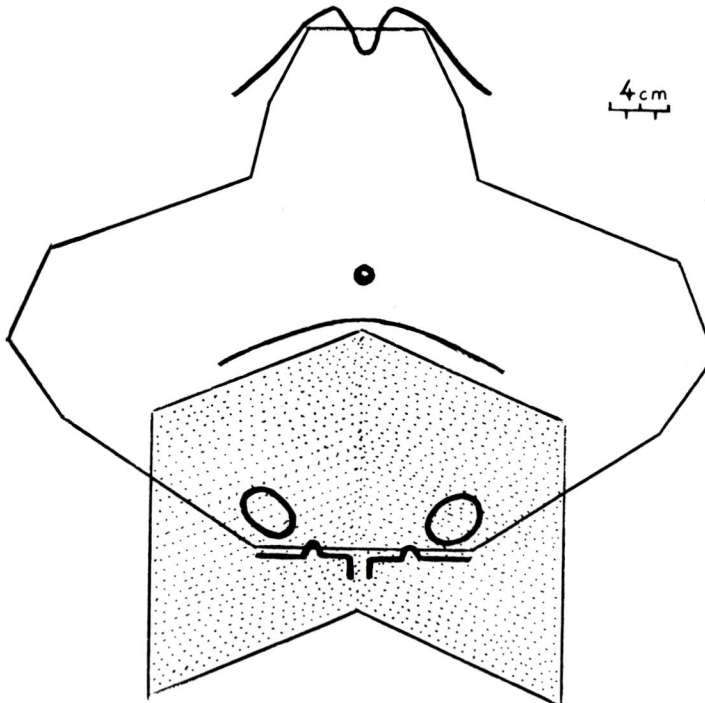

Figure 10-6. Schematic superposition of our chevron-shaped prosthesis over the plane projection of the retrofascial–preperitoneal cleavable space. The chevron-shaped pattern of the prosthesis provides better centering and broader overlapping of the two musculopectineal openings. (See also Fig. 10-11.)

Goñi-Moreno.[18] General anesthesia is usually used, as is spinal or peridural anesthesia in patients at respiratory risk. Some useful surgical instruments are: mounted swabs for the retroparietal cleavage, two straight retractors (6-and 10-cm long) for the abdominal wall, Ombrédanne forceps or tape for handling the cord, a sterilized scale and scissors for measuring and cutting the prosthesis, and long, curved Rochester forceps for no-touch handling of the prosthesis.

The Operation

Medial Preperitoneal Approach

The patient is placed supine in a light Trendelenburg position. The surgeon is on the opposite side of the hernia. An adhesive field is applied as the usual protection against skin contamination. A median subumbilical incision is made, and the umbilicoprevesical fascia is cut with Mayo scissors (Fig. 10-7). The pre-

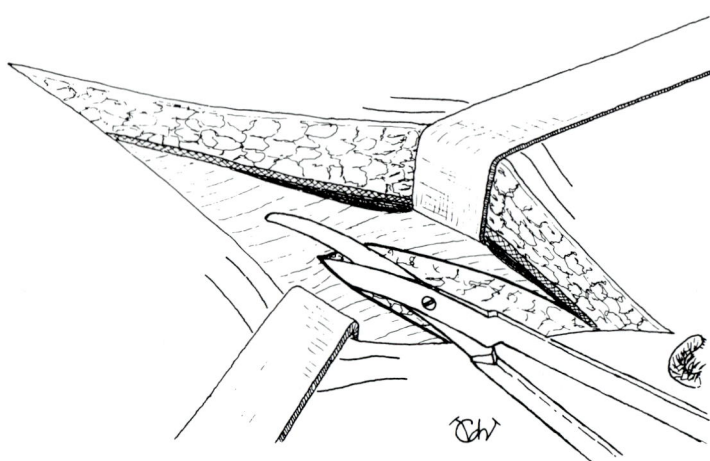

Figure 10-7. The section downward of the umbilicoprevesical fascia, with Mayo scissors.

peritoneal cleavage starts from the lower portion on the median line in the retropubic space of Retzius. It continues laterally, posteriorly to the rectus abdominis muscle on the far side of the operator, and proceeds behind the epigastric vessels. The dissection advances downward in front of the bladder, up to the prostatic compartment, and then outward behind the iliopubic ramus in the space of Bogros. Thus is the hernial pedicle isolated (Fig. 10-8), and the spermatic cord is either united to or distinct from the hernial sac, depending on the type of hernia. This dissection does not necessitate a difficult search even in recurrent hernias, which is pleasing for all operators regardless of their experience. The iliac vessels and crural nerve in their sheath do not incur any injury.

Single or multiple hernial sacs are treated in different ways, according to their volume and degree of adherence to the musculopectineal orifice. They are freed by continued moderate traction, incision, resection, and suture in first-time procedures on direct hernias of moderate size; for multirecurrent, indirect, or inguinoscrotal hernias with wide defects and parietal sclerosis, however, the surgeon may use a scalpel or scissors, guided by a finger inserted into the peritoneal infundibulum, to free the adherent sac. The preperitoneal approach opens a large exposure of the whole region and uncovers other clinically nonapparent hernias (eg, obturator hernias). The peritoneum is closed after resection of the hernial sac, and the preperitoneal dissection continues rapidly and without difficulty under the external iliac vessels and laterally to the ureter. It is not necessary to pursue the dissection above the Douglas linea arcuata where the peritoneum is adherent or may tear. When an iliac ap-

pendectomy scar is present, dissection may become somewhat difficult but is easily overcome with scissors. On the whole, the surgeon can perform the dissection of the spaces of Bogros and Retzius quickly and easily without bleeding, using a single straight retractor under the inner wall while depressing the peritoneal sac with the left hand.

Joining the constituting elements of the spermatic cord with the pelvic wall simplifies placement of the large prosthesis and eliminates the need to cut it for passage of the spermatic cord. The cord is seized in its retroparietal course with an Ombrédanne forceps or a tape, with moderate traction applied, so that the scissors and a blunt swab may dissociate the different elements of the cord from the peritoneal sac. At the end of the dissection, one finds a triangular cellular spread (Fig. 10-9) with a posterosuperior base, the sides of which contain the deferent canal, on its medial side, and the spermatic vascular pedicle on its lateral side. When they are released, as when the Ombrédanne forceps are opened, the elements of the spermatic cord join by gravity with the posterior wall so that no element now crosses the preperitoneal prevesical space. During this operative time, preperitoneal and cordal lipomas should be suppressed in the aim to avoid the deceiving cough-impulsion of a false recurrence. To perform the retroparietal dissection on the other side, the operator and assistant change sides and proceed in the same manner as for the first side.

Placement of the Prosthesis

Unilateral Patch. Rives, who routinely uses the inguinal approach for prosthetic repairs, scarcely uses

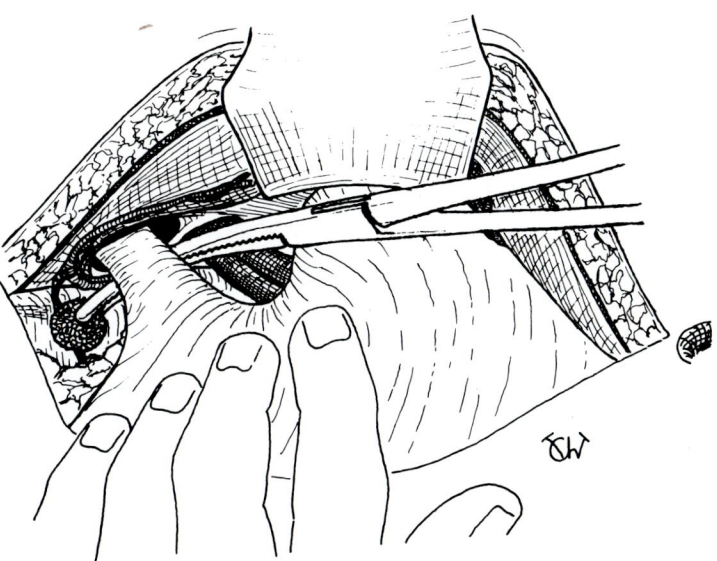

Figure 10-8. The right indirect hernial pedicle lifted on a forceps with a small swab.

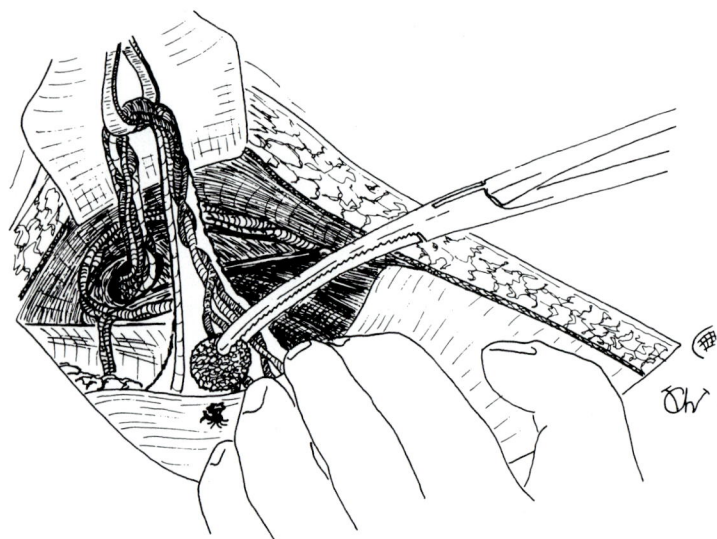

Figure 10-9. Representation of the right cord seized with an Ombrédanne forceps after its separation from the peritoneum and bladder.

the preperitoneal approach for the placement of a unilateral piece of mesh. In this case, he places two to three stitches to close the musculopectineal orifice, joining the arch to the Cooper ligament. Then, a 10-cm² piece of Dacron mesh is cut up and inserted in the angle formed by the abdominal wall and the fascia iliaca (Fig. 10-10). The prosthesis is usually split to let the cord through, then attached to the wall of the inguinal region by a few carefully executed sutures. If a hernia exists on the opposite side, the operator changes sides and proceeds in the same manner as for the first side; in this situation, two symmetric pieces are placed.

Wantz, whose technique is presented later, places a 12-cm² piece of Dacron mesh unilaterally, without

splitting it (for the passage of the cord), owing to the parietalization of the cord elements (the same maneuver as mentioned earlier).

Large Bilateral Prosthesis. This technique, which I have used for 25 years, does not require any attempt at repair of the hernial orifice. The size of the prosthesis is measured on the patient. The correct transverse dimension is equal to the distance between both anterior superior iliac spines minus 2 cm, the height of the prosthesis being equal to the distance between the umbilicus and the pubis. The mean values are 24 cm transversally and 16 cm vertically; the extreme values are 20 to 30 cm and 14 to 19 cm. The prosthesis is cut with straight scissors, using a no-touch tech-

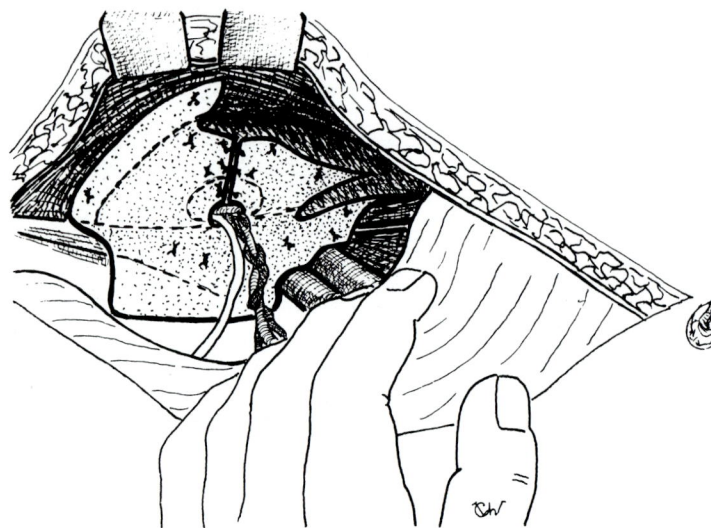

Figure 10-10. Schematic anteromediolateral view of a unilateral prosthesis placed by the medial preperitoneal approach. The operator's left hand depresses the peritoneal sac. The prosthesis, split to let the cord pass through, is sewn to the parietal wall, the Cooper ligament, the femoral sheath, and the fascia iliaca.

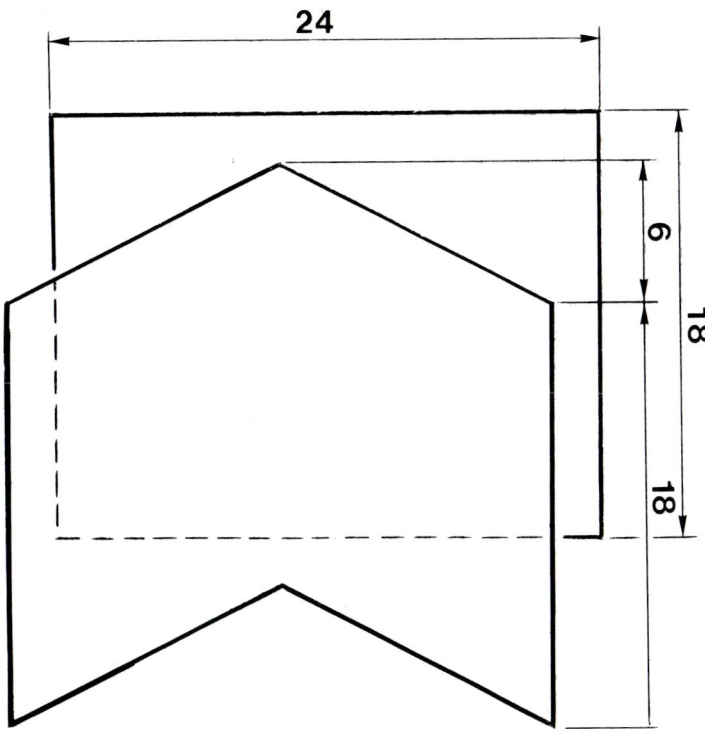

Figure 10-11. The chevron-shaped prosthesis is cut with regard to the mean dimensions of the rectangle measured on the patient.

nique, taking into account the main dimensions, which are chevron-shaped, so that its lateroinferior angles will later be placed far down behind the two pelvic obturator frames (Fig. 10-11) and its superior convex border will fit to the concavity of the line of Douglas.

The patch is then seized by all angles and by the middle of the lateral borders with long Rochester forceps that facilitate placement (Fig. 10-12). The patch is first placed on the opposite side of the operator. The assistant retracts the parietal wall up as the operator depresses the peritoneal sac with his or her left hand, pulling it upward; this opens the parietoperitoneal cleavage space. The prosthesis is then pushed into this space with the Rochester forceps. The inferior median forceps is first placed between the pubis and bladder, followed by the inferior angle forceps, median lateral forceps, and superior angle forceps, while pushing them as far as possible. This maneuver unfolds the prosthesis on all points of the parietoperitoneal cleavage space, surrounding the part of the visceral sac opposite the operator (Fig. 10-13). Every time one of the forceps is pushed into its correct place, the assistant immobilizes it until the operator releases the visceral sac with his or her left hand, which enables it to take its place. The valve is removed from under the parietal wall. The forceps used to place the prosthesis are then delicately removed at the same an-

gle in which they were placed, while passing along the inner facet of the parietal wall.

The operator and the assistant again change sides and perform the same maneuvers on the opposite side (Fig. 10-14). The Dacron mesh prosthesis is fully unfolded and inserted to surround the visceral sac, generously overlapping the hernial orifices and protecting the median subumbilical incision (Fig. 10-15). Then, the middle of the superior border of the prosthesis is fixed with a synthetic absorbable suture to the inferior border of the Richet umbilical fascia. No other stitch is used for fixation of the prosthesis, simplifying the technique. No antibiotic but only antiseptic agents are used in the surgical wound.

Closure and Drainage
The parietal suture is made with slowly absorbing synthetic suture material, the subcutaneous fat is padded with small sutures, and the skin is sewn with fine nylon. When suction drainage tubes are necessary, they are placed in front of the prosthesis.

Postoperative Care
The patient is encouraged not to restrict activity. Recovery of activity is usually not a problem because postoperative discomfort is minimal. Nevertheless, slow-acting heparin is used for a few days. Prophylactic antibiotic therapy is never used. Eventual suction

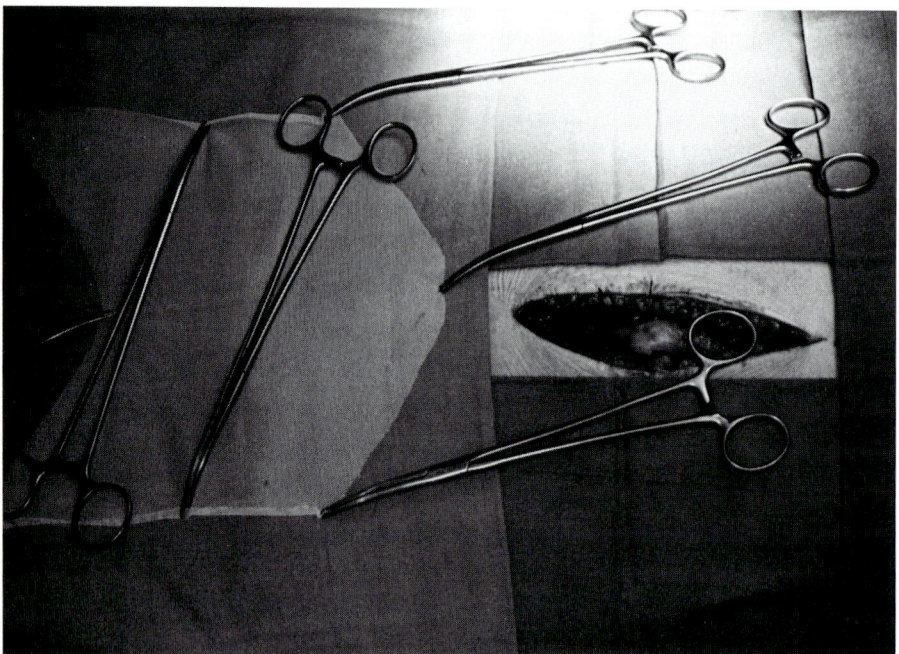

Figure 10-12. The large chevron-shaped Dacron mesh prosthesis, cut to the correct dimensions, has been seized by eight long Rochester forceps for no-touch handling. (*Right*) The subumbilical midline incision.

drainage and dressings are discontinued on the second postoperative day. Hospital discharge occurs between the third and the fifth day.

Miscellaneous Remarks

A huge inguinoscrotal sac may be freed by an associated direct inguinal approach, leaving the lower por-

tion of the sac adherent to the scrotal fundus, with the possible risk of hematoma formation not regularly avoided despite careful suction drainage.

In unilateral hernias, one must carefully observe the clinically uninvolved side. A tip of hernia is frequently discovered, usually when the hernia being operated on is direct or large or when preperitoneal li-

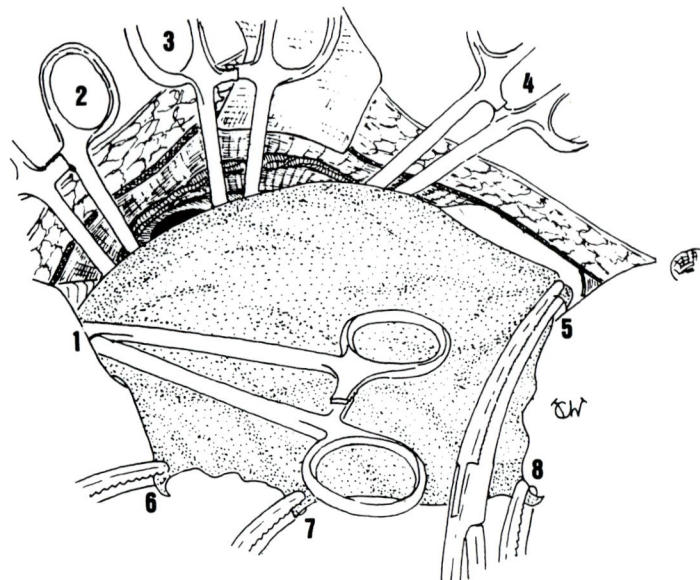

Figure 10-13. The right part of the giant bilateral mesh prosthesis has just been pushed, with no. 8 Rochester forceps, into the right part of the parietoperitoneal cleavage space. The numbers (1 to 8) show the order in which the forceps have been used (*right side,* 1–5) or will be used (*left side,* 6–8).

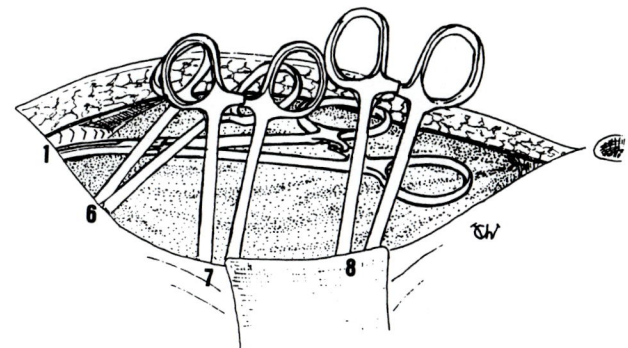

Figure 10-14. The mesh prosthesis has been pushed into the two sides of the parietoperitoneal cleavage space. Forceps 6 to 8 have just pushed the left side of the prosthesis and still have not been removed. Forceps 1 is the medioinferior (prevesical) one still in place. A single stitch is visible at the upper part of the incision (*right*), fixing the medial point of the superior border of the mesh prosthesis to the Richet umbilical fascia.

pomas exist. One may be tempted to use a unilateral patch, but for patients older than 50 years of age, we routinely insert a large bilateral prosthesis because of the frequent later appearance of a contralateral hernia.

The Trendelenburg position is helpful in obese patients. It is impossible not to recognize other hernias when the preperitoneal approach is used.

Hernias in unusual locations are identified precisely from the inner hernial orifice and easily treated, no matter what the location—laterofemoral, prevascular, mediofemoral, or obturator. The same is true for low eventration.

Most problems related to sliding hernias are solved by the preperitoneal approach. One obtains the correct diagnosis by opening the sac at the appropriate level. Reduction of the contents and eventual limited resection of the sac are performed without difficulty. The prosthetic repair abolishes the hazards resulting from the large hernial orifice.

Although hernias in elderly patients have a low recurrence rate in our experience,[67] when the hernias are bilateral, elderly patients profit from a large prosthetic repair, which can be done quickly.

We have developed a prosthetic repair by the preperitoneal approach for multirecurrent hernias. This technique is irreplaceable when previous attempts by the inguinal approach have destroyed the Poupart and Cooper ligaments. The preperitoneal approach also avoids the difficult dissection by the inguinal approach of modified groin structures and saves time.

In technique, associated pelvic abdominal intraperitoneal or extraperitoneal lesions can be treated if no potentially septic maneuver is required.

One may summarize our method in the following way: The *giant bilateral prosthesis* repair is the placement of a wide piece of Dacron mesh in the large bilateral cleaved space. The prosthesis has large dimensions; thus, its stability is excellent without any fixation, and there is no need for a direct repair of the wall. The surgeon's only concerns are to separate the retroparietal cellular spaces, to cut a prosthesis of the needed size, and to surround the visceral sac while at the same time reinforcing the endoabdominal fas-

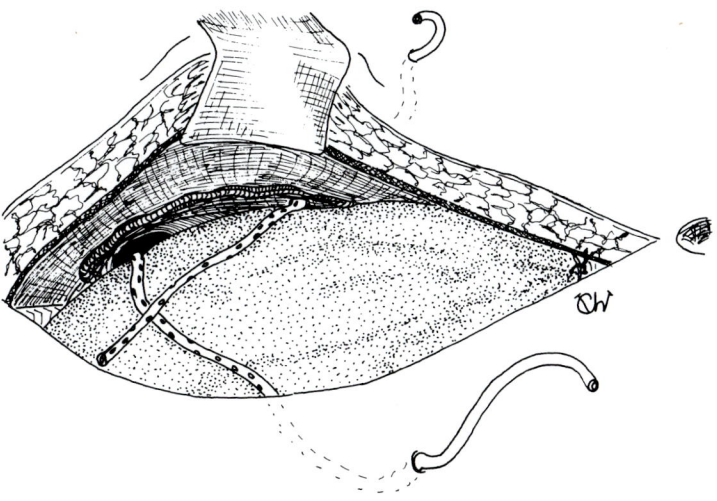

Figure 10-15. The large prosthesis, bilaterally overlapping the hernial orifices, protecting the subumbilical midline incision. Note the suction drains.

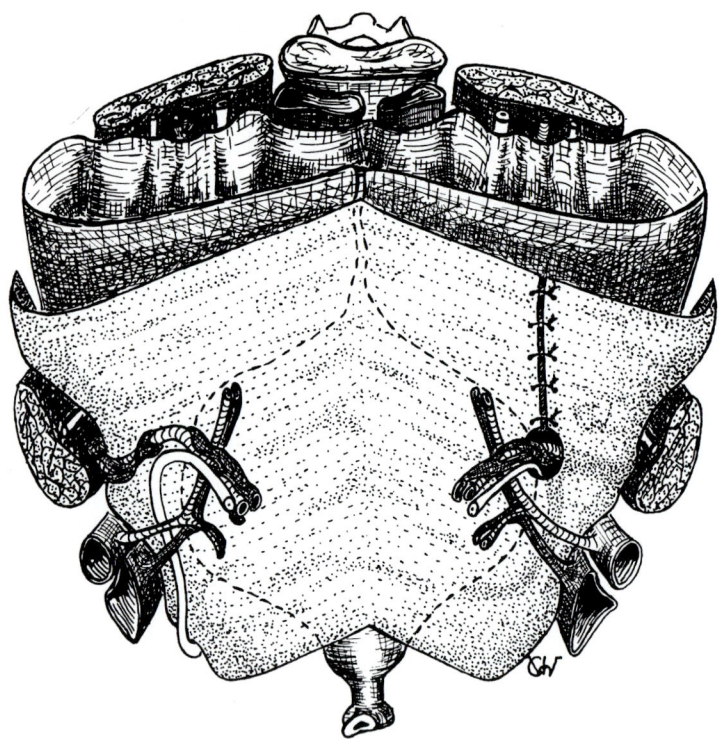

Figure 10-16. Schematic anteroposterior view of the giant bilateral Dacron mesh prosthesis surrounding the inferior part of the visceral sac as an artificial endoabdominal fascia (the tight layer of the abdominal wall). The spermatic cord may either pass through the slit prosthesis (*right,* wrong technique) or be parietalized (*left,* best solution).

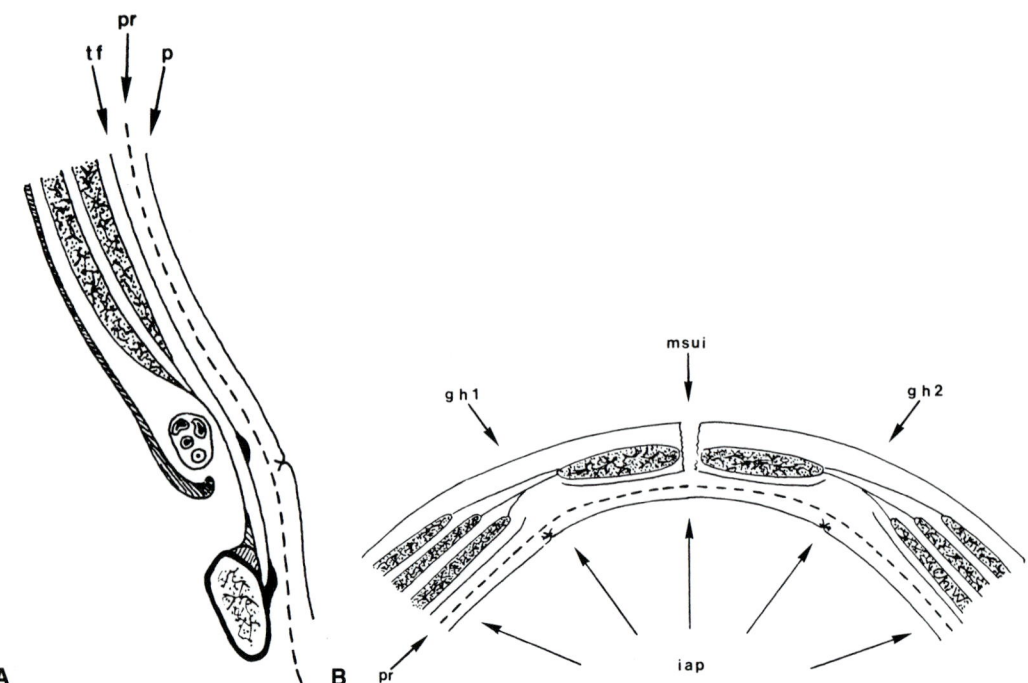

Figure 10-17. Schematic representations of the giant bilateral prosthesis at the end of the operation. (*A*) Sagittal paramedian cross section of the inguinal wall showing the deep position (underlay) of the mesh (pr) between peritoneum (p) and transversalis fascia (tf). (*B*) Horizontal cross section of the abdominal wall, at the level of the inguinal regions, showing how intraabdominal pressure (iap), acting in all directions (*arrows*) and following Pascal's hydrostatic principle, fixes the prosthesis (pr), which involves the peritoneal sac, rendering it inextensible, and at the same time reinforces the endoabdominal fascia. msui, midline subumbilical incision; gh1 and gh2 arrows indicate the locations of two groin hernias. (Adapted from Nyhus LM, Baker RJ, eds. Mastery of surgery, ed 2, vol 2. Boston, Little, Brown, 1992)

cia by placing the mesh barrier across the different hernial orifices and the midline laparotomy wound so that there is no possibility of recurring hernia or eventration (Figs. 10-16 and 10-17). The operative time is short (30–40 minutes), which is important for elderly patients and those at risk.

DO PREPERITONEAL PROSTHESES CARRY SPECIAL RISKS?

We have not found prosthetic repair by the preperitoneal approach to be a risky or complex procedure. The most elaborate herniorrhaphies (eg, the Shouldice technique) require thorough dissection, which is useless in our method. Moreover, certain complicated hernias, such as huge, sliding, bilateral, or recurrent hernias, are more easily treated by a preperitoneal prosthetic repair than by a standard herniorrhaphy. They are also treated more quickly and more reliably. In addition, the preperitoneal prosthetic repair avoids some rather frequent and medicolegal complications of inguinal herniorrhaphies—femoral vein thrombosis, testicular atrophy, and persistent pains.[12,62–64] Like any technique, however, this hernial repair must be well studied and well understood before it is well executed.

Septic complications are more disagreeable when they occur after prosthetic repair than after nonprosthetic approaches. The suppurations observed do not represent rejection, but are the consequences of bacterial contamination. Thus, rigorous vigilance before, during, and after operation is imperative. Before operation, the patient's skin must be carefully and extensively disinfected. No attempt at Dacron repair should be made in the presence of an obstinate dermatosis. During operation, the no-touch technique and the frequent use of antiseptic agents should be followed. During the postoperative course, no dressing should be applied to the wound to allow better observation. A superficial inflammation requires an early and generous opening of the skin incision. In the case of a deep infection related to the prosthesis, fortunately a rare occurrence, the wound must be opened widely. On the other hand, one must not remove the prosthesis immediately; when the drainage is done precociously and correctly, the prosthesis can be penetrated and covered by the connective tissue, and healing can take place.

The inclusion of the prosthesis between wall and peritoneum does not impede subsequent operations on the abdomen, which can be performed with the usual blade and sutured normally, as in a primary laparotomy, and normal healing should occur. In our experience, several patients have had to undergo subsequent operations for prostatectomy or intra-abdominal diseases, mostly colonic cancers, without any disadvantage. Three patients have withstood transprosthetic peritoneal dialysis for later renal insufficiency.

RESULTS

Personal Experience

In my contribution to the third edition of this text, my staff and I reviewed a series of 1522 patients with 2108 groin hernias operated on from 1970 to 1984. We compared, using a computerized study of 140 items, the results of four techniques in our hands—the Bassini operation (BO), Cooper ligament repair (CLR), inguinal patch (IP), and our preperitoneal prosthetic repair (PPR). Patients were 16 to 103 years of age, the median ages being 55.8 years for men and 61.5 years for women. The sex ratio was 5.32 men to 1 woman. The anatomic and clinical breakdown of types of hernia was 40.1% indirect hernias, 30% direct hernias, 6.6% groin eventrations, 6.3% femoral hernias, and 17% diverse hernias; 12.6% of the hernias were recurrent; 9.7% of the operations were for acute complications. The breakdown by techniques was 99 BO, 549 CLR, 213 IP, and 604 PPR; 42 modified Shouldice operations were also performed.

Postoperative Course
Uncomplicated courses were followed in 91 BOs (92.1%), 525 CLRs (95.1%), 191 IPs (89.9%), and 572 PPRs (94.7%); that is, each of the techniques had a similarly favorable success rate. (Note that BO was used for some complicated hernias and PPR for the most unfavorable instances.)

Hematoma rates were 2.2% after BO, 2.8% after CLR, 4% after IP, and 3.2% after PPR; there was no important difference between the techniques.

Sepsis rates were 5.6% after BO, 2.2% after CLR, 6.1% after IP, and 2.1% after PPR (BO was used in complicated hernias).

Other complications reported were 16 chest infections (8 after herniorrhaphies, 7 after PPR, 1 after IP), 4 instances of phlebitis (3 after CLR, 1 after PPR), and 2 pulmonary embolisms (1 after CLR, 1 after PPR).

Twenty deaths occurred during the first postoperative month (1.3%), related to 14 herniorrhaphies (2%) and 6 PPRs (0.7%) in elderly patients and complicated operations.[67]

Lengths of hospitalization are reported in Table 10-1. The results show that using Dacron does not much lengthen the median hospital stay, especially when taking into account the use of PPR in the most unfavorable situations. Incidentally, these lengths of

Table 10-1. Comparison of Length of Hospital Stay for Patients Operated on by the Four Techniques of Hernial Repair (N = 2108)

Time (days)	Technique			
	BO (%)	CLR (%)	IP (%)	PPR (%)
<7	68.4	57.9	30.5	19.4
8–12	25.5	37.1	57.7	68.3
>13	6.1	5.9	11.9	12.2
Median length of stay	7.3 days	7.7 days	9.2 days	9.7 days

BO, Bassini operation; CLR, Cooper ligament repair; IP, inguinal patch; PPR, preperitoneal prosthetic repair.

hospitalization will probably startle our North American colleagues; although French surgeons aim to reduce the length of the postoperative hospital stay for economic reasons, they have to consider different problems. These data are changing, however: since 1985, 97.3% of operated patients are discharged between the third and fifth postoperative day in my department.

Comparison of off-work periods for each of the operations is reported in Table 10-2, which shows that prostheses are responsible not only for the higher rate of shorter off-work periods but also for the lower proportions of the longer off-work periods.

Follow-up Data

Of 1522 patients reviewed in 1984, 1330 (87.4%) had their repairs intact 1 to 10 years after the operation. One hundred thirteen (8.5%) had recurrences: 22.5% after BO, 15.3% after CLR, 10.7% after IP, and 1.4% after PPR. The recurrences after PPR were caused by prostheses that were too small or that had split. Of the recurrences after 1 year, 27.8% were after BO and 31.4% after CLR, whereas there was no worsening of results after Dacron herniorrhaphy. The sequelae observed were four testicular atrophies and two hydroceles, all occurring after an inguinal approach. The

late migration into the bladder of a preperitoneal prosthesis placed during a prostatectomy emphasizes that septic gestures and prosthetic herniorrhaphy should not be associated with each other. The computerized study of our 1984 series demonstrates the favorable results of the preperitoneal prosthetic repair of groin hernias when compared with other techniques. These are emphasized by my 1989 control of another 529 PPR personal series, which has found the following recurrence rates: 1.1% for recurred hernias and 0.56% for primary repairs.

Results Reported in the Literature

Tables 10-3 and 10-4 report results obtained by other surgeons using diverse prosthetic repair techniques. The results found in these studies do not contradict our own good results with prosthetic repair. Most interestingly, Nyhus's report[27] demonstrated "a dramatic difference in recurrence rates when prosthetic material is used and particularly if the operative approach is preperitoneal or posterior."

PATIENT SELECTION FOR PREPERITONEAL PROSTHETIC REPAIR

It is often said that the treatment of hernias must be as simple as possible, restoring the wall with the support of a perfect knowledge of regional anatomy and technical details, with the aim of opposing the mechanisms of herniation and avoiding recurrence. The preperitoneal prosthetic repair fits these principles, but one should keep in mind the potential of septic accidents. Thus, a logical attitude includes selective indications for repairs with prostheses and careful attention to the prevention of septic complications. If the surgeon makes efforts to avoid septic risk, he or she cannot do much more than use Dacron to im-

Table 10-2. Comparison of Time Off From Work for Patients Operated on by the Four Techniques (N = 2108)

Time (wk)	Technique			
	BO (%)	CLR (%)	IP (%)	PPR (%)
1–4	23.8	33.9	32.7	42.3
5–8	57.1	50.3	44.9	45.5
>9	19.1	15.8	22.4	12.2

BO, Bassini operation; CLR, Cooper ligament repair; IP, inguinal patch; PPR, preperitoneal prosthetic repair.

Table 10-3. Recurrence Rates After Inguinal Patch

Authors	Techniques	No. Hernias Operated On	Control Rate (%)	Follow-up Duration (y)	Recurrence Rate (%)
Bapat*	Steel	95	84.2	0.5–5.5	1.0
Barthes (1971)[6]	Nylon	273		3	9.9
Cerise*	Dacron	100	100.0	1–4.5	1.0
Courtot*	Rhodergon	31		1	7.0
Martin*	Marlex	365		1–10	0.0
Nahas*	Nylon	51			2.0
Notaras*	Dacron	246		1–8	0.4
Piper*	Skin	246	67.7		12.2
Rives et al. (1978)[42]	Dacron	65			0.0
Rives et al. (1982)[41]	Dacron	183	66.1	1–9	1.6
Saliba*	Dacron	204			0.0
Snidjers*	Teflon	150	93.0	1–8	2.7
Warlaumont (1982)[67]	Dacron	208	87.3	1–10	10.9
Usher*	Marlex	541	44.4	1	10.2
Zagdoun (1959)[68]	Nylon	185	80.0	1–7	7.0

*Cited in Stoppa and Houdard, 1984.[50]

prove the strength of a weakened transversalis fascia. Reasonably, the respective indications for repairs using prostheses must be founded on the evaluation of the recurrence risk, restricting prosthetic repairs to hernias with high risks of recurrence. As are many others,[29] we are still trying to finalize recurrence risk by a classification of groin hernias through their morphologic characteristics; but rational arguments have to be assessed by consistent results.

Contraindications to prosthetic repair occur when septic risk cannot be controlled and when general or spinal anesthesia cannot be used. We do not consider

a previous median laparotomy a contraindication, nor do we consider the sequelae of an iliocaval thrombosis (the supply shunts do not embarrass the midline) contraindications. However, one must be extremely selective in using prostheses in emergency operations or when treating strangulated hernias.

The practical indications for the preperitoneal prosthetic repair include the following:

1. The patient is preferably a man who is not younger than 40 years of age.
2. The hernia is intricate, as are some types of

Table 10-4. Recurrence Rates After Preperitoneal Prosthetic Repairs

Authors	Techniques	No. Hernias Operated On	Control Rate (%)	Follow-up Duration (y)	Recurrence Rate (%)
Blondiaux et al. (1979)[9]	Teflon, mid. ap.	91	52.7	0.5–3.5	0.0
Brismoutier*	Silicone, mid. ap.	101		4	6.0
Calne (1967)[10]	Dacron, Pfannenstiel	30		1–7.5	13.3
Detrie*	Nylon, mid. ap.	50		0.5–4	0.0
Fagot*	Dacron, mid. ap.	29	100.0	0.5–3	1.3
Gosset (1972)[19]	Rhodergon-Velvet, mid. ap.	7		2	0.0
Read (1975)[37]	Marlex, mid. ap.	83		4	7.0
Rignault et al. (1983)[38]	Dacron, Pfannenstiel	658	86.3	4	4.6
Saint Julien†	Dacron, mid. ap.	309	63.0	0.5–6	2.9
Stoppa et al. (1973)[51]	Dacron, mid. ap.	168	88.1	1–7	3.3
Warlaumont (1982)[67]	Dacron, mid. ap.	285	91.3	1–10	1.2

*Cited in Stoppa and Houdard, 1984.[50]
†Cited in Salinier, 1983.[49]
mid. ap., midline approach.

groin hernia, bilateral hernia, and hernia associated with single or multiple lower eventrations.

3. The hernia is complicated by nature, as in sliding hernias, enormous inguinoscrotal hernias, and recurrent or multirecurrent hernias; when a recurred hernia is associated with a destroyed Poupart or Cooper ligament, it is the last resort.
4. The hernia is femoral prevascular.
5. The hernia has recurred after repair by an inguinal patch.
6. The conditions are such that the surgeon must aim for a guaranteed result. Obesity, advanced age, and cirrhotic disorders are such conditions.
7. The operation must be performed quickly, as in bilateral hernias or in elderly or high-risk patients.
8. Ehlers-Danlos or Marfan disease with multirecurrent hernia is present.[66]

RECURRENCE

The six recurrences in my series occurred because the prostheses used were too small. Thus, the recurrent sac made its way through the insufficient fascia under the lower edge. Because of these recurrences, we now cut the piece of mesh into a chevron shape, which results in a larger downward interposition. A reoperation by the inguinal approach has allowed us to suture the displaced lower edge of the prosthesis to the Cooper ligament. Satisfactory results have been obtained in all patients. Failure of the inguinal patch can easily be eliminated by a large prosthesis inserted by the preperitoneal approach.

CONCLUSION

Prosthetic repairs are an important development in herniology because of their excellent results. When I hear "prosthetic repair," I think of reinforcement or replacement of the transversalis fascia; this means the interposition of a synthetic mesh underlay between muscles and peritoneum for the restoration of the tightness of the abdominal wall against intraabdominal pressure. Not all synthetic materials are equally efficient; Dacron mesh is the best fitting one for giant prosthesis repair. The midline preperitoneal approach allows the surgeon to reach the deep hernial orifice quickly and easily and with a wide exposure while also managing a deep cleaved site for the place-

ment of a large bilateral prosthesis. Large prostheses are kept in place by intraabdominal pressure; they need not be fixed or associated with a repair of the hernial orifice. It is an easy operation that allows repair of badly damaged inguinal walls in multirecurrent hernias.

Because of the disagreeable septic accidents that can occur after prosthetic repair (neither to be neglected nor exaggerated), the indications for the procedure must be selective. The operation may be used logically and reservedly in instances in which other techniques may fail, usually recurrences and re-recurrences.

In regard to the future of preperitoneal prosthetic repairs, we do not believe that randomized studies comparing the diverse techniques will lead us to an exclusive choice because hernias are polymorphous lesions. The time lag factor also presents difficulty in randomized studies; although a prosthesis gives virtually immediate definitive results, repairs must be intact 20 years after the operation. As for socioeconomic concerns, I believe that using a prosthesis when a hernia is expected to recur fits to a good socioeconomic plan. Finally, the remarkable possibilities offered by prostheses have been an important and gratifying attainment in my technologic look out in the field of hernia surgery.

ACKNOWLEDGMENTS

I would like to express my sincere thanks to Dr. Christian Warlaumont, hernia surgeon and friend, for having thoroughly studied one of my series in his excellent medical thesis and provided his talent in the illustrations of this chapter.

REFERENCES

1. Acquaviva DE, Bourret P, Corti F. Considerations sur l'emploi des plaques de nylon dites crinoplaques comme matériel de plastie pariétale. 52e Congrès Fr. de Chirurgie. Paris, Masson, 1949:453–457.
2. Ami G. Le canal inguinal chez l'homme. Thèse Méd. Lyon, no. 73, 1964.
3. Anson BJ, Morgan E, McVay C, et al. The anatomy of hernia regions: inguinal hernia. Surg Gynecol Obstet 1949;89:417.
4. Anson BJ, Reimann AF, Swigard LL, et al. The anatomy of hernia regions: femoral hernia. Surg Gynecol Obstet 1949;89:753.
5. Arnaud JP, Eloy R, Weill-Bousson M, et al. Résistance et tolérance biologique de 6 prothèses "inertes" utilisées dans la reparation de la paroi abdominale. J Chir 1977;113:85.

6. Barthes JN. Traitement des hernies et éventrations par une prothéses de nylon: la crinoplaque à propos de 420 cas personnels. Thèse Méd. Paris, no. 91, 1971.

7. Berliner SD. Adult inguinal hernia: pathophysiology and repair. Surg Annu 1983;15:307.

8. Berliner SD. An approach to groin hernia. Surg Clin North Am 1984;64:197.

9. Blondiaux JV, Verheyen V, Colard M, et al. Cure des hernies inguinocrurales par voie médiane prépéritoneale et prothèse en Téflon. Acta Chir Belg 1979; 5:317.

10. Calne RY. Repair of bilateral hernias with Mersilene mesh behind the rectus abdominus (*sic*). Arch Surg 1967;109:532.

11. Chevrel JP, ed. Chirurgie des parois de l'abdomen. Berlin, Springer-Verlag, 1985.

12. Chevrel JP, Gatt MT, Sarfati E, et al. Les névralgies résiduelles apres cure de nernie inguinale. Groupe de Recherche et d'Etude de la paroi abdominale (GREPA), 4e réunion, St. Tropez, Boulogne-Billancourt, Bruneau, 1982:29–31.

13. Condon RE. The anatomy of the inguinal region. In: Nyhus LM, Condon PE, eds. Hernia, ed. 2. Philadelphia, JB Lippincott, 1978:14–53.

14. Condon RE, Nyhus LM. Complications of groin hernia and of hernia repair. Surg Clin North Am 1971;51:1325.

15. Fruchaud H. Anatomie chirurgicale des hernies de l'aine. Paris, Doin, 1956.

16. Fruchaud H. Traitement chirurgical des hernies de l'aine. Paris, Doin, 1957.

17. Gaston EA. The internal oblique muscle in inguinal herniorrhaphy. Am J Surg 1964;107:366.

18. Goñi-Moreno I. The rational treatment of hernias and voluminous chronic eventrations: preparation with progressive pneumoperitoneum. In: Nyhus LM, Harkins HN, eds. Hernia, ed 1. Philadelphia, JB Lippincott, 1964:688.

19. Gosset J. La cure des hernies inguino-crurales récidivées avec effondrement de l'aine (laparotomie médiane et prothèse sous-péritonéale en velours siliconé). J Chir 1972;104:493.

20. Iles JD. Specialisation in elective herniorrhaphy. Lancet 1965;2:751.

21. Iles JD. The management of elective hernia repair. Ann Plast Surg 1979;6:538.

22. Koontz AR, Kimberley RC. Tissue reaction to tantalum mesh and wire. Ann Surg 1948;131:666.

23. Koontz AR, Kimberley RC. Tantalum and Marlex mesh (with a note on Marlex thread): an experimental and clinical comparison. Preliminary report. Ann Surg 1960;151:796.

24. Levasseur JC, Lehn E, Rignier P. Réflexion sur l'utilisation du treillis résorbable de polyglactine 910 dans le traitement des hernies et de l'éventration. J Chir 1980;117:563.

25. McVay CB. Groin hernioplasty: Cooper ligament repair. In: Nyhus LM, Condon RE, eds. Hernia, ed. 2. Philadelphia, JB Lippincott, 1978.

26. McVay CB, Anson BJ. Inguinal anal femoral hernioplasty. Surg Gynecol Obstet 1949;88:473.

27. Nyhus LM. The recurrent groin hernia: therapeutic solutions. World J Surg 1989;13:541.

28. Nyhus LM, Condon RE, Harkins HN. Clinical experiences with preperitoneal hernia repair for all types of hernia of the groin. Am J Surg 1960;100:234.

29. Nyhus LM, Klein MS, Rogers FB. Inguinal hernia. Curr Probl Surg 1991;28:403.

30. Odimba BFK, Stoppa R, Laude M, et al. Les espaces clivables sousparietaux de l'abdomen. J Chir 1980; 117:621.

31. Palumbo LT, Shape WS. Primary inguinal hernioplasty in the adult. Surg Clin North Am 1971; 51:1293.

32. Panou de Faymoreau T. Les plasties locales par plaque de nylon dans la cure chirurgicale des hernies inguinales et des éventrations. Thèse Méd, Nantes, no. 174, 1976.

33. Peacock EE. Biology of hernia. In: Nyhus LM, Condon RE, eds. Hernia, ed 2. Philadelphia, JB Lippincott, 1978.

34. Petit J, Stoppa R. Evaluation expérimentale des réactions tissulaires autour des prothèses de la paroi abdominale en mesh de Dacron. J Chir 1974;107:667.

35. Radojevic S. Contribution à l'étude de l'étiologie de la hernie inguinale. J Méd Bordeaux 1958;135:1223.

36. Read RC. Preperitoneal exposure of inguinal herniation. Am J Surg 1968;116:653.

37. Read RC. Recurrence after pre-peritoneal herniorrhaphy in the adult. Arch Surg 1975;110:666.

38. Rignault D, Dubois C, Andre H. Hernioplasties inguinales avec interposition prothétique (950 cures dont 226 récidives). Chirurgie 1983;109:841.

39. Rignault D, Dumeige F. Pose de deux plaques par voie de Pfannenstiel pour hernie bilatérale. J Chir 1981;118:673.

40. Rives J. Surgical treatment of the inguinal hernia with Dacron patch: principles, indications, technic and results. Int Surg 1967;47:360.

41. Rives J, Flament JB, Delattre JF, Palot JP. La chirurgie moderne des hernies de l'aine. Cah Méd 1982; 7:1205.

42. Rives J, Fortesa L, Drouard F, et al. La voie d'abord abdominale sous-péritonéale dans le traitement des hernies de l'aine. Ann Chir 1978;32:245.

43. Rives J, Hibon J. Hernies de l'aine. Encycl Méd Chir Paris 1974;9:90095.

44. Rives J, Lardennois B, Flament JB, Convers G. La pièce en tulle de Dacron, traitement de choix des hernies de l'aine de l'adulte: a propos de 183 cas. Chirurgie 1973;99:564.

45. Rives J, Lardennois B, Flament JB, Hibon J. Utilisation d'une étoffe en Dacron dans le traitement des hernies de l'aine. Acta Chir Belg 1971;70:284.

46. Rives J, Lardennois B, Hibon J. Traitement moderne des hernies de l'aine et de leurs récidives. Encycl Méd Chir Paris 1974;3:40090.

47. Rives J, Nicaise H. A propos des hernies de l'aine et de leurs recidives. Semin Hop Paris 1966;31:1932.

48. Rives J, Stoppa R, Fortesa L, Nicaise H. Les pièces en Dacron et leur place dans la chirurgie des hernies de l'aine. Ann Chir 1968;22:159.

49. Salinier L. Etude comparative du traitement des hernies inguinales par prothese: a propos de 309 observations. Thèse Méd. Bordeaux II, no. 233, 1983.

50. Stoppa R, Houdard C. Le traitement chirurgical des hernies de l'aine. Paris, Masson, 1984.

51. Stoppa R, Petit J, Abourachid H. Procede original de plastie des herniese de l'aine: l'interposition sans fixation d'une prothese en tulle de Dacron par voie mediane sous-peritoneale. Chirurgie 1973;99:119.

52. Stoppa R, Quintyn M. Les déficiences de la paroi abdominale chez le sujet agé: colloque avec le praticien. Semin Hop Paris 1969;45:2182.

53. Stoppa RE, Rives JL, Warlaumont CR, et al. The use of Dacron in the repair of hernias of the groin. Surg Clin North Am 1984;64:269.

54. Stoppa RE, Warlaumont CR. The preperitoneal approach and prosthetic repair of groin hernia. In: Nyhus LM, Condon RE, eds. Hernia, ed 3. Philadelphia, JB Lippincott, 1989.

55. Stoppa RE, Warlaumont CR. The midline preperitoneal approach to and the prosthetic repair of groin hernias. In: Nyhus LM, Baker RJ, eds. Mastery of surgery, ed 2. Boston, Little Brown, 1992.

56. Stoppa RE, Warlaumont C, Henry X. Socio-économie de la chirurgie des hernies. Bull Acad Nat Méd 1983;167:333.

57. Stoppa R, Warlaumont C, Verhaeghe P, et al. Les prothèses dans le traitement des hernies de l'aine: Pourquoi? Comment? Quand? Paris, Entretiens de Bichat L'Expansion Scientifique Francaise, 1982: 36–40.

58. Van Damme JP. A preperitoneal approach in the prosthetic repair of inguinal hernia. Int Surg 1985; 70:223.

59. Wagh PV, Read RC. Collagen deficiency in rectus sheath of patients with inguinal herniation. Proc Soc Exp Biol Med 1971;137:382.

60. Wagh PV, Read RC. Defective collagen synthesis in inguinal herniation. Am J Surg 1972;124:819.

61. Wagh PV, Read RC. Defective collagen synthesis in inguinal herniation. Rev Surg 1973;30:394.

62. Wantz GE. Testicular atrophy as a risk of inguinal hernioplasty. Surg Gynecol Obstet 1982;154:570.

63. Wantz GE. Complications of inguinal hernial repair. Surg Clin North Am 1984;64:287.

64. Wantz GE. L'atrophie testiculaire, un risque de la hernioplastie inguinale. Chirurgie (Mém. de l'Académie de Chirurgie) 1991;117:645.

65. Wantz GE. Giant reinforcement of the visceral sac. Surg Gynecol Obstet 1989;169:408.

66. Wantz GE. Atlas of hernia surgery. New York, Raven Press, 1991:102.

67. Warlaumont C. Les hernies de l'aine: place des prothèses en tulle de Dacron dans leur traitement (a propos de 1236 hernies opérées). Thèse Méd Amiens, no. 127, 1982.

68. Zagdoun J, Sordinas A. L'utilisation des plaques de nylon dans la chirurgie des hernies inguinales. Mém Acad Chir 1959;85:747.

Editor's Comment

New concepts are rare in hernial surgery. The concepts presented by Stoppa represent a bold extension of the preperitoneal approach to ventral abdominal and groin hernias, both primary and secondary. The application of Pascal's hydrostatic principle, allowing placement of large sheets of prosthetic material without the necessity for sutures, must be considered revolutionary. Wantz (see Special Comment) confirms the use and effectiveness of this technique.

The reader should carefully review the discussion of the types of prosthetic material used and the pros and cons of their use. Although my colleagues and I are wed to polypropylene mesh, I know that other materials are satisfactory.

L.M.N.

Special Comment

Personal Experience With the Stoppa Technique
George E. Wantz

René E. Stoppa's operation—the operation he calls giant prosthetic reinforcement of the visceral sac (GPRVS)*—is the solution to the difficult problem of recurrent and re-recurrent inguinal herniations and selected other hernias of the groin at high risk for recurrence. Conceptually, it is correct. Recurrences are inconceivable. Personal experiences with it are gratifying.[3]

I gave up the Shouldice repair of re-recurrent inguinal hernias when an analysis of my personal experience revealed an unacceptably high recurrence rate, averaging 13.25%, and instead adopted the posterior approach to this truly difficult problem.[6]

The preperitoneal access of Nyhus and colleagues[1] was chosen, and the repair was reinforced with a triangular piece of polypropylene mesh sutured in place as described by Read[2] (Fig. 10-18A). This approach has important advantages. It reduces the chances of testicular atrophy by avoiding redissection of the spermatic cord; it provides an unexcelled

---

*La grande prothese de renforcement du sac visceral.

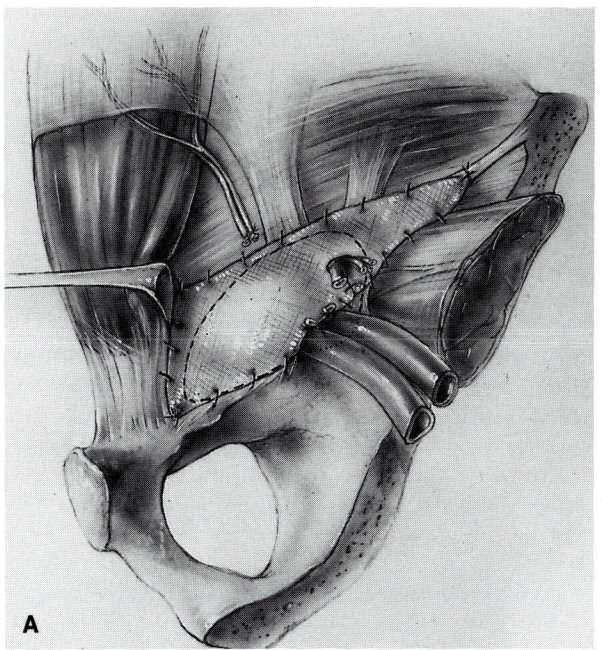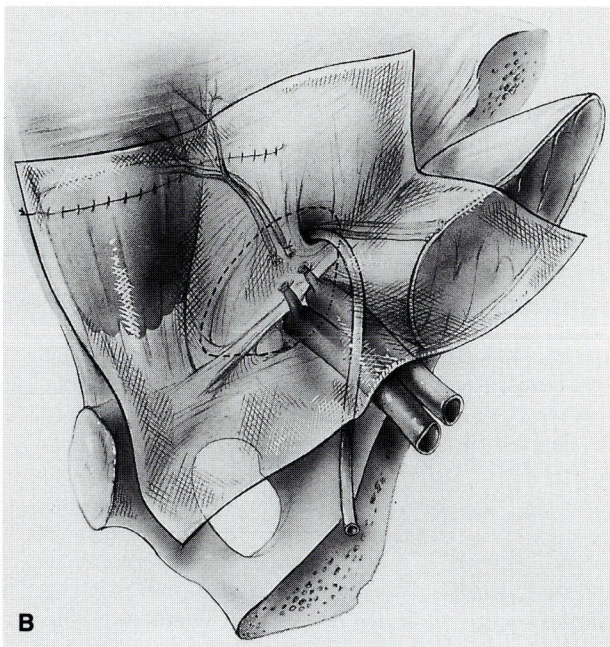

Figure 10-18.   Patch preperitoneal hernioplasty (*A*) is contrasted with unilateral giant prosthetic reinforcement of the visceral sac (GPRVS) (*B*). With patch prosthetic repair, hernias recur through the unrepaired portion of the myopectineal orifice and at the borders of the prosthetic suture attachment. With GPRVS, recurrent herniation is difficult to conceive. (Wantz GE. Atlas of hernia surgery. New York, Raven Press, 1991:105)

view of the wall of the posterior inguinal canal; it is the ideal site for the prosthesis; and the repair can still be done with local anesthesia.

Sixty-eight operations for re-recurrent inguinal herniations were performed. There were five recurrences, for a rate of 7.4%. Although this rate is the same as reported by Read in his patients with mesh, it was again discouragingly high when it became evident. The recurrences were at the sutured edge of the mesh and were of the following types: two indirect, one femoral, and two through the oblique muscles lateral and superior to the mesh. They would not have occurred had the mesh been larger.[5]

At about the time the disappointing results became known, I became aware of Dr. Stoppa's operation, and a patient coincidentally sought my help who was a perfect candidate for it. The patient, with multiple recurrences, had Ehlers-Danlos syndrome and was cured by the operation. No other operation would have worked in this patient in whom sutures would not hold. I became an immediate enthusiast for the Stoppa operation.

Early in my experience with GPRVS, I used knitted polypropylene mesh and even Gore-Tex, which are synthetic prosthetic soft tissue materials favored by American surgeons. I had no experience with Mer-

silene and failed to appreciate the importance this mesh plays in the success of GPRVS.[5]

Mersilene is the preferred prosthesis for GPRVS. It is a knitted, lace-like, supple mesh composed of loosely braided fine fibers of pure uncoated Dacron (polyester). It has a texture that grips the tissue and prevents slippage. Fibroblastic infiltration is fast and does not cause the mesh to crinkle or curl at the edges. Buckling when bent in two directions at once is minimal. Consequently, the Mersilene is able to conform readily without distortion to the complex curvatures of the pelvis. Contrary to the fears of many surgeons, Mersilene is tolerant of infection. Surgeons distrustful of Dacron forget the enormous success of Dacron aortic prostheses.

To date, 121 of Stoppa's bilateral GPRVS have been successfully performed. Unfortunately, most of these patients require 1 or 2 days of hospitalization, and this fact has restricted its routine use. Its chief indication is for patients with bilateral recurrent inguinal hernias.

A reliable ambulatory surgical procedure for recurrent hernias and other hernias at high risk for recurrence was needed. The procedure developed was unilateral preperitoneal hernioplasty with a large piece of Mersilene. It evolved from my experience with Read's preperitoneal patch repair and Stoppa's preperitoneal GPRVS. By combining the operations, unilateral GPRVS was born[5,6] (see Fig. 10-18).

TECHNIQUE OF UNILATERAL GIANT PROSTHETIC REINFORCEMENT OF THE VISCERAL SAC

The preperitoneal space is accessed by a lower-quadrant transverse incision similar to that of Nyhus. The preperitoneal space is widely cleaved in all directions, and the elements of the spermatic cord are parietalized as described by Stoppa (see Fig. 10-18*B*). The inferior epigastric vessels are usually preserved. Parietal defects are not closed. When necessary, the dead space of a direct hernia sac can be minimized by withdrawing the transversalis fascia, which envelops the peritoneal sac in the abdominal wall, and suturing it to the abdominal wall. Surplus preperitoneal fat should be cleared away from the abdominal wall. Closed-suction drainage is needed if hemostasis is incomplete or dead space from a large retained indirect sac remains.

The prosthesis is arranged so that the material stretches transversely. The prosthesis is shaped somewhat like a diamond (Fig. 10-19). The width of the superior edge of the prosthesis equals the distance from the midline to the anterior superior iliac spine minus 1 cm. The vertical distance is about 14 cm. Distances of the inferolateral corner increase the mea-

sured dimensions by 2 to 4 cm. The exaggerated elongated lateral inferior corner ensures a solid prosthetic grip on the lateral visceral sac. The shape of the mesh is different from that described in the original publication.

The prosthesis is secured to the abdominal wall 2 to 3 cm above the incision by three absorbable synthetic sutures appropriately placed along the upper border of the mesh (Fig. 10-20). The inferior portion of the mesh is implanted with the aid of three long clamps, which grasp the two corners of the middle lower edge. Retracting the abdominal wall opens the properitoneal space, enabling the clamps to unfold the mesh and slide it into place: medially deep into the space of Retzius and in front of the bladder; inferiorly over the peritoneum facing the superior ramus of the pubis, the obturator foramen, and the iliac vessels; and laterally up into the iliac fossa and over the peritoneum facing the deep ring (Fig. 10-21). Wrinkling of the mesh occurs with clamp removal if the preperitoneal space is insufficiently cleaved or the prosthesis incorrectly positioned. After inspecting the position of the prosthesis and the closed-suction drain, if used, the incision is closed without tension.

RESULTS OF EXPERIENCE

Three hundred and forty patients with 358 hernias of the groin at high risk for recurrence after classic repair were treated by unilateral GPRVS. There were 16 recurrences. Mostly, the recurrences were the result of technical errors and were corrected with experience with this new procedure: two resulted (presumably) from hematomas displacing the mesh, one was an overlooked interstitial hernia near the anterior superior iliac spine, one resulted from mesh displacement due to premature disruption of a large parietal defect closed with excess tension, three were pseudo recurrences and consisted of fat only, and eight were due to errors in the shape and size of the mesh.

PREVENTION OF RECURRENCE

Because most of the recurrences were technical, it is important that the procedure be carried out correctly to avoid pitfalls. The preperitoneal space must be cleaved sufficiently to center smoothly the prosthesis over Fruchaud's myopectineal orifice. Previous preperitoneal dissection, and especially suprapubic prostate surgery, inhibits a wide cleavage. Previous preperitoneal prostate or bladder surgery may be a contraindication for unilateral GPRVS. Dissection of the space of Retzius may be difficult or impossible,

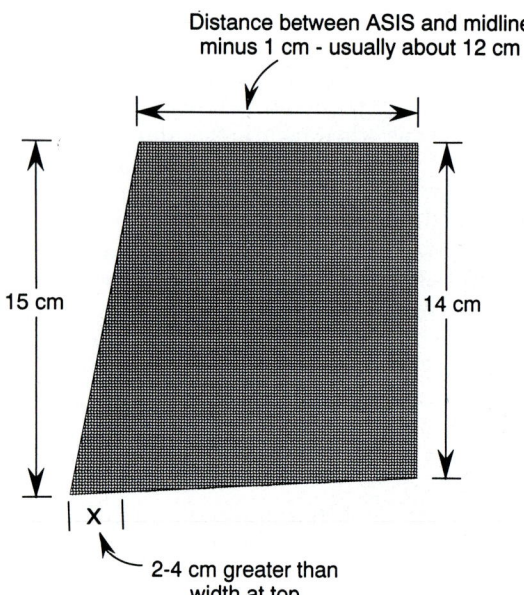

Figure 10-19. Diagram illustrating the size and shape of the permanent prosthesis.

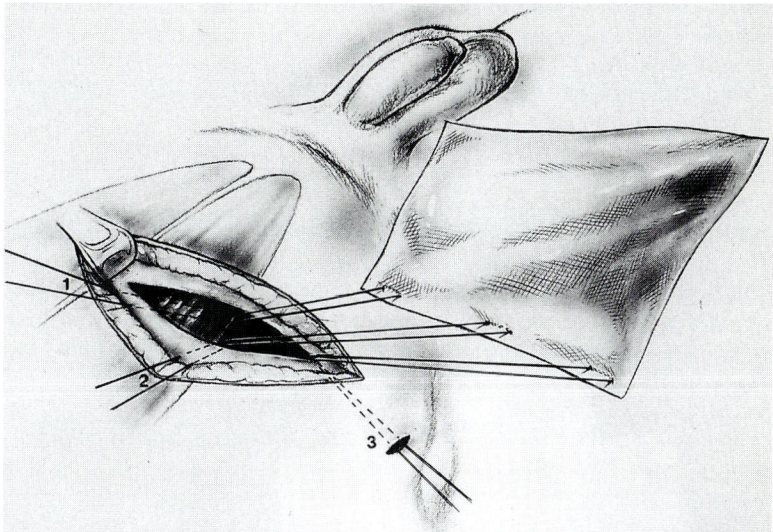

Figure 10-20. The mesh is drawn into the superior retromuscular space by three absorbable sutures. One suture attaches the mesh to the linea alba 2 to 3 cm above the incision and another at the semilunar line 2 to 3 cm above the incision; a third is placed in the oblique muscles 2 to 3 cm lateral and above the incision. (Adapted from Wantz GE. Atlas of hernia surgery. New York, Raven Press, 1991:141)

and there is a good chance of unintentionally opening the bladder.

Large parietal defects should not be closed. Invariably, there is tension that becomes excessive when the lower-quadrant access incision is closed. Also, surplus preperitoneal fat and large lipomas of the cord need excision to prevent the fat from passing in and out of small aponeurotic defects or the deep ring and mimicking a peritoneal protrusion.

Finally, the original suggested rectangular shape of the mesh may prove inadequate and is no longer recommended. Repair of the recurrence and review of pelvic anatomy revealed why this was so. The pelvic contours make the distal mesh twist and deflect medially, thereby exposing the lateral border of the myopectineal orifice and inadequately retaining the peritoneum in this region. This flaw in the original procedure was corrected by elongating the inferior

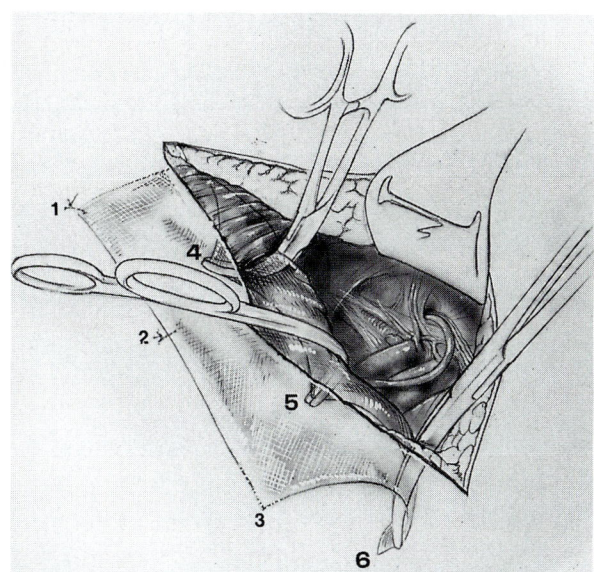

Figure 10-21. The distal portion of the mesh is slid into place with three long clamps. (Wantz GE. Atlas of hernia surgery. New York, Raven Press, 1991:148)

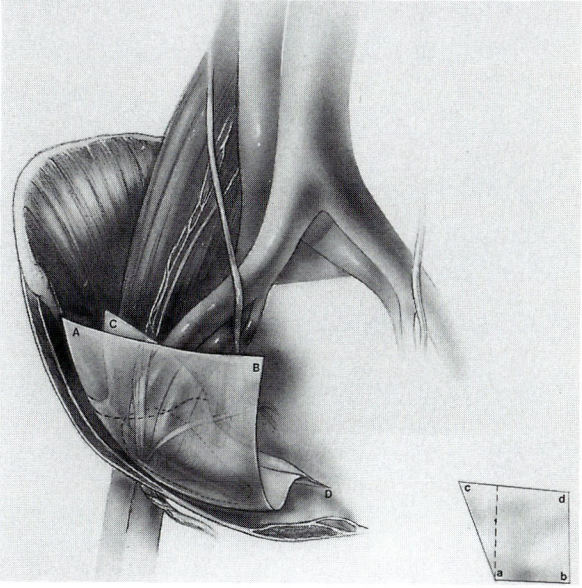

Figure 10-22. The illustration demonstrates the complex curves to which a prosthesis must conform. It also shows that the diamond-shaped prosthesis adequately covers the myopectineal orifice, whereas a rectangular prosthesis might not.

lateral corner of the mesh, which allows it to be implanted up into iliac fossa, cover adequately the myopectineal orifice, and retain visceral sac (Fig. 10-22). No recurrences have occurred since the prosthesis was enlarged and reshaped.

REFERENCES

1. Nyhus LM, Condon RE, Harkins HN. Clinical experiences with preperitoneal hernial repair for all types of hernia of the groin. Am J Surg 1960;100:234.

2. Read RC. Bilaterality and the prosthetic repair of large recurrent inguinal hernias. Am J Surg 1979;138:788.

3. Wantz GE. Personal experience with the Stoppa technique. In: Nyhus LM, Condon RE, eds. Hernia, ed 3. Philadelphia, JB Lippincott, 1989.

4. Wantz GE. The Canadian repair of inguinal hernia. In: Nyhus LM, Condon RE, eds. Hernia, ed 3. Philadelphia JB Lippincott, 1989:236–248.

5. Wantz GE. Giant prosthetic reinforcement of the visceral sac for the management of hernias of the groin at high risk for recurrence. Surg Gynecol Obstet 1989;169:408.

6. Wantz GE. Atlas of hernia surgery. New York, Raven Press, 1991.

Hernia, Fourth Edition, edited
by Lloyd M. Nyhus and Robert E. Condon.
J.B. Lippincott Company, Philadelphia © 1995.

Chapter 11

Groin Hernias: A Personal Approach

H. Brendan Devlin

THE PROBLEM

Groin hernias continue to excite the interest of health care planners, surgeons, and patients in the United Kingdom. Health care planners are most interested in the variations in the provision and outcome of hernia surgery; surgeons are more interested in the techniques available, in recurrence rates, and in short-term complications of hernia surgery; and patients are most interested in access to specialists, return to work and to full social activity, pain-free convalescence, and a well-healed wound.[28] For all three constituencies, elective groin hernia repair is a safe surgical procedure that can be performed under general, local, or regional anesthesia. All three constituencies are concerned with the variability of clinical decision making, with problems of deciding whether the benefits of surgery outweigh the benefits of conservative or nonoperative management, and with patient preferences for treatment. An estimated 40,000 trusses are sold annually in the United Kingdom, 75% of these being distributed through ordinary retail outlets rather than through hospitals.[6] These facts suggest that patients are unsure of the benefits of surgery in some cases or that there may be some problems with access to surgical care.

All categories of groin hernia can be treated easily by surgery. The clinical diagnosis of most of these hernias is simple for an experienced clinician, and elective surgery gives considerable benefits; no lump, pain, or uncomfortable sensations from the hernia; and above, all no likelihood of incarceration or strangulation. The risks of strangulation, particularly with femoral and recent indirect inguinal hernias, are considerable. In the elderly, despite emergency surgical intervention, they continue to be a cause of premature mortality.[2]

MORBIDITY

In 1990, 330 deaths were recorded in England as a result of strangulation or obstruction of groin hernias: 210 adults died as a result of complications of inguinal hernias, and 120 died from complications of femoral hernias. Ten percent of these strangulated hernias presented with no prior known history. The risks of bowel infarction, metabolic disturbance, and mortality increase if the diagnosis is delayed. Groin hernias represent 8.2% of general surgical operations in England. These patients occupy 5% of all hospital beds and account for 18% of general surgical waiting lists. In the calendar year 1989 to 1990, about 58,000 elective and emergency operations were performed in adults in National Health Service (NHS) hospitals in England. In addition, about 16,000 operations were performed privately in England and Wales. Of the operations, 92.7% were for inguinal hernias (6000 of these were primary and 3500 recurrent), and a further 5400 operations were for femoral hernias. Hernias in children accounted for a further 7000 operations, with 10% of these cases presenting as emergencies. The proportion of adult patients treated as day cases was 5.5% in 1989 to 1990.[14] This is in contradistinction to the policy in the United States whereby most cases are treated on a day-case basis. The standardized surgical waits, for instance, of England vary considerably in different districts, between 0.57 and 24 per 10,000 population for primary repairs and 0.16 and 2.3 per 10,000 population for primary femoral hernia repairs.[1] Overall, the rate of operation for groin hernia in the United Kingdom is less than half the rate in the United State (10 per 10,000 population in the United Kingdom versus 28 per 10,000 in the United States).[8]

PATIENT SELECTION

In the United Kingdom, patients come to surgeons with groin hernias after previously consulting their general practitioner or family doctor or sometimes after previously consulting a physician (internist). There is cause for concern that general practitioners do not refer all the cases they see, neither do physicians. The reluctance of colleagues to refer cases for what is straightforward surgery may be due, in part, to a perception of the overburdened workload of general surgeons and a failure to understand the benefits that can accrue from elective surgery. In a general practitioner morbidity study conducted in 1981–1982, only 42% of patients who were consulted for inguinal hernia were referred for surgical treatment in the NHS. Such misinformation about the benefits of surgery is commonplace.

SURGICAL OUTCOME

The outcome of surgery is dominated by surgical follow-up of hernia operations rather than by a purely epidemiologic process looking at the functional improvement and relief of symptoms or satisfaction to the patient. Optimal published results of surgeons indicate recurrence rates of between 1% and 2% over a 5- to 10-year period.[4] However, this is not the universal pattern of care in the United Kingdom, where many elective operations are undertaken by junior staff with varying levels of experience and quality of training and supervision. Outcomes in such circumstances are rarely studied, and the results are even more rarely published. However, 5-year recurrence rates of between 10% and 30% overall were reported. In one study of junior surgeons, 61.2% did not specify the technique of operation, and 38.8% used darns. At follow-up, 31% of these hernias recurred after 3 years, 14.3% developed a wound infection, 6.3% developed a deep sinus, 16.3% had pain, and 6.6% of patients developed testicular atrophy. Only 53% of patients were satisfied.[27] Clearly, there is room for audit and improvement of results here.

ELECTIVE HERNIA REPAIRS

One area of controversy that appears to be resolved now is whether the increasing numbers of elective hernia repairs have resulted in a fall of the number of patients presenting with complications of hernias.[25] There are two facts: (1) there has been no significant change overall in the frequency of groin hernia strangulation over a 12-year period in England, but groin hernias as a proportion of all cases of intestinal obstruction have fallen from about 50% of cases in 1932 to 20% in 1987;[10] and (2) there has been a progressive increase in the rate of elective hernia repairs, particularly for elderly men and women, which might indicate either changed clinical policy or fulfillment of a need already in the population. Whereas in 1931 the perioperative mortality rate for strangulated hernias varied from 5.95% to 13.6%, this figure remains the same, although 40% of the patients who now have

strangulations are older than 75 years of age, compared with 15% in 1931. Overall, the English national figures for all cases of mortality with strangulated inguinal or femoral hernias declined between 1975 and 1990, but there is wide variation between different parts of the country.[9] The issue that English health care planners face is how to bring consistency into the rates of diagnosis, the rates of operation, and the outcomes of hernia operations in different parts of the United Kingdom.

VARIATION OF OPERATIVE APPROACHES

Variations among different districts in England have been investigated exhaustively, and results have shown that there is little correlation between the variations of operation rates and the outcome of health care. Variations in operation rates within the NHS previously were ascribed to supply-side factors, that is, the government control over NHS expenditures; but more robust information refutes this. There are coefficients of correlation of under 0.05 in most cases when availability of funding, operating teams, and surgeons are set against operating rates. The key problem appears to be in explaining these variations in clinical practice, a similar problem to that identified by Wenneberg and Gittlesohn in the United States.[26] The lack of agreed surgical diagnostic definitions, the lack of agreed criteria for treatment, the uncertainty about operation techniques, and the lack of information on the part of practitioners about the expected outcomes of hernia surgery all contribute to this professional confusion. Epidemiologic studies show little evidence of unmet demand in the United Kingdom. There is, however, evidence that patients do not perceive hernias as a health problem and do not present for surgical treatment. Many patients who seek advice are given a truss by a general practitioner and no specific surgery. Surgeons may decline elective surgery on the grounds of comorbidity or age. Patients are bewildered by the differing modes of treatment and advice offered by different specialists. Patients often cannot understand why they stay in the hospital for 7 days under the care of one surgeon and have a day case operation under the care of another surgeon, often in the same hospital.[12] Again, patients have a bewildering choice of surgeons, and little information is given to patients about the qualities of the different surgeons, about the different techniques of operation, or about the outcome of these operations. Freedom of information is a nebulous concept in the English situation at present. The arrival on the scene of laparoscopic hernioplasty has added further to this bewilderment, particularly with the manufacturers and some surgeons pushing the exaggerated benefits of this innovation.

DETAILS OF THE SURGICAL APPROACH

From a surgical perspective, all patients should be offered surgery. With day surgery and local anesthesia so easily available, operation is almost mandatory for every case of hernia. Surgery should be offered to relieve the patient of an uncomfortable mass, to prevent strangulation, and to dispense with a truss if one is worn. This view may be modified somewhat by the elderly male patient who has a direct, broad-necked, freely reducible hernia. The risk of strangulation in these cases is extremely small, and therefore some judgment is allowed about whether to offer these patients surgery. The risk of these patients' hernias strangulating and subsequently needing emergency surgery is so remote as to be not part of the calculus of surgical decision making. The problem of making an accurate diagnosis of a direct broad-necked hernia can be solved by modern imaging, especially contrast herniography.[7]

Among surgeons in England, the options of repair techniques differ widely. A study of 240 consultant surgeons in four selected regions of England was reported in 1991. The most popular repair technique is some variant of the Maloney darn used by 83 surgeons (35%), usually using nylon suture material. A variety of suture materials are still in vogue, and some surgeons were using absorbable polymer. Pure Bassini operations, without development and suturing of the fascia transversalis, were used by 62 surgeons (26%), and layered techniques, based on the Shouldice model, account for no more than 20% of the techniques used. Archaic techniques still persist in some centers.[13] The best results reported in the United Kingdom are from centers that use Shouldice-type operations, which record recurrence rates of well under 2% at 5 years. The use of prosthetics in primary hernia repair is uncommon. General anesthesia is the preferred option for most surgeons. There is a national drive to change these habits and particularly to recommend Shouldice-type operations for primary hernia repairs; to recommend the use of monofilament, nonabsorbable sutures; to recommend day-case surgery in up to 30% of cases; and to expand the use of local anesthesia. All these principles have been embodied in the recent clinical guidelines published by the Royal College of Surgeons of England[20] and the Audit Commission[1] and the guidelines for day cases published by the Royal College of Surgeons of England.[19]

CONCEPTS OF GROIN HERNIATION

Modern concepts of groin herniation stress the laminar musculoaponeurotic structure of the groin region and the musculoaponeurotic fenestration, which allows the vessels to the genitalia or to the thigh to penetrate this structure, the concept of Fruchaud. Disruption or stretching of the fascia or parts of these laminae give rise to groin hernia. The essential goal of hernia repair is therefore to restore the functional integrity of these layers. In the groin, inguinofemoral hernias result from a breakdown of the fascia transversalis, which is the investing fascia of the deep surface of the transversalis muscle, including its aponeurotic tendon of insertion into the pubis and the posterior wall of the inguinal canal.[3,15]

A direct inguinal hernia is a weakening of the transversalis fascia in the posterior wall of the inguinal canal medial to the deep epigastric vessels (Hesselbach triangle). This type of hernia generally is acquired. Chronic cigarette smokers exhibit circulating proteoses of pulmonary origin, giving rise to increased serum elastolytic activity. This is associated with a qualitative defect in the inhibitory capacity of α_1-antitrypsin. In these patients, there are changes in the fascia transversalis lamina (the metastatic emphysema of Read) leading to direct inguinal herniation.[16]

An indirect hernia is due to a dilation of the fascia transversalis at the deep ring. Failure of closure of the processus vaginalis allows abdominal contents, omentum, and small gut to move into it. The deep ring then becomes stretched repeatedly. Inguinal hernia is due to a congenital defect. This may be exacerbated later by the raised abdominal pressure pushing abdominal contents into the sac and leading to stretching of the deep ring. A similar phenomenon as stretching can occur in patients on chronic ambulatory peritoneal dialysis, when the dialysis fluid can fill up an otherwise empty sac and stretch the deep ring.

A femoral hernia is caused by atrophy or dilation of the femoral ring. This allows the fascia transversalis, which impinges on the ring from above, to be forced into it. As the fascia transversalis stretches and traverses the femoral canal, extraperitoneal fat and peritoneum follow to give the classic thick-walled, fatty, femoral hernia sac, which is often compromised by ischemia in the tissues, and fibrosis occurs as a consequence.

Injury is an uncommon cause of hernias, although many hernias present with pain immediately after straining. Sometimes, the patient in retrospect remembers a strain that "caused" the hernia. Immediate operation in these cases does not reveal any evidence of tissue damage. Furthermore, fractured pelvises are rarely associated with any form of inguinal herniation. Other rare causes of herniation are related to osteotomies of the pubic bones or orthopedic operations on the hip. Again, these are due to distortion of the fascia transversalis by the surgery.

CONCEPTS OF REPAIR

Therefore, any concept of repair of these hernias must be firmly based on repairing or reinforcing the fascia transversalis. The fascia transversalis can be repaired by suturing, which must be done sensibly so as not to throw undue strain on one part of the fascia transversalis, causing it to disrupt further, or by replacing the fascia transversalis with a nonabsorbable mesh. Based on these two principles, two methods of hernia repair command our attention.[4] First are the suturing techniques based on the work of Bassini, refined and formalized by Shouldice—this is the repair I recommend for all primary inguinal hernias. However, I do not think it is necessary to divide completely the posterior wall of the inguinal canal in cases in which there is no stretching of the deep ring, such as in children younger than 15 years of age when a simple herniotomy will suffice or in young adults when the hernia is of recent origin and at operation there is no great stretching of the deep ring. On these occasions, division of the medial part of the deep ring and resuturing with nonabsorbable material is all that is required. Therefore, in Nyhus type I and type II hernias, a full-scale posterior wall repair is unnecessary.[15] When the deep ring is grossly dilated with displacement of the deep epigastric vessels, in a scrotal hernia and in cases of sliding hernia, particularly in hernias in which the contents are persistently in the hernia sac (Nyhus type IIIB), the principle of Shouldice, completely dividing the posterior wall of the inguinal canal, is essential. Similarly, in all direct hernias (Nyhus type IIIA), a Shouldice operation is appropriate. Suturing should be with nonabsorbable material, the suturing of bites should be small and broken in line so that there is not undue stretching on the individual fibers of the fascia transversalis, and there should be an overlap to spread the load on the fascia. The femoral canal should always be examined in these cases at operation, and if it is in any way stretched or dilated, it should be repaired from above. Simultaneous bilateral repairs of inguinal hernias are generally inadvisable except in the elderly in whom the risk of long-term recurrence is not a major factor when compared with life expectancy. Similarly, with femoral hernias, the repair of the femoral canal from above is preferable in all but the smallest hernias and the thinnest of women.

RECURRENT HERNIAS

For recurrent hernias, the extraperitoneal repair with mesh, popularized by Stoppa in France and by Nyhus and Wantz in the United States, has much to commend it. This can be done either bilaterally at one time or unilaterally using horizontal incisions about the level of the anterior superior iliac spine. To do this operation satisfactorily is difficult, particularly for the tyro, and my recommendation is that these patients have the hernia defect identified, both recumbent and standing, before operation and carefully marked out. Then, at operation, the area of the patch needed should be marked on the skin before to any incision. It is important that the Marlex patch overlap the sites of defect, the whole musculoaponeurotic fenestra, by 2 cm or more. Therefore, a double chevron bilaterally or a single parallelogram piece of Marlex should be marked on the skin and measured appropriately before any incision. The marking before operation is important because at operation the entire tissues and their dimensions are distorted by the dissection. I always fix the Marlex into place with a solitary suture to the iliopectineal ligament (Cooper ligament) to prevent its moving, particularly when the wound is being closed.

Using these methods, it is easy to obtain recurrence rates and morbidity rates similar to those published in the literature. Wound infection is the most immediate complication, and this must be avoided at all costs. With primary repairs using the Shouldice operation, careful skin handling and tissue handling with clean sharp dissection is important. The avoidance of hematomas and of any trauma to the tissues is a key to success. Wound infection rates of under 1% over large numbers of patients should be accomplished. With adequate repair of the posterior wall of the inguinal canal, recurrence rates of under 1% at 5 years are easily achievable. When placing mesh in an extraperitoneal repair, particularly of the complex recurrent hernia, it is essential to avoid tissue trauma and damage. The avoidance of sepsis is paramount, and the administration of a bolus dose of prophylactic antibiotic at the start of the operation is recommended.

ISCHEMIC ORCHITIS

Longer-term complications that must be avoided at all costs include ischemic orchitis, the cause of much litigation in the United Kingdom at present, and long-term neurologic complications from an entrapment syndrome or nerve damage.

It is not customary in the United Kingdom to warn of the risk of any surgical catastrophe that is likely to occur in under 1% of patients. With primary inguinal hernia repairs, the incidence of ischemic orchitis should be well under 1%, so no warning usually is given.[18] However, the reported 6% incidence of ischemic orchitis and a report from Israel of testicle atrophy associated with previous hernia surgery in army recruits is changing attitudes.[29] There are known risk factors, including a previous clumsy vasectomy, previous scrotal surgery, concomitant scrotal surgery, and dissection of a scrotal indirect sac, which disrupt the blood supply and collateral supply of the testicle and cord. A scrotal indirect sac should never be dissected out of the scrotum; it should be divided in the upper part of the inguinal canal, its proximal peritoneal part closed flush with the peritoneum and its distal part just left open and in situ.[5] Accurate dissection of the cord and the deep ring in the canal is important in the Shouldice operation. Such accurate dissection, resection of the cremaster muscle with preservation of the cord vasculature, reduces the risk of testicular ischemia. A young man who is still fertile and expecting to reproduce should never have bilateral repairs of hernias carried out together.

Recurrent hernias present an even greater risk of up to 5% of testicular ischemia if anterior repairs are done. This is a consequence of the difficulties of dissecting the cord and its collateral vasculature in the canal. Therefore, anterior repairs in recurrent hernias are to be avoided. Patients who have recurrent hernias repaired should be warned of the risks of testicular ischemia, and they should always be advised to have an extraperitoneal approach to the repair carried out.

The problems of persistent neurologic pains after inguinal hernia repair are rare but must be taken seriously.[24] Every year in the United States, some 400,000 inguinal hernias are repaired, and yet even the biggest series of reports of pain after inguinofemoral hernia from the United States are only of 17 or 23 cases. Therefore, this must be a remote hazard of surgery, and as such, patients should not be warned about it. If persistent pain does occur, it may be due to an entrapment syndrome with local somatic pain along the ilioinguinal, iliohypogastric, or genitofemoral nerve; these nerves can be successfully blocked with a local anesthetic, which should give pain relief. An alternative explanation of persistent pain after any incision is the deafferentation pain that occurs most commonly after thoracotomy scars. This pain is not restricted to the area of a peripheral nerve and is not altered by movement. The explanation of this pain is unknown, but it cannot be blocked by local anesthetic injections. Somatic (nociceptive) pain, which can be blocked by a local anesthetic, is often characterized by pain when the nerve is tapped, similar to the Tinel sign in regenerating nerves. The solution applied by orthopedic surgeons to such pain is repeated trauma with a hammer to tire the nerve; subsequently, the pain disappears. This usually works with ilioinguinal and iliohypogastric nerve pain. However, if the pain persists and is blocked by a local anesthetic, resection of the affected nerve may be carried out, although this should not be recommended lightly because any reexploration of the nerve may make the pain worse or add other hazards to the previous surgery.

In summary, within the United Kingdom, there is an appreciation nationally that hernias constitute a big burden for both our private health insurers and for the NHS. Our rates of operation are lower than elsewhere in the developing world. We have in the NHS a problem with waiting lists, which, when analyzed in detail, really consist of an excessive wait for surgery of up to 8 weeks. Rates of operation remain low, and rates of recurrence remain high. Every year, 10% of all hernias operated on in the United Kingdom require a second operation, and this course of treatment is clearly uneconomical. We have many surgeons operating on inguinal hernias, and the possibility of confining these cases to specialist units is being considered. The success of American freestanding hernia centers and day centers is so blatantly apparent that, even in the bureaucratized Merry Olde England, the message is getting across.

REFERENCES

1. Audit Commission for Local Authorities and the National Health Service. A short cut to better services: day surgery in England and Wales. London, HMSO, 1990.
2. Campling EA, Devlin HB, Hoile RW, Lunn J. Report of the National Confidential Enquiry Into Perioperative Deaths: 1991–1992. London, 1993.
3. Devlin HB. The management of abdominal hernias. London, Butterworths, 1988.
4. Devlin HB. Groin hernias. Surgery 1993;114:385.
5. Fong Y, Wantz G. Prevention of ischaemic orchitis during inguinal hernioplasty. Surg Gynecol Obstet 1992;174:399.
6. Goldman M. Trusses. Br Med J 1991;302:238.
7. Gullmo A, Broome A, Snedburg S. Herniography. Surg Clin North Am 1984;64:229.
8. Ham C. Research report. Health care variations: assessing the evidence. London, The King's Fund Institute, 1988.
9. Holland WW. European community atlas of avoidable deaths. Oxford, Oxford University Press, 1991.
10. McEntee G, Pender D. Current spectrum of intestinal obstruction. Br J Surg 1987;74:976.
11. Morbidity statistics from general practice: third na-

tional study. Royal College of General Practitioners and Office of Population, Census and Surveys: 1981–1982. London, HMSO, 1986.

12. Morgan M, Paul E, Devlin HB. Lengths of stay for three common surgical procedures: variations between districts. Br J Surg 1987;74:884.

13. Morgan M, Reynolds A, Swan AV, Beech R, Devlin HB. Are current techniques of inguinal hernia repair optimal? A survey in the United Kingdom. Ann R Coll Surg Engl 1991;73:341.

14. Mortality statistics: Office of Population Census and Surveys. London, HMSO, 1991.

15. Nyhus LM. Iliopubic tract repair of inguinal and femoral hernia: the posterior (preperitoneal) approach. Surg Clin North Am 1993;73:487.

16. Peacock EE, Madden JW. Studies on the biology and treatment of recurrent inguinal hernia: II. Morphological changes. Ann Surg 1974;179:567.

17. Read RC. Attenuation of the rectus sheath in inguinal herniation. Am J Surg 1970;120:610.

18. Reid I, Devlin HB. Testicular atrophy as a consequence of inguinal hernia repair. Br J Surg 1994; 81:91.

19. Royal College of Surgeons of England. Commission on the provision of surgical services: guidelines for day case surgery. London, RCS, 1992.

20. Royal College of Surgeons of England. Clinical guidelines on the management of groin hernia in adults. London, RCS, 1993.

21. Stoppa R, Warlaumont CR, Verhaeghe PJ, Odimba BKFE, Henry X. Comment, pourquoi, quand utiliser les prostheses de tulle de Dacron pour traiter les hernies et les eventrations. Chirurgie 1982;108:570.

22. Tons Ch, Kupczyk-Joeris D, Pleye J, Rotzscher VM, Schumpelick V. Cremasterresektion bei Shouldicereparation. Eine Prospektiv Kontrollierte Bicenter-Studie. Chirurg 1990;61:109.

23. Wantz G. Atlas of hernia surgery. New York, Raven Press, 1991.

24. Wantz G. Testicular atrophy and chronic residual neuralgia as risks of inguinal hernioplasty. Surg Clin North Am 1993;73:571.

25. Watkins D. Which adult patients should be operated upon electively for groin hernia and with what urgency? Ann Roy Coll Surg Engl (in press).

26. Wenneberg JE, Gittlesohn A. Variation in medical health care delivery. Science 1982;182:1102.

27. Williams MH (unpublished, 1992). See: Corson RJ. Management of groin hernias in adults. Bull Roy Coll Surg Engl 1993;125.

28. Williams M, Frankel S, Nanchahal K, Coast J, Donovan J. Epidemiologically based needs assessment: report 13. Hernia repair. NHS Management Executive. London, HMSO, 1992.

29. Yavetz H, Harash B, Yogev L, Homonnai ZT, Paz G. Fertility of men following inguinal hernia repair. Andrologia 1991;23:443.

Editor's Comment

Devlin leads the United Kingdom in concern over quality care considerations. During the spring of 1993, we spent two work-filled days at the Royal College of Surgeons (London) discussing matters of importance in the care of the patient suffering from various types of hernia.

The brief discussion of femoral hernia and its causes deserves comment. Devlin suggests that transversalis fascia leads the preperitoneal fat and peritoneum through the femoral ring into the upper thigh. Actually, the posterior inguinal wall (transversalis fascia analogue) inserts into the descending ramus of the pubis as the iliopubic tract (ligamentum Condoni), thus leaving an unprotected opening—the femoral ring. Our explanation (the Monsen concept) about the causes of femoral hernia is given in Chapter 9.

I applaud Devlin for his recommendation that we use a selective approach relative to type of operation for different hernia problems. This individualization of operative approaches is further documented in chapter 8.

L.M.N.

Hernia, Fourth Edition, edited
by Lloyd M. Nyhus and Robert E. Condon.
J.B. Lippincott Company, Philadelphia © 1995.

Chapter 12

The Shouldice Repair

Robert Bendavid

The study of hernias never ceases to present a myriad of challenges. Knowledge of the anatomy (no mean task) must be succinct. The mechanics of the muscles, ligaments, and sling (the shutter of Keith) require a logical aptitude. The formation and evolution of hernias, which imply the presence of aberrant tissue physiology, must impose a preemptive attitude in the choice of treatment. Eminent authors of the past have considered it a worthy intellectual and academic endeavor to devote their life to understanding the many facets that hernias present. Some of these authors have left an indelible mark: Astley Cooper (1768–1841), Henry Marcy (1837–1924), Edoardo Bassini (1844–1924), Chester B. McVay (1911–1987). Edward Earle Shouldice (1890–1965) belongs to this pantheon. His unique fascination with the treatment of abdominal wall hernias in the 1930s culminated in 1945 in the establishment of a hospital where more than 215,000 operations have been performed to date, providing a wealth of anatomic, clinical, and statistical observations.

HISTORICAL SYNOPSIS

An interesting parallel often has been pointed out between the Shouldice and Bassini repairs. Wantz refers to the procedure as the Bassini-Shouldice repair. In 1887, Bassini presented a personal series of 42 patients at the Fourth Assembly of Italian Surgeons in Genoa. His textbook was published in 1889 and remained essentially unknown. It was Bassini's pupil, Attilio Catterina, who authored a superb monograph that appeared in Berlin (1933), Paris (1934), London (1934), and Madrid (1935). For some reason, publication in North America never took place. In the late 1930s, E.E. Shouldice's interest in hernias resulted in the presentation of 272 cases at the annual meeting of the Ontario Medical Association (September 1944). Modifications to his original repair were introduced and, by 1952, the operation had taken on the final character that we know today. Although similarities exist between the two procedures, so do differences, and these are appreciated best by gleaning through the improved results of many authors.

Certain steps in the operation, which are considered crucial, have been associated with eminent contributors to the field of hernia surgery. These steps are (1) resection of the cremaster (Bassini, Shouldice); (2) ligation of the indirect hernial sac (Championnier, Marcy, Bassini, Shouldice); (3) incision of the entire posterior wall of the inguinal canal (Marcy, Bassini, Shouldice); (4) reconstruction of the inguinal floor (Marcy, Bassini, Halsted, Shouldice, Condon); and (5) incorporation of the iliopubic tract of Thomson in the reconstruction of the posterior inguinal floor (Bassini, Condon, Shouldice).

GENERAL PRINCIPLES

The Shouldice operation involves the use of local anesthesia, as well as a 48- to 72-hour period of convalescence in the hospital, which is described more accurately as a period of active rehabilitation during which patients ambulate early and perform exercises as a group. Because 7500 operations are carried out yearly at the Shouldice Hospital by full-time surgeons, an extensive experience has been acquired that translates into well-founded principles and practices. These have been corroborated and confirmed by others, and merit discussion here.

Weight Control

Controversy surrounding the ideal weight of a patient has polarized surgeons. Whereas obesity is agreed on as a major factor in the recurrence of incisional hernias, the same cannot be said of groin hernias. If anything, the overweight patient seems to have a protective mechanism, as can be seen in the follow-up studies of Abrahamson, Abramson, Thomas and Barnes, DeWilt, and Wantz. Disagreement has been expressed by Pietri, Sitzman, Stoppa, Weinstein, and Zimmerman. There is no doubt, however, that surgery on a thin patient is easier, a lesser volume of local anesthesia is required, a smaller incision is needed, and ambulation takes place sooner.

Local Anesthesia

In 1900, the use of local anesthesia already had been reported by Cushing, Halsted, and Bloodgood during 200 operations, 49 of which were herniorrhaphies. The reasons, now as then, include safety in elderly patients and those whose cardiac, pulmonary, and renal function is compromised. By its nature, local anesthesia also implies a benign procedure to patients who fear general anesthesia. An added advantage is that the patient retains the ability to cooperate during surgery and can strain on request to reveal secondary hernias and allow the surgeon to assess the quality of the tissues and the repair. Table 12-1 presents the age distribution of patients undergoing the Shouldice operation.

Early Ambulation

Early resumption of normal activities is not associated with an increased incidence of hernia recurrence. This was noted initially by Herzfeld in 1938 and subsequently confirmed by Blodgett, Ryan, Iles, Palumbo, and Kingsworth. The most comforting aspect of early ambulation was the disappearance of deep-vein thrombophlebitis and pulmonary complications in the postoperative period.

Ligation of the Hernial Sac

Ligation of the hernial sac has been well established for indirect sacs, but not for direct ones. Resection of an indirect sac is not an absolute necessity, as demonstrated by Glassow, Lichtenstein, and Welsh. It is essential, however, that the indirect sac be freed from the cord and the surrounding tissue layers deep to the internal ring (transversus aponeurosis, transversalis fascia, and posterior lamina) so that it disappears into the preperitoneal space of Bogros.

Incision of the Transversalis Fascia

Incision of the transversalis fascia is of paramount importance and was emphasized by Marcy, Bassini, and Shouldice. It allows exploration and detection of femoral, interstitial, prevesical, and smaller direct inguinal hernias. This maneuver also exposes the myoaponeurotic layers needed for an adequate repair. Incision of the transversalis fascia is not as crucial in women. In a review of 27,870 external abdominal wall hernias, Glassow reported the use of this incision in 0.2% of cases. Still, the lateral third of the floor should be incised to allow examination of the femoral ring and assessment of the integrity of the posterior wall.

Reconstruction of the Internal Ring

Reconstruction of the internal ring was the mainstay of the Marcy repair and, combined with reconstruction of the entire posterior wall, it formed the basis of the Bassini, Condon, and Shouldice repairs. Marcy used only the transversalis fascia, but this tissue is relatively weak. Therefore, the transversus myoaponeurotic arch subsequently was included for re-creation of the posterior inguinal wall.

Sliding Hernias

The various operations described for the treatment of sliding inguinal hernias have become historical footnotes. In a series of more than 3000 cases, Ryan and Welsh provided conclusive evidence that simply freeing a sac and reducing it in the preperitoneal space is adequate. They recorded 11 recurrences, only one of which was a true recurrence of the previous repair, the others being femoral and direct inguinal hernias.

Relaxing Incisions

The relaxing incision, first described in 1892 by Wölfler, is an important adjunct to all repairs. This was emphasized by Tanner in 1942 and endorsed by Read

Table 12-1. Patient Population Older Than 50 Years (of 7159 Operations in 1990)

Age Group (y)	No. of Patients	No. of Operations	Percentage (%)
50–59	1116	1369	19.1
60–69	1330	1533	21.4
70–79	603	689	9.6
80–89	124	144	2.0

and McLeod, Rutledge, Postlethwait, and Griffith. I believe fervently in using relaxing incisions if they are necessary. I have never seen a recurrence take place through what may have been identified as a relaxing incision.

Resection of the Cremaster

The longitudinal incision of the cremaster between the internal ring and the pubic crest is a crucial maneuver that ensures the detection of an indirect inguinal hernia. Overlooking such a defect is a significant technical error that has been reported by Obney and Chan to account for 37% of the recurrences identified in patients referred to the Shouldice Hospital.

Subsequent resection of the medial and lateral leaves of the cremaster exposes the posterior inguinal wall and allows accurate assessment of a direct inguinal hernia, if one is present. A peritoneal protrusion on the medial aspect of the spermatic cord always should be identified, freed, and reduced into the preperitoneal space. This practice rules out the presence of an indirect sac and removes any possibility of this protrusion becoming a lead point for a recurrence.

The Cribriform Fascia

At the upper medial end of the thigh, the fascia lata extends as a thin cribriform fascia. This fascia is incised routinely from the level of the femoral vein to the pubic crest for two reasons: (1) to allow examination of the femoral opening below the inguinal ligament, and (2) to free the lowermost fibers of the external oblique aponeurosis medially so that they may cover the medial aspect of the floor of the canal (a site that is known for its tendency to break down) during the inguinal repair. This practice results in a 2-cm lateral displacement of the superficial inguinal ring.

Stainless Steel Wire

Stainless steel wire has been a tradition, if not a trademark, of the Shouldice repair. Since it first was introduced in 1941 by Jones, it has been endorsed by both Abel and Goligher. It is an ideal material, elicits no inflammatory response, may remain in situ in case of infection, does not cause granulomas, and has a modest price. It is not a difficult suture to handle, but does require some practice.

Continuous Suture

The use of continuous rather than interrupted sutures needs no further support from the surgical literature. Wantz was able to obtain better results after converting to the use of continuous sutures. Poole demonstrated a decided improvement in bursting pressure as well as a better distribution of tension. Bartlett reported that excessively tight sutures may contribute to the development of pressure necrosis and wound dehiscence, and recommended that tissue layers be approximated gently. Jenkins estimated that the length of a suture used should be four times the length of the incision to allow for adequate give. In the Shouldice Hospital experience, the continuous suture also has sealed fascial edges better, preventing a lead point for herniation, which may occur between interrupted sutures.

Search for Multiple Hernias

The search for secondary hernias must be sedulous. Our statistics reveal that 13.5% of patients have more than one hernia. Hernias that are overlooked are a source of both early recurrence and embarrassment.

TECHNICAL ASPECTS

Sedation

All patients are given diazepam, 10 to 20 mg orally, 90 minutes before surgery and pethidine hydrochloride, 25 to 100 mg, 45 minutes before surgery.

Local Anesthesia

A solution of 1% procaine hydrochloride is used, to a maximum dose of 10 to 15 mg/kg, or about 1000 mg. Infiltration of the skin is carried out along a line joining the anterior superior iliac spine and the pubic spine. This step requires 30 to 40 mL of procaine. When the skin incision has been made, another 15 to 30 mL is infiltrated deep to the external oblique aponeurosis. After the latter is incised, the ilioinguinal, iliohypogastric, and genitofemoral nerves are identified, and each is infiltrated again with 1 mL of procaine. Some sympathetic pain fibers are present along the transversus arch deep to the transversalis fascia, and 5 mL of procaine is injected at this site. The deep inguinal ring also is given 3 to 5 mL of procaine, and the loose areolar tissue of the spermatic cord near the internal ring receives another 2 to 5 mL. If an indirect

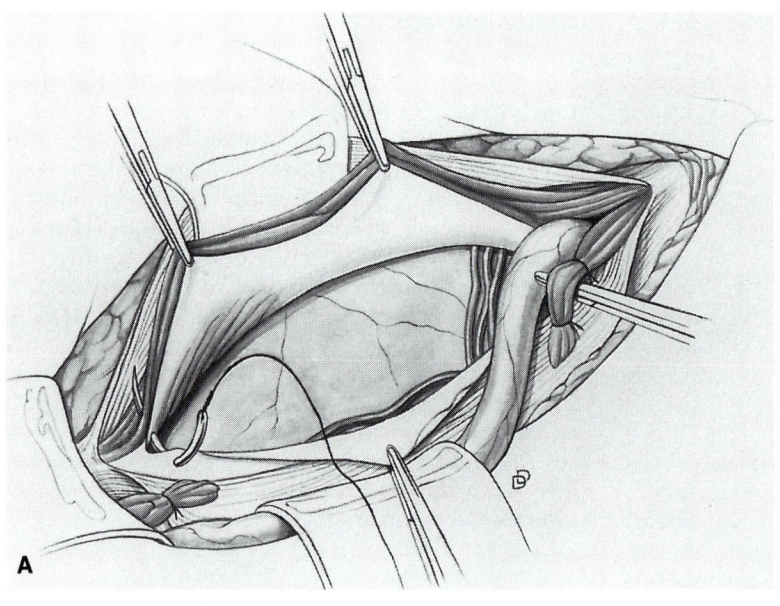

A

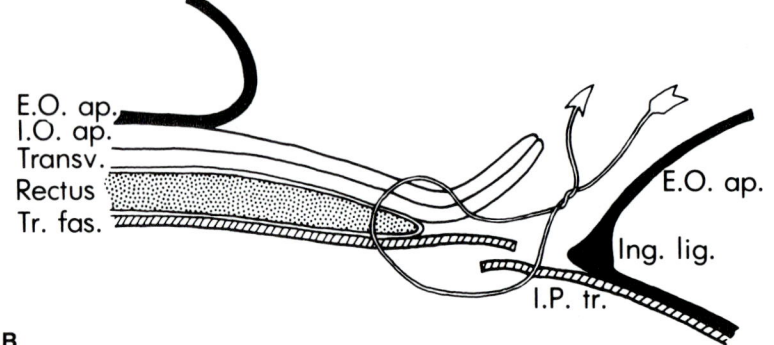

E.O. ap.
I.O. ap.
Transv.
Rectus
Tr. fas.

E.O. ap.

Ing. lig.

I.P. tr.

B

Figure 12-1. (*A*) Dissection completed. Note the cremasteric stump and iliopubic tract laterally. Medially, the first suture incorporates the transversalis fascia, lateral border of the rectus, transversus abdominis, and internal oblique. (*B*) Cross section at the site of the first suture. Laterally, the iliopubic tract (I.P. tr.) is being incorporated. Medially, the transversalis fascia (Tr. fas.), the lateral edge of the rectus, transversus abdominis (Transv.), and internal oblique are incorporated. E.O. ap., external oblique aponeurosis; Ing. lig., inguinal ligament; I.O. ap., internal oblique aponeurosis.

inguinal sac is present, a few milliliters of procaine are injected around the base of the sac as well as within it.

Dissection

The skin incision is made along a line joining the anterior superior iliac spine and the pubic crest, and should extend to the pubic crest to expose eventually the medial aspect of the posterior inguinal floor. The external oblique aponeurosis is incised along the direction of its fibers from the superficial inguinal ring to a point 2 to 3 cm lateral to the deep inguinal ring. The medial flap of the external oblique aponeurosis is freed from its underlying loose areolar adhesions, as far as the rectus sheath. Laterally, the fibers of the cremaster are freed from the underlying inguinal sulcus. The cremaster is incised along the direction of the muscular fibers from the level of the deep inguinal ring to the pubis, and is separated from the contained spermatic cord. This results in medial and

lateral muscular flaps. The lateral flap, which contains the external spermatic vessels and the genital branch of the genitofemoral nerve, is divided between two clamps, creating two stumps, a medial one near the pubis and a lateral one at the level of the internal ring. Each stump is doubly ligated with an absorbable tie. The medial flap of the cremaster near the transversus arch usually is less substantial and also is resected. If an indirect sac is present, it will become evident now and should be dissected free from the cord at the internal ring and deeper.

At this point, some surgeons resect the sac. It is essential to ascertain that the peritoneal sac is freed thoroughly of all attachments at the internal ring, so that the stump retracts deep to the plane of the deep inguinal ring.

The next step consists of incising the transversalis fascia. To accomplish this without injuring the deep inferior epigastric vessels, the transversalis fascia is picked up with a hemostat on the superomedial aspect of the internal ring. A gentle snip of the scissors will

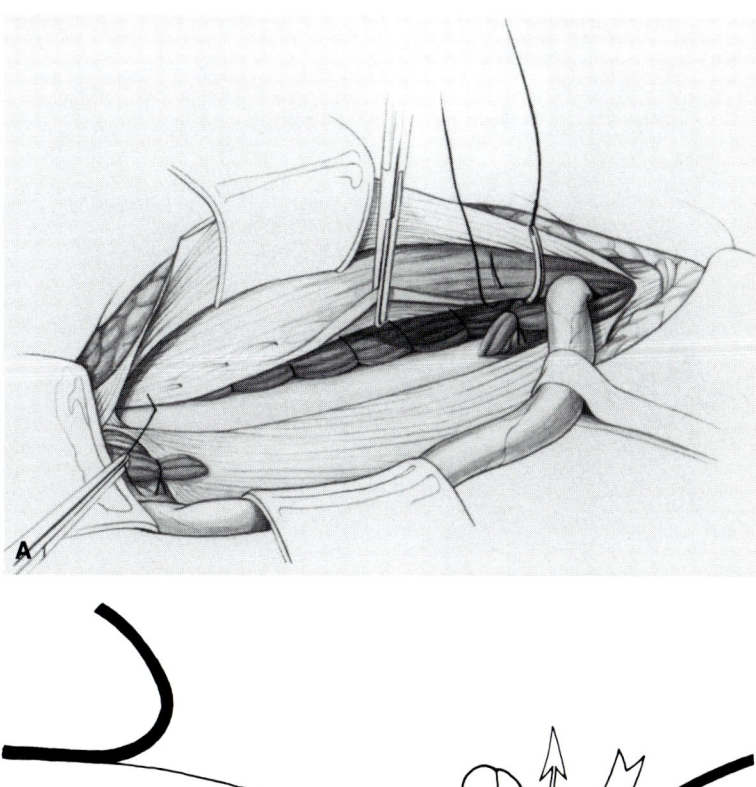

Figure 12-2. (*A*) The first line of suture has approximated the iliopubic tract laterally to the full thickness transversus arch (ie, the transversalis fascia, transversus abdominis, and internal oblique). The cremasteric stump laterally is also carried deep to the transversus arch before the first line of suture reverses to become the second line. (*B*) Cross section at the level of the internal ring when the first line is being inserted. Note that the lateral edge of the rectus no longer is incorporated because it has become too medial and too distant.

reveal a yellowish, diaphanous layer; this posterior lamina is incised and reveals the glistening, yellow preperitoneal fat situated in the space of Bogros. The incision is extended inferomedially to the level of the pubis. Medial to the longitudinal incision, the preperitoneal fat is separated from the posterior aspect of the myoaponeurotic transversus arch. Laterally, the preperitoneal fat also is separated from the posterior aspect of the transversalis fascia. More laterally, the transversalis fascia can be seen to thicken and dip posteriorly as the iliopubic tract or bandelette of Thomson.

At this stage, the cribriform fascia of the thigh is incised below the inguinal ligament, from the level of the femoral vein to the pubis. It then is possible to examine the femoral ring from above the inguinal ligament and the femoral orifice from below. A fat pad lying in the femoral fossa should not be disturbed because this may set the stage for a femoral hernia.

Deep to the iliopubic tract, the iliopubic vein, which sometimes is paired, is identified and avoided carefully because it may be the source of bleeding and hematoma.

The dissection is terminated and the internal oblique, transversus abdominis, and transversalis fascia can be identified medially, with the lateral border of the rectus in a deeper and more medial plane. Laterally, the iliopubic tract can be seen free, leading to the cremasteric stump.

Reconstruction of the Inguinal Region

The floor of the inguinal canal is reconstructed using stainless steel wire (gauge 32 or 34). Two strands of wire are required, each of which will provide two lines. The first strand approaches the lateral aspect of the iliopubic tract near the pubis, without ever includ-

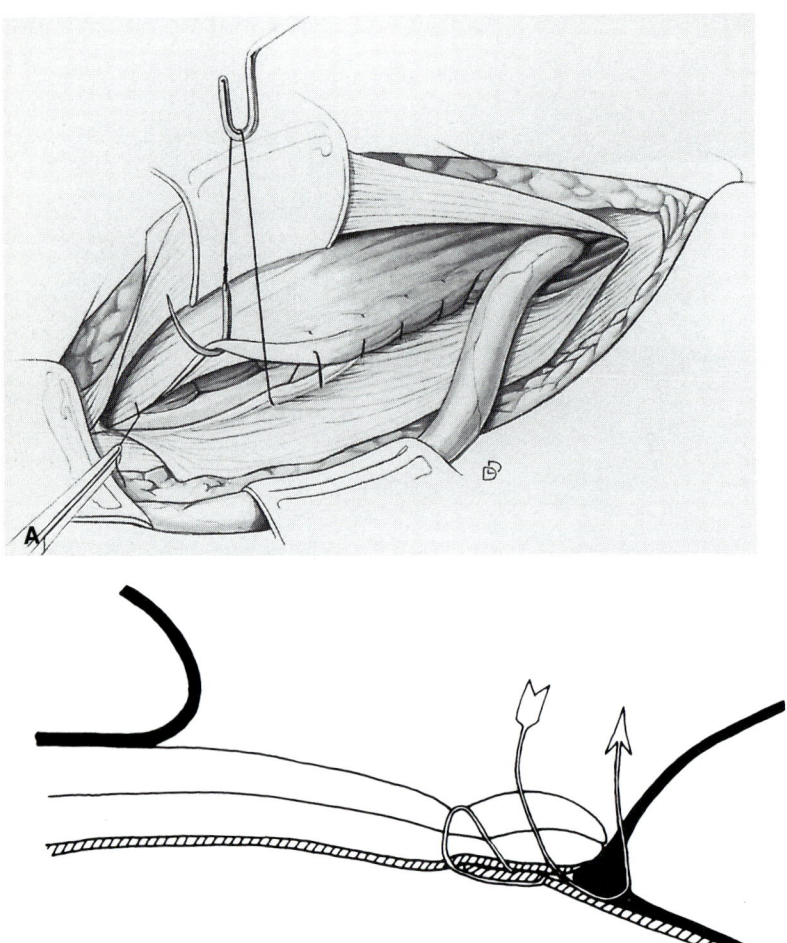

Figure 12-3. (*A*) The second line of suture, approximating the free border of the transversus arch to the inguinal ligament. A knot is tied at the level of the pubic crest. (*B*) Cross section showing the second line, which now incorporates the inguinal ligament and causes the free border of the transversus arch to abut against the inguinal ligament, thus filling the inguinal sulcus.

ing the periosteum, and crosses over to the full-thickness abdominal wall (Fig. 12-1). This wall consists of the transversalis fascia, the lateral edge of the rectus, the transversus abdominis, and the internal oblique. A knot is tied and the longer wire becomes the continuous suture that will form the first line. This suture line is continued toward the deep ring, picking up alternately the iliopubic tract laterally and the full-thickness transversus arch medially, leaving a free edge to this arch. Halfway between the pubis and the deep inguinal ring, the edge of the rectus becomes too distant and is abandoned. Near the internal ring, this first suture line incorporates the cremaster stump and carries it across to form a new deep inguinal ring (Fig. 12-2). The suture now reverses itself, as the second line, and advances toward the pubic crest. To do this, it picks up the free edge of the transversus arch, approximating it to the inguinal ligament all the way to the pubic crest. Near the latter, the two ends of the wire are tied (Fig. 12-3).

The next strand of wire will become the third and fourth lines. The third line begins near the internal ring, goes through the internal oblique and transversus abdominis medially, then crosses to the inner aspect of the external oblique aponeurosis, creating an artificial inguinal ligament adjacent to the true one (Fig. 12-4). This line continues to the pubic crest before reversing itself as the fourth line toward the internal ring (Fig. 12-5). Near the pubic crest, the medial 2 cm of the external flap of the external oblique aponeurosis is used to cover the medial end of the floor of the canal before proceeding along yet another artificial inguinal ligament superficial to the previous one. At the internal ring, the two ends of the wires are tied. Each suture line, as it is added on, serves the purpose of reducing tension on the previous one.

The spermatic cord is replaced in its usual anatomic bed and the external oblique aponeurosis is reapproximated with an absorbable suture. The medial cremasteric stump is anchored near the pubis to

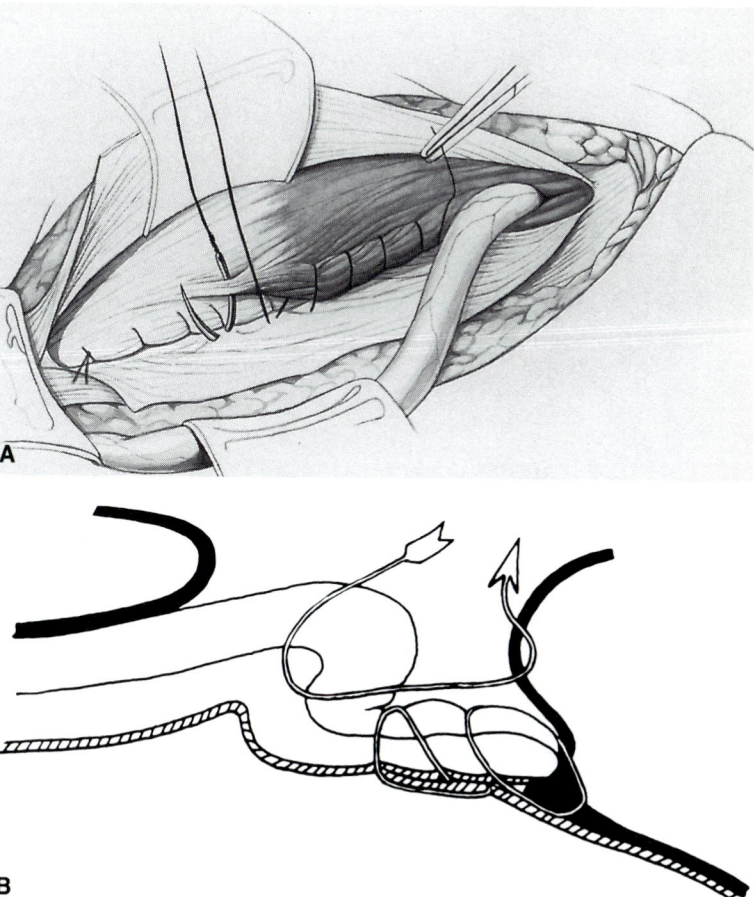

Figure 12-4. (*A*) The third line of suture begins near the internal ring and advances toward the pubic crest, approximating the internal oblique and the deeper transversus to the external oblique aponeurosis along a line parallel to the inguinal ligament. (*B*) Cross section of the third line. The suture approximates the transversus and internal oblique medially and the external oblique aponeurosis laterally. Gentle traction eliminates the dead space in between.

prevent a low-lying testicle, which could become excessively pendulous with time.

The subcutaneous tissues are approximated with fine, absorbable sutures and the skin edges are approximated with Michel clips. Half these clips are removed in 24 hours and the remainder in 48 hours. When surgery is terminated, the patient stands away from the table and walks to the recovery room.

POSTOPERATIVE PERIOD

Patients are allowed to remain in bed for 4 hours to allow the effect of preoperative drugs to dissipate. At that point, ambulation is encouraged. The first meal after surgery is brought to the hospital room, but all subsequent meals are eaten in a cafeteria. Patients are brought together daily for a session of light physical exercises. Discharge from the hospital takes place 48 to 72 hours after surgery.

RESULTS

More than 215,000 Shouldice operations have been performed. The rate of recurrence depends on the length of follow-up (Table 12-2). After a short follow-up period, recurrence may be less than 1%. In a group of patients from 1955 who were followed up for 35 years, however, the rate of recurrence was 1.46% (Table 12-3). These results have been duplicated, supporting the efficacy of this operation (Table 12-4).

Many of the patients referred to the Shouldice Hospital have recurrent groin hernias. The number varies from 900 to 1300 cases per year and amounts to 12% to 16% of the yearly total. For most patients, a standard Shouldice herniorrhaphy is adequate. Our statistics before 1983, however, reveal an average global repeated recurrence rate of 2.3% for the first recurrent hernia and 11.4% for the third through the sixth recurrent hernias. These high recurrence rates are the result of extensive tissue destruction and the

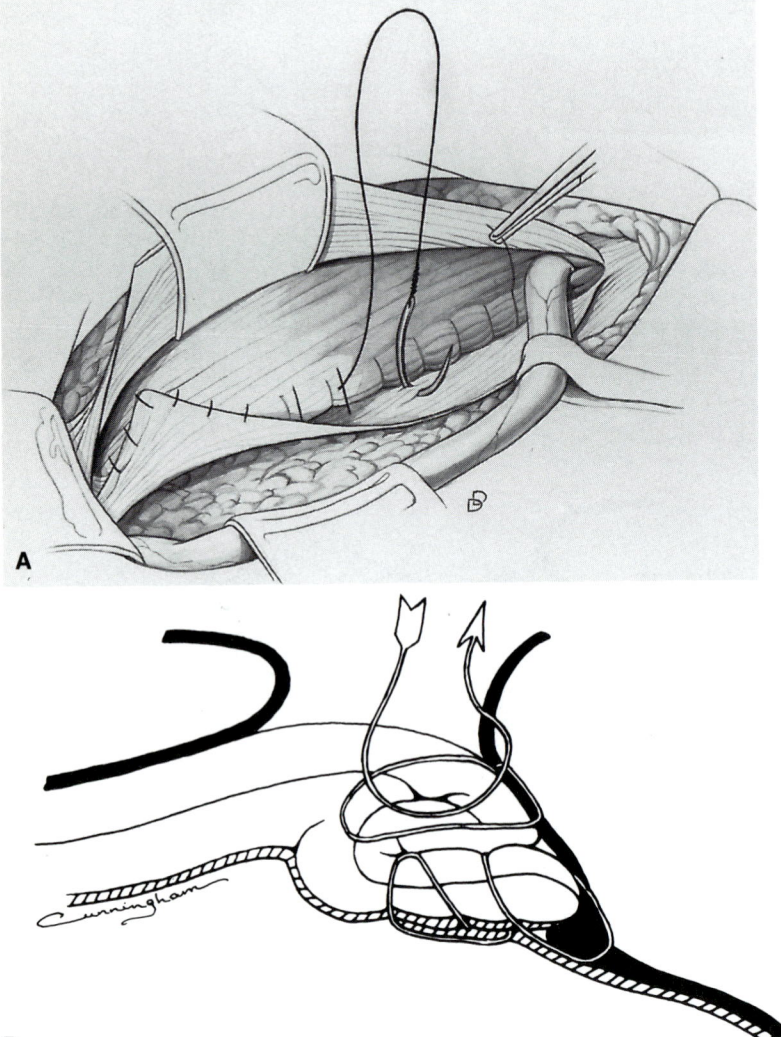

A

B

Figure 12-5. (*A*) Fourth line showing apposition of the medial 2 cm of the external oblique aponeurosis on the medial portion of the inguinal floor and continuing laterally along a line parallel to the inguinal ligament. The two suture ends are tied at the level of the internal ring. (*B*) Cross section with the fourth line in place showing the superimposition of two myoaponeurotic layers forming the new inguinal floor and sulcus.

absence of an intact inguinal ligament. Such cases now are treated by the insertion of prosthetic mesh, which produces better results and is associated with a recurrence rate of 2.2%.

COMPLICATIONS

The combination of local anesthesia, a short hospital stay, and a simple but effective herniorrhaphy through an anterior approach has created the belief that hernias are a minor surgical problem. This is true in most cases, and is supported further by the fact that complications are few and rarely life-threatening (Table 12-5).

Testicular Atrophy

Benign testicular and scrotal swelling is common after inguinal herniorrhaphy. Testicular atrophy can occur, however, and usually is characterized by a firm,

Table 12-2. Recurrences: Their Timing

Years	No. of Patients	Percentage
0–4	27	65.8
5–8	7	17.1
9–13	7	17.1

Table 12-3. 35-Year Follow-up of 2748 Repairs on 2270 Patients Operated on in 1955 (Recurrence Rate, 1.46%)

Year	No. of Recurrences Discovered	Percentage Follow-up	Cumulative Total
1955	3	—	3
1956	4	95.6	7
1957	1	92.4	8
1958	3	88.9	11
1959	3	84.8	14
1960	2	81.0	16
1965	8	—	24
1975	7	—	31
1990	9	—	40

woody, enlarged testicle 2 to 3 times its normal size, associated with severe pain and a low-grade fever. This complication arises within 24 to 48 hours. The pain resolves in 3 to 6 weeks, but the atrophy may be present for months. The manifestations of testicular atrophy vary; atrophy has been documented with no associated pain or swelling. In some cases, what appears to be threatening testicular atrophy resolves with no adverse sequelae. Atrophy never should be predicted until a year has elapsed. The Shouldice Hospital reports the incidence of testicular atrophy to be about 0.1% after repair of a primary inguinal hernia and 0.9% after repair of recurrent inguinal hernias.

Hematomas

Hematomas are found in the preperitoneal or subcutaneous space. Preperitoneal hematomas are rare: only two have occurred in the last 15 years. Subcutaneous hematomas have been noted in 0.3% of 5762

patients. They are a minor complication and should be treated with evacuation and a careful search for the source of bleeding.

Infections

The rate of wound infection after surgery at the Shouldice Hospital has always been low (< 1%) because we avoid contamination. Any patient known to harbor an infection (eg, cutaneous, pulmonary, draining sinus) is not admitted to the hospital until antibiotic treatment has been administered. This practice effectively limits the incidence of nosocomial infection.

Dysejaculation

Dysejaculation is a syndrome characterized by severe burning and pain on ejaculation. Its incidence is probably 0.25%. Seventeen cases were reported in April 1993 and another 6 cases have been identified since then. Most patients improve without active treatment, although symptoms may persist for as long as 5 years.

Hydrocele

Hydrocele is seen occasionally after herniorrhaphy; Obney reported an incidence of 0.7% after 14,442 hernia operations. He also pointed out that lipomas around the spermatic cord should be dissected cleanly and resected, ligatures about the cord should be kept to a minimum, and both deep and superficial inguinal rings should not be too snug.

Table 12-4. Recurrence Rate After the Shouldice Operation for Primary Inguinal Hernias, as Reported by Various Authors

Author	No. of Cases	Percentage Follow-up	Years Follow-up	Recurrence (%)
Shearburn	550	100	13	0.2
Volpe	415	50	3	0.2
Wantz[1]	2087	—	5	0.3
Bocchi	1640	84	5	0.6
Myers	953	100	18	0.7
Devlin	350	—	6	0.8
Flament	134	—	6	0.9
Wantz[2]	3454	—	1–20	1.0
Moran	121	—	6	2.0
Berlin	591	—	2–5	2.7

Table 12-5. Summary of Postoperative Complications

Complication	Affected Patients
Infection	1.0%
Hematoma	0.3%
Hydrocele	0.7%
Dysejaculation	0.25%
Recurrence	1.46%
Phlebitis	Practically nonexistent as a result of early ambulation and exercise
Atelectasis	
Pneumonitis	
Pulmonary embolism	
Cerebrovascular accident	5 patients
Coronary thrombosis	12 patients
Intestinal obstruction	4 patients
Acute mesenteric thrombosis	1 patient
Perforated duodenal ulcer	1 patient
Spontaneous rupture of gallbladder	1 patient
Pancreatitis	1 patient
Death	20 patients (0.009%)

Mortality

Since 1945, 20 patients have died within 30 days of surgery. This represents a mortality rate of 0.009%. The diagnosis clinically or at autopsy was myocardial infarction in 15 patients (average age, 70 years; range, 56 to 85 years), cerebrovascular accident in 1 patient (age 66 years), and undetermined in 4 patients (ages 56, 66, 70, and 78 years).

CONCLUSION

No doubt exists in any surgeon's mind that a well-executed primary herniorrhaphy will yield excellent results. Good technique does not mean legerdemain, but a good understanding of the anatomy and the procedure. The Shouldice repair lends itself to easy execution with confirmed good results, but above all, to near perfection in terms of safety.

SELECTED READING LIST

Abel AL, Hunt AU. Stainless steel wire for closing abdominal incisions and for the repair of hernias. BMJ 1948;2:379.

Bartlett LC. Pressure necrosis is the primary cause of wound dehiscence. Can J Surg 1985;28:27.

Bendavid R. The Shouldice method of inguinal herniorrhaphy. In: Nyhus LM, Baker RJ, eds. Mastery of surgery, ed 2. Boston, Little, Brown & Company, 1992:1584.

Blodgett JB, Beattie EJ. The effect of postoperative rising on the recurrence rate of hernia. Surg Gynecol Obstet 1947;84:716.

Bocchi P. Bassini, the man, the soldier, the surgeon. Postgraduate General Surgery 1992;4:175.

Cushing H. The employment of local anaesthesia in the radical cure of certain cases of hernia, with a note upon the nervous anatomy of the inguinal region. Ann Surg 1900;31:1.

Glassow F. Inguinal hernia in the female. Surg Gynecol Obstet 1963;116:701.

Glassow F. High ligation of the sac in indirect inguinal hernia. Am J Surg 1965;109:460.

Goligher JC, Irvin TT, Johnston D, de Dombal FT, Hill GI, Horrocks JC. A controlled clinical trial of three methods of closure of laparotomy wounds. BMJ 1975;62:823.

Griffith CA. The Marcy repair of indirect inguinal hernia: 1870 to the present. In: Nyhus LM, Condon RE, eds. Hernia, ed 3. Philadelphia, JB Lippincott, 1989:106–118.

Herzfeld G. Hernia in infancy. Am J Surg 1938;39:422.

Iles JDH. Specialisation in elective herniorrhaphy. Lancet 1964;1:751.

Iles JDH. Convalescence after herniorrhaphy. JAMA 1972;219:385.

Jenkins TPN. Incisional hernia repair: a mechanical approach. Br J Surg 1980;67:335.

Jones TE, Newell ET, Brubaker RE. The use of alloy steel wire in the closure of abdominal wounds. Surg Gynecol Obstet 1941;72:1056.

Kingsworth AN, Britton BJ, Morris PJ. Recurrent inguinal hernia after local anaesthetic repair. Br J Surg 1981;68:273.

Lichtenstein IL. Herniorrhaphy. A personal experience with 6321 cases. Am J Surg 1987;153:553.

Marcy HO. The anatomy and surgical treatment of hernia. New York, D Appleton & Company, 1892:100.

Obney N. Hydrocoeles of the testicle complicating inguinal hernias. Can Med Assoc J 1956;75:733.

Obney N, Chan CK. Repair of multiple time recurrent inguinal hernias with reference to common causes of recurrence. Contemporary Surgery 1984;25:25.

Palumbo LT, Sharpe WS. Primary inguinal hernioplasty in the adult. Surg Clin North Am 1971;51:1293.

Poole GV Jr, Meredith JW, Kon ND, Martin MB, Kawamoto EH, Myers RT. Suture techniques and wound bursting strength. Am Surg 1984;50:569.

Postlethwait RW. Recurrent inguinal hernia. Ann Surg 1985;202:777.

Read RC, McLeod PC. Influence of a relaxing incision on suture tension in Bassini's and McVay's repairs. Arch Surg 1981;116:440.

Rutledge RH. Cooper's ligament repair: a 25 year experience with a single technique for all groin hernias in adults. Surgery 1988;103:1.

Ryan EA. Recurrent hernias: an analysis of 369 consecutive cases of recurrent inguinal and femoral hernias. Surg Gynecol Obstet 1953;96:343.

Ryan EA. An analysis of 313 consecutive cases of indirect sliding inguinal hernias. Surg Gynecol Obstet 1956; 102:45.

Shouldice EE. Surgical treatment of hernia. In: Annual Meeting of Ontario Medical Association, District Number 9, September 10, 1944. 3–28.

Wantz G. The operation of Bassini as described by Attilio Catterina. Surg Gynecol Obstet 1989;168:67.

Welsh DRJ. Bilateral sliding inguinal hernias. Postgraduate General Surgery 1992;4:114.

Special Comment

The Shouldice Repair

George E. Wantz

Some aspects of the Shouldice hernioplasty merit discussion. In common with all hernioplasties, it consists of a dissection and a repair, both of which are equally important for a successful outcome. The important steps in the dissection are division of the cremaster muscle and division of the posterior wall of the inguinal canal. Only by dividing these structures can the surgeon correctly assess the innermost aponeuroticofascial layer of the abdominal wall.

Division of the cremaster muscle and posterior wall of the inguinal canal, however, are not unique to the Shouldice repair. Many surgeons at the forefront of hernia surgery have stressed their importance. They are essential components of the original Bassini hernioplasty, according to Attilio Catterina, a colleague of Bassini's who described and depicted this operation in a beautiful atlas.[3] Numerous surgeons, however, still perform the Bassini operation without dividing the cremaster muscle and the floor of the inguinal canal. Perhaps this is because Bassini did not actually describe these steps in his original papers, and because Catterina's atlas, although it was pub-

lished in many languages in the early 1930s in Europe, never was published in North America. It is possible that popular demand for the Shouldice hernioplasty played a role in surgical education.

The Shouldice Hospital repair also resembles the Bassini repair in that the same structures are approximated. In the Bassini procedure, his "triple layer" consisting of the internal oblique and transverse abdominal muscles and the transversalis fascia is sutured with interrupted sutures to the inguinal ligament and iliopubic tract. In the Shouldice hernioplasty, the same structures are approximated, but in a more refined and precise manner. Perhaps the Shouldice hernioplasty should be called the Shouldice-Bassini hernioplasty.

The classic Shouldice hernioplasty includes a to-and-fro, continuous suture uniting the internal oblique abdominal muscle and the inguinal ligament. Most surgeons, including me, do not place this suture, and consider it superfluous.

The Shouldice repair has been criticized by many. McVay claimed that the medial portion of the iliopubic tract is not a true anatomic structure and is seen only in patients with direct inguinal hernias. It is, therefore, illusional and not strong enough to ensure a long-lasting hernioplasty. The Shouldice hernioplasty, however, is not a purely anatomic transverse aponeurotic repair and does not rely solely on the iliopubic tract. That portion considered insufficient is overlapped and reinforced by healthy transverse aponeurosis, which is attached, for the most part, to the lacunar portion of the inguinal ligament, which inserts in turn onto the bony pectin.

McVay also argued that the inguinal ligament is not a suitable structure for the repair of inguinal hernias because it is movable and attached to the fascia lata by only the flimsy innominate fascia of Gallaudet. Furthermore, attaching any structure other than the aponeurosis of the external abdominal oblique muscle to the inguinal ligament is "unanatomic."

This criticism, originally directed at the Bassini hernioplasty, also applies to the Shouldice repair. Although it may be illogical and "unanatomic" for an inguinal hernioplasty to rely on the inguinal ligament, it unquestionably works. In both the Canadian hernioplasty and the authentic Bassini operation, the inguinal ligament is not the sole structure on which the seam of the hernioplasty depends, because the iliopubic tract is an integral structure in both repairs. This makes both the Shouldice and the Bassini hernioplasty anatomic, therefore, because the defect between the iliopubic tract and the transverse aponeurotic arch is closed.

The Shouldice hernioplasty has been rightly criticized because it does not address the femoral canal. Primary femoral hernias in men are rare, however, and femoral hernias in women are repaired successfully by the Bassini method from below the inguinal ligament, despite the objections of many.

Femoral hernias after Shouldice hernioplasty are uncommon, but well known. In my experience, they typically occur a few months after the primary repair. This observation has been used by critics of the procedure to justify a routine Cooper ligament repair. Whether a recurrent femoral hernia actually is an overlooked hernia or a result of the procedure itself has not been ascertained with certainty. In any case, recurrent femoral hernias are nearly unheard of after the Bassini repair, in which sutures are attached only to the inguinal ligament. This suggests that recurrent femoral hernias after a Shouldice repair are not undetected hernias, but new hernias induced by tension on the femoral sheath.

BILATERAL HERNIAS

Surgeons at the Shouldice Hospital do not repair hernias in each groin at the same time. I no longer follow this custom, and routinely correct bilateral direct inguinal hernias simultaneously with unassisted local anesthesia in day surgery as long as the first hernioplasty was easy. Patients prefer this. They tolerate ambulatory bilateral hernioplasty well and recover as quickly as do patients undergoing a single hernia repair.

I caution against the simultaneous repair of two indirect inguinal hernias, especially in men in their reproductive years. Ischemic orchitis is associated with the removal of indirect sacs from a spermatic cord. The complications can be nearly eliminated if the distal portion of an indirect hernial sac is not dissected from the cord. In this case, two indirect inguinal hernias can be repaired simultaneously. Left-sided, large indirect hernias are operated on first, because sliding hernias necessitating sac excision are most common on the left. If a hernial sac must be dissected from the cord, repair of a hernia on the opposite side should be delayed until it is certain that ischemic orchitis has not occurred.

OBESITY

Surgeons at the Shouldice Hospital do not repair hernias in obese patients and require some weight loss even in those who are only slightly overweight. This policy excludes many patients. Hernioplasty in an obese individual is difficult and usually requires general anesthesia. I no longer adhere to this attitude and do not withhold hernioplasty from a patient simply because of obesity. In addition, in my experience, obe-

sity is not an etiologic factor for inguinal hernia recurrence.

RECURRENCE

An in-depth analysis of my experience has been reported and updating that report is superfluous because it does not change the conclusions or significantly alter the percentages.[1] For the record, however, the raw recurrence rate of 5483 primary Shouldice hernia repairs followed up for 2 to 20 years is 1.6%. Recurrence rates are not the measure of a hernioplasty, and they should not be used to compare the worth of different techniques. Too many variables exist.

Nevertheless, additional data regarding recurrence are illuminating. Recurrences were placed into two categories: those attributable to the hernioplasty and those attributable to deterioration of the patient's tissues. Hernias recurring within the first year and the well-known pubic tubercle recurrences were considered the result of the hernioplasty and the others were not.

Patients operated on before 1981 were compared with those operated on thereafter because the surgical technique was modified slightly in 1981. To reduce tension on the suture line at the pubic tubercle, the first continuous suture was started by anchoring it only in the lateral aponeuroticofascial segment near the pubic tubercle, rather than beginning as an interrupted bite approximating the two aponeuroticofascial segments. It was theorized that this type of recurrence might be eliminated by this technique. In addition, relaxing incisions were used with increasing frequency and now are routine.

In the years between 1970 and 1980, a total of 1697 primary Canadian hernioplasties were performed. Forty-six (2.7%) recurred. Of these, 8 (0.5%) were at the pubic tubercle and 15 (0.9%) occurred in the first year. In the years between 1980 and 1990, 3786 primary Canadian hernioplasties were performed and 34 (0.9%) recurred. Among these recurrences, only 1 was at the pubic tubercle and 9 (0.2%) occurred in the first year.

These improved results related to experience and, possibly, attention to surgical detail are striking. The results confirm the surgical opinion that the outcome of inguinal hernioplasty depends more on the skills and experience of the surgeon than on the type of repair performed, and explains the astoundingly low recurrence rates obtained at the Shouldice Hospital.

Only 6 (0.14%) recurrences were femoral hernias, of which only 5 occurred in the femoral canal and developed within a few months of the hernioplasty. The remaining femoral hernia was prevascular and occurred 3 years after surgery. This number of femoral hernias is insignificant and does not justify routine use of the McVay Cooper ligament hernioplasty.

The unassigned recurrences (a total of 49, including the prevascular femoral hernia) occurred more than a year after the repair and were considered, rightly or wrongly, not to be the result of surgical technique. The resulting recurrence rate, 0.9%, indicates that the Shouldice repair is a superb inguinal hernioplasty, and that recurrence rates of less than 1% are theoretically possible.

The Shouldice hernia repair was used to repair 639 initially recurrent and repeatedly recurrent inguinal hernias. Forty-six (7.2%) hernias recurred. This recurrence rate is unsatisfactory and unacceptable, especially if the recurrent hernia is coupled with the complication of testicular atrophy, which may not be preventable for recurrent hernioplasty and for which the incidence always is high and unpredictable. Consequently, the preperitoneal approach with a synthetic prosthesis is preferred for nearly all patients with recurrent hernias.[2]

REFERENCES

1. Wantz GE. The Canadian repair of inguinal hernias. In: Nyhus LM, Condon RE, eds. Hernia, ed 3. Philadelphia, JB Lippincott Co, 1989:236.
2. Wantz GE. Giant prosthetic reinforcement of the visceral sac. Surg Gynecol Obstet 1989;169:408.
3. Wantz GE. The operation of Bassini as described by Attilio Catterina. Surg Gynecol Obstet 1989;168:67.

Special Comment

The Toulouse Experience With the Shouldice Hernia Repair
Franck Lazorthes

"Are the results obtained by the Shouldice surgeons the consequence of the technique itself, or are they the result of the experience and exclusive specialization of this team?" This was the question we asked in the preceding edition of this book, and the question we will attempt to answer in light of our experience with more than 2500 Shouldice hernia repairs.

LOCAL ANESTHESIA

After a short learning period, we have used local anesthesia to accomplish our hernia repairs in nearly

every case. Only rarely have we needed to convert to general anesthesia. In our opinion, recurrent hernia alone requires another type of anesthesia because the operation may be long and the position difficult for the patients to support.

Many of our patients prefer to undergo local anesthesia for primary hernia repair, and it can be used in the occasional cases in which other types of anesthesia are contraindicated. Although we tend to believe, as does Wantz,[4] that local anesthesia contributes fully to the success of this operation, we will admit that this has not been proved.

Figures 12-6 through 12-12 give an overview of the Shouldice technique.

DISSECTION

Adequate dissection is essential. Regardless of the surgical technique used, the repair will not be satisfactory unless all the structures have been identified correctly and dissected free before suturing.

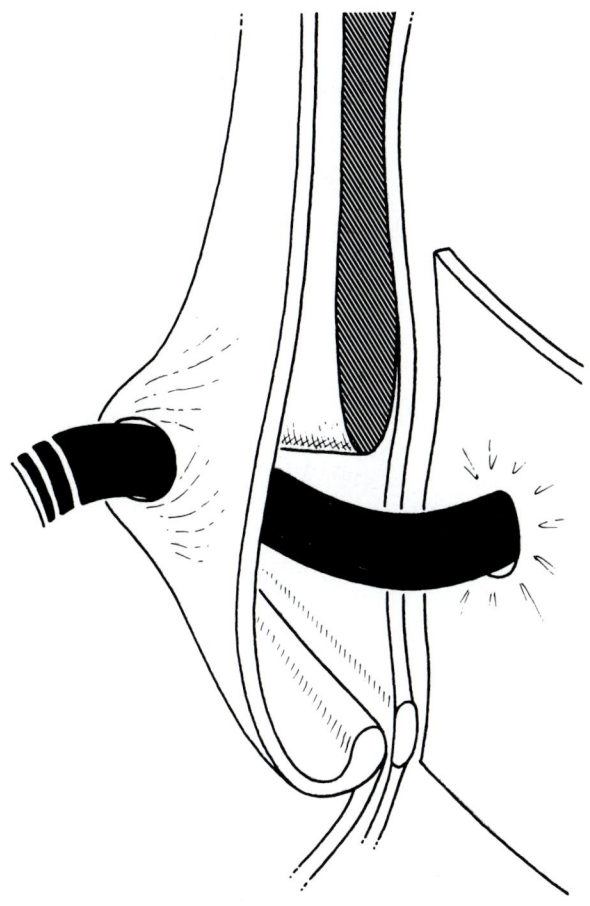

Figure 12-6. Parasagittal section, left side.

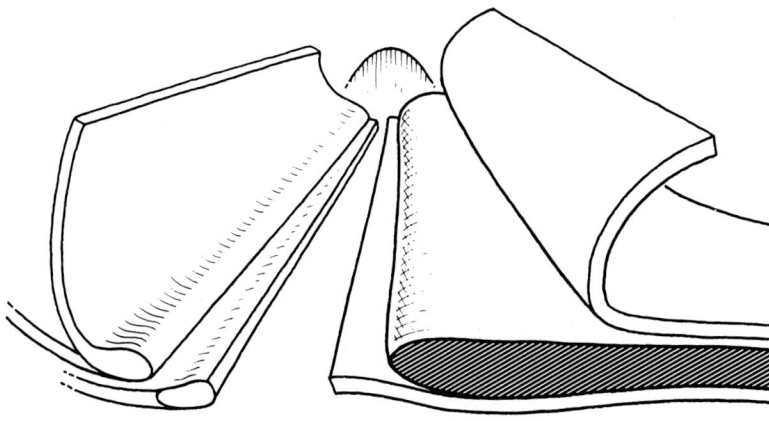

Figure 12-7.   Division of transversalis fascia.

RESECTION OF THE CREMASTERIC MUSCLE

The principal objective of resection of the cremasteric muscle fibers is to provide adequate visualization of the deeper structures that are needed for the repair. Although this objective is justified completely, it is not necessary to resect the entire muscle. Adequate exposure may be obtained simply by dividing the perimeter of the cremasteric muscle at its origin on the internal oblique muscle without resecting it. This circular division resembles the division that will be made later on, more deeply, on the prolongation of the transversalis fascia on the spermatic cord.

INCISION IN THE TRANSVERSALIS FASCIA

The incision in the transversalis fascia usually is made from the medial aspect of the internal ring to the pubic tubercle. We prefer to incise the fascia starting from the lower edge of the internal ring. Before making this incision, however, the lower flap of the cremasteric muscle, which later will help to calibrate the size of the internal ring, is dissected up to its origin at the level of the internal oblique and freed from the Poupart arch for several millimeters. For correct visualization of this area, the flap can be raised up after a stitch has been passed through it with the suture material that will be used later on. The transversalis fascia then is opened at the lower edge of the internal ring between the low iliopubic tract, which remains clearly visible at this level, and the high transversalis fascia reflection of the spermatic cord. This incision is prolonged along the upper edge of the iliopubic tract to the pubic tubercle. At this level, the inferior epigastric vessels may be cleaved easily. This procedure is especially useful in direct hernia because it separates the iliopubic tract, which is resistant, from the fascia, which is weakened by the hernia.

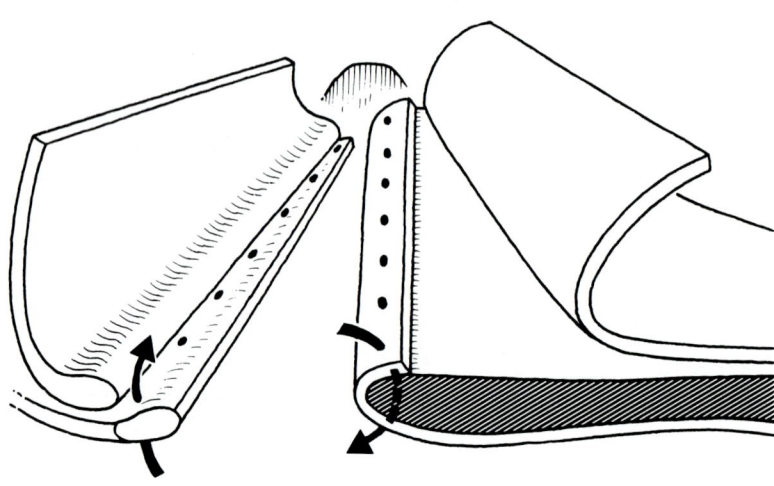

Figure 12-8.   First suture line.

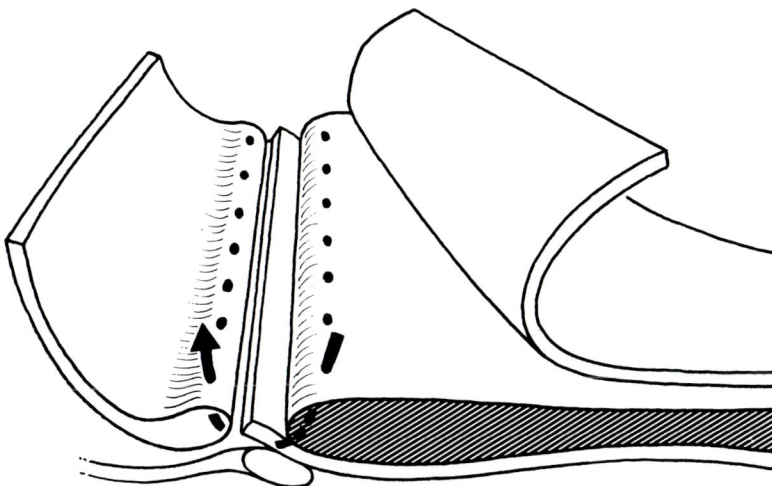

Figure 12-9.   Second suture line.

Resection of the cremasteric muscle and opening of the transversalis fascia are not specific to the Shouldice repair. These steps are an integral part of many other techniques, including the Bassini repair, at least in its original description. Of importance is the fact that the Shouldice team has made surgeons "rediscover" this practice in their approach to hernia repair, and has made them aware that it helps to reduce the rate of recurrence. The technical details in the performance of these steps may vary, but their importance does not.

REPAIR

Plication of the Transversalis Fascia

"The essence of the repair is the overlap of the divided transversalis."[2] This definition is justified, because it supports the concept that "a groin hernia results anatomically from a disruption or relaxation of transversalis fascia," but it can be a source of confusion. The transversalis fascia never should be sutured

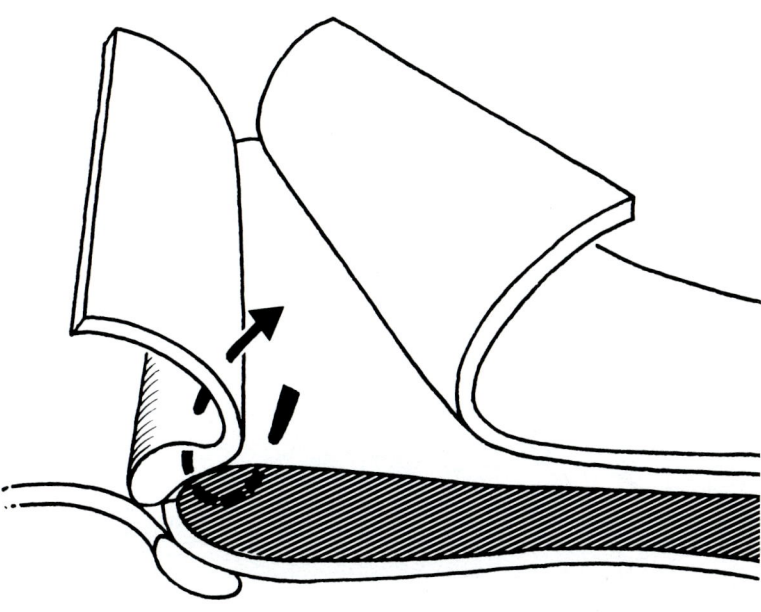

Figure 12-10.   Third suture line.

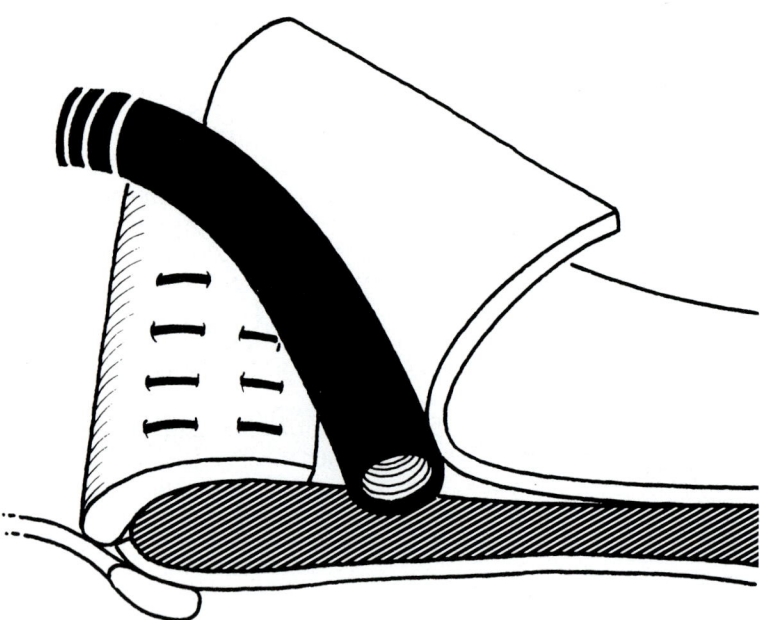

Figure 12-11. Fourth suture line.

alone. Moreover, the transversalis fascia of a patient with a hernia, especially a direct hernia, often is weak. The repair consists of two layers, each made with a continuous suture composed of two suture lines. The first line of sutures involves not only the transversalis medially, but also the rectus sheath, the aponeurotic arch of the transversalis muscle, and, more deeply, the internal oblique muscle. Laterally, the suture line involves the reinforced part of the transversalis fascia

(ie, the iliopubic tract) from its insertion on the pubis up to the internal ring. Although this term is not mentioned in the Canadian description (in which it is called the "lower flap"), this is the true structure involved. We always have been able to identify it, whether the hernia was direct or recurrent, and are convinced of its solidity. The first line of sutures involves the same tissues as does the iliopubic tract repair.

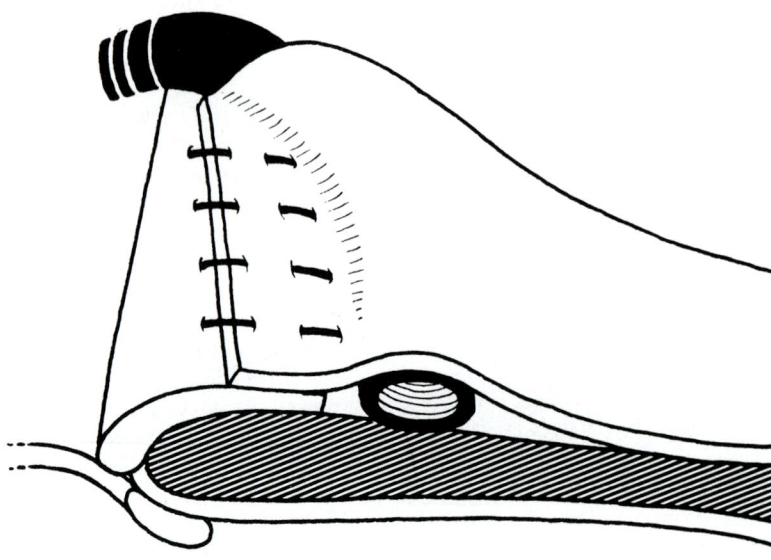

Figure 12-12. Fifth and sixth suture lines.

The second line of sutures involves the free edge of the transversalis fascia and the muscular arch of the internal oblique muscle above, and the Poupart ligament below.

Calibration of the Internal Ring

Calibration of the internal ring is difficult. An excessively tight closure may cause ischemia or venous stasis in the testis, whereas insufficient closure may result in recurrence. The Canadian authors do not recommend (and they are right) calibration with the fingertip; they prefer to use the reintegration test of the spermatic cord. Calibration should be performed during plication of the transversalis fascia, a step in which the tightening of the internal ring can be excessive. If the cremasteric stump is large, we prefer not to use it in this step because it may form a sleeve that can hinder the reintegration of the cord even if there is no real stenosis. We use the stump at the beginning of the third line of sutures by sewing it to the lower edge of the internal oblique arch, thus creating a complete muscular ring.

The Second Line of Continuous Sutures

The construction of the second line of continuous sutures is the most difficult part of the operation to understand. It may be conceived of as the lowering of the muscular arch of the internal oblique muscle onto the inguinal ligament. As described by Brendan Devlin and colleagues,[1] "the conjoint tendon is sutured to the inguinal ligament ... using a double breasting technique." This second layer of sutures actually is plastic surgery of the aponeurosis, and should not be considered to represent the lowering of one structure to another, but the apposition of two musculoaponeurotic surfaces. The lower flap of the external oblique aponeurosis is raised back to its normal position, consequently without tension, with its deep surface joined by a double continuous suture to the superficial surface of the internal oblique aponeurosis.

This part of the repair has been debated widely. Wantz,[4] who does not perform this step routinely because he considers that sutures on muscle tend to be necrotic, has obtained the same results as the group at Shouldice Hospital. It is true that the internal oblique muscle is mostly muscular, but its lower and most medial part usually is aponeurotic. This corresponds to the weak point of the repair, because most recurrences take place near the pubic tubercle. The usefulness of this second layer of sutures, therefore, remains a subject of discussion, and a study comparing a one-layer repair with a two-layer repair would be welcome.

MORBIDITY AND CONVALESCENCE

We encourage our patients to get up on the evening of surgery and to leave the hospital the next day. They are instructed to return to work or to physical exercise as soon as they wish, as in the Shouldice Hospital technique.

Conversely, our wound abscess rate has been higher than that reported at the Shouldice Hospital. This may be because our surgical activity is not limited to hernia repair, and because other patients, occasionally infected patients, are hospitalized in the same ward. This prompted us to use antibiotics with the local anesthesia solution, and wound abscesses no longer occur.[3]

RECURRENCE

In attempting to evaluate our rate of recurrence, we found it difficult to obtain follow-up on a large group of patients over a long period. Surveillance by questionnaire is uncertain and does not allow for accurate data collection; nevertheless, this is the method that seems best adapted to this common pathology, and it allows comparison with other published results.

Among 2500 hernia repairs performed, we noted 22 recurrences (nearly 1%), making our results comparable to those of the Shouldice Hospital. In considering only those patients for whom follow-up was sufficient (ie, the 922 patients who underwent surgery between 1980 and 1987), 143 were lost to follow-up because they did not answer the questionnaire or moved away without providing their new address. Among the 779 remaining patients, who underwent 856 operations and were followed up for 3 to 12 years, there were 17 recurrences (1.9%). These results are less spectacular than those of the Shouldice Hospital, but satisfactory nonetheless because these patients were operated on by several different surgeons, some of whom were in training, and it was our policy to use the Shouldice repair for all types of hernia surgery, irrespective of the size, bilateral nature, or primary character of the hernia.

Our approach to the treatment of recurrent hernia has changed because of the degree of technical difficulty encountered during surgery. These operations occasionally were simple, similar to primary hernia repair. At other times, considerable difficulty was encountered, and there was no way of predicting this before surgery. Difficult operations typically were long. Because adequate repair with the Shouldice technique was uncertain, the use of a prosthetic reinforcement was considered. If a prosthetic mesh is used, the inguinal route should be avoided. Therefore, we prefer to use a giant prosthetic mesh placed through a preperitoneal route for recurrent hernia.

In conclusion, for primary hernia repair, the Shouldice technique corresponds to the objectives we have set for ourselves: nearly routine use of local anesthesia, a short hospital stay, quick return to work, and a low rate of recurrence. Because data are not yet available from controlled, randomized trials (several of which are under way), however, the clear superiority of the Shouldice repair over other techniques remains to be proved.

REFERENCES

1. Brendan Devlin H, Russel IT, Muller D, et al. Short-stay surgery for inguinal hernia. Lancet 1977;1:847.
2. Glassow F. The Shouldice repair for inguinal hernia. In: Nyhus LM, Condon RE, eds. Hernia, ed 2. Philadelphia, JB Lippincott, 1978:163–173.
3. Lazorthes F, Chiotasso P, Massip P, et al. Local antibiotic prophylaxis in inguinal hernia repair. Surg Gynecol Obstet 1992;175:569.
4. Wantz GE. The Canadian repair of inguinal hernia. In: Nyhus LM, Condon RE, eds. Hernia, ed 3. Philadelphia, JB Lippincott, 1989:236–247.

Special Comment

Bassini Versus Shouldice: Original Methods and Physiologic Variants

Matthias Kux

"The imbrication of a weak fascia on top of a weak fascia, a strong fascia it doesn't make!" This statement by McVay[4] epitomizes the numerous theoretic objections against the Shouldice technique for inguinal hernia repair. Ever since it first was described in the surgical literature in the late 1960s, the Shouldice repair has been defined erroneously as overlap or imbrication of the transversalis fascia.[1] In the third edition of this text, Wantz[6] termed the imbricated layers *transverse aponeuroticofascial fibers*. The surgeons at the Shouldice Hospital, however, use full-thickness stitches that include the transversalis fascia, transversalis muscle, and internal oblique muscle—in fact, Bassini's triple layer (see discussion in preceding chapter).

At the centenary of Bassini's publication, Wantz[7] showed that the original Bassini method long has been corrupted in North America by omission of the transversalis fascia from the repair. This author has qualified the Shouldice technique as the inadvertent North American reinvention of the authentic, uncorrupted Bassini method.[7] At about the same time, Nyhus and associates[5] questioned the entire concept of the Bassini-Shouldice repair, which restricts natural inguinal musculoaponeurotic movement and may account for impaired sphincter and shutter mechanisms. Other dangers associated with transfixion of the internal oblique muscle with nonabsorbable sutures (ie, muscle necrosis and infection, nerve entrapment, orchitis, and testicular atrophy) have intrigued proponents of the Bassini-Shouldice technique for some time. In the previous edition of this book, Wantz[6] stated that the third and fourth rows of the Shouldice method "should probably be left out because sutures in muscle do not hold and may, in fact, damage it." Reflecting a similar concern, the nonabsorbable suture material used in the original Bassini method largely has been replaced with slowly absorbable sutures.[2]

In 1985, a prospective trial was begun at our institution specifically to address the following questions: Are the recurrence rates for the original, "uncorrupted" Bassini and Shouldice repairs identical? Are there dangers inherent in transfixing the internal oblique muscle with permanent sutures? Can the excellent results of specialist centers be reproduced in routine general surgery? Is any single method adequate for all types of hernia?[3]

For this purpose, 750 consecutive inguinal hernia repairs were assigned to one of four groups:

Group A—Bassini with absorbable sutures (polyglycolic acid)
Group B—Bassini with nonabsorbable sutures (polyester)
Group C—Shouldice with four rows of polypropylene sutures
Group D—Shouldice with two rows of polypropylene sutures

After the enrollment of 150 repairs for group A, recruitment for this group was closed because actuarial recurrence rates were unacceptably high; 200 repairs were allocated each to groups B, C, and D. Three board-certified surgeons and six residents were involved in the trial. The dissection phase was identical for all groups, as illustrated in the respective reference descriptions.[1,2,5,6] In the Bassini repair, the triple layer consisting of divided transversalis fascia, transversalis muscle, and internal oblique muscle was apposed to the inguinal ligament with 6 to 8 interrupted sutures of slowly absorbable material in group A and nonabsorbable material in group B. In the Shouldice repair, the first continuous suture approxi-

Table 12-6. Absolute Figures for Local Complications in Combined Groups A and D (No Permanent Suture Material at Internal Oblique Muscle) and Groups B and C (With Permanent Sutures in Oblique Musculature)

Complication	Groups A and D	Groups B and C
Abscess	3	5
Sinus	0	6
Neuralgia	2	5
Scrotal swelling	3	7
Testicular atrophy	0	2
Total*	8 of 350	25 of 400

*$P < .05$.

mated the undersurface of the transverse aponeurotic arch to the iliopubic tract; the second continuous suture attached the free edge of the transverse aponeurotic arch to the inguinal ligament. Full-thickness stitches, including the internal oblique muscle, were not used for the first two rows. In the original Shouldice method (group C), two additional continuous suture lines approximated the flesh of the internal oblique muscle to the inguinal ligament. In the modified Shouldice repair (group D), the suture lines into the internal oblique muscle were omitted. The recurrence rate was determined through clinical examination by hospital staff surgeons for 93.6% of surviving patients. Independent prognostic risk factors were studied by logistic regression.

When herniorrhaphy is performed under local anesthesia and the patient is requested to perform a Valsalva strain, it is immediately obvious that tension is distributed more evenly by the two-row Shouldice technique (group D) than by any of the other operations, all of which interfere grossly with the subtle muscle play that protects the inguinal floor from a rise in intraabdominal pressure. Accordingly, postoperative edema and pain were reduced and recovery was more prompt among patients who underwent the two-row Shouldice technique. In the other groups, some pain usually persisted for several weeks, about the time that it takes slowly absorbable suture material to resorb. The formidable sequelae of chronic ilioin-

guinal pain, and infectious and testicular complications were reduced significantly in combined groups A and D, in which suturing of the internal oblique muscle with nonabsorbable suture material was avoided (Table 12-6). In addition, there were four cases of litigation or reoperation for neuralgia and two cases of litigation for testicular atrophy in combined groups B and C, but none in groups A and D.

The overall recurrence rate for groups C and D (Shouldice repair) combined was 3.0%, a highly significant improvement over the rate of 10.4% for groups A and B combined (Bassini repair). Even when group A (Bassini repair with absorbable sutures), which had the highest recurrence rate, is excluded, significant differences still exist between group B (original Bassini repair) and groups C and D (Shouldice repair) considered either separately or together (Table 12-7). Overall differences were related to differences in repair of primary hernias: 7.5% for Bassini versus 2.0% for Shouldice. For repair of recurrent hernias, the superiority of the Shouldice technique was not statistically significant: the repeated recurrence rate was 7.6% versus 13.5% for the Bassini technique. Compared to the two-row Shouldice technique, the risk of recurrence was increased fourfold among patients undergoing the original Bassini procedure with nonabsorbable suture material.

Before the significant differences in recurrence became apparent, the most striking feature of the study was diminished pain and shortened recovery in group C and, particularly, group D (Shouldice repair). This indicates that *what* is sutured together is more important than *how* it is sutured. Musculoaponeurotic movement is restricted significantly by the interrupted mass sutures in the Bassini technique, which exert traction and fixation in the vertical direction (the plane of highest tension). In addition, the sutures invariably are tied too tightly, causing pain and postoperative reflex immobilization. Early mobilization probably is as important for good results as is technique itself!

The crisscross arrangement of Shouldice sutures allows for more freedom of movement and sliding in-

Table 12-7. Overall Recurrence Rates for Bassini and Shouldice Techniques With Permanent Suture Material (Groups B, C, D)*

Technique	No. of Patients	Recurrences	Percentage
Bassini (Mersilene)	184	16	8.7
Shouldice (4 rows)	194	7	3.6
Shouldice (2 rows)	172	4	2.3

*$P = .012$.

terfaces between suture lines. The dangers inherent in suturing the internal oblique muscle, however, were documented clearly in this trial. We believe that these sutures are of particular concern for surgeons with less experience than those at the Shouldice Hospital, where meticulous attention and testing under local anesthesia help to avoid nerve entrapment. We strongly recommend omitting the third and fourth suture lines of the original Shouldice method. The fact that this not only reduces local complications, but also preserves the sphincter and shutter mechanisms, has been demonstrated well under local anesthesia. Using the two-row modification of the original Shouldice method (ie, an anterior iliopubic tract repair using the Shouldice suture technique), we obtained results equal to those of specialist centers without an extensive learning curve.

The transverse aponeurotic arch and iliopubic tract are the layers best suited for reconstruction of the inguinal floor. But is incision and repair of a normal inguinal floor appropriate for all hernias? We agree with Nyhus and colleagues[5] that high ligation of the sac and closure of the defect at the internal ring probably is sufficient for type I and type II hernias, and we include this repair in our protocol. Without opening the inguinal floor, however, adequate exposure of the internal ring is not a simple and straightforward undertaking. Conversely, no suture technique can confer structural integrity to deficient and used-up tissues. Prostheses have a place in the repair of these often recurrent and more complex hernias. If a surgeon decides to use only one method for all hernias, the two-row Shouldice modification should be the first choice. It can be recommended as safe and practicable for the nonspecialized general surgeon.

REFERENCES

1. Glassow F. The Shouldice repair for inguinal hernia. In: Nyhus LM, Condon RE, eds. Hernia, ed 2. Philadelphia, JB Lippincott, 1978:163–173.
2. Houdard Cl, Stoppa R. Le traitment chirurgical des hernies de l'aine. Paris, Masson, 1984.
3. Kux M, Fuchsjäger N, Schemper M. Shouldice is superior to Bassini inguinal herniorrhaphy. Am J Surg 1994;168:15.
4. McVay CB. Cited by: Madden JL. Abdominal wall hernias. Philadelphia, WB Saunders Company, 1989:110.
5. Nyhus LM, Klein MS, Rogers FB. Inguinal hernia. In: Wells SA, ed. Current problems in surgery, vol 28. St Louis, Mosby-Year Book, Inc, 1991:403–450.
6. Wantz GE. The Canadian repair of inguinal hernia. In: Nyhus LM, Condon RE, eds. Hernia, ed 3. Philadelphia, JB Lippincott, 1989:236–248.
7. Wantz GE. The operation of Bassini as described by Attilio Catterina. Surg Gynecol Obstet 1989;168:67.

Editor's Comment

Chapter 12, with its Special Comments, might be considered a mini-symposium on the Shouldice approach to hernia repair. Bendavid provides a clear enunciation of the classic Toronto method. Wantz, the student, helps to bring the subject into proper perspective. It is exciting to have the prospective study comparing the classic Bassini and Shouldice operations by Kux.

These presentations will help both neophyte and experienced surgeons understand the seeming similarities and also the real differences between the Bassini and Shouldice operations.

L.M.N.

Hernia, Fourth Edition, edited
by Lloyd M. Nyhus and Robert E. Condon.
J.B. Lippincott Company, Philadelphia © 1995.

Chapter 13

The Tension-Free Repair of Groin Hernias

Irving L. Lichtenstein, Alex G. Shulman, and Parviz K. Amid

It was well over 100 years ago that Bassini described the first true herniorrhaphy. It was believed then, and for many decades thereafter, that immobilization and bed rest enhanced wound healing and were necessary for the successful outcome of the operation. It was only after venous stasis was recognized as the primary culprit in the genesis of fatal pulmonary emboli that early ambulation was suggested. Nevertheless, it still often is recommended that patients remain in the hospital 4 to 5 days after their herniorrhaphy and not return to full activity for at least 6 weeks.

One of many projects we undertook in the animal research laboratory was the study of wound healing. We wondered why wounds remained intact days after surgery, even after vigorous retching, when there had been little time for the reparative processes to ensure the wound's integrity. A review of the world literature failed to provide a satisfactory answer.

It required 5 years of experimentation and the lives of many rabbits before we could come up with a satisfactory answer. It was the strength of the suture material and the strength of the tissues holding the sutures that gave the wound its strength for the first several months after operation.[6] With unbreakable sutures approximating strong tendinous structures, a wound was 70% as strong as normal tissue the moment surgery was completed. This figure remained constant for 2 months. Why then, we questioned, was it necessary to restrict a patient's activity for 6 weeks, when it was apparent that the wound gained little or no strength during that period?

Publication of this work failed to impress most of our surgical colleagues.[4] Despite many publications and lectures throughout the country, surgeons were reticent to accept new concepts when their own results appeared to be equally effective.

More than 700,000 groin hernia repairs are performed each year in the United States. Of these, more than 70,000 are for recurrent inguinal hernia. A national study performed in 1983 by the Rand Corporation[10] concluded that at least 10% of all primary hernia repairs will fail. Hernia was estimated to result in the loss of a minimum of 10 to 15 million workdays each year in this country. The high incidence of recurrent hernia revealed the enormous impact of hernia surgery on health care costs. Reliable statistics largely are flawed for the following reasons:

1. The dissatisfied patient with a recurrence is likely to seek a new surgeon if the previous operation failed.
2. Accurate follow-up data are difficult to obtain because of the expense involved, the time required, and the change in address or lack of cooperation of patients.
3. Written questionnaires have only a 50% reliability factor.
4. Surgical methods and individual surgical techniques differ between surgeons.
5. Because 50% of recurrences appear 5 or more years after the original operation, and 20% are discovered first as long as 15 to 25 years after surgery, inadequate follow-up is the rule rather than the exception.
6. Confusion exists regarding the anatomy and pathophysiology of the groin. The best example of this is the substitution of the term *transversalis fascia* for the *transversus abdominis tendon,* two entirely different structures that have different strengths and arise in different layers.

CAUSES OF RECURRENT GROIN HERNIA

Early Recurrence (Mechanical)

Early recurrence develops within the first 2 years after the initial operation. The prime cause of early failure is tension on the suture line. The fibroblasts require sufficient oxygen tension for proper hydroxylation of proline and lysine. In 1984, Berliner[2] properly cautioned that "total absence of tension on the suture line is the sine qua non for the (hernia) repair. An operation that regularly requires a relaxing incision is not physiologically appropriate."

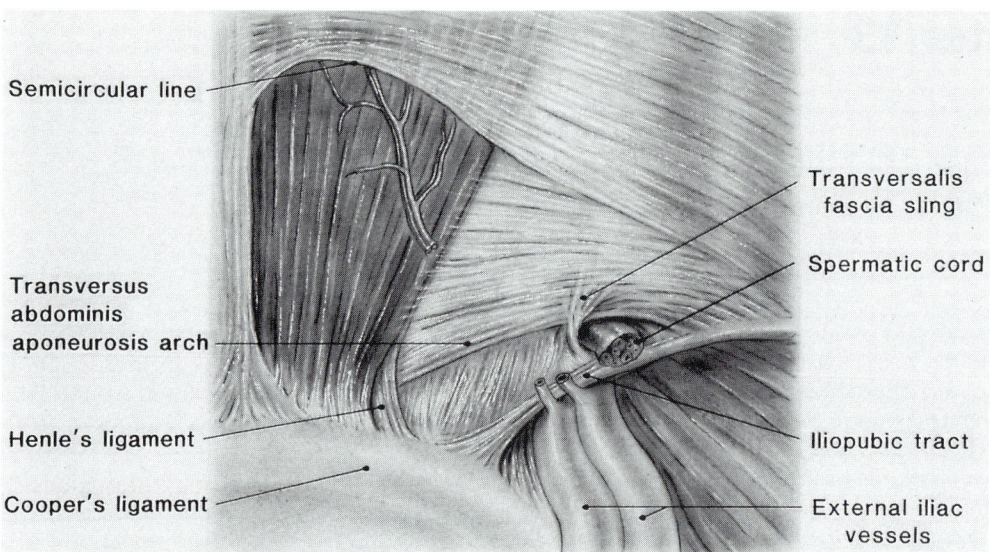

Semicircular line

Transversus
abdominis
aponeurosis arch

Henle's ligament

Cooper's ligament

Transversalis
fascia sling

Spermatic cord

Iliopubic tract

External iliac
vessels

Figure 13-1.   The normal structures of the inguinal region viewed from the internal aspect.

To create a hernia repair without tension, it is necessary to review some anatomic concepts:

1. Transversalis fascia: The canal floor is covered only by transversalis fascia, a structure of insignificant strength. It cannot be depended on in hernia repair because it contains a variable number of aponeurotic fibers from the overlying transversus abdominis tendon. This fascia inserts into the Cooper ligament.

2. Conjoined tendon: The transversus abdominis tendon is the only aponeurotic structure cephalad to the canal floor and ordinarily inserts into the rectus sheath. The so-called "conjoined tendon" includes the internal oblique, which is muscular in the groin and, therefore, of poor value in reparative surgery.

3. Hernia sac: The peritoneal sac consists of a single layer of transparent mesothelium, and its presence never caused or cured an adult hernia. Its ligation and excision contributes little to the strength of the wound and may add to the postoperative discomfort.

4. Direct versus indirect herniation: The differential diagnosis of direct versus indirect inguinal hernia is of little practical importance. The defect always is located in the transversalis fascia, regardless of whether it is medial or lateral to the epigastric vessels.

Many centuries ago, mankind's ancestors began to forego walking on all fours for reasons of the three "f's" (food, flight, and fight). As a result, we suffer from architectural deficiencies (eg, back pathology, hemorrhoids, varicose veins, hernias). A unique problem was created in that our upright posture produced an Achilles heel in the groin (the only area of the abdominal wall without muscular aponeurotic support).

The closest tendinous structures around this defect are the transversus abdominis tendon above and the Poupart or Cooper ligament below. These semimobile structures may be situated as far apart as 2 cm (Fig. 13-1). Nevertheless, since Bassini's time, virtually all repairs have depended on approximation of these divergent structures, which normally are not in apposition. The conjoined muscle tendinous arch is stretched down forcibly and sutured to the inguinal ligament in this technique. The resulting suture line always is under tension, regardless of the use of a relaxing incision (Fig. 13-2). Because the insertion of the transversus abdominis tendon into the rectus sheath is essentially inelastic, placement of the suture line any significant distance from the pubic tubercle explains why most recurrences first appear at this point.[3] At the internal ring (the second most common site of recurrence), complete approximation of tissue is prevented by the spermatic cord.

Therefore, any attempt to approximate forcibly the transversus tendon to the rigid tubercle, the ilio-

Figure 13-2.   (*A* and *B*) Transversus abdominis aponeurotic curtain. A, internal oblique muscle; B, rectus sheath; C, transversus abdominis aponeurosis. (Lichtenstein IL. Hernia repair without disability, ed 2. St Louis, Ishiyaku EuroAmerica, 1986:102)

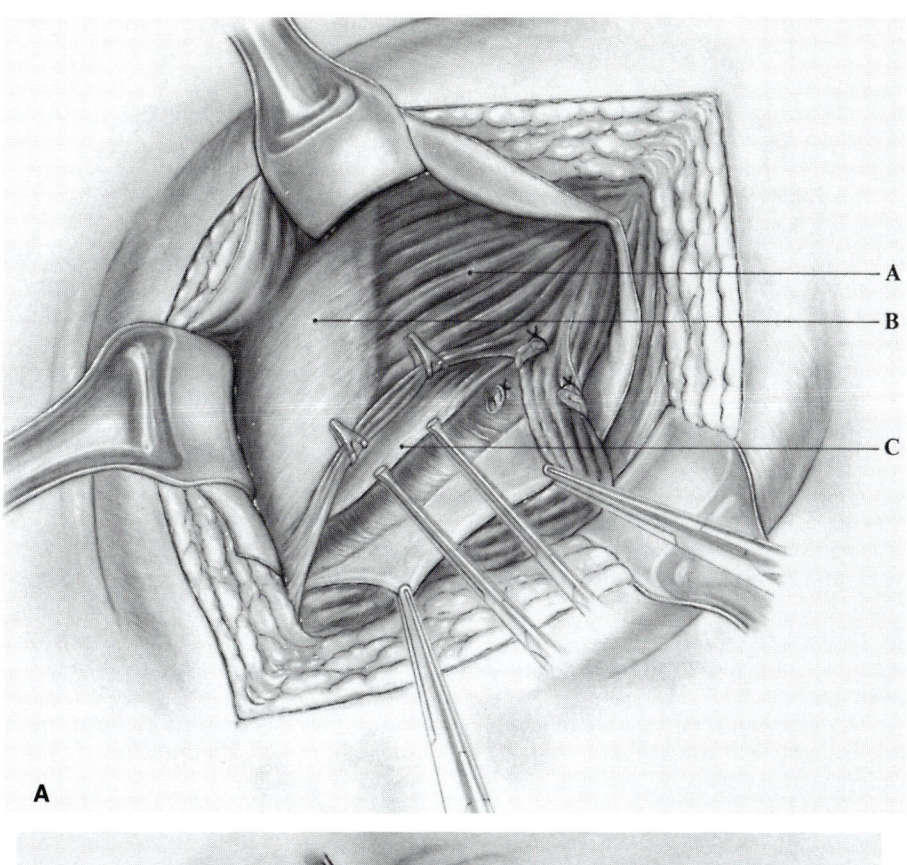

A

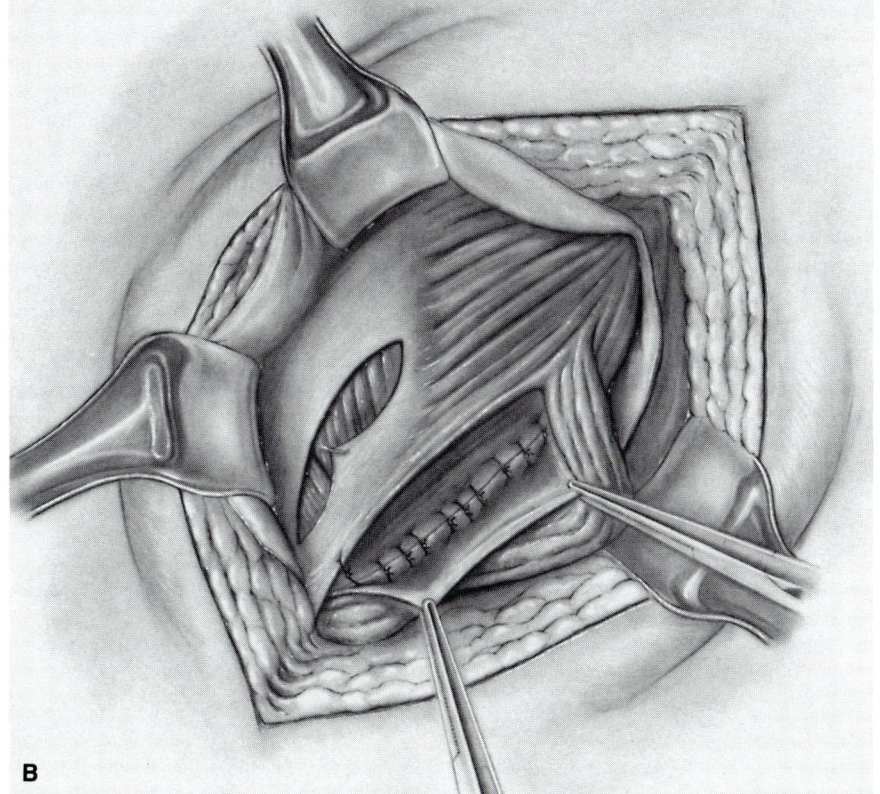

B

pubic tract, or the Poupart or Cooper ligament, whether it be by the Shouldice repair (a modification of the Bassini technique) or the McVay approach, inevitably results in distortion of the anatomy and severe tension on the suture line. In addition, because the iliopubic tract and Poupart ligament form the anterior border of the femoral canal, forced approximation of these structures can cause dilation of the femoral opening and create a postoperative femoral hernia. It has been reported that as many as 45% of all femoral hernias are formed as the result of a previous inguinal herniorrhaphy.

Late Recurrence (Metabolic)

It long has been recognized that the incidence of hernia increases with age. In more recent studies,[9] the cause has been established to be defective collagen metabolism, either increased destruction or decreased formation. This problem is critical as it pertains to the canal floor in the groin, because only transversalis fascia protects this area. It has become apparent in connective tissue diseases such as the Ehlers-Danlos syndrome that some permanent reinforcement is necessary to prevent recurrence of the hernia.

The development of appropriate synthetic materials has solved this problem. In addition to providing permanent reinforcement for the floor of the canal, the mesh or screen can eliminate tension on the suture line.

TECHNIQUE OF TENSION-FREE REPAIR OF PRIMARY GROIN HERNIAS[8]

Tension-free repair of primary groin hernias is performed in an outpatient setting using local anesthesia. It is essential to avoid any initial discomfort so that the patient retains confidence undiminished by distress during the procedure and can cooperate more fully.

Field-block injections have proven unnecessary. Epidural anesthesia is required only in exceptional cases, such as extreme obesity, simultaneous bilateral hernioplasty, some multiple recurrent hernias, and large, irreducible scrotal hernias. General anesthesia is needed only for hernias with suspected bowel incarceration and for the rare cases in which it is decided, at the time of operation, to revert to an open preperitoneal approach. (Stoppa and Warlaumont, 1989; Wantz, 1989)

The presence of a qualified anesthesiologist is preferable for many reasons, but especially to recognize unanticipated emergencies. Many anesthesiologists prefer to administer intravenous medications,

particularly for anxious patients. A small bolus of propofol, a short-acting amnestic hypnotic, can induce an immediate brief sleep that wears off in a few minutes. This elegant refinement spares the patient the pain of the first needle stick of the skin. Although no drug is essential, small increments of fentanyl, a narcotic hypnotic, or the sedative midazolam, contribute to the patient's comfort. In spite of these additions, patients can be assured of being awake and fully responsive at the end of the operation, usually with an amnestic effect that removes any possible stressful memory of the procedure.

Local infiltration of a mixture of one half 2% lidocaine and one half 0.5% bupivacaine without epinephrine is injected into the skin and subcutaneous tissues, permitting immediate incision. A window is established through the subcutaneous tissues at the lateral end of the wound, exposing the external oblique aponeurosis (Fig. 13-3). Through this window, 8 to 10 mL of the anesthetic mixture is injected beneath the external oblique aponeurosis to block all three nerves in the inguinal canal. Other sensitive sites, which require additional 3- to 5-mL increments, are the tissues over the pubic bone and the peritoneum at the internal ring, including the indirect sac. For a routine elective groin hernia, 40 to 50 mL of anesthetic is sufficient. This amount is well within the safe range for toxicity and avoids the risks and complications that often are associated with more complicated anesthetic routines.

In addition to the iliohypogastric and ilioinguinal nerves, we are convinced that it is essential to preserve the genital branch of the genitofemoral nerve if at all possible.[5] Care should be exercised when lifting the spermatic cord to use the avascular space between the pubic tubercle and the cord itself to avoid injury to the floor of the canal, damage to testicular blood flow, and crushing of the genital nerve, which always lies in juxtaposition to the external spermatic vessels (Fig. 13-4). On rare occasions, sacrifice of this nerve can cause inordinate and incapacitating neuralgia for years.

To thin the spermatic cord and remove any lipoma present, the cremaster fibers are incised transversely at the level of the internal ring over a clamp, thus avoiding the nerves. Complete excision of the cremaster fibers from the spermatic cord is unnecessary and may result in injury to the vas deferens, increasing the likelihood of postoperative neuralgia and ischemic orchitis.

Indirect hernia sacs always are opened and digital exploration is performed to detect any other defects or the presence of a femoral hernia. The sac simply is inverted into the abdomen without excision, suture, or ligation, which not only is unnecessary, but may be

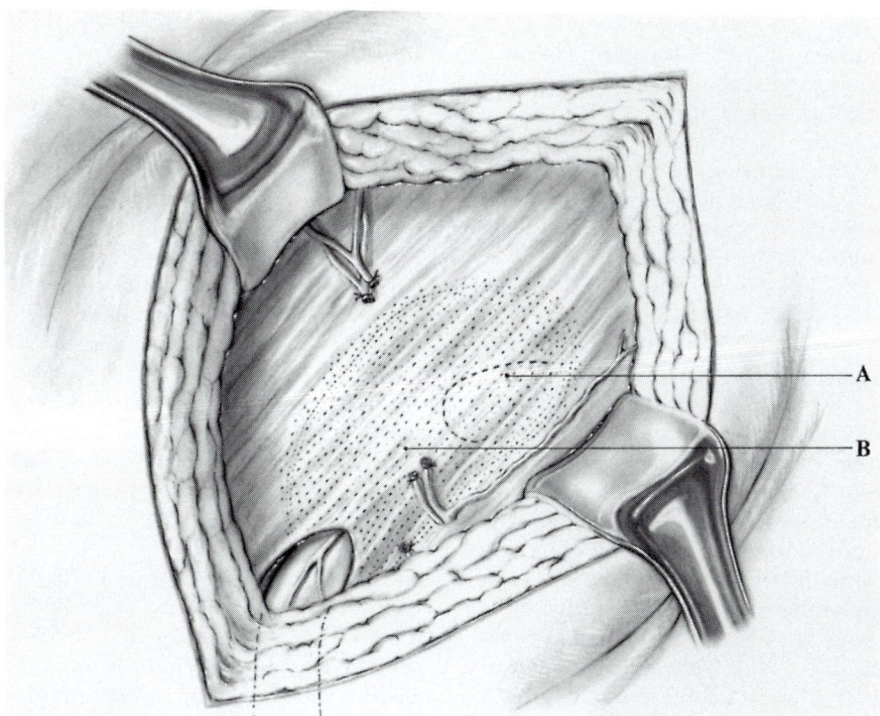

Figure 13-3. Internal ring (A) and anesthetic solution surrounding cord beneath aponeurosis (B). Lichtenstein IL, Hernia repair without disability, ed 2. St Louis, Ishiyaku Euro-America, 1986:57.

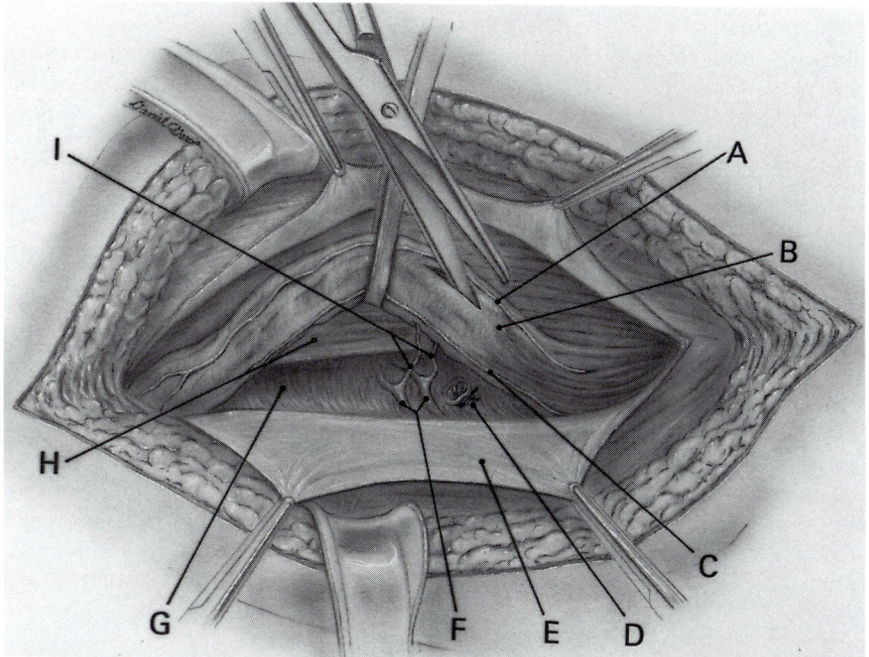

Figure 13-4. To elevate the cord and its coverings completely, the cremaster vessels arising from the epigastric vessels must be sacrificed, because the clamps easily may crush the nearby genital nerve. A, ilioinguinal nerve; B, cremaster covering of cord; C, genital nerve; D, ligated sac at the internal ring; E, external oblique aponeurosis; F, epigastric vessels giving off external spermatic branches to the cremaster muscle; G, transversalis fascia; H, transversus aponeurosis; I, external spermatic vessels.

responsible for some postoperative discomfort. To prevent postoperative hydrocele formation, complete scrotal sacs are transected at the mid-point of the canal, with the distal section left in place after incising the anterior wall of the sac. With direct hernias, the femoral ring is evaluated through a small opening in the floor of the inguinal canal. In the event of a large direct hernia, the sac is invaginated with an absorbable imbricating suture to achieve a flat surface over which to lay the synthetic screen. The external oblique aponeurosis is separated from the underlying internal oblique muscle at a point high enough to accommodate a patch measuring 6 × 8 cm.

A precut sheet of Marlex mesh from the manufacturer measures about 8 × 16 cm and is trimmed as necessary so that the patch overlaps the internal oblique muscle and aponeurosis by at least 2 cm above the border of the Hesselbach triangle. The medial portion of the mesh is rounded to the shape of the medial corner of the inguinal canal. The mesh is sutured to the aponeurotic tissue over the pubic bone, overlapping the bone to prevent any tension or weakness at this critical point. The same suture is continued along the lower edge, attaching the patch to the shelving portion of the Poupart ligament to a point just lateral to the internal ring with a running suture.

A slit is made at the lateral end of the mesh, creating a wider tail above the cord and a narrower one below. This maneuver positions the cord between the two tails of the mesh and avoids the keyhole opening, which is less effective and results in an occasional reported recurrence (Fig. 13-5). The upper edge of the patch is sutured to the internal oblique aponeurosis or muscle using a few interrupted absorbable sutures. Sharp retraction of the upper leaf of the external oblique from the internal oblique is important, because it provides the appropriate amount of laxity for the patch. When the retraction is released, a true tension-free repair is taken up when the patient strains on command during the operation or resumes an upright position afterward. Using a single nonabsorbable, monofilament suture, the lower edges of the two tails are fixed to the shelving margin of the Poupart ligament just lateral to the completion knot of the lower running suture. Thus, a new internal ring of mesh is created.

The excess patch on the lateral side is trimmed, leaving 3 to 4 cm beyond the internal ring. This is tucked underneath the external oblique aponeurosis and the aponeurosis is closed with a continuous absorbable suture. Patients are discharged from the outpatient department within a few hours of their operation. Postoperative discomfort is minimal and treated with mild analgesics. Unrestricted activity is encouraged and patients usually return to their normal occupations 2 to 7 days after surgery.

RESULTS OF TENSION-FREE REPAIR OF PRIMARY HERNIAS

The series from the Lichtenstein Hernia Institute includes 3125 consecutive patients who underwent primary inguinal hernia repair. Only the tension-free technique was used. The follow-up period ranged from 1 to 8 years and the follow-up rate was 87%. Four recurrences resulting from technical errors occurred in patients who were operated on early in the evolution of this technique. No recurrences have occurred among patients who underwent operation in the past 5 years.

We have conducted a multicenter study involving five groups of surgeons with a special interest in hernia surgery. Using the "tension-free" technique, they obtained recurrence rates ranging from 0% to 0.77%, a rejection rate of zero, and an infection rate of less than 0.5%.

A multicenter survey of 70 different surgeons without a special interest in hernia surgery who performed 22,300 "tension-free" hernioplasties showed similar results with regard to rates of recurrence, rejection, and infection, and length of recovery period.

The results obtained by surgeons with a special interest in hernia surgery were virtually identical to those obtained by surgeons without such an interest, and are testimony to the simplicity, safety, and effectiveness of primary "tension-free" hernioplasty.

It must be emphasized that the use of mesh alone does not always guarantee success. The mesh must be large enough and secured without tension for a good outcome. Recurrences through the mesh are unknown.

PREVENTION OF RECURRENT GROIN HERNIA

Before the treatment of recurrent groin hernia is discussed, it is useful to review the steps necessary for its prevention:

1. Fascia never should be used for the repair of inguinal hernias. The mere presence of the hernia is proof that the fascia is inadequate. Only tendinous or aponeurotic structures are used in the reconstructive process. The mesh patch is inserted between the two oblique muscles.
2. Direct and indirect inguinal hernias differ only in that they are either medial or lateral to the epigastric vessels, and they should be treated in a similar fashion. The entire canal floor always should be reinforced in adults with an inguinal hernia.

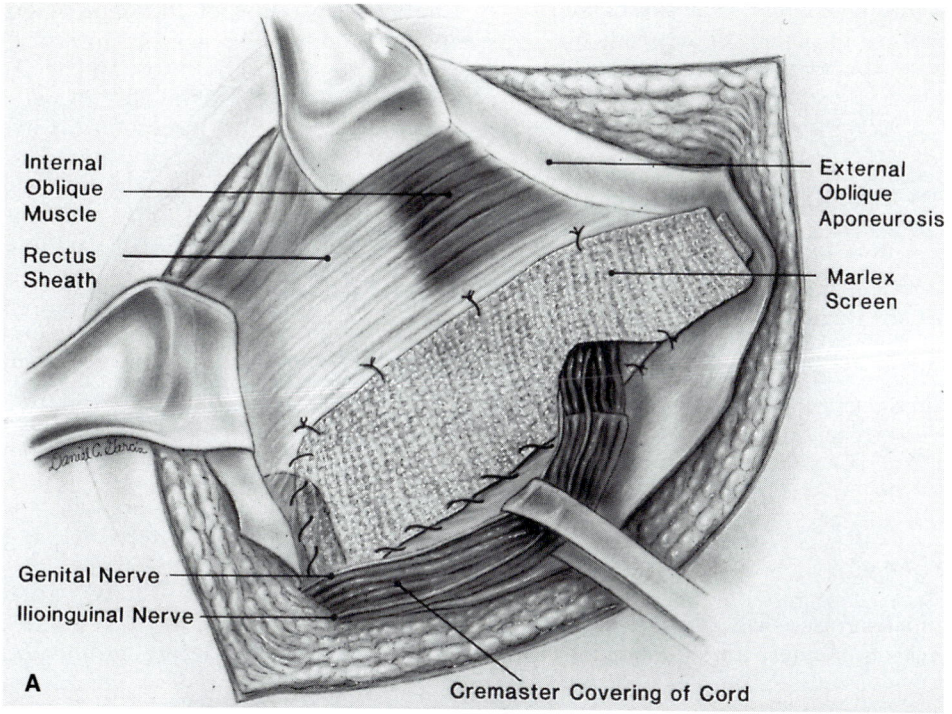

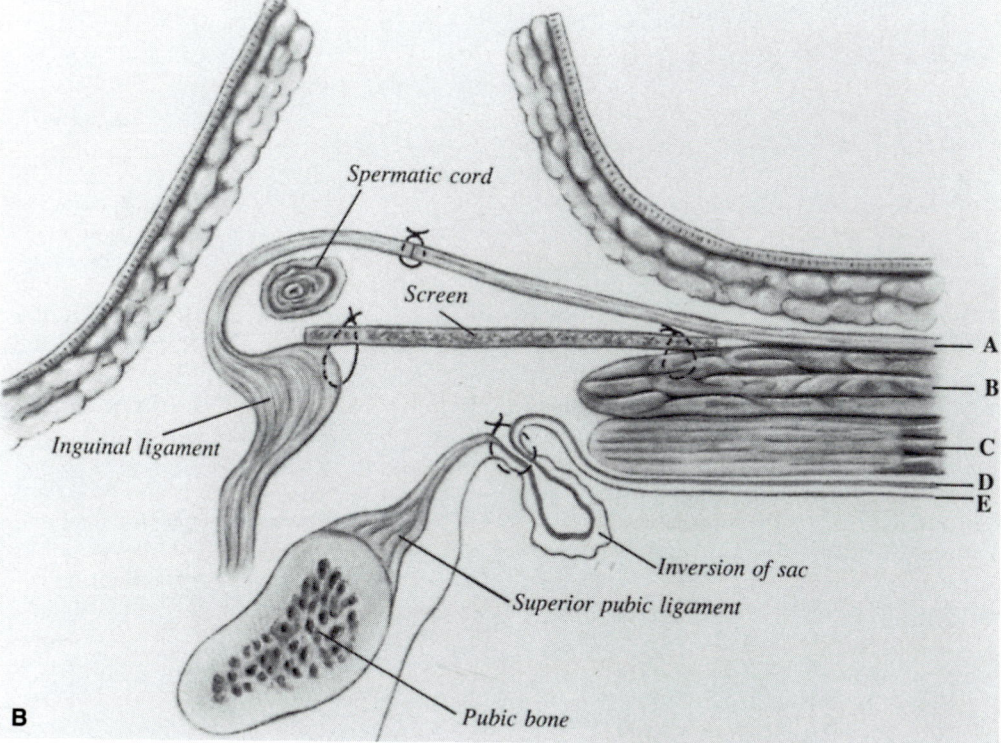

Figure 13-5. (*A*) The mesh prosthesis sutured in place. (*B*) The implanted mesh viewed in a parasagittal section. A, external oblique aponeurosis; B, internal oblique muscle; C, transversus muscle and aponeurosis; D, transversalis fascia; E, peritoneum. (Lichtenstein IL. Hernia repair without disability, 2nd ed. St Louis, Ishiyaku EuroAmerica, 1986)

3. Tension must be avoided on all suture lines.
4. Permanent reinforcement with a synthetic mesh always should be used to avoid both late recurrence and tension. Our preference is Marlex—a polypropylene screen.

TECHNIQUE OF TENSION-FREE REPAIR OF RECURRENT INGUINAL HERNIA

Depending on the conditions found at surgery, three different repairs are available to the surgeon:

Plan A—"Plug" repair for defects less than 4 cm.
Plan B—Patch repair for large defects.
Plan C—Preperitoneal repair for cases involving excessive scarring and anatomic destruction of the entire groin area.

Plan A—Plug Repair

Recurrent inguinal hernias usually are found at either the pubic tubercle or the internal ring. In almost 90% of cases, there is only one defect and it is 4 cm or smaller.[11] Dissection of the entire inguinal floor is counterproductive because it converts a small defect into a larger one using scarred and devascularized tissue for the repair. For the past 20 years, the "plug" has been used at our institution for most recurrent inguinal hernia repairs, with gratifying success.

Lichtenstein[7] introduced the plug in 1968 and reported on it in 1974. The technique since has been modified to form a firmer plug to eliminate the hole in the center and prevent future shrinkage (Fig. 13-6).

It is essential that the exact position of the bulge in regard to the pubic tubercle be determined preoperatively. Nothing is more embarrassing to the surgeon than to find the recurrent hernia still present several days after surgery. The bulge ordinarily disappears when the patient lies supine and may be difficult to locate during the operation.

The sac may be discovered either beneath the flattened cord or over it. In either case, it is dissected carefully from the cord and freed to the fascial level until firm scar tissue is discovered. Finger exploration of the floor of the canal through the opening is performed to check for a rare second defect.

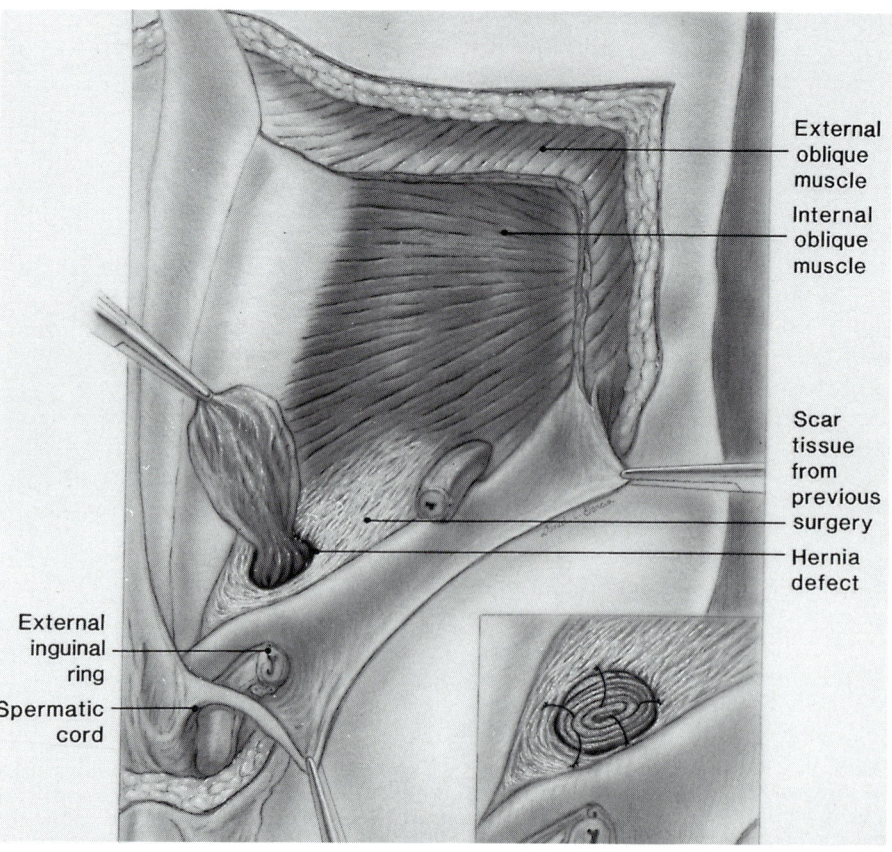

Figure 13-6. Typical recurrence at the pubic tubercle treated with a "plug" (*inset*).

A strip of Marlex mesh measuring 2 × 20 cm (or longer, depending on the size of the defect) is rolled into the shape of a solid cylinder (Fig. 13-7). The plug is inserted snugly into the defect. The firmness of the plug prevents the possibility of future shrinkage, which can result in eventual recurrence of the hernia.

Only a small rim of scar tissue must be cleared around the defect, because the plug itself fills the hole. Several anchoring sutures are all that is required. Before the sutures are tied, the effectiveness of the repair is tested by having the patient cough or strain.

The usual defect lends itself to repair by the plug technique, which is preferable to the patch for the following reasons:

1. Its slight extension into the preperitoneal space prevents the protrusion of omentum or bowel into the cul-de-sac that an onlay patch may create.
2. Laying down a secure flat patch requires a wider dissection of tissue that may endanger the spermatic cord as well as destroy the intact portion of the previous repair.
3. The plug itself is a stronger barrier to recurrence than is the single layer in the flat patch technique.
4. The plug is associated with less postoperative discomfort, rapid rehabilitation, insignificant complications, and excellent results, and it can be performed on an outpatient basis. It is recommended, therefore, for the treatment of most recurrent inguinal hernias.

Results

More than 1500 recurrent inguinal hernias have been observed for 3 to 20 years, with a follow-up rate exceeding 80%. The defect was at the pubic tubercle in 46% of cases and at the internal ring in 40%. The entire floor was absent in 13%, and these required the patch repair. One of five recurrent cases had a history of two or more previous repairs. Including all the multiple recurrences, our failure rate for recurrent hernias was 1.6%. This compares favorably with the rate of more than 25% that is achieved with conventional methods. Our own failures resulted from a plug that was too small or too loose in 12 patients, too few sutures in 2 patients, and an unrecognized second defect in 4 patients. In the past 5 years, only two failures have occurred among 390 recurrent hernia repairs (< 1%).

Plan B—Patch Repair

Patch repair was described in the section on tension-free repair of primary inguinal hernias.

Plan C—Preperitoneal Repair

Stoppa, of France, strongly advocates a preperitoneal repair and is supported in this by Wantz,[12] of New York. This technique involves the insertion of a large sheet of Mersilene mesh into the preperitoneal space to act as a broad barrier to the entire groin area. In our experience, this approach rarely is required and has several disadvantages:

1. Local anesthesia usually is not sufficient.
2. The procedure can be made more difficult by previous operations in the same area resulting in scarring and obliteration of anatomic planes.
3. Drains are required and the procedure generally cannot be performed on an outpatient basis.
4. Several days of hospitalization usually are necessary.

FEMORAL HERNIAS (THE TENSION-FREE PLUG TECHNIQUE)

There are four conventional techniques for the repair of femoral hernias, all of which are associated with tension on the repair site and an unacceptable rate of recurrence:

1. The Bassini repair, in which the inguinal ligament is sutured to the pectineal fascia.
2. The Bassini-Kirshner repair, in which the inguinal ligament is sutured to the Cooper ligament.

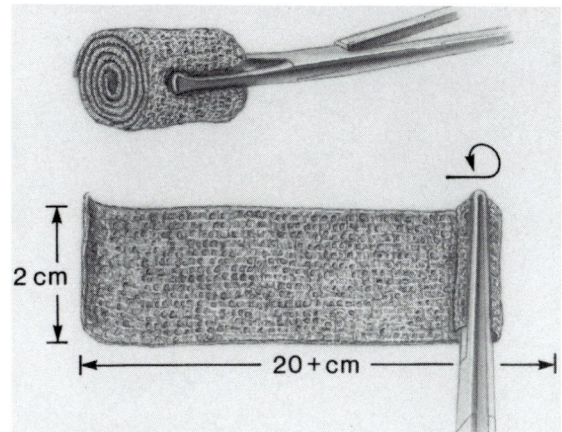

2 cm

20 + cm

Figure 13-7. Formation of the "plug."

3. The Moschcowitz repair, in which the iliopubic tract is sutured to the Cooper ligament.
4. The Lotheissen-McVay repair, in which the transversus abdominis tendon is sutured to the Cooper ligament.

In the Lichtenstein plug repair, no anatomic structures are sutured together. A plug of Marlex simply acts as an obturator in the femoral canal to prevent recurrence (Fig. 13-8). The plug repair is the only one that avoids all suture line tension, accounting for its minimal recurrence rate. It is simple, rapidly performed in the outpatient department, associated with minimal discomfort, and effective.

More than 200 femoral hernias, both primary and recurrent, were repaired using the plug technique and the patients were followed up for 1 to 15 years. There were two recurrences resulting from inadequate plug size.

COMPARISON OF MODERN SYNTHETIC MATERIALS

The search for the ideal artificial support for hernia repair has been under way for decades. Materials evaluated have ranged from gold filigree to ox tendon, cutis grafts, and metal plates. The appropriate material should meet the following criteria:

1. Permanent.
2. Inert.
3. Monofilament.
4. Nononcogenic.
5. Resistant to infection.

6. Stimulates the growth of fibroblasts through its interstices, permitting a strong layer of collagen deposition.
7. No crevices or pores less than 10 μm in diameter.
8. Fixed rapidly in place by the patient's fibrin glue.

Over the years, we have had the opportunity at our institution to study, compare, and use in thousands of cases all the popular meshes. Only the monofilament polypropylene screens of Prolene or Marlex fulfill all the requirements listed above.

Mersilene is popular in France, but is not a monofilament and does not stimulate sufficiently the growth of fibroblasts through its interstices, as does Marlex. The internodal architecture of Gore-Tex (Fig. 13-9) contains an infinite number of pore sizes, providing innumerable spaces in which bacteria can hide and proliferate. They are protected from neutrophilic granulocytes (about 12 to 14 μm in diameter), which are unable to reach the offending organism, diminishing the body's defenses against infection. This material also fails to stimulate an intense fibroblastic response and it is not fixed in place rapidly.

Therefore, for the past few decades, we have used Marlex (Fig. 13-10) exclusively for the repair of adult groin hernias. The screen is infiltrated rapidly with fibroblasts and fixed in place by fibrin so that it is impossible to remove or even identify the patch after several weeks have passed. Of hundreds of cases referred to our institution with existing multiple recur-

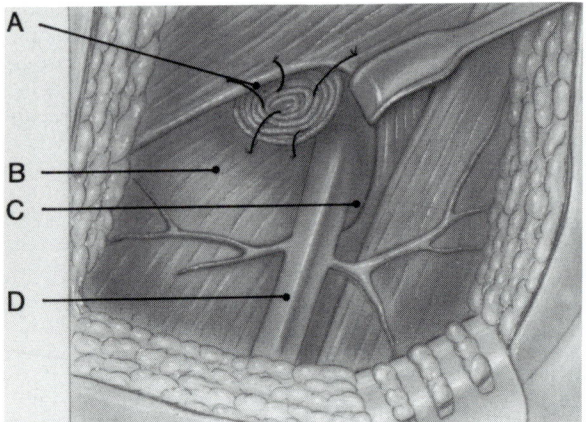

Figure 13-8. Subinguinal approach to femoral inguinal repair. A, falciform edge of fascia lata; B, pectineus fascia; C, femoral vein; D, saphenous vein.

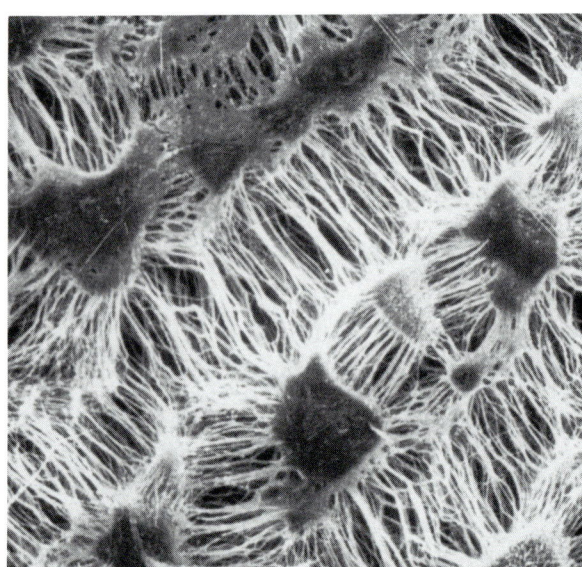

Figure 13-9. Gore-Tex soft tissue patch (magnified).

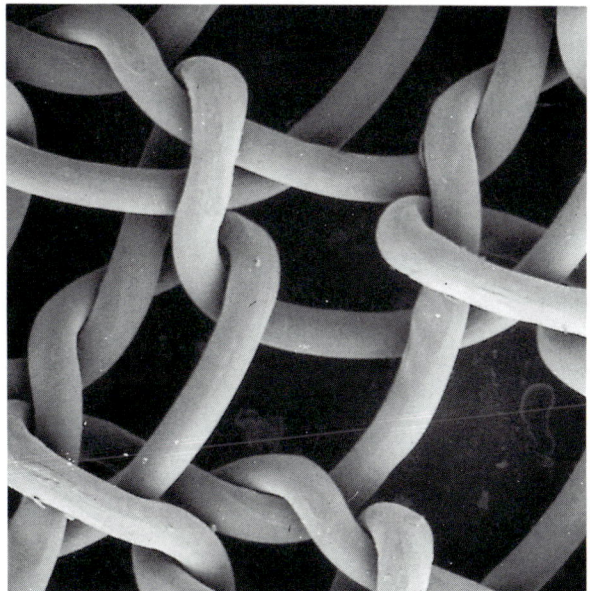

Figure 13-10. Polypropylene (Marlex, magnified).

rent groin hernias, only twice was removal of the previously inserted mesh required. In both cases, it was found to be floating in a sea of pus along with other necrotic material. It usually is not necessary to remove the polypropylene screen in the presence of infection, because it is a monofilament. Opening and draining the incision (as for any infected wound) will cure the problem without the necessity of removing the mesh.

Polypropylene (Marlex) is the preferred biomaterial for the repair of groin hernias at the Lichtenstein Hernia Institute. Concern remains regarding its use in ventral hernias, however, because of the possible formation of intraabdominal adhesions and intestinal fistulas. Available synthetic meshes are plagued by this problem.

Based on our animal experiments in the research laboratory, the use of nonabsorbable mesh with an absorbable layer on the peritoneal surface to prevent adhesions is not a satisfactory solution. Adhesions appear shortly after the absorption is complete, although it may take many weeks for this to occur. Because adhesion of the intestine to the biomaterial is the first stage of prosthetic mesh–related intestinal fistula formation, its prevention is a logical step toward the elimination of this complication. A biomaterial developed in our laboratory by Amid has the selective property of allowing infiltration of the fibroconnective tissue of the abdominal wall into one side, yet preventing the bowel from adhering to the other side. We are exploring the feasibility of clinical application of this mesh.

CONCLUSIONS

Despite numerous advances, the recurrence rate for groin hernia repair remains depressingly high for such a simple operation. The cure rate for recurrent herniation is even more distressing. With increased understanding of the anatomic physiology of the groin and the routine use of a synthetic prosthesis in tension-free primary hernia repair, it is hoped that results will improve markedly. In addition, the plug technique offers a simplified, more effective attack on recurrence, the bête noire of all hernia surgeons.

REFERENCES

1. Amid PK, Shulman AG, Lichtenstein IL. Selecting synthetic mesh for repair of groin hernia. Postgraduate General Surgery 1992;4:150.
2. Berliner SD. An approach to groin hernia. Surg Clin North Am 1984;64:197.
3. Condon RE. The anatomy of the inguinal region. In: Nyhus LM, Harkins HN, eds. Hernia. Philadelphia, JB Lippincott, 1964.
4. Lichtenstein IL. Hernia repair without disability, ed 1. St Louis, CV Mosby, 1970.
5. Lichtenstein IL. Hernia repair without disability (introducing tension-free herniorrhaphies), ed 2. St Louis, Ishiyaku EuroAmerica, 1986.
6. Lichtenstein IL, Herzikoff S, Shore JM, Jiron MW, Stuart S, Mizuno L. The dynamics of wound healing. Surg Gynecol Obstet 1970;130:685.
7. Lichtenstein IL, Shore JM. Simplified repair of femoral and recurrent inguinal hernias by a "plug" technic. Am J Surg 1974;128:439.
8. Lichtenstein IL, Shulman AG, Amid PK, Montllor MM. Tension-free hernioplasty. Am J Surg 1988; 157:188.
9. Peacock EE. Wound repair, ed 3. Philadelphia, WB Saunders Co, 1984.
10. Rand Corporation of Santa Monica, CA. Conceptualization and measurement of physiologic health for adults, vol 15. Santa Monica, CA, Rand Corporation, 1983.
11. Shulman AG, Amid PK, Lichtenstein IL. Plug repair of 1,402 recurrent inguinal hernias. Arch Surg 1990; 125:265.
12. Wantz GE. Atlas of hernia surgery. New York, Raven Press, 1991.

Editor's Comment

The Lichtenstein "tension-free" repair is one of the two really successful nonanatomic approaches to the treatment of groin hernias (the other is the Shouldice repair). The major features of the Lichtenstein method are that local anesthesia is used, the sac is not excised, the primary hernia defect is not sutured or repaired, and a prosthesis is used routinely.

This technique has been adopted widely by surgeons, particularly those with no special interest or talent in the repair of groin hernias. It has proven to be popular because it succeeds about as well in the hands of generalists as it does in the hands of its originator, and that success rate—as detailed in this chapter—is excellent.

One could quibble with the "one-size-fits-all" approach of the Lichtenstein repair, or with its use of mesh in every case—a maneuver that the experience of other surgeons demonstrates to be unnecessary as a routine. One cannot argue, however, with the results of the "tension-free" repair. "Rien ne réussit comme le succès."

R.E.C.

Special Comment

The No-Tension Repair of Groin Hernias
Arthur I. Gilbert

Excess tension between approximated tissues is the most destructive element of all traditional hernia repairs. There has never been a text written that could teach a surgeon how much tension is too much. This is learned only by personal operating experiences and diligent long-term correlation of techniques with one's own successes and failures. The same principles apply regarding currently used prosthetic grafts. The disappointing consequence of suture line tension between grafts and surrounding tissues is a failed repair.

In 1892, the earliest of tension-relieving procedures was introduced. Devised by Wölfler, improved by Tanner and Halsted, and popularized by McVay, relaxing incisions have been used to facilitate and improve the outcomes of every eponymic technique of inguinal hernia repair. With some extremely large defects, however, even multiple relaxing incisions often prove helpless. Excess tension on tissues caused by a single suture or an entire line results in ischemic necrosis and failed repairs.

Read[5] compared the benefit of relaxing incisions by measuring the reduction of suture line tension in Bassini (Poupart ligament) and McVay (Cooper ligament) repairs of indirect and direct inguinal hernias. Before and after the development of relaxing incisions for indirect and direct hernias, the Bassini repair was associated with measurably less tension than was the McVay technique. After relaxing incisions began to be used for McVay repairs, direct hernias benefited more than did indirect hernias. Because of stretching of the posterior wall in a full-floor direct hernia, the relaxing incision afforded a greater "slide" effect. Reduction of tension was most significant in the middle third of the suture line, yet it was notable that most recurrent direct hernias presented nearer the pubic tubercle. Excess pull on tissues in any direction creates future failures, either in recurrence of original hernias or in development of new adjacent hernias. The higher incidence of femoral hernias, which develop subsequently in relationship to the upward pull of the Poupart ligament in the Bassini and Shouldice repairs, must be compared to the high incidence of recurrent direct inguinal hernias that follow failures of McVay repair as a result of excess downward tension on the transversus aponeurotic arch to the rigid Cooper ligament.

A numeric measure of tension that is detrimental to a hernia repair has never been established. It is literally impossible to approximate tissue layers without creating some amount of tension, minor as it may be. Regarding the "tension-free repair" designed by Newman and popularized by Lichtenstein,[4] curious surgeons have wondered how the posterior wall of a direct hernia can be invaginated, or how a prosthetic graft can be sutured in place completely free of tension. Qualitative evaluation of excess tissue stress resulting from suture line tension is essentially one's own appraisal while observing the patient perform functional activities such as coughing and straining on request. Whether the Lichtenstein repair is absolutely free of tension is moot, because of the commendably low failure rate of 0.2% reported from five diverse surgical centers where this technique was used.[6]

Two repairs that are completely free of tension have been described. Both have the same denominator: no sutures are used. Stoppa's technique is performed through the posterior approach. After dissecting the preperitoneal space on both sides, a large Dacron mesh is positioned between the peritoneum and the endopelvic fascia. Defects in the myopectineal orifices are left unsutured, as is the mesh. The mesh is compressed between tissue layers by intraabdominal pressure alone, affording the entire pelvis protection from anterior wall herniation. Stoppa's procedure is superb for complicated recurrent groin hernias and large bilateral primary hernias.

In 1987, I described the "sutureless repair" technique for inguinal hernia. I recognized that the internal ring is a natural window through which a prosthetic graft could be placed into the preperitoneal space.[2] This procedure is accomplished through the anterior approach, and a local anesthetic is used in 95% of cases. Patients exercise and ambulate immediately after the operation; they are discharged from the hospital 2 hours later. All patients are encouraged to resume regular activities immediately. This repair is ideal for indirect hernias (types I, II, and III) and occasionally for diverticular direct hernias (type V).[1] In the past 5 years, I have used this repair in 989 patients. Only two failures have occurred, both with type III hernias with peritoneal sacs of scrotal proportion. In each case, to avoid injuring the testicle, I divided the large peritoneal sac at its neck, ligated the proximal end, and left the distal sac undisturbed. The overlay grafts initially used alone proved insufficient to protect the internal ring, and both cases recurred as indirect hernias. The error in both cases was not to have protected the internal ring. I now use a single Marcy suture in type III hernias to secure the internal ring after I have inserted the umbrella plug; then I apply the overlay graft.

The strategy of this repair is similar to that of Stoppa's technique: principally, once the internal ring has been cleared of the neck of the peritoneal sac, access to the ring by the peritoneum can be occluded by positioning an intervening mesh. By applying traction on the head of the sac, its neck and "shoulders" are freed of adhesions, allowing the potential preperitoneal space to be actualized (Fig. 13-11). This is akin to Henry's[3] description of the false neck and true neck of the peritoneal sac. Dissection of the shoulders I describe for the graft to be placed is performed in an area of greater radius from the internal ring than is

Henry's description of the true neck. This repair is accomplished instantaneously by inserting an umbrella plug of polypropylene mesh through the internal ring into the newly developed preperitoneal space. There, it opens between the invaginated peritoneal sac and the endopelvic fascia that surrounds the ring. Hydrostatic pressure conveyed through the peritoneal sac deep to the graft immediately fixes it in place against the anterior abdominal wall (the Pascal principle). The greater the pressure generated by natural stresses (ie, coughing, straining), the firmer the bond becomes. The functional energy of this repair is to capture and use the same force that created the hernia to repair it. Because it has memory to return to its flat contour, polypropylene mesh is the only available prosthetic material suitable for this repair.

The second aspect of this repair provides protection of the canal's normal posterior wall from future development of an incipient direct hernia. This important step is accomplished without cutting or repositioning existing normal tissues, as traditionally is done in the Bassini repair and all its modifications. A swatch of mesh placed flat against the posterior wall is covered and secured by the external oblique aponeurosis closed above it. Because suturing the mesh is unnecessary, technical mistakes described as errors of commission are avoided.

Of all current repairs for indirect inguinal hernias, none can be done more simply, with less expense, and with better results than the "sutureless repair." For complex, more challenging, large, or recurrent hernias, Stoppa's repair has proven most effective.

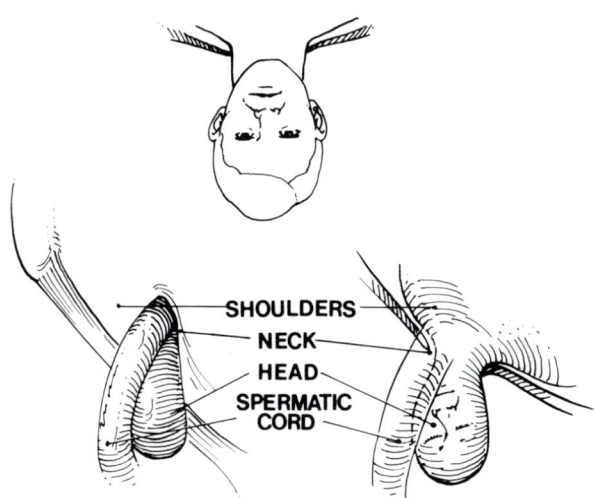

Figure 13-11. The peritoneal sac is analogous to the head, neck, and shoulders of a human figure. The potential space between the shoulders of the peritoneum and the endopelvic fascia is actualized by a high surgical dissection. After invaginating the peritoneum, prosthetic mesh is passed through the internal ring and positioned in this actualized preperitoneal space.

SHOULDERS
NECK
HEAD
SPERMATIC CORD

REFERENCES

1. Gilbert AI. An anatomic and functional classification for the diagnosis and treatment of inguinal hernia. Am J Surg 1989;157:331.
2. Gilbert AI. Sutureless repair of inguinal hernia. Am J Surg 1992;163:331.
3. Henry AK, Dub MB. Operation for femoral hernia by a midline extraperitoneal approach: with a preliminary note on the use of this route for reducible inguinal hernia. Lancet 1936;1:531.
4. Lichtenstein IL. Hernia repair without disability, ed 2. St Louis, Ishiyaku EuroAmerica, 1986.
5. Read RC. Influence of a relaxing incision on suture tension in Bassini's and McVay's repairs. Arch Surg 1981;116:440.
6. Shulman AG, Amid PK, Lichtenstein IL. The safety of mesh repair for primary inguinal hernias. Am Surg 1992;58:255.

Hernia, Fourth Edition, edited
by Lloyd M. Nyhus and Robert E. Condon.
J.B. Lippincott Company, Philadelphia © 1995.

Chapter 14

Groin Hernia Surgery in an Office-Based Surgical Suite

Ira M. Rutkow and Alan W. Robbins

Along with many other cost-saving approaches in modern health care, specialized surgical care provided in single-specialty institutions is becoming a widely accepted economic concept. Coincidentally, there have been recent discussions in the surgical literature regarding presumably better short- and long-term results obtained by specialized hernia surgeons or services in comparison to those obtained by general surgeons.[3,5] Whether we, as a profession, should promote this novel idea as the most effective means of obtaining presumably better operative results is an intriguing question, but one that is fraught with numerous pitfalls.

Yet, in full recognition of this super-specialist concept, a growing number of surgeons in North America have developed a special interest in hernia surgery, and some have built their own facilities exclusively for this purpose. The most prominent example of this unique approach to hernia repair is the Shouldice Hospital in Toronto, Canada.[10] In a medical facility devoted entirely to a single class of surgical operations, preoperative, operative, and postoperative protocols can be standardized more easily. Standardization should have a positive effect on the results and cost-effectiveness of surgery.

There are no inpatient facilities strictly dedicated to the repair of abdominal wall hernias in the United States. Surgeons at The Hernia Center in Freehold, New Jersey, however, have begun to offer office-based herniorrhaphy in a private ambulatory surgical suite.[1,2,4] Although the concept of office-based surgery is regarded as a recent phenomenon, it actually harkens back to a pre–World War II era of surgical health care delivery. During that period, it was common for old-time general practitioners/surgeons to perform numerous operations, including tonsillectomy, adenoidectomy, and groin hernia surgery, within the confines of their own offices. Costs were reduced and the physician enjoyed great time savings and increased overall practice efficiency.

It was during the 1980s that the concept of ambulatory surgery again became widely accepted in the United States. Many privately owned office-based operating suites were built during this decade, primarily by ophthalmologists and plastic surgeons. This trend now is spreading to other surgical specialties, including general surgery. For instance, The Hernia Center houses what is believed to be the country's first Medicare-approved and state-inspected office-based operating suite dedicated solely to the ambulatory repair of abdominal wall hernias (Figs. 14-1 through 14-4). The 5800–sq ft facility includes two operating suites, a three-bed recovery room, and a six-bed post-recovery area.[8]

By moving away from the hospital, the office-based operating suite provides the surgeon with greater control over his or her practice and time usage. The patient also has a more pleasant experience, including the scheduling of the operation. Turnaround time between procedures in an office-based operating room is a fraction of that at a hospital. Inefficient hospital practices can be eliminated in the office without sacrificing quality of care. Most important from an economic standpoint, the overall cost of a hernia repair can be reduced strikingly by decreasing the facility charges.

As a consequence, global packages (ie, surgeon, anesthesiologist, and facility fees grouped together) can be offered to managed-care plans, health maintenance organizations, large employers, labor unions, and others at reduced rates compared to existing charges for a "standard" hospital-based herniorrhaphy. This reduces the payer's overall medical costs and should result in more referrals to the office-based operating surgeon.

At The Hernia Center, our caseload of about 500 to 1000 groin hernias per year made it financially tenable for us to construct a facility dedicated to ambulatory hernia surgery. Since moving into our surgical suite, we have been able to increase our efficiency such that we normally complete five hernioplasties by 1:00 PM. Using epidural anesthesia and a tension-free mesh plug repair, our patients are discharged routinely within 2 hours of completion of their operation.[6,9]

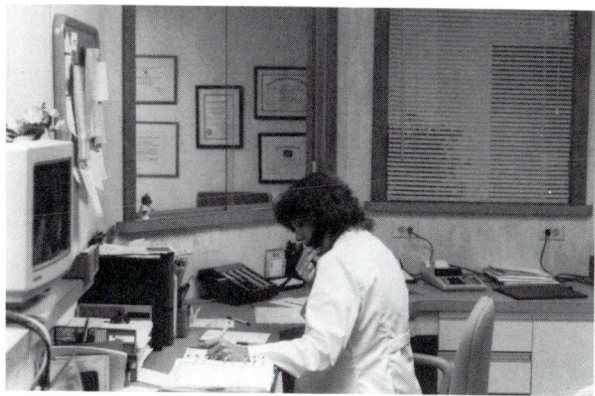

Figure 14-1. Reception area serving both the physician's office and the surgical suite.

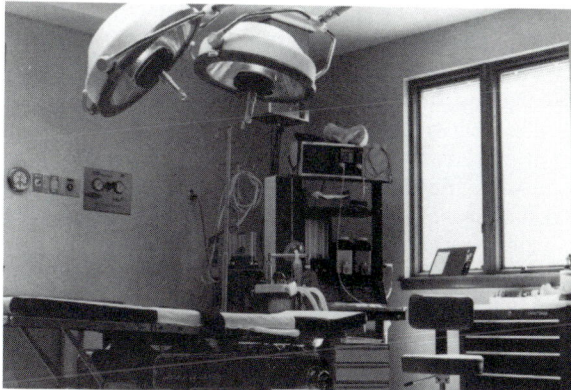

Figure 14-3. One of The Hernia Center's two operating rooms.

Costs for disposable items—for example, gloves, drapes, gowns, epidural trays, sutures—and for the Marlex mesh plug have remained less than $200 per case. This monetary efficiency permits us to remain financially solvent even in the face of ever-decreasing reimbursements for our facility. For example, our Medicare facility reimbursement in mid-1993 averaged $650 for all recurrent and primary groin hernia repairs.

For the office staff at The Hernia Center, the construction of our own surgical facility has brought about much greater office efficiency. Both new and old patients now are scheduled for examination during the turnaround breaks between cases. This better use of office time permits the staff to complete their usual workday by 2:00 to 3:00 PM.

Many health care officials and lawmakers are concerned about the quality of care that patients receive in privately owned, freestanding centers and office-based facilities. There is a special urgency to their anxiety, because studies by the Inspector General of the Department of Health and Human Services and by the United States General Accounting Office show that many out-of-hospital surgery centers, particularly those owned by individual physicians, complete their activities with little or no special licensing or certification. They are, in effect, practicing surgery in a virtually unregulated environment. Such conditions should not be allowed, and surgeons should be legally, if not morally and ethically, restrained from practicing in such a facility.

To ensure quality of care, the following steps must be undertaken if a surgeon wishes to perform hernia repairs within the confines of a private office. The operating room facility must be licensed or certified by the state as a medical facility. It is absolutely essential that Medicare certification be received, as well as accreditation by other professional groups that set standards. Among these are the Joint Commission on Accreditation of Health Care Organizations and the Accreditation Association for Ambulatory Health

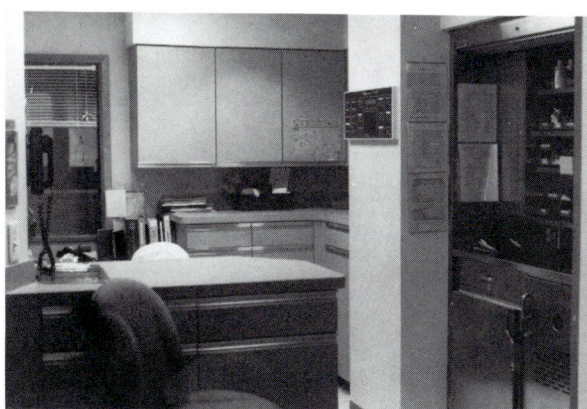

Figure 14-2. Nurses' station in the surgical suite.

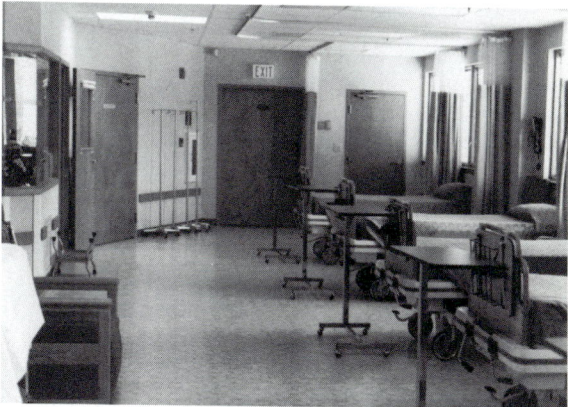

Figure 14-4. The six-bed postrecovery area.

Care. Even if local anesthesia is the anesthetic of choice, it is helpful if a certified nurse-anesthetist or even an anesthesiologist is present. The legal risks of not having such coverage, despite the admirable intent of decreasing health care costs, are too significant in our overly litigious society. Any individual who administers anesthesia that is other than local in an office-based surgical suite should be fully trained and certified in this specialty. Emergency plans and equipment, including full resuscitation capabilities, must be available in the facility in case medical or surgical problems arise. Finally, the availability of a bona fide patient transfer plan to a full-service acute-care hospital is an absolute necessity. Accordingly, any surgeon who wishes to perform hernia surgery in the office must continue to maintain admitting privileges to a nearby acute-care hospital.

The ever-changing socioeconomic environment in which American surgeons practice requires new approaches to maintaining quality of care while controlling costs. The advent of groin hernia surgery conducted in an office-based surgical suite will be among these important new changes.[7]

REFERENCES

1. Crane M. Does a practice need a gimmick to survive today. Medical Economics 1986;132.
2. Crane M. What $1 million in advertising can buy. Medical Economics 1992;87.
3. Deysine M, Grimson R, Soroff HS. Inguinal herniorrhaphy: reduced morbidity by service standardization. Arch Surg 1991;126:628.
4. Holden JM. MD's find market niche with N.J. hernia center. AMA Med News 1988;17.
5. Iles JD. Specialization in elective herniorrhaphy. Lancet 1965;1:751.
6. Robbins AW, Rutkow IM. The mesh-plug hernioplasty. Surg Clin North Am 1993;73:501.
7. Rutkow IM. Laparoscopic hernia repair: the socioeconomic tyranny of surgical technology. Arch Surg 1992;127:1271.
8. Rutkow IM, Robbins AW. Demographic, classificatory, and socioeconomic aspects of hernia repair in the United States. Surg Clin North Am 1993;73:413.
9. Rutkow IM, Robbins AW. "Tension-free" inguinal herniorrhaphy: a preliminary report on the "mesh plug" technique. Surgery 1993;114:3.
10. Welsh DRJ, Alexander MAJ. The Shouldice repair. Surg Clin North Am 1993;73:451.

Hernia, Fourth Edition, edited
by Lloyd M. Nyhus and Robert E. Condon.
J.B. Lippincott Company, Philadelphia © 1995.

Chapter 15

Laparoscopic Herniorrhaphy
Eric B. Rypins

The clinical use of therapeutic laparoscopy has grown exponentially since the incorporation of video technology. The ability to perform common procedures under laparoscopic control has resulted in its application to a wide variety of surgical problems. The advantages of laparoscopic cholecystectomy in reducing postoperative pain, length of hospital stay, and disability are well documented and accepted. The laparoscopic repair of inguinal hernia, however, remains controversial. The rationale for using the laparoscopic approach for hernia repair is the same as for other laparoscopic procedures, namely small incisions, less postoperative pain, and a shorter period of disability. Weighed against it are the disadvantages: lack of a standard technique, potential for intraabdominal injury and adhesion formation, necessity of general anesthesia, unknown long-term outcome with respect to recurrence, and increased costs related to materials and supplies used. Since the first report, various techniques have been described, and have either evolved or been discarded.

Inguinal herniorrhaphy through an anterior open approach is a time-tested, safe, and well-understood operation that has a reasonably high success rate. It can be performed using general, regional, or local anesthesia, and in either an inpatient or an outpatient setting with acceptable and reproducible results. Understandably then, there is a great deal of resistance to laparoscopic herniorrhaphy, because many surgeons see no reason to adopt a new, more expensive procedure when the standard one works well.[18,22] In addition, because there is considerable profit to be made from the sale of the high-technology products that are used in therapeutic laparoscopy, some have expressed their distress regarding the intrusion of commercial interests into the surgical decision- and policy-making processes.[27]

One of the primary concerns regarding laparoscopic herniorrhaphy are recurrence rates. Unfortunately, patients undergoing laparoscopic herniorrhaphy have not been followed up for 5 years, and most reports have average follow-up periods of less than 1 year. This makes it difficult to predict with any accuracy the ultimate incidence of recurrence. Some

techniques already have shown an unacceptably high recurrence rate within the first year, however, causing them to be modified or discarded.

Despite the controversy, there is a lively interest in laparoscopic herniorrhaphy, and the early results of various procedures have been reported. In addition to reports from individual surgeons and centers, a large multicenter trial is under way to assess the results of several different laparoscopic repairs. This chapter draws these data together in an attempt to put the current status of laparoscopic herniorrhaphy into perspective.

HISTORY OF LAPAROSCOPIC HERNIORRHAPHY

Ger[12] is credited with the first laparoscopic approach to hernia. In this initial series, hernias were repaired using Michel clips placed at open operation for problems other than the hernia. One patient in this series was described as having the procedure performed under laparoscopic guidance. Subsequently, Ger and colleagues[13] reported the repair of indirect hernias using a stapling instrument (Herniostat) developed for this purpose.

An intraabdominal suture repair has been described by Gazayerli,[11] who performs this technique through a transperitoneal approach. After everting the hernia sac and trimming away excess peritoneum, a sutured repair is carried out between the transversus abdominis aponeurotic arch and the iliopubic tract. If excessive tension is present, a relaxing incision is made in the transversalis fascia parallel and cephalad to the suture line. After the repair is completed, the peritoneum is reapproximated.

Other surgeons have taken a different approach and used prosthetic material to repair the defect. Schultz and associates[30] reported using a mesh plug technique and were one of the first groups to describe a series of patients with laparoscopically treated hernias. The plug and patch techniques described by Schultz[30] and Corbitt,[6] which involved the insertion of rolls of prosthetic material into the hernia defect, have been abandoned by both authors because of a high recurrence rate and patient complaints regarding migration of the plug into the scrotum. Over the last 4 years, laparoscopic hernia repair has evolved from simple closure of a small indirect hernia, to the placement of mesh plugs and a small mesh patch over the internal ring, to the current use of large pieces of prosthetic material to reinforce the lower abdominal wall.

The use of large mesh sheets placed into the preperitoneal space was foreshadowed by the open preperitoneal hernia repair reinforced with prosthetic mesh. This approach has been successful in the treatment of recurrent hernia.[24,26,33] Because this problem is associated with the highest rates of repeated recurrence, the success rates achieved by these authors have been cited frequently as a rationale for the laparoscopic techniques using large prosthetic mesh repairs. Most surgeons place a single large patch that covers the entire myopectineal orifice.[10] This area is an oval space formed by the rectus abdominis muscle and the pubic tubercle medially, the transversus abdominis arch superiorly, the psoas muscle laterally, and the Cooper ligament inferiorly.

Although a variety of laparoscopic repairs have been described, they can be categorized in general according to the approach used to expose the defect. Three exposures are used: the intraperitoneal approach in which the prosthesis is placed as an inlay graft over the peritoneum, the transabdominal preperitoneal repair, and the purely extraperitoneal approach.

Initial attempts at laparoscopic hernia repair were complicated by the need for suturing. The introduction of multiple-firing, angling, and rotating stapling devices has simplified the procedure greatly, decreasing operating times and increasing surgeon acceptance. The trade-off is that these devices increase the cost of the procedure significantly and require the use of larger trocar sheaths.

MATERIALS

Nonabsorbable prosthetic materials such as polypropylene (Prolene, Marlex) are the most popular choices for laparoscopic repair when the mesh is placed in the preperitoneal position. These materials are strong, easily stapled, and have interstices that allow for tissue ingrowth. They have been used extensively in the past, particularly for open anterior and posterior repairs, and are known to be durable and relatively resistant to infection.

If the prosthesis is exposed to the peritoneal cavity, as in intraperitoneal inlay repairs, e-polytetrafluoroethylene (e-PTFE) is the material of choice.[34,35]

This material comes in sheets either 1 or 2 mm thick. The 1-mm sheets are preferred because they are thin enough to be stapled. The 2-mm e-PTFE prosthesis must be sutured into place. PTFE is thought to be less likely than polypropylene to form adhesions to intraperitoneal structures.

ANATOMY OF THE INGUINAL CANAL— INTRAPERITONEAL LANDMARKS

All techniques of laparoscopic herniorrhaphy require a thorough understanding of the anatomy of the posterior inguinal canal. Visualization of the structures of the inguinal area is facilitated if the patient is placed in the Trendelenburg position and if a 30- or 45-degree, angled telescope is used. The lateral umbilical ligaments are useful landmarks for orienting the surgeon immediately on inspection of the pelvis. These structures are the remnants of the obliterated umbilical arteries, although they occasionally may contain a patent vessel. They originate at the internal iliac vessels and course anteriorly toward the umbilicus. After the umbilical ligaments have been located, the surgeon should inspect the internal rings. These often can be found by identifying the spermatic vessels and the vas deferens (Fig. 15-1). The spermatic vessels frequently are visible through the peritoneum, entering the internal ring from its lateral aspect. The vas deferens courses medially over the pelvic brim upward toward the internal ring, and joins the spermatic vessels as they enter the internal ring. Between these two structures lie the external iliac artery and vein. In normal patients, the internal inguinal ring is a dimple in the peritoneum where the vas deferens and spermatic vessels merge into the spermatic cord. The inferior epigastric vessels generally extend upward from the external iliac artery and vein, coursing along the medial side of the internal ring and then cephalad between the rectus abdominis muscle within its posterior sheath (Fig. 15-2).

By dissecting the peritoneum off the abdominal wall, additional structures are exposed. The pubic tubercle frequently is obscured by the lateral umbilical ligaments and preperitoneal fat. It is an important landmark, however, and can be palpated with the tip of a blunt instrument. It is important to identify the pubic tubercle early in the dissection because it is the point of insertion of the transversus abdominis arch, the iliopubic tract, and the Cooper ligament. The Cooper ligament is identified easily as a shiny, firm structure that can be palpated using a blunt probe. Following it inferolaterally from the pubic tubercle will lead to the external iliac vessels. Transversalis fascia analogues such as the iliopubic tract and the medial and lateral crura of the internal ring are

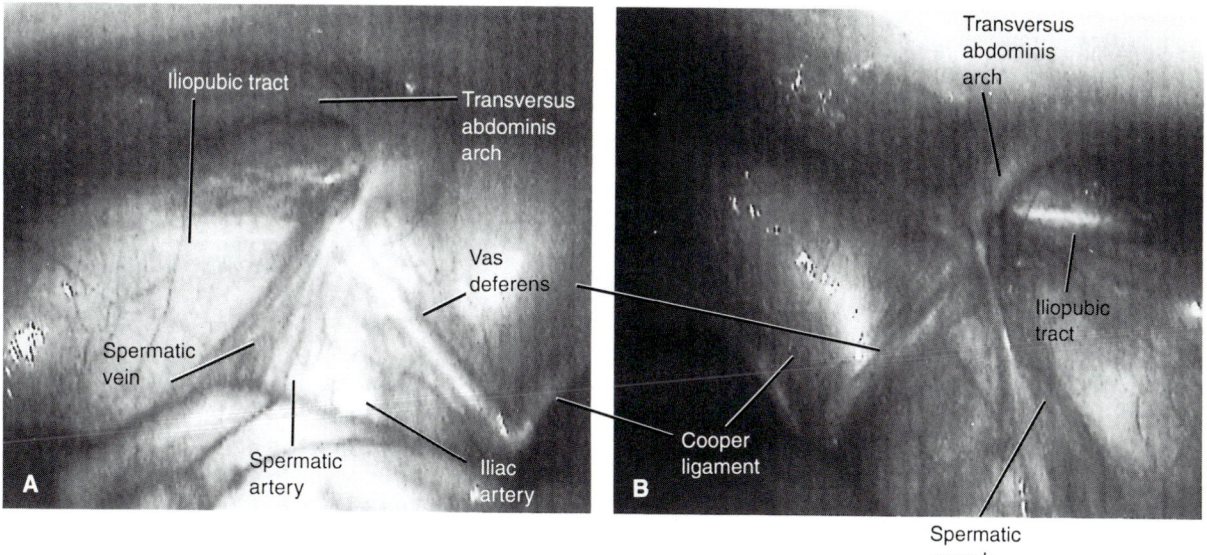

Figure 15-1.   (*A* and *B*) Laparoscopic view of bilateral indirect hernias in a thin patient. The vas deferens can be seen entering the medial edge of the hernia defect and the spermatic vessels can be seen entering more laterally. The external iliac artery and vein lie in the triangle formed by the vas deferens and the spermatic vessels. A portion of the iliopubic tract can be seen extending laterally from beneath the spermatic vessels.

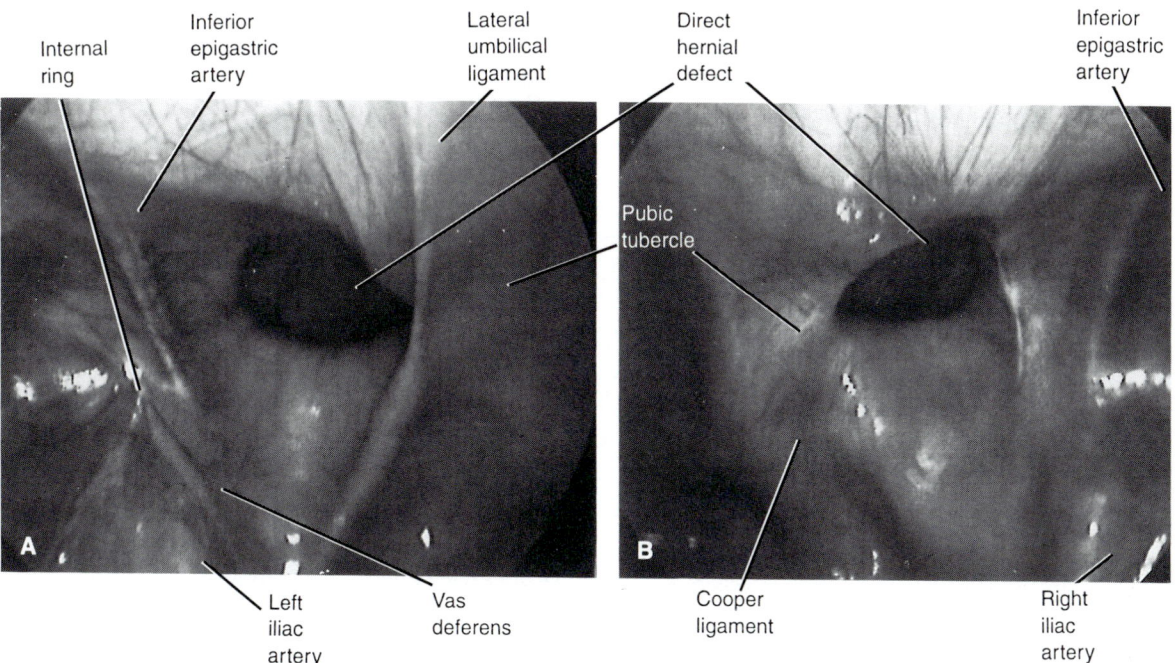

Figure 15-2.   Laparoscopic view of bilateral direct hernias. (*A*) The defect is between the inferior epigastric vessels and the lateral umbilical ligament. The internal ring can be found to the left of the epigastric vessels, with the vas deferens entering from the bottom of the picture. (*B*) A mirror image view. Here, the epigastric artery is displayed particularly well, arching upward from the external iliac artery along the edge of the rectus muscle.

identified more readily after stripping away the peritoneum. The medial iliopubic tract crosses the inferior border of the internal ring and separates the inguinal canal from the femoral canal. This structure usually is easy to see through the laparoscope and is an important landmark. The pubic branch of the inferior epigastric artery often can be seen immediately below the medial portion of the iliopubic tract. The junction of the transversus abdominis arch, the iliopubic tract, and the Cooper ligament at the pubic tubercle is an excellent orientation point. These structures can be followed superiorly, laterally, and inferiorly, and represent potential areas of fixation for mesh repairs of the inguinal canal. The lateral aspect of the iliopubic tract joins with transversus abdominis muscle fibers to create the lateral border of the internal ring. Following the iliopubic tract laterally will lead to the anterior superior iliac spine.

The nerves in the area of dissection include the genitofemoral nerve, the femoral nerve, and the lateral femoral cutaneous nerve. The genitofemoral nerve arises from the first and second lumbar nerves, and courses through the psoas muscle before emerging on its ventral surface. It commonly divides into a femoral and a genital branch proximal to the internal ring. The genital branch continues along the psoas major, perforates the iliopubic tract, and joins the spermatic cord at the internal inguinal ring. It supplies sensory innervation to the scrotal skin and medial thigh, and motor innervation to the cremaster muscle. The femoral branch of the genitofemoral nerve follows the psoas muscle more laterally and continues under the iliopubic tract, supplying sensation to the proximal anterior thigh in the femoral triangle.

The femoral nerve arises from the lumbar plexus (L2, L3, and L4) and emerges through the fibers of the psoas major muscle at the distal part of its lateral border. From there, it passes between the psoas and the iliacus, lying lateral and deep to the external iliac artery, and then passes under the iliopubic tract and breaks up into branches in the upper thigh. Its sensory branches in the thigh are the intermediate cutaneous nerve and the medial cutaneous nerve. These nerves supply sensation to the anterior and medial thigh from below the femoral triangle to the knee.

The lateral femoral cutaneous nerve arises from L2-3 and travels through the psoas major muscle. It emerges from the mid-portion of the psoas along its lateral border and runs across the iliacus obliquely toward the anterior superior iliac spine. It then passes under the lateral portion of the iliopubic tract. This nerve supplies sensation to the lateral aspect of the thigh and injury to it produces the syndrome of meralgia paresthetica. The ilioinguinal and iliohypogastric nerves exit the abdominal cavity above the iliac crest and usually are not within the limits of dissection.

OPERATIVE EXPOSURES FOR LAPAROSCOPIC HERNIORRHAPHY

Three different operative exposures are used for laparoscopic hernia repair: purely intraperitoneal exposure with intraperitoneal repair or inlay graft, transabdominal preperitoneal exposure with preperitoneal repair, and purely extraperitoneal exposure.

Intraperitoneal Inlay Prosthesis

In the intraperitoneal repair with an inlay graft, the prosthesis is placed within the peritoneal cavity.[29,34,35] The operation described here is the one used by Toy and Smoot.[35] After insufflation of the abdominal cavity and insertion of the laparoscope, two additional trocars are placed under direct vision. The medial umbilical ligament is incised to expose the Cooper ligament and pubic tubercle. An e-PTFE prosthesis 1 mm thick, 7.5 cm wide, and 10 cm long is placed on a patch spreader and fixed with staples medially to the pubic tubercle, inferiorly to the Cooper ligament (stopping medial to the vas deferens), anteromedially to the posterior rectus sheath, anteriorly to the transversalis fascia, and laterally to the endoabdominal fascia just lateral to the cord structures. The prosthesis is left exposed within the peritoneal cavity. Toy and Smoot noted that, of the first 75 patients who underwent this procedure, 4 required conversion to open herniorrhaphy when they were discovered to have large, direct sliding hernias with bladder making up the medial wall of the sac.

Filipi and coworkers[7] have used this approach selectively for smaller indirect hernias, but recommend the transabdominal preperitoneal approach for direct and sliding indirect hernias. Compared to the transabdominal preperitoneal approach, the intraperitoneal inlay technique has the advantages of being less time-consuming to perform and requiring less dissection of the preperitoneal space, decreasing the risk of hematoma formation. The mesh must be anchored firmly, however, so that it does not migrate into the hernia sac. Moreover, this approach has the disadvantage of leaving prosthetic material exposed within the peritoneal cavity.

Transabdominal Preperitoneal Prosthetic Repair

The transabdominal preperitoneal prosthetic repair is one of the most popular approaches used for laparoscopic herniorrhaphy. The abdomen is insufflated with CO_2 and the laparoscope is introduced through an umbilical incision. Two accessory trocars are used to provide access for dissecting instruments and the stapler. After both groins have been inspected, the hernia defect is exposed by making a second incision in the pelvic peritoneum several centimeters above the hernia defect. The peritoneum is dissected bluntly away from the abdominal wall, allowing the hernia sac to be inverted and dissected free of underlying adherent tissue. Alternatively, the neck of the sac may be incised and separated from the peritoneum with the scrotal component of the sac left in place. After the peritoneum has been dissected away from the abdominal wall, preperitoneal fat is removed to allow identification of the transversus abdominis arch, the pubic tubercle, the iliopubic tract, and the Cooper ligament. A prosthetic mesh of sufficient size (usually at least 10 × 12 cm) is inserted and fixed in place with sutures or staples so that it covers the entire myopectineal orifice. The peritoneum is closed over the mesh with staples or suture. This approach has the advantage of permitting inspection of the abdomen in general, and of the opposite side in particular, enabling bilateral repairs to be performed if necessary. In addition, exposure usually is excellent. The disadvantage is that a wider dissection is required to accommodate the mesh than is used in the intraperitoneal inlay approach. In addition, the intraabdominal incision presents the possibility of injury to intraperitoneal structures, and a second peritoneal incision in the groin increases the potential for adhesion formation and late bowel obstruction.

Preperitoneal Approach[2,21,25,37]

The preperitoneal approach is a laparoscopic adaptation of the open posterior preperitoneal approach first described by Annandale.[1] It has been modified and adapted for the treatment of recurrent hernia using prosthetic mesh, with superior results.[24] In the preperitoneal technique, the laparoscope is introduced into the preperitoneal space through an incision in the umbilicus. Some surgeons perform a brief laparoscopic examination of the abdomen and both groins before withdrawing the laparoscope and beginning the preperitoneal repair. The peritoneum is dissected toward the symphysis pubis, the Cooper ligament, and the iliac vessels using a blunt probe or clamp. CO_2 is insufflated into the preperitoneal space to maintain exposure. Care must be taken to avoid entering the peritoneum; if this occurs, loss of pressure in the preperitoneal space results and exposure is lost. A prosthetic mesh is used to reconstruct the inguinal floor and is fixed to the Cooper ligament, along the iliopubic tract, and to the edge of the rectus sheath using staples or sutures. In cases of indirect hernia, the sac usually is reduced. Typically, the mesh

is slit so that it can be placed around the cord in the preperitoneal space. Proponents of this procedure note that the insufflation pressure must be kept at less than 12 mmHg to avoid widespread subcutaneous emphysema. This approach avoids the risk of intraperitoneal adhesions while maintaining the advantages of minimally invasive surgery. The operating space is more limited than in transabdominal preperitoneal repairs, however, and the procedure can be more tedious and time-consuming.

COMPLICATIONS OF LAPAROSCOPIC HERNIORRHAPHY

Recurrence after repair of groin hernia is a commonly reported complication of anterior inguinal wall repairs. Rydell[28] reported an overall complication rate of 7% in a series of 961 hernia operations. Rates of recurrence and several other complications of open inguinal hernia repair are shown in Table 15-1. One of the lowest recurrence rates in the literature has been reported by Lichtenstein and colleagues[19] in a large series of patients undergoing open herniorrhaphy in which prosthetic mesh was used routinely. Their long-term follow-up and remarkable success with the "tension-free repair" has provided much of the stimulus for the development of laparoscopic methods that use prosthetic mesh.

A report of a large multicenter trial reviewed the complications of laparoscopic herniorrhaphy in 762 patients with 841 inguinal hernias.[20] This was a nonrandomized study in which the surgical techniques of the participants were not regulated strictly. The report has provided some data that allow conclusions to be drawn regarding the efficacy of several types of repair, and has produced some insight into the way in which laparoscopic herniorrhaphy has evolved in the larger centers. In this series, hernia repairs were classified as follows:

Type I: High ligation of an indirect sac and closure of the inguinal ring in patients with indirect hernias. The sac was not removed and the ring was closed with either staples or suture.

Type II: The "plug and patch" repair of indirect hernias in which the sac was disconnected from the peritoneum, the defect was plugged with nonabsorbable prosthetic material, and a small piece of mesh was used to cover the defect.

Type III: Repair in which a direct or indirect herniorrhaphy was performed by suture approximation of the transversalis fascia to the iliopubic tract or the Cooper ligament. This

Table 15-1.   Complications of Open Herniorrhaphy

Recurrence rates: (Nyhus et al, 1991[23]; collected series)
  Indirect: 1%–7%
  Direct: 4%–10%
  Femoral: 0%–7%
  Recurrent: 1.7%–35%
Urinary retention: 0.2%–15% (Finley et al, 1991[8]; Kozol et al, 1992[16])
Ischemic orchitis and testicular atrophy: 0.03%–0.65% (Fong and Wantz, 1992[9])
Wound infection: (Condon and Nyhus, 1989[5])
  Primary repair: 1%
  Recurrence: 3%
Neuroma of ilioinguinal or genitofemoral nerves: < 1%.

essentially was a standard type of repair performed laparoscopically from a posterior approach.

  Type IV: Repair using a large, nonabsorbable mesh prosthesis to cover the myopectineal orifice. Within this classification, there were three subclassifications, depending on whether the mesh was placed as an intraperitoneal inlay, through a transabdominal preperitoneal exposure, or outside the peritoneum.

During the course of their review, the authors noted that the type II repair (plug and patch) was abandoned by the surgeons who initially had used it because of significant complications and high recurrence rates. They also observed that type III repairs were described as being technically challenging and were associated with more complications. With regard to type IV repairs, they noted that the size of the mesh used increased progressively as the surgeon gained experience. This led them to conclude that the best results were achieved by covering the entire myopectineal orifice with the prosthesis. They noted that recurrences usually occurred early in the surgeon's experience and in cases involving smaller pieces of

mesh. These authors recommend using a patch that is 10 × 12 cm or larger, and reinforcing the abdominal wall from the pubic tubercle to the anterior superior iliac spine and from above the transversus abdominis arch to the Cooper ligament.

  Surgical complications and recurrence rates are summarized in Table 15-2. Specific complications reported after type I repairs included testicular pain (2) and two cases of recurrence. Recurrence was the most common complication after type II repairs (6), followed by palpable mesh in the scrotum (4), bladder injury (1), and hydrocele (1). After type III repairs, there were two cases of recurrence, one bladder injury, and one hydrocele, and two procedures were converted to open approaches because of inability to visualize adequately the iliopubic tract.

  The complications associated with intraperitoneal placement of a prosthesis included six cases of recurrence (3.2%; including two "retained hernias" that did not disappear postoperatively, although patients remained asymptomatic), three scrotal hydroceles, two bladder injuries, thigh pain, urinary retention, hematomas in the scrotum or in the trocar site puncture wounds (3%), hydrocele, and pain or numbness in the anterior or lateral aspect of the thigh. In this series, MacFadyen and coworkers[20] mention that, although no case of bowel obstruction occurred, they did receive a personal communication describing the occurrence of this complication after an intraperitoneal inlay prosthesis repair. Arregui and associates[3] reported an infection of an intraperitoneal inlay graft associated with dense adherence of the cecum to the prosthesis, obliteration of the appendix, and an associated abscess. Although this may have been the result of an episode of acute appendicitis, their group has decided to stop using the intraperitoneal inlay technique pending long-term follow-up results of patients who underwent intraabdominal inlay graft repairs.

  Among the patients who underwent transabdominal preperitoneal repair with mesh, 11 had hematomas (7 scrotal, 2 trocar site, 2 retroperitoneal), 8 had thigh numbness (2.2%), and 7 had urinary retention

Table 15-2.   Complications of Laparoscopic Herniorrhaphy

	Average Age (y)	No. of Patients/Hernias	Total Complications, Including Recurrence	Recurrence (average mo. follow-up)
Type I	< 50	87/98	2.2%	2.2% (24)
Type II	< 50	74/84	13.5%	6.8% (8)
Type III	< 55	28/30	19.8%	6.6% (6)
Type IV (all types)	48	563/635	9.0%	1.4% (5.6)
Intraperitoneal	48	182/186	7.3%	3.2% (<5)
Transabdominal preperitoneal	52	328/359	9.3%	0.8% (5)
Extraperitoneal	45	53/90	7.7%	0.0% (7)

(MacFadyen BV Jr, Arregui ME, Corbitt JD Jr, et al: Complications of laparoscopic herniorrhaphy. Surg Endosc 1993;7:155)

(2.0%). There were three cases of recurrence in this group (0.84%).

Among patients who underwent extraperitoneal repair, there were no cases of recurrence, six cases of postoperative hematoma (five in the inguinal canal and one in the abdominal wall), and one case of testicular pain. All the hematomas resolved spontaneously in less than 4 weeks.

Initially, it was believed that laparoscopic herniorrhaphy would result in fewer nerve injuries because the ilioinguinal and iliohypogastric nerves were outside the operating field. Almost all series report nerve injuries associated with laparoscopic herniorrhaphy, however, although most are transient. Two recent abstracts presented at the 1993 Scientific Session of the Society of American Gastrointestinal and Endoscopic Surgeons addressed the problems of nerve injury associated with laparoscopic herniorrhaphy.[17,31] Reports of lateral and anterior thigh numbness are consistent with irritation or injury to the lateral femoral cutaneous nerve and the femoral branch of the genitofemoral nerve, respectively. Although most of these complications resolve in 3 to 4 weeks, a few persist for months and are associated with significant disability. These nerves lie in close approximation to the lateral iliopubic tract and may be injured by sutures or staples placed either into the iliopubic tract lateral to the internal ring or into the psoas muscle. The genital branch of the genitofemoral nerve courses through the lateral aspect of the internal ring and can be injured at this point, resulting in numbness or causalgia of the scrotum. Testicular pain occurring after laparoscopic hernia repair has been attributed to dissection of an indirect hernia sac from the cord structures, because this has not been seen in patients undergoing intraperitoneal inlay prosthetic repair or procedures in which the hernia sac is divided at its neck.

Injury to the iliac vein and artery is possible during laparoscopic hernia repair, although this did not occur in the large series cited earlier. Spaw and associates[32] have pointed out the pertinent anatomic landmarks for identifying the iliac vessels, and describe a "triangle of doom" to avoid in dissecting the inguinal canal. This area is identified as a triangle created by the vas deferens medially and the spermatic vessels laterally. Arregui and colleagues[4] recommend that the triangle of doom be extended to include the lateral iliopubic tract and be renamed the "triangle of peril" because of the likelihood of nerve entrapment when sutures or staples are placed in this area.

The most common complications seen in this series were hematomas found in the scrotum, along the spermatic cord, or in trocar sites. Although they were not mentioned in MacFadyen's[20] series, trocar site hernias have been reported after laparoscopic operations when trocars larger than 10 mm in diameter are

used and the fascia is not closed.[15] Most of these have resulted in omental incarceration, but bowel obstruction is possible. At our institution, a Richter hernia occurred in a trocar site stab wound 5 weeks after a gynecologic procedure requiring open laparotomy and bowel resection.

COST FACTORS

The cost of the procedure is another important factor. A procedure that requires general anesthesia and high-technology equipment undeniably is more expensive. The increased cost may be offset, however, by a more rapid recovery and shorter period of disability. No randomized, prospective trial of laparoscopic versus open herniorrhaphy has been published that compares the cost of the two procedures and also analyzes disability. An abstract has been published comparing the costs of unilateral, nonrecurrent hernia repair using laparoscopic and open techniques.[14] Based solely on average charges for operating time, supplies, and the total hospital bill, the authors found laparoscopic hernia repair to be 135% more expensive than open hernia repair at their institution. They noted that the quality of laparoscopic herniorrhaphy is unknown, and that morbidity, recovery time, and recurrence rates must be evaluated to determine whether the higher cost of supplies is warranted.

CONCLUSIONS

The future of laparoscopic herniorrhaphy is not entirely certain, and considerable debate surrounds its place in the treatment of inguinal hernia. Questions regarding long-term outcome and late complications cannot be answered without additional information. The necessity of general anesthesia represents a significant disadvantage as well. Based on the results of the multicenter trial reported earlier, laparoscopic herniorrhaphy is feasible and can be performed with acceptably low early recurrence rates. The best results have been obtained when a large prosthetic mesh is used to reinforce the myopectineal orifice. The advantages of shorter disability periods and less postoperative pain are difficult to prove.

Laparoscopic herniorrhaphy may have distinct advantages in the treatment of bilateral or recurrent inguinal hernias. The incidence of complications is likely to be lower and the recovery period shorter when it is used for these indications. Whether laparoscopic repair is better than standard anterior repair for uncomplicated inguinal hernias, however, is debatable. It is more expensive than open hernia repair, requires additional training and expertise beyond that required for laparoscopic cholecystectomy, and has a less dramatic advantage in terms of length of disability. Moreover, failure of a hernia repair generally is defined by recurrence; because about 50% of recurrences occur after 5 years, long-term follow-up is required to identify this complication. Randomized, prospective trials are necessary to show the benefits of laparoscopic over conventional hernia repair and the relative merits of different techniques of laparoscopic repair. Despite these concerns, laparoscopic herniorrhaphy repair is a reasonably safe procedure that can be performed with a low incidence of early recurrence and complication rates similar to those reported for anterior hernia repair. Future technologic advances may reduce the requirement for general anesthesia and lower the cost of materials. To represent a significant advance, however, laparoscopic herniorrhaphy should be able to duplicate the results of open herniorrhaphy performed in the outpatient setting using local anesthesia.

REFERENCES

1. Annandale T. Case in which a reducible oblique and direct inguinal and femoral hernia existed on the same side and were successfully treated by operation. Edinburgh Med J 1876;27:1087.
2. Arregui ME, Davis CJ, Yucel O, Nagan RF. Laparoscopic mesh repair of inguinal hernia using a preperitoneal approach: a preliminary report. Surg Laparosc Endosc 1992;2:53.
3. Arregui ME, Fitzgibbons RJ, Schultz LS. Laparoscopic hernia repair: experts discuss the best technical approach. Insights Today 1993;3:1.
4. Arregui ME, Navarrete J, Davis CJ, Castro D, Nagan RF. Laparoscopic inguinal herniorrhaphy. Techniques and controversies. Surg Clin North Am 1993;73:513.
5. Condon RE, Nyhus LM. Complications of groin hernia. In: Nyhus LM, Condon RE, eds. Hernia, ed 3. Philadelphia, JB Lippincott, 1989:253–269.
6. Corbitt JD. Laparoscopic herniorrhaphy. Surg Laparosc Endosc 1991;1:23.
7. Filipi CJ, Fitzgibbons RJ Jr, Salerno GM, Hart RO. Laparoscopic herniorrhaphy. Surg Clin North Am 1992;72:1109.
8. Finley RK Jr, Miller SF, Jones LM. Elimination of urinary retention following inguinal herniorrhaphy. Am Surg 1991;57:486.
9. Fong Y, Wantz GE. Prevention of ischemic orchitis during inguinal hernioplasty. Surg Gynecol Obstet 1992;174:399.
10. Fruchaud H. Anatomie chirurgicale des hernies de l'aine. Paris, Doin, 1956.
11. Gazayerli MM. Anatomical laparoscopic hernia repair of direct or indirect inguinal hernias using the transversalis fascia and iliopubic tract. Surg Laparosc Endosc 1992;2:49.
12. Ger R. The management of certain abdominal hernias by intraabdominal closure of the neck. Ann R Coll Surg Engl 1982;64:342.
13. Ger R, Monroe K, Duvivier R, Mishrick A. Management of indirect inguinal hernias by laparoscopic closure of the neck of the sac. Am J Surg 1990;159:370.
14. Gill BD, Traverso LW. Continuous quality inventory: open versus laparoscopic groin hernia repair. (Abstract) Surg Endosc 1993;7:116.
15. Jenkins DM, Paluzzi M, Scott TE. Postlaparoscopic small bowel obstruction. Surg Laparosc Endosc 1993;3:139.
16. Kozol RA, Mason K, McGee K. Post-herniorrhaphy urinary retention: a randomized prospective trial. J Surg Res 1992;52:111.
17. Kraus MA. Laparoscopic identification of preperitoneal nerve anatomy in the inguinal area. (Abstract) Surg Endosc 1993;7:114.
18. Lichtenstein IL, Shulman AG, Amid PK. Laparoscopic hernioplasty. Arch Surg 1991;126:1449.
19. Lichtenstein IL, Shulman AG, Amid PK, Montllor MM. The tension-free hernioplasty. Am J Surg 1989;157:188.
20. MacFadyen BV Jr, Arregui ME, Corbitt JD Jr, et al. Complications of laparoscopic herniorrhaphy. Surg Endosc 1993;7:155.
21. McKernan BJ, Laws HL. Laparoscopic repair of inguinal hernias using a totally extraperitoneal prosthetic approach. Surg Endosc 1993;7:26.
22. Nyhus LM. Laparoscopic hernia repair: a point of view. Arch Surg 1992;127:137.
23. Nyhus LM, Klein MS, Rogers FB. Inguinal hernia. Curr Probl Surg 1991;28:407.
24. Nyhus LM, Pollak R, Bombeck CT, Donahue PE. The preperitoneal approach and prosthetic buttress repair for recurrent hernia. Ann Surg 1988;208:733.
25. Phillips EH, Carroll BJ, Fallas MJ. Laparoscopic preperitoneal inguinal hernia repair without peritoneal incision: technique and early clinical results. Surg Endosc 1993;7:159.
26. Rignault DP. Properitoneal prosthetic inguinal hernioplasty through a Pfannenstiel approach. Surg Gynecol Obstet 1986;163:465.
27. Rutkow IM. Laparoscopic hernia repair. The socioeconomic tyranny of surgical technology. Arch Surg 1992;127:1271.
28. Rydell WB Jr. Inguinal and femoral hernias. Arch Surg 1963;87:493.
29. Salerno GM, Fitzgibbons RJ Jr, Filipi CJ. Laparoscopic inguinal hernia repair. In: Zucker KA, ed. Surgical laparoscopy. St Louis, Quality Medical Publishing, 1991:281–293.
30. Schultz L, Graber J, Pietrafitta J, Hickock D. Laser laparoscopic herniorrhaphy: a clinical trial preliminary results. J Laparoendosc Surg 1990;1:41.
31. Seid AS, Ruhalter A. Significance of groin nerve anatomy for laparoscopic hernia repair. (Abstract) Surg Endosc 1993;7:115.
32. Spaw AT, Ennis BW, Spaw LP. Laparoscopic hernia repair: the anatomic basis. J Laparoendosc Surg 1991;1:269.

33. Stoppa RE, Warlaumont CR. The preperitoneal approach and prosthetic repair of groin hernia. In: Nyhus LM, Condon RE, eds. Hernia. Philadelphia, JB Lippincott, 1989:199–225.
34. Toy FK, Smoot RT Jr. Toy-Smoot laparoscopic hernioplasty. Surg Laparosc Endosc 1991;1:151.
35. Toy FK, Smoot RT Jr. Laparoscopic herniorrhaphy update. J Laparoendosc Surg 1992;2:197.
36. Wantz GE. Atlas of hernia surgery. New York, Raven Press, 1991:4–5.
37. Willis IH, Sendzischew H. Laparoscopic preperitoneal prosthetic inguinal herniorrhaphy. J Laparoendosc Surg 1992;2:183.

Special Comment

Laparoscopic Repair of Recurrent Groin Hernias

Edward L. Felix

Fifty thousand recurrent hernias are repaired each year in the United States.[7] The surgical techniques used vary widely, but most are fixed through an anterior approach. As many as one third of all the repairs that are performed fail.[5] Reviews by Nyhus and colleagues[8] and by Stoppa[17] suggest that a mesh-buttressed posterior approach may reduce the rate of recurrence to less than 3%. When Schapp and associates[14] altered their technique by using only small pieces of mesh or no mesh at all, however, their recurrence rate reached 33%, suggesting that the extent of dissection and the size of the mesh are crucial. In an effort to reduce the morbidity and recovery time associated with the traditional posterior approach, but still achieve its low recurrence rate, we extended the original principles of a total mesh-buttressed repair to a laparoscopic approach. This approach was shown to be technically reliable for the repair of primary hernias. The recovery time was shorter and postoperative discomfort reduced. Therefore, we extended this laparoscopic approach to the repair of recurrent groin hernias.

MATERIALS AND METHODS

Over an 18-month period, 54 recurrent groin hernias were repaired in 50 patients, 48 men and 2 women. Patient age ranged from 12 to 86 years, with a mean of 55 years. Forty-six recurrent hernias were unilateral and 4 were bilateral. In only 10 patients was the contralateral side normal. Twenty-seven had a previous repair on the opposite side and 13 had a new contralateral hernia, 7 of which were repaired. The recurrent hernias consisted of 25 direct hernias, 19 indirect hernias, 10 pantaloon hernias, and 2 hernias with a femoral component. It was the first recurrence in 39 patients, the second in 10 patients, the third in 4 patients, and the fourth in 1 patient.

A transabdominal preperitoneal technique was used in all patients. The men were repaired using a double-buttress technique and the women were repaired using only a single sheet of mesh. The peritoneum was incised from lateral to medial and the preperitoneal space was opened. Both the medial and lateral floors were exposed. The hernia sac was dissected out of the recurrent defect using blunt and scissors dissection, with unipolar cautery applied as needed. Any persistent lipoma of the cord was removed. In the double-buttress repair, an oval mesh with a slit for the cord structures was cut from a 4- × 2½-inch polypropylene sheet. The wings of the slit were brought around the cord medially and stapled to the Cooper ligament. The upper part of the mesh was stapled to the transversalis fascia and the lower part to the iliopubic tract. A larger piece of mesh cut from a 6- × 6-inch polypropylene sheet was placed over the first piece to repair the direct floor and secure the area over the slit. It also was stapled in place with a multiple-firing hernia stapler. In the women, only the latter piece was used, and the round ligament was divided. The peritoneum was closed with a running Gore-Tex suture or staples in all patients. The fascial incisions were closed and Steri-strips were applied to the skin. Patients were discharged from the short-stay area and instructed to resume normal activity as tolerated.

RESULTS

Laparoscopic hernia repair was completed in all 50 patients explored. Examination of the patients took place at 1 week, 3 months, 6 months, and every 6 months thereafter. Follow-up ranged from 1 to 18 months, with a mean of 8 months. No recurrences have been found and none of the patients in this small group have been lost to follow-up. The most common complication was seroma formation, which occurred in 10% of the patients. The seroma resolved spontaneously in most cases and was aspirated successfully in the others. One small-bowel injury resulted from lysis of adhesions in a patient with a history of a previous ruptured appendix. This was repaired through the lateral port site. The patient has done well and shows no evidence of infection or recurrence more than 1 year after his operation. Other complications included urinary retention in one patient and a lateral cutaneous neuralgia in another patient who was undergoing his fourth repair for an incarcerated hernia. The pain and paresthesia lasted almost 6 months, but then resolved completely. Several patients have had transient scrotal discomfort with hyperesthesia after surgery, but all experienced spontaneous resolution.

DISCUSSION

Bassini's anterior floor repair was introduced a little more than 100 years ago and revolutionized inguinal herniorrhaphy. Recurrence rates were reduced to 10%, but have remained at this level to this day except in a few specialty centers. Several factors appear to be involved in the failure of primary hernia repair. Forty percent to 59% of recurrences are indirect, and 24% of these are the result of overlooked hernias.[9,10] Technical errors such as not dissecting or finding the sac, leaving too long a peritoneal stump, and closing the hernial orifice incorrectly lead to early indirect failure.[4,13] Thirty percent to 53% of recurrences are direct.[6] Most of these are the result of repairs made under tension, which cause holes, usually near the pubic tubercle.[9] Failure to identify and repair coexisting floor defects also results in early direct recurrence. Femoral hernias represent about 4% of recurrences and result from either overlooked hernias or upward traction on the iliopubic tract. In addition, studies have shown that intrinsic fascial weakness caused by abnormal collagen may play some role in influencing the fate of the hernia repair.[1] Eighty percent of the patients we saw for a recurrent hernia had bilateral disease, either previously repaired or new, suggesting that an intrinsic floor defect may be partially responsible for the failure of the primary repair.

Once a hernia repair has failed, the results of further efforts to correct the problem are even worse than with the first repair. Recurrence rates as high as 39% have been reported for repair of previously repaired groin hernias.[15] Improved results have been described with the use of mesh-buttressed repairs and a posterior approach.[8,12,18] Given the causes of recurrence (overlooked hernias, tension-disruption, intrinsic collagen weakness, and the late development of a new defect), improved results seem logical. The posterior or preperitoneal approach avoids previous scar and dissects the entire inguinal floor. It identifies clearly the hernia and any other potential sites of failure. This technique should eliminate overlooked hernias; Stoppa's only reported failures were technical and occurred within 1 year after surgery.[17] Open posterior repair, however, is associated with an uncomfortable recovery that may take as long as 6 weeks.

Laparoscopic preperitoneal hernioplasty, which was developed to shorten the recovery period, failed to heed the lessons taught by the open preperitoneal approach. Early investigators used small pieces of

mesh or none at all and failed to expose the entire floor.[16] Consequently, they obtained a high early recurrence rate. Other investigators, who used a larger mesh buttress, dissected the entire floor to avoid overlooking subtle defects, and stabilized the mesh with staples, have noted low early recurrence rates.[2,3]

The present study applied these principles to the laparoscopic repair of recurrent hernias. A double-buttressed repair, as described in this report, was used to ensure adequate closure of the internal ring and complete coverage of the entire floor. As in other studies using the laparoscopic approach to inguinal hernia repair,[20] recovery time and postoperative pain were reduced. The average time required for patients to return to normal daily activities was 1 week. No early recurrences were seen on close follow-up. Recurrence rates ranging from 4% to 11% at 1 year were noted in several studies using the open hernia repair and represented 25% to 50% of their long-term recurrence rate.[11,17] Although the mean follow-up period of our study was short (8 months), the absence of early recurrence appears to make it meaningful. It is almost certain that the words of Stoppa and coworkers,[19] "A hundred years after the famous Bassini, it is not possible these days to ignore the extraordinary possibilities offered by prostheses in groin hernia surgery," will be applied to the laparoscopic approach to inguinal hernioplasty for the repair of recurrent hernias.

REFERENCES

1. Clear J. Ten year statistical study of inguinal hernia. Arch Surg 1976;46:70.
2. Felix E, Michas C. The double-buttress laparoscopic herniorrhaphy. J Laparoendosc Surg 1993;1:1.
3. Ferzli GI, Massad A, Albert P. Extraperitoneal endoscopic inguinal hernia repair. J Laparoendosc Surg 1992;2:281.
4. Glassow F. Recurrent inguinal and femoral hernia. BMJ 1970;1:215.
5. Glassow F. Inguinal hernia repair: a comparison of the Shouldice and Cooper ligament repair of the posterior inguinal wall. Am J Surg 1976;131:306.
6. Marsden AJ. Recurrent inguinal hernia: a personal study. Br J Surg 1988;75:263.
7. Nyhus L. Recurrent groin hernia. World J Surg 1989;13:541.
8. Nyhus LM, Pollak R, Bombeck CT, Donahue P. The preperitoneal approach and prosthetic buttress repair for recurrent hernia. Ann Surg 1988;208:722.
9. Postlethwait RW. Causes of recurrence after inguinal herniorrhaphy. Surgery 1971;69:772.
10. Postlethwait RW. Recurrent inguinal hernia. Ann Surg 1985;207:277.
11. Read R. Recurrence after preperitoneal herniorrhaphy in the adult. Arch Surg 1975;110:666.
12. Rignault DP. Preperitoneal prosthetic inguinal her-

niorrhaphy through a Pfannenstiel approach. Surg Gynecol Obstet 1986;163:465.

13. Ryan EA. Recurrent hernias: an analysis of 369 consecutive cases of recurrent inguinal and femoral hernias. Surg Gynecol Obstet 1953;96:343.

14. Schapp HM, Van de Pavoordt HD, Bast TJ. The preperitoneal approach in the repair of recurrent inguinal hernias. Surg Gynecol Obstet 1992;174:460.

15. Shulman AG, Amid PK, Lichtenstein I. The safety of mesh repair for primary inguinal hernias: results of 3019 operations from five diverse surgical sources. Am Surg 1992;58:255.

16. Shultz L, Graber J, Pietrafitta J, Hickok P. Laser laparoscopic herniorrhaphy: a clinical trial: preliminary results. J Laparoendosc Surg 1990;1:41.

17. Stoppa R. The treatment of complicated groin and incisional hernias. World J Surg 1989;13:545.

18. Stoppa RE, Rives JL, Warlaumont CR, et al. The use of Dacron in the repair of hernias of the groin. Surg Clin North Am 1984;64:269.

19. Stoppa RE, Warlaumont CR, Verhaeghe PJ, et al. Prosthetic repair in the treatment of groin hernias. Int Surg 1986;71:154.

20. Voeller GR, Mangiante EC, Britt LG. Preliminary evaluation of laparoscopic herniorrhaphy. Surg Laparosc Endosc 1993;3:100.

Special Comment

Laparoscopic Hernia Repair Using the Dudai Butterfly With or Without Mesh, According to Nyhus Hernia Type

Mosha Dudai

Our approach to hernia repair is based on the distinction between small and large hernias. We have developed a completely new technique for small hernias (Nyhus types I and II) that is under investigation and still controversial (Fig. 15-3). For large hernias (Nyhus types III and IV), on the other hand, our recommended technique is based on experience that we and others have accumulated over recent years.[1-3]

The objective is to exploit the advantages of laparoscopy, compared to the anterior approach to hernia repair, to obtain a better surgical result. The basic strategy is to customize the repair technique to the hernia type, as classified by Nyhus, using the technique that is most appropriate for each class.[5]

Nyhus type I and II hernias are small, congenital defects in the internal ring, with an otherwise intact pelvic floor. The strength and integrity of the pelvic floor are not compromised, and a tension-free closure of the defect alone is sufficient. It is totally unnecessary, and potentially harmful, to repair the entire pelvic floor. Patients with these hernias usually are young and have strong abdominal walls and intact inguinal canal shutter mechanisms. In these patients, the anterior approach can cause structural damage. In addition, most surgeons add some form of plastic repair of the inguinal canal floor. In the laparoscopic approach, the defect is identified and repaired without injury to these abdominal structures. We suggest creating a small peritoneal opening behind the internal ring and performing minimal dissection around the ring, then achieving a tension-free closure of the defect using a small Dudai Butterfly (DB) (Figs. 15-4 and 15-5). The process takes only 15 to 20 minutes, trauma is minimal, the risk of damage to neurovascular structures is small, and unimpeded recovery is rapid. The incidence of recurrence is inconsequential.

Nyhus type III and IV hernias, however, have two components: a large defect in the abdominal wall (di-

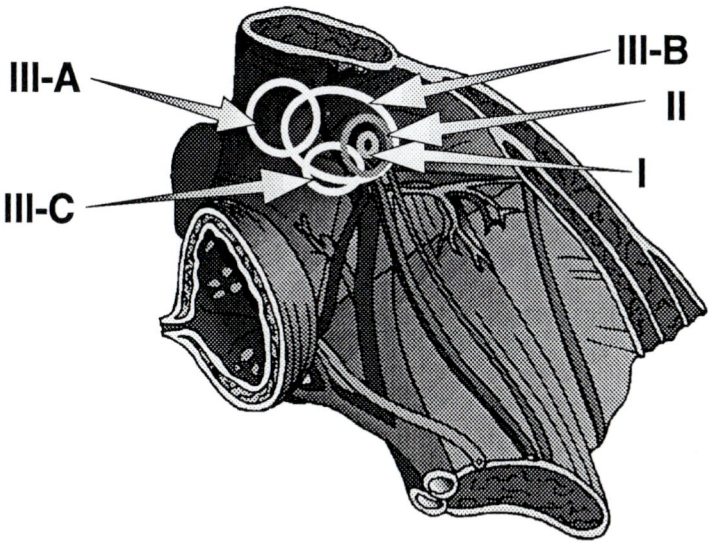

Figure 15-3. Hernia type according to Nyhus classification.

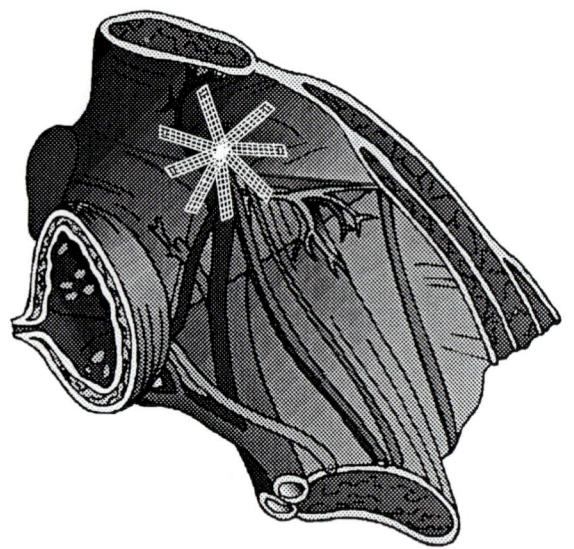

Figure 15-4. Small hernia: Nyhus type I and II. Repair by tension-free closure of the defect using a Dudai butterfly.

rect, indirect, and femoral), and weakening of the entire pelvic floor stemming from the large defect. In these hernias, repairing the defect is not sufficient; the entire pelvic floor must be repaired and reinforced. Neglecting this defect leaves the area weak in relation to the rest of the pelvic floor. This allows the covering mesh to invaginate the defect, sometimes resulting in recurrent hernias. Two-layer repairs prevent recurrence of these hernias. We believe that laparoscopy is superior to the anterior approach. Recurrence rates of 2% to 3% for large hernias are unacceptable. Nyhus[4] and Stoppa and Warlaumont,[6] using their procedures, have obtained better results. Two-layer repairs in large hernias achieve recurrence rates of less than 1%; this cannot be accomplished with one-layer repairs.

To repair the first layer, we recommend using the DB, which is easy to position and provides a tension-free closure and support of the defect. The DB also stimulates fibroblast proliferation. The subsequent placement of mesh gives the pelvic floor additional strength by creating uniform support for the entire area, including the hernia defect previously closed by the DB (see Fig. 15-5*B* and *C*).

Our approach can be summarized briefly as follows: small hernia, small repair; large hernia, large repair. In small hernias, we use only tension-free closure with the DB. In large hernias, we use a two-layer repair, with the DB as the first layer covered by a wide mesh that serves as the second layer.

METHODS

Small Hernia—Nyhus Types I and II (see Figs. 15-3 and 15-4)

Step 1. A small opening is made in the peritoneum behind the ring at its upper level. The sac is everted to the abdominal cavity.

Step 2. The upper flap is deperitonealized. Both sides of the internal ring are dissected, exposing the internal oblique muscle (including the iliopubic tract) laterally and the medial aspect of the inferior epigastric vessels (IEV) on the Hesselbach triangle medially.

Step 3. The lower flap is deperitonealized. The peritoneum is separated from the cord elements, exposing the vas deferens and the spermatic vessels.

Step 4. A small DB is inserted and stapled to the abdominal wall at five fixed points, avoiding the "neurovascular triangle." The points of fixation are (1) lateral to the IEV in the anterior abdominal wall, (2) on the internal oblique muscle, (3) above the iliopubic tract, (4) medial to the IEV on the Hesselbach triangle, and (5) on or close to the Cooper ligament. The remaining three arms are left unstapled on the cord and at each of its sides.

Step 5. The peritoneum is closed with ordinary laparoscopic clips using the same "step-by-step" maneuver used to staple the skin closure.

Large Hernia—Nyhus Types III and IV (Fig. 15-6)

Step 1. The peritoneum is opened at the upper level of the defect from a point 2 cm medial to the anterior superior iliac spine to the medial umbilical ligament. By using this incision, we avoid the lateral femoral cutaneous nerve and the bladder. The sac undergoes "ring excision" as appropriate.

Step 2. The upper flap is deperitonealized. The entire pelvic floor undergoes a wide dissection laterally, exposing the internal oblique muscle and the iliopubic tract. The anterior abdominal wall is dissected medially, exposing the Hesselbach triangle, rectus muscle, pubic tubercle, and Cooper ligament. In large hernias, we divide the IEV, yielding free margins of the hernia defect and wide exposure of the pelvic floor for mesh fixation.

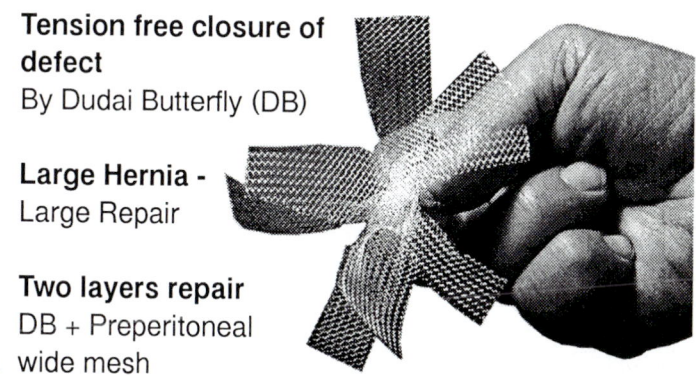

Small Hernia - Small Repair

Tension free closure of defect
By Dudai Butterfly (DB)

Large Hernia -
Large Repair

Two layers repair
DB + Preperitoneal
A wide mesh

DB1 = Dudai Butterfly

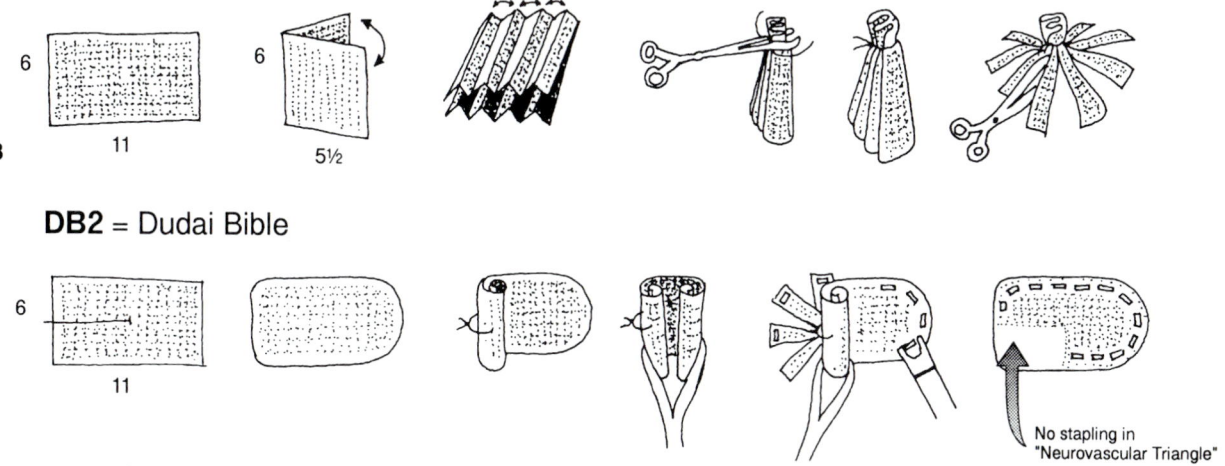

DB2 = Dudai Bible

No stapling in "Neurovascular Triangle"

Figure 15-5. (*A*) Concept and application of Dudai butterfly (DB). (*B*) Preparation of DB. (*C*) Preparation of Dudai "bible." The second layer of mesh is used for type III and IV hernias.

Step 3. The lower flap is deperitonealized. The peritoneum is separated from cord elements, exposing the vas deferens and spermatic vessels and the lateral aspect of the iliopubic tract. A space is created to allow the mesh to be inserted between the peritoneum and structures of the pelvic floor.

Step 4. A large DB is inserted and stapled to the abdominal wall in five fixed points, avoiding the "neurovascular triangle." The points of fixation are (1) the anterior abdominal wall above the defect, (2) the internal oblique muscle, (3) above the iliopubic tract, (4) the Hesselbach triangle, and (5) the Cooper ligament. The remaining three arms are left unstapled on the cord and at each of its sides.

Step 5. A wide mesh is positioned to cover the entire pelvic floor from the symphysis pubis to a point medial to the superior anterior iliac spine. The length of mesh needed (on the average, 6 × 10 cm) is measured by a thread of chromic catgut held between two grasping instruments. The mesh is stapled at the Cooper ligament, pubic tubercle, rectus muscle, anterior abdominal wall, and internal oblique muscle above the iliopubic tract, avoiding the "neurovascular triangle."

Step 6. The peritoneum is closed with ordinary laparoscopic clips using the same "step-by-step" maneuver used to staple the skin closure.

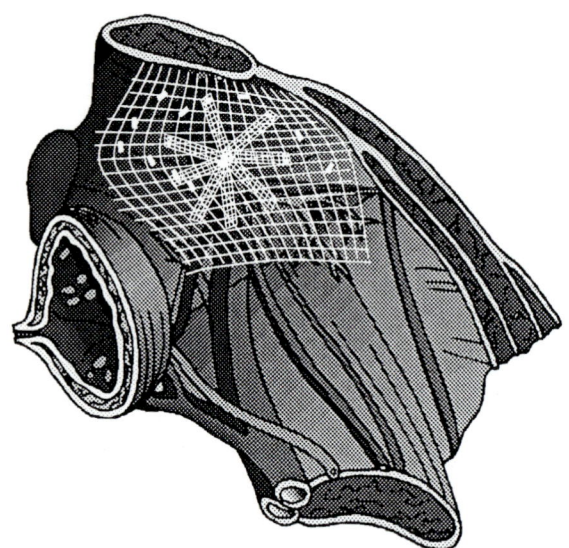

Figure 15-6. Double layer of mesh for type III and IV hernias. Repair by two layers: Dudai butterfly in the defect and wide mesh covering the entire pelvic floor.

RESULTS

During the 2-year period from September 1991 to September 1993, we performed 332 laparoscopic hernia repairs on 245 patients, 87 of whom had bilateral hernias (Table 15-3). The mean age was 43.8 years (range, 14–87 years). The distribution of hernias by Nyhus classification was as follows: type I—9, type II—93, type III—194 (subtypes A—84, B—101, C—9), and type IV—36. It is noteworthy that three fourths of the hernias were large and bilateral. This is relevant information, because it is important to know when checking recurrence rates, for example, whether an assessed rate of 0.5% occurred in large or in small hernias. It is of fundamental importance to report results in accordance with the Nyhus classification to facilitate the comparison of results from different centers.

At the conclusion of the procedure, we inject bupivacaine (Marcaine) 0.25% into both the preperitoneal space and the skin at the sites of penetration. No narcotics are administered postoperatively. Only 186 patients received simple analgesics for pain relief; 38 of them asked for a second dose.

With only a few exceptions, the patients were discharged from the hospital the morning after the operation. The average postoperative stay was 1.09 days (range, 1–7 days). In our follow-up questionnaire, we assess only partial and full recovery compared to presurgical functional ability. We never ask about return to work, because this is difficult to evaluate. Most patients resume partial activity after 2 days and achieve full recovery in 3 to 8 days (mean, 3.8 days). Patient follow-up is conducted by physicians at the outpatient clinic at 2 weeks, 3 months, 6 months, 1 year, and 2 years after surgery.

Nine of the patients had subcutaneous hematomas. One large hematoma resulted from bleeding of the rectus muscle. There was only one wound infection at the trocar site, and 14 "groin hematomas" in patients who underwent ring excision of scrotal hernia sacs. At first, we aspirated these hematomas, but later we let them resorb spontaneously. One patient had entrapment of the lateral femoral cutaneous nerve as a result of firm adhesions of the mesh to the nerve. Repeated laparoscopy 1 week later ruled out stapling injury. We recommend that the peritoneum not be dissected 2 cm medial to the superior anterior

Table 15-3.   Results: September 1991 to September 1993

Total no. of hernia repairs	332
No. of patients	245
Bilateral hernia	87
Average age (y)	43.8 (14–87)
Hernia types:	I: 9
	II: 93
	III: 194 (A–84, B–101, C–9)
	IV: 36
Postoperative narcotics	0
Postoperatives analgesics	186 (148, 1 time; 38, 2 times)
Postoperative stay (d)	1.09 (1–7)
Full recovery (d)	3.8 (3–8)
Subcutaneous hematoma	9
"Groin hematoma" (ring excision)	14
Wound infection	1
Entrapment of left femoral cutaneous nerve	1
Bladder injury	1
Recurrence	2 (0.59%)

Table 15-4. Complications in Laparoscopic Hernia Repair and Their Prevention

Nerve injury	No stapling in the "neurovascular triangle"; peritoneal dissection starting 2 cm medial to superior anterior iliac spine
Bladder injury	Peritoneal dissection medially up to medial umbilical cord
Intestinal obstruction	Closure of the peritoneum above the mesh; closure of penetrating trocar port 10 mm and larger
Recurrence	Use of nonabsorbable mesh; fixation of the mesh; adequate size of mesh; two layers of repair in type III and IV hernia; wide deperitonealization of lower peritoneal flap from cord elements

iliac spine, and that the mesh not be extended beyond this point. In one of our early patients, the bladder was injured as a result of medial excision of the peritoneum to the medial umbilical cord. In the two patients with recurrent hernia, a review of the videotapes demonstrated our mistakes. One type III-B hernia recurred 3 months after surgery because of an inadequate dissection of the lower flap of peritoneum resulting in recurrence behind the mesh. A type III-A hernia recurred 1 month after surgery because of a limited dissection of the pubic tubercle and mesh placement that resulted in invagination of the mesh into the defect. Both cases were repaired successfully by completion of the dissection and laparoscopic placement of additional mesh. All of our complications occurred in the first 50 cases, which can be attributed to learning experience. A summary of common hernia complications and means for their prevention is presented in Table 15-4.

Early hernia recurrence after laparoscopic repair occurs in the first 3 months and is related to technical mistakes that can be avoided or corrected. Thanks to the technique of tension-free closure, we believe that early and late recurrence rates will be similar. We also believe that two-layer repair for large hernias will restrict recurrence rates to less than 1%.

Among the benefits of our procedure are minimal pain and morbidity, early recovery and full activity, and low complication and recurrence rates. These advantages make our approach superior to the anterior approach for large hernias, recurrent hernias, and bilateral hernias.

Our indications for the laparoscopic approach are summarized in Table 15-5.

We conclude that large hernias require a large, laparoscopic two-layer repair, which is superior to the anterior approach. We recommend considering a small, laparoscopic tension-free repair, which does not affect adversely the integrity of the anterior abdominal wall, for the repair of small hernias.

REFERENCES

1. Arregui ME, Navarrete J, Davis CJ, Castro D, Nagan RF. Laparoscopic inguinal herniorrhaphy, techniques and controversies. Surg Clin North Am 1993;73:513.
2. Felix EL, Michas C. Double-buttress laparoscopic herniorrhaphy. J Laparoendosc Surg 1993;3:379.
3. Geis WP, Crafton WB, Novak MJ, Malago M. Laparoscopic herniorrhaphy. Results and technical aspects in 450 consecutive procedures. Surgery 1993;114:765.
4. Nyhus LM. Iliopubic tract repair of inguinal and femoral hernia: the posterior (preperitoneal) approach. Surg Clin North Am 1993;73:487.
5. Nyhus LM. Individualization of hernia repair: a new era. Surgery 1993;114:1.
6. Stoppa RE, Warlaumont CR. The preperitoneal approach and prosthetic repair of groin hernia. In: Nyhus LM, Condon RE, eds. Hernia. Philadelphia, JB Lippincott, 1989:199–255.

Editor's Comment

Interest in laparoscopic techniques is escalating. The "plug" method, although originally touted as the answer, has fallen into disrepute because of an early and unacceptable incidence of recurrent hernias.

Table 15-5. Indications for Laparoscopic Groin Hernia Repair

Mandatory (Absolute Indication)	Recommended (Relative Indication)	Open (Under Investigation)
Type III (large hernia)	Combined with other laparoscopic procedure	Type I (small)
Type IV (recurrent hernia) Bilateral hernia	Physically active people	Type II (moderate)

Today, there is enthusiasm for high ligation of the hernial sac with posterior prosthetic patching over the Hesselbach triangle and internal abdominal ring. The fascial defects are not closed; the mesh is kept in place by staples and intraabdominal pressure.

Laparoscopic herniotomy plus patching of the posterior inguinal wall may be acceptable for type I, type II, and type III-C (femoral) hernias. Most recurrent groin hernias treated at my clinic are medial defects and are relatively small (type IV-A). The laparoscopic patch method should be effective for these hernias as well.

The prosthetic patch alone may be inadequate for controlling type III-A and III-B hernias (sliding, pantaloon, and very large hernias). When laparoscopic suturing techniques evolve to perfection, the laparoscopic approach could become another acceptable method for these complex hernias.

Unfortunately, the proponents of the laparoscopic method are placing too much emphasis on how well patients accept the procedure (ie, patients complain of less pain and return to work earlier than if they had undergone a standard repair). As experience increases, the complications reported to occur after the laparoscopic procedure mirror those seen after all invasions of the body cavity: infections, incisional hernias, seromas, hematomas, bladder injuries, and nerve damage.

I have watched innumerable videotapes of laparoscopic procedures and have been surprised to observe the blunt dissection in the preperitoneal space extend far beyond that found to be necessary in the classic open approach. The learning curve is still extant. As experience increases, the current broad opening of tissue spaces lateral to the internal abdominal ring and posterior to the psoas muscle or the obturator foramen should be reduced. Contraction of the area of operative dissection will decrease the incidence of complications without diminishing the effectiveness of the procedure.

Of greatest concern is injury to one or more of the cutaneous nerves that traverse the lower abdominal wall. The blind placement of staples lateral to the internal abdominal ring to attach the prosthetic mesh has caused severe pain in the distribution of the ilioinguinal, iliohypogastric, femoral, and genitofemoral nerves. I hope that this serious complication can be prevented as we learn new and better ways to apply laparoscopic skills.

Unfortunately, enthusiasts for laparoscopic hernia repair are attempting to make this approach common to all types of hernias. As with standard repairs, each patient must undergo the operative approach and repair best suited to cure the specific type of hernia encountered.

L.M.N.

Hernia, Fourth Edition, edited
by Lloyd M. Nyhus and Robert E. Condon.
J.B. Lippincott Company, Philadelphia © 1995.

Chapter 16

Complications of Groin Hernia

Robert E. Condon and Lloyd M. Nyhus

Half a million Americans each year undergo repair of a groin hernia. Fortunately, complications are uncommon. An overall complication rate of only 1% would affect 5000 patients each year, however, and a complication rate of 10%, which is more likely, would involve 50,000 patients each year. The magnitude of the problem is apparent.

Certain complications are well recognized; others are not. Our purpose in this chapter is to review many of the common and uncommon complications that are associated with groin (indirect and direct inguinal, and femoral) hernias. Many of the considerations outlined here for groin hernias apply as well to hernia repair in other anatomic sites (ie, ventral, lumbar, and pelvic hernias).

PREOPERATIVE COMPLICATIONS

Misleading Lumps

The possibility that an apparent hernial mass actually is something else should be kept in mind as the patient is examined. A variety of rounded, elastic, and movable lumps can be found, particularly in the femoral area. Most misleading lumps readily can be identified as such. Nonetheless, even the most careful surgeon occasionally makes an error in diagnosis. The problem in differentiation most commonly involves a suspected femoral hernia. An enlarged lymph node, a lipoma, a saphenous varix, or a psoas abscess may mimic a femoral hernia.

The presence of a single, greatly enlarged lymph node is unusual. Lymph nodes usually are multiple, are attached to the superficial fascia in the region of the fossa ovalis, and are equally mobile in all directions. In contrast, a femoral hernia has less mobility in a transverse direction than does a femoral lymph node. Inguinal buboes are uncommon today. They may be caused by lymphogranuloma venereum, syphilis, tuberculosis, or plague. Veterans who have served overseas may have been exposed to these diseases, so the presence of a femoral lump in such a patient

should arouse suspicion that the process may be something other than a femoral hernia.

Lipomas in the subcutaneous fat usually can be lifted free from the underlying fascia and the absence of a neck of a hernial sac progressing under the inguinal ligament confirmed. A saphenous varix can be confusing, because the varix undergoes apparent reduction on pressure and transmits a cough impulse. It also mimics a hernia in that it appears when the patient is upright and reduces spontaneously when the patient lies down. The feature of a saphenous varix that usually allows it to be differentiated from a femoral hernia is the extremely soft consistency of the mass. Eventually, as the saphenous varix enlarges, it displaces subcutaneous fat and appears beneath the skin as a blue discoloration; at this stage, diagnostic confusion evaporates.

Psoas abscess is uncommon today, but continues to cause diagnostic confusion despite the fact that it possesses none of the clinical characteristics of a femoral hernia. A psoas abscess often is softer than a femoral hernia and has ill-defined borders, in contrast to the more sharply defined margins of the hernia. The major differentiating feature, however, is the fact that a psoas abscess lies lateral to the femoral artery, not medial to it.

New Symptoms From an Old Hernia

Changes in intraperitoneal pressure dynamics may transform an otherwise asymptomatic hernia of years' duration into a hernia causing real annoyance. In an older patient who suddenly, after years of procrastination, desires surgical correction of a hernia, the possibility that something is going on within the abdominal cavity always must be considered. It is well recognized that obstructive uropathy and chronic pulmonary disease may be related to worsening of the hernia and must be treated before an elective operation. It is not so well recognized that carcinoma of the pancreas or colon, or cirrhosis with subclinical ascites, may produce an increase in intraabdominal pressure sufficient to cause symptoms in a previously asymptomatic groin hernia. Indeed, the development of symptoms may be sufficiently severe to produce strangulation.

In the evaluation of such patients, particular attention must be paid to the system review and history, as well as to the performance of a particularly careful physical examination. Sigmoidoscopy should be performed and barium enema given in all older patients. A routine barium enema in every patient with a groin hernia is unnecessary, because the yield of abnormal examinations is relatively small. In an older patient with new symptoms relating to a long-standing hernia, however, a thorough search for an occult carcinoma or another intraabdominal lesion is indicated. Terezis and colleagues[11] documented this phenomenon as it relates to the colon. In an analysis of 107 consecutive men with clinically proven cancer of the large intestine, 17% first sought medical assistance because of symptoms referable to an inguinal hernia.

Intestinal Obstruction

Failure to look for evidence of a groin hernia is a sure way to make an erroneous diagnosis in a patient who has not had a previous abdominal operation and who has complaints related to an intestinal obstruction. If careful examination of the inguinal-femoral region fails to disclose evidence of an incarcerated or strangulated hernia, one also should think of the less common hernial causes of intestinal obstruction, such as (1) internal hernias: periduodenal, mesenteric, retroanastomotic, interparietal, supravesical, and herniation into the foramen of Winslow; (2) pelvic hernias: obturator, sciatic, and perineal; and (3) ventral hernias: umbilical, epigastric, spigelian, lumbar, and incisional. A partial enterocele or Richter hernia is particularly treacherous, because it does not cause intestinal obstruction early. The partial incarceration progresses insidiously to necrosis of a portion of the wall of the intestine; only then does surrounding inflammation produce intestinal obstruction.

Incarceration

Incarceration is a relatively common finding in patients with indirect inguinal or femoral hernia. The incidence is about 10% in indirect inguinal hernia and about 20% in femoral hernia. Incarceration implies inability to reduce the hernial mass into the abdomen. Incarceration is an important finding because, in a proportion of patients in whom it is present, it progresses to intestinal obstruction and strangulation, with a consequent increase in the patient's risk of

morbidity and mortality. An attempt to reduce an apparently incarcerated hernia is worthwhile, because the information gained from the maneuver may be of some diagnostic help. If the hernia can be partially reduced but a portion of the mass remains protruded, the surgeon should suspect that the patient has a sliding hernia. The sliding component of an inguinal hernia is irreducible, but not incarcerated.

Reduction of an incarcerated hernia also has an advantage in that it permits the inflammatory response in and around the hernia to subside. Early repair then is carried out, with a better prognosis for permanent cure of the hernia. The incidence of recurrence is higher after the repair of an incarcerated hernia than that of a nonincarcerated hernia, the difference resulting in large part from the inflammatory state of the tissues around the hernia.

If, in the process of vigorous attempts with external pressure to reduce an apparently incarcerated hernia, the mass seems to disappear all at once, rather than slipping away bit by bit with loud gurgles, the occurrence of reduction en masse should be suspected. This is a rare event, the mechanisms of which are not entirely understood.[8] If reduction en masse is suspected, the patient should undergo an early exploratory operation.

Strangulation

Strangulation means that the blood supply to the herniated tissues is compromised. The process usually begins with angulation or constriction of the neck of an indirect inguinal or femoral hernia. Outflow of lymphatic fluid from the hernial mass is impeded, and the herniated tissues become edematous. The consequent increase in the size of the hernial mass leads to a further increase in the degree of constriction at the neck of the hernial sac. A vicious circle of accumulating edema begins. The patient also will have early signs of intestinal obstruction.

Pain and tenderness, produced by the accumulating edema and increased pressure in the herniated tissues, are characteristic of beginning strangulation. Any patient whose hernia is apparently irreducible (incarcerated) and who complains of pain or tenderness associated with the hernia should be suspected of having strangulation and should undergo an urgent operation aimed at relief of the constriction at the neck of the hernial sac and, if appropriate, repair of the hernia.

If the progressing chain of edema, pressure, and inflammation is not interrupted by an operation, tissue pressure in the hernia eventually exceeds venous pressure. Venous obstruction and thrombosis ensue, producing tissue necrosis. Venous hemorrhagic infarction is a vicious form of strangulation and, if uncorrected, leads to hypovolemic and septic shock. There is an increase in pain and tenderness, higher fever ensues, and there is a shift in the differential leukocyte count and an increase in the total leukocyte count in most patients. Patients in whom strangulation is suspected need an emergency operation, with particular precautions taken to prevent the dissemination of strangulation fluid.

Truss-Related Problems

An inguinal truss often is advised for an older patient with a hernia in whom, without real justification, the risks of hernia repair are believed to be excessive. It must be remembered, and emphasized to those non-surgeons who often advise elderly patients with a hernia, that hernia repair does not involve a major opening into a body cavity, manipulation of viscera, or risk of significant blood loss. Repair of a groin hernia, therefore, is a procedure of low mortality risk at all ages. Wearing a truss does not guarantee that an indirect inguinal or femoral hernia will remain reduced. In fact, a truss rarely is successful in maintaining continuous reduction of these types of hernias.

It also must be remembered that wearing a truss is not an adequate substitute for surgical repair of the hernia, and actually increases the patient's susceptibility to complications that will require emergency surgical relief. The many complications associated with wearing a truss are well recognized, but two deserve particular emphasis. In the patient with a small hernia, the pressure of the overlying truss on a protruding hernial mass *enhances the chances of strangulation* by obstructing lymphatic and venous drainage. In a patient with a large direct inguinal hernia, the constant overlying pressure of the truss pad on the margins of the hernial defect eventually *leads to atrophy of the fascial and aponeurotic structures,* enlarging the hernial orifice, promoting the growth of the hernia, and making subsequent surgical repair a far more difficult task.

SURGICAL COMPLICATIONS

Hemorrhage

Serious hemorrhage during repair of a groin hernia is unusual, but may occur after trauma to (1) the pubic branch of the obturator artery, the so-called corona mortis; (2) the deep circumflex iliac vessels; (3) the inferior deep epigastric vessels; (4) the cremasteric artery; or (5) the external iliac vessels. Damage to the first three is troublesome, particularly if the hernia is

being repaired through the inguinal canal. The exposure should be extended sufficiently to approach the vessels directly; they may be ligated with impunity. Damage to the cremasteric artery is more of an annoyance; it is managed easily intraoperatively. The more usual problem is that this vessel goes unligated or the ligature slips, resulting in a postoperative scrotal ecchymosis or hematoma.

The deep circumflex iliac vessels may be injured by placement of sutures too deeply through the iliopubic tract, particularly during repair at the lateral side of the deep inguinal ring. The suture should be removed and pressure applied until hemostasis is achieved. Because the deep circumflex iliac vessels are small and bleeding almost always is venous in origin, these maneuvers usually are sufficient to achieve control.

Placement of sutures too deeply into the anterior femoral sheath, iliopubic tract, or inguinal ligament may result in injury to the external iliac artery or vein. If sutures are to be placed into the fascial structures bridging these important vessels, the fascia should be tented up and the point of the needle passed flatly along the axis of the iliac vessels to reduce the chances of injury to them. If the vessels are injured, immediate bleeding will be noted. There always is a tendency to tie the suture and then apply pressure, hoping that the bleeding will stop. Placement of the suture through the vessel wall, particularly through the wall of the iliac vein, only maintains bleeding. The suture should be removed and pressure then applied. Arterial bleeding responds more readily than does venous bleeding. If pressure does not control the situation, the femoral sheath should be opened widely and the vascular defect approached directly. Adequate exposure may allow effective local tamponade, or the vascular wound may require closure with fine suture. The external iliac vessels must not be ligated.

Transection of the Spermatic Cord

The spermatic cord is cut, usually deliberately, in occasional repairs of indirect inguinal hernias. The maneuver allows complete closure of the deep inguinal ring and, it is assumed, lessens the chances of subsequent repeated recurrence. Although this maneuver is performed much less frequently today than in the past, it still is required occasionally. In addition, there are rare instances in which unintentional transection of the spermatic cord occurs during an operation.

Fever, and tenderness and swelling of the testis follow in two thirds of patients, but cause few symptoms in the rest. In patients with symptoms, the fever may be spiking in nature, suggesting the presence of an abscess, but it usually resolves after a few days without antibiotic therapy.

Although testicular atrophy or a hydrocele may ensue in as many as one third of patients with a transected spermatic cord, routine orchiectomy is unnecessary.

Severance of Nerves

The ilioinguinal and iliohypogastric nerves, and both the genital and femoral branches of the genitofemoral nerve, are vulnerable to injury during groin hernia repair. The ilioinguinal and iliohypogastric nerves penetrate the internal oblique muscle in the lateral third of the groin and then lie between the internal oblique and external oblique aponeuroses. The ilioinguinal nerve provides sensory innervation to the base of the penis, and to the upper scrotum and adjacent thigh. Because the ilioinguinal nerve lies just beneath the external oblique aponeurosis and overlies the spermatic cord in the inguinal canal, it is particularly vulnerable to injury when the external oblique aponeurosis is opened.

The iliohypogastric nerve, located 1 to 2 cm above the inguinal canal, provides sensation to the suprapubic area. This nerve is endangered during the course of hernia repair when a relaxing incision is made in the rectus sheath, or during the medial exposure of the musculoaponeurotic layers of the groin in the conduct of a preperitoneal approach to hernia repair.

The genitofemoral nerve, arising from the sacral plexus, lies on the surface of the iliopsoas muscle and divides into its genital and femoral branches just internal and lateral to the deep inguinal ring. The genital branch perforates the internal oblique muscle at the origin of the cremaster muscle and provides both motor innervation to the cremaster muscle and sensory innervation to the skin of the penis and scrotum. The femoral branch is sensory to the skin of the upper lateral thigh. This branch lies deeper and is less vulnerable to injury, but it may be traumatized during dissection on the lateral side of the deep inguinal ring.

Fortunately, there are multiple cross-connections between peripheral nerves in the groin and considerable central segmental overlap in their sensory representation. Prolonged anesthesia of the skin generally does not follow injury to one of these nerves. Anesthesia that may be present in the immediate postoperative period after nerve injury generally regresses by the sixth postoperative month. Patients rarely complain of loss of sensation or of loss of cremasteric or scrotal contractile response, even if nerves are injured in the conduct of hernia repair. On occasion, a patient will note, after transection of the genital branch of the genitofemoral nerve, that the testis on the side operated on rests in a somewhat more dependent position.

If these nerves are severed during hernia repair, it is impractical to attempt anastomosis. The nerve ends should be ligated to close the neurolemmal sheath and enforce development of the inevitable posttraumatic neuroma within the continuity of the nerve sheath. Preventing attachment of regenerating neurofibrils to surrounding musculoaponeurotic structures reduces the incidence of symptomatic neuroma after nerve injury.

Entrapment of a nerve by postoperative scar formation or by a suture is likely to result in prolonged postoperative symptoms. Such entrapped nerves may be a source of pain or, at least, of discomfort associated with movement of the lower abdominal wall or upper thigh. The only way to avoid nerve entrapment is to identify nerves during the dissection for primary hernia repair, and thus protect them. Unfortunately, that is easier said than done because some nerves, particularly the genitofemoral, have fine branches in the groin, and others, such as the femoral nerve, are not easily seen because they are covered by fascia.

Severance of Testicular Blood Supply

The internal spermatic or testicular artery arises from the abdominal aorta and is the main arterial supply to the testis. This artery joins the cord structures just internal to the deep inguinal ring. The external spermatic artery, a branch of the inferior epigastric artery, joins the spermatic cord by either passing through the deep inguinal ring or perforating the iliopubic tract immediately adjacent to the ring. This artery supplies the cremaster muscle. A small arterial branch accompanies the vas deferens. In addition, a small cremaster branch arises directly from the femoral artery and perforates the iliopubic tract or inguinal ligament at the origin of the cremaster muscle.

A potentially rich collateral circulation exists at the upper end of the testis between end branches of the vesical and prostatic arteries and the internal spermatic and deferential arteries (Fig. 16-1). The scrotal branches of the internal and external pudendal arteries also have free anastomotic connections to vessels of the spermatic cord just external to the superficial inguinal ring.

Every precaution must be taken to prevent damage to the major vessels of the spermatic cord during repair of an inguinal hernia. Despite care, however, laceration of small arterial and venous vessels does occur, and, repair being impractical, ligation is necessary. Ligation even of the major artery to the testis at the level of the deep inguinal ring does not necessarily result in atrophy or necrosis of the testis as long as the external collateral circulation is undisturbed. This collateral circulation is preserved by avoiding dissection

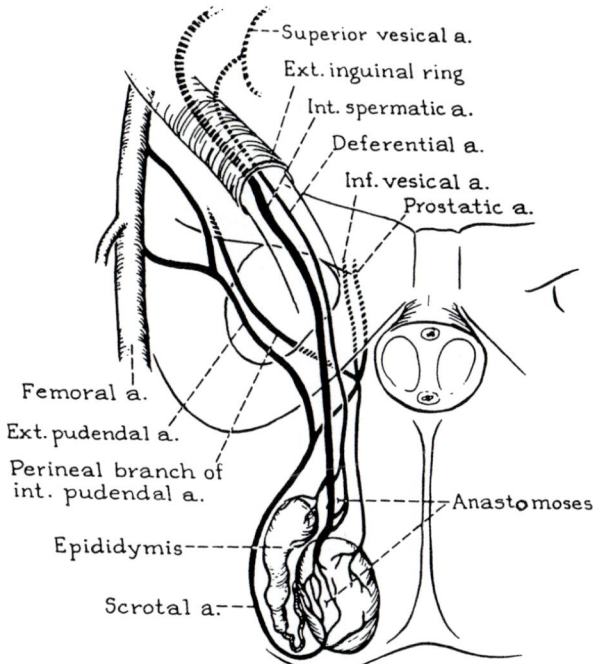

Figure 16-1. The primary and collateral blood supply of the testis. The collateral communications are mainly external to the superficial inguinal ring. If the testis and distal spermatic cord are not mobilized during a hernial repair, the potential collateral circulation is not disturbed.

of the testis from the scrotum during hernia repair. Combined with interruption of the internal spermatic artery, dissection of the testis from the scrotum may result in postoperative atrophy or necrosis of the testis. Such damage is more likely to occur in the process of treating a recurrent inguinal hernia.

Severance of the Vas Deferens

Because there are two vasa deferentia, transection of a single vas may be considered of minimal importance by some surgeons, but rarely is so considered by the patient. Unless permission for transection of the cord, including the vas, has been obtained preoperatively, repair of an injured vas deferens should be undertaken if it is traumatized in the course of a hernia repair. Although it is difficult to evaluate the results after repair of the vas on one side, about 50% usually are considered to function.

The cut ends should be trimmed cleanly and approximated with interrupted sutures of fine catgut or silk (Fig. 16-2). If loupes or an operating microscope are available, they can aid in the construction of an accurate anastomosis. Placement of an internal splint, using a fine monofilament steel wire suture brought out through the wall of the vas at a distance from the repair, usually facilitates accurate reapproximation and maintenance of the lumen. This splint can be maintained for some days postoperatively, but its immediate removal after the anastomosis is just as satisfactory.

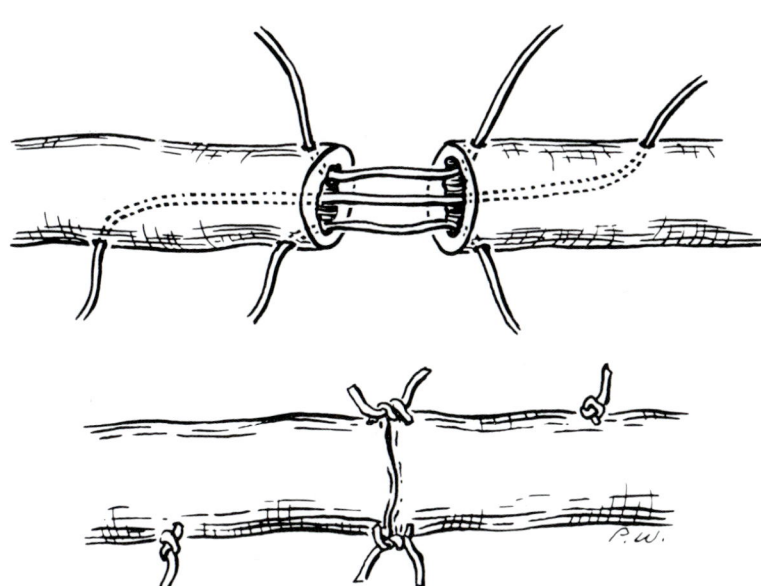

Figure 16-2. Technique of repair of severed vas deferens using a fine, plain catgut internal stent and sutures of chromic catgut to approximate the ends of the vas. Alternatively, the anastomosis can be made over a monofilament suture of wire or plastic that is pulled out later. To preserve the blood supply, only a few catgut sutures (two or three at most) should be used to approximate the stumps of the vas deferens.

Damage to the Intestine

Meticulous attention must be given to suture placement during high ligation of the sac of an indirect inguinal hernia. Blind suturing is never acceptable because of the possibility of incorporating a loop of intestine within the suture, leading to subsequent development of a fecal fistula, an abscess within the intestinal wall, or intestinal obstruction. The sutures for high ligation may be placed in a pursestring manner or may be individual interrupted sutures, but they always must be placed through the peritoneum under direct vision, which, in turn, necessitates adequate exposure.

In repair of a sliding hernia, two complications arise with some frequency. Before the existence of a sliding type of hernia is recognized, the intestine may be entered unintentionally or the intestinal wall may be devascularized. Because the hernial sac in sliding hernias usually is anterior, dissection of any hernial sac should be started from this aspect. Rarely, a sliding hernia occurs without a sac; this situation usually is the result of acute trauma and not the consequence of a chronic hernia. If the hernial sac seems excessively thickened, extreme caution must be exercised until it is certain that one is not dealing with the wall of the intestine.

Because the blood supply to the intestine enters at the posterior aspect of a sliding hernia, incautious dissection in this area may result in hemorrhage or compromise of the vascular supply, leading to necrosis of the intestinal wall. This potential problem is handled by beginning the incision of the peritoneum about 1 inch anterior and medial to the sliding component. Mobilization and dissection then are carried completely around the intestine with direct visualization of the mesentery and blood supply, allowing preservation of the vascular supply on the posterior aspect of the sliding hernia.

If the colon is entered, careful two-layer closure using catgut in the mucosa and interrupted nonabsorbable sutures in the seromuscular layer must be performed. Closure of the intestine is followed by irrigation of the wound with large volumes of saline or antibiotic solution, and the hernia repair is continued. Compromise of intestinal vascularity may be more difficult to ascertain. If there is any question as to whether devascularization of the intestine has occurred, the individual situation will dictate the course of action, which may include (1) wedge resection, primary closure, and temporary proximal diversion by colostomy or ileostomy; (2) an in-continuity exteriorization of the Mikulicz type; or (3) colectomy and primary anastomosis with or without proximal decompression of the intestine.

Injury to the Urinary Bladder

The medial side of a direct inguinal hernia often contains a sliding portion of bladder wall. The presence of the bladder usually is detected by identification of perivesical fat. Injury to the bladder is not associated with a marked increase in morbidity if the damage is recognized intraoperatively, repaired appropriately, and the bladder drained through a Foley catheter. It is the unrecognized or ignored bladder injury that leads to trouble.

Strangulated Intestine

There are two problems associated with the management of necrotic intestine in the course of treating a hernia: (1) determining intestinal viability, and (2) preventing the escape of lymphatic-venous and peritoneal fluid.

Accurate determination of intestinal viability is difficult. The large number of tests suggested to aid in this decision is indicative that none is completely reliable. Fortunately, most intestine is recognizable clinically as viable by such criteria as the rapid return of good color and serosal shine, the presence or return of peristalsis, pulsation in the mesenteric blood vessels, and refilling of both arterial and venous vessels after stripping. Tests such as arteriography or the injection of fluorescein followed by examination under a Wood's lamp are difficult to conduct in the course of the usual operation.

The best method of determining intestinal viability remains careful observation. If there is any continuing doubt about viability, the best course is to resect the affected segment. If questionable intestine is returned into the peritoneal cavity, the patient must be observed closely after the operation for any evidence of peritoneal irritation. If even minimal symptoms of peritonitis appear, or metabolic acidosis persists, reexploration of the abdomen and resection of the questionable bowel loop is necessary.

The presence of necrotic bowel in a femoral or inguinal hernia approached from within the peritoneal cavity or the preperitoneal space should be suspected if manipulation of the bowel produces subserosal petechiae in the normal bowel adjacent to the hernial orifice. In the presence of necrotic intestine associated with a strangulated hernia, control and interruption of the lymphatic and venous drainage need to be achieved before reduction of the hernia. If this is not done, lymphatic fluid and venous blood containing large amounts of endotoxin as well as viable bacteria may enter the general circulation, with consequent endotoxic shock. It is better to resect if there is a question of necrosis being present.

In addition, the surgeon must ensure that a loop of nonviable intestine does not slip away into the peritoneal cavity. Transection of the constricting band at the neck of a hernial sac in strangulated hernias may release the entrapped necrotic intestine with great rapidity. Unless the surgeon is alert to this possibility, intestine may disappear suddenly into the peritoneal cavity. The dilemma in such situations is apparent. Is the intestine viable or not? No definite answer can be given unless the intestine can be observed.

If the hernia has been approached through the inguinal canal and a questionable loop is lost into the peritoneal cavity, laparotomy is mandatory to recover the intestine. The involved intestine must be visualized and its viability ascertained. It is not sufficient to observe the patient for developing signs of intestinal necrosis.

If the hernia has been approached through the preperitoneal space, the intestine proximal to the neck of the hernial sac usually has been controlled before the hernia is reduced, and loss of a loop of intestine into the peritoneal cavity is less likely. In addition, the preperitoneal approach provides direct access to the peritoneal cavity; in the unlikely event that a loop of intestine does slip from the operator's grasp, exploration of the peritoneum and recovery of the loop can be accomplished through the same operative wound used to approach and repair the hernia.

Femoral Vein Constriction

The femoral vein may be constricted by sutures placed during the course of hernia repair. This is particularly so if the sutures are placed in the Cooper ligament for repair of a large indirect or direct inguinal hernia. If the sutures are placed too far laterally and impinge on the femoral vein, constriction will ensue. In addition, excessively tight approximation of the Cooper ligament and the femoral sheath by a "transition suture" also may bring about constriction of the femoral vein.

The incidence of this problem is unknown because routine venography is not obtained in patients who have undergone groin hernia repair. It is likely that the constriction is minimal and clinically unrecognized in most patients. Major complications can ensue from femoral vein constriction, however. Of the six patients described by Nissen,[9] pulmonary embolism was the initial symptom in four and usually appeared early in the postoperative course. Deep venous thrombosis occurred in three patients; its onset typically was at the end of the first postoperative week.

If a patient has clinical symptoms of possible pulmonary embolus, or signs of deep venous thrombosis, a venogram should be obtained. If constriction is noted on the medial side of the femoral vein, consideration should be given to reoperation and removal of the offending suture.

Incidental Appendectomy

The removal of a normal appendix during an intraabdominal operation for some other purpose is a common practice. The reasons for performing incidental appendectomy are that appendicitis is a common disease associated with an appreciable morbidity and some mortality risk, and that the appendix is a dispensable organ. The objection to routine incidental appendectomy during right inguinal hernia repair centers around the concern that appendectomy may be associated with an increased risk of wound infection. Infection of the wound in a patient in whom repair of a hernia was the primary reason for operation is undesirable, because the wound infection may lead to breakdown of the repair and recurrence of the hernia.

Despite apprehension regarding wound infection, studies have indicated that appendectomy concurrent with repair of a right inguinal hernia is associated with only a slightly increased risk of wound infection or other morbidity if appropriate conditions are met.[3,4] The two conditions are (1) that there is no complicating disease that contraindicates the 5- to 10-minute prolongation of operative time for the incidental appendectomy, and (2) that the entire appendix, from tip to base, can be delivered easily into the wound so that the appendix can be amputated and the base secured without enlargement of the incision.

The possible risks and benefits of incidental appendectomy should be considered in relation to the age-dependent and progressively diminishing future risk of the development of appendicitis. In patients older than 30 years, the future overall risk of appendicitis is about 1%. The risk of wound infection after incidental appendectomy is increased by about 1%. Thus, there is no clear rationale for incidental appendectomy in most adults.

Loss of "Right of Domain"

In dealing with massive hernias, those in which large segments of the intestine have resided in the hernia and outside the abdominal cavity for some time, intraoperative reduction of the intestine into the peritoneal cavity may be difficult or impossible without appropriate preoperative preparation. In such circumstances, resection of the intestine occasionally has been performed to allow wound closure. This rarely should be necessary, however.

Preoperative preparation of the patient with a massive hernia by means of progressively induced pneumoperitoneum was suggested initially by Goñi Moreno.[5] The pneumoperitoneum gradually enlarges the abdominal cavity to provide room for intraoperative reduction of the herniated intestine. We have used this method of preparation in the past in patients with massive hernias in whom the intestine cannot be reduced preoperatively. Today, we simply return all the intestines to the peritoneal cavity, even if this increases abdominal pressure, and proceed with hernia repair. The patient remains intubated and on ventilator support for 1 to 4 days after the operation, until the tissues adjust, the diaphragm returns to a relatively normal position, and the need for respiratory support no longer is present. We have never had to resect intestine to permit wound closure.

POSTOPERATIVE COMPLICATIONS

General Complications

Systemic complications occur at a rate comparable to that seen after other surgical procedures of the same magnitude. Atelectasis and pneumonitis are most frequent, followed by thrombophlebitis and urinary retention. A wide variety of miscellaneous complications have been reported, including cholecystitis, intestinal obstruction, gastrointestinal hemorrhage, renal calculus, herpes zoster, liver necrosis, gout, and acute psychosis.

The anesthetic technique used for hernia repair sometimes is invoked to explain the occurrence of certain postoperative complications. Postoperative complications occur with similar frequency, however, in patients receiving either spinal or general anesthesia. Local anesthesia often is recommended in the treatment of aged, high-risk patients. Whether this technique is associated with a lower incidence of postoperative complications has not been established. Local anesthesia is no different from general anesthesia in terms of its impact on cardiorespiratory function.[1]

Urinary Retention

Urinary retention occurs in as many as one third of patients undergoing inguinal hernia repair, and is related directly to the dose of opioids used for postoperative analgesia. Two groups of patients seem to be affected—older men with prostatic obstructive disease and young, healthy, muscular men. If this complication does not respond to such simple measures as assumption of the upright position, prompt catheterization of the urinary bladder is indicated. Catheterization always should be undertaken if urinary retention persists beyond 12 hours to prevent overdistention and damage to the urinary bladder. Placement of a retention (Foley) catheter is preferable to repeated episodes of catheterization for continued inability to void. We treat urinary retention by placing a Foley catheter in the first instance, maintaining it in place for at least 24 hours, and testing return of detrusor function by having the patient void through the catheter before it is removed.

In patients who have even minimally symptomatic prostatic obstruction, transurethral resection of the prostate should be conducted before the hernia is repaired. In a study by Cramer and colleagues,[2] adherence to this policy resulted in no episodes of incarceration or strangulation in patients awaiting hernia repair after prostatectomy and reduced the incidence of urinary tract infection after hernia repair. Thus, accomplishing prostatectomy first does not expose the patient to any additional risk related to the inguinal hernia.

Scrotal Ecchymosis

It is distressing to both the surgeon and the patient to find on the first or second postoperative day that the skin of the scrotum has become discolored by a dark purple ecchymosis. This complication results from dissection of blood from the inguinal canal into the scrotum following the path of the spermatic cord. There usually is little or no hematoma palpable in the scrotum or the inguinal canal; a small amount of blood can produce a surprisingly large ecchymosis. The usual cause of scrotal ecchymosis is a small vessel overlooked during the operation. There are no serious sequelae, and the ecchymosis resolves spontaneously within the first few weeks after surgery.

Swollen Testis

Swollen testis after repair of an inguinal hernia most commonly results from tight closure of the tissues of the deep inguinal ring around the spermatic cord. Less frequently, the venous and lymphatic vessels have been interrupted during dissection of an indirect inguinal hernia sac or of the spermatic cord as it passes through the deep inguinal ring, or the pampiniform plexus has undergone thrombosis. Collateral lymphatic and venous channels usually develop in this situation, and the swelling eventually subsides. Treatment involves supporting the swollen testis and restricting the patient's activity to alleviate discomfort.

Testicular Atrophy

Koontz[7] made the important observation that "atrophy of the testicle sometimes follows a simple primary operation for inguinal hernia repair, in which neither the collateral nor primary circulation has been molested as far as the surgeon is aware."

This complication usually develops after episodes of postoperative testicular swelling induced by either interruption of the testicular blood supply or a hernia repair tight around the spermatic cord. Testicular atrophy is especially prone to occur after repair of an indirect complete scrotal hernia.[12,13]

Although atrophy of one testis does not diminish a patient's fertility or sexual potency, such reassurances often are not completely satisfying to many patients. The likelihood of testicular atrophy can be reduced by nontraumatic dissection of the spermatic cord, by attention to preservation of venous and lymphatic drainage, and by avoidance whenever possible of dissection of the testis and the distal portion of the spermatic cord from the scrotum.

Hydrocele

A collection of fluid in the scrotum or along the spermatic cord may result if a portion of the distal hernia sac is left in situ. Hydrocele-like collections of fluid also may form if lymphatic or venous drainage is unduly interrupted in the course of hernia repair. Finally, in some patients in whom a Marlex prosthesis is inserted in the course of the hernia repair, fluid collection within the inguinal canal as well as the scrotum may be noted postoperatively. Most patients with hydrocele or other forms of fluid collection respond to simple aspiration of the fluid by syringe, on repeated occasions if necessary. Such collections practically never require secondary operative intervention.

Wound Infection

The overall incidence of wound infection after primary repair of a groin hernia is about 1%, even though the incision is in an area carrying a high burden of skin bacteria. The risk also is influenced by host defense factors and the duration of the operation. The incidence of infection after repair of a recurrent hernia is slightly higher.

If the deep tissues beneath the external oblique aponeurosis are involved (ie, the infection extends below the external oblique aponeurosis), the risk of hernia recurrence is high. Wound infections after hernia repair are treated as they are in other surgical situations—by early recognition, reopening of the wound to permit drainage, and appropriate local care. Systemic administration of antibiotics in the treatment of an established wound infection is indicated only if there is evidence of continued invasive sepsis as reflected by high or spiking fever or spreading tenderness or inflammation.

Neuroma

Ilioinguinal or femoral neuritis caused by nerve entrapment by sutures, or the actual formation of a symptomatic neuroma after section of a nerve in this region can occur. Patients complain bitterly when afflicted with this complication. Most such syndromes resolve spontaneously without specific treatment. Those that cause persistent symptoms can be treated by local nerve blocks after the first postoperative month.

In a few patients, persistent and disabling symptoms necessitate reexploration of the wound. In such instances, accurate preoperative localization of the point source of pain may help in finding the elusive offending suture or neuroma. After the suture has been removed or the neuroma excised, any open ends of nerve must be ligated so that any further neuroma will form within the nerve sheath, thereby reducing the likelihood of symptoms.

Genitofemoral neuralgia is a syndrome characterized by chronic pain and paresthesia in the region of the distribution of the genitofemoral nerve.[6,10]

Missed Hernia

A missed hernia is one that was present but unrecognized at the time of a primary hernia repair and subsequently appears as a new hernia. An associated direct inguinal hernia may be obvious during repair of an indirect inguinal hernia, but the diagnosis of a femoral hernia may be subtle. During repair of a direct inguinal hernia, a small indirect inguinal hernia or a femoral hernia may be overlooked easily. Careful palpation of the deep inguinal ring, the femoral canal, and the region of the Hesselbach triangle at the time of primary hernia repair keeps the incidence of missed hernia at a minimum.

Recurrence

There is no question that both thorough knowledge of inguinal-femoral anatomy and skilled technical accomplishment of hernia repair are essential to successful surgical therapy for groin hernias. The anatomic and technical operative considerations relating to hernia repair are presented in detail elsewhere in this volume. One technical point, however, deserves particular emphasis: *Absence of tension in the completed hernia repair is essential to success.*

Although not commonly thought of as a complication of hernia repair, recurrence of the hernia is a form of morbidity and should be viewed as a complication. Reported recurrence rates vary from less than 1% to 7% for indirect inguinal hernias, from 4% to 10% for direct inguinal hernias, from 1% to 7% for femoral hernias, and from 5% to 35% for recurrent hernia repair.

Although recurrence of a hernia is related in a small group of patients to inadequacy of fascial structure, technical failure is the cause in most cases. A hernia repaired under tension does not heal normally and is subject to disruption throughout the period of wound healing. Tension usually can be relieved easily through the use of a relaxing incision. We use a relaxing incision whenever a groin hernia, other than the smallest femoral or indirect inguinal hernia, is repaired.

If the hernia is repaired adequately, using strong fascial margins, and a relaxing incision is used to eliminate tension, then considerations such as the strength of the suture material, straining during the early postoperative period, and external trauma to the inguinal area after the operation are much less important than if the hernia is repaired under tension and depends on the strength of sutures or the absence of additional strain for integrity in healing. If primary approximation of strong tissue cannot be accomplished without tension, insertion of a prosthesis is indicated.

REFERENCES

1. Behnia R, Hashemi F, Stryker SJ, Ujiki GT, Poticha SM. A comparison of general versus local anesthesia during inguinal herniorrhaphy. Surg Gynecol Obstet 1992;174:277.
2. Cramer SO, Malangoni MA, Schulte WJ, Condon RE. Inguinal hernia repair before and after prostatic resection. Surgery 1983;94:627.
3. Eiseman B, Fowler WG, Robinson JM. Appendectomy during right inguinal herniorrhaphy. Ann Surg 1959;149:110.
4. Eiseman B, Robinson RM, Brown FH. Simultaneous appendectomy and herniorrhaphy without prophylactic antibiotic therapy. Surgery 1962;51:578.
5. Goñi Moreno I. The rational treatment of hernias and voluminous chronic eventrations: preparation with voluminous pneumoperitoneum. In: Nyhus LM, Condon RE, eds. Hernia, ed 2. Philadelphia, JB Lippincott, 1978:536–550.
6. Harms BA, De Haas DR Jr, Starling JR. Diagnosis and management of genitofemoral neuralgia. Arch Surg 1984;119:339.
7. Koontz AR. Atrophy of the testicle as a surgical risk. Surg Gynecol Obstet 1965;120:511.
8. Mings H, Olson JD. Reduction "en masse" of groin herniae. Arch Surg 1965;90:764.
9. Nissen HM. Constriction of the femoral vein following inguinal hernia repair. Acta Chir Scand 1975;141:279.
10. Starling JR, Harms BA, Schroeder ME, Eichman PL. Diagnosis and treatment of genitofemoral ilioinguinal entrapment neuralgia. Surgery 1987;102:581.
11. Terezis NL, Davis WC, Jackson FC. Carcinoma of the colon associated with inguinal hernia. N Engl J Med 1963;268:774.
12. Wantz GE. Testicular atrophy as a risk of inguinal hernioplasty. Surg Gynecol Obstet 1982;154:570.
13. Wantz GE. Testicular atrophy as a sequela of inguinal hernioplasty. Int Surg 1986;71:159.

Special Comment

Genitofemoral Neuralgia

James R. Starling

Irrespective of the technique used, most cases of primary inguinal herniorrhaphy are executed successfully, with excellent patient satisfaction and return to normal activity. A myriad of esoteric complications can occur, but fortunately these are rare. Persistent pain (neuralgia) and pricking, burning sensations (paresthesias) in the inguinal region caused by ilioinguinal, iliohypogastric, or genitofemoral nerve entrapment after herniorrhaphy are exceedingly rare, but may result in severe patient morbidity.

That peripheral nerve trauma can occur despite optimal caution is demonstrated by the observation that 10% to 15% of patients have neurapraxia and hypesthesia after herniorrhaphy that may last for as long as 6 months. In addition, pain in the distribution of the peripheral nerves can persist for weeks after the incisional pain abates. This unwelcome extended pain pattern in the inguinal region subsides in most cases.

In the performance of inguinal herniorrhaphy through a conventional anterior inguinal incision, it has been emphasized routinely that the ilioinguinal nerve should be identified as the primary peripheral sensory nerve. The iliohypogastric nerve is mentioned sparingly. Few references before 1984 emphasized the branches of the genitofemoral nerve or the fact that this nerve can be involved by entrapment neuropathy. Only recently have some surgeons mentioned attention to the genital branch of the genitofemoral nerve in their description of operative technique.[4,10]

Genitofemoral neuralgia is an unusual clinical entity resulting in severe pain and paresthesia in the distribution of the genitofemoral nerve. The syndrome of genitofemoral neuralgia (causalgia) first was reported by Magee[6] in 1942 and by Lyon[5] in 1945. Of the 10 cases of genitofemoral neuropathy reported by these authors, 8 occurred after an appendectomy, 1 after a psoas abscess, and 1 after blunt groin trauma. Genitofemoral neurectomy effectively alleviated symptoms in 8 of the patients.

The ilioinguinal or iliohypogastric nerve can become entrapped by sutures, adhesions, or actual formation of a cicatricial neuroma after transection, resulting in severe, debilitating postoperative pain. Occasionally, it may be necessary to reexplore a postoperative hernia incision to perform a neurectomy of the ilioinguinal (iliohypogastric) nerve or to excise the neuroma. The common differential diagnosis of ilioinguinal (iliohypogastric) neuralgia includes entrapment of neighboring nerves.

The surgical literature infrequently mentions genitofemoral neuralgia. Patients with this syndrome previously may have undergone repeated groin exploration for ilioinguinal or iliohypogastric entrapment, or may have received therapy for chronic pain with repeated local injections, nerve stimulators, or pain and antidepressant medications. Symptoms usually occur immediately after the primary operation.

Since 1981, 29 patients have undergone retroperitoneal genitofemoral neurectomy at the University of Wisconsin Clinical Science Center and the Veterans Administration Hospital. In 20 patients, the condition was diagnosed after primary inguinal herniorrhaphy. The other 9 patients had stigmata of genitofemoral entrapment after a perforated appendix, blunt trauma, or nephrectomy.

ANATOMY

The inguinal region, which includes the inguinal canal, spermatic cord, and surrounding skin and subcutaneous tissue (including the femoral triangle of Scarpa), receives sensory innervation from the 11th and 12th thoracic nerves and the ventral divisions of

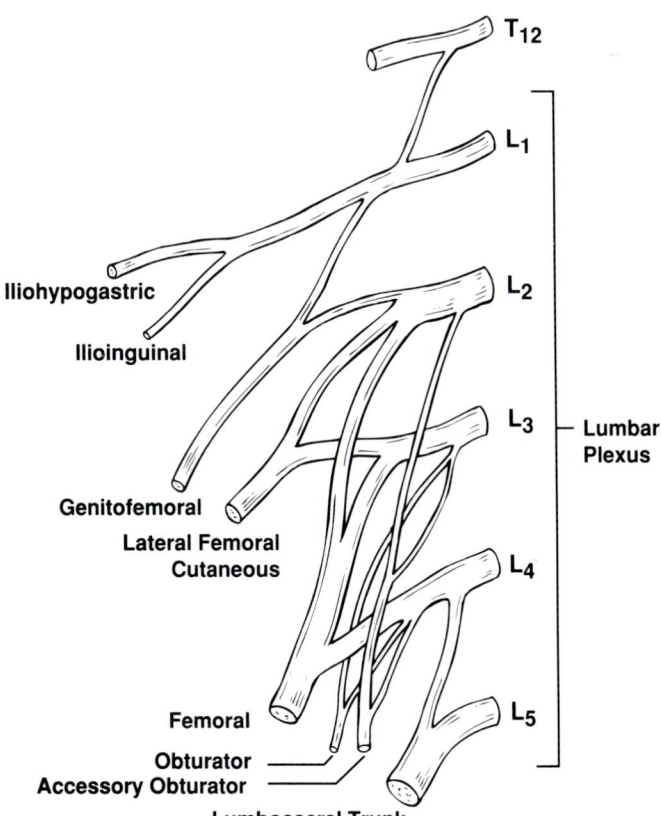

Figure 16-3. Origins of the ilioinguinal, iliohypogastric, and genitofemoral peripheral nerves.

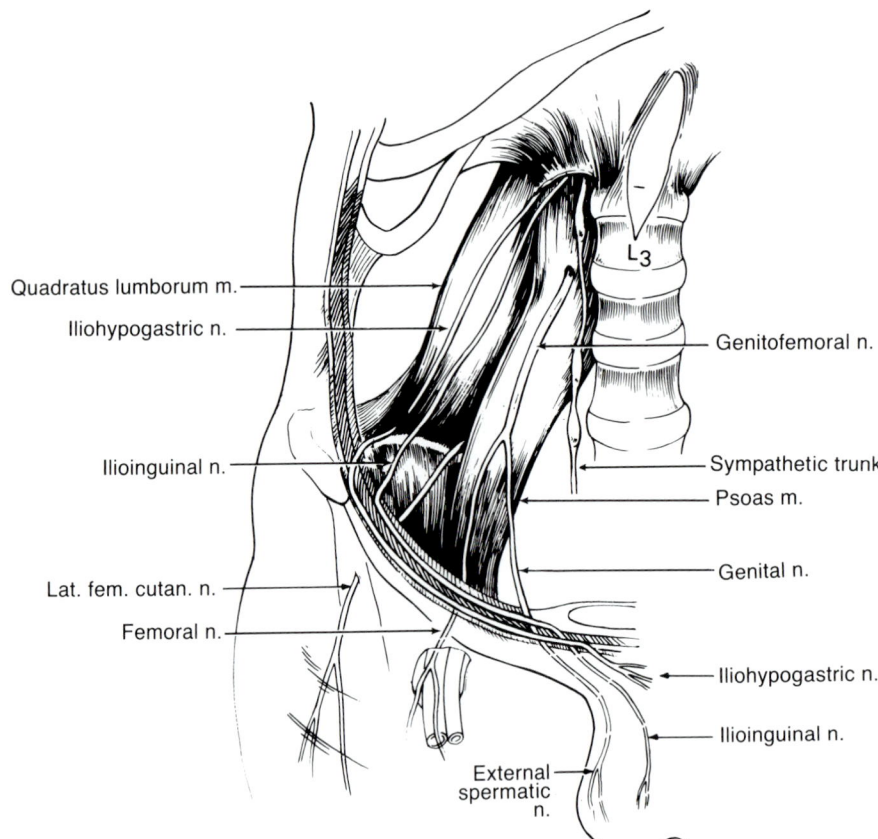

Quadratus lumborum m.

Iliohypogastric n.

Ilioinguinal n.

Lat. fem. cutan. n.

Femoral n.

External
spermatic
n.

L₃

Genitofemoral n.

Sympathetic trunk

Psoas m.

Genital n.

Iliohypogastric n.

Ilioinguinal n.

Figure 16-4. Course of the ilioinguinal, iliohypogastric, and genitofemoral nerves.

the 1st and 2nd lumbar spinal nerves. The cutaneous branches of the lumbar plexus include the iliohypogastric, ilioinguinal, genitofemoral, lateral femoral cutaneous, and obturator nerves (Fig. 16-3). The spermatic sympathetic plexus contains the sensory fibers for the testes.

The genitofemoral nerve arises from the 1st and 2nd lumbar vertebral plexus and consists mainly of sensory fibers with a motor component to the cremaster muscle (cremasteric reflex). It lies within the fascial lining of the abdomen by piercing the psoas muscles and the psoas fascia near its medial border opposite the 3rd or 4th lumbar vertebra (Fig. 16-4). It descends under the peritoneum on the surface of the psoas major muscle, crossing obliquely behind the ureter. At a variable distance above the inguinal ligament, the nerve divides into the genital (external spermatic) and femoral (lumboinguinal) branches. Great variation of nerves is not unusual, with free communication between branches of the genitofemoral nerve or the ilioinguinal and iliohypogastric nerves. The femoral branch (lumboinguinal) is the cutaneous nerve to the femoral triangle. Branches of the femoral nerve descend laterally to the external iliac artery, behind the

inguinal ligament, through the fascia lata, and into the femoral sheath. The femoral nerve supplies the skin over the upper part of the femoral triangle and communicates with the intermediate cutaneous nerve of the thigh. The genital branch (external spermatic) crosses the lower end of the external iliac artery and enters the inguinal canal through the internal inguinal ring. It supplies the cremaster muscle and traverses the inguinal canal to the end of the skin of the scrotum. In women, the genital branch accompanies the round ligament of the uterus and ends in the skin of the mons pubis and labium majus.

The ilioinguinal and iliohypogastric nerves are formed by branches of the 12th thoracic and 1st lumbar nerves. The ilioinguinal nerve runs under the peritoneum at first and then pierces the transversus abdominis muscle. The iliohypogastric nerve passes between the internal oblique and transversus abdominis muscles. The ilioinguinal and iliohypogastric nerves gradually pierce the internal oblique muscle and lie between it and the external oblique muscle as they near the internal inguinal ring. Within the inguinal canal, they usually lie on the anterior surface of the spermatic cord. A frequent anatomic variation is an aberrant inguinal sensory trunk of the ilioinguinal nerve, which descends with the genital branch of the genitofemoral nerve.

DIAGNOSIS

The clinical features of genitofemoral neuralgia consist of intermittent or constant pain in the inguinal region with radiation of pain to the genitalia and upper thigh. Pain can be aggravated by walking, stooping, or hyperextension of the hip and may be helped by recumbency and flexion of the thigh. Tenderness along the inguinal canal or the inguinal ring may be detected, and hyperesthesia in the distribution of the nerve may be present. The major differential diagnosis of genitofemoral neuralgia includes entrapment of or damage to the ilioinguinal or iliohypogastric nerves. The latter condition usually is characterized by burning pain over the lower abdomen that radiates down into the inner portion of the upper thigh and into the scrotum or labia majora. The pain occasionally can be reproduced by gently tapping over an area of point tenderness (Tinel sign) or by extending the thigh or hip.

Because communication between the genitofemoral and ilioinguinal (iliohypogastric) nerves causes overlap of sensory innervation, local or specific blocks should be done to attempt to determine whether the ilioinguinal or genitofemoral nerve is specifically entrapped. If a local entrapment or neuroma is responsible for the pain, a local block of the ilioinguinal (iliohypogastric) nerve should alleviate the symptoms. If the pain is not relieved, the 1st and 2nd lumbar nerve plexus can be blocked through a paravertebral route with 0.5% bupivacaine and 0.75% lidocaine with epinephrine at a ratio of 1:200,000. By performing separate blocks and observing for pain relief, the distinction between genitofemoral and inguinal neuropathy can be made in most instances.

We are especially cautious in recommending remedial surgery in those patients who have severe coexisting ipsilateral testicular pain.

SURGICAL TREATMENT

If an ilioinguinal nerve block provides complete or substantial relief of pain, surgical exploration of the inguinal incision and identification of the ilioinguinal (iliohypogastric) nerve is indicated. If the ilioinguinal nerve block does not relieve pain, then a 1st and 2nd lumbar nerve block should be performed. If this results in pain relief, surgical exploration of the genitofemoral nerve should be considered. If pain is re-

lieved partially with both blocks, staged surgical exploration of both nerves should be contemplated.

The genitofemoral nerve classically is approached through a transverse flank incision similar to that used for lumbar sympathectomy.[3] The incision is made several centimeters lateral to and above the umbilicus, extending to the anterior axillary line. The external and internal oblique and transversus abdominis muscles are divided if necessary. The retroperitoneum is exposed and the psoas muscle and ureter are identified. The ilioinguinal and iliohypogastric nerves course lateral to the psoas muscle on the quadratus lumborum muscle. The genitofemoral nerve can be identified as it penetrates the psoas muscle, usually as a single trunk along the medial edge. A 4- to 5-cm section of the genitofemoral nerve is excised to include the bifurcation. Because of frequent abnormal variation in the site of nerve bifurcation, both branches of the genitofemoral nerve must be identified to ensure transection of the proximal genitofemoral nerve trunk. Respective distal branches are too small to be identified precisely. Hypesthesia of the scrotum (or labium majus), skin over the femoral triangle, and loss of the cremasteric reflex are the only side effects of genitofemoral neurectomy and have not caused significant morbidity. There have been a few anecdotal reports of laparoscopic genitofemoral neurectomy, and this technique may become a viable alternative to the conventional approach.

COMMENT

Severe pain and paresthesia in the inguinal region, scrotum, or proximal medial thigh after inguinal herniorrhaphy are rare, given the number of herniorrhaphies performed each year. Severe postoperative pain, however, can lead to severe debilitation and occupational incapacitation. With the exception of postoperative ilioinguinal entrapment and neuromas, little has been written about entrapment of other peripheral sensory nerves that supply the inguinal region.[1] A singular exception is trauma-induced entrapment of the lateral femoral cutaneous nerve, which may result in meralgia paresthetica. Although initially there was considerable enthusiasm for neurolysis or neurectomy of the lateral femoral cutaneous nerve, the operation seldom is performed today because of dysesthesia.

Before the article my associates and I published in 1984,[2] only 12 cases of genitofemoral neuralgia treated by neurectomy had been reported.[3,5–7] Our present series consists of 29 patients who underwent retroperitoneal resection of the genitofemoral nerve. Our results are unchanged from those of our previous publications, with 70% of patients experiencing total or significant improvement.[8,9] All patients had sensory loss in the nerve distribution without dysesthesia. One failed case, in which the patient had undergone two previous lumbar disk operations in addition to an inguinal herniorrhaphy, probably involved pain of radicular origin. Continued pain in another patient may have been caused by the rectus abdominis syndrome.[1] Most patients who are not afforded pain relief by remedial surgery are classified with chronic pain or myofascial pain syndromes.

REFERENCES

1. Dawson DM, Hallett M, Millender LH. Entrapment neuropathies. Boston, Little, Brown, 1983.
2. Harms BA, DeHaas DR, Starling JR. Diagnosis and management of genitofemoral neuralgia. Arch Surg 1984;119:339.
3. Laha RK, Rao S, Pidgeon CN, Dujovny M. Genitofemoral neuralgia. Surg Neurol 1977;8:280.
4. Lichtenstein IL, Shulman AG, Amid PK, Montllor MM. Cause and prevention of postherniorrhaphy neuralgia: a proposed protocol for treatment. Am J Surg 1988;155:786.
5. Lyon EK. Genitofemoral causalgia. Can Med Assoc J 1945;53:213.
6. Magee RK. Genitofemoral causalgia (a new syndrome). Can Med Assoc J 1942;46:326.
7. O'Brien MD. Genito-femoral neuropathy. BMJ 1979;1:1052.
8. Starling JR, Harms BA. Diagnosis and treatment of genitofemoral and ilioinguinal neuralgia. World J Surg 1989;13:586.
9. Starling JR, Harms BA, Schroeder ME, Eichman PL. Diagnosis and treatment of genitofemoral and ilioinguinal entrapment neuralgia. Surgery 1987;102:581.
10. Tons HWCh, Kupczyk-Joeris D, Rotzscher VM, Schumpelick V. Chronic inguinal pain following Shouldice repair of primary inguinal hernias. Contemp Surg 1990;37:24.

Special Problems

Part Three

Hernia, Fourth Edition, edited
by Lloyd M. Nyhus and Robert E. Condon.
J.B. Lippincott Company, Philadelphia © 1995.

Chapter 17

Strangulating External Hernia

Jack Marshall Bergstein

DEFINITIONS

A discussion of strangulating hernias that did not encompass incarceration and obstruction would be incomplete. The three problems are related and often present in the same patient. As the name implies, strangulating hernias are choked or throttled; the blood supply of the hernia contents is restricted or cut off entirely. By definition, they present danger of tissue death. They invariably are incarcerated (irreducible), but the converse is not true (ie, incarcerated hernias are not always strangulating). Likewise, obstruction usually, but not always, is present with strangulation. Strangulating hernias are ischemic, but the ischemia may be reversible (ie, the bowel may be viable). Gangrenous hernias are those with frankly necrotic contents or irreversible ischemia.

IMPORTANCE

Although strangulating hernias are uncommon, they are the most important type of hernia because of their high morbidity and mortality risk. Serious illness invariably ensues if a strangulating hernia is neglected. These defects are responsible for nearly all the serious infections and deaths that occur after hernia repair. Strangulation also limits the options for definitive repair, making prosthetic mesh placement risky, at best.

Incarcerated hernia is a relatively frequent cause of bowel obstruction, accounting for most cases of acute bowel obstruction in nearly all series of patients without previous operations.[15,37]

INCIDENCE

About one fourth of all cases of bowel obstruction result from hernias and, in most series, they are the leading cause of this condition in patients without prior operations.[6,15,24]

Inguinal hernias comprise about half of all obstructing hernias.[37] Of strangulating hernias, 43% to 62% are inguinal, 19% to 46% are femoral, 9% to 19% are umbilical, and less than 5% are incisional and other types.[1,14,22] The prevalence of strangulating inguinal hernias probably is related to the prevalence of inguinal hernias in general, rather than to a propensity to strangulate. The overall rate of incarceration is 6% to 10%,[1,32,42] whereas that of femoral hernias is 14% to 56%.[7,26,28,36]

In children, the incidence of incarcerated hernia is greatest in infancy and decreases steadily thereafter. Frank strangulation is rare.[40,42]

PATHOPHYSIOLOGY

Incarceration

Incarceration usually requires entrapment by a narrow fascial opening, often by a shutter mechanism preventing the bowel or other tissue from returning whence it came. The tissue generally becomes somewhat traumatized and edematous, and the swelling ensures irreducibility. The extent of scarring of the hernial sac at the level of the fascia varies, but may be severe and contribute further to entrapment.

Because they require a narrow but rigid fascial defect, incarceration and strangulation usually occur in femoral or small indirect inguinal hernias, or in abdominal wall hernias such as an umbilical hernia.

Incarceration in an adult is considered a surgical emergency because of the frequent presence of complete bowel obstruction and the high likelihood of progression to strangulation, with its attendant increase in morbidity and mortality.

Obstruction

Bowel obstruction occurs frequently with hernia strangulation, but is less common when the hernia sac contains omentum, preperitoneal fat, mesentery, or a solid organ. Even if bowel is present in the sac, obstruction may not occur if the hernia strangulates only a contained appendix, a Meckel diverticulum (Littre hernia), or only part of the circumference of the bowel (Richter hernia).

Whenever bowel obstruction is diagnosed, hernias must be sought as a potential cause, especially in patients without a history of abdominal operations. When obstruction and hernia coexist, they usually are causally related.

Strangulation

If the blood supply to the hernia contents becomes occluded, strangulation ensues. This may involve occlusion of a mesenteric blood vessel, but more commonly is a local phenomenon, with bowel ischemia or necrosis extending exactly to a line of clear demarcation at the edge of the fascial defect. Usually only a short segment of small intestine is involved, but on occasion the hernia may include several contiguous or noncontiguous segments of small or large bowel (eg, a Maydl hernia, or hernia-en-W).[29] Often, particularly with umbilical or incisional hernias, the strangulated tissue is omental or extraperitoneal fat.

The rate of strangulation in incarcerated hernias is related to the duration of incarceration (not to the duration of the hernia). The mortality rate is related directly to strangulation.[1,7,22,34,36]

Gangrene

Lack of blood supply results rapidly in gangrene (necrosis) because the ischemia usually is acute and local in nature. Any potential collateral vessels also are occluded by the compression at the edge of the fascia. The bowel appears dark blue, green, or black, and often has a foul or feculent smell. At this stage, restoration of blood flow cannot salvage the intestine, because of tissue death and occlusion of microvasculature by thrombus. The mucosal barrier to bacterial invasion breaks down, allowing gram-negative aerobic and anaerobic bacteria and endotoxin to invade tissue and blood. Segments of intestine that are returned to the abdomen in this condition usually perforate within 48 hours. If perforation does not occur, they often heal by fibrous tissue formation, resulting in a stricture.[2] Fortunately, the profoundly abnormal appearance of bowel at this stage usually prevents its inadvertent return to the abdomen.

Perforation

Strangulated bowel eventually perforates as bacterial invasion and tissue autolysis proceeds. This releases the stagnant bowel contents, which contain actively proliferating gram-negative aerobic and anaerobic bacteria, into the surrounding soft tissue. This may occur spontaneously, resulting in spontaneous reduction followed by diffuse peritonitis, or in abscess with necessitation and bowel fistula.[12] Perforation also occurs when the thinned-out bowel is handled at operation and, having the strength of wet tissue paper, perforates almost immediately, spilling infectious material over the entire wound. Having thus decompressed and decreased the tissue volume, the perforated bowel now may slip back into the abdomen. The surgeon must make an abdominal incision to scoop out collections of succus entericus or stool.

Infection

Infection may occur at almost any stage of a strangulating hernia. With bowel obstruction comes the potential for vomiting and aspiration pneumonia. Bacteria proliferate, reaching concentrations in the small bowel equivalent to those in the colon.

It is uncommon for strangulating hernia to present late enough that an infection already is established. Strangulation with or without perforation, however, increases the risk of infection after operation. Surgical site infection may occur in as many as 50% of patients with gangrenous bowel[37] (Table 17-1). A substantial number are gram-negative enteric bacterial infections. This is in contrast to an elective hernia repair operation, in which wound infection is unusual and, when it does occur, is likely to be caused by a gram-positive organism. In this setting, as in others, gram-negative infection tends to release endotoxin, causing severe sepsis and, potentially, multisystem organ failure and death.

Mortality is increased in the presence of discolored peritoneal fluid, especially if it is red, red-black, black, cloudy, or purulent. Such fluid contains high concentrations of enteric bacteria because it accompanies hemorrhage and gangrene of the bowel wall and loss of bacterial barrier function.[22]

Mortality

Mortality is particularly high in incarcerated femoral hernia; rates of 18% to 50% have been reported. Several factors contribute to the significant mortality rate, including a high incidence of gangrene, delayed presentation and treatment (see Strangulation and Infection), improper treatment, and advanced age of the patients. McNealy and coworkers[26] reported 60% mortality in gangrenous femoral hernia. In 70% of the fatal cases, error in diagnosis led to delay in operative treatment of 1 to 8 days. In Andrews'[1] series,

Table 17-1. Infections and Mortality in Hernias Causing Small-Bowel Obstruction

Type	No. Hernias (%)	No. Gangrenous Wounds (%)	No. of Wounds Closed (%)	No. of Wounds Infected (%)	No. of Deaths (%)
Inguinal	31 (54)	10 (32)	6 (19)	2 (33)	0
Femoral	8 (14)	6 (75)	2 (25)	2 (100)	0
Umbilical	9 (16)	1 (11)	0	0	0
Incisional	8 (14)	3 (38)	1 (13)	1 (100)	0
Diaphragmatic	1 (2)	1 (100)	—	—	1 (100)
Total	57	21 (37)	10	5 (50)	1 (1.8)

(Stewardson RH, Bombeck CT, Nyhus LM. Critical operative management of small bowel obstruction. Ann Surg 1978;187:189)

strangulating hernia occurred most often in patients aged 70 to 75 years.

DIAGNOSIS

History

Most patients give a history of a previously reducible mass that suddenly has become enlarged, hard, tender, and irreducible. Many, however, have new onset of a mass or painful tender area. Femoral hernia strangulation often presents with abdominal pain; Jens and Adelaide[20] reported lower abdominal pain (usually colicky) in 76% of cases, but pain over the hernia in only 26% of cases. Nausea, vomiting, and abdominal distention are common. These findings suggest bowel obstruction, although strangulation may occur without obstruction. A history of fever or oliguria should be sought, as well as signs of sepsis. A review of the past surgical history, with specific attention to previous abdominal operations and hernia repairs, is essential. In particular, patients should be asked whether they have any synthetic material in place.

Physical Examination

The patient should be disrobed for an adequate hernia examination. Hernia should be sought in all patients with bowel obstruction. The general aspects of the physical examination for hernia are detailed elsewhere in this book. Incarcerated inguinal hernia presents as a firm, often tender mass in the inguinal canal or groin. A femoral hernia presents as a tender lump medial to the femoral pulse and is not always appreciated by the patient. Often, by the time the surgeon sees the patient, several other examiners have attempted to reduce the hernia. Nonetheless, an incarcerated hernia without strangulation should not have overlying redness or severe tenderness. Such findings

indicate possible strangulation. If the patient has been vomiting, the chest examination should not be overlooked.

A complete abdominal examination is essential, seeking distention, the presence and character of bowel sounds, and abdominal tenderness or rebound. When examining a patient who complains bitterly of pain in a large, tender mass, it is easy to overlook or minimize other physical findings. This probably is why peritonitis coexisting with strangulating hernia rarely is diagnosed before surgery. Under these circumstances, the standard hernia incision (eg, groin) may contribute to inadequate exploration and treatment, and thus the high mortality of this condition (15%–40%).[12,33] If the results of a rectal examination are positive for gross or occult blood, strangulation, gangrene, or a coincident gastrointestinal malignancy may be present.

Because of the potential for both bowel obstruction with attendant fluid sequestration and septic shock, careful attention should be given during the physical examination to the state of the patient's hydration and perfusion. Such criteria as urine output and skin turgor should be evaluated. Cool skin, oliguria, tachycardia, confusion, and lethargy all are ominous findings and warrant further attention to resuscitation, as well as fluid administration and possible invasive monitoring in the intensive care unit.

Laboratory and Roentgenographic Evaluation

Objective diagnostic aids such as laboratory and roentgenographic evaluation have only an adjunctive role in the diagnosis of strangulating hernia. Patients may have substantial physiologic derangements with strangulating hernia, including septic shock, electrolyte abnormalities, vomiting, ketoacidosis (in diabetics), and substantial volume deficits. Therefore, electrolyte levels, blood counts, and blood gas vol-

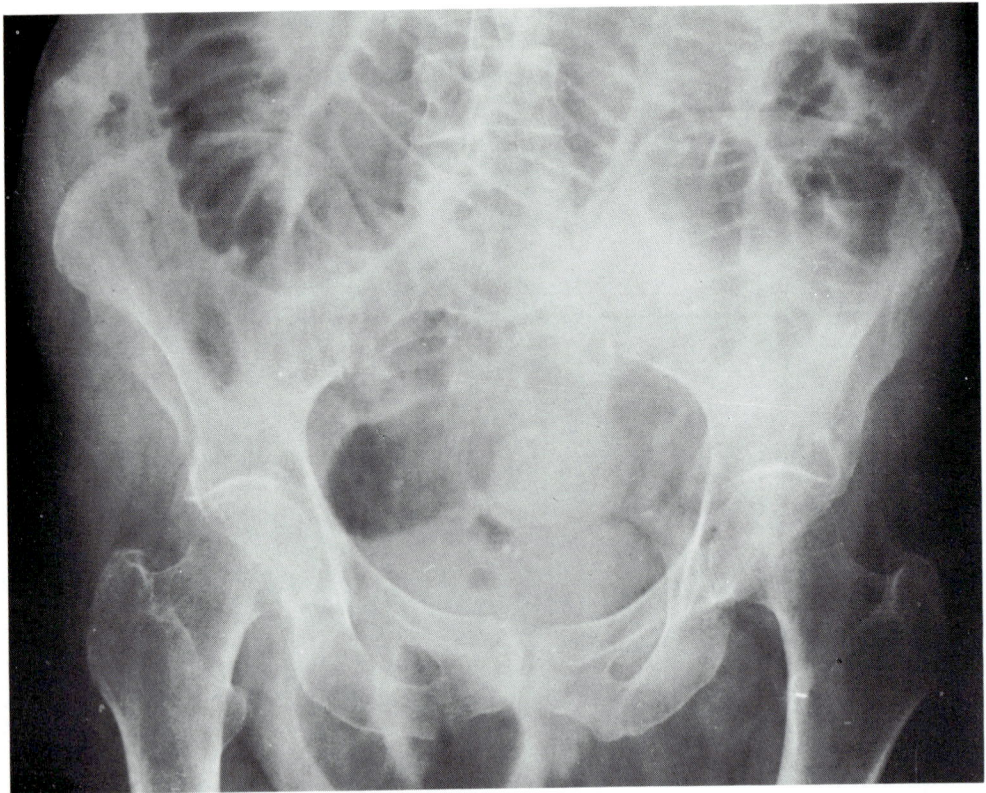

Figure 17-1. Abdominal roentgenogram, demonstrating an air-filled loop of small bowel in the inguinal region.

umes should be determined if there is a suggestion of physiologic abnormalities.

Metabolic acidosis and elevation of the serum potassium level both are strongly suggestive of dead gut. They usually are not associated with bowel necrosis resulting from strangulation, however, because the same constricting band that prevents blood flow to the bowel prevents the return of mesenteric venous blood with its load of potassium, lactic acid, and endotoxin.

Ultrasonography may help in detecting obscure inguinal or abdominal wall masses. Occasionally, an interstitial hernia may require ultrasound or computed tomographic (CT) scanning for diagnosis. A plain film of the abdomen may demonstrate a gas-filled structure in the area of a mass, confirming the diagnosis of hernia (Fig. 17-1). In addition, roentgenographic evidence of bowel obstruction should be apparent. A lateral film may demonstrate that the structure lies anterior to the anterior abdominal fascia. A chest roentgenogram should be obtained if there is a history of vomiting, to determine whether aspiration pneumonia is present.

CT scanning generally is sensitive and specific for hernia, and on occasion is the test that first demonstrates the abnormality. Certain interstitial hernias may be difficult to diagnose accurately with any other modality. Most of the hernias diagnosed by CT, however, were overlooked during the physical examination.

TREATMENT—GENERAL CONSIDERATIONS

Attempts at Reduction

Several authors advocate attempting to reduce incarcerated hernias ("taxis") in an effort to convert a surgical emergency into an elective operation and thereby decrease the mortality risk.[21] Others, citing the possibilities of reducing dead bowel into the abdomen or of reducing the mass still strangulated by a fibrous ring adherent to the hernia sac neck (reduction en masse [Fig. 17-2]), abhor reduction attempts.

Although gangrenous strangulation can occur in as few as 5 hours, a hernia that has been incarcerated for less than 24 hours is unlikely to contain dead bowel; if it does, gentle attempts at reduction probably will not be successful. Furthermore, reduction en masse is uncommon and may not be prevented by

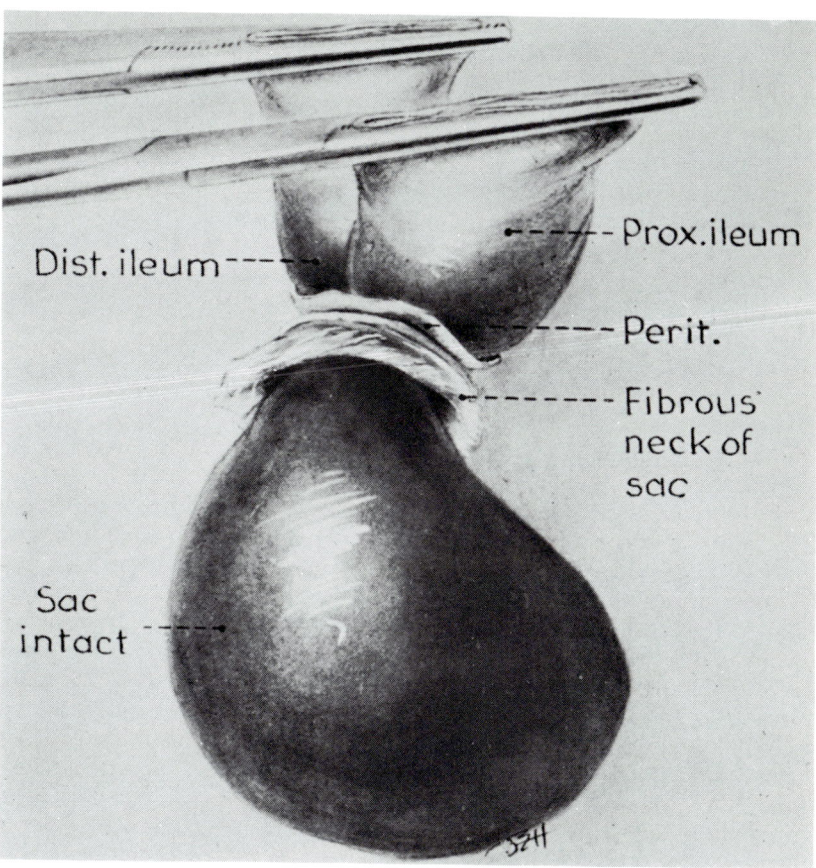

Dist. ileum

Prox. ileum

Perit.

Fibrous
neck of
sac

Sac
intact

Figure 17-2. Loop of small bowel with adherent, obstructing fibrous ring. When this is reduced with the ring intact (reduction en masse), the strangulation is not relieved, only hidden.

avoiding taxis, because it can occur with spontaneous reduction.[27,44]

Patients with an incarcerated hernia generally come to the emergency department within a few hours of initial incarceration. Preliminary attempts to reduce the hernia often are made by inexperienced physicians with the patient upright or straining. In these cases, however, reduction often is simple. Assumption of the Trendelenburg position is helpful and may result in "spontaneous" reduction if the patient is left alone for about 10 minutes. If not, gentle pressure with or without *light* sedation often is successful. If reduction occurs and the patient's symptoms are relieved, herniorrhaphy should be scheduled as soon as possible to prevent repeated incarceration (the next operating day if possible, but definitely within the week). If gentle attempts at reduction are not successful, more forceful maneuvers are *not* indicated; emergency operation should be undertaken.

No attempt should be made to reduce the hernia if any of the following are present: diffuse abdominal tenderness, red or purple discoloration of the mass, signs and symptoms of systemic sepsis, or extraluminal air (on roentgenography). If the mass has been irreducible for more than 24 hours, the likelihood of strangulation is increased and reduction should be attempted warily, if at all.

Resuscitation

Patients with strangulating hernia occasionally require significant resuscitation before surgery is undertaken. They are at risk of bowel obstruction, which may cause dehydration of 10% to 20% of body water through vomiting or fluid sequestration in the bowel wall or lumen.[9] The presence of abscess or intraabdominal infection, necrotic tissue, or infarcted bowel may lead to bacterial translocation, endotoxemia with systemic sepsis, or frank septic shock.

Induction of anesthesia under these conditions almost always leads to cardiovascular collapse. A scramble results to perform in 5 minutes the resuscitation that should have taken place over a few hours, and can fail by being inadequate or by "drowning" the patient, but is almost certain to be less satisfactory than preoperative resuscitation.

Signs of shock should be sought, even in normotensive patients. Urine output should be monitored, remembering that the volume of an initial specimen is not useful because the length of time since the bladder was last emptied is not known. Tachycardia should be considered prima facie evidence of shock, and should prompt further monitoring as well as initiation of fluid resuscitation.

In a young and previously healthy patient who responds to an initial fluid challenge with normalization of the heart rate and urine output, no further monitoring may be necessary. If the initial response is not as expected, additional information should be obtained. A central venous pressure monitor may suffice, particularly if a low central venous pressure confirms a clinical suspicion of hypovolemia. In any patient older than 65 years, or with a history of heart, lung, or kidney disease, invasive monitoring with a flow-directed pulmonary artery (Swan-Ganz) catheter is necessary.

Most patients are somewhat dehydrated; this usually can be confirmed by a low to low-normal pulmonary artery occlusion pressure ("wedge" pressure). Cardiac output may be in the normal range, but this may be the result of compensatory reflexes. The surgeon should be particularly wary of the patient with tachycardia and an elevated systemic vascular resistance; the inherent vasodilative effects of anesthetic agents may result in the well-known hypotensive "crash on induction." Most patients require staged fluid administration (5–10 L may be necessary), occasionally followed by inotropic agents or vasodilators.

When physiologic parameters have been brought as close to normal as possible, the patient is ready for operation, and further delay should be avoided because it allows time for further deterioration. It should be remembered, however, that some patients may not normalize until the pathologic process is treated and abnormal tissue is resected.

Treatment of Obstruction

Bowel obstruction should be treated as is any complete mechanical obstruction. Gastric decompression and fluid resuscitation are mandatory. Nonoperative therapy has no place in the treatment of strangulating, obstructed hernia. Because strangulation cannot be ruled out until the bowel is examined in the operating room, continued nonoperative therapy may allow a strangulated loop of bowel to perforate.

Timing of Operation

Operation for strangulating hernia should be considered a true emergency. Once the patient is resuscitated adequately, as evidenced by such criteria as sufficient urine output, absence of postural hypotension, and normal cardiovascular parameters on Swan-Ganz catheterization, operative exploration and repair must proceed without delay. Even an hour may make the difference between dead and viable bowel, and between perforated and intact bowel.

Patients who have had an incarcerated hernia reduced by a physician in the emergency department should be scheduled for elective operation at the earliest possible date, to prevent recurrence and even more disastrous results.

Antibiotic Therapy

Because the presence of dead or perforated bowel must be presumed in patients with strangulating hernia, broad-spectrum intravenous antibiotics should be administered during the operation, ideally beginning at least 15 minutes before the induction of anesthesia. Coverage should be adequate for a colon operation (ie, gram-negative aerobes, such as *Escherichia coli,* and anaerobes such as *Bacteroides fragilis,* must be attacked adequately). In most cases, antibiotics need not be administered after the first postoperative day because no advantage of more prolonged antimicrobial therapy can be demonstrated. In patients with a prosthetic device, either preexisting (eg, a heart valve) or implanted as part of the hernia repair, a longer course of antibiotics (as much as 5 days) may be warranted.

Operative Therapy

There are four goals of surgery for strangulating hernia: (1) to remove gangrenous tissue, (2) to prevent further sepsis, (3) to relieve obstruction, and (4) to repair the hernia defect. Of these, hernia repair is least important. All four goals must be considered in planning the operation, because an approach may be required that differs substantially from the optimal approach for a nonstrangulating hernia. For example, it is important to use an operative approach that incorporates initial control of the bowel to avoid the possibility that necrotic or perforated bowel will slip out of sight through the inguinal canal, spreading bacteria, stool, and endotoxin as it goes. Thus, any approach used for an incarcerated (possibly strangulating) hernia must include access to the abdominal cavity.

It also should be remembered that other serious conditions may masquerade as a strangulating hernia, including hemorrhagic pancreatitis, peritonitis of various causes, and internal strangulation. Red, black, or cloudy peritoneal fluid (or pus) found in the hernia sac, even in the presence of otherwise normal contents, should prompt immediate celiotomy, through an incision that allows inspection of the entire peritoneal cavity.

Prosthetic Mesh

The use of prosthetic material should be tempered by the knowledge that the risk of infection is increased in strangulating hernia, especially in the presence of any gangrenous bowel, perforation, or red, black, purulent, or cloudy peritoneal fluid.

Prosthetic materials have been used successfully for years, and some experts recommend them routinely. Certain guidelines must be followed, however. Mesh should be placed in uncontaminated abdominal or preperitoneal locations, if possible. Polypropylene (Marlex) mesh is preferable to polytetrafluoroethylene (Gore-Tex) mesh for its greater tolerance of infection. If the latter becomes infected, it must be removed completely, whereas the former may incorporate despite infection. When prosthetic substances are used in a potentially contaminated field, a 5-day

course of prophylactic antibiotics is advisable. Permanent prosthetic materials should *not* be placed in a space that has been frankly infected because the foreign body usually precludes cure of the infection. In such cases, it is safest to resect the bowel, control the infection, and leave the repair of the fascial defect for another day. Bioabsorbable meshes (Vicryl, Dexon) may be useful temporarily, but the hernia usually recurs when the mesh resorbs, so later definitive repair should be planned. If the hernia has an immediate tendency to recur and strangulate again, other options include immediate repair with a fascial or musculofascial flap, or enlargement of the defect (to eliminate its ability to strangulate) followed by later repair.

TREATMENT OF GROIN HERNIAS

The preperitoneal approach is ideal for strangulating inguinal hernia because it allows easy access to the abdomen for control and resection of the bowel and pre-

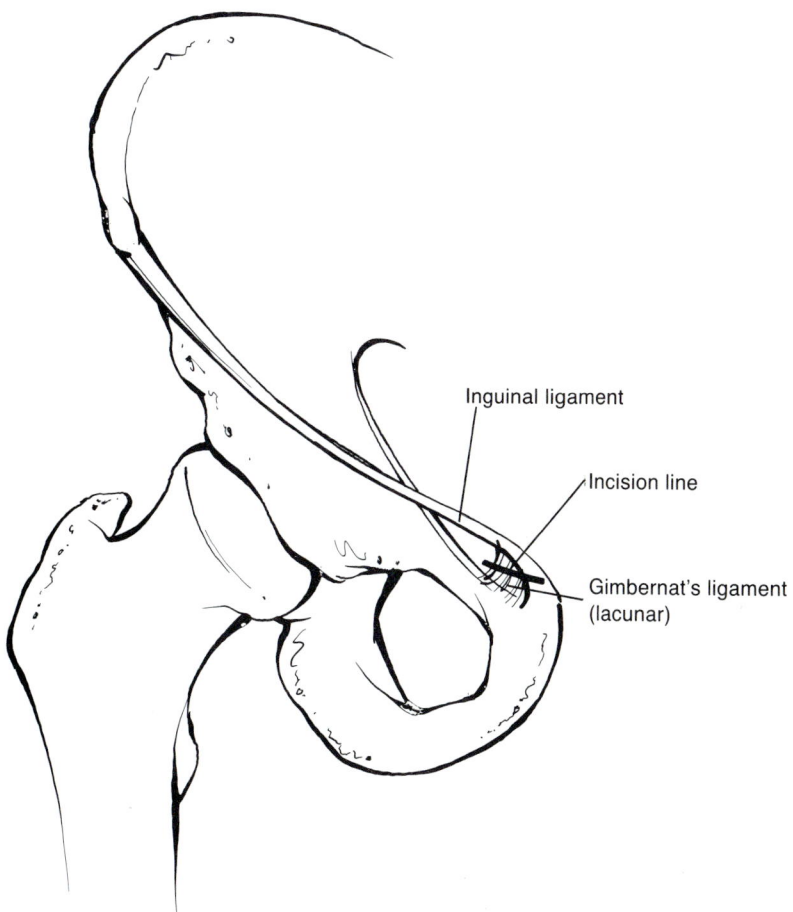

Figure 17-3. Medial incision of Gimbernat ligament and, if necessary, inguinal ligament to relieve incarceration of femoral hernia. (Redrawn from McNealy RW, Lichtenstein ME, Todd MA. The diagnosis and management of incarcerated strangulated femoral hernia. Surg Gynecol Obstet 1942;74:1005)

Inguinal ligament

Incision line

Gimbernat's ligament (lacunar)

liminary control of the vasculature, as well as excellent exposure for treatment of the hernia without requiring the abdominal counterincision that is necessary in an anterior approach.

Once the peritoneum is incised, the neck of the entrapped viscus is inspected for petechiae, which suggest strangulation. If none are present, temporary control of the bowel and vascular pedicle is secured with noncrushing clamps, the bowel is reduced manually, and the hernia is repaired. In some cases, it may be necessary to incise the medial margin of the deep inguinal ring or the femoral canal (the Gimbernat ligament), or the inguinal ligament (Fig. 17-3). If petechiae are present, strangulation must be assumed. The bowel is controlled and resected without reducing the hernia contents, and anastomosis is performed. The peritoneum then is closed and the strangulated bowel is removed from the inguinal canal along with the hernia sac. A surgical stapling device used to divide the bowel neatly and securely prevents spillage from either end, which is difficult if bowel clamps are used to pass an end of infarcted bowel through a hernia opening. If an indirect hernia is entrapped by the external ring, it is easy to lift a skin flap to expose the area.[16,25a]

Femoral hernias are treated most easily by the preperitoneal approach. Alternative approaches include the anterior (inguinal canal) and inferior (thigh) routes, which may require an abdominal counterincision for bowel resection and risk losing control of a loop of gangrenous or perforated bowel into the abdominal cavity. Some surgeons use a transperitoneal approach routinely. This affords excellent bowel control and easy hernia repair, but not all patients require laparotomy because reduction sometimes can be accomplished simply by allowing viable bowel to slip back in.

In the presence of signs and symptoms of diffuse peritonitis or other intraabdominal pathology, laparotomy is mandatory. A midline incision provides ample exposure for repair of groin or femoral hernias, as well as access to the entire abdomen. The principles described above for indirect inguinal hernia apply here as well. Control of the bowel is assured before reduction of the hernia.

TREATMENT OF OTHER HERNIAS

Treatment principles for umbilical, incisional, and ventral strangulating hernias are the same as outlined above. If the bowel is clearly gangrenous, intraabdominal control of viable bowel with preliminary resection offers the best chance of avoiding subsequent intraab-

dominal infection. If the hernia appears to be a simple, early incarceration, direct incision over the hernia will reveal whether the contents are viable, and can be followed by counterincision or extension if necessary.

Ventral and incisional hernias, because of their size, have the potential to strangulate most of the intestine. This is a special problem, because as much intestinal length as possible must be preserved to avoid short-bowel syndrome, yet unresected nonviable gut threatens the patient's life. Pink color and peristalsis are strong predictors for bowel segment survival. Intestine that appears dusky and flaccid but has a pulse in mesenteric vessels may be delineated by using Doppler ultrasound to examine mural blood flow[43] or by examining the intestine under ultraviolet (Wood's) light after fluorescein injection. In an animal model, a diffuse reticular fluorescent pattern predicted survival of the segment, whereas a pattern of patchy nonfluorescence required reexamination 24 hours later. At that time, all segments appeared grossly nonviable. Segments that retained fluorescein from the initial injection died. Others again showed the patchy pattern on repeated injection, and all segments survived, although 5 of 15 had localized perforation.[38]

NEW TREATMENTS—LAPAROSCOPY

Although laparoscopic hernia repair has become popular in many medical centers, it is unlikely to play much of a role in the treatment of strangulating hernia. Bowel obstruction is a relative contraindication to laparoscopy, because distended loops impair visualization of the abdominal cavity. Surgeons who are familiar with laparoscopy know that it is not well suited to emergency operations because of the complexity of the instruments and video setup, which usually requires a special operating room team that may not be available for an emergency case. Even more important, laparoscopic bowel-handling instruments are still somewhat crude, and will never match the sophistication and delicacy of the human finger in handling strangulated bowel; control and delicacy are paramount considerations.

SUMMARY

Strangulating hernias demand special attention because of the urgent way in which they present, the extreme distress they cause, and the dire consequences they inflict. Treatment must be directed at the potential complications: bowel gangrene, obstruction, infection, sepsis, and death. With these problems in mind, the hernia can be treated with maximum likelihood of success.

REFERENCES

1. Andrews NJ. Presentation and outcome of strangulated external hernia in a district general hospital. Br J Surg 1981;68:329.
2. Barry HC. Fibrous stricture of the small intestine following strangulated hernia. Br J Surg 1942;30:64.
3. Boley SJ, Cahn D, Lauer T, Weinberg G, Kleinhaus S. The irreducible ovary: a true emergency. J Pediatr Surg 1991;26:1035.
4. Bowesman C. Reduction of strangulated inguinal hernia. Lancet 1951;1:1396.
5. Cheatle GL. An operation for the radical cure of inguinal and femoral hernia. BMJ 1920;2:68.
6. Chifan M, St. Georgescu T, Tircoveanu E, Niculescu D, Bordea M. Surgical aspects of intestinal obstruction in the elderly. Rev Med Chir Soc Med Nat Iasi 1989;93:711.
7. Dean GO. Strangulated femoral hernia. Arch Surg 1942;44:933.
8. Dennis C. Oblique, aseptic, end-to-end ileac anastomosis, procedure of choice in strangulating small bowel obstruction. Surg Gynecol Obstet 1943;77:225.
9. Dennis C, Varco RL. Femoral hernia with gangrenous bowel. Surgery 1947;22:312.
10. Douglas DM. Strangulated hernia: a consideration of some factors affecting mortality. BMJ 1942;1:354.
11. Dunphy JE. The diagnosis and surgical management of strangulated femoral hernia. JAMA 1940;114:394.
12. Ekwueme O. Strangulated external hernia associated with generalized peritonitis. Br J Surg 1973;60:930.
13. Fashakin EO. Experience with 103 cases of intestinal gangrene in Ile-Ife, Nigeria. Trop Doct 1989;19:25.
14. Frankau C. Strangulated hernia: a review of 1487 cases. Br J Surg 1931;19:176.
15. Fuzun M, Kaymak E, Harmancioglu O, Astarcioglu K. Principal causes of mechanical bowel obstruction in surgically treated adults in Western Turkey. Br J Surg 1991;78:202.
16. George SM Jr, Mangiante EC, Voeller GR, Britt LG. Preperitoneal herniorrhaphy for the acutely incarcerated groin hernia. Am Surg 1991;57:139.
17. Gibson LD, Gaspar MR. A review of 606 cases of umbilical hernia. Int Abstr Surg 1959;109:313.
18. Gillespie RW, Glas WW, Mertz GH, Musselman MM. Richter's hernia: its etiology, recognition and management. Arch Surg 1956;73:590.
19. Glicklich M, Eliasoph J. Incarcerated obturator hernia: case diagnosed at barium enema fluoroscopy. Radiology 1989;172:51.
20. Jens J, Adelaide MB. Strangulated femoral hernia. Lancet 1943;1:705.
21. Kauffman HM Jr, O'Brien DP. Selective reduction of incarcerated inguinal hernia. Am J Surg 1970;119:660.
22. Laufman H, Daniels J. Clinical factors affecting mortality in strangulated hernia. Arch Surg 1951;62:365.
23. Lichtenstein IL, Shore JM. Exploding the myths of hernia repair. Am J Surg 1976;132:307.
24. Liu My, Lin HH, Wu CS. Etiology of intestinal obstruction—4 years' experience. Chang Keng I Hsueh 1990;13:161.
25. MacKenzie I. Management of strangulated hernia. Surg Clin North Am 1960;40:1367.
25a. Malagoni MA, Condon RE. Preperitoneal repair of acute incarcerated and strangulated hernias of the groin. Surg Gynecol Obstet 1986;162:65.
26. McNealy RW, Lichtenstein ME, Todd MA. The diagnosis and management of incarcerated strangulated femoral hernia. Surg Gynecol Obstet 1942;74:1005.
27. Mings H, Olson JD. Reduction "en masse" of groin herniae. Arch Surg 1965;90:764.
28. Moran B. Strangulated external hernia. (Letter) Trop Doct 1988;73.
29. Moss CM, Levine R, Messenger N, Dardik I. Sliding colonic Maydl's hernia: report of a case. Dis Colon Rectum 1976;19:636.
30. Nemir P Jr, Hawthorne HR, Cohn I Jr, Drabkin DL. The cause of death in strangulation obstruction: an experimental study. Ann Surg 1949;130:857.
31. Nomikos IN, Papaioannou AN. Experience with the intra-abdominal approach for complicated hernias of the inguinal region. Int Surg 1992;77:232.
32. Nyhus LM, Condon RE, Harkins HN. Clinical experiences with preperitoneal hernial repair for all types of hernia of the groin. Am J Surg 1960;100:234.
33. Pfeffermann R, Freund H. Symptomatic hernia: strangulated hernia combined with acute abdominal disease. Am J Surg 1972;124:60.
34. Requarth W, Theis FV. Incarcerated and strangulated inguinal hernia. Arch Surg 1948;57:267.
35. Rizk TA, Deshmukh N. Obturator hernia: a difficult diagnosis. South Med J 1990;83:709.
36. Rogers FA. Strangulated femoral hernia: a review of 170 cases. Ann Surg 1959;149:9.
37. Stewardson RH, Bombeck CT, Nyhus LM. Critical operative management of small bowel obstruction. Ann Surg 1978;187:189.
38. Stolar CJ, Randolph JG. Evaluation of ischemic bowel viability with a fluorescent technique. J Pediatr Surg 1978;13:221.
39. Stoppa RE. The treatment of complicated groin and incisional hernias. World J Surg 1989;13:545.
40. Thorndike A Jr, Ferguson CF. Incarcerated inguinal hernia in infancy and childhood. Am J Surg 1938;39:429.
41. Watts GT. Fallacies: a hernia has an expansile impulse on coughing except when strangulated. Lancet 1986;1:261.
42. Wiklander O. Incarcerated inguinal hernia in childhood. Acta Chir Scand 1951;101:303.
43. Wright CB, Hobson RW. Prediction of intestinal viability using Doppler ultrasound technics. Am J Surg 1975;129:642.

44. Wright RN, Arensman RM, Coughlin TR, Nyhus LM. Hernia reduction en masse. Am Surg 1977; 43:627.
45. Zarins CK, Skinner DB, Rhodes BA, James AE Jr. Prediction of the viability of revascularized intestine with radioactive microspheres. Surg Gynecol Obstet 1974;138:576.

Editor's Comment

Strangulating hernias, those in which compromise of the blood supply to the hernial contents has led to gangrene, are responsible for most of the deaths that occur as a direct consequence of an abdominal hernia. Bergstein indicates that the mortality risk may be as high as 40% in hernias that involve strangulation. Although this may be true in parts of the Third World, it does not reflect current experience in the United States, even in those centers that treat predominantly the indigent and disadvantaged among our population.

The essential substrate that permits the development of a strangulating hernia is the presence in the abdominal wall of a small opening with rigid margins. It is not surprising, therefore, that femoral and umbilical hernias are associated more commonly with strangulation than are other types of hernia. The primary objectives of operative therapy for a suspected strangulating hernia are to prevent the release of toxin-loaded blood and lymph from the gangrenous herniated tissues into the systemic circulation, and to prevent the spill of contaminated material from the necrotic intestine in the hernia into the peritoneal cavity.

For more than 20 years, I have been examining candidates on the oral examinations of the American Board of Surgery. In this context, I have posed to hundreds of examinees a question regarding the treatment of strangulating hernia. I outline, in an obese 70-year-old woman, the clear presence for more than 48 hours of a small-bowel obstruction, coupled on examination with the additional finding of a tender mass in the right upper thigh just below the inguinal ligament and medial to a palpable femoral pulse. Less than 10 of the hundreds of candidates examined have been able to outline a satisfactory approach to this clinical situation that recognizes the important principles of therapy: preoperative resuscitation, initial proximal control of involved bowel, resection and anastomosis before reduction of the hernia contents, reduction and removal of the gangrenous loop of bowel without spillage onto tissue, use of appropriate antibiotics and other drugs to mitigate postoperative complications, and repair of the hernia despite the presence of inflammation or infection.

The failure of most of the candidates I have examined to be able to outline successful treatment of a strangulating hernia is, in my view, a major failure of surgical pedagogy. I hope that future generations of surgeons will avail themselves of the cogent advice contained in this chapter by Bergstein.

R.E.C.

Hernia, Fourth Edition, edited
by Lloyd M. Nyhus and Robert E. Condon.
J.B. Lippincott Company, Philadelphia © 1995.

Chapter 18

Sliding Inguinal Hernia

Michael J. Demeure

Sliding inguinal hernia remains a problem for many surgeons despite the excellent treatises written on the subject over the past 70 years. Failure to recognize a sliding hernia appears to be the principal cause of difficulty. Although most of these defects may be repaired well through the inguinal approach that is used for other types of hernia, an occasional large sliding hernia may require combined abdominal and inguinal incisions.

A sliding inguinal hernia is defined as one in which a viscus or its mesentery forms a portion of the wall of the hernia sac. The term often is applied incorrectly to hernias in which the viscus simply is attached to the sac by adhesions. Once the adhesions are lysed, however, such a hernia may be reduced and repaired as any other hernia.

Indirect sliding hernias are the most common type, but femoral and direct sliding inguinal hernias also occur. A sliding hernia on the left side usually contains the sigmoid colon and one on the right side contains the cecum. Typically, these organs comprise the posterolateral wall of the hernia sac. A variety of other organs, however, including the female adnexa, ileum, appendix, ureter, or bladder, may be part of a sliding hernia. The greatest danger presented by failure to recognize the presence of a sliding hernia is that the viscus or its mesenteric vasculature may be injured during the course of surgical repair. The vas deferens and spermatic vessels also are at risk of inadvertent injury during dissection of a sliding hernia because the hernia tends to lie between the vas deferens and the spermatic artery.

Sliding hernias may be classified as one of three types: (1) intrasaccular sliding hernia, in which the sliding component is free except that the peritoneum of its mesentery is contiguous with that of the hernia sac; (2) parasaccular or intramural sliding hernia, in which the sliding component lies in the wall of the hernia sac and cannot be separated from the peritoneum of the sac without injury to the organ; or (3) extrasaccular sliding hernia, also called sac-less because the sliding viscus may be separated completely from the hernia sac or there may be no sac at all. Anatomically, the bladder is the only organ in position to

comprise the rare third type of hernia. Of these three groups, the parasaccular type is by far the most common, accounting for about 95% of all sliding inguinal hernias.

As the treatment of sliding inguinal hernias has evolved with a better appreciation of their pathogenesis, anatomy, and natural history, surgeons have adopted a simplified operative approach through an inguinal incision. The combined inguinal and abdominal approach now generally is reserved for large or strangulated sliding inguinal hernias. In the early literature, recurrence rates were reported to be higher for repaired sliding inguinal hernias than for repaired nonsliding inguinal hernias.[11] This claim has been repudiated in more recent reports, which have demonstrated that use of the inguinal approach alone results in recurrence rates at least as low as those associated with the repair of other inguinal hernias.[24]

INCIDENCE

The relative rarity of sliding inguinal hernias may be one reason that they have remained somewhat enigmatic for many surgeons. Sliding hernias are more common in men than in women, and their incidence increases with advancing age. Most reports indicate that sliding hernias account for 3% to 6% of all inguinal hernias (Table 18-1), but the incidence is higher in series composed primarily of elderly patients. By most accounts, bilateral sliding hernias are distinctly uncommon. Barrow[2] found only one in 1000 male military recruits. Burton[4] encountered only two during the course of 2614 hernia operations. In contrast, Piedad and associates[21] reported that 10% of sliding hernias were bilateral.

The largest single series of sliding inguinal hernias included 313 patients seen over an 8-year period. In this series, Ryan[25] reported many demographic data. Almost all the patients had indirect sliding inguinal hernias; 3 had direct hernias and 1 had a sliding femoral hernia of the sigmoid colon. The left side was involved 4.5 times more often than was the right side. Eight patients (2.6%) had bilateral sliding her-

Table 18-1. Incidence of Sliding Inguinal Hernia

	Total No. of Hernias	Sliding Hernias	Incidence (%)
Gibson and Felter (1930)	1,878	56	3.0
Fallis (1936)	1,600	53	3.3
Parsons (1937)	702	27	3.8
Longacre (1939)	925	29	3.1
Sensenig and Nichols (1955)	1,200	59	4.9
Ryan (1956)	6,188	313	5.1
Giuseffi and McSwain (1957)	1,457	50	3.4
Estes (1960)	400	36	9.0
Maingot (1961)	1,000	64	6.4
Palumbo and Sharpe (1971)	3,572	99	2.8
Piedad et al. (1973)	1,080	60	5.6
Obney (1984)	107,854	9,599	8.9

nias. Men, particularly obese men, were more prone to have a sliding hernia than were women. The likelihood of an indirect sliding hernia increased with age from a low of 0.44% in the third decade of life to more than 13% in the eighth decade (average, 6.7%). The mean age at presentation with a sliding hernia was 59 years compared to 51 years for a nonsliding hernia. A factor that may favor the development of a sliding hernia is the long-standing presence of a hernia. The average duration of the condition before operation was 11.8 years for a sliding hernia compared to 7.4 years for hernias with no sliding component.

Sliding hernias are infrequent in adult women; there were none among Ryan's 313 patients, and Longacre[15] reported only one woman among 29 patients with sliding hernias. Sliding hernias do occur in female infants, however. Up to 28% of all inguinal hernias in female infants contain sliding elements composed of fallopian tube and broad ligament with or without the ovary. Although they can and do occur, sliding hernias are rare in male infants. In contrast to adult sliding hernias, which appear to be acquired, sliding hernias in infants have been attributed to a congenital malformation.[6]

DIAGNOSIS

A sliding hernia is difficult to diagnose before operation and usually is not discovered until the time of hernia repair. This type of hernia typically is partially, but not completely, reducible. Ryan, however, reported that all but 2.9% of the sliding hernias in his series were completely reducible. One feature that should arouse suspicion is intolerance to a truss. A truss may be particularly unsuitable for a sliding her-

nia because the bowel is not completely reduced. The truss puts pressure on the viscus, not only causing discomfort, but possibly injuring the bowel. Based on the physical examination, a sliding component may be suspected if the hernia is bulky, large, and extends into the scrotum. Because the internal inguinal ring is large, obstruction, incarceration, and, consequently, strangulation are rare. Therefore, bowel resection almost never is necessary in the repair of a sliding hernia. A preoperative barium enema may demonstrate the sigmoid colon or cecum within the hernia sac, suggesting a sliding hernia. Such a finding is not conclusive, though, because it could be associated with a nonsliding hernia if the viscus merely resides in the hernia sac. Although the diagnosis of a sliding hernia ultimately is made at the time of operation, suspicion should be aroused if the patient is an elderly man with a large inguinal hernia of long duration that extends well into the scrotum.

ANATOMY AND PATHOGENESIS

In 1925, Moschcowitz gave his description of the pathogenesis of sliding indirect inguinal hernia, noting with seeming frustration that "The literature appertaining to the subject of sliding inguinal hernia may be divided into three classes, good, bad and indifferent. The number of the good articles alone is, however, so large that the ignorance which still prevails is more than surprising."

Moschcowitz identified a basic two-part phenomenon comprised of what he termed a *pulling mechanism* and a *pushing mechanism*. The pulling mechanism occurs when traction is applied to the parietal peritoneum by the enlarging hernia sac through an enlarged internal ring, until some part of the retroperitoneal viscus is pulled into the sac (Fig. 18-1). In this case, the anterior wall of the hernia sac is free peritoneum, whereas the posterior wall is comprised of the viscus or its mesentery. Conversely, an anteriorly located viscus, such as the bladder, may be pushed or may protrude through a defect to become part of the hernia sac. The resultant hernia is known as an extrasaccular sliding hernia.

The ultimate result of either mechanism is that a previously retroperitoneal organ becomes the content of a hernia. It was predicated further that only such

an organ can become a sliding hernia. Moschcowitz observed that the ascending colon and descending colon, normally retroperitoneal structures, are attached loosely to the posterior abdominal wall by their peritoneal connections. Their blood and nerve supplies are from relatively midline structures that would not restrict downward traction if this force were applied over a long period.[17] Therefore, as force is applied gradually over months to years, the viscus moves downward into the hernia defect and becomes part of a steadily enlarging sac. Moschcowitz could not reconcile the observation that the sigmoid colon typically

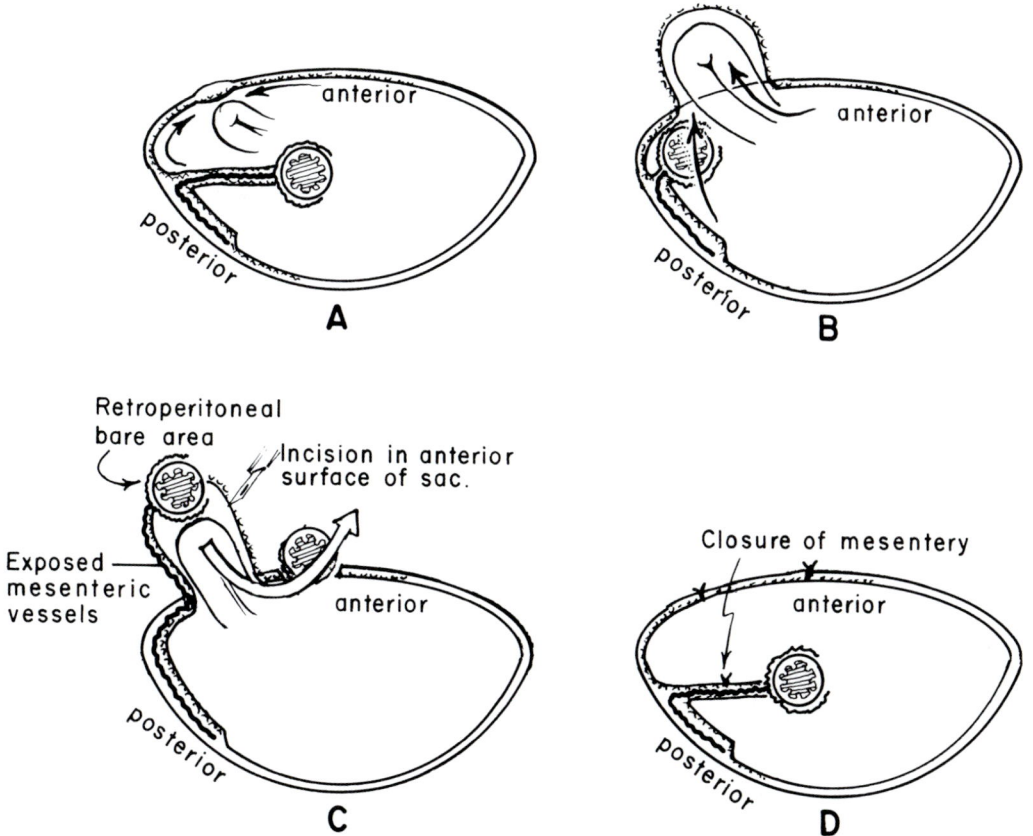

Figure 18-1. Pathogenesis of sliding inguinal hernia. (A) Elevated abdominal pressure forces the small intestine against the parietal peritoneum at the widened internal ring, causing the peritoneum from anterior and posterior peritoneal surfaces to be pushed through the internal ring. The contribution from the posterior peritoneum comes from the peritoneum covering the mesocolon. (B) The progressive enlargement of the hernial sac results in displacement of large intestine downward to the internal ring. As this occurs, the mesentery unfolds and the two peritoneal surfaces are peeled away from each other into medial and lateral leaves. (C) The intestine has now been pulled through the internal ring and has become incorporated as part of the hernial sac. Posteriorly, the exposed mesenteric vessels and retroperitoneal surface of the intestine are indicated. Anteriorly, the peritoneal surface is free of any vital structure and can be incised with impunity. The arrow indicates the direction of inversion and reduction of the intestine through a separate abdominal incision when the Moschcowitz method is used. (D) The intestine returned to its normal place. The opening in the anterior surface of the sac has now become a rent in the mesentery, which is shown repaired with a suture.

is invested completely with peritoneum and yet is the most commonly involved viscus in a left-sided sliding hernia. It was Graham[10] who later explained a mechanism whereby the sigmoid colon could become involved in a sliding hernia. As the left-sided indirect hernia develops, traction causes one of the leaves of the mesentery covering the sigmoid mesocolon to separate and peel apart from its companion leaf.

REPAIR OF A SLIDING INGUINAL HERNIA

The Early Attempts by Hotchkiss, Moschcowitz, and LaRoque

The early methods of repairing sliding hernias were complex compared to current approaches. Each of the methods was designed to re-form a peritoneal covering over the involved viscus and mesentery to re-store the abdominal contents to their normal relationships within the abdomen. The techniques described by Hotchkiss and Moschcowitz were the standard repairs for many years. Their techniques were derived from the prevailing understanding of the pathogenesis of sliding inguinal hernia. The gradual development of the enlarging sliding hernia requires the peritoneum forming the hernia sac to receive contributions from anterior and posterior peritoneal surfaces, as well as from the peritoneum that originally covered the mesentery and serosa of the enclosed viscus. The anterior contribution is made easily because there is no organ involvement. A different situation exists posteriorly, because the posterior peritoneum may be the serosa of the cecum or sigmoid colon or it may cover the mesentery of these organs. The anterior border of such a sliding hernia is relatively avascular and may be opened for inspection of the contents of the hernia sac. It is the posterior border of

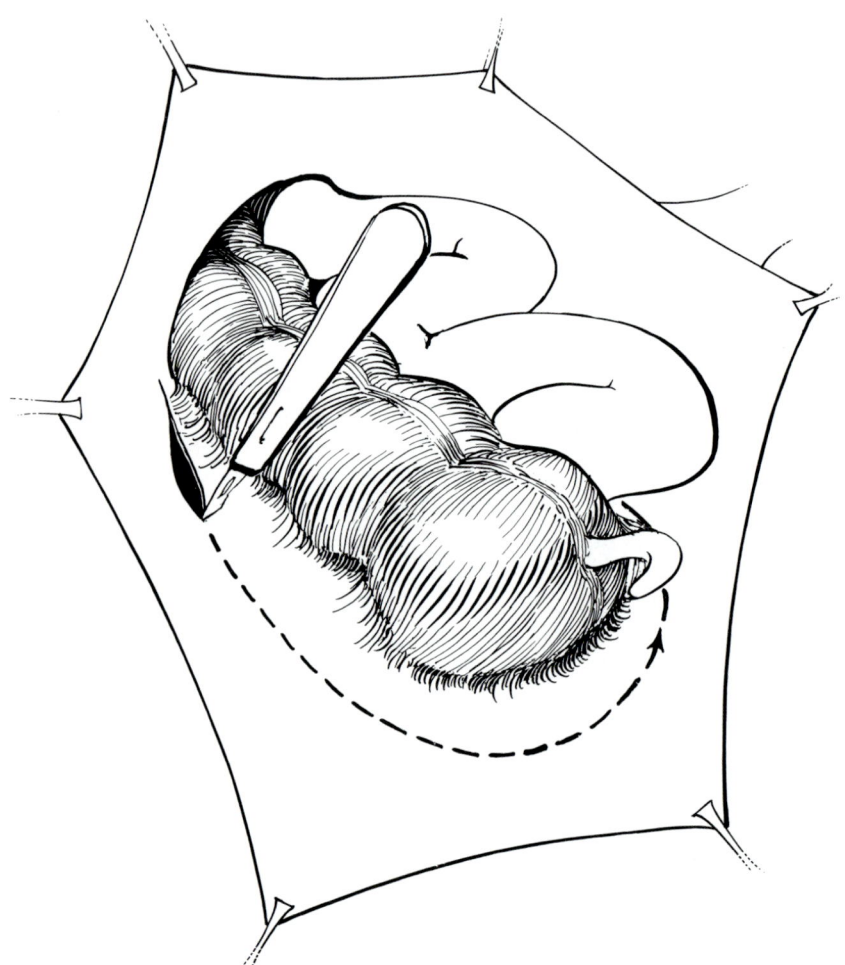

Figure 18-2. Hotchkiss technique for repair of a sliding hernia containing the right colon, showing an incision in the sac immediately distal to the colon.

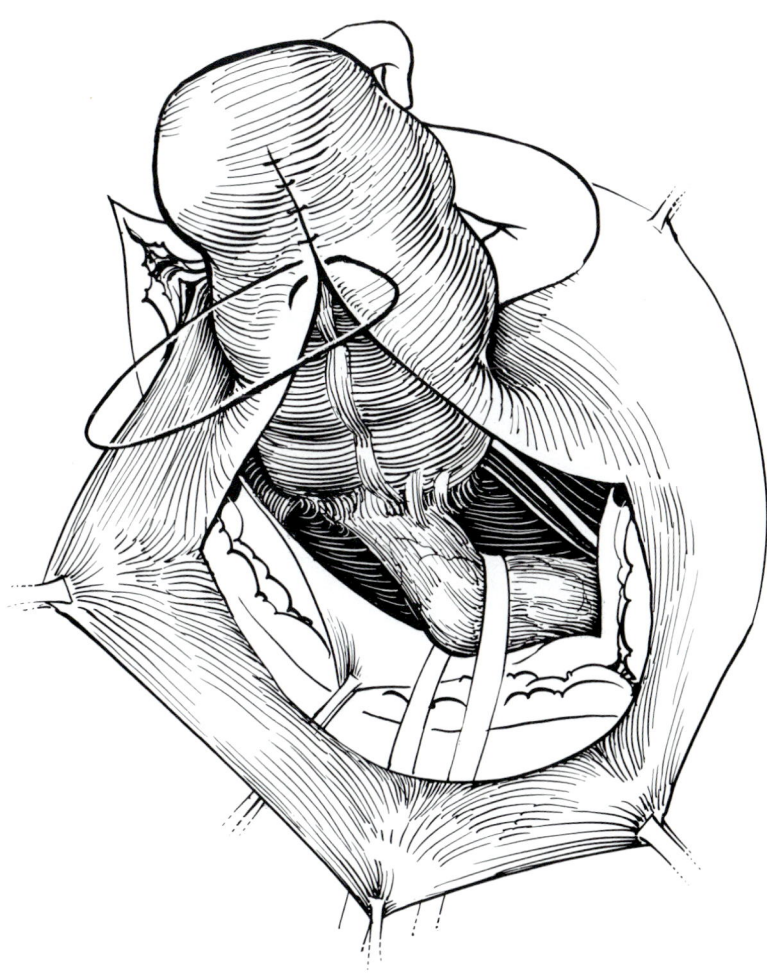

Figure 18-3. Hotchkiss technique for repair of a sliding hernia, showing the posterior, bare surface of the colon reperitonealized by suturing together the cut edges of the peritoneum.

the sac that contains all the mesenteric vessels and also is devoid of a peritoneal covering.

The repair described by Hotchkiss[12] was designed to address a large traction sliding hernia of the sigmoid colon (Figs. 18-2 through 18-5). Hotchkiss observed that sliding hernias were unlikely to strangulate because of a wide internal ring, but by definition were not completely reducible because the mesocolon or viscus was an essential part of the posterior wall of the hernia sac. He predicated that any repair of a sliding sigmoid hernia must accomplish complete reduction without injuring the blood supply of the involved viscus. Hotchkiss felt that repair was impaired further because the patients tended to be old men and the tissues were likely to be "fatty, feeble and atrophied." He found on opening the hernia sac that, after the contents are reduced as far as possible, one is left with the sigmoid colon attached posteriorly to the hernia sac by a short mesocolon. Hotchkiss believed that this

precluded any simple repair or ligation of the peritoneal defect. High ligation of the hernia sac was felt to be fundamental to the repair of all indirect hernias. Consequently, Hotchkiss constructed an elongated mesosigmoid from the tissues of the hernia sac to permit a facile reduction of the sigmoid into the abdomen. The internal opening of the sac then could be ligated easily. To accomplish the elongated mesosigmoid, the sac is opened anteriorly and those contents that can be, are reduced into the abdomen. The incision in the sac is extended upward to the internal ring and downward to the lowermost point of attachment of the mesosigmoid on its posterior wall. Thus, the sac wall can be everted by grasping and gently pulling the adherent sigmoid colon forward. The resultant new mesentery is completed by suturing together the free edges. The sigmoid colon now could be reduced without difficulty. The remaining defect in the anterior abdominal wall was closed with a pursestring suture

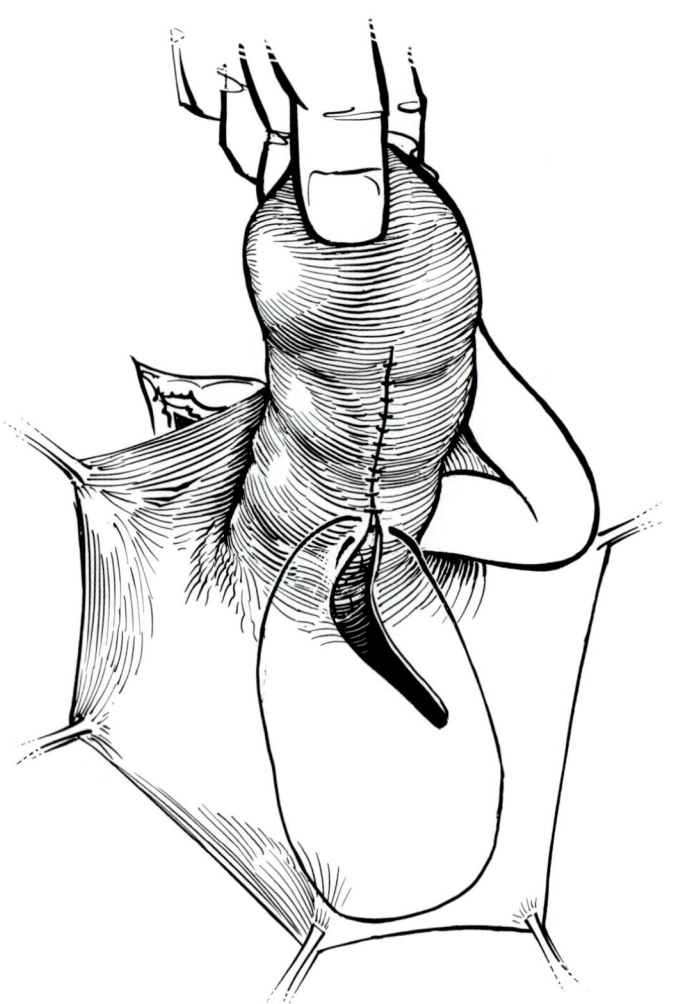

Figure 18-4. Hotchkiss technique for repair of a sliding inguinal hernia. The cut edges of the peritoneum are completely reapproximated, forming a new mesentery for the colon. This allows simultaneous closure of the sac with either single or multiple pursestring sutures (Bevan, 1935) and inversion of the intestine into the abdominal cavity.

or by any other suitable technique. Modifications of this technique later were used by Bevan[3] and by Sensenig and Nichols.[26]

Moschcowitz[18] developed a different approach largely because he was dissatisfied with that espoused by Hotchkiss. Similar to Hotchkiss, however, Moschcowitz stressed the danger of failing to recognize a sliding hernia. Liberation of the viscus risked injury to nutrient vessels and inadequate repair, portending a high recurrence rate. Moschcowitz recommended a separate incision through which the hernia could be reduced and replaced in the peritoneal cavity. The accessory incision he used for small hernias was an upward extension of the inguinal skin incision. Through this incision, a McBurney muscle-splitting incision was made above the internal ring (Fig. 18-6), similar to the LaRoque operation described below. For larger

hernias, Moschcowitz used a completely separate vertical incision, usually paramedian in location. An incision then was made in the anterior wall of the sac through the separate incision and the hernia sac with its contents could be inverted through the internal ring and out through the separate incision (Fig. 18-7). By this maneuver, the hernia sac actually is turned outside in so that the retroperitoneal surfaces of the intestine and the peritoneum can be reapproximated (Figs. 18-8 and 18-9). The remaining anterior defect is a small hernia sac and may be only a slit in the anterior peritoneum that is amenable to easy closure with suture. The replaced intestines then were anchored to the posterior parietal peritoneum for added security. The McBurney incision was closed, and the inguinal floor and internal ring were repaired in a suitable fashion. Graham[10] agreed with the perfor-

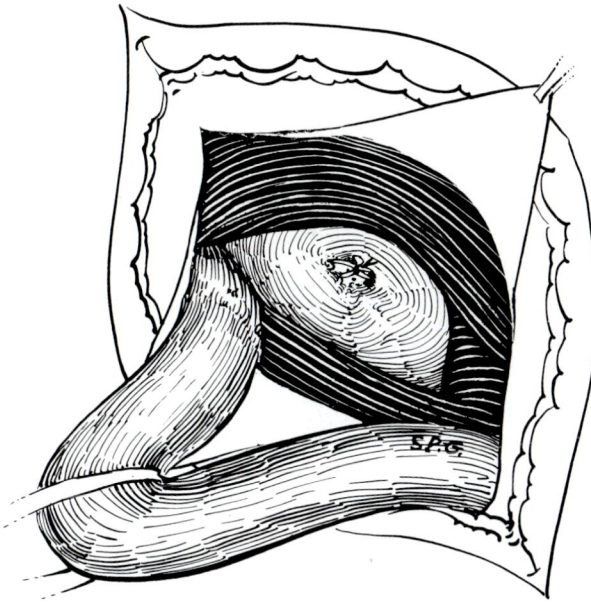

Figure 18-5. Hotchkiss technique for repair of a sliding inguinal hernia. The sac has been closed with pursestring sutures and the intestine inverted into the peritoneal cavity.

mance of a separate laparotomy for sliding hernia, stating that this facilitated reduction of the herniated viscus while reducing the hazard of injury to the nutrient vessels.

In a 1919 report, LaRoque[13] advocated the use of a muscle-splitting incision above the internal ring to approach such hernias. He further adapted this approach to sliding hernias in a later writing.[14] An excellent summary of this technique has been provided by Williams.[27] The usual inguinal incision is made, the external abdominal oblique muscle is opened into the external ring, and the sac is exposed and dissected free from the spermatic cord. The sac is opened anteriorly to expose the involved sliding viscus. The internal abdominal oblique and transversus abdominis muscles are opened transversely about 1 inch superior to the internal ring, with care taken to avoid injury to the iliohypogastric nerve. The transversalis fascia is incised and the muscles are retracted. The peritoneum then is opened to expose the contents of the hernia entering the internal ring. The sac now can be dissected free from the cord and the colon mobilized, with care taken not to damage the vasculature of the mesocolon, which lies posteriorly. Once the colon and mesocolon are pulled back into the abdominal cavity, it can be appreciated that the anterolateral portion of the sac is the outer leaf of the mesocolon. The excess peritoneum is excised, the

mesocolon is closed with suture, and the bowel is returned to the abdomen. The transversalis fascia frequently is strong enough that it can be sutured so as to provide support, superiorly, for the reconstructed internal ring. The internal oblique and transversus abdominis muscles are sutured, and the hernia repair can proceed in any manner desired to repair the inguinal defect.

Recent Approaches

Although the early repairs of Hotchkiss and Moschcowitz were based on a sound understanding of the pathogenesis of sliding hernias, and were aesthetically successful in that the anatomic defects were corrected, these procedures were tedious and unnecessarily complex. Current approaches follow the observations and reports of surgeons such as Ryan, Maingot,[16] and Zimmerman and Anson,[28] who found that simplified repairs through an inguinal approach alone yielded excellent results.

Ryan concluded that the important feature of the sliding hernia operation was to repair the defect in the abdominal wall through which the hernia sac protruded. He found the large size of many such sliding hernias to be no hindrance and was able to conduct successfully all his repairs through an inguinal incision. Furthermore, Ryan saw no need to resect the hernia sac if it could be dissected from the spermatic cord and replaced deep to the repaired transversalis fascia. Using this approach, he obtained a recurrence rate of less than 1%.

Maingot, as well as Zimmerman and Anson, also espoused simplified approaches through a single inguinal incision. These surgeons resected a portion of the hernia sac and closed it with a pursestring suture placed as high as possible on the anterior margin and, on the posterior aspect, at the reflection of the peritoneum onto the viscus (Fig. 18-10). As the pursestring suture is pulled taught, the bowel is turned upward and the sac is closed. The sac then is freed from the cord structures and the entire mass is reduced into the abdomen (Figs. 18-11 and 18-12). Bevan[3] invaginated the sac by a series of three or four pursestring sutures. The overlying fascial defect then could be repaired. On occasion, enlargement of the internal ring was necessary for reduction of a massive sliding hernia; this was accomplished by incising the internal oblique muscle. These authors also reported low recurrence rates, indicating that a procedure involving an inguinal incision and inversion of the hernia sac was preferable to the more complex approaches advocated by their predecessors.

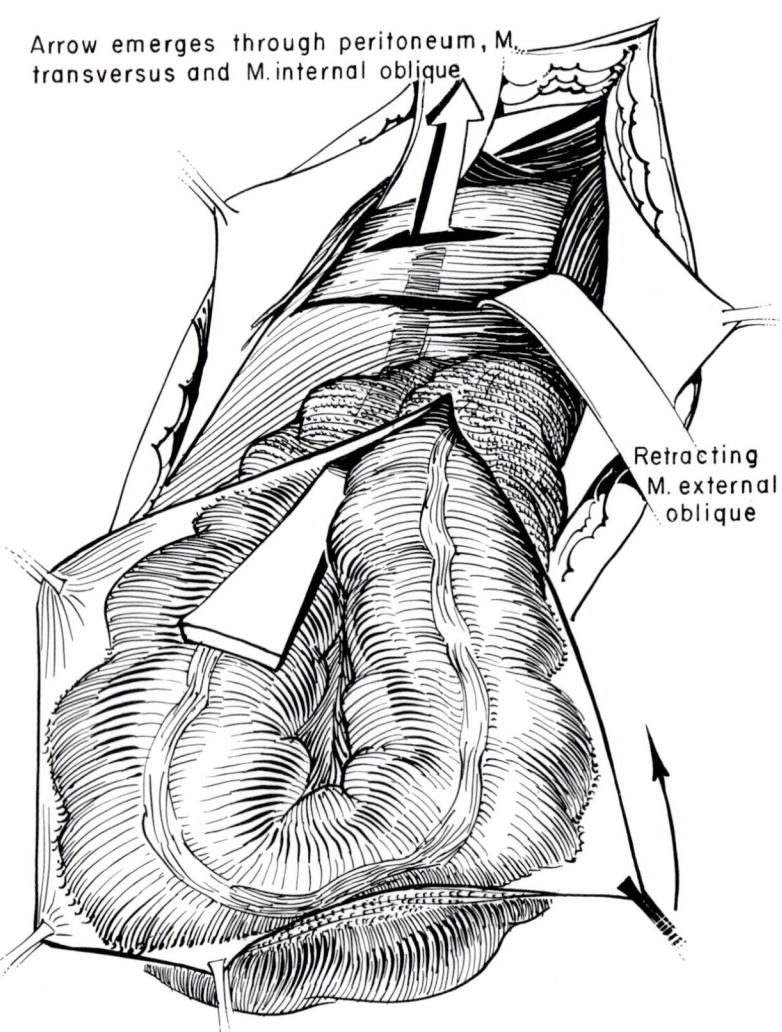

Arrow emerges through peritoneum, M. transversus and M. internal oblique

Retracting M. external oblique

Figure 18-6. Moschcowitz technique for repair of a sliding inguinal hernia of the sigmoid colon. The hernial sac has been opened anteriorly and a separate muscle-splitting incision has been made through the external oblique muscle above the internal ring. The external oblique is shown retracted, and an incision has been made through the internal oblique muscle, the transversus abdominis muscle, and the peritoneum. The arrow shown emerging through this incision indicates the direction in which the intestine is moved when the sac is inverted into the abdominal cavity and then pulled out through the accessory incision.

Ponka[22] described a simplified method of repair applicable to most sliding hernias. His technique was based on his conclusion that a sliding hernia of the cecum or sigmoid colon is "really a variety of indirect inguinal hernia, no more, no less." If a sliding hernia is seen or felt on exploration of the groin, Ponka recommended dissecting the entire hernia sac from the spermatic cord by severing the areolar tissues between these structures. It is important to continue dissection just deep to the transversalis fascia to delineate the internal ring and facilitate later reconstruction. Division of the hypertrophied cremasteric muscle at this point is helpful in further delineating the anatomy in this area. In the interest of safety, the hernia sac is opened superiorly and anteriorly, because the viscus or mesocolon forms the posterior aspect of the sac.

Ponka's innovation was to incise the sac medially and laterally to separate the bowel from the remaining sac (Fig. 18-13). The bowel then could be reduced into the abdominal cavity. The complete peritoneal ring is reconstructed and a routine high ligation is performed. This maneuver illustrates the observation that such a sliding hernia is in effect a variety of acquired indirect inguinal hernia. The redundant sac is excised and the floor is reconstructed using any of the suitable standard repairs. Any repair, however, should accomplish snug reconstruction of the internal ring around the spermatic cord. To prevent compromise of the spermatic artery and vein, which results in ischemic swelling followed by atrophy of the testis, care should be taken not to injure the testicular vessels or to create an internal ring that is too tight.

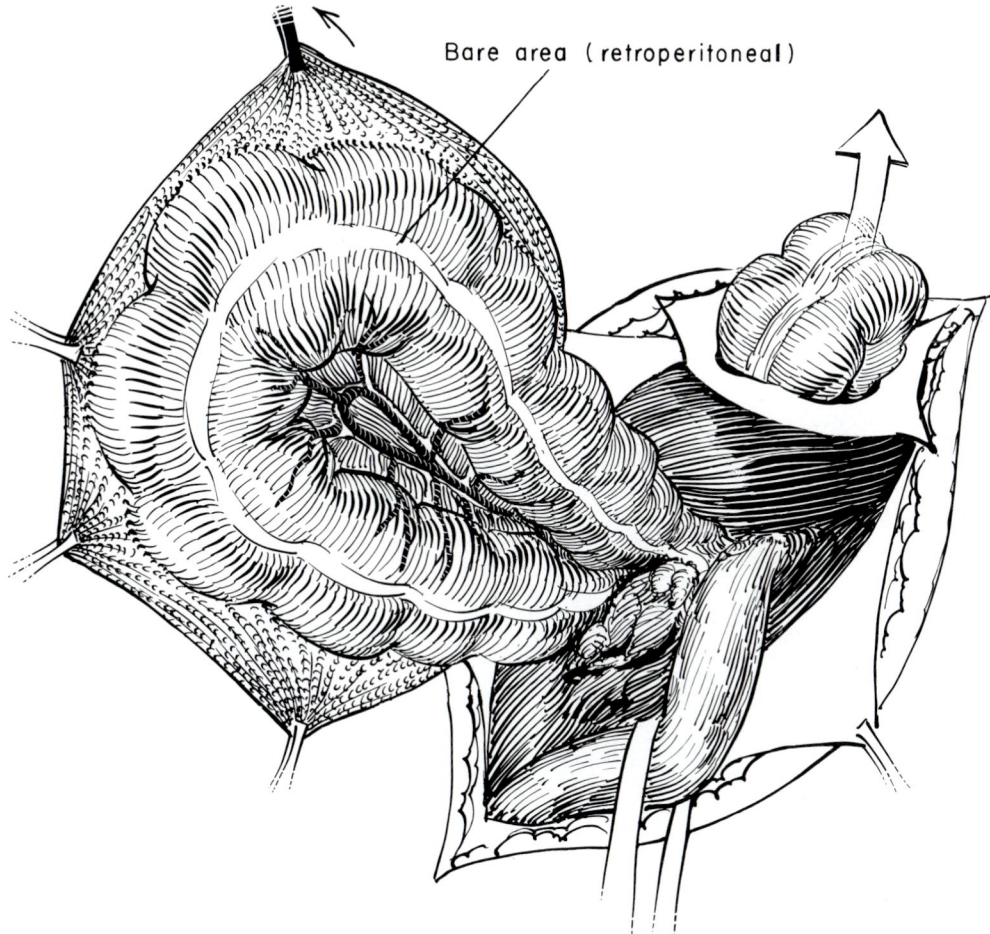

Figure 18-7. Moschcowitz technique for repair of a sliding inguinal hernia of the sigmoid colon. The hernial sac with its contained intestine has been lifted up to demonstrate the retroperitoneal bare area of the colon and to show the mesenteric vessels that emerge through this posterior portion of the hernial sac. The colon is also shown emerging through the separate abdominal incision as inversion and reduction of the hernial sac are begun.

Even simpler approaches are satisfactory in most cases. These techniques involve return of the viscus to the peritoneal cavity with closure of the peritoneum on its external aspect. In essence then, reduction of the sliding hernia through a "stuffing maneuver" or the creation of a peritoneal flap (Fig. 18-14) suffices for most sliding hernias provided the internal ring and inguinal floor are reconstructed properly.[19]

Urinary System Sliding Hernias

The urinary bladder sometimes forms a part of the sac wall in a direct sliding hernia or a large indirect inguinal hernia. In describing his handling of sliding hernias of the bladder, Moretz[17] stated that this entity generally poses no particular problem as long as it is recognized. It is important, however, because the bladder may be injured if it is mistaken for a sac or is caught by a pursestring suture used to ligate the neck of a sac. The surgeon may notice that the bladder has been entered only after detecting the escape of urine. Little harm is likely if the injury is recognized and closed primarily, and the bladder is decompressed with a Foley catheter for several days. If the injury is overlooked, however, a serious wound infection may develop. If a sliding hernia that incorporates the bladder is encountered, it usually is possible to dissect the bladder free from the peritoneum and treat the sac in the usual manner. If necessary, a patch of peritoneum

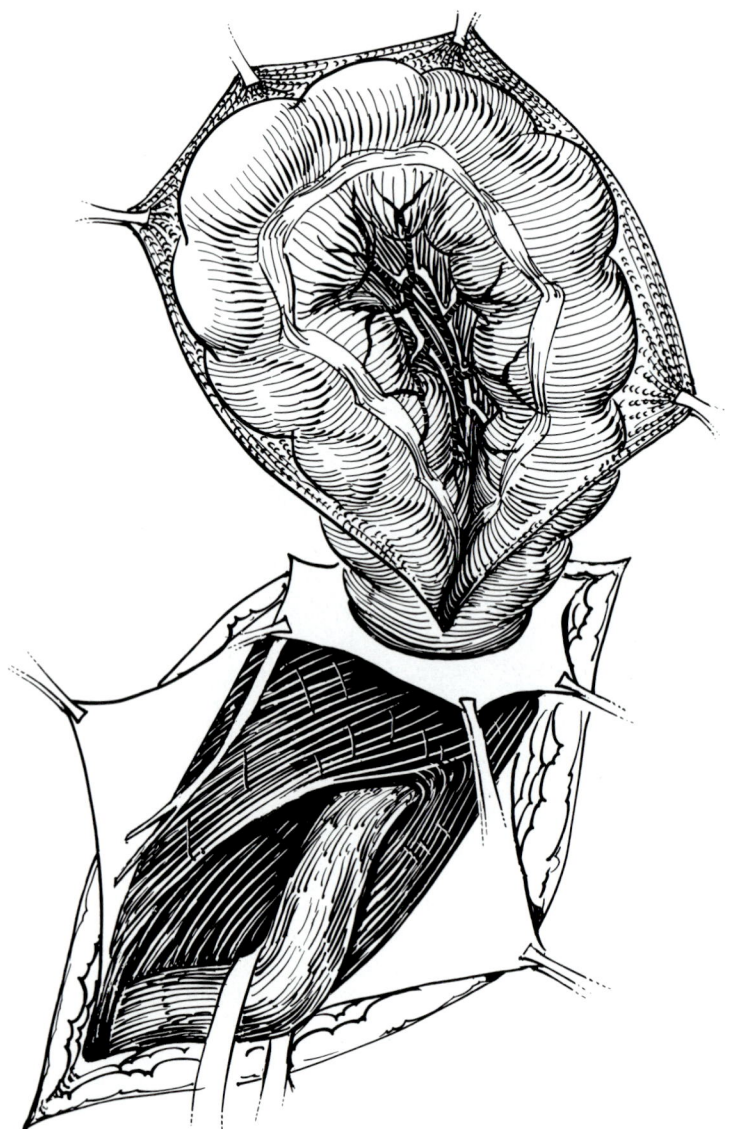

Figure 18-8. Moschcowitz technique for repair of a sliding inguinal hernia of the sigmoid colon. The hernial sac and contained intestine have been completely inverted and pulled up and through the separate abdominal incision. The stippled surface of the peritoneum is now shown to be the inside of the hernial sac. Before reduction and inversion, it was the outer surface of the hernial sac.

may be left attached to the bladder by cutting it free of the sac, leaving a hole in the sac that can be repaired. The sac then is handled as any other.

If the ureter is involved, it usually may be reduced with the bladder, taking care to avoid kinking.[20a] Patel and colleagues[20] postulated that the ureter attained its position within the sliding hernia as a result of traction caused by an adherent layer of posterior parietal peritoneum. The redundant ureter and surrounding inflammation frequently is dilated, lacks peristalsis, and is matted in adhesions. Ballard and associates[1] consequently were concerned that simply replacing the ureter from behind the peritoneum could lead to

ureteral necrosis or worsening of the ureteral obstruction. They concluded that each case should be handled on an individual basis, but that a diseased ureter should be excised and anastomosis performed again over a stent.

RESULTS OF OPERATIONS TO REPAIR SLIDING HERNIAS

The classic treatises by Hotchkiss,[12] Moschcowitz,[18] Bevan,[3] and other early reports dealt with only a few patients. The reports provided eloquent and detailed

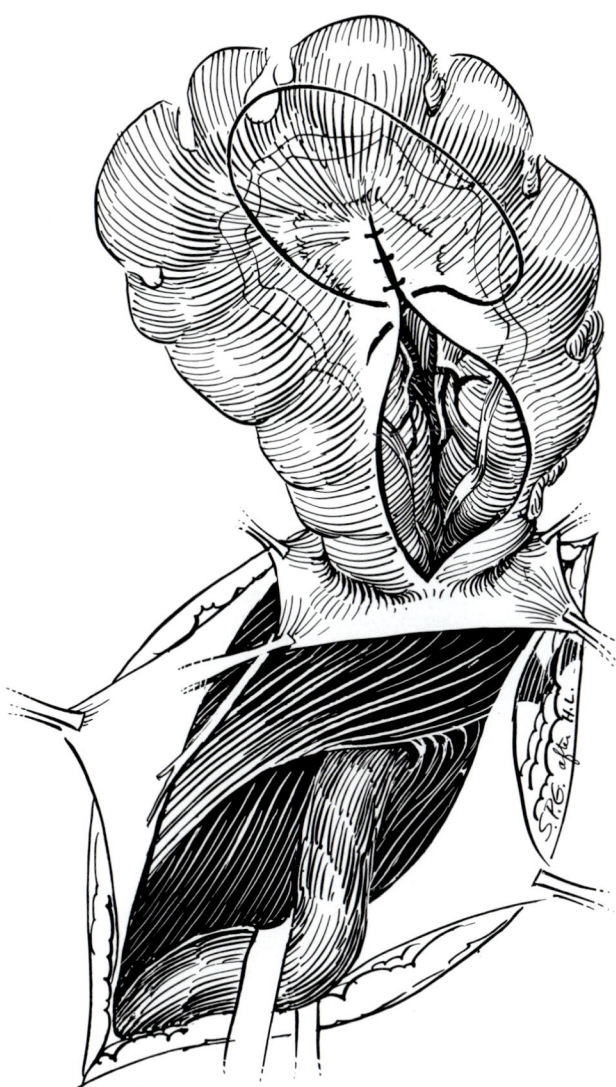

Figure 18-9. Moschcowitz technique for repair of a sliding inguinal hernia of the sigmoid colon. The peritoneal surfaces are brought together, forming a new mesenteric leaf, and serve to cover the bare portions of the colon. This closure brings together the two edges of the peritoneum that initially were the incision in the anterior surface of the hernial sac.

involving many patients report low recurrence rates using only inguinal incisions and simple handling of the sliding hernia sac. Two points of caution should be heeded in interpreting statistics regarding recurrence. First, many studies report the incidence of recurrence after 2 years, because most recurrences are said to occur within this time frame. Both Fallis[7] and Clear,[5] however, noted that one third of all recurrences may take place after 2 years. Second, many patients have no symptoms and are unaware of their recurrent hernia. Therefore, any good study must include a surgeon's examination of all patients to detect possible recurrences.

Longacre[15] reported a 15.3% recurrence rate for repair of sliding inguinal hernia. It is unclear which techniques were used to repair the hernias, because the report included the experience of many surgeons at one hospital. Longacre did note that the urinary bladder was injured accidentally in two of four patients in whom the sac included the bladder. Piedad and colleagues[21] repaired 43 sliding inguinal hernias during a 7-year period using either a simple repair or a counterincision. They had seven recurrences, all in young men who had returned to work after a simple repair. Based on these results, they concluded that young patients warranted a more "aggressive" repair, presumably with a counterincision. Sensenig and Nichols[26] reported their results repairing 53 sliding inguinal hernias. Five of the patients were asymptomatic and had no knowledge of their recurrence. In 25 of the cases, the sliding inguinal hernia was repaired through a single inguinal incision, but the authors did reconstruct the mesentery of the involved bowel to cover it with peritoneum, followed by high ligation of the sac. Sensenig and Nichols examined each patient after 2 years and found seven recurrences. They concluded that an inguinal approach was satisfactory in that it was associated with a lower recurrence rate and less morbidity than was hernia repair done through an abdominal incision.

Ryan's[25] large series of patients operated on at the Shouldice Clinic for sliding hernia was the first important series providing data on operative results. He reported only four recurrences in 313 patients, for a recurrence rate of 1.3%. Two recurrences were not of the original sliding hernia. Ryan used local anesthesia and repaired the floor of the inguinal canal using a classic Shouldice repair, which essentially imbricates the transversus abdominis fascia. No counterincisions were used and the hernia sac was handled by simple reduction or excision. In a subsequent report from the Shouldice Clinic, Glasgow[8] reported his personal series involving almost 15,000 patients with inguinal hernia in which the recurrence rate was 0.6%. This series included 704 patients with a sliding hernia,

descriptions of operative technique, but little information regarding results. In particular, no statistics were provided on recurrence rates. Although no prospective, randomized trials comparing complex and simple repairs of sliding hernias have been performed, most surgeons now concede that a simple approach is preferable if satisfactory results are obtained, believing that fewer operative complications are associated with simpler procedures. Several series

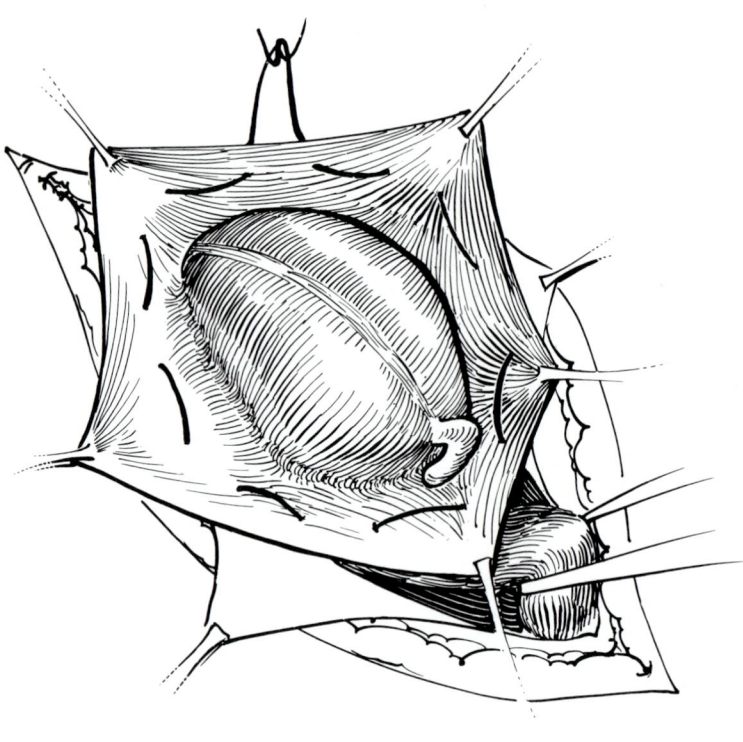

Figure 18-10. Zimmerman technique for repair of a sliding inguinal hernia. The hernial sac has been opened and the excess has been trimmed away. A pursestring suture is shown being placed near the intestine.

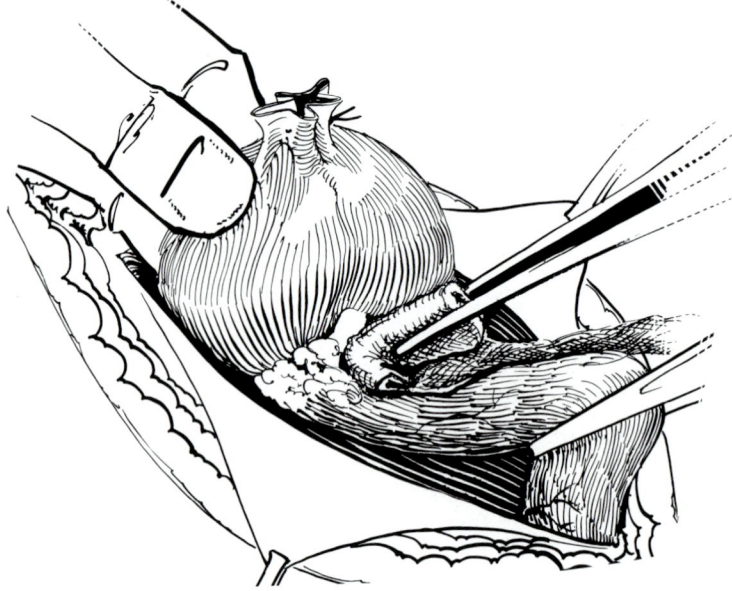

Figure 18-11. Zimmerman technique for repair of a sliding inguinal hernia. A pursestring suture has been tied, and the hernial sac is carefully freed from the cord sutures that lie posteriorly.

none of which had a recurrence. These hernias were repaired using the standard Shouldice technique with no special accommodations made for the sliding hernia sac. In a later report, Glassow[9] reported a 0.8% recurrence rate in more than 20,000 hernia repairs,

but did not comment specifically on sliding hernias except to note that the sac usually need not be opened and that they pose no particular difficulty. In a recent report from the Shouldice Clinic, Kingsnorth, Gray, and Nott (1992) compared recurrence rates between

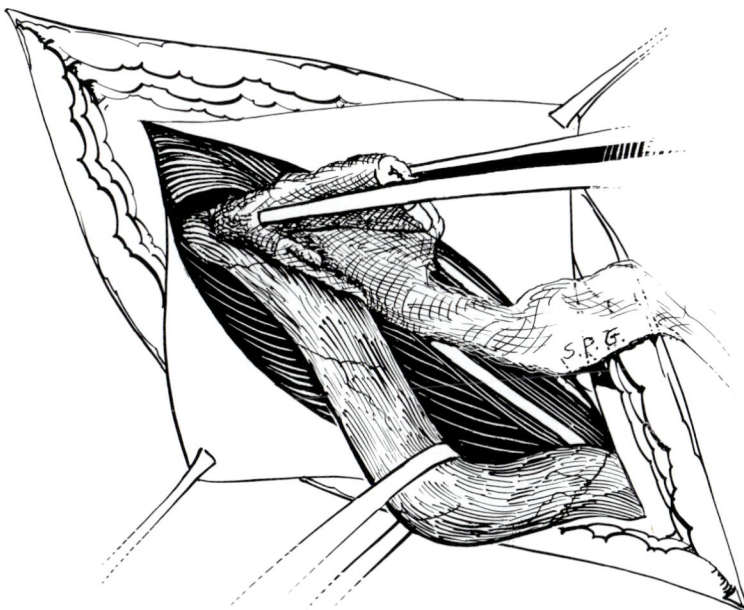

Figure 18-12. Zimmerman technique for repair of sliding inguinal hernia. The hernial sac has been reduced beneath the transversalis fascia in preparation for repair of the internal ring and the floor of the inguinal canal.

experienced surgeons and resident surgeons. After at least 2 years of follow-up, the overall recurrence rate was 3.5% for the Shouldice repair and 2.3% for a plication darn. The number of sliding hernias in each group was similar, and sliding hernias did not seem to portend an increased rate of recurrence, although they were not the focus of the study.

Smaller series by other authors also seem to justify simple handling of the sliding inguinal hernia, with adequate reconstruction of the internal ring and inguinal floor. A contemporary of Longacre, Fallis[7] reported a recurrence rate of only 1.5% among 53 patients with a sliding hernia. He did not detail the techniques used at his institution, but did state that they did not ever find it necessary to resort to intraabdominal fixation of the pelvic colon or to the Moschcowitz operation. After a 5-year follow-up period, Estes (1960) reported one recurrence among 36 patients who underwent repair of a sliding hernia. He did not open the hernia sac, but simply reduced it and repaired the floor using a Cooper ligament repair. Maingot[16] claimed a low, but unspecified, recurrence rate in his series of 64 sliding hernias repaired by his technique of simple reduction and reconstruction of the internal ring. Zimmerman and Laufman (1942) recommended applying a pursestring suture to the neck of the sliding hernia sac as high as possible on the anterior free portion of the surface of the sac and close to the colon posteriorly. As the pursestring is

tied, the bowel is turned upward and the sac invaginates on itself. The sac, with its contents, then can be dissected from important spermatic cord structures and returned to the abdominal cavity. The internal ring is reconstructed by suturing the transversalis fascia snugly around the cord, and the remainder of the floor is repaired in any suitable fashion. These researchers recorded no recurrences in 24 patients treated with this method. Age need not affect the results adversely. Using a simple inguinal approach, Ponka and Brush[23] reported the repair of 62 sliding inguinal hernias in 60 patients older than 70 years, with only one recurrence.

CONCLUSIONS

As the operative repair of sliding hernias has evolved, two conclusions have become evident. First, it is imperative that sliding hernias be recognized to avoid inadvertent injury to the involved viscus or its blood supply. Second, the key to a satisfactory repair is the recognition that almost all sliding hernias simply are an acquired variant of an indirect hernia. Complex repairs rarely are necessary. Replacement of the involved viscus into the abdominal cavity using any one of several maneuvers, followed by careful reconstruction of the internal ring and inguinal wall, provides a satisfactory repair with a low rate of recurrence.

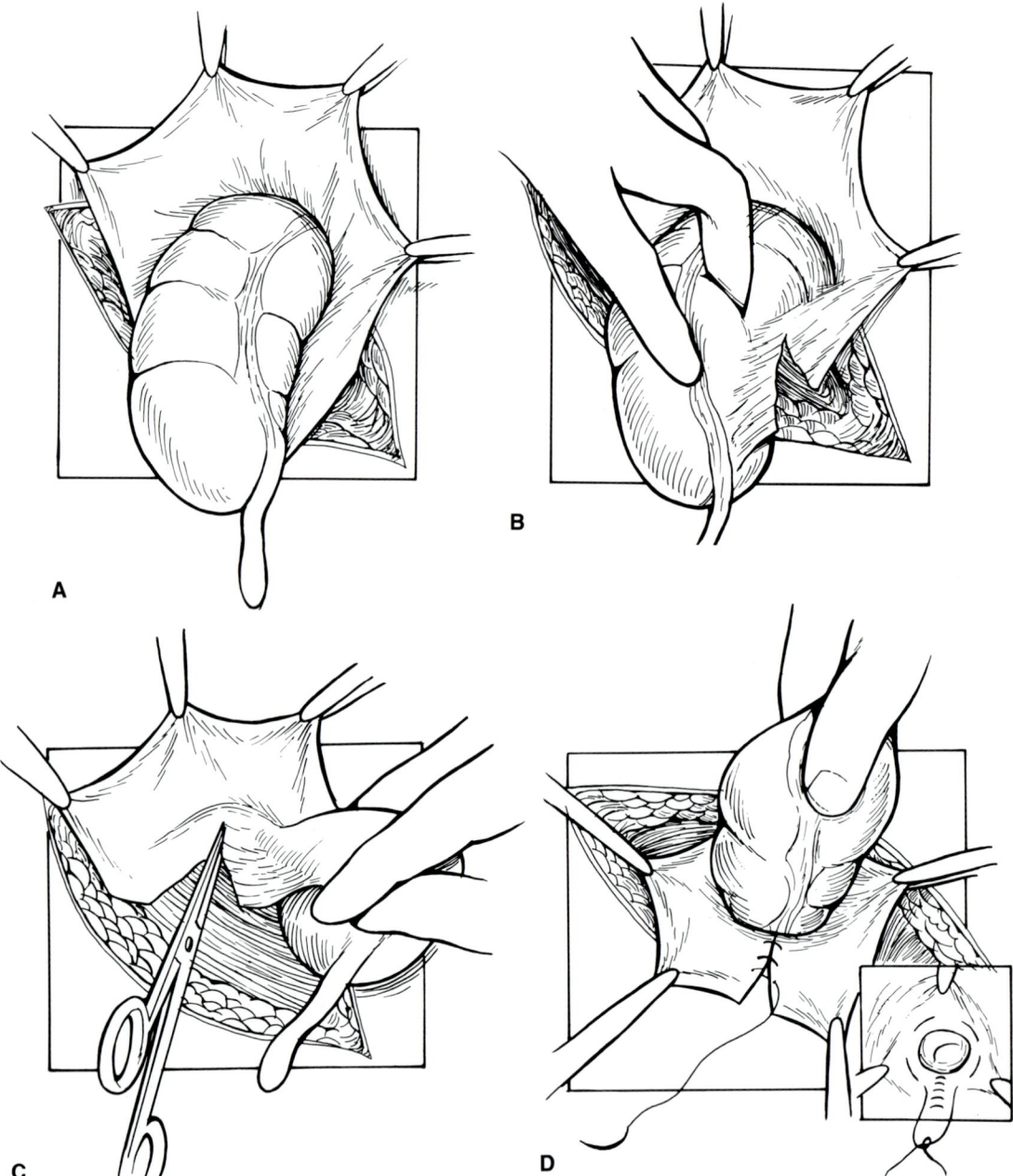

Figure 18-13. (*A* through *D*) Ponka's method of repair reconstructs the complete peritoneum so that a routine high ligation can be done. The sac is incised medially and laterally to separate the bowel from the remaining sac. The bowel is then reduced into the abdominal cavity. This maneuver illustrates the observation that such a sliding hernia is, in effect, a variety of acquired indirect inguinal hernia. (Ponka J. Surgical management of large bilateral indirect sliding inguinal hernias. Am J Surg 1966;112:55)

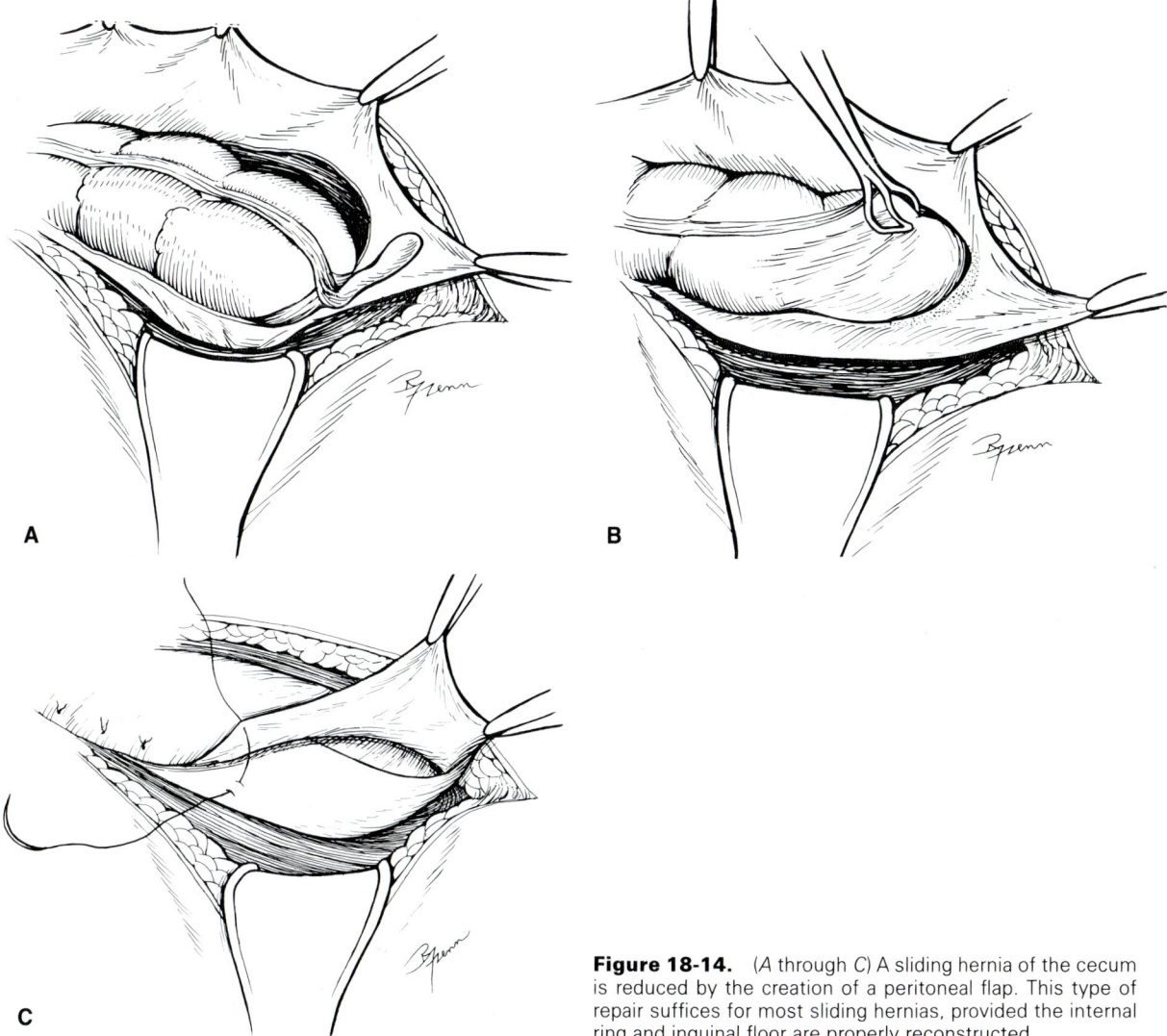

Figure 18-14. (*A* through *C*) A sliding hernia of the cecum is reduced by the creation of a peritoneal flap. This type of repair suffices for most sliding hernias, provided the internal ring and inguinal floor are properly reconstructed.

REFERENCES

1. Ballard JL, Dobbs RM, Malone JM. Ureteroinguinal hernia: a rare complication of sliding inguinal hernias. Am Surg 1991;57:720.
2. Barrow DW. Bilateral sliding hernia. Am J Surg 1954;87:932.
3. Bevan AD. Sliding hernias of the ascending colon and caecum, the descending colon and sigmoid and of the bladder. Ann Surg 1930;92:754.
4. Burton CC. Large bowel hernia. Ann Surg 1942; 39:116.
5. Clear JJ. Ten year statistical study of inguinal hernias. Arch Surg 1951;62:70.
6. David VC. Sliding hernias of the cecum and appendix in children. Ann Surg 1923;77:438.
7. Fallis LS. Inguinal hernia: report of 1,600 operations. Ann Surg 1936;104:403.
8. Glassow F. Inguinal hernia repair: a comparison of the Shouldice and Cooper ligament repair of the posterior inguinal wall. Am J Surg 1976;131:306.
9. Glassow F. The Shouldice Hospital technique. Int Surg 1986;71:148.
10. Graham RR. The operative repair of sliding inguinal hernia of the sigmoid. Ann Surg 1935;102:784.
11. Hagan WH, Rhoads JE. Inguinal and femoral hernias: a follow-up study. Surg Gynecol Obstet 1953; 96:226.
12. Hotchkiss LW. Large sliding hernias of the sigmoid colon. Ann Surg 1909;50:470.
13. LaRoque GP. The permanent cure of inguinal and femoral hernia. Surg Gynecol Obstet 1919;29:507.

14. LaRoque GP. The intra-abdominal method of removing inguinal and femoral hernias. Arch Surg 1932;24:180.

15. Longacre AB. Follow-up of hernia repair. Surg Gynecol Obstet 1939;68:238.

16. Maingot R. Operations for sliding herniae and for large incisional herniae. Br J Clin Pract 1961;15:993.

17. Moretz WH. Sliding inguinal hernia. In: Nyhus LM, Harkins HN, eds. Hernia, ed 1. Philadelphia, JB Lippincott, 1964:128–145.

18. Moschcowitz AV. The rational treatment of sliding hernia. Ann Surg 1925;81:330.

19. Nyhus LM. Editor's comment on sliding inguinal hernia. In: Nyhus LM, Condon RE, eds. Hernia, 3rd ed. Philadelphia, JB Lippincott, 1989:299.

20. Patel PH, Rao SS, Gallagher JJ. Bilateral ureteral herniation into the scrotum. A case report and review of the literature. Del Med J 1979;51:143.

20a. Percival WL. Ureter within a sliding inguinal hernia. Can J Surg 1983;26:283.

21. Piedad OH, Stoesser PN, Wels PB. Sliding inguinal hernia. Am J Surg 1973;126:106.

22. Ponka JL. Surgical management of large bilateral indirect sliding inguinal hernias. Am J Surg 1966;112:52.

23. Ponka JL, Brush BE. Sliding inguinal hernia in patients over 70 years of age. J Am Geriatr Soc 1978;26:68.

24. Rhoads JE, Mackie JA. Comments on sliding inguinal hernias. In: Nyhus LM, Harkins HN, eds. Hernia, 1st ed. Philadelphia, JB Lippincott, 1964:148–149.

25. Ryan EA. An analysis of 313 consecutive cases of indirect sliding hernias. Surg Gynecol Obstet 1956;102:45.

26. Sensenig DM, Nichols JB. Sliding hernias. Arch Surg 1955;71:756.

27. Williams C. Repair of sliding inguinal hernia through the abdominal (LaRoque) approach. Ann Surg 1947;126:612.

28. Zimmerman LM, Anson BJ. Special forms of hernia. In: Zimmerman LM, ed. Anatomy and surgery of hernia, ed 2. Baltimore, Williams & Wilkins, 1967:202–215.

29. Zimmerman L, Laufman H. Sliding hernia. Surg Gynecol Obstet 1942;75:76.

Editor's Comment

The important component of this comprehensive review by Dr. Demeure is this: simple techniques for mobilizing and reducing the sliding portion of the hernia can be used in nearly every case. The complex repairs using counterincisions and similar maneuvers that were described in the past are not really needed. In essence, a sliding hernia is simply a variant of indirect inguinal hernia. The sliding component constitutes the posterolateral wall of the hernia, and extraperitoneal dissection into the preperitoneal space allows mobilization and inversion of the herniated viscus. The peritoneum is brought over the viscus and sutured on its lateral side, thus restoring the formerly sliding viscus to an intraperitoneal position.

A second important observation is that a preoperative diagnosis of sliding inguinal hernia can be made in most cases. The clue is that the hernia is partially reducible, but not completely so. Such a combination otherwise is unusual. An incarcerated hernia is not reducible at all, and other varieties of indirect hernia that are reducible usually can be reduced completely. Thus, if a portion of the contents of a hernia sac can be reduced but a residual component persists, the presence of a sliding hernia is probable.

R.E.C.

Hernia, Fourth Edition, edited
by Lloyd M. Nyhus and Robert E. Condon.
J.B. Lippincott Company, Philadelphia © 1995.

Chapter 19

Richter and Littre Hernias

William A. Tito and Alejandra Perez-Tamayo

*It will be impossible to determine by any general description what those are that ought to be
opened, and what those are that ought not; that must be left in a great measure to the
discretion of the surgeon, when once he is master of the arguments on both sides.*
 John Hunter: A Treatise on the Blood, Inflammation and Gunshot Wounds, 1794

Richter hernia and Littre hernia are separate entities
that share common histories. Some authors equated
the two as little as 50 years ago, but in historical perspective they are different conditions. In the more
common Richter hernia, less than the full circumference of the intestinal lumen protrudes through a hernial orifice. Strangulation may take place without
complete obstruction, and early physical examination
may be deceptively benign. Littre hernia, on the other
hand, is a rare entity that features protrusion of a
Meckel diverticulum as the sole content of a hernial
sac. Neither term has been supplanted by functional
or anatomic definitions, and the eponyms persist as
most descriptive.

HISTORY

In 1598, Fabricius Hildanus attended a 63-year-old
woman who had suffered from a groin hernia for 17
years. After apparent reduction en masse, the hernia
became abscessed and a fecal fistula resulted. Within
2 months, the fistula had closed, and Hildanus concluded that only part of the intestinal lumen involved
itself with the strangulation process. Little was said
about the concept of partial herniation for almost 100
years until Lavater implied the possibility with a
vague reference that was largely ignored.

In 1700, the French surgeon Alexis Littre (1658–
1726) published autopsy findings on three patients
with groin masses.[15] One body had decomposed to an
extent that prevented reasonable study, but the other
two harbored what most historians regard as ileal diverticula. Because such diverticula were not recognized as entities separate from the small bowel proper,
Littre proposed that they were lesions acquired from
traction by the hernial sac. On the basis of this assumption, some authors defined Littre hernia as a
partial enterocele. Recognition of the unique identity

of Littre hernia awaited the work of Johann Meckel.[18]
Partial herniation was described again by Mery[19] in
1701, and Littre described similar involvement of the
colon in 1714. Before 1800, eight more authors described similar findings. Most notable was August
Gottlieb Richter (1742–1812) in Göttingen. In 1785,
he reviewed partial enteroceles occurring mainly from
the umbilicus to the xiphoid process, but also in the
inguinal and femoral areas.[26]

Finally, two important events occurred in 1809.
Antonio Scarpa of Milan demonstrated the mechanism for obstruction with partial enterocele in an experimental model. He showed that constriction of two
thirds or more of the intestinal lumen in autopsy specimens produced universal obstruction, but that compromise of one third or less produced no such con-
stancy. The amount of obstruction, Scarpa reasoned,
depended on the proportion of intestinal lumen involved in the hernia. No published verifications of
Scarpa's experiments have appeared, but the simplicity of his observations remains attractive in explaining
the variable degrees of obstruction encountered with
partial herniation of the intestinal wall. Assumptions
that his mathematical proportions are correct have
been challenged by Bissel[1] and others, yet most workers accept Scarpa's general principles regarding partial obstruction.

Also in 1809, Johann Friedrich Meckel (1781–
1833) described the diverticulum that bears his
name.[10] Although Littre, Mery, and Ruysch[28] all had
described it 100 years previously, Meckel postulated
its congenital origin and described its presence as a
variant of normal development.

By the end of the 19th century, another dozen
authors, including Sir Astley Cooper and Valpeau,
had described partial herniation of the intestinal
wall. Most important among these was Sir Frederick
Treves[31] (1853–1923) of London. He collected 50 records of partial enteroceles and defined the condition

as strangulation of part of the circumference of the intestinal wall within a hernial orifice. This he distinguished from herniation of a Meckel diverticulum, which was described classically by Littre. Treves' work is a scholarly triumph and cornerstone to modern understanding. To August Richter, Sir Frederick Treves credited the distinction of "establishing the individuality of this lesion." Treves named it Richter hernia to distinguish it from the congenitally acquired Meckel herniation described by Littre. Nonetheless, Fowler[7] in 1899 and Rhodes[25] in 1928 used the terms Richter hernia and Littre hernia interchangeably. They contended that Littre had described both types of hernia and that Richter was more concerned with supraumbilical hernias than with groin hernias. Modern authorities such as Cattell[4] and Keynes,[13,14] however, agree with Treves' assessment. Thus evolved the distinction between the hernias of Richter and Littre.

RICHTER HERNIA

Pathology

Any part of the large or small intestine may participate in a Richter hernia, although the distal ileum is involved most commonly. The hernial orifice may be any conceivable one within the abdomen, but usually involves the femoral canal. To satisfy the requirements of a Richter hernia, the antimesenteric border of the intestine must protrude into the hernial sac, but never to the point of involvement of the entire circumference of the intestine (Fig. 19-1). Thus, the mesenteric portion of the herniating intestine should not be expected to participate in the contents of the hernial sac. Omentum is encountered infrequently.

Unless they are compromised by strangulation, Richter hernias usually are small and easy to overlook on physical examination. Because the contents of the sac are minimal, reduction generally is simple unless chronicity effects scarification and incarceration. Thus, muscular or anesthetic relaxation may produce spontaneous reduction, and the true incidence of occurrence is never known.

Incidence and Site of Hernia

Recent publications have contributed little to modify concepts regarding the sites and incidence of Richter hernia. The classic reports of Treves,[31] Frankau,[8] Gillespie,[9] and others remain the best sources for data on its incidence and distribution (Table 19-1). Patients with Richter hernias typically are in their sixth or seventh decade of life and most frequently are women with femoral hernias. Richter hernias constitute 5% to

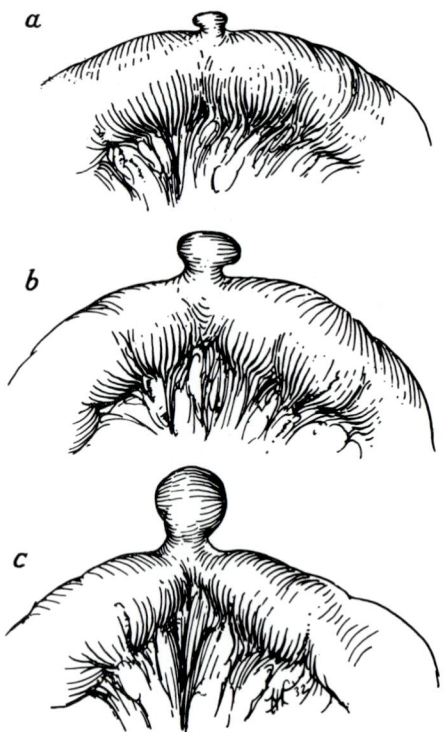

Figure 19-1. Richter hernia. (a) Only a small part of the circumference of the antimesenteric wall of the small intestine has been nipped. There is no intestinal obstruction, but gangrene can occur. (b) With a larger constriction of the circumference, partial obstruction may occur. (c) When there is greater involvement (two thirds, or more, of the circumference), there is kinking of the intestine and the obstruction is likely to be complete. (Cattell RB. Surg Gynecol Obstet 1933;56:700)

15% of the strangulated hernias encountered in large series. The true incidence of this hernia may never be known, however, because of spontaneous reduction with any relaxation and the paucity of adhesions in uncomplicated cases.

In addition to the common groin and umbilical sites, Richter hernia has been described in incisional hernias,[13,25] in obturator hernias,[5] in epigastric and ventral hernias, and through the lumbar triangle of Petit.[22] Keynes[13] reported a supravesical hernia in 1956. In 1977, Bourke[3] reported the first Richter-type herniation through a laparoscopy incision and Botsford[2] implicated a sacral foramen as a site of herniation.

Clinical Presentation and Diagnosis

Richter hernia may proceed along an asymptomatic or a life-threatening course. Critical to recognition are the degrees of obstruction effected and the presence

Table 19-1. Sites and Incidence for Richter Hernia

Author	No. of Richter Hernias (%)	Median Age (y)	Site
Treves (1887)	38		Femoral
	13		Inguinal
	2		Ventral
Frankau (1931)	15 (2.2)		Inguinal
	77 (11.3)		Femoral
	2 (1.3)		Umbilical
Jens (1943)	7 (7)		Femoral
Lyall and Luomanen (1948)	15	61	Femoral
	2		Inguinal
Gillespie et al. (1956)	11	70	Femoral
	5		Ventral
	4		Inguinal

or absence of strangulation. As obstructive symptoms intensify, colicky abdominal pain referable to the distribution of visceral afferent nerves manifests. Distention and borborygmi parallel the extent of obstruction. Hence, minimally obstructing lesions may cause only vague abdominal pain or nausea, whereas a complete obstruction yields more recognizable features associated with adhesive obstruction. Physical examination can frustrate the examining physician. Most Richter hernias occur in the femoral canal, where the small hernia may be masked by body fat or mistaken for inflamed lymph nodes. The key to recognition of these lesions remains a high index of suspicion on the examiner's part and a willingness to explore suspicious groin masses.[27]

Most critical to patient survival are intestinal integrity and viability. A notable feature of a Richter hernia is the propensity to effect intestinal necrosis in the presence of aboral intestinal function. Minimally obstructing lesions can cause necrosis of the intestinal walls with grossly normal intestinal motion until peritonitis produces ileus. Frankau[8] noted that 60% of patients endured more than 2 days before surgical intervention, and mortality exceeded 20%. Clearly, early recognition is key to minimizing the morbidity associated with inappropriate attempts at nonoperative reduction and with strangulation obstruction.

Gillespie and coworkers[9] subdivided patients into three groups on the basis of clinical response. In the first group, mechanical obstruction dominated the clinical picture. One third[7] to one half[11] of patients presented in this manner, and they generally did well because surgical intervention occurred before strangulation. Another third of the patients[9] had intestinal necrosis and little else. Initial examinations with or without contrast roentgenography failed to reveal impending disaster. Subsequent resection and postoperative sepsis were the price for delayed diagnosis and

explained the higher mortality in this group. The third and smallest group (15%)[9] experienced localized necrosis with intestinal-cutaneous fistulization, similar to that described by Hildanus 400 years earlier. Because the septic process was contained and self-limiting, these patients improved with time.

Throughout the literature assembled on Richter hernia, the most constant physical finding remains tenderness and swelling over the common sites of hernias. Treves[31] and Governale[11] noted this in 50% of patients, whereas Gillespie[9] observed the same in 90%. Overlying erythema should heighten the index of suspicion. As in all patients with obstructed intestine, early therapy to avoid resection is mandatory, even if complete obstruction has not manifested itself.

Treatment

Once the diagnosis of Richter hernia is made, timely and aggressive resuscitation should precede operative therapy.[24] There is no place for closed reduction, because the viability of the hernial sac cannot be guaranteed without direct inspection. If the hernial sac recedes during preoperative preparations, a laparotomy should be performed to ensure intestinal viability.

Modern preoperative resuscitation should allow for isotonic rehydration and broad-spectrum antibiotic therapy while hemoglobin, hematocrit, and serum electrolyte levels are measured. Electrocardiograms and chest roentgenography are done routinely. The need for invasive monitoring should be determined on an individual basis according to the specific situation. Preoperative preparations should take no longer than 6 to 12 hours except in unusual circumstances.

Most incarcerated Richter hernias involve the groin, and the favored approach to this area is through the preperitoneal space. This approach affords the surgeon excellent access to repair the hernia defect and to inspect the bowel through one incision. If sanguinous fluid involves the peritoneal cavity, or if the intestine reduces itself in the process of anesthetic induction, it is a simple matter to incise the peritoneum for a direct look inside.

The approach is made through a transverse incision overlying and just lateral to the rectus abdominis muscle about 4 cm above the inguinal ligament. The full thickness of the three musculoaponeurotic layers of the abdominal wall is incised, with care taken to stay cephalad to the internal ring and above the preperitoneal fat and the subjacent peritoneum. The femoral, direct, and indirect groin hernial orifices can be seen readily by blunt dissection. Sharp dissection through the medial border of the femoral canal should free any stubborn attachments of the femoral hernial sac and spare its contents.

If the intestine remains viable, nothing need be done except repair the hernia. Antibiotics should not be given beyond the preoperative dose, and the patient's prognosis is excellent. If necrotic or marginally viable intestine is encountered, resection with primary anastomosis is preferred. In extreme circumstances, exteriorization of the resected intestine may be necessary, but this should be rare in modern surgical practice.

No data have been published concerning the safety and efficacy of laparoscopic surgery in the treatment of Richter hernia. The same concerns relative to the assessment and treatment of nonviable intestine need to be addressed with a technique that is still developmental and relies on prosthetic material for hernia repair.

LITTRE HERNIA

Defined strictly by the guidelines proposed by Treves,[31] Davis,[6] Keynes,[13,14] and others, the sole content of a Littre hernia sac is a Meckel diverticulum. Other viscera associated with a Meckel diverticulum preclude the hernia from being designated a Littre hernia. Thus, it is a relatively rare entity, with fewer than 50 cases documented during this century.

Pathology

A Meckel diverticulum is a remnant of the vitelline duct, which normally becomes involuted during the seventh week of fetal existence. It is present in about 2% of the population, occurring twice as often in males as in females. Gastric or pancreatic tissue may line the lumen of the diverticulum in about 25% of affected individuals.[17] Most commonly, the structure is found within 2 ft of the ileocecal valve on the antimesenteric border of the intestine. Before Meckel's[18] publication in 1809, the diverticulum was considered a traction phenomenon occasioned by a hernia.

Incidence

Littre hernia has been found in every age group.[6] Early confusion about the nature of a true Littre hernia exaggerated the number of patient reports involving this relatively rare entity, but in Frankau's[8] review of 1487 strangulating hernias, its frequency was 0.3%. Keynes noted that half the described Littre hernias were inguinal, 25% to 30% were umbilical, and 20% to 25% were femoral. Most clinical problems occur before the patient reaches 30 years of age.

Clinical Presentation and Diagnosis

Peculiar to Littre hernia is the near-total absence of mechanical obstruction with incarceration or strangulation. Properly defined, Littre hernia excludes participation of the small intestine in its sac. Hence, symptomatic Littre hernia presents much as does Gillespie's third classification of Richter hernia—with abscess or fistulization from undiagnosed strangulation.[32] Obstruction has been described, but is distinctly unusual.

Symptomatic Littre hernias present with a mass over a hernial site. Visceral afferent stimulation can cause anorexia, nausea, and, rarely, vomiting. With necrosis, fever and leukocytosis occur. Obstruction rarely happens, and intestinal function remains relatively normal. The correct preoperative diagnosis seldom is rendered unless lower gastrointestinal hemorrhage dominates the clinical presentation of a young patient. Some success has been reported with nuclear Meckel scanning, but indications for operation do not depend on preoperative diagnosis of the Meckel diverticulum.

Treatment

Treatment is surgical. If a Meckel diverticulum is discovered incidentally in the course of hernia repair for an asymptomatic lesion, Perlman and associates[23] recommend avoiding resection in patients older than 30 years of age. In younger patients and those with symptoms, resection is advised. Local excision with transverse closure should suffice for narrow diverticula. If the base is wide, Keynes[13,14] recommends local ileal resection with end-to-end anastomosis. Severe intercurrent illness may militate against resection in patients with symptoms, but excision of the diverticulum does not complicate subsequent hernia repair. Theoretic objections exist toward laparoscopic resection of a Meckel diverticulum and subsequent use of mesh to repair the hernia, but the literature contains no reports of laparoscopic surgery for Littre hernia.

1808	Percival Pott: Chirurgical Works, Vol. ii, p. 164, London.
1809	Antonio Scarpa: Sull' Ernie, Milano.
1809	P.J. Roux: Melanges de Chirurgie, Paris.
1812	Benjamin Travers: Injuries of the Intestines, London.

Richter Hernia: A Bibliography in Chronological Order

1606	Fabricius Hildanus: Cent. I. Obs. Chir. 55, 1606.
1672	J.H. Lavater: Dissert. de intest. compress (quoted by Defaut).
1700	Littre, Memoires de l'Academie royale des Sciences (Recueil le Memoires, Dijon, 1754, I, pp. 616–622), p. 300. "Observation sur une nouvelle espece de Hernie."
1701	Mery: Same reference, p. 272. (This was a strangulated Meckel diverticulum.)
1707	Ruysch: Thesaurus Anat., Amsterdam.
1710	Verheyen: Corporis Human Anat., Vol. I, p. 51.
1714	Littre: Memoires de l'Academie royale des Sciences, p. 200. "Sur une Hernie rare" (part of colon wall).
1731	Le Dran: Observation de Chirurgie, t. ii, p. 37, Paris.
1741	Morgagni: Adversaria Anatomica, English edition, vol. ii, Bd. Art. 15, p. 136.
1744	Gunz: De Herniis, Lips. p. 6.
1749	George Arnaud: Traite des Hernies, Paris.
1757	Louis: Memoires de l'Academie royale de Chirurgie, t. viii, p. 16.
1761	Morgagni: De Sedibus et Causis Morborum, Venet. Epist. 34. p. 18.
1761–1775	Antonius de Haen: Ratio Medendi Lugd. Bat.
1778–1785	Augustus Gottlob Richter: Abhand-lung von den Bruchen.
1788	A.G. Richter: Traite des Hernies, traduit de l'Allemand sur ed, par J.C. Rougemont, 4° Bonn, 1788.
1788	Adolpus Murray: Animadvers in hernias incompletas casu singulari Il-lust., Upsal, 1788 (quoted by Loviot).
1797	Wrisberg: Loder's Journal für die Chirurgie, Band i, p. 182; also Band iii, S. 92, pp. 101–108.
1806	Manikhoff: Ueber die Bruche, Loggers, Leyden (original Dutch). German translation, Leipsig, 1806, Theil ii, pp. 224–225.

REFERENCES

1. Bissel AH. Richter's hernia. Am J Surg 1929;7:864.
2. Botsford TW. Richter hernia in a sacral foramen: new site for Richter hernia. Arch Surg 1977;112:304.
3. Bourke JB. Small intestinal obstruction from a Richter's hernia at the site of insertion of a laparoscope. BMJ 1977;2:1393.
4. Cattell RB. Richter's hernia. Surg Gynecol Obstet 1933;56:700.
5. Cook MD, Yarrington CD Jr. Strangulated Richter's hernia of the obturator canal: report of two cases. American Practitioner 1962;13:115.
6. Davis CE Jr. Littre's hernia. Ann Surg 1954;139:370.
7. Fowler RS. Partial enterocele. Ann Surg 1899;29:533.
8. Frankau C. Strangulated hernia: a review of 1487 cases. Br J Surg 1931;19:176.
9. Gillespie RW, Glas WW, Mertz GH, Musselmann MM. Richter's hernia. Arch Surg 1956;73:590.
10. Gluecklich B. Johann Friedrich Meckel, the younger (1781–1833). Am J Surg 1976;132:384.
11. Governale SL, Markiewicz SS, Rotondi AJ. Strangulated Richter's femoral hernia, with report of a case. J Int Coll Surg 1941;4:160.
12. Jens J. Strangulated femoral hernia: review of 100 cases. Lancet 1943;1:705.
13. Keynes WM. Richter's hernia. Surg Gynecol Obstet 1956;103:496.
14. Keynes WM. Richter's and Littre's hernias. In: Nyhus LM, Condon RE, eds. Hernia, ed 2. Philadelphia, JB Lippincott, 1978:320–326.
15. Littre A. Observation sur une nouvelle espece de hernie. Memoirs Acad R Soc Paris 1700:300.
16. Lyall D, Loumanen R. Richter's hernia. Am J Surg 1948;75:828.
17. Matt JG, Timpone PJ. Peptic ulcer of Meckel's diverticulum: case report and review of literature. Am J Surg 1940;47:612.
18. Meckel JF. Uber die Divertikel am Darmkanal. Arch Physiol Riel Autenrieth 1809;9:421.
19. Mery J. Observations sur les hernies. Memoirs Acad R Soc Paris 1701:273.
20. Meyerowitz BR. Littre's hernia. BMJ 1958;1:1154.
21. Middlebrook MR, Eftekhari F. Sonographic findings in Richter's hernia. Gastrointest Radiol 1992;17:229.
22. Millard DG. Richter's hernia through the inferior lumbar triangle of Petit. A radiographic demonstration. Br J Radiol 1959;32:693.
23. Perlman JA, Hoover HC, Safer PK. Femoral hernia with strangulated Meckel's diverticulum (Littre's hernia). Am J Surg 1980;139:286.

24. Pualwan F. Operative aspects of Richter's hernia. Surg Gynecol Obstet 1958;106:358.
25. Rhodes RL. Partial enterocele; Richter's, Littre's herniae. Trans South Surg Assoc 1928;61:175.
26. Richter AG. Abhandlung von den Bruchen. Gottingen, JC Dieterich, 1785:597–624.
27. Rowe PH, Hunter-Craig C. Richter's hernia in a direct inguinal sac in a female. J R Coll Surg Edinb 1984;29:264.
28. Ruysch F. Thesaurus anatomicus septimus. Amsterdam, Jansson-Waesberg, 1726.
29. Sackier JM. Future horizons of minimal access surgery. In: Berci G, Nyhus LM, eds. Problems in general surgery, vol 8, no 3. Philadelphia, JB Lippincott, 1991:507–511.
30. Salerno GM, Fitzgibbons RJ, Filipi CJ. Laparoscopic inguinal hernia repair. In: Surgical laparoscopy. St Louis, Quality Medical Publishing, 1991:292–293.
31. Treves F. Richter's hernia or partial enterocele. Med Chir Tr 1887;52:149.
32. Weinstein BM. Strangulated Littre's femoral hernia with spontaneous fecal fistula. Ann Surg 1938;108:1076.
33. Zuniga D, Zupanec R. Littre hernia. JAMA 1977;237:1599.

Hernias of the Abdominal Wall

Part Four

Hernia, Fourth Edition, edited
by Lloyd M. Nyhus and Robert E. Condon.
J.B. Lippincott Company, Philadelphia © 1995.

Chapter 20

Incisional Hernia
Robert E. Condon

This chapter discusses acquired epigastric and trau-matic hernia, as well as incisional ventral hernia. Peri-stomal hernia is discussed in Chapter 21. The inci-dence of the various abdominal wall hernias varies enormously from one institution to another. On our surgical services, the incidence of incisional ventral hernia (including those caused by penetrating abdom-inal trauma or previous hysterectomy) is less than 5% of all anterior abdominal wall incisions. Hernias in the flank or in a subcostal wound used for cholecystec-tomy, although uncommon, are next in frequency. Spontaneous epigastric hernia and diastasis recti oc-cur less often. A "blowout" abdominal wall hernia re-sulting from blunt trauma is rare.

With the laparoscope being used increasingly to conduct intraabdominal operations, small hernias oc-casionally are found through the wounds created for laparoscopic access. Similarly, hernias sometimes oc-cur through the punctures used to insert peritoneal dialysis catheters, particularly in patients with poorly treated renal failure associated with uremia and poor connective-tissue healing. These small hernias are subject to all the problems of ventral hernias. Because of their small size, they may lead early in their course to incarceration of fat or of a knuckle of bowel, with the expected consequences; left untreated, they pro-gressively enlarge.

EPIGASTRIC HERNIA AND DIASTASIS RECTI

Epigastric hernia and diastasis recti usually appear during adulthood and are associated with multiple pregnancies or with obesity. The notion that epigas-tric hernias, especially when they are multiple, are the result of incomplete fetal fusion of the linea alba in the epigastrium is attractive. Because most of these hernias are not present at birth and do not appear until after childhood, however, such an etiologic ex-planation is not tenable. Diastasis recti is related to a slow spreading apart of the medial borders of the rec-tus abdominis muscles, with a diffuse bulge of the thinned-out linea alba between. Other than the un-

toward cosmetic appearance, diastasis recti does not lead to any complications.

In contrast, spontaneous epigastric hernias fre-quently are associated with incarceration of fat and resultant pain. These hernias also are related to mul-tiple pregnancies and to obesity, although they occa-sionally are truly spontaneous, with no recognizable antecedent factors. The presence of a spontaneous epigastric hernia should be suspected in any patient who has well-localized midline tenderness in the epi-gastrium.

The treatment of diastasis recti is complicated by recurrence because of continued deterioration of the connective tissue in the midline of the abdomen. Pa-tients should be discouraged from undergoing repair until etiologic factors, such as pregnancy or obesity, are no longer operative. Simple running plication of the margins of the rectus abdominis muscle has been advocated, but often results in a recurrence. It is more successful to open the midline, dissect laterally in the extraperitoneal plane beneath the rectus muscle for a distance of 5 to 6 cm, and then close the midline again after placing mattress sutures for a single-layer, prosthetic-reinforced repair (see later).

Small epigastric hernias are repaired by amputat-ing the protruding preperitoneal fat. They rarely con-tain a peritoneal sac, but if one is present, it is mobi-lized from the margins of the hernia defect and reduced into the abdominal cavity, usually without opening it. The hernia defect then is sutured primar-ily with a few interrupted sutures, oriented so that the closure is in the vertical midline. If an epigastric her-nia is associated with marked diastasis recti, the entire epigastric linea alba should be repaired at the first op-eration; if this is not done, the patient will be at sig-nificant risk for the development of subsequent addi-tional epigastric hernias. In patients with wide diastasis recti associated with an epigastric hernia, the linea alba should be opened from just above the um-bilical ring to the tip of the xiphoid. The peritoneum and extraperitoneal fat should be dissected away from the posterior surface of the rectus sheath and the sub-cutaneous tissues should be dissected away from the anterior surface for a distance of 5 or 6 cm. Mattress sutures are placed in two rows on each side of the opened midline and the thinned-out tissues of the linea alba are sutured, pulling the two rectus muscles more toward the midline. I prefer to use a running monofilament nylon suture for this task. An onlay, one-layer prosthetic repair then is conducted (see later).

VENTRAL HERNIA

Etiologic Factors

Several factors may influence the occurrence or affect the progression of the acquired ventral incision abdominal wall hernias that are encountered in adults. Some of these factors can be ameliorated by changes in life-style or by technical maneuvers made during the repair. Many others cannot be controlled, however, and their continued presence influences surgical judgment regarding the technique of hernia repair.

Obesity

Among the many other problems that afflict the markedly obese, a tendency toward ventral incisional hernia clearly is present. Excessive fat in the omentum and the subcutaneous tissue results in increased strain on the wound with all body movements in the early postoperative period. Associated poor muscle tone and lack of muscle mass also are causative factors in the development of ventral incisional hernias.

Many surgeons recommend a program of weight reduction in such patients and will not undertake an operation for repair until the patient has lost weight. It is my experience that most patients either do not lose weight or promptly regain it once it has been lost, and I have given up weight reduction as a precondition for operative repair of ventral hernia. Surgery in an obese patient is associated with an increased potential for postoperative pulmonary complications, wound infection, pulmonary embolus, and similar risks, and these should be discussed with the patient. Reapproximation of the thick layer of subcutaneous fat should not be accomplished with sutures during wound closure. It is better to insert subcutaneous closed-suction drainage catheters, which are brought out through small stab wounds remote from the incision and are kept on suction for a few days after the operation until the wound is stable.

Pregnancy

The increase in abdominal pressure accompanying pregnancy is variable, depending not only on the frame of the woman, but also on the size to which the uterus and the contained fetus grow. In many cases,

the increase in abdominal pressure is sufficiently great to place appreciable strain on the anterior abdominal wall. In these circumstances, diastasis recti or epigastric hernia may occur, or an incisional ventral hernia may develop in a previously healed incision. Hernia repair in such patients should be deferred, if possible, until future pregnancies are unlikely to occur.

Location and Direction of Abdominal Incisions

It has been taught in the past that vertical midline incisions are excessively prone to the development of subsequent ventral hernia. An incidence of postoperative herniation as high as 25% has been reported. Although it is widely thought that transversely oriented incisions heal more solidly and with a lower incidence of herniation, that has not been our experience. We recently examined our experience with the use of vertical midline incisions for both elective and emergency operations, a proportion of which had been opened on multiple occasions, and determined that the incidence of incisional hernia 2 years after the last wound closure was only 4%. The incidence of incisional hernia was influenced adversely by expected factors such as contaminated operation in an injured patient, obesity, and the use of postoperative chemotherapy.

It is our view that most major abdominal operations are improved by the adequate exposure that can be obtained rapidly through a vertical midline incision, and we do not hesitate to use this incision in preference to other incisions that either take longer to open and close or provide more restricted exposure of the abdominal viscera.

Sutures and Suture Technique

The continued use of relatively rapidly absorbed suture material, such as chromic catgut, for closure of the fascia in an abdominal wound is a practice that is difficult to understand. These sutures do not maintain their integrity long enough for the wound to achieve sufficient strength to resist the forces generated by the patient's ordinary daily activities. Nonabsorbable or slowly absorbable sutures (polyglyconate [Maxon]; lactomer 9-1 [Polysorb]) are preferable to catgut or to sutures that are absorbed relatively rapidly (polyglactin [Vicryl]; polyglycolate [Dexon]).

The purported advantage of rapidly absorbable suture material—the absence of foreign material that could serve as a nidus of infection—never was a good argument for the use of such sutures and now has been obviated completely by the development of excellent synthetic suture materials. Of these preferred nonabsorbable materials, stainless-steel wire was the standard some years ago, but has been largely discarded in favor of monofilament nylon and polypropylene sutures, which are equally resistant to infection, are well tolerated by tissues, are much easier to tie, and do not break as readily.

Wound closure of the fascia using a running technique also has been a matter of controversy. Most surgeons use and recommend an interrupted suture technique, and often use a near–far technique for fascial closure of a vertical midline abdominal wound. Our experience indicates that running closure is just as effective as is interrupted closure. Running closure has the advantage that the tension in the tissues along the line of closure is adjustable to some degree so that tissues are less ischemic than when they are approximated comparably with multiple interrupted sutures. We not only recommend using a vertical midline incision, but also advise that it be closed with a running suture technique. The sutures should be placed well back into strong tissues, encompassing a bite of at least 2 cm on each side of the wound.

Infection/Sepsis

The most common causative factor in the development of a wound hernia is wound infection that leads to impaired wound healing. Although the infection usually drains gross pus and is clinically obvious, a subclinical wound infection, associated with prolonged wound erythema and tenderness but without frank discharge of pus, also can lead to impaired wound healing and the subsequent appearance of a hernia. Wound infection interferes with normal healing, resulting in a wound that contains less collagen and in which the collagen is not as highly cross-linked as in a normally healed wound. This weakness sets the stage for later postoperative ventral herniation.

In wounds that are subject to intraoperative contamination, the incidence of subsequent infection can be reduced (although not eliminated) by the administration of appropriate antibiotic prophylaxis. Patients whose abdomens already are contaminated as a result of trauma or primary infection should be given parenteral antibiotics as early as possible during their resuscitation and preparation for operation. The objective is to establish and maintain in the tissue antibiotic levels that are higher than the level necessary to kill the bacteria that are contaminating the peritoneal cavity and will invade the wound. In addition, adherence to principles of exquisite and gentle tissue dissection; the use of minimal amounts of suture material or of electrocautery; avoidance of drains or a stoma through the wound; irrigation of the wound during closure to remove debris, blood clot, and any foreign matter; and meticulous hemostasis all improve wound healing and reduce the risk of ventral hernia development.

Age

There is no question that incisional hernia becomes more frequent as the age of the patient increases. Wound healing in older patients is retarded as compared with young adults, but the differences do not appear to be so appreciable as to account fully for the subsequent development of a hernia. It may be that the apparent effect of age simply is a reflection of the fact that the extent of dissection and the potential for intraoperative contamination are greater in operations conducted in older patients (ie, extensive resection for cancer).

Debility and Malnutrition

Malnourished patients, particularly those who have lost a significant amount of weight over a relatively short period before operation, and whose levels of serum albumin and other proteins reflect a state of malnutrition, are at higher risk for poor wound healing and the subsequent development of an incisional hernia. It usually is not possible to delay an indicated operation until these nutritional deficits have been fully corrected. Furthermore, studies have indicated that short-term preoperative parenteral alimentation does not alter the serum albumin concentration or other indicators of malnutrition, and does not decrease the subsequent incidence of incisional hernia.

Postoperative Pulmonary Complications

The effects of postoperative coughing and straining are much overdone as etiologic factors for subsequent incisional hernia. Occasionally, however, "bucking" during the termination of general anesthesia or, vigorous coughing while sedated, literally tears the sutures in the wound. The patient often is aware of the fact that the sutures have torn or "popped." In many instances, either the early appearance of a subcutaneous mass or leakage of fluid through the cutaneous wound heralds the presence of dehiscence and mandates an immediate return to the operating room for repeated repair of the incision. Sometimes the dehiscence is not associated with such signs; the wound breakdown is occult, although the patient often can remember a sensation of suture popping or tearing.

In occasional patients, secure closure without undue tension cannot be obtained at the completion of the initial operation because of bowel distention with fluid and gas, or because of marked edema in the intraabdominal tissues. Under such circumstances, rather than performing closure under tension, which is likely to lead to ischemia and poor wound healing, temporary closure should be obtained with an artificial bur or a similar device and the wound should be repaired again after a day or two.

Steroids

The use of steroids is detrimental to wound healing. Patients who have received long-term steroid therapy have an increased incidence of ventral hernia. The short-term use of even high doses of steroids in the few days immediately preceding an operation, however, is not associated with an excess incidence of herniation caused by poor wound healing as long as the drugs are discontinued in the early postoperative period. Wounds heal poorly in patients receiving long-term steroid therapy because the normal inflammatory responses that are necessary to initiate wound healing are blunted, with consequent impaired deposition and polymerization of collagen in the wound.

Chemotherapy

The early postoperative administration of chemotherapy for cancer is associated with impaired wound healing and an increased incidence of subsequent incisional herniation. There is a dilemma inherent in the treatment of patients who require chemotherapy after resection of their cancer. It is preferable to delay such treatment for several weeks to permit maximal wound healing. Chemotherapeutic agents, however, are most likely to be maximally effective in the first days after operation, when the burden of residual cancer cells may be minimal. There is no good answer to this problem. Our practice has been to delay the initiation of postoperative chemotherapy for 3 to 4 weeks; the subsequent incidence of incisional hernia is about doubled.

Ascites

Patients with cirrhosis and ascites not only have increased abdominal pressure caused by the peritoneal fluid, but also often are severely malnourished. An umbilical hernia is the usual consequence, although the development of a hernia in any previous abdominal incision, even one long healed, is recognized. Patients with ascites should be treated nonoperatively with marked salt restriction and the administration of spironolactone and diuretics. If ascites cannot be controlled by these measures, consideration should be given to the placement of a peritoneovenous shunt. It is pointless to attempt hernia repair in these patients unless the ascites can be brought under control, because the relative risk of recurrence is so high. The only exception is patients with skin necrosis and rupture, in whom repair must be carried out even though the prognosis is less salutary than it would be in the absence or reduction of ascites.

Peritoneal Dialysis

Abdominal hernias are noted with increased frequency in patients undergoing peritoneal dialysis. Although some of these defects may present initially in the groin, the development of a hernia in a preexisting abdominal wound also is possible. The factors that contribute to the development of abdominal wall hernias in patients undergoing continuous ambulatory peritoneal dialysis include uremia, obesity, marked anemia, and chronically elevated intraperitoneal pressure caused by the presence of the dialysate.

Miscellaneous Factors

An etiologic factor cannot be identified in every patient with a ventral incisional hernia. The role of ascorbic acid, zinc, and manganese in extracellular fluid has not been established definitively, although they are thought to influence the maintenance of connective-tissue integrity. Anticoagulants such as warfarin sodium (Coumadin) can have an adverse effect on fibrinogenesis. Both warfarin and heparin increase the incidence of postoperative wound hematoma, which may increase modestly the risk of incisional hernia development.

Clinical Manifestations

Patients with incisional hernia usually complain of a diffuse, enlarging bulge in a previously healed incision. If the patient is obese, it may be difficult to diagnose an epigastric ventral hernia with certainty. Sometimes, exploration of the subcutaneous tissues under local anesthesia is appropriate as a preliminary step in repair. If an incisional hernia is not repaired, it enlarges progressively. What may have begun as a relatively linear defect, caused by a suture under tension tearing through tissues, gradually assumes an ovoid to round shape.

Another presenting complaint, particularly in older patients, may be signs and symptoms of small-bowel obstruction. The obstruction may result from the incarceration of small bowel in the hernia sac. More commonly, it is related to adhesions immediately around the hernia orifice that entrap and kink the bowel. The obstruction is at or immediately adjacent to the neck of the sac, and sometimes is under the fascial rim at a small distance away from the hernia orifice. Colonic obstruction is less common, although a Richter-type colonic hernia may occur as an incisional hernia.

External rupture of a large incisional hernia is uncommon, and usually is preceded by ischemia and necrosis of thinned-out skin overlying a grossly enlarged hernia. Right of domain of the bowel and omentum contained in the hernia sac typically is lost, adding to the difficulty of treatment. Patients with ulceration of the skin overlying a hernia should undergo urgent repair of the hernia. If the ulcerated skin is infected, absorbable prostheses provide temporary control of the hernia, enabling treatment of the cutaneous infection followed by definitive repair of the hernia primarily or with an implanted prosthesis in a few months. In some cases, the ulcerated skin can be excised as the initial step in an operation, and the abdomen can be prepared again and the hernia repair conducted as a clean operation with the insertion of a permanent prosthesis at the initial procedure.

Timing of Operation

Most hernias of the abdominal cavity can be repaired on an elective basis. The major exception is an incisional hernia that occurs in a previously infected wound. Whenever infection has been present, prosthetic hernia repair should be deferred until at least 6 months after all signs of infection have subsided. A delay of 1 year is preferable. When such hernias are explored with the intention of prosthetic repair, if any residual evidence of possible infection is encountered (such as pus in and around a suture from the previous repair), a Gram stain of the apparently purulent material should be obtained. If the Gram stain shows any bacteria, the offending focus of infection should be cleaned up and the definitive hernia repair deferred further. A prosthesis should not be inserted in any wound that continues to harbor bacteria from a preceding infection unless the clinical situation absolutely dictates such action. The likelihood of recurrent infection in such circumstances is high and may vitiate completely the effectiveness of the prosthetic repair.

Loss of Domicile

In some patients with large hernias of the abdominal wall, most of the intestines, together with omentum, may come to reside in the hernia sac rather than in the abdominal cavity. When the viscera are returned to the abdominal cavity and the hernia aperture is repaired, the resulting increased tension in the abdominal cavity may impair diaphragmatic motion, enhancing the possibility of postoperative pulmonary complications. Venous return from the lower extremities also may be impaired because of compression of the vena cava. To enlarge the abdominal cavity and promote restoration of the right of domicile, decompression of the small intestine with a long tube and induction of preoperative pneumoperitoneum

have been recommended. Although I formerly used these adjuncts freely, I have found that modern management of respiratory function with positive-pressure assisted respiration has largely obviated the need for such measures, and I no longer use them often. They remain valuable in some cases, however, and should be kept in mind as therapeutic alternatives in selected patients.

Instead, after the abdominal contents are returned to the abdomen (typically during prosthetic repair of the hernia), the patient is maintained postoperatively with the endotracheal tube in place and receiving respirator support for a few days. During this time, the tension in the abdominal cavity is relieved, the diaphragm returns to a more normal position, pressure within the vena cava readjusts, and the patient can be extubated without difficulty. In an occasional patient with essentially all the abdominal contents outside the abdominal cavity, pneumoperitoneum still may be a useful maneuver to provide preoperative stretching of the residual and retracted musculature of the abdominal wall, and to reduce the need for intubation and respirator support after the operation.

Preparation for Operation

Many patients with a large ventral hernia have poor cutaneous hygiene in skin folds below the hernial mass. This problem requires intensive attention during the preoperative period to control smoldering cutaneous infection. The organisms involved are both fungi and aerobic bacteria, usually coliforms. The patient should shower twice a day with a germicidal soap, clotrimazole or another effective antifungal cream should be applied to the affected skin, and talcum powder should be used to help keep the skin dry. In extreme cases, it may be necessary to admit the patient to the hospital or to a nursing home for appropriate skin care to clear chronic infection.

Certain other general principles apply to all types of abdominal wall hernia repair. Although spinal or epidural anesthesia often provides adequate muscle relaxation and analgesia, well-conducted general anesthesia is safer for high-risk patients. Because of the wide dissection of tissue planes that usually is required to repair all but the smallest ventral hernias, subcutaneous suction drainage catheters should be used postoperatively, brought through small stab wounds remote from the main hernia repair incision, to reduce the risk of postoperative hematoma or seroma formation. Nonabsorbable permanent suture materials should be used for the repair. I prefer nylon sutures, although polypropylene, Dacron, and similar permanent sutures are acceptable.

Antibiotic Prophylaxis

The presence of prosthetic materials always disables the normal host defense mechanisms within the wound enough to increase the risk of infection. This risk can be ameliorated with appropriate antibiotic prophylaxis. Parenteral antibiotics should be administered when anesthesia is induced and continued postoperatively until 12 hours after the drains have been removed. A first-generation cephalosporin antibiotic is the agent of choice for this purpose.

Absorbable Prostheses

Complex glycolic acid meshes developed from the use of these materials as sutures. Polyglycolic acid (Dexon) and polyglactin (Vicryl) are complex molecules based on repetitive strings of glycol moieties. Both meshes are supplied as a broadcloth that is useful as a temporary prosthesis in covering hernia defects. Polyglycolic acid also is supplied as a loose mesh that can be used to wrap up an injured spleen. Both materials are absorbed within 3 to 4 weeks, leaving behind a thin film of connective-tissue scar. Because they are absorbed relatively quickly, these prostheses are not useful in the permanent repair of a hernia. In the past, they were used as the internal layer of a two-layer prosthetic repair in selected circumstances. Today, these absorbable prostheses find their greatest utility in excluding small bowel from the pelvis (using the prosthesis as a temporary dam) in patients who are to undergo postoperative irradiation.

Gelatin film is relatively brittle and inflexible, and is not easy to suture. Because it dissolves within a few days, it finds occasional use as a temporary barrier between the intestines and more permanent prosthetic materials when the omentum or the peritoneum is absent. Although it is useful as a supplemental material in the prosthetic repair of abdominal wall hernias, gelatin film cannot be used as the only prosthesis in such repair.

Permanent Prostheses

Polypropylene mesh (Marlex, Prolene) is the most widely used prosthetic material. It is formed of knitted, monofilament plastic fibers and has minimal elasticity or stretch capacity. Polypropylene elicits an intense desmoplastic reaction in tissue, accompanied initially by serous exudation and resulting eventually in the formation of a sheet of scar that uses the mesh as a scaffold for its formation. The mesh thus becomes densely incorporated in the scar. Polyester mesh (Dacron) is a similar material, but it stimulates less marked formation of connective tissue and is used less widely today.

Expanded polytetrafluoroethylene (Gore-Tex) is supplied as a felted sheet in which fibers randomly interlace. It is more flexible than polypropylene, but otherwise has minimal elasticity or stretch. It elicits little reaction by tissues, but eventually is encased by a surrounding layer of scar tissue to which the polytetrafluoroethylene fabric is loosely attached. This material has been introduced into surgical practice only recently, and experience with it is insufficient to define its liability to infection or its future role in hernia repair.

Metal meshes (stainless steel, tantalum) are woven from monofilament wire and were used widely as prostheses in the past. As might be expected, metal meshes have no elasticity, are relatively stiff, and result in only a modest inflammatory reaction by tissues so that the resulting layer of new scar is relatively thin. They are subject to fatigue fracture of the metal over time because of repeated bending induced by body motion. The use of these meshes in surgical practice today is limited.

Reinforced silicone elastomer (Silastic) is a relatively thick and stiff material that initiates only a minimal inflammatory reaction. It has proven to be useful in the temporary closure of abdominal wall defects in infants (gastroschisis, omphalocele) and, occasionally, as the deep component of a two-layer prosthetic repair of abdominal wall defects in adults.

Fascia lata is natural tissue harvested from the lateral aspect of the thigh. It is strong and flexible, although minimally elastic. The use of fascia lata as a prosthetic material in hernia repair previously was widespread, but largely has been abandoned. The amount of fascia lata available is limited, even when it is harvested from both lower extremities, and additional incisions are necessary in the thigh to excise this tissue.

Incision and Initial Dissection

The choice of incision for repair of a ventral hernia is governed by the orientation of the defect. In most patients, the incision will reopen or excise the scar of the incision used for the original operation, extending it somewhat beyond the margins of the recurrent hernia orifice so as to approach the margin of the hernia and the hernia sac through fresh subcutaneous tissue. Once the skin incision is completed, the skin edges and subcutaneous fat are retracted and the dissection is continued down to the hernia sac and out to healthy fascia at the edges of the hernia defect. Flaps of skin and subcutaneous tissue are dissected to a point beyond the margins of the hernia defect. Any connective tissue overlying the hernia sac is opened and trimmed back to firm fascial margins. After normal fascia is identified at one aspect of the border of the hernia, the dissection is continued all around the hernia, raising the skin and subcutaneous fat for a distance of 5 to 6 cm from the margin of the hernia defect. Next, the peritoneum is mobilized from the margins of the hernia orifice and the extraperitoneal plane internal to the muscular abdominal wall is dissected widely. If the hernia sac is redundant, it is entered and the contents are reduced; any adjacent adhesions are taken down to reduce the risk of postoperative obstruction. Any excess peritoneum is amputated and the sac is closed. If peritoneum is not redundant, the hernia sac simply is maintained in a reduced position with external pressure as the repair is completed.

The extraperitoneal plane beneath the abdominal wall fascia is developed by dissection beginning at the margin of the hernia defect, freeing the underside of the fascia for a distance of 4 to 5 cm completely around the circumference. Thinned-out fascia and connective tissue at the margins of the defect are excised so that there is strong fascia at all margins.

Skin with a large hernia probably is redundant, but the excision of excess skin should be deferred until the completion of the hernia repair, when both viability and the true degree of excess can be judged more accurately.

Avoidance of Counterincisions

A variety of counterincisions made parallel to and at a distance from the margins of the hernial aperture are recommended by others as part of their technique of hernia repair. The objective of these incisions is to make a bipedicled flap of fascia or of fascia and muscle that slides toward the center of the hernial opening and allows a primary closure. Even when counterincisions are extensive, however, they often do not mobilize tissue sufficiently to allow primary approximation without undue tension. Prosthetic repair of a hernia using tissue replacement techniques is preferable to the use of counterincisions, flaps of rectus fascia, and similar maneuvers. The exception to this principle is the use of a relaxing incision in the anterior rectus fascia during primary repair of a groin hernia. Even in this instance, though, careful attention must be paid to ensure the absence of undue

tension and a prosthesis must be used if any doubt exists.

Direction of Closure

A hernia that begins as a slit-like aperture changes progressively into an ovoid and then rounder aperture as the hernia enlarges. The reason for this change in shape relates to the physics of tissue resistance. A circle is most resistant to the application of external force, and becomes the shape that the aperture of most hernias eventually assumes. Therefore, the direction in which closure is made is not important. There is no inherent advantage in transverse as compared with vertical closure, for example, of a ventral incisional hernia. Closure should be accomplished in the direction that causes the least tension on the repair.

Choosing the Technique for Repair

The probable direction of primary closure of the hernia is determined by placing Kocher clamps on the proposed mid-point of opposite margins and pulling the clamps toward each other. The tension necessary to approximate the margins of the hernia is determined; if the margins can be approximated with less than 3 lb of force, successful primary repair of the hernia with interrupted sutures probably is possible. Three pounds of pull is the limit for a tension-free repair. This is equivalent to the effect of suspending a plastic 1-qt jug full of water from the index finger. This is not much weight, so there should be a low threshold for the use of prosthetic reinforcement (one-layer repair) or the replacement of missing tissue (two-layer repair).

If the fascial margins can be approximated without undue tension, but appear to be intrinsically weak, reinforced repair with a one-layer onlay polypropylene prosthesis should be performed. If undue tension cannot be avoided, the hernia is repaired using a two-layer prosthetic technique, with Gore-Tex used for the internal layer and polypropylene mesh used for the external layer.

Primary Repair

In a primary repair, sutures are inserted 2 to 3 cm from the free margin of the hernia and 1 to 2 cm apart. When all the sutures for closure have been placed, they are pulled up and tied serially and then the wound is closed.

Onlay (One-Layer) Reinforced Repair

If onlay reinforced repair is necessary (Fig. 20-1), the fascia must be cleared on both the superficial and internal aspects for a distance of 6 to 7 cm from the edge of the hernia defect. A series of 0 braided nylon mattress sutures are placed through the full thickness of the fascia 5 to 6 cm from the margin of the hernia defect. Each mattress suture should encompass about a 1-cm bite of the full thickness of the musculoaponeurotic abdominal wall. The long ends of the sutures are in the space between the subcutaneous fat and the superficial aspect of the fascia; on the internal surface of the musculoaponeurotic layers of the abdominal wall, these sutures are carried in the extraperitoneal plane. The ends of the sutures are left long and are collected in hemostats.

The hernia defect then is closed primarily with interrupted or running sutures. After the primary closure, a piece of polypropylene mesh 1 cm wider than the circle of mattress sutures is cut. The ends of all the mattress sutures and of some of the sutures used for primary closure are brought through the prosthesis in appropriate locations so that the prosthesis lies flat against the abdominal wall. The mattress sutures are pulled up and tied successively. Suction drains are placed over the prosthesis and brought out through remote stab wounds. The skin and subcutaneous portion of the wound is closed.

Tissue Replacement (Two-Layer) Prosthetic Repair

In tissue replacement prosthetic repair (Fig. 20-2), the hernia margins are not closed. Both the subcutaneous plane superficial to the musculoaponeurotic abdominal wall and the extraperitoneal plane immediately in-

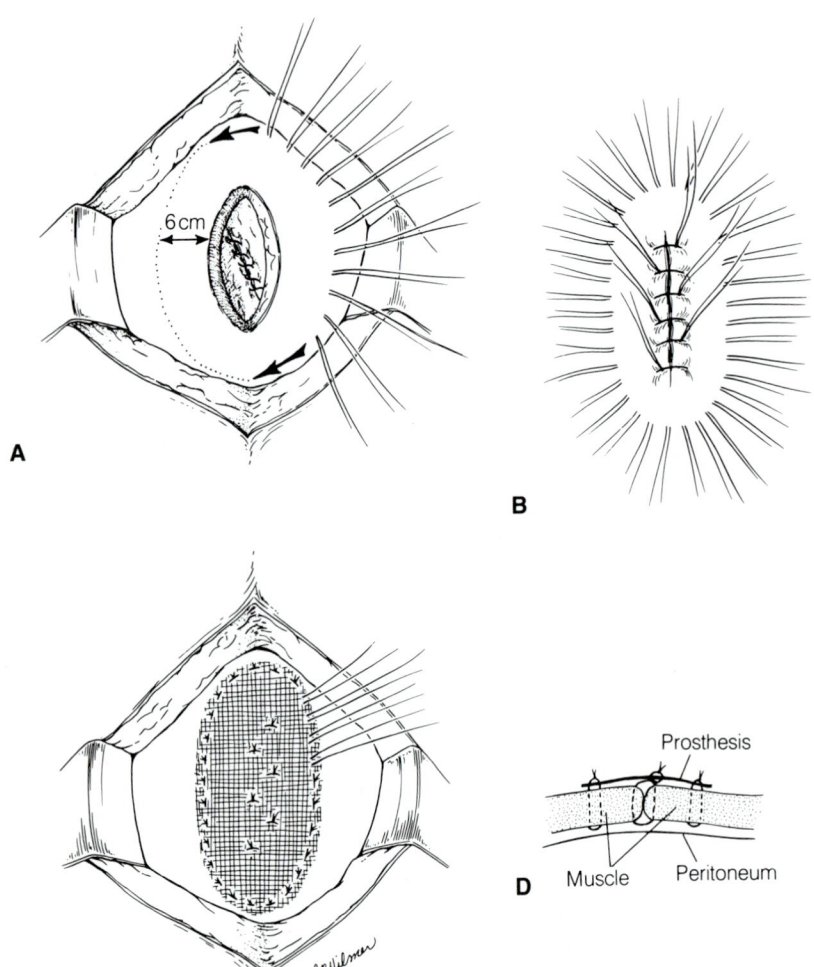

Figure 20-1. One-layer, onlay, prosthetic-reinforced repair of a recurrent ventral hernia. (*A*) Mattress sutures are placed through the muscular abdominal wall. (*B*) The hernia is closed with interrupted sutures. (*C*) The ends of all sutures are brought through the prosthesis and tied. (*D*) The completed repair in cross section.

ternal to this wall are dissected for 6 to 7 cm from the margins of the hernia.

In the two-layer prosthetic technique, the superficial and internal aspects of the musculoaponeurotic wall are cleared and a piece of Gore-Tex about 6 cm wider in all dimensions than the hernia aperture is cut. For the largest hernias, more than one piece of Gore-Tex may be needed to bridge the entire defect; in these exceptional cases, the pieces of Gore-Tex are sutured to each other to maintain continuity of the internal layer of the prosthesis. It should be kept in mind that the primary functions of the internal layer of this prosthesis are to maintain the hernia in a reduced position and to provide a secure anchor for the mattress sutures that hold the external layer of the prosthesis. The strength of the repair derives primarily from the strength of the external polypropylene mesh prosthesis.

In a two-layer repair, mattress sutures of 0 braided nylon are placed 1 to 2 cm back from the margins of the hernia defect. Suturing is begun at the external aspect of the musculoaponeurotic abdominal wall and carried into the extraperitoneal plane. Sutures then are placed through the Gore-Tex prosthesis about 1 cm from the margin and encompassing about 1 cm of the prosthesis, and are returned from the extraperitoneal plane back to the subcutaneous plane. Placing sutures around the entire circumference of a ventral incisional hernia is tedious, but necessary. All sutures should encompass 1-cm bites of tissue in the internal prosthesis, should be placed 1 to 2 cm back from the margin of the hernia defect, and should be situated about 1 cm apart.

The size of the prosthesis should be rechecked for fit as each suture is placed, pulling the prosthesis into position in the extraperitoneal plane and then pulling

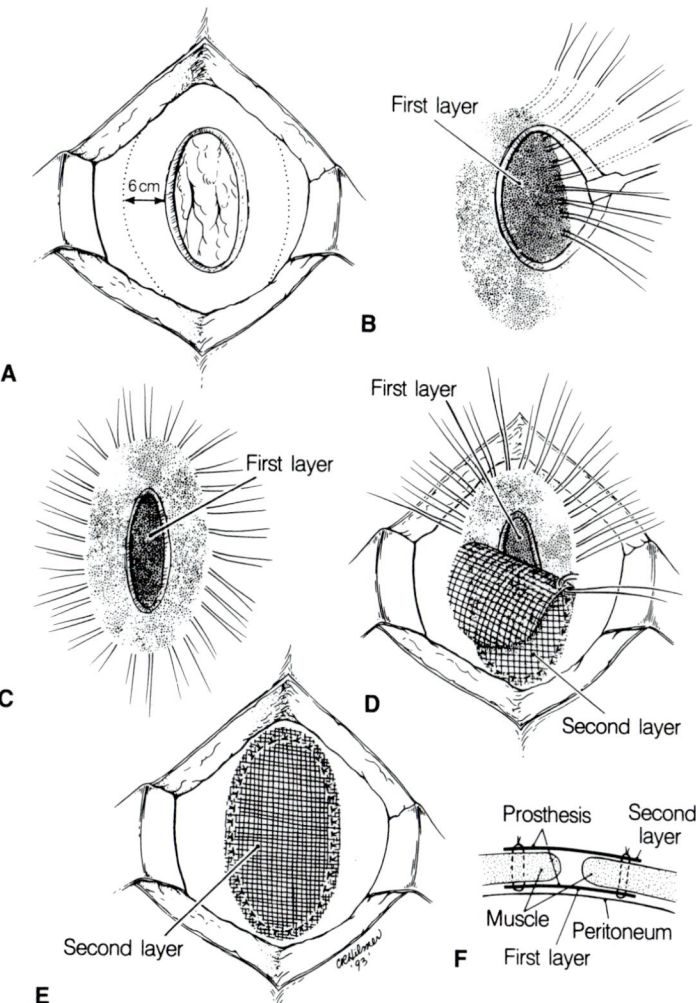

Figure 20-2. Two-layer prosthetic repair of a recurrent ventral hernia. (*A*) The hernia orifice is not sutured. Sutures will be placed around the hernia and about 6 cm from its margin. (*B*) Sutures are first placed in half the circumference of the prosthesis and are then brought through the full thickness of the muscular abdominal wall. (*C*) Completion of placement of sutures for the first (deep) layer of the prosthesis. (*D*) A second (superficial) layer of mesh prosthesis is placed, and the ends of all sutures are brought through it. (*E*) The completed repair. (*F*) Cross section of the completed repair.

it out again into the main wound for placement of the next suture. Improperly placed sutures should be removed and replaced in appropriate positions.

Once all the mattress sutures have been placed, they are pulled up and maintained on traction. Placing a hemostat on the end of each suture and gathering groups of sutures on a ring forceps helps to keep the sutures under appropriate tension. We have tried various spring clips and other devices as suture holders and do not find them as satisfactory as racking hemostats on a ring forceps.

When the first layer of this repair is complete, the prosthesis should lie flat in the extraperitoneal plane. It may be under slight tension, but it is not necessary to pull the margins of the hernia aperture together. If the prosthesis is not snug and lying flat, sutures be repositioned as appropriate.

The external layer of polypropylene mesh is trimmed so that it is similar in size to the internal Gore-Tex layer. The ends of each pair of mattress sutures are brought through the polypropylene mesh all around its circumference and about 1 cm from the margin of the prosthesis. The prosthesis then is pressed against the superficial aspect of the musculoaponeurotic abdominal wall, bridging the hernia aperture, and is checked for appropriate fit. The position of sutures is readjusted as necessary. The superficial polypropylene mesh prosthesis should lie flat and snug against the external aspect of the musculoaponeurotic abdominal wall.

Once both layers of prosthetic material have been placed properly, the mattress sutures are pulled up and tied successively. The free edge of the superficial layer of polypropylene mesh is tacked down to the superficial fascia with interrupted 3-0 polyglycolic sutures.

Two closed-suction drains are placed on top of the prosthesis and brought out through stab wounds away from the main operative incision. The wound is irrigated, hemostasis is secured, the skin is closed with running 3-0 monofilament nylon suture, and a dressing is applied. Alternatively, subcuticular closure can be performed with running 3-0 polyglycolic suture. Suction is maintained on the drains as long as more than 30 mL of serous fluid is aspirated daily from either drain.

REFERENCES

1. Hesselink VJ, Luijendijk RW, de Wilt JH, Heide R, Jeekel J. An evaluation of risk factors in incisional hernia recurrence. Surg Gynecol Obstet 1993;176:228.
2. Monaghan RA, Meban S. Expanded polytetrafluoro-ethylene patch in hernia repair: a review of clinical experience. Can J Surg 1991;34:502.
3. Santora TA, Roslyn JJ. Incisional hernia. Surg Clin North Am 1993;73:557.

Special Comment

Expanded Polytetrafluoroethylene Prosthetic Patches in Repair of Large Ventral Hernia
James R. DeBord

The history of prosthetic repair of abdominal wall hernias began in 1984 with Phelps' use of silver-wire coils placed on the floor of the groin to incite an inflammatory fibrosis to augment the repair.[16] The evolution of modern prosthetics in hernia repair has been extensively reviewed.[5] Practice has focused on the use of polypropylene mesh, polyester mesh, and the expanded polytetrafluoroethylene (e-PTFE) patch. In this discussion, I review my personal experience, along with that of my associates, with the use of large e-PTFE patches (Gore-Tex Soft Tissue Patch, W.L. Gore and Associates, Inc., Flagstaff, AZ) to repair large ventral incisional hernias.

The Gore-Tex Soft Tissue Patch (STP) is manufactured in sheets measuring up to 20 × 30 cm, or larger, and 1 or 2 mm in thickness. The e-PTFE patch is composed of pillar-shaped nodes of polytetrafluoroethylene (PTFE) that are connected by fine fibrils of PTFE with a multidirectional arrangement of the fibrils in the surface view, which imparts balanced strength to the patch in all directions (Fig. 20-3). The average internodal fibril length (ie, "pore size") is 20 to 25 µm, and this unique porous microstructure provides a conformable biomaterial that is flexible, soft, and nonfraying. The microstructure allows cellular infiltration and tissue incorporation into the patch and promotes a monolayer of cells on the peritoneal surface of the patch, creating a pseudoperitoneum that retards adhesions to the patch (Figs. 20-4 and 20-5). The material strength of e-PTFE has been documented as adequate for safe clinical use. Industrial testing methods have shown the Gore-Tex STP to be stronger than Marlex, Prolene, or Mersilene mesh, and its strength in terms of suture retention to be equivalent to that of these materials.[13,25]

The first clinical study using Gore-Tex STP in hernia repair was that of Wool and colleagues in 1985.[26] They reported 30 hernia repairs with no recurrences and no infections, but follow-up was short in this preliminary report. Further clinical reports by Hamer-Hodges and Scott,[8] Bauer and coworkers,[2]

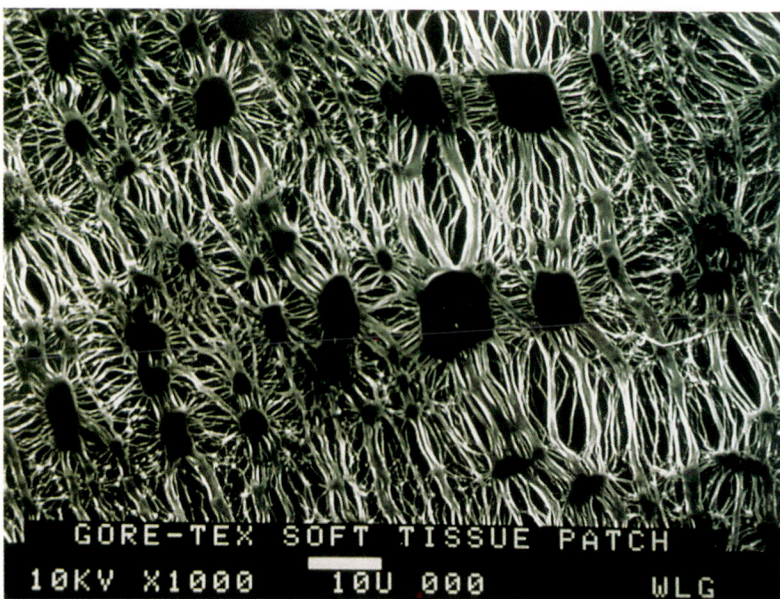

Figure 20-3. Surface view of expanded polytetrafluoroethylene (e-PTFE) patch showing nodes of polytetrafluoroethylene (PTFE) connected by multidirectional fibrils of PTFE.

Antonini and coworkers,[1] Van der Lei and coworkers,[23] Pailler and coworkers,[15] Colombo and coworkers,[4] Deysine,[7] and DeBord and coworkers[6] have documented the efficacy of Gore-Tex STP repair of ventral incisional hernias.

MATERIALS AND METHODS

The ideal prosthetic material should be strong and inert, should provide a lattice for incorporating connective tissue while resisting the formation of adhesions, and should be stable in the presence of infection. Because e-PTFE appears to meet many of these criteria, we used e-PTFE patches to repair large ventral incisional hernias in 62 patients. Over an 8-year period (1983–1991), we repaired unusually large and difficult ventral incisional hernias in 30 females and 32 males whose average age was 57.8 years. Patients were selected on the basis of primary repair being unrealistic, either because tissue was insufficient or because tension would have been too great on a primary closure. All patients were given preoperative antibiotics (cefazolin, 1 g). The hernia sac was excised, and the fascial margins were débrided of attenuated fascia and cleared of any underlying adhesions and overlying subcutaneous tissue. Inability to close the fascia without excessive tension was confirmed, and an appropriately sized, 2-mm-thick e-PTFE patch repair was performed.

Two methods of repair, involving polypropylene or e-PTFE suture, were used in this series. The first method consisted of full-thickness replacement of the abdominal wall defect by the e-PTFE patch, with edge-to-edge, patch-to-fascia suturing. The second method consisted of full-thickness repair with a wide underlay at the margins (usually about 4–6 cm), with U-sutures placed through the healthy fascia at the edge of the patch underlay (Fig. 20-6). Whenever possible, with the patch underlay technique, the attenuated fascia was preserved and closed above the e-PTFE patch to increase the opportunity for tissue incorporation into the patch and to provide an additional tissue layer between the patch and the overlying skin and subcutaneous tissue. Closed-suction drainage was normally used for 4 to 6 days postoperatively, and intravenous antibiotics were continued until the drains were removed.

RESULTS

Average follow-up was 24.4 months, with a range of 1 to 82 months. Sixty-nine percent of the repairs were on recurrent hernias. The average size of the e-PTFE patch required for the repair was 168 cm² or approximately 11 × 15 cm. The largest defect measured 600 cm² and required three patches to be sewn together to achieve an adequate repair. Many patients required several patches to be sewn together to repair the large defect present (Fig. 20-7).

Seroma, the most common complication, occurred in nine (14.5%) of the patients. Infections developed in six (9.6%) of the patients and led to patch

(text continues on p. 332)

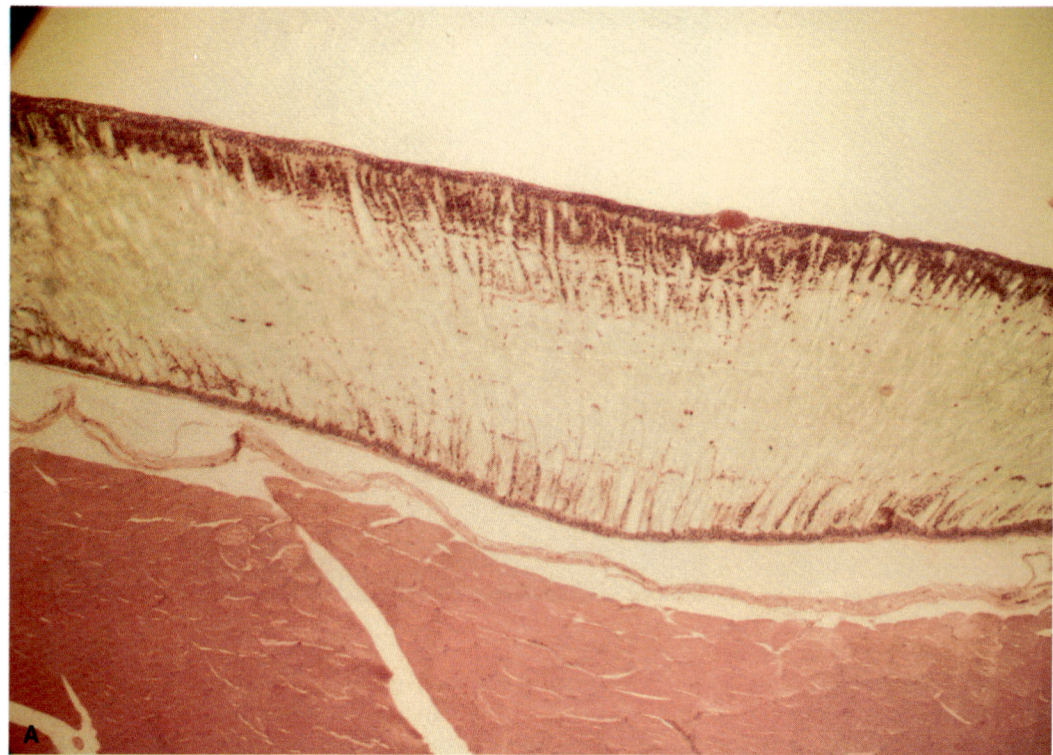

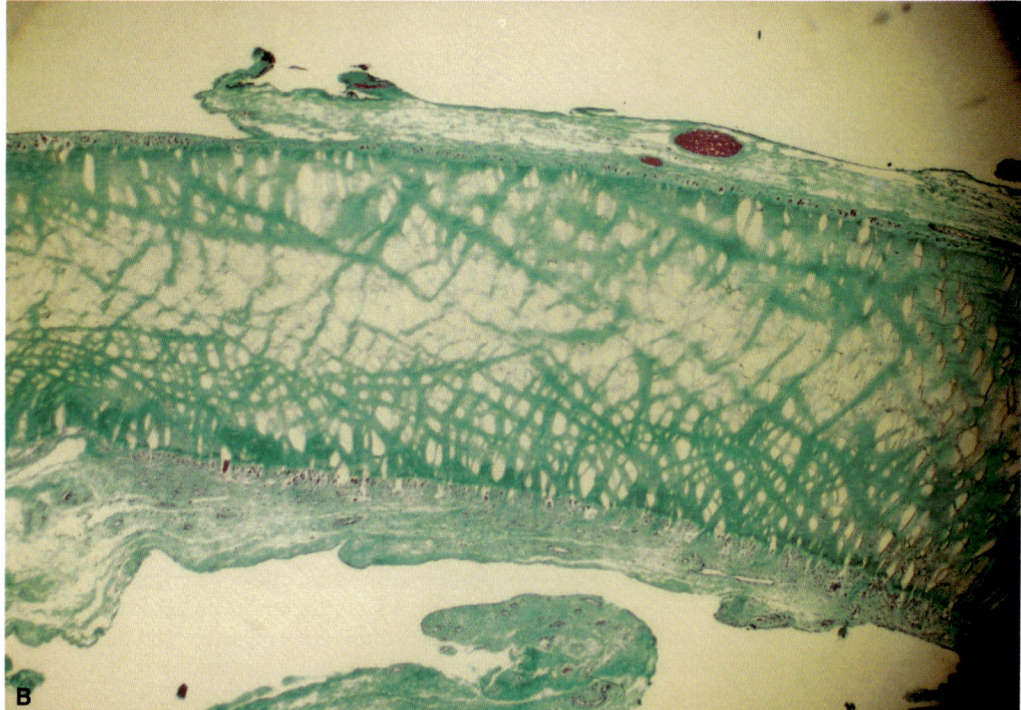

Figure 20-4. (*A*) Gore-Tex Soft Tissue Patch (STP) (W.L. Gore and Associates, Inc., Flagstaff, AZ) with cellular ingrowth into the interstices of the e-PTFE occupying the entire width of the patch (hematoxylin–eosin). (*B*) Collagen deposition throughout the STP with attachment of vascularized fibrous tissue to the external surface (Milligan trichrome).

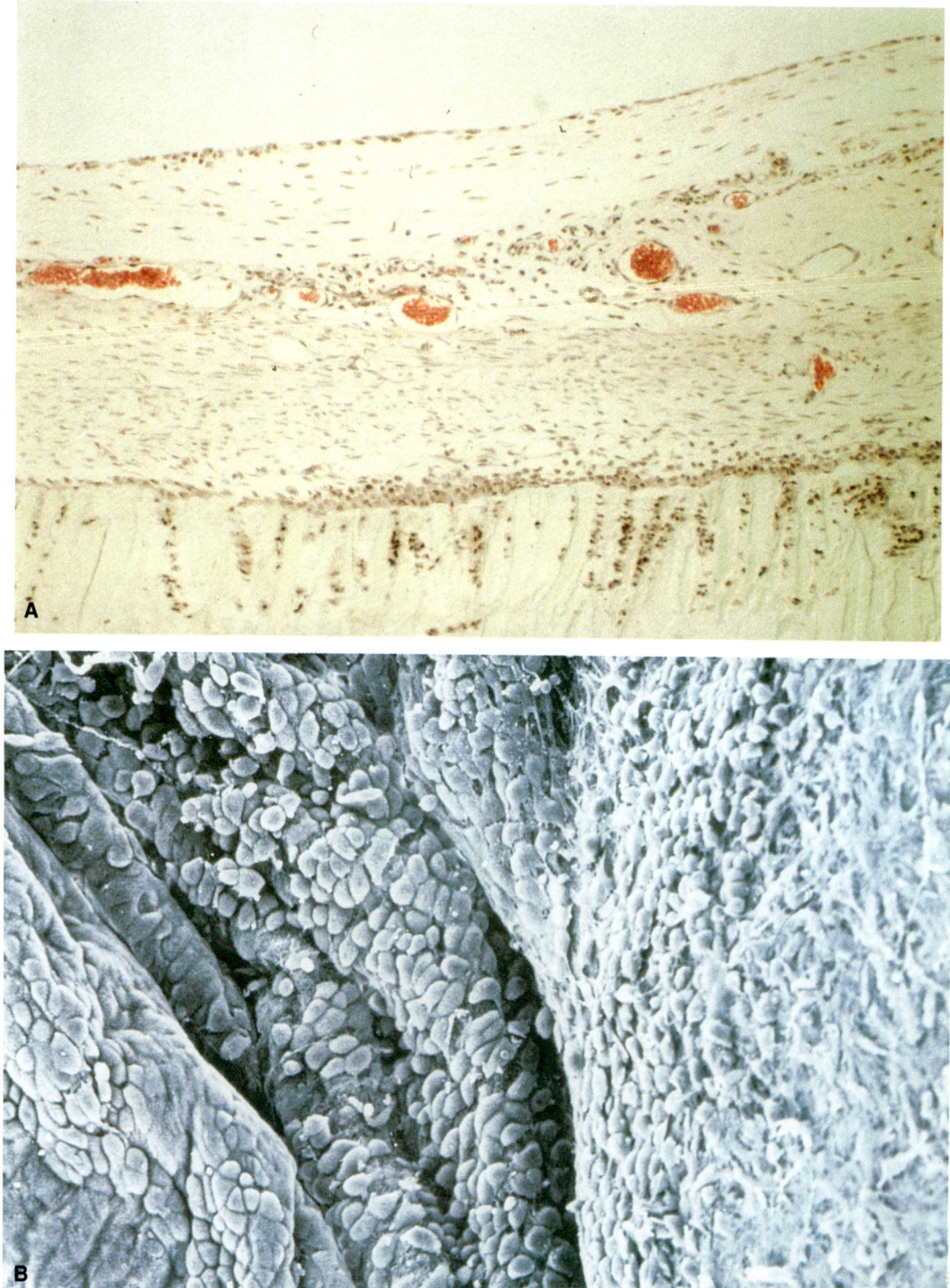

Figure 20-5. (*A*) A flat monolayer of neomesothelial cells forms a pseudoperitoneum above areolar tissue at peritoneal surface of the e-PTFE patch. (*B*) Scanning electron micrograph of the junction between the peritoneum (left) and the STP (right), showing that mesothelial cells having migrated from the peritoneum to the surface of the patch.

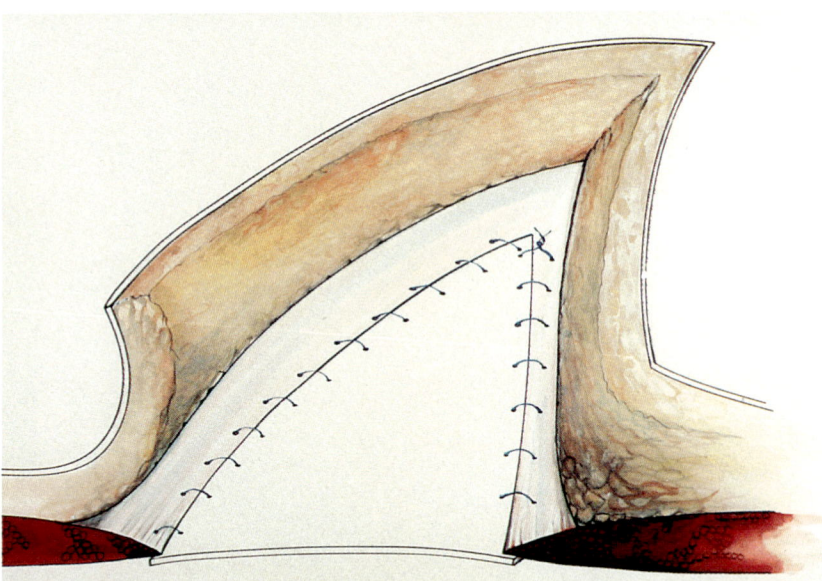

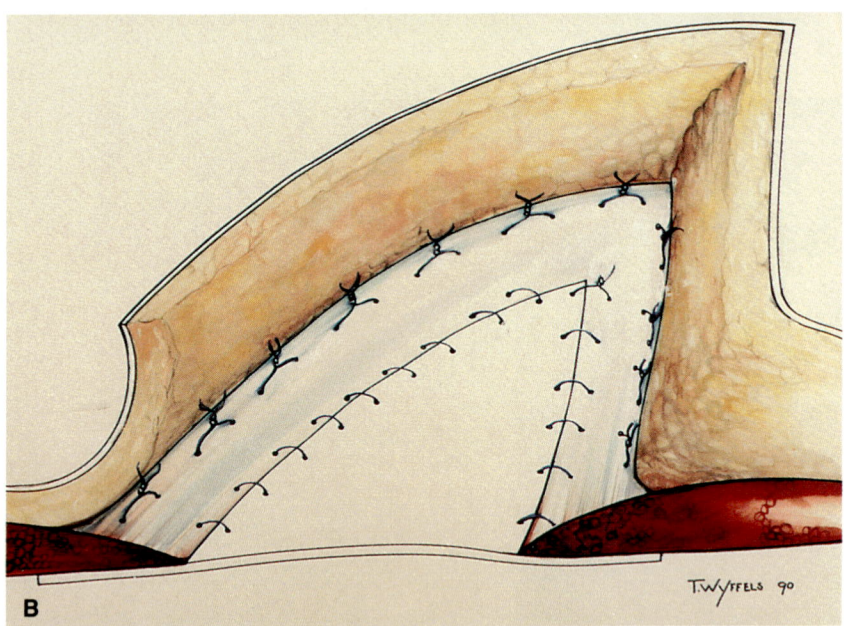

Figure 20-6. (*A*) Edge-to-edge, patch-to-fascia repair. (*B*) Patch repair with wide underlay technique. (Reprinted from DeBord et al. Postgraduate General Surgery 1992;4:156–160. Copyright 1992 R.G. Landes Company.)

repair failure in five patients. One infected patch was salvaged with long-term antibiotic therapy and local wound care. No cases of adhesive small-bowel obstruction, enterocutaneous fistula, or patch extrusion occurred during the follow-up period. Three additional patch failures (recurrent herniation) that developed were unrelated to infection. These recurrences were due to new defects in the fascia lateral to the repair and appeared to be the result of suture material pulling through the fascia (Fig. 20-8). Thus, the overall recurrence rate in this series of large abdominal wall defect repairs using e-PTFE patch was 12.9% (8 of 62 repairs).

DISCUSSION

The ideal prosthetic should be biologically inert to reduce or prevent foreign body reaction. It should be strong yet pliable, should maintain its form after im-

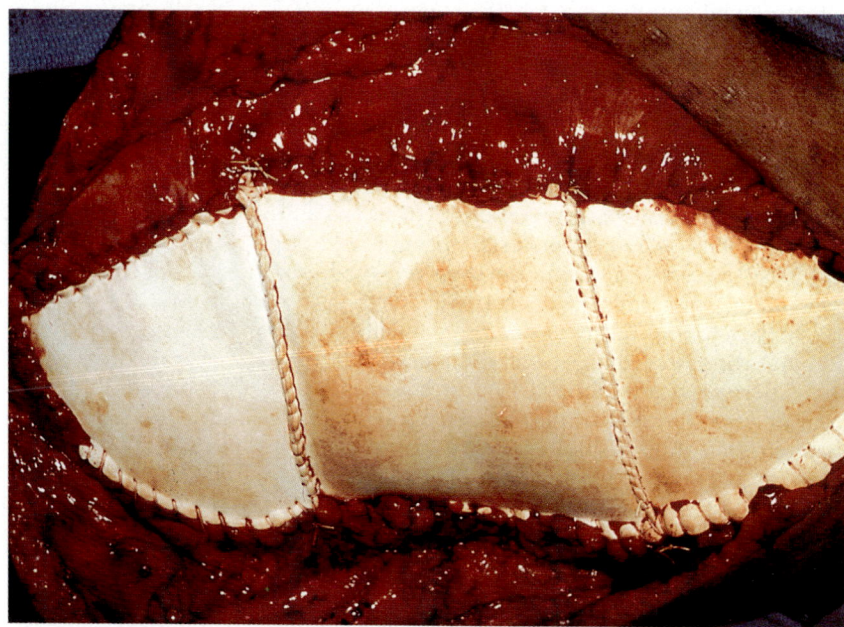

Figure 20-7. Repair of giant ventral hernia with multiple patches sewn together. (Reprinted from DeBord et al. Postgraduate General Surgery 1992;4:156–160. Copyright 1992 R.G. Landes Company.)

plantation, and should resist the formation of adhesions while supporting fibrous ingrowth of connective tissue (particularly when a portion of the entire abdominal wall is being replaced.)

Polypropylene mesh has been the most widely used prosthetic material in hernia repair since it was first introduced in 1963.[19,21] However, clinical experience with polypropylene mesh indicates a variety of complications that may be related to the physical properties of the mesh, including enteric fistula, erosion into intraabdominal organs, and mesh extrusion.[9,18,24]

In contrast, e-PTFE produced fewer adhesions in animal models.[10,14] Fewer adhesions were also found in the presence of infection.[3] The e-PTFE patch is biologically inert and produces little or no inflammatory reaction, and its porous microstructure provides a lattice for the incorporation of connective tissue.[2,8,10]

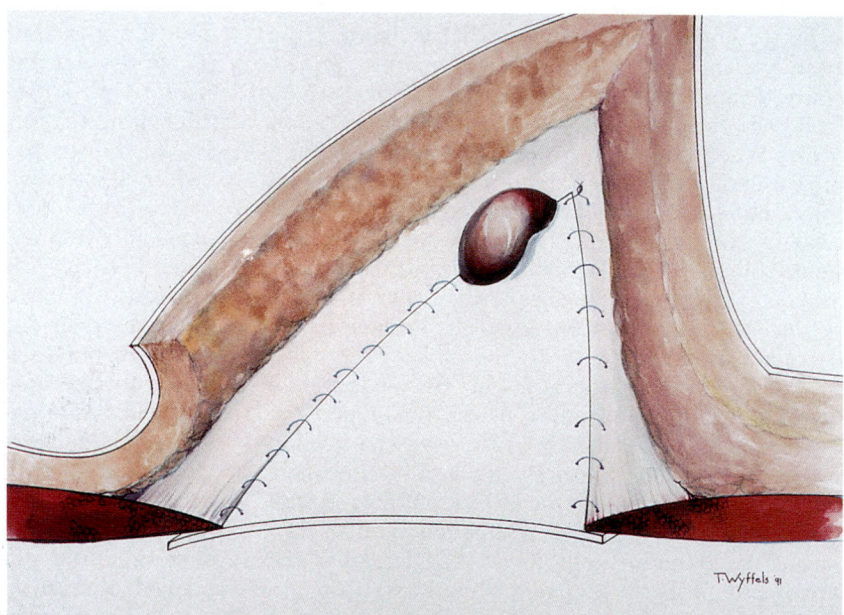

Figure 20-8. Hernia recurrence lateral to the patch due to excess tension, with sutures tearing through the fascia. (Reprinted from DeBord et al. Postgraduate General Surgery 1992; 4:156–160. Copyright 1992 R.G. Landes Company.)

Experimental results with full-thickness wall defect repairs indicate a statistically significant reduction in adhesion formation with the e-PTFE patch.[3,14] These findings are also supported by clinical results, which indicate that adhesions bind less firmly and densely to the relatively smooth, pliable surface of the e-PTFE patch than to the individual fibers of both absorbable and nonabsorbable mesh materials.[10,17] The e-PTFE patch exhibits adequate material strength (22 kg/cm).[25] No material failures have been reported, and none occurred in this series.

In general, we did not attempt to shield intraabdominal contents from the patch material. We have not experienced any difficulties with bowel obstruction, enterocutaneous fistula, or extrusion of patch material. In a study that included 28 patients, Bauer and associates noted a similar lack of these complications.[2] These particular attributes of the e-PTFE patch become more important in the repair of large abdominal wall defects, because of the large surface area of patch exposed to the viscera.

Seroma was the most common complication occurring in nine (14.5%) of the patients. This complication is a chronic one and has plagued prosthetic repair of large ventral incisional hernias since its inception.[22] The major factor in seroma development is most likely the large dead space that is inevitable with defects as large as those reported here. Closed suction drainage and pressure dressings seem to be reasonable measures to reduce seroma collections, but they are not uniformly successful. It has been proposed that polypropylene mesh is a more porous material than e-PTFE and should allow for better drainage of seroma collections into the peritoneal cavity; however, evidence suggests that the peritoneal cavity is sealed within 12 hours of surgery even when polypropylene mesh is used.[3] Aspiration of the seroma may be necessary if large amounts accumulate; however, these fluid collections often resorb if left alone for a few weeks. When aspiration is necessary, adherence to a strict aseptic technique is required—we believe that one of our patch infections was directly related to repeated seroma aspiration. The omentum can be used on occasion to help eliminate large areas of dead space between the patch and the skin when it can be technically brought out on a pedicle away from the actual hernia defect.[6]

Infection in the wound led almost invariably (5 out of 6 instances) to failure of the repair and the need for patch removal, although one patch infection healed and remained healed with local wound care and antibiotic treatment. One infection occurred with a large ventral hernia repair in a patient with a colostomy. Even though the stoma site was lateral to the repair and properly prepared and draped, the increased risk was noted, and a complicating infection

in the wound developed despite precautions. In these large abdominal wall defects, the occurrence of wound infections is not surprising, given the large area of foreign biomaterial in the wound and the associated large dead space between the patch and the skin. Our 9.6% incidence of infection is too high but may be attributable in some respects to this unique group of patients, who had an average patch size of 168 cm^2. *Staphylococcus aureus* and *S. epidermidis* were the major pathogens involved in these infections; however, *Escherichia coli* was cultured from the wound abscess in the colostomy patient. The same factors of large patch size and degree of dead space that may have increased the chances for infection were probably responsible for the failure of local care measures and antibiotics to salvage the infected prostheses.

The more successful experience of vascular surgeons in managing infected e-PTFE vascular grafts and hemodialysis access grafts might lead one to expect better results in cases of smaller e-PTFE patch infections in areas where more healthy surrounding soft tissue and less dead space are present (smaller ventral hernias and inguinal hernias). No biomaterial, however, can really be considered infection-proof, and continued investigation in the area of antibiotic incorporation into biomaterials and other developments are needed to improve the management of these difficult clinical problems. In experiments using rats, Law and Ellis concluded that polypropylene mesh is preferable to e-PTFE patch for repair of contaminated abdominal wall defects.[11]

Although polypropylene mesh is a tested material in the repair of difficult hernias, we prefer the e-PTFE patch for its ease in handling, its inherent softness and pliability, its strength, and, primarily in this group of large abdominal wall defects, its lack of complications related to direct exposure to the abdominal viscera. An 87% success rate was achieved in these 62 difficult hernia repairs using the e-PTFE patch.

To reduce the amount of dead space associated with these repairs, and thus the complications associated with this dead space, we have used a new technique in the prosthetic repair of large ventral incisional hernias. Taking our cue from the laparoscopic surgeons who claim that a prosthesis can be successfully tacked up against the inside of the abdominal wall with only a few shallow staples,[12] we have repaired three large ventral incisional hernias and created essentially no dead space in the process. Using the technique reported by Stoppa,[20] the hernia is entered directly through the defect (usually a midline incision). The underlying adhesions to the abdominal wall and hernia sac are lysed, but no subcutaneous dissection on the anterior surface of the fascia is performed. Several small cuts are made in the skin and subcutaneous tissue circumferentially and widely beyond the hernia defect. The oversized Gore-Tex STP prosthesis is then placed intraperitoneally and secured with U-sutures of heavy monofilament suture. The sutures are placed through the full thickness of the abdominal wall at the small cuts in the skin beyond the periphery of the defect and then pass through and back out of the prosthesis, returning through the full thickness of the abdominal wall to exit from the same small skin cut at which the suture

entered. Four corner anchoring sutures are placed, and then a few others are put between each corner suture to secure the prosthesis firmly against the inner abdominal wall. None of these sutures are tied until they are all placed, and then they are all carefully tied to avoid catching a loop of bowel or omentum between the patch and the abdominal wall. The prosthesis is now well secured, and the hernia repaired, with Pascal's principle providing additional support in

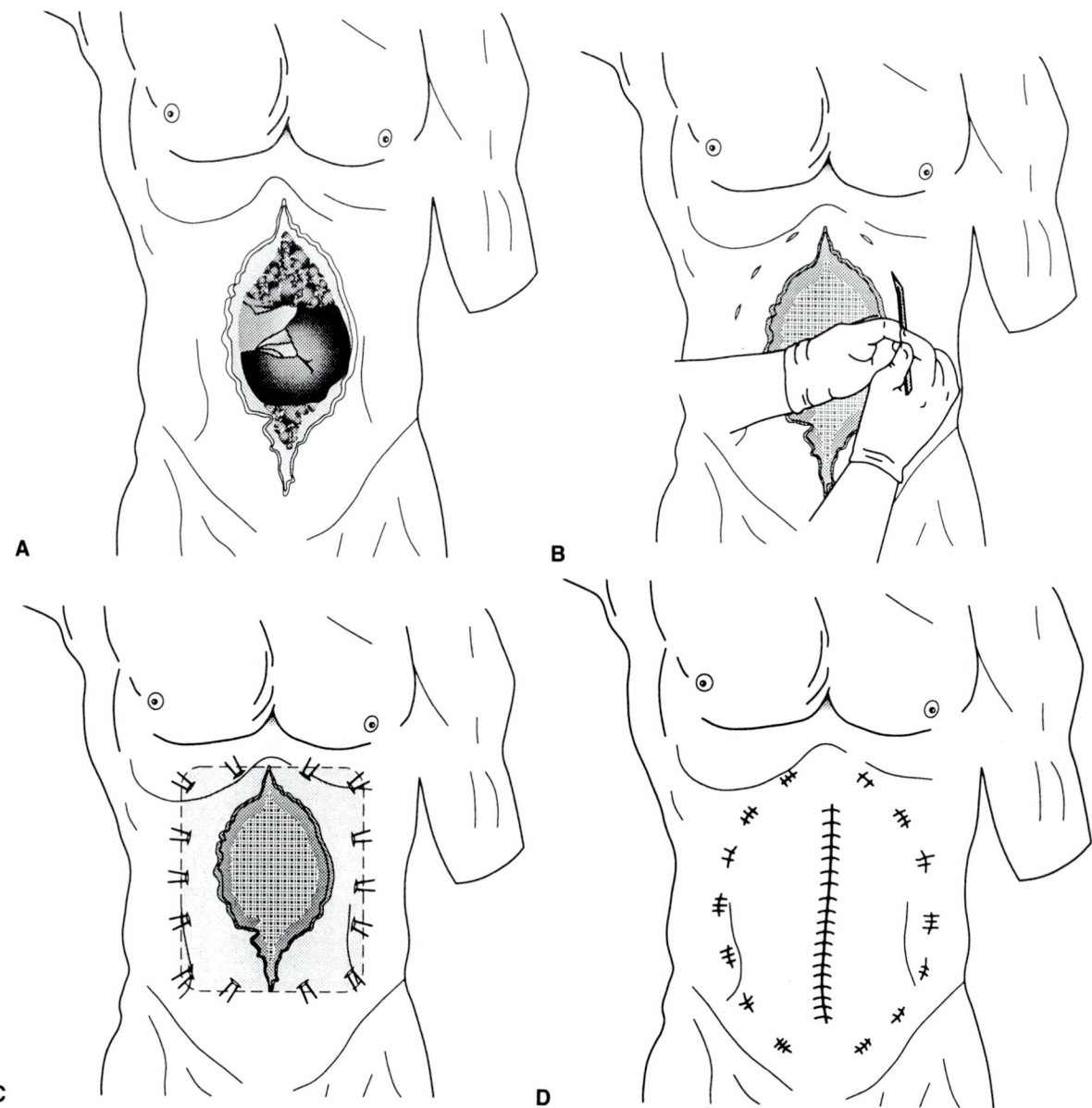

Figure 20-9. (*A*) Large ventral incisional hernia. (*B*) Small skin incisions widely surrounding the edge of the fascial defect for placing sutures. (*C*) Wide underlay of e-PTFE patch secured with full-thickness monofilament sutures. (*D*) Wounds closed; hernia repaired with minimal dead space.

securing the patch in place. The midline attenuated fascial tissues are trimmed if necessary and closed over the patch, as are the subcutaneous tissue and skin, leaving essentially no dead space beneath the wound (Fig. 20-9). No drains are necessary, and there have been no wound complications in the three patients so far treated in this way. One might reasonably consider the 1-mm-thick e-PTFE patch to be more than adequate for this repair, so that the use of the thicker 2-mm patch, as reported here, may not be necessary.

Since its first clinical use in 1983, the Gore-Tex STP has been found to be an effective biomaterial for a wide array of clinical problems requiring prosthetic buttressing, bridging, or augmentation of the human body. Its unique properties distinguish it from all previous mesh prostheses, which are macroscopically composed of a coarse weave or knit that is freely permeable to air and liquid. In contrast, the soft, smooth surface of e-PTFE patch is nonabrasive, elicits minimal foreign-body response, and is able to support a layer, on the peritoneal surface of the patch, of neo-mesothelial cells, which results in a low incidence of postoperative visceral adhesion formation and a reduction in long-term bowel complications. The role of this biomaterial in modern surgical practice is still evolving, and long-term follow-up data have yet to become available.

REFERENCES

1. Antonini R, Biandrate F, Piccolini M, Pesenti A, Francia L. Nostra esperienza sull'utilizzo di un materiale protesico (P.T.F.E.) nel trattamento di laparoceli voluminosi ed iterativi. Acta Chir Mediterranea 1988;4:537.
2. Bauer JJ, Salky BA, Gelernt IM, Kreel I. Repair of large abdominal wall defects with expanded polytetrafluoroethylene (PTFE). Ann Surg 1987;206:765.
3. Brown G. Comparison of prosthetic materials for abdominal wall reconstruction in the presence of contamination and infection. Ann Surg 1985;201:705.
4. Colombo PL, Roveda S, Belisomo M, Bianchi C, Pulviventi A, and Tinozzi S. Considerzioni sui grandi laparoceli abdominal, l'utilizzo di protesi. Minerva Chir 1992;47:161.
5. DeBord JR. Prosthetics in hernia surgery: the evolution of the ideal biomaterial. In: Bendavid R, ed. Prostheses in abdominal wall surgery. Austin, RG Landes (in press).
6. DeBord JR, Wyffels PL, Marshall JS, Miller G, Marshal WH. Repair of large ventral incisional hernias with expanded polytetrafluoroethylene prosthetic patches. Postgrad Gen Surg 1992;4:156.
7. Deysine M. Hernia repair with expanded polytetrafluoroethylene. Am J Surg 1992;163:422.
8. Hamer-Hodges DW, Scott NB. Replacement of an abdominal wall defect using expanded PTFE sheet (Gore-Tex). J R Coll Surg Edinb 1985;30:65.
9. Kaufman Z, Engelberg M, Zager M. Fecal fistula: a late complication of Marlex mesh repair. Dis Colon Rectum 1981;24:543.
10. Law NW, Ellis H. Adhesion formation and peritoneal healing on prosthetic materials. Clinical Materials 1988;3:95.
11. Law NW, Ellis H. A comparison of polypropylene mesh and expanded PTFE patch for the repair of contaminated abdominal wall defects—an experimental study. Surgery 1991;109:652.
12. LeBlanc KA, Booth WV. Laparoscopic repair of incisional abdominal hernias using expanded polytetrafluoroethylene: preliminary findings. Surg Laparosc Endosc 1993;3:39.
13. McClurken ME, McHaney JM, Colone WM. Physical properties and test methods for expanded polytetrafluoroethylene (PTFE) grafts. In: Kambic HE, Kantrowitz A, Sung P, eds. Vascular graft update: safety and performance, ASTM, STP 898. Philadelphia, American Society for Testing and Materials, 1986.
14. Murphey JL, Freeman JB, Dionne PG. Comparison of Marlex and Gore-Tex to repair abdominal wall defects in the rat. Can J Surg 1989;32:244.
15. Pailler JL, Essoussi H, de Calan L. Eventrations post opératoires: les prothèses. Moniteur Hospitalier. No. 27. Juillet-Août, 1990.
16. Phelps AM. A new operation for hernia. New York Med J 1894;60:291.
17. Reisfeld D, Schechner R, Wetzel W. Traumatic lumbar hernia. Surg Rounds 1989;12:69.
18. Schneider R, Herrington JL Jr, Granada AM. Marlex mesh in repair of a diaphragmatic defect later eroding into the distal esophagus and stomach. Am Surg 1979;45:337.
19. Smith RS. The use of prosthetic materials in the repair of hernias. Surg Clin North Am 1971;51:1387.
20. Stoppa RE. The treatment of complicated groin and incisional hernias. World J Surg 1989;13:545.
21. Usher FC. Hernia repair with knitted polypropylene mesh. Surg Gynecol Obstet 1963;117:239.
22. Usher FD. Hernia repair with Marlex mesh. In: Nyhus LM, Condon RE, eds. Hernia, ed 2. Philadelphia, JB Lippincott, 1979:561–571.
23. Van der Lei B, Bleichrodt RP, Simmer-Macher RKJ, Van Schilfgaarde R. Expanded polytetrafluoroethylene patch for the repair of large abdominal wall defects. Br J Surg 1989;76:803.
24. Voyles CR, Richardson JD, Bland KI. Emergency abdominal wall reconstruction with polypropylene mesh: short-term benefits versus long-term complications. Ann Surg 1981;194:219.
25. WL Gore and Assoc, Inc, Patch Project, Work Plan #215.
26. Wool NL, Strauss AK, Roseman DL. Clinical experience with the Gore-Tex Soft Tissue Patch in hernia repair: a preliminary report. Proc Inst Med Chicago 1985;38:33.

Hernia, Fourth Edition, edited
by Lloyd M. Nyhus and Robert E. Condon.
J.B. Lippincott Company, Philadelphia © 1995.

Chapter 21

Peristomal Hernia
Robert E. Condon

A hernia occurring adjacent to or surrounding a colostomy or ileostomy is distressing to the patient because it makes fitting of a stoma appliance unreliable. A peristomal hernia is equally distressing to the surgeon charged with its repair because the presence of the stoma in the operative field presents a potential for infection. Because the sac usually contains omentum and small intestine, and because it exerts sufficient pressure on the stoma, hernias associated with stomas also may functionally obstruct the bowel traversing the abdominal wall.

Factors that lead to the formation of a hernia around an intestinal stoma are placement of the stoma outside the sheath of the rectus abdominis muscle, poor tone of the abdominal wall musculature related to a sedentary way of life, long-term use of steroids, denervation of the abdominal wall musculature during placement of the original stoma, infection occurring around the stoma any time after an earlier operation, and obesity and other factors that increase abdominal strain.

Before operation, the hernia should be examined by palpation through the peristomal skin as well as through the stoma. Such a maneuver usually reveals the extent of the defect. It is important to determine whether the hernia is present only eccentrically on one margin of the stoma or more or less surrounds the entire stoma.

MOVING THE STOMA

The simplest way to correct a peristomal hernia is to move the stoma to a new site on the abdominal wall and then to close completely the wound through which the old stoma and the hernia exited. If possible, a new stoma should be brought through the midportion of the rectus abdominis muscle and its sheath, because this provides the most secure site of bowel egress to protect against the possibility of recurrent herniation.

PRIMARY STOMAL HERNIA REPAIR

If the stoma cannot be moved, primary repair in situ is appropriate in those cases in which the hernia orifice is relatively small and elliptic, and involves no more than one third of the circumference of the stoma. The incision is placed 6 cm from the margin of the stoma, to avoid scar in the skin to which the stoma appliance needs to be attached, and is made over the apex of the hernia bulge. Dissection is carried down through the subcutaneous tissues to expose the hernia sac, and the exact extent of herniation is determined by palpation and dissection, as necessary. If the hernia proves to be larger than was appreciated preoperatively, such that prosthetic stomal hernia repair (see later) is appropriate, the stoma should be mobilized completely to permit its extraction back into the peritoneal cavity and the hernia should be approached by reopening the old abdominal incision.

If in situ primary repair appears to be appropriate, the sac should be freed from the musculofascial layers of the abdominal wall and opened, the intestine reduced, redundant peritoneum mobilized from the deep surface of the musculoaponeurotic layers, excess sac excised, and the peritoneum closed. The stoma is not mobilized from those tissues to which it remains firmly attached. Only that aspect of the stoma that is on the margin of the hernia is dissected. The fascial opening then should be closed in a single layer with interrupted nonabsorbable sutures. Typically, the old stoma is at the medial end of the closure. The fascial closure should be made so that the new aperture is no larger than 2 cm as judged with a finger in the lumen of the bowel (slightly larger than the average second digit at the proximal interphalangeal joint). The edge of the loop of bowel exiting through the reconstructed stoma should be fastened to the peritoneum and to the fascia with interrupted absorbable sutures.

A closed-suction drain is placed in the subcutaneous hernia cavity and brought out through a stab wound well remote from both the stoma and the operative wound. In selecting the site of the stab wound, it is important to be able to fit a collecting device to the stoma with which the dressings of the main operative wound or the drainage stab wound will not interfere. The main operative wound is closed with running monofilament nylon suture to the skin. A plastic sheet with adhesive along one margin is used to isolate the operative wound from the stoma. The wounds are dressed and then covered loosely with the plastic (towel drape No. 1010, 3M Manufacturing Company). Last, the stoma is fitted with a temporary collecting device.

IN SITU PROSTHETIC STOMAL HERNIA REPAIR

Preoperative preparation of the intestine should be undertaken with oral neomycin-erythromycin in patients who have a stomal hernia around a colostomy or distal ileostomy. The stoma initially is freed by incising the skin–mucosa margin without appreciable enlargement of the stoma aperture in the skin (Fig. 21-1). Dissection into the subcutaneous tissue frees the stoma so that it may be closed by suture, or by the application of a Stone clamp, before the abdomen is

opened. The abdominal cavity is opened, usually through the old incision but occasionally through a new incision made at a distance from the existing stoma. Adhesions of omentum and intestine are taken down and the intestine in the peristomal hernia is freed. Next, the fascial attachments of the stoma are cut, and the stoma is mobilized further from the musculoaponeurotic layers of the abdominal wall and withdrawn into the abdomen.

The peritoneum is mobilized in the extraperitoneal plane, beginning from the main wound margin nearest the hernia and continuing to encompass the peritoneal hernia sac and the former site of the exit of the intestine through the body wall. Redundant peritoneum is excised and the old peritoneal stoma site usually is sutured closed with running absorbable suture.

The intestine leading to the stoma now is mobilized further to provide sufficient additional length (typically 3 to 5 cm) to permit eventual amputation of the end of the old stoma. The skin and subcutaneous tissue are dissected in the plane immediately above the fascia from the margin of the main wound to and around the site of the former stoma, exposing 6 to 8

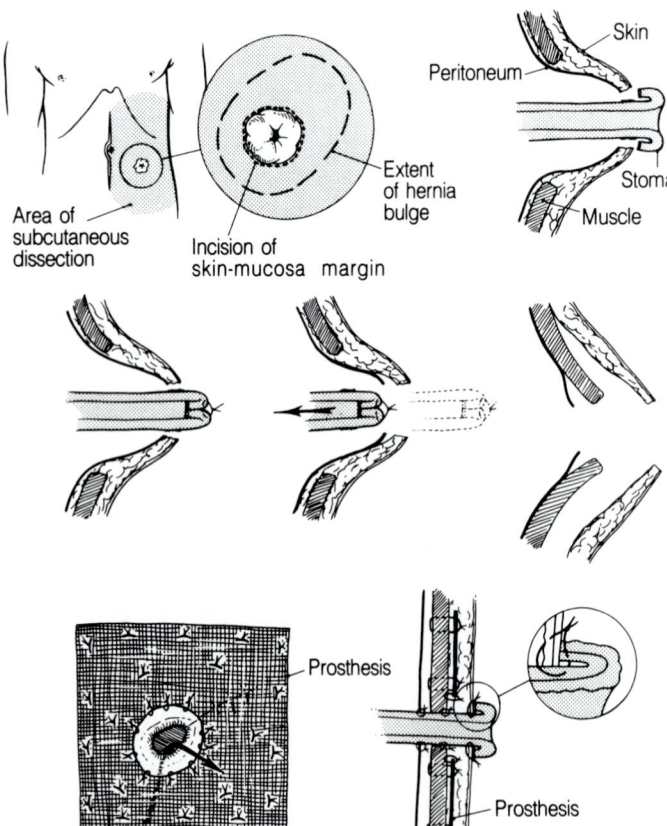

Figure 21-1. Peristomal hernia repair with prosthetic reinforcement. (*A*) The bowel segment forming the stoma is mobilized and closed. The peritoneal cavity is reopened. A wide area around the stoma and hernia is dissected in the subcutaneous plane. (*B* through *E*) The bowel segment traversing the abdominal wall is mobilized, closed, and withdrawn into the peritoneal cavity. The peritoneal sac is reduced and excised. (*F*) The old hernia site in the abdominal wall is partially closed by suture to fashion a new stoma orifice. An onlay prosthesis is sutured in place to reinforce the repair. (*G*) The bowel is drawn through the reconstructed aperture and matured.

cm of fascia around the old stoma site. The fascial margins of the old stoma site and the hernia aperture are cleaned of scar and tags of connective tissue, preserving a firm and healthy fascial margin.

The margins of the hernial aperture are sutured together with interrupted 3-0 or 2-0 braided nylon sutures to create a new aperture in the muscular abdominal wall that is no greater than 2 cm in diameter. A polypropylene mesh prosthesis is cut with a 2.5- to 3-cm aperture in its center. This prosthesis is fixed in place as an onlay on the external aspect of the musculofascial layers of the abdominal wall with interrupted, full-thickness, extraperitoneal mattress sutures of 0 or 2-0 braided nylon. Each of these mattress sutures encompasses a 1-cm, full-thickness bite of the prosthesis and of the muscles and fascia of the abdominal wall. Sutures are placed in a row, about 1 cm apart and 1 cm from the free margin of the new stoma. Additional sutures are scattered in the prosthesis between the stomal aperture and the outer margin of the prosthesis. Finally, a row of sutures is placed 1 cm from the free margin of the prosthesis all around its periphery.

A new aperture is made in the peritoneum, and the intestine and old stoma are drawn successively through the new peritoneal aperture, the reconstructed orifice in the musculoaponeurotic abdominal wall, the prosthesis reinforcement, and the old skin aperture. The exiting loop of bowel is sutured internally to the peritoneum with absorbable suture. The fascia is sutured to the intestine as it exits through the repaired stoma. These sutures encompass only a partial thickness of the intestinal wall and do not engage the prosthesis. It is important that a small rim of tissue be interposed between the margin of the prosthesis and the exiting loop of bowel to prevent the hard edge of the prosthesis from cutting into the bowel.

A closed-suction drain is placed in the cavity between the subcutaneous fat and the muscular abdominal wall, and is brought out through a stab wound. The stab wound exit site for the suction drain should be selected so that it will not interfere with postoperative placement of a stoma collection device. The remainder of the wound closure follows the steps used in the closure of a primary repair. The stoma site is isolated from the main abdominal wound with an adhesive plastic sheet (towel drape No. 1010, 3M Manufacturing Company). The main operative wound is closed using running 0-loop nylon to the fascia and running 3-0 monofilament nylon for the skin. Dressings to the main wound are applied and covered lightly with the plastic sheet.

Last, the closed end of the bowel loop exiting through the new stoma site is amputated, and the stoma is primarily matured to the skin using Dexon suture. A temporary collecting device is fitted to the stoma.

REFERENCES

1. Sjodahl R, Anderberg B, Bolin T. Parastomal hernia in relation to site of the abdominal stoma. Br J Surg 1988;75:339.
2. Sugarbaker PH. Peritoneal approach to prosthetic mesh repair of paraostomy hernias. Ann Surg 1985; 201:344.
3. Williams JG, Etherington R, Hayward MW, Hughes LE. Paraileostomy hernia: a clinical and radiological study. Br J Surg 1990;77:1355.

Hernia, Fourth Edition, edited
by Lloyd M. Nyhus and Robert E. Condon.
J.B. Lippincott Company, Philadelphia © 1995.

Chapter 22

Omphalocele

Timothy G. Canty

The term *omphalocele* refers to herniation of the abdominal viscera into the tissues of the umbilical cord. The hernia sac, therefore, has an internal lining of peritoneum and an external covering of thinned amnion that makes up the covering of the umbilical vessels within the cord. The resulting abdominal wall defect varies considerably in size from no larger than a normal umbilical stump to a defect that appears to involve the entire ventral abdominal wall (Figs. 22-1 and 22-2). Although most omphaloceles involve herniation of the abdominal viscera, more extensive forms may involve complex malformations of the pelvic viscera with exstrophy of the bladder (cloacal exstrophy, vesicointestinal fissure) or the thoracic viscera, as well as a sternal cleft and ectopia cordis.[3] Cryptorchidism and brain malformations are known to join omphalocele in a triad. A careful evaluation of the central nervous system should be performed whenever a child with omphalocele and cryptorchidism is examined.[16] This discussion is limited to defects that involve the abdominal viscera exclusively. Other anomalies and complex chromosomal defects also may be present.

EMBRYOLOGY AND PATHOGENESIS

Although controversy continues regarding whether omphalocele, ruptured omphalocele, and gastroschisis are varying expressions of the same embryologic defect, many pediatric surgeons consider omphalocele and gastroschisis to be distinctly different clinical entities. This opinion is supported by the clear epidemiologic differences between the two conditions.

In the early weeks of gestation, the embryo consists of a dorsal plate containing all three primitive germ layers sitting atop the nourishing yolk sac in communication with the developing midgut. As development continues, a complex series of events involving ventral migration of the caudal, cephalic, and lateral folds results in the formation of the embryologic coelom. The communication with the yolk sac becomes smaller and smaller (omphalomesenteric

duct) until it closes completely. The apices of the folds come together at the umbilical ring, which continues to contract, leaving the umbilical cord as a vascular communication with the placenta. This last series of events takes place rapidly during the 5th to 10th weeks of embryologic life. As the abdominal viscera develop, the midgut elongates more rapidly than does the embryologic coelom, and the viscera lie outside the confines of the coelom in the umbilical stump. As the coelom then enlarges, not only do the viscera return to it, but the gastrointestinal tract undergoes an intricate process of rotation and fixation to the dorsal parietes, resulting in the normal antenatal configuration. These events are completed by the 10th to 12th gestational week.

In omphalocele, there is a delay in the formation of the coelom caused by failure of the fold to advance normally, the viscera do not return to the intraembryonic coelom, or both these events occur.[8,13,17] The stage at which delay or developmental arrest occurs may relate to the size of the defect. It is thought by some that early rupture of a small herniation of the umbilical cord with resultant healing of the medial skin surrounding the insertion of the cord is responsible for the condition that is commonly termed gastroschisis.[27] In almost all these defects, the intestine is not fixed properly to the posterior parietes and has not undergone the usual normal rotational sequence.

INCIDENCE

The incidence of abdominal wall defects, including small and large omphaloceles, intact or ruptured, and gastroschisis, probably is between 1:3000 and 1:6000 live births.[19,24] It is difficult to determine the relative incidence of the individual defects because of the continued controversy regarding classification. Early series did not recognize gastroschisis as a separate entity, but as an antenatal ruptured omphalocele.[15] More recent reports have attempted to differentiate the two conditions, and in these, gastroschisis is by far more common.[4,11,18,20] The differentiation probably has little practical importance because the principles

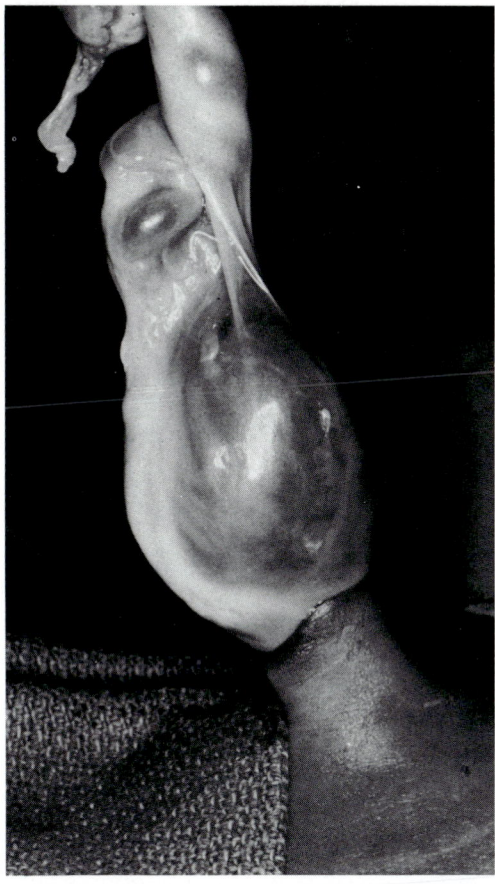

Figure 22-1. Small intact omphalocele (hernia into the umbilical cord) was repaired with one-stage primary closure of the abdominal wall defect.

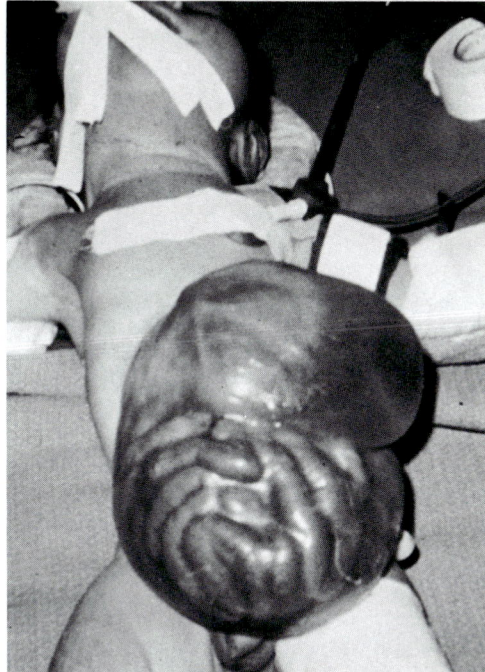

Figure 22-2. Giant omphalocele that contained the entire liver, spleen, gonads, and gastrointestinal tract. The abdominal wall defect extends from flank to flank and from xiphoid to pubis. With the staged method, using silicone rubber sheets that were sewn to the skin flaps, after 4 weeks it finally was possible to make a ventral hernia covered with the patient's own skin.

of treatment are similar, although the outcome in each group may vary.

ASSOCIATED ANOMALIES

One of the more convincing arguments for the separate classification of omphalocele and gastroschisis is the wide discrepancy in epidemiologic observations. Gastroschisis tends to occur as an isolated defect with a higher preponderance in small and premature babies. In contrast, omphalocele is more common in full-term babies, but is associated with other serious anomalies or as part of recognized syndromes (Beckwith-Wiedemann syndrome), chromosomal aberrations (trisomy D and E), and the previously mentioned vesicointestinal fissure and pentalogy of Cantrell.[3] In other newborns, the abdominal wall defect may be associated with additional gastrointestinal tract abnormalities (Meckel diverticulum, intestinal atresia, anorectal malformations), congenital heart lesions (tetralogy of Fallot, atrial or ventricular septal defects, hypoplastic left heart syndrome),[22,24] and diaphragmatic hernia.[31] Much of the morbidity and mortality of omphalocele is related to the severity of these defects rather than to the abdominal wall defect itself.

CLINICAL FEATURES IN UTERO

Recent experience with maternal sonography for study of the pregnant uterus has led to relatively precise antenatal imaging of abnormal and normal fetal anatomy from 15 to 16 weeks' gestation to term.[5,6]

Fetal abdominal wall defects usually are not subtle and have been visualized as early as 15 weeks' gestation. On ultrasound examination, an omphalocele appears as fluid-filled loops of intestine anterior to the normal fetal abdominal wall well contained in the smooth, contoured sac. The liver also is seen easily, with its distinct dense sonographic appearance often traceable from the external sac into the abdominal cavity. Other anomalies that may complicate postnatal care, such as diaphragmatic hernia and hydronephrosis, may be noted as well. In contrast, gastroschisis appears as fluid-filled loops of bowel anterior to the abdominal wall that are not contained in a sac and usually are not accompanied by the liver.[5,6] In patients whose sonographic findings are equivocal, measurement of amniotic fluid α-fetoprotein and acetylcholinesterase levels may be helpful. Normal levels may be more consistent with the diagnosis of omphalocele.[32] Glick and coworkers[12] described the visualization of an intact omphalocele sac at 27 weeks' gestation, only to detect its rupture 7 weeks later. At birth, the infant had the obvious clinical appearance of gastroschisis. This type of sonographic data may supply the "missing link" in the long-standing controversy regarding similar or different causes for these two conditions.

CLINICAL FEATURES AT BIRTH

The appearance of an intact omphalocele at birth varies considerably, depending on the size of the abdominal wall defect and the size of the sac, which are not necessarily related. Schuster[24] has subdivided omphaloceles into those with a fascial defect less than or greater than 4 cm. The former are termed *herniation of the umbilical cord.* It is believed that this represents a later embryologic defect of failure of closure of the umbilical ring rather than failure of migration of the folds related to the larger defects. In smaller defects, a single loop of intestine may not be obvious, and ligation of what was thought to be a normal umbilical cord will result in transection of the intestine, leaving the embarrassing problem of an umbilical-enteric fistula.[9]

In most defects, both large and small, the umbilical cord is at the apex of a thinned, avascular, two-layer translucent sac. The umbilical vessels run between the layers of the sac to the abdominal wall. The surrounding skin may advance upward on the sac for a short distance. The sac usually is moist and shiny at birth, but if it is left exposed for any length of time, it becomes opaque, dry, and brittle, and may rupture with handling. In large defects, the liver, spleen, stomach, pancreas, colon, or bladder also may be seen through the membrane. The intestine lies freely mobile within the intact sac without evidence of adhesions or inflammation. In contrast, the liver has dense adhesions to the sac, a fact that must be considered carefully during surgical repair.

Babies with an isolated omphalocele defect usually are robust full-term infants. Early or immediate clinical deterioration suggests one of the important life-threatening associated anomalies, most com-

monly congenital heart disease, or another lethal syndrome. Because of the significant potential for heat and water loss from the eviscerated intestine, these babies quickly can become cold, dehydrated, and acidotic.

Antenatal ruptured omphalocele may present with a large abdominal defect, bits and remnants of the ruptured sac attached to the intestine, and varying degrees of thickening of the visceral coverings similar to gastroschisis. In those in whom rupture has occurred late (ie, during or soon after delivery), the intestine appears normal. In these cases, expedient stabilization, transport, and repair is critical.

THERAPY

Prenatal Therapy

With the discovery of a serious congenital anomaly before birth, especially early in gestation, several potential management decisions arise. When an omphalocele is discovered as an almost incidental defect in a more complex syndrome or chromosomal anomaly that is incompatible with extrauterine life, the issue of termination of pregnancy arises. In the isolated finding of an omphalocele, the potential for benefiting the overall care of the pregnant mother, and eventually the child, is obvious. I strongly believe that this abnormality, as well as most other surgically correctable anomalies discovered before birth, are handled best by expeditious treatment after normal vaginal delivery. Advanced knowledge of the defect, however, can allow for appropriate planning to meet both the mother's and the child's needs at the time of birth.

One of the most important contributors to the morbidity and mortality of isolated abdominal wall defects is the delay between delivery and appropriate repair that is occasioned by transportation to a suitable tertiary care institution. Antenatal knowledge of the existence of an omphalocele can allow for birth of the child at or near the institution where the infant will be cared for, with the appropriate neonatal and pediatric surgical personnel standing by.[6,21] The best vehicle for neonatal transport is not an incubator and ambulance, but a pregnant mother.

The issue of elective or nonelective cesarean section in antenatally discovered omphaloceles is not resolved. In giant omphaloceles in which dystocia or rupture may occur at the time of vaginal delivery, cesarean delivery may be advantageous. The superiority of the routine use of cesarean section in smaller defects, with the attendant increased risks to mother and child, has not been proven.[5,21,29] In my experience, obstetricians often make this decision in favor of cesarean section without consulting the surgeons who will care for the infant. This method of management needs further careful scrutiny.

Therapy At Birth

Preoperative management is directed at keeping the baby warm and hydrated, and bringing him or her to the operating room in stable condition as rapidly as possible. Gentleness and care must be used in handling the sac to avoid rupture or twisting of the sac in relation to the abdominal torso. The sac or extruded viscera are wrapped in moist, sterile gauze and covered with impervious plastic sheeting. Aluminum foil also is suitable for this purpose. Placing the lower torso of the infant in a plastic "bowel bag" also serves well to prevent heat and water loss. These babies often excrete both urine and stool while awaiting operation, however, further contaminating the bag and its contents.

A brief, thorough physical examination and chest and abdominal roentgenograms are carried out to detect other associated anomalies. If indicated, cardiac echography also can be performed. A peripheral intravenous line for hydration is placed at the time of blood sampling, and broad-spectrum antibiotics and vitamin K are administered. The gastrointestinal tract is decompressed with nasogastric suction.

Definitive Treatment

Several alternatives for the treatment of omphalocele have been described over the past 35 years, and each has enthusiastic supporters. The wide variation of opinion reflects not only changes in surgical techniques, but also parallel developments in anesthesia, general neonatal care, fluid management, and, especially, nutritional therapy and methods of mechanical ventilation. It was only a decade and a half ago that a newborn infant who could not breathe or eat spontaneously would die. Many of the methods that were described early, therefore, were limited by the ability to care for the infant postoperatively. A discussion of any method must take into consideration the time at which it was proposed.

Before the use of mechanical ventilation, initial attempts at primary closure of all but the smallest omphaloceles were almost universally fatal because of sepsis, ventilatory compromise, or vena caval compression caused by increased abdominal pressure.[15] Thus emerged a variety of skin flap or skin escharification techniques followed by later closure of

the resultant ventral hernia.[14,15,30] This reduced the initial mortality of these large or ruptured defects from virtually 100% to about 50%. Unfortunately, the anticipated increase in size of the abdominal cavity over time often did not occur, and the ventral hernia sac itself merely grew. Secondary ventral hernia closure later was hampered by the same problems encountered in newborn infants in addition to often tenacious adhesions between the skin and the underlying viscera. Alternatives to this form of treatment remained nonexistent for almost 20 years.

Schuster[23] proposed using a prosthetic ventral hernia sac that could be reduced gradually in size, forcing the abdominal cavity to enlarge to allow the return of the herniated viscera. This technique initially was applied to children undergoing secondary ventral hernia closure, and later was used in newborn infants.[1] This further reduced the initial mortality of the large defects to less than 50%. Moreover, it was learned that the abdominal cavity, when encouraged, would enlarge rapidly such that the prosthetic material usually could be removed in 3 to 7 days. This greatly reduced the complications of sepsis, sac dehiscence, prolonged ileus, and the need for multiple operative procedures. Many surgeons today believe that this is the optimal method of therapy for all but the smallest of omphaloceles, with a reduction in mortality to less than 25%.[11,26]

Stimulated by the observations with the Schuster technique and the parallel advent of safe maximal muscle paralysis and mechanical ventilation, other observers began to advocate the initiation of abdominal enlargement in the operating room by vigorous abdominal wall stretching and reduction of the volume of the abdominal contents by gentle evacuation of the gastrointestinal tract proximally and distally. Coupled with paralysis and ventilation after surgery, this allowed for primary closure of most omphaloceles with relative ease. The initially tense abdomen softened readily over the ensuing 1 to 3 days and the child could be weaned from the ventilator and extubated. This technique virtually eliminated the problems of sepsis around a foreign body, sac dehiscence, and the need for multiple operative procedures. It further decreased the hospital stay and the prolonged ileus that prevented early initiation of oral feeding.[4,10,25]

I favor enlarging the abdomen and reducing its contents in most cases. There still are infants who have such enormous visceroabdominal disproportion that they require the use of the prosthetic silo with staged reduction, and others who have serious associated anomalies, prematurity, or instability and require skin flap closure or escharification. Each of these techniques is described briefly, and my primary closure technique is described in detail.

Nonoperative Therapy

Nonoperative therapy is appropriate for premature infants with a gigantic intact sac or those in whom associated anomalies make survival of a major operation unlikely.

The intact sac is painted carefully each day with a desiccating antiseptic solution, such as merbromin (Mercurochrome), benzalkonium, or alcohol. If the painting is successful and infection is avoided, an eschar eventually forms over the sac and skin, and granulation grows in from the periphery. The remaining ventral hernia then can be repaired later by either primary closure or staged repair. This form of treatment requires prolonged hospitalization (1–3 months) for skin coverage to occur. In addition, the risks of infection or sac rupture always are present. The inability to inspect the abdomen for other anomalies also limits this form of therapy.

Skin Flap Closure

The original technique of skin flap closure involved wide mobilization of skin flaps laterally with closure over the intact omphalocele sac.[15] This does not allow for inspection of the intraabdominal viscera to detect other potentially life-threatening intestinal anomalies that may need correction. Alternatively, the sac can be trimmed away carefully and the intraabdominal contents inspected. The skin is freed from the fascial edges and undermined laterally. The umbilical vessels are ligated, or one artery is cannulated and transplanted to the lower abdomen to be used for monitoring. The skin flaps are approximated in the midline over the viscera with simple sutures (Fig. 22-3). The ventral hernia then is closed primarily or by staged procedures months or even years later when it appears that the abdominal cavity has enlarged sufficiently.[30]

Staged Closure

There are many variations of the original technique of staged closure using different prosthetic sheeting materials or preformed silo devices.[1,23,28] Initial trials of this technique proceeded slowly, and the process often took 3 to 4 weeks. The complication rate from infection or sac dehiscence was high. Using a cloth mesh that allowed for tissue ingrowth as originally suggested by Schuster[23] and others is helpful, but does not eliminate these complications. With aggressive daily sac reduction, closure usually can be accomplished with reduced morbidity and mortality within 3 to 5 days. In these instances, the prosthesis is not present long enough for tissue ingrowth to occur, and it matters little what prosthetic material is used, including one of the spring-loaded, preformed devices that may be inserted without suturing.[28]

The infant is brought to the operating room and the entire abdomen is prepared and draped. The sac is trimmed carefully from the skin edge, and the skin is separated further from the fascial edge all the way around. The prosthetic material then is sewn with interrupted nonabsorbable sutures circumferentially to the full thickness of the musculofascial abdominal wall. If two sheets of material are used, they are joined to each other in the midline, forming a ventral pocket. If a single sheet is used, a cylinder (silo) results when the two edges of the prosthetic material are sutured together along one side. The top of the silo can be closed with further sutures or simply gathered and tied with a piece of umbilical tape. The entire prosthetic pouch is wrapped with gauze soaked in antiseptic and then with a dry gauze dressing to support the pouch without kinking or tension. Further support is provided by attaching an umbilical tape to the apex of the sac and suspending this above the abdomen.

At daily intervals, without anesthesia and usually in the nursery, the pouch is unwrapped under absolutely aseptic conditions and inspected for signs of sepsis or dehiscence. The viscera are pushed gently into the abdomen while the infant is observed for signs of increased abdominal pressure. The sac is tied or sutured at the reduced level and covered with an antiseptic dressing as before. When the sac is flush or nearly flush with the abdominal wall without tension, the infant is returned to the operating room and placed under general anesthesia. The final bit of prosthetic material is removed and primary fascial closure with interrupted nonabsorbable sutures is performed. Standard skin closure over the fascia completes the procedure (Fig. 22-4). Infection and sac dehiscence are disastrous complications, often requiring a secondary skin flap closure or simple covering with biologic dressings until infection subsides and another attempt at closure can be made. For this reason, systemic antibiotics are used routinely during the closure period and every effort is made to remove the sac as rapidly as possible.

Amniotic inversion is a recently described variation of staged closure that warrants further study. With this technique, the prosthetic material is sutured to the intact skin–amnion junction, and progressive reduction is performed as described earlier. The final stage involves inversion of the freed intact amnionic sac into the abdomen as the fascia and skin are closed. Proponents of this technique report a lower incidence of infection and delayed adhesive obstruction as advantages.[7,34]

Primary Closure

Primary fascial closure of an omphalocele is the superior approach when feasible, achieving definitive treatment with a single operation and eliminating the

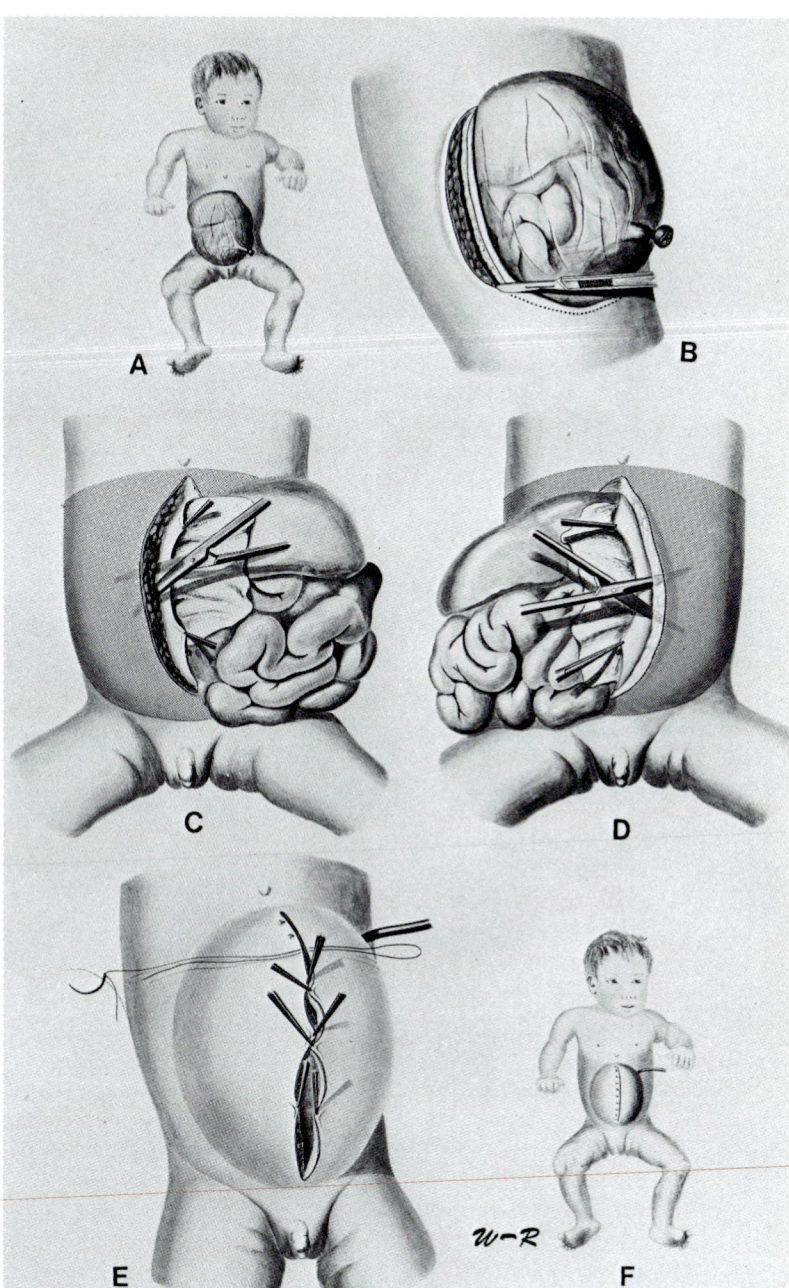

Figure 22-3. Operative technique for skin closure over the omphalocele (A). The cuff of skin at the base of the sac is incised circumferentially (B). The umbilical vein and arteries are ligated, and the sac with the attached small rim of skin is removed. After a thorough abdominal exploration, the skin and subcutaneous tissues are cut free on both sides and sufficiently undermined into each flank and over the lower abdomen, but not above the level of the xiphoid (C and D). Then the cutaneous flaps are approximated without tension over the exposed viscera (E) to create a ventral hernia covered with skin (F).

problems of infection and sac separation. Current technique can be applied safely to most omphaloceles with favorable results.

The infant, in stable condition, is brought to the operating room in a warm, sterile environment with the intestines or intact sac covered with warm dressings and plastic sheeting. Once anesthesia has been induced and stabilized, including maximal paralysis with muscle relaxants, the dressings are removed and the skin is prepared quickly around the body from neck to toes with warm povidone-iodine solution. The infant then is placed on a sterile sheet and draped.

The sac is cut away from the skin edge and the skin is dissected from the underlying fascia. One umbilical artery is cannulated and transplanted to the appropriate lower quadrant of the abdomen through a small stab wound, and the other two vessels are ligated. The upper margin of the sac frequently is ad-

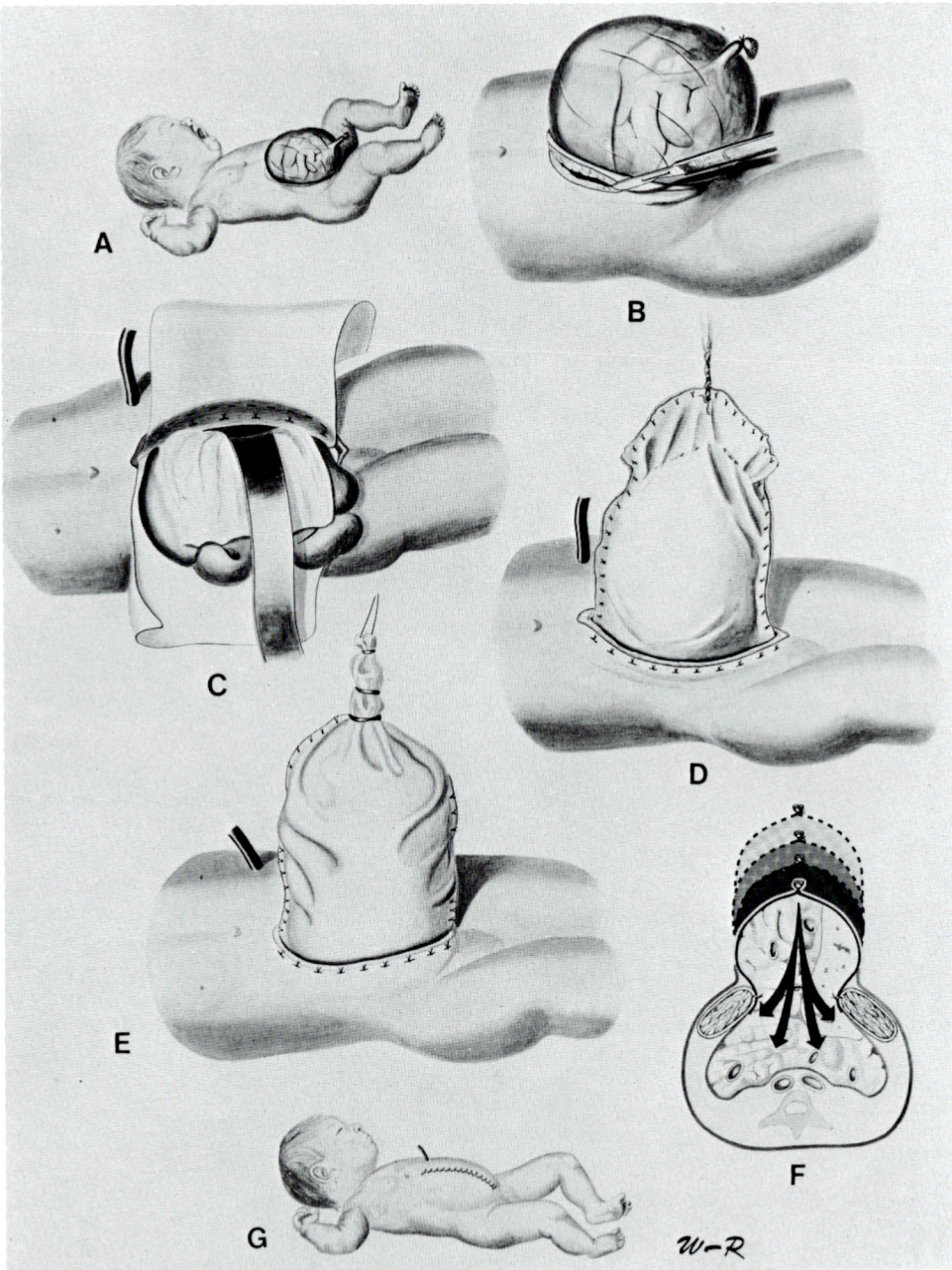

Figure 22-4. Method for the staged primary repair of a large omphalocele (*A*). A circumferential incision is made around the base of the omphalocele sac (*B*), the umbilical vein and arteries are ligated, and the sac with a small rim of the adjacent skin is removed. After abdominal exploration and performance of gastrostomy, two silicone rubber sheets are sewn to the full thickness of the abdominal wall around the margins of the defect (*C*). The sheets are approximated over the viscera as the excess sheeting is removed (*D*). Postoperatively, the size of the prosthesis is reduced progressively at intervals of 1 to 3 days. This is done by squeezing off and tying the sac (*E*) to reduce its size and to increase the size of the true intraabdominal space (*F*). At the final stage, all remaining excess sheeting is removed and the abdominal wall is closed anatomically (*G*) without producing excessive intraabdominal pressure.

herent to the liver and is dissected carefully from the liver capsule. The diaphragmatic attachments of the liver are taken down completely to allow increased mobility. The intestine and remainder of the abdomen are examined thoroughly for additional anomalies. Because most of these infants exhibit various degrees of nonrotation of the intestine, the area of the duodenum is inspected carefully for obstructive bands and kinks that may require correction. The intestine then is evacuated totally of fluid and meconium both proximally, with a nasogastric tube, and distally, through the anus. The abdominal wall is stretched gradually and repeatedly by hand in quadrants. With gentleness and perseverance, the abdominal cavity usually can be more than doubled in volume. This maneuver, as well as replacing the viscera into the abdominal cavity, is simplified greatly by the absence of a gastrostomy tube. The viscera are replaced into the abdomen, usually with moderate tension.

An advantageous method of fascial closure is the use of several far-near/near-far pulley stitches of 00 nonabsorbable material. These stitches overcome excess tension without tearing, and multiple simple 000 nonabsorbable sutures are placed between them. When the pulley stitches are pulled up gradually, bringing the fascial edges together, the simple sutures are tied, followed by the pulley stitches. This maneuver greatly simplifies what often seems to be an impossible task of approximating the fascial edges. Whether vertical or horizontal closure is used depends largely on the surgeon's determination of the best fit under the least tension. Most often, fascial closure is vertical, especially in larger defects, although there are occasions when transverse closure is obtained more easily. After the fascia is closed, the abdomen is tense and hard, and the infant's hemodynamic status should be assessed for evidence of vena cava compression. Intragastric or other methods of intraabdominal pressure monitoring may be of value in this regard.[33]

The method of skin closure has evolved gradually in an attempt to provide a satisfactory facsimile of a normal umbilicus, a minor and frequently overlooked cosmetic aspect. At the completion of the fascial closure, there commonly is excess skin with ragged edges. Nonviable skin is trimmed from the edge and a nylon suture is run in and out through the edge circumferentially in a true pursestring manner such that, when it is drawn taut, it brings the skin together in the position of the normal umbilicus. A small rubber-band drain is left in the center of the pursestring for 1 to 2 days. Initially, this closure looks puckered and irregular. The stitch is removed in about 10 days, and in 1 to 2 months, this closure looks much like a normal umbilicus as the puckers and wrinkles resolve[4] (Fig. 22-5).

Postoperative Care

The infant is returned to the intensive care nursery and maintained in a warm, clean environment with appropriate supplemental oxygen as necessary. Monitoring of intravenous fluid requirements includes the use of arterial blood gas determinations, urine output, blood pressure measurements, and clinical determinations of overall perfusion. Nasogastric decompression is maintained with an indwelling suction catheter, and broad-spectrum antibiotics are administered for at least the first 7 days or until the prosthetic material is removed. Intravenous alimentation usually

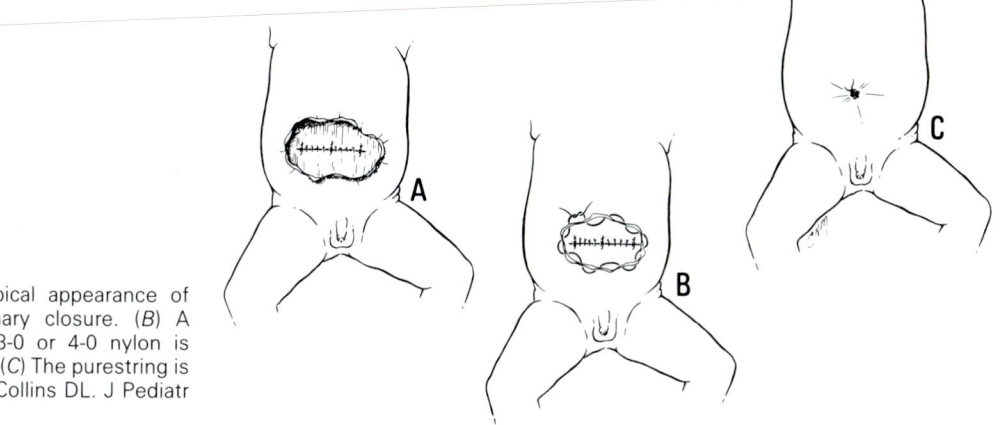

Figure 22-5. (A) Typical appearance of skin defect after primary closure. (B) A pursestring suture of 3-0 or 4-0 nylon is placed in the skin edge. (C) The purestring is pulled taut. (Canty TG, Collins DL. J Pediatr Surg 1983;18:707)

is begun on the second postoperative day and continued until gastrointestinal function returns, the nasogastric tube is removed, and oral feeding is initiated. The infant is discharged from the hospital once adequate nutrition and weight gain can be maintained by oral feeding alone.

Infants who are treated by primary fascial closure require specialized postoperative care. All these babies are kept paralyzed with nondepolarizing neuromuscular blocking agents for varying periods after surgery. To eliminate problems with incipient respiratory failure in a nonventilated patient, no attempt is made to base the decision for initial paralysis and ventilation on an attempt to assess the degree of abdominal tension. Over the ensuing 24 to 72 hours, the abdomen softens, paralysis is eliminated, and the patient is weaned rapidly from the ventilator and extubated. Standard blood gas measurements made through the indwelling umbilical artery catheter are used for ventilatory management. Fluid needs initially are met with simple Ringer's lactate and 5% albumin solutions given as 1.5 to 2 times maintenance for the first 12 to 24 hours after operation. Urine output often is scanty at first because of increased abdominal pressure, but increases dramatically as the abdomen softens. Edema of the lower extremities is common during the first 72 hours and resolves quickly as abdominal tension decreases. Elimination of nasogastric decompression, institution of oral feeding, and preparation for discharge are the same as in the other methods of closure.

CLINICAL RESULTS

A review of my experience at Children's Hospital of San Diego revealed 103 consecutive infants, including 76 with gastroschisis and 28 with omphalocele. Five infants with omphalocele underwent closure using staged reduction of prosthetic material. Two infants with associated large diaphragmatic hernias and pulmonary hypoplasia died shortly after repair. One infant had severe necrotizing enterocolitis and died before reduction was completed. One premature infant also died with multiple additional anomalies and pulmonary hypoplasia. One infant survived complete staged reduction and is alive and well at the age of 11 years.

Twenty-three patients with omphalocele underwent primary closure by the technique outlined earlier. There were three deaths in this group, each of which was caused by associated severe congenital anomalies, including pentalogy and heart disease, severe respiratory distress syndrome, and Beckwith-

Wiedemann syndrome. Of interest is that the omphalocele was small and easily closed in all three cases. Twenty patients were long-term survivors. In the past 15 years, all patients with omphalocele closed primarily have survived. Using the treatment scheme outlined, ventilatory assistance with paralysis was required for an average of 3 days after operation. One patient required prolonged ventilatory assistance because of congenital heart disease, which required palliative shunting in the first week of life. The average length of time before feeding was begun was 5 to 7 days. The hospital stay averaged 26 days (range, 5–87 days). There were no complications of sepsis or the use of mechanical ventilation and paralysis. One patient had gastroduodenal obstruction from hepatic compression after primary closure that required surgical correction.[2] Follow-up results to as long as 23 years have shown no other sequelae.[4]

The results of this review compare favorably with those of many others who also advocate primary fascial closure.[10,25] The most important aspects of this form of therapy are definitive treatment of the problem with one operation, a shortened hospital stay, a decreased incidence of long-term postoperative complications, and rapid return of gastrointestinal function. Although the need for mechanical ventilation and paralysis is considered by some to be a complication or negative factor, we believe it to be essential in this method of treatment.[4]

Whatever method of therapy is used for infants with omphalocele, there will continue to be improvement in the overall morbidity and mortality of this important pediatric surgical condition. These infants must be cared for in a tertiary center with a neonatal intensive care unit as well as expertise in pediatric surgery and anesthesiology. Advances in general neonatal care already have done much to reduce the morbidity and mortality of this and many other serious, surgically correctable anomalies.

REFERENCES

1. Allen RG, Wrenn EL. Silon as a sac in the treatment of omphalocele and gastroschisis. J Pediatr Surg 1969;4:3.
2. Bruce J, Afshani E, Karp MP, Jewett TC Jr. Omphalocele with pyloroduodenal obstruction by extrinsic hepatic compression: a case report. J Pediatr Surg 1988;23:1018.
3. Cantrell JR, Haller JA Jr, Ravitch MM. A syndrome of congenital defects involving the abdominal wall, sternum, diaphragm, pericardium and heart. Surg Gynecol Obstet 1958;107:602.

4. Canty TG, Collins DL. Primary fascial closure in infants with gastroschisis and omphalocele: a superior approach. J Pediatr Surg 1983;18:707.

5. Canty TG, Leopold GR, Wolf DA. Maternal ultrasonography for the antenatal diagnosis of surgically significant neonatal anomalies. Ann Surg 1981;194:353.

6. Canty TG, Leopold GR, Wolf DA. Ultrasonography of pediatric surgical disorders. New York, Grune & Stratton, 1982:9.

7. DeLorimier AA, Adzick NS, Harrison MR. Amnion inversion in the treatment of giant omphalocele. J Pediatr Surg 1991;26:804.

8. Duhamel G. Embryology of exomphalos and allied malformations. Arch Dis Child 1963;38:142.

9. Ehrenpreis T. Omphalocele. In: Nyhus LM, Harkins HN, eds. Hernia, ed 1. Philadelphia, JB Lippincott, 1964:322.

10. Gierup J, Olsen L, Lundkvist K. Aspects on the treatment of omphalocele and gastroschisis: twenty years' clinical experience. Kinderchirurgie 1982;35:3.

11. Gilbert MG, Mencia LF, Brown WT, Linn BS. Staged surgical repair of large omphaloceles and gastroschisis. J Pediatr Surg 1968;3:702.

12. Glick P, Harrison M, Scott N, et al. The missing link in the pathogenesis of gastroschisis. J Pediatr Surg 1985;4:406.

13. Gray SW, Skandalakis JE. Embryology for surgeons. Philadelphia, WB Saunders, 1972:409.

14. Grob M. Conservative treatment of exomphalos. Arch Dis Child 1963;138:148.

15. Gross RE. A new method for surgical treatment of large omphaloceles. Surgery 1948;24:277.

16. Hadziselimovic F, Duckett JW, Snyder HM III, Schnaufer L, Huff D. Omphalocele, cryptorchidism, and brain malformations. J Pediatr Surg 1987;22:854.

17. Izant RJ, Brown F, Rothmann BF. Current embryology and treatment of gastroschisis and omphalocele. Arch Surg 1966;93:49.

18. Johnson AH. Omphalocele and related defects. Am J Surg 1966;114:279.

19. Mahour GH, Weitzman JJ, Rosenkrants JG. Omphalocele and gastroschisis. Ann Surg 1973;177:478.

20. Moore TD. Gastroschisis and omphalocele: clinical differences. Surgery 1977;82:561.

21. Nakayama DK, Harrison MR, Gross BH, et al. Management of the fetus with an abdominal wall defect. J Pediatr Surg 1984;19:408.

22. Nishimura M, Taniguchi A, Imanaka H, Taenaka N. Hypoplastic left heart syndrome associated with congenital right-sided diaphragmatic hernia and omphalocele. Chest 1992;101:263.

23. Schuster SR. A new method for the staged repair of large omphaloceles. Surg Gynecol Obstet 1967;125:837.

24. Schuster SR. Omphalocele, hernia of the umbilical cord and gastroschisis. In: Ravitch MM, Welch KJ, Benson CD, Aberdeen E, Randolph JG, eds. Pediatric surgery, vol 2. Chicago, Year Book Medical Publishers, 1979:778.

25. Schwaitzberg SD, Pokorny WJ, McGill CW, et al. Gastroschisis and omphalocele. Am J Surg 1982;144:650.

26. Schwartz MZ, Tyson KR, Milliorn K, Lobe TE. Staged reduction using a Silastic sac is the treatment of choice for large congenital abdominal wall defects. J Pediatr Surg 1983;6:713.

27. Shaw A. The myth of gastroschisis. J Pediatr Surg 1975;10:235.

28. Shermeta PW, Haller JA. A new preformed transparent silo for the management of gastroschisis. J Pediatr Surg 1975;10:973.

29. Sipes SL, Weiner CP, Sipes DR 2d, Grant SS, Williamson RA. Gastroschisis and omphalocele: does either antenatal diagnosis or route of delivery make a difference in perinatal outcome. J Obstet Gynecol 1990;76:195.

30. Thompson J, Fonkalsrud EW. Reappraisal of skin flap closure for neonatal gastroschisis. Arch Surg 1976;111:684.

31. Tucci M, Bard H. The associated anomalies that determine prognosis in congenital omphaloceles. Am J Obstet Gynecol 1990;163:1646.

32. Tucker JM, Brumfield CG, Davis RO, et al. Prenatal differentiation of ventral abdominal wall defects. Are amniotic fluid markers useful adjuncts? J Reprod Med 1992;37:445.

33. Yaster M, Scherer TL, Stone MM, et al. Prediction of successful primary closure of congenital abdominal wall defects using intraoperative measurements. J Pediatr Surg 1989;24:1217.

34. Yokomori K, Ohkura M, Kitano Y, Hori T, Nakajo T. Advantages and pitfalls of amnion inversion repair for the treatment of large unruptured omphalocele: results of 22 cases. J Pediatr Surg 1992;27:882.

Special Comment

Omphalocele
Janet L. Meller

Caring for an infant with omphalocele is a multidisciplinary challenge. Surgical correction of the anomaly often is the least difficult part of treatment. It is our experience that these patients exhibit a wide spectrum of conditions, ranging from small defects without other problems to large defects accompanied by chromosomal, neurologic, and cardiac anomalies.

Before any patient with an omphalocele is operated on, therefore, a detailed evaluation must be performed. This evaluation should include cardiac and renal ultrasound; consultation with a neonatologist and, possibly, a geneticist regarding the possibility of a lethal chromosomal defect; and discussion of the pulmonary status of the patient.

If a surgeon is fortunate enough to be consulted based on the results of a prenatal ultrasound, many important questions may be answered before the baby is born. The most important of these concerns is the genetic work-up. Operating on an infant with a chromosomal anomaly that is incompatible with life (ie, trisomy 13) is futile. Some information also may be available regarding the cardiac, renal, and pulmonary status, and whether the spine is closed.

In the absence of other conditions, omphalocele alone generally is not sufficient indication for a cesarean delivery.[3] Parents should be counseled regarding the probability of other anomalies and allowed to make their own decision regarding the status of the pregnancy.

Infants with omphalocele can be maintained without surgery as long as the sac remains intact. Nonoperative therapy may be chosen, especially in infants with associated life-threatening anomalies. Even if the sac has ruptured, the infant may be observed while questions regarding his or her stability are answered. After all these issues have been resolved, surgical closure should be attempted.

Problems associated with the closure of omphaloceles center around the size of the defect and the amount of intestine/liver that is present in the defect. We have used several strategies to address these issues. The most important factor in the closure of an omphalocele is whether venous return will be compromised unduly by compression of the vena cava. If the closure seems tight, we use intragastric pressure measurement as described by Wesley and colleagues.[4] This technique involves advancing a feeding tube filled with saline into the stomach. The tube then is connected to a pressure line and a manometer. The abdomen is closed temporarily and the pressure is measured. A pressure less than 19 cm H_2O is felt to be compatible with safe closure. Pressures greater than 19 cm H_2O are believed to indicate the need for staged closure.[1,2] It is important to note that we, along with many other investigators, have noted no increase in morbidity with staged closure.

In the event that staged closure is necessary, a silo made of Marlex mesh is sutured to the full thickness of the abdominal wall and the top is closed with a row of sutures. This technique allows full-thickness stretching of the abdominal wall. Daily reduction of intraabdominal contents is accomplished in the neonatal intensive care unit under aseptic conditions by direct compression from the top of the silo downward. A row of sutures is placed at the superior margin of the visceral contents. The mesh is supported by wrapping it in gauze and suspending the entire wrapping from the top of the incubator or warmer. Suspension also allows for more efficient stretching of the abdomen and reduction of the intestinal contents.

It almost always is possible to reduce completely all the contents and achieve closure of the abdomen within 7 days. If the closure at this time seems tight, the intragastric pressure should be measured. Occasionally, a patient with a giant omphalocele will not be stretched sufficiently to enable closure even after several weeks of silo treatment. In such cases, a Gore-Tex graft may be placed to bridge the fascial defect completely. A skin flap then can be developed over the graft. This technique prevents growth of the liver outside the coelom. If this is not possible, the liver itself eventually may cover the defect or the bowel may become sufficiently adherent that the silo can be removed and the wound allowed to granulate.

Ventral hernias develop in most patients with congenital abdominal wall defects, regardless of how they are closed. It is important not to close these too early. The defect usually becomes smaller with time, and better fascia will be available for closure and the risk of recurrence will decrease as the child grows. We generally delay closure of these secondary hernias until the age of 4 to 5 years. In some children with especially large ventral hernias, it may be better to wait until the age of 7 years. By this time, many of these defects can be closed primarily, although some require prosthetic materials.

At the time of reexploration, consideration should be given to performing a Ladd procedure and appendectomy. Most patients with abdominal wall defects have malrotation. It is unusual for these infants to have a midgut volvulus, but their appendix may have an aberrant location that would complicate diagnosis if appendicitis ever developed. In general, appendectomy is not performed at the time of primary closure of the abdominal wall. This information also may be useful to general surgeons, who may treat these patients as they reach adulthood.

In a recent review of our experience with omphalocele, we found that 31% of affected infants were premature and 19% were small for their gestational age. Twenty percent had cardiac anomalies. Most patients were treated with primary closure, with only 12% requiring placement of a silo. The mortality rate for patients with omphalocele was 30%, reflecting the high incidence of associated congenital anomalies.[2]

Although the surgical treatment of omphalocele can be challenging, the primary consideration in the care of these infants should be the diagnosis and treatment of associated anomalies. The limiting factor in the long-term survival of these infants is not the type of omphalocele surgery performed, but the severity of associated cardiac, pulmonary, neurologic, and chromosomal anomalies. Therefore, a multidisciplinary approach is essential and must bridge the prenatal and postnatal periods.

REFERENCES

1. Hatch EI Jr, Baxter R. Surgical options in the management of large omphaloceles. Am J Surg 1987;153:449.
2. Meller JL, Reyes HM, Loeff DS. Omphalocele and gastroschisis. Clin Perinatol 1989;16:113.
3. Sipes SL, Weiner CP, Sipes DR II, et al. Gastroschisis and omphalocele: does either antenatal diagnosis or route of delivery make a difference in perinatal outcome? Obstet Gynecol 1990;67:195.
4. Wesley JR, Drongowski R, Coran AG. Intragastric pressure measurements: a guide for reduction and closure of the Silastic chimney in omphalocele and gastroschisis. J Pediatr Surg 1981;16:264.

Hernia, Fourth Edition, edited
by Lloyd M. Nyhus and Robert E. Condon.
J.B. Lippincott Company, Philadelphia © 1995.

Chapter 23

Gastroschisis

Eric W. Fonkalsrud

The word *gastroschisis* originally referred to all congenital malformations of the abdominal wall, and is derived from the Greek word that literally means *cleft belly*. Calder[4] is given credit for describing the first detailed reported case of gastroschisis in 1733. Little progress was made in either the understanding or the treatment of abdominal wall defects until the modern era. In 1940, Bernstein[2] accurately described the gastroschisis anomaly and distinguished it from omphalocele by the complete absence of a sac and the presence of an intact umbilical cord.

The gastroschisis abdominal wall defect rarely measures more than 3 cm in diameter and characteristically is situated to the right of the umbilical cord. It usually is immediately adjacent to the cord, but, on rare occasions, is separated from it by a narrow strip of skin. In most instances, the entire small intestine and the colon down to the sigmoid are extruded from the abdomen (Fig. 23-1). The stomach, the testes, and, rarely, the ovaries may be outside the abdomen. There is neither a peritoneal covering sac nor evidence of sac remnants.

In infants with gastroschisis, fixation of the small intestine and colon to the posterior abdominal wall is incomplete, and malrotation always is present; the cecum is situated on the left side of the abdomen. The intestine often is bound together with fibrinous adhesions and appears to be shortened compared with that of normal infants. It is believed that the irritating effects of prolonged exposure of the fetal intestine to amniotic fluid are a major factor in causing it to swell and mat together. In addition, further congestion of the intestine may result from partial lymphatic and venous obstruction in the mesentery that passes through the small abdominal wall defect. In most cases, the arterial blood supply and the number of arcades to the intestine are normal. Infants with gastroschisis defects are much more subject to prolonged ileus and delay in absorption than are those with omphalocele, in which the viscera is unexposed. It has been demonstrated in the fetal rabbit model that experimentally produced gastroschisis is associated with a decrease in fetal weight, presumably caused in part by failure of in utero intestinal absorption of sub-strates from the amniotic fluid.[17] This situation may contribute to the large number of small-for-gestational-age infants with gastroschisis.

Associated anomalies occur in about one third of all cases; however, most do not cause major complications. Intestinal atresia or stenosis occurs in about 15% of patients.[10] Intestinal necrosis or perforation is uncommon. Within a few weeks after the abdomen has been closed and the intestine covered, the edema subsides and the intestine gradually assumes normal length and resumes peristaltic activity and normal mucosal absorption.[16] The abdominal cavity is small, and appears scaphoid on examination. Three forms of gastroschisis have been described based on the appearance of the intestine relative to the duration of evisceration and exposure to amniotic fluid: antenatal, perinatal, and intermediate.[15]

The actual frequency of gastroschisis is believed to be about 1 in 3000 live births. Familial occurrences are rare, and the genetic aspects are poorly understood. Gastroschisis anomalies are almost twice as common as are omphalocele defects. Moore[14] reported a 59% incidence of prematurity in 273 infants with gastroschisis. Mothers of babies with gastroschisis tend to be younger than those of infants with omphalocele. More than 60% are younger than 20 years, and more than 50% are primigravid.

Both gastroschisis and large omphalocele defects may be identified during the early third trimester by maternal ultrasonography (Fig. 23-2). Prenatal diagnosis of the condition alerts the obstetrician to take extra precautions during the delivery to avoid traction on the eviscerated intestine. Although there is controversy regarding the desirability of performing cesarean section on involved infants, we have not found this to be necessary in most cases.

The embryologic origin of gastroschisis remains unclear. Duhamel[7] and others concluded that this condition results from a mesenchymal defect that occurs after the eighth week of gestation. Shaw[21] considers gastroschisis to be a consequence of intrauterine rupture of the amniotic membrane at the base of the hernia of the umbilical cord. De Vries[6] suggests that gastroschisis results from a rupture of the paraumbil-

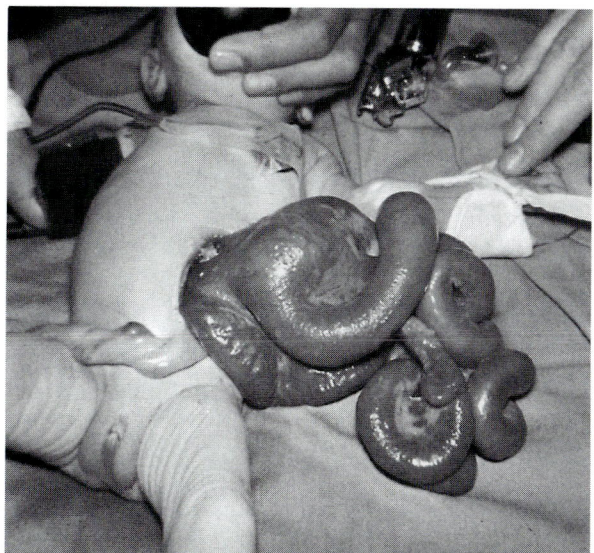

Figure 23-1. Newborn infant with gastroschisis showing moderate visceroabdominal disproportion. The intestine is thick and edematous, and it appears shortened as a result of exposure to amniotic fluid.

ical somatopleure, but does not represent a ruptured omphalocele. Moreover, gastroschisis may represent a mechanical accident rather than a teratogenic occurrence. Although the embryonic distinction between gastroschisis and omphalocele remains controversial, the clinical differentiation is useful.[6,21] Infants with

omphalocele have more than twice as many associated anomalies as do those with gastroschisis.[13] Patients with gastroschisis rarely have other life-threatening anomalies and virtually always are candidates for definitive surgical repair. In contrast to infants with large omphalocele defects, patients with gastroschisis most often have the entire liver within the abdominal cavity at birth. Furthermore, the rectus muscles are in the midline, making repair of the anomaly technically more feasible than in infants with large omphalocele defects, in which the medial border of the rectus muscle may reside as far lateral as the mid-axillary line.

PREOPERATIVE CARE

Gastroschisis is a complex emergency that is treated best in a tertiary neonatal center. Hypothermia is the most important immediate problem because exposure of the intestine to the ambient environment leads to rapid heat loss. The intestine should be wrapped with thin plastic sheeting and the infant placed either in an incubator or a plastic bag up to the neck (Fig. 23-3). The placement of warm, moist gauze directly on the intestinal surface leads to rapid cooling of the infant after the gauze attains ambient temperature, and the gauze also may become adherent to the intestine and injure the muscularis when it is removed. Heat lamps should be used cautiously because of the danger of desiccating the intestine. A nasogastric tube should be inserted immediately after birth, and an intravenous

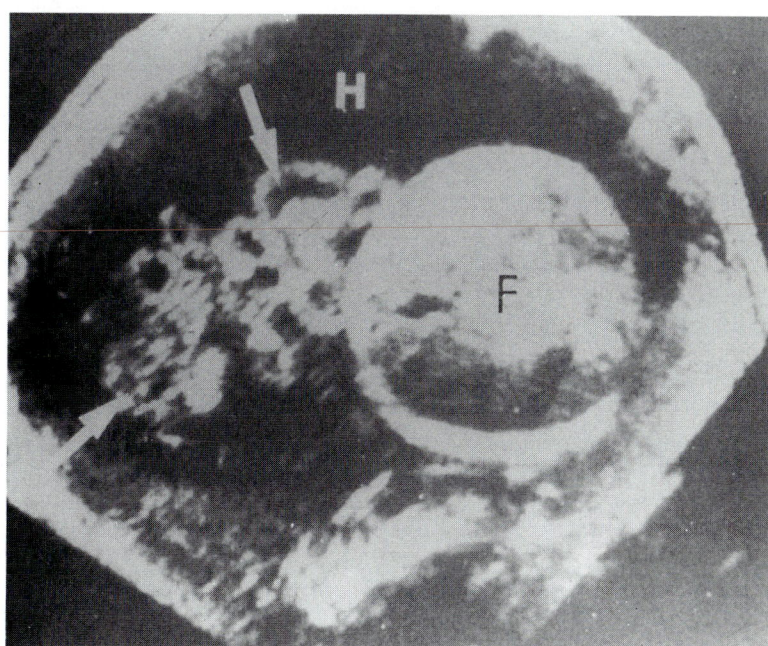

Figure 23-2. Maternal ultrasound study performed at 30 weeks' gestation, showing appearance of characteristic gastroschisis abdominal wall defect. F, fetus; H, amniotic fluid. Arrows point to eviscerated intestine.

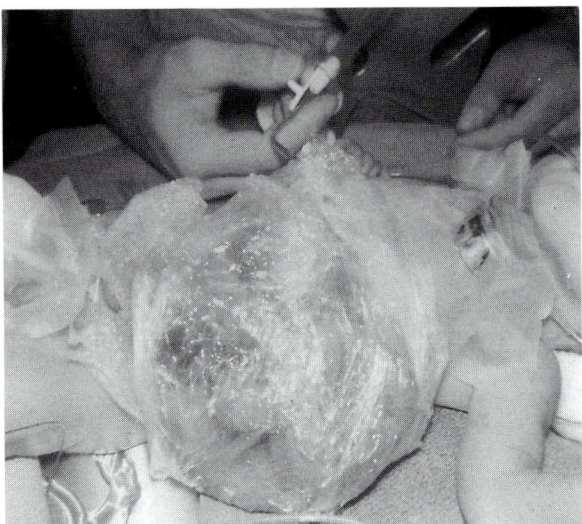

Figure 23-3. Newborn infant with gastroschisis abdominal defect showing Silastic sheet over viscera to maintain body heat and prevent injury to intestine as the infant is transported to the operating room.

route established for restoring adequate hydration. Intravenous antibiotics (ampicillin and gentamicin) are given soon after birth. The infant should not be transferred to another hospital without these precautions.

Before surgery, the infant should receive 0.5 to 1.0 mg of vitamin K intravenously. Because these newborns frequently are hypoglycemic, as well as dehydrated, a solution containing 10% glucose should be given intravenously at a rate of 25 to 50 mL/kg every 24 hours, in addition to the maintenance fluids of 5% dextrose and 0.25% normal saline solution given at a rate of 100 mL/kg every 24 hours. An evaluation for cardiac and other anomalies should be performed, but operation should not be delayed for more than a few hours after birth.

OPERATIVE THERAPY

Until about 1970, the mortality of infants with gastroschisis exceeded 50%. Since that time, the mortality has declined steadily to its present level of less than 10% in most major children's centers, largely because of improved operative techniques and close attention to the details of preoperative and postoperative care. Successful surgical repair of a gastroschisis defect by primary fascial closure first was reported by Watkins[22] in 1943. Before the development of adequate mechanical ventilation for newborn infants, primary closure was considered hazardous because of respiratory and vascular compromise from increased intraabdom-

inal pressure and elevation of the diaphragm. In an attempt to delay reduction while still providing coverage of the viscera, Gross[11] in 1948 reported a method of skin flap coverage for omphalocele and gastroschisis defects. Although this approach was used frequently for the next two decades, alternative methods of repair have been devised and are used more often now. In 1967, Schuster[19] described a technique of reducing omphalocele and gastroschisis defects by using polytetrafluoroethylene (Teflon) mesh. This approach subsequently was modified to form a prosthetic silo or chimney covering for the intestine, with gradual reduction of the intestine downward into the abdomen every 1 to 3 days.[1] Raffensperger[18] in 1974 diminished the mortality further by stretching the abdominal wall before primary closure. Advances in neonatal intensive care, particularly mechanical ventilation and parenteral nutrition, have been instrumental in increasing the survival rate of infants with gastroschisis during the past 25 years, to its current level of more than 90% in most large children's medical centers.

The choice of primary fascial closure, skin coverage with subsequent fascial closure, or use of a temporary prosthetic silo depends on the surgeon's subjective assessment of the abdominal wall tension during the surgical repair. Although some authors suggest that almost all infants may undergo safely a snug primary closure, increased pressure within the abdomen may cause the intestine to tear, with occasional resultant fistulas and sepsis. Our clinical experience,[8,9] as well as that of Harrison and colleagues,[12] and Caniano and associates,[5] indicates that the severity of intestinal edema and the disparity between the size of the eviscerated intestine and the abdominal cavity determine which operative technique is best suited for an individual patient.

General anesthesia with endotracheal intubation, using halothane and muscle relaxants, is preferred. Monitoring of airway resistance and ventilatory volume is helpful in determining the amount of pressure applied to the diaphragm during the surgical closure. Continuous monitoring of the rectal temperature, heart rate, blood pressure, and electrocardiogram are routine.

The eviscerated loops of intestine are washed lightly with warm antibiotic solution (cephalosporin). While an assistant elevates the loops of intestine, the surgeon passes a soft rectal catheter and washes away meconium with warm saline irrigations, because deflation of the intestine helps to achieve closure of the abdomen. The abdominal wall defect then is enlarged with 1- to 2-cm incisions in the midline directed toward both the pubis and the xiphoid. The umbilical arteries and vein, and the urachal remnant, are ligated and the remaining cord structures are excised.

Fibrinous material on the surface of the intestine is removed gently if feasible, with care taken to avoid injury to the edematous mesentery and muscularis.

The intestine is inspected carefully for atresia or perforation (Fig. 23-4). In patients with mild intestinal edema in whom there is not a large disparity between the size of the proximal and distal atretic ends, primary anastomosis using an end-to-oblique-end technique may be feasible with interrupted 5-0 monofilament sutures (Maxon). In infants with more severe visceroabdominal disproportion (VAD) and edema, or a disparity between the diameter of the proximal and distal ends, no attempt is made to repair the atresia at the initial operation. A secondary laparotomy, usually at the time of secondary fascial closure of the abdomen, will reveal the intestinal edema to have disappeared almost completely, making repair of the intestinal atresia a technically easier, and safer, undertaking.[20] Although a diverting enterostomy with mucous fistula was used in the past, this technique is used rarely today.

The lateral and anterior abdominal wall is stretched firmly by the surgeon's index finger. This maneuver almost doubles the size of the abdominal cavity. The upper and lower ends of the intestine should be manipulated slightly to encourage enteric contents to drain through the rectal catheter or the nasogastric tube. The bladder is decompressed gently to provide more space in the abdominal cavity. The viscera are examined for other anomalies, such as undescended testes, Meckel diverticulum, and duodenal bands.

In our experience, VAD is sufficiently mild that primary fascial closure can be performed readily at the initial operation in about one third of affected infants[9] (Fig. 23-5). If the rectus muscles cannot be approximated with mild to moderate tension, primary fascial closure is abandoned in favor of a Silastic chimney. The prosthesis is sutured to the skin and underlying muscle with interrupted, nonabsorbable stitches (Fig. 23-6). The upper end of the chimney is supported from the top of the crib warmer with a rubber band and umbilical tape. Povidone-iodine ointment or solution is placed on the base of the prosthesis twice daily. The intestine is encouraged to retreat into the abdominal cavity, assisted by mild pressure from above as new ligatures are placed on the upper end of the sac every 12 to 24 hours. In most patients, the entire intestine is reduced into the abdominal cavity within 7 to 10 days. The Silastic prosthesis then is removed under general anesthesia in the operating room and the rectus muscles and overlying skin are closed.

In our clinical experience, about 25% of infants with gastroschisis have severe VAD. In these cases, initial repair with a Silastic chimney, followed by one or more subsequent staged reconstructive operations during the ensuing weeks, appears to be the safest

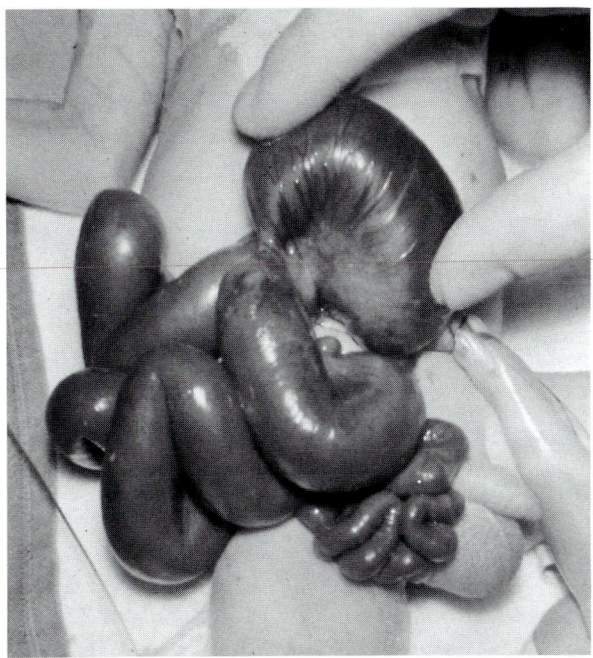

Figure 23-4. Newborn male infant with gastroschisis defect and low jejunal atresia.

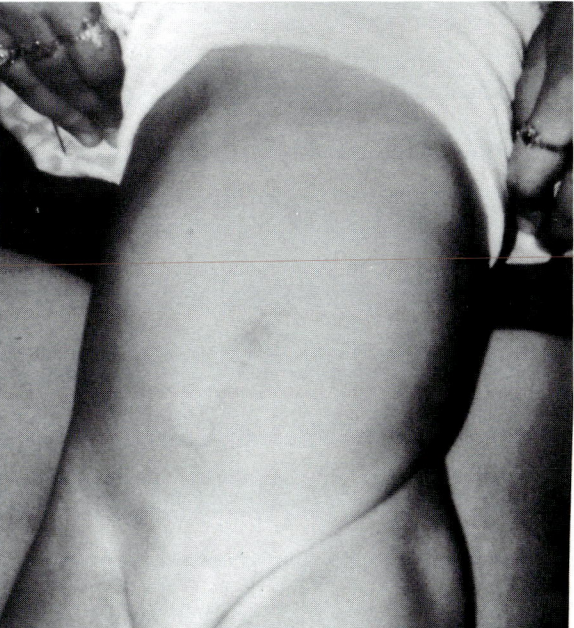

Figure 23-5. Primary fascial repair of gastroschisis with minimal intestinal edema or visceroabdominal disproportion. A small cutaneous scar with simulated umbilicus is constructed.

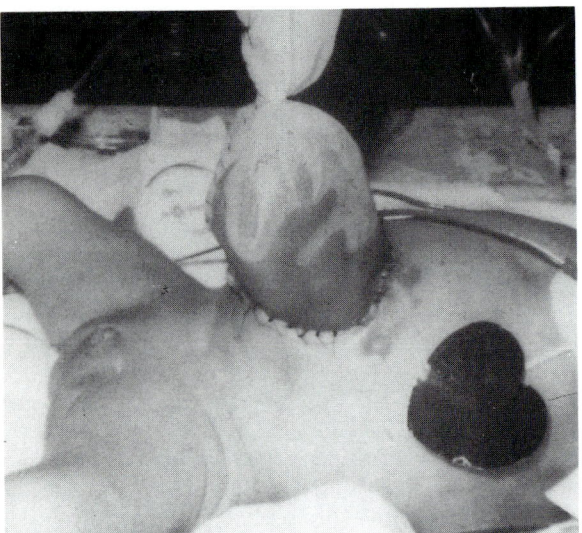

Figure 23-6. Prosthetic Silastic chimney attached to skin and muscle to contain eviscerated intestine until edema subsides and the abdomen enlarges.

method of achieving complete closure (Fig. 23-7). During the past few years, we increasingly have performed minor abdominal wall reconstruction in the neonatal intensive care nursery using intravenous analgesics and muscle relaxants. In those infants in

whom the remaining skin defect has been allowed to epithelialize over the intestine, it has been remarkably easy to close surgically the muscles and skin 6 to 8 weeks later. When complete fascial closure is delayed for more than 4 months, the rectus muscles often contract into narrow bands that become more difficult to approximate in the midline and cause a permanently narrow waist with an hourglass configuration.

Although skin flap closure was used with good outcome in most infants until about 1980 (Fig. 23-8), there has been an evolution during the past decade toward use of the Silastic chimney technique for almost all infants in whom primary closure is not feasible. Skin flap closure continues to have a role in treating occasional infants in whom the prosthesis cannot be removed completely after 2 to 3 weeks. The placement of a Silastic prosthesis between the rectus muscles and beneath the skin flaps may permit earlier hospital discharge than might otherwise be possible in selected patients with severe VAD.

POSTOPERATIVE CARE

After operative repair, the infant is placed under an overhead warmer in a neonatal intensive care facility. In cases in which respiratory function is compromised

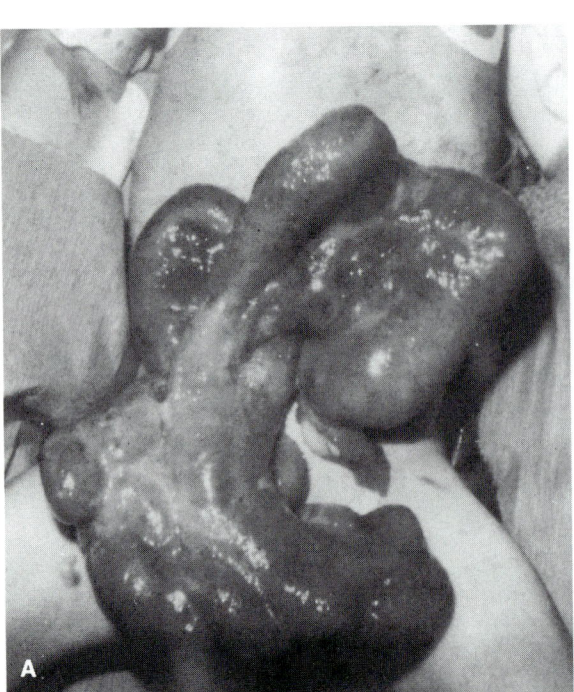
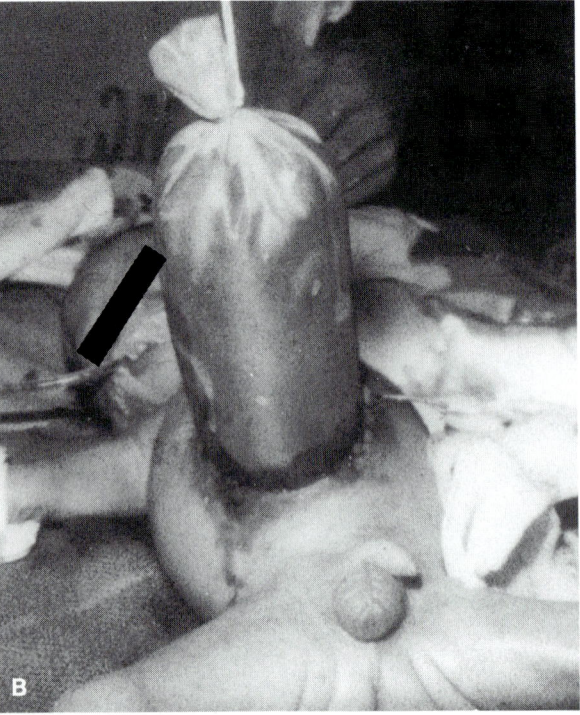

Figure 23-7. (A) Newborn infant with severe visceroabdominal disproportion requiring three operative procedures and 28 days before complete closure. (B) Large prosthetic silastic chimney as first stage of repair.

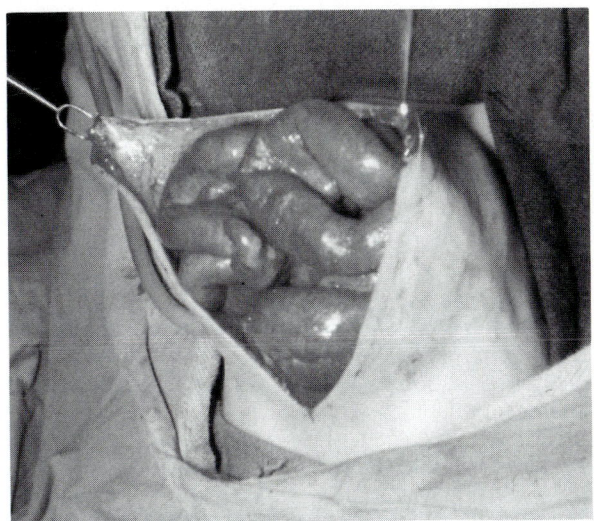

Figure 23-8. Elevation of skin flaps from each side of the abdomen to cover eviscerated intestine when primary fascial closure is not feasible. The linea alba is open 2 to 3 cm above and below the original defect.

by a tight closure, the endotracheal tube is left in place and the patient is managed with a mechanical ventilator or with continuous positive airway pressure.[3] The respiratory status should be monitored with serial arterial pH and blood gas determinations. The period of postoperative mechanical ventilation in our clinical experience has ranged from 4 hours to 21 days. When patients with complications were excluded, the average period of ventilation was 3.5 days.

Intravenous fluid infusions of 10% glucose in 0.25% saline solution are delivered at a rate of about 125 to 150 mL/kg/d. Because of the edema in the tissues and the loss of fluid from the eviscerated intestine, patients with gastroschisis require larger volumes of fluid than do other newborns during the first few days after surgery. The fluid administered is reduced after the third to fifth day, depending on urine output. Gastric aspirate from either a nasogastric or an orogastric tube should be replaced according to volume with 5% dextrose and 0.5% normal saline solution. Antibiotics are continued for about 7 days, or until the prosthesis is removed.

Although we previously used gastrostomy routinely, we rarely have done so during the past 10 years, when the Silon chimney technique has been used more often. Nonetheless, gastrostomy continues to be helpful in patients with short-bowel syndrome or other conditions requiring long-term parenteral nutrition.

In an effort to shorten the hospital stay, there has been a progressive trend toward the routine use of central venous parenteral nutrition and home parenteral nutrition for infants with severe VAD or short-bowel syndrome. All patients in our recent clinical experience received parenteral nutrition postoperatively until the ileus resolved and complete enteral nutrition was tolerated. The average duration of parenteral nutrition was 33 days. The severity of the ileus correlated closely with the degree of intestinal edema and the severity of VAD. Percutaneously placed, fine, Silastic central venous catheters inserted through the basilic vein were used in more than two thirds of the infants, and Broviac single-lumen catheters were inserted by cutdown in the saphenous veins of the remaining infants, who required longer periods of parenteral nutrition.

Because parenteral nutrition increases the risk of catheter sepsis and occasionally may cause cholestasis, particularly in the young infant with an immature liver, enteral nutrition should be initiated as early as considered feasible. The development of the cholestatic liver syndrome appears to be variable among neonates, and sometimes may lead to rapidly progressive cirrhosis with hepatomegaly and portal hypertension. Thus, total parenteral nutrition, although it is a helpful adjunct, must be monitored closely because it has the potential for producing serious, and even fatal, complications.

Enteral nutrition with breast milk or formula first was tolerated successfully after a mean of 20 days (range, 5–67 days) in our experience. The length of hospitalization averaged 39.4 days (range, 12–161 days). No significant difference was noted in the time of the initial feeding between patients who had Silastic chimney repair and those who had skin flap repair, although the former were hospitalized for longer periods largely because this group included most of the infants with severe VAD. Infants with initial primary closure began feeding earlier (mean, 15.6 days) and had a shorter hospital stay (mean, 27.6 days).

During the past few years, we have used continuous epidural analgesia during the postoperative period for most infants with moderate to severe VAD for as long as 7 days. Both the period of mechanical ventilation and respirator support, as well as the time for abdominal wall closure, have been decreased through the use of epidural analgesia. Furthermore, the requirement for pancuronium bromide (Pavulon), fentanyl, and intravenous or muscular analgesic medications has been reduced, with a resultant decrease in both peripheral and pulmonary edema, compared to infants not receiving epidural analgesics. We have recorded no complications from this technique.

In our clinical experience, almost all postoperative complications (27%) occurred in those infants with severe VAD. Major complications included pneumonia, septic episodes, intestinal necrosis and perforation, necrotizing enterocolitis, wound separation,

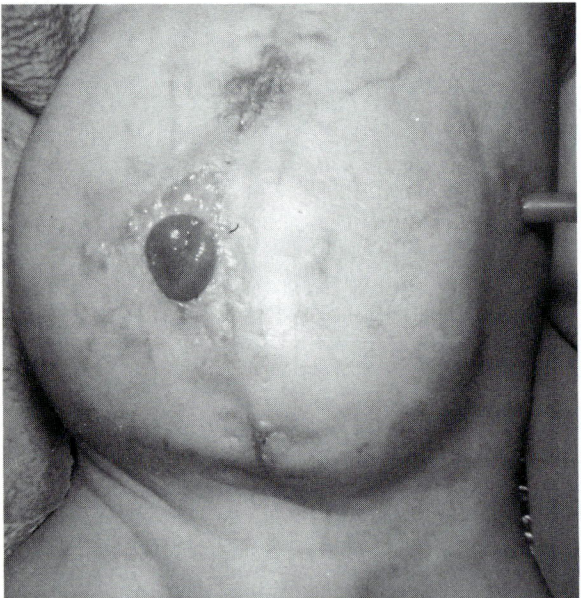

Figure 23-9.   Enterocutaneous fistula resulting from closure of gastroschisis abdominal defect with severe visceroabdominal disproportion. The abdominal wound was closed under moderate tension. Five weeks later, the fistula was resected and the intestine was reanastomosed. Complete abdominal wall closure was feasible at that time.

parenteral nutrition cholestasis, and symptomatic gastroesophageal reflux (Fig. 23-9). Each of the surviving patients is progressing well, with nearly normal growth and development. Mortality in our series of 82 patients was 4%. The long-term outlook is excellent for infants who survive repair of gastroschisis, exceeding 90% in most centers. Three decades ago, their survival was only 10%.

REFERENCES

1. Allen RG, Wren EL Jr. Silon as a sac in the treatment of omphalocele and gastroschisis. J Pediatr Surg 1969;4:3.
2. Bernstein P. Gastroschisis: a rare teratological condition in the newborn. Arch Pediatr 1940;57:503.
3. Bower RJ, Bell MJ, Ternberg JL, Cobb ML. Ventilatory support and primary closure of gastroschisis. Surgery 1982;91:52.
4. Calder J. Medical essays and observations. Edinburgh, 1733:203.
5. Caniano DA, Brokaw B, Ginn-Pease ME. An individualized approach to the management of gastroschisis. J Pediatr Surg 1990;25:297.
6. De Vries PA. The pathogenesis of gastroschisis and omphalocele. J Pediatr Surg 1980;15:245.
7. Duhamel B. Embryology of exomphalos and allied malformations. Arch Dis Child 1963;38:138.
8. Fonkalsrud EW. Selective repair of neonatal gastroschisis based on degree of viscero-abdominal disproportion. Ann Surg 1980;191:139.
9. Fonkalsrud EW, Smith MD, Shaw KS, Borick JM, Shaw A. Selective management of gastroschisis according to degree of viscero-abdominal disproportion. Ann Surg 1993;218:742.
10. Grosfeld JL, Weber TR. Congenital abdominal wall defects: gastroschisis and omphalocele. Curr Probl Surg 1982;19:159.
11. Gross RE. A new method for surgical treatment of large omphaloceles. Surgery 1948;24:277.
12. Harrison MW, Campbell TJ, Campbell JR. Selective management of gastroschisis. Am Surg 1986;203:214.
13. Hollabaugh R, Boles T. The management of gastroschisis. J Pediatr Surg 1973;8:263.
14. Moore TC. Gastroschisis and omphalocele: clinical differences. Surgery 1977;82:561.
15. Moore TC, Stokes GE. Gastroschisis: report of two cases treated by a modification of Gross' operation for omphalocele. Surgery 1953;33:112.
16. O'Neill JA, Grosfeld JL. Intestinal malfunction after antenatal exposure of viscera. Am J Surg 1974;127:129.
17. Phillips JD, Kelly RE Jr, Fonkalsrud EW, Mirzayan A, Kim CS. An improved model of experimental gastroschisis in fetal rabbits. J Pediatr Surg 1991;26:784.
18. Raffensperger JC, Jona JC. Gastroschisis. Surg Gynecol Obstet 1974;138:230.
19. Schuster SR. A new method for the staged repair of large omphaloceles. Surg Gynecol Obstet 1967;125:837.
20. Shah R, Woolley MM. Gastroschisis and intestinal atresia. J Pediatr Surg 1991;26:788.
21. Shaw A. The myth of gastroschisis. J Pediatr Surg 1975;10:235.
22. Watkins DE. Gastroschisis. Virginia Med Month 1943;78:42.

Special Comment

Gastroschisis

Jayant Radhakrishnan

Gastroschisis is an abdominal wall defect to the right of the umbilical cord through which the entire small intestine and parts of the colon are eviscerated from the abdomen. Although these babies often are premature, they have few associated anomalies and always are candidates for surgical repair. Today, more than 90% of these infants should be expected to survive. Now that mortality has been controlled by advances in perioperative care such as improved respiratory and nutritional support, it has become apparent that the major cause of morbidity in these infants is prolonged ileus resulting from damage to the intestinal wall (Fig. 23-10). The eviscerated intestines always are edematous and adjacent loops often are adherent to each other, being covered by a thick yellow pellicle and bound together by fibrinous adhesions. In spite of obvious external damage, atresia, necrosis, and perforation are uncommon. Because abdominal wall defects now can be identified by maternal ultrasonography in the third trimester of pregnancy, it seems logical to attempt to control intestinal damage.

In a retrospective review of 24 cases of gastroschisis, Lenke and Hatch[5] noted an absence of "bowel peel" and edema in babies born by cesarean section, thus permitting closure of the defect more often than was possible in infants born vaginally. They felt that all babies with gastroschisis should be born by cesarean section. Meizner and Bar-Ziv[6] also recommended routine cesarean delivery based on three theoretic concerns regarding vaginal delivery: (1) possible damage to eviscerated bowel, which could become ischemic; (2) dystocia caused by eviscerated bowel; and (3) predisposition of the abdominal viscera to infection. The data from their study, however, did not support this recommendation. Subsequently, Sipes and colleagues[7] studied 61 pregnancies complicated by either fetal gastroschisis (33 cases) or omphalocele (28 cases). In their retrospective review, there were no fetal deaths and no instances of dystocia or bowel ischemia. Thirty-one of the 33 fetuses with gastroschisis survived (1 fetus was aborted and 1 baby died at 3 months of age). With the exception of a significantly lower umbilical pH level in fetuses diagnosed at birth,

no other differences were noted between those born vaginally and those born by cesarean section.

Crabbe and associates[2] carried out a retrospective review of 47 infants with gastroschisis. Their patients were analyzed in two groups according to gestational age: group A consisted of 21 infants born at 26 to 38 weeks' gestation and group B consisted of 26 infants born at 39 to 40 weeks' gestation. They further analyzed a subgroup of 9 infants born at 36 weeks' gestation because they considered the optimum gestational age for delivery of infants with gastroschisis. The mean duration of postoperative ileus for their series was 14.1 days, with no statistically significant difference between the two groups. On evaluating the subgroup born at 36 weeks' gestation, the mean duration of ileus was found to be 11.3 days, but this difference just failed to reach statistical significance. The mean duration of hospitalization also was not significantly different between the two major groups or those born at 36 weeks' gestation. In this series, 11 of the 47 neonates were delivered by cesarean section for obstetric reasons rather than the presence of gastroschisis. The mean duration of hospitalization in these infants was slightly shorter, but the duration of ileus was slightly longer.

Langer and coworkers[4] attempted to develop objective sonographic criteria for predicting outcome. They conducted a retrospective and prospective review of 24 consecutive fetuses. They found that a maximal bowel wall thickness greater than 3 mm was associated with an increase in time to oral feeding, but this difference was not statistically significant. They did note that a bowel diameter of at least 18 mm was

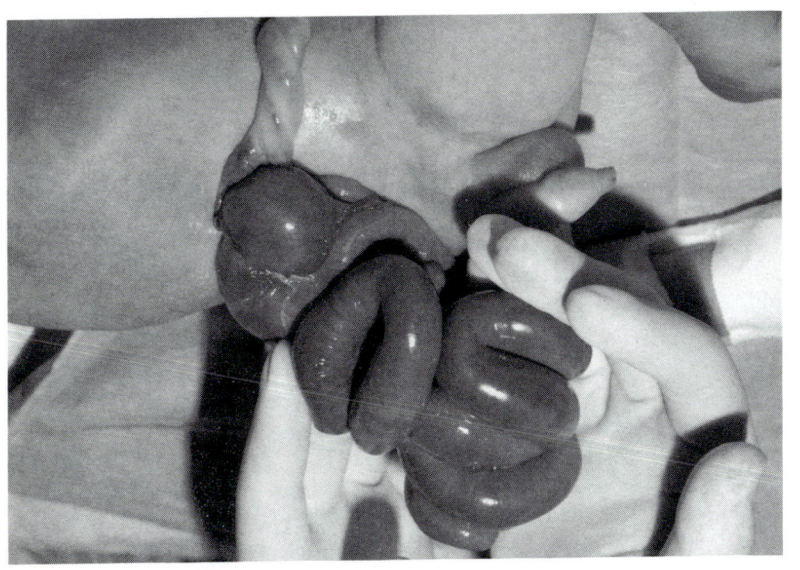

Figure 23-10. A typical case of gastroschisis. The eviscerated intestines demonstrate edema, bowel dilation, and a layer of fibrinous adhesions.

associated with a significantly longer time to oral feeding, and also with a significantly greater need for
bowel resection. By plotting gestational age against
bowel diameter, they were able to generate a "threshold" line above which all patients had prolonged hypoperistalsis and below which only 30% demonstrated
hypoperistalsis. Two infants in their series were born
at 35 weeks' gestation and both had complications related to prematurity, compared to only 1 of 22 infants
born after 33 weeks' gestation. It is interesting that
their threshold line permits a larger bowel diameter
at early gestational ages and implies that late onset of
dilation may be of greater concern. This may be explained on the basis that associated intestinal atresia
would cause larger bowel diameters in early pregnancy without necessarily being indicative of a poor
outcome.

While most researchers were concentrating on
the size of the bowel wall, Crawford and colleagues[3]
carried out morphometric measurements in a retrospective review of 24 consecutive cases of gastroschisis. Their studies indicate that fetal gut measurements are not the only criterion affecting the timing
and mode of delivery. In addition to fetal morphometric measurements and the ultrasonic appearance
of fetal bowel, they also evaluated fetal well-being by
cardiotocography, measurement of the amniotic fluid
volume, and a full biophysical profile score. They
found that half the babies in their series were small
for gestational age at birth. Gut dilation was noted to
be an indicator of either antenatal or intrapartum fetal distress, but it did not correlate with poor neonatal
surgical outcome. They suggested that close antenatal
surveillance of fetal well-being always is necessary in
cases of gastroschisis because, in addition to growth
retardation, many fetuses demonstrated evidence of
distress and 12.5% were stillborn even though they
had grown appropriately.

Coughlin and associates[1] observed that bowel
changes characteristic of gastroschisis occur after
birth and are not the result of antenatal exposure to
amniotic fluid. They compared 13 infants born by
elective cesarean section who had their abdominal
wall defect repaired in the delivery suite within 15
minutes of birth to another 19 infants, whose condition was also diagnosed before birth and who were
born by cesarean section at other institutions. Because
these patients had to be transferred, their repair was
delayed for a few hours (mean, < 6 hours after cesarean section). In general, both groups of babies were
comparable. In the group that underwent immediate
repair, 73% had fascial closure; in the group that was
transferred to another hospital, only 37% underwent
successful primary closure. When term infants without associated anomalies in the two groups were compared, the patients who received immediate repair
were extubated sooner, tolerated enteral feeding earlier, and had a shorter hospital stay. The researchers
attribute the difference between the two groups to
their observation that the bowel of babies operated on
immediately did not have the characteristic edematous, matted appearance that was noted in the group
of patients in whom surgery was delayed.

Therefore, it appears that antenatal morphometric evaluation and assessment of bowel wall thickness
and bowel diameter are important, but that immediate surgical correction may be the most significant
means of controlling morbidity. Fetal morphometric
measurements and bowel thickness and dilation determinations can be of value in carrying out a pre-
planned cesarean section with immediate repair of the
defect.

REFERENCES

1. Coughlin JP, Drucker DEM, Jewell MR, Evans MJ, Klein MD. Delivery room repair of gastroschisis. Presented at the Central Surgical Association meeting March 4–6, 1993, Cincinnati, Ohio.
2. Crabbe DCG, Thomas DFM, Beck JM, Spicer RD. Prenatally diagnosed gastroschisis: a case for preterm delivery? Pediatr Surg Int 1991;6:108.
3. Crawford RAF, Ryan G, Wright VM, Rodeck CH. The importance of serial biophysical assessment of fetal wellbeing in gastroschisis. Br J Obstet Gynaecol 1992;99:899.
4. Langer JC, Khanna J, Caco C, Dykes EH, Nicolaides KH. Prenatal diagnosis of gastroschisis: development of objective sonographic criteria for predicting outcome. Obstet Gynecol 1993;81:53.
5. Lenke RR, Hatch EI Jr. Fetal gastroschisis: a preliminary report advocating the use of cesarean section. Obstet Gynecol 1986;67:395.
6. Meizner I, Bar-Ziv J. Prenatal ultrasonic diagnosis of anterior abdominal wall defects. Eur J Obstet Gynecol Reprod Biol 1986;22:217.
7. Sipes SL, Weiner CP, Sipes DR II, Grant SS, Williamson RA. Gastroschisis and omphalocele: does either antenatal diagnosis or route of delivery make a difference in perinatal outcome? Obstet Gynecol 1990;76:195.

Hernia, Fourth Edition, edited by Lloyd M. Nyhus and Robert E. Condon. J.B. Lippincott Company, Philadelphia © 1995.

Chapter 24

Umbilical Hernia

Jayant Radhakrishnan

A heretic . . . is a fellow who disagrees with you regarding something neither of you knows anything about.

William Cowper Brann (1855–1898)

Umbilical hernias occur in both children and adults, but the mode of presentation, natural history, and treatment strategy are different in the two groups.

HISTORY

The Hindu physician Charaka described umbilical hernias in his writings dated AD 1 or earlier, but he believed they were abdominal tumors. The ancient Jews recognized umbilical hernias and treated them conservatively.[45] Celsus, in the first century AD, treated umbilical hernias with an elastic suture, and Soranus (AD 98–117) described a technique of strapping.[60] Antonio Benivieni (1443–1502) probably was the first to treat an incarcerated hernia in a child; he ligated the hernia. Once the mortified flesh fell off, the child "regained perfect health."[23] In 1737, Queen Caroline of England had an incarcerated hernia that eventually was lanced to permit drainage of intestinal matter. She succumbed to her illness, however, because surgical treatment had been delayed for 3 days while she was treated with polypharmacy, enemas, aperients, and bleeding.[20] In his *Anatomy of the Human Body*, published in 1740, William Cheselden describes a patient with an incarcerated umbilical hernia in whom he amputated the protruding mass of "mortified bowel and left the end of the sound gut hanging out of the navel to which it afterwards adhered: she recovered and lived many years after, voiding excrement through the intestine at the navel."[23] Credit for modern surgical treatment of umbilical hernias is given to William J. Mayo,[41,42] who repaired these de-

fects by overlapping fascia downward from above ("vest-over-pants").

EMBRYOLOGY AND ANATOMY OF THE UMBILICUS

The complex embryology of the umbilical region can be simplified as follows. Fascial margins of the umbilical defect are formed by the 3rd week of fetal life when the four folds of somatopleure tend to fold inward. An umbilical cord is produced in the 5th week. By the 10th week of embryonic life, abdominal contents return from their location outside the coelom into the developing abdominal cavity. The vitelline duct and the allantois regress by the 15th to 16th week. If any of these processes are defective, umbilical malformations occur.[17]

At birth, the umbilical arteries and the vitelline vein become thrombosed, and the vitelline duct and the allantois already have been obliterated. The umbilical ring then scars and contracts. The obliterated umbilical vein (round ligament) usually is attached to the inferior border of the umbilical ring along with remnants of the urachus and the two obliterated umbilical arteries. The round ligament, by crossing and partially covering the umbilical ring, may protect against herniation. In instances where the ligament divides and inserts in the upper part of the umbilical ring without crossing it, a potential weakness is present. The umbilical fascia of Richet also reinforces the umbilical ring. If the Richet fascia is absent, located outside the limits of the umbilical ring, or only partially covers the ring, the area appears much weaker.[46] Askar[2] believes that variations in decussation of aponeurotic fibers in the midline have a role in the occurrence of umbilical and paraumbilical hernias.

CLASSIFICATION

Umbilical hernia may be classified as one of the following types: (1) infantile umbilical hernia, (2) acquired umbilical hernia, (3) paraumbilical hernia (supraumbilical or infraumbilical), or (4) umbilical hernia in adults.

Infantile Umbilical Hernia

In children, umbilical hernias may be the third most common surgical disorder after hydroceles and inguinal hernias. They occur in about one in every five births.[60] Blumberg[7] is the only published author who believes that there is no racial predisposition to umbilical hernias. In his report from Johannesburg, South Africa, 23% of black and 19% of white children had umbilical hernias. The incidence was 25% for black females and 21% for white females. Among males, blacks had an incidence of 22%, whereas whites had an incidence of 17%. In contrast, James[31] reported from Cape Town, South Africa, that 19.8% of Xhosa infants and children had umbilical hernias. All reports from the United States indicate that the incidence of umbilical hernia is as much as eight times higher in black infants as in white infants. Both sexes seem to be affected equally.[16,22,55] Jelliffe,[33] reporting from the West Indies, found that 58.5% of children of African origin had umbilical hernias, compared to 8% of white children, 3.3% of "East Indian" children, and 1.3% of children of Chinese origin. In East Africa, 60% of black infants have umbilical hernias compared to only 4% of Asian infants.[38] In the United States, 32% to 42% of black infants have umbilical hernias.[16,22] The reason for the increased incidence of umbilical hernia in black infants is not clear. Mahorner[99] attributes it to a lack of umbilical fascia. Jelliffe[33] believes it is related to the "skin type" of the umbilicus in which the cord stops $1/4$ to $3/4$ of an inch from the abdomen, being joined there by a tubular projection of peritoneum-lined integument. Crump[16] and Woods[60] have blamed rickets, malnutrition, poor prenatal and postnatal care, colic, and constipation for the development of umbilical hernias, without convincing supportive evidence.

Prematurity and low birth weight are known to predispose to umbilical hernias.[16] Vohr and colleagues[57] studied a group composed almost entirely of white infants at 3 months of age and found umbilical hernias in 75% of those who weighed less than 1500 g at birth; all the hernias resolved spontaneously by 12 months of age. They felt that there was an association between the diagnosis of respiratory distress syndrome in the immediate postnatal period and the development of umbilical hernias, possibly related to the effect of increased intraabdominal pressure associated with the respiratory distress syndrome on inadequately developed anterior abdominal muscle and fascia. Evans[22] found the incidence of umbilical hernia to be 84% in babies weighing between 1000 and 1500 g, 38% in those weighing between 1500 and 2000 g, and 20.5% in those weighing between 2000 and 2500 g at birth. Woods[60] noted an increased incidence of umbilical hernias in infants with a birth weight of more than 3200 g. He postulated that the large size of the umbilical cord in these infants may predispose to persistence of the defect. A study performed by Sibley and coworkers,[55] however, do not support such a correlation. An unexplained higher incidence of umbilical hernias has been reported in Jamaican children with delayed closure of the anterior fontanelle.[14] Umbilical hernias also are common in children with Down syndrome, hypothyroidism, mucopolysaccharidoses (particularly Hurler syndrome), Beckwith syndrome, and trisomy 13 and 18.[6,60] The tendency to spontaneous resolution is maintained in patients with Down syndrome. There also appears to be a 9% to 12% familial predisposition to umbilical hernias.[1,16,55,60] but no genetic pattern of inheritance has been identified and the incidence is difficult to evaluate statistically. In sets of identical twins, both children invariably are affected.[31,60]

Diagnosis

Although there may be a history of vague intermittent abdominal pain, most children with umbilical hernia are seen for the obvious cosmetic defect. The hernia results in a cone-like protrusion at the umbilicus that bulges every time the child cries or strains (Fig. 24-1). The size of the facial defect must be evaluated, and this is done best with the patient supine. A collar of fibrous tissue typically is found at the neck of the sac. It should be determined whether the defect is circular or elliptic and, if it is elliptic, whether the long axis is transverse or vertical. The linea alba immediately above the umbilicus also should be evaluated to identify a coexisting paraumbilical hernia or diastasis recti.

Differential Diagnosis. Umbilical hernia must be differentiated from hernia of the umbilical cord, which consists of a small umbilical defect through which intestines herniate into the base of the cord. This defect is covered with peritoneum and does not have skin coverage. It is particularly important to identify this lesion at birth and to avoid clamping or

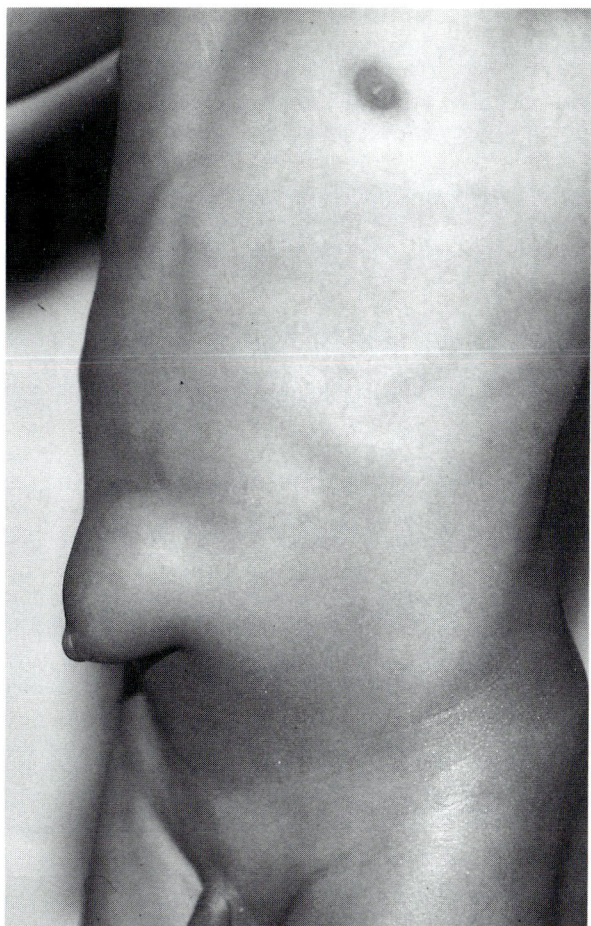

Figure 24-1. A 6-year-old black male with a large infantile umbilical hernia. The typical conical shape is maintained, although it is starting to droop downward.

dividing the wide base of the cord, which results in inadvertent enterectomy. An umbilical granuloma is a subacute infection at the umbilicus that is treated with the application of silver nitrate. If two to three applications do not result in resolution of the problem, an umbilical polyp (which is covered with pinched-off intestinal mucosa), an omphalomesenteric duct, or a urachus must be considered. Remnants of the omphalomesenteric duct and urachus also can produce cystic masses within the umbilicus. In addition, the fact that metastatic tumor nodules (Sister Joseph's nodules) occur at the umbilicus should be kept in mind.[53] An incarcerated umbilical hernia may be simulated by an abscess of the obliterated umbilical artery[40] or by primary bacterial peritonitis.[10] We have seen patients with peritonitis caused by infected ventriculoperitoneal shunts who had tender, erythematous umbilical hernias. Finally, patients with bowel obstruction from

other causes may have an irreducible umbilical hernia that is not truly incarcerated.

Natural History

There is general agreement that infantile umbilical hernias tend to resolve spontaneously. Unfortunately, no prospective, longitudinal studies of a stable population followed up from infancy to adulthood are available to provide clear guidelines. Blumberg[7] flatly states that all infantile umbilical hernias close by the age of 3 to 4 years. In his opinion, only "indirect" or adult-type umbilical hernias do not resolve spontaneously. Woods,[60] Sibley and coworkers,[55] and Walker[59] have observed that umbilical hernias persisting after the age of 5 to 6 years are unlikely to close spontaneously, and Crump[16] found no cases of umbilical hernia in children older than 7 years. Hall and associates[26] carried out a statistical evaluation of black children between 4 and 11 years of age, and estimated that half the hernias present at 4 to 5 years closed spontaneously by 11 years. Although his is not a longitudinal study, it does offer indirect evidence that spontaneous closure of umbilical hernias continues, even after the age of 5 years. Mack[38] has reported healing of umbilical hernias until puberty, but not after.

The size of the umbilical ring appears to have a direct influence on the spontaneous resolution of umbilical hernias. Walker[59] observed 314 black children over a 6-year period and found that 96% of hernias with a fascial ring of less than 0.5 cm at the age of 3 months healed spontaneously, usually within 2 years. If the ring had a diameter greater than 1 cm, it did not close until after the age of 4 years, and none of the defects that had a ring larger than 1.5 cm resolved spontaneously by the age of 6 years. The possibility that defects larger than 1.5 cm may persist into adult life was suggested by Jackson and Moglen[30] in a retrospective study. Heifetz and colleagues[28] observed over a 4-year period 78 infants with umbilical hernias that had a fascial ring exceeding 0.5 cm in diameter. Seventy-two hernias disappeared spontaneously, 31 in the first year of life, 20 in the second year, 16 in the third year, and 5 after more than 3 years. He observed that these hernias disappeared by gradual contraction of the ring until there no longer was room for intraabdominal contents to protrude. More than 30% of the rings began to close in the first month. The remainder did not start to close for varying periods, but once closure started, it continued at a rate of 18% of the area per month and occlusion occurred almost invariably in less than a year. Thus, larger defects took longer to close than did smaller ones, but closure always was complete within less than a year, and often within 6 months. He also found that hernial protrusions did not change in volume until just before resolution, when they disappeared almost overnight.

Coupled with the natural tendency to closure of the fascial ring is the fact that complications of infantile umbilical hernias are extremely uncommon. Morgan and associates[44] observed only 7 incarcerated infantile umbilical hernias over a 14-year period during which he saw 101 incarcerated umbilical hernias in adults. In western countries, complications have been reported only in the study by Lassaletta and coworkers.[35] In a series of 590 children, he found a 5.1% incidence of complications, which included incarceration, strangulation, and evisceration. In my experience of the past 15 years, only three cases have required emergency surgery, two for incarceration of the transverse colon caused by inspissated feces (Fig. 24-2) and one for strangulated omentum (Fig. 24-3). Although they are rare, complications of umbilical hernias have been reported and consist of strangulation of the omentum,[52,55] strangulation of the intestine,[32] and evisceration.[8,50,54] The reported incidence of complications has been higher in studies from Asia[11,13] and the Middle East[18] than in those from western countries.

Treatment

In a child with no physical or psychological symptoms and a fascial defect less than 1.5 cm in diameter, we recommend that herniorrhaphy be delayed until the age of 5 years in anticipation of spontaneous closure. A child with a proboscoid hernia often is subjected to ridicule, however, and because the hernial defect usually is larger than 1.5 cm in diameter, repair at the age of 3 years is appropriate. If a child has a tender hernia, even if it is reduced, we recommend early surgical correction. It is possible that, given enough time, all umbilical hernias would resolve.[26,28] In the meantime, though, the child must live with an obvious deformity. We believe that umbilical herniorrhaphy definitely should be carried out by the time the child is in first grade, for psychological reasons. Patients who have a defect in the ring but no protuberance can be observed until the age of 9 or 10 years, or even longer.

Taping of umbilical hernias seems to have no value and actually may result in maceration of the underlying skin or even death if umbilical binders are extremely tight.[21] There are those who believe that strapping prevents local stress, which seems to be an important factor in promoting the muscular and fascial strength required for spontaneous closure of the umbilical orifice.[7] Furthermore, the placement of a coin in the defect before strapping actually provides an obturator in the defect and prevents contraction of the cicatrix. A coin placed in the umbilicus also has been blamed for maceration of skin and rupture of the umbilical hernia.[55] Finally, strapping does not prevent strangulation of the hernia under the strap.[1]

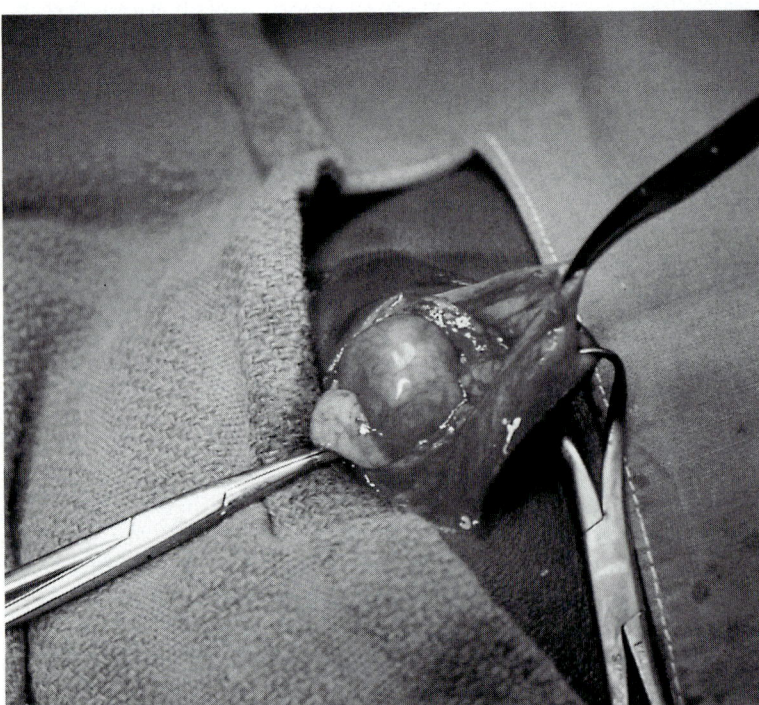

Figure 24-2. Incarcerated but viable transverse colon in an infantile umbilical hernia resulting from inspissated feces.

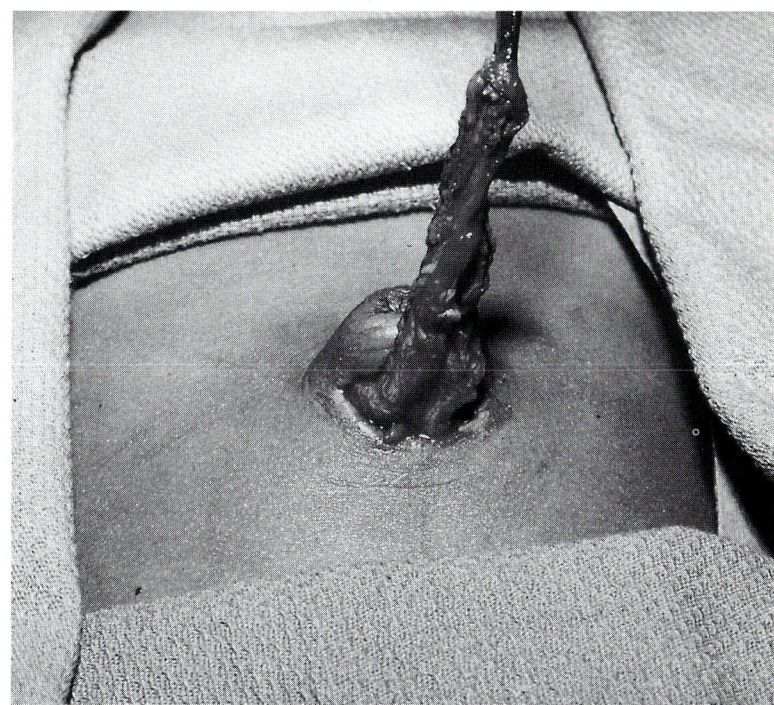

Figure 24-3. Incarcerated infantile umbilical hernia with strangulated omentum that was adherent to the undersurface of the cicatrix.

Operative Technique

Elective repair of umbilical hernias in children is performed on an outpatient basis using general anesthesia. With the patient in the supine position, the apex of the umbilicus is elevated with a towel clip and a curvilinear "smile" incision is made within a skin fold on the inferior aspect of the hernia. The incision is carried through subcutaneous fat to expose the caudad aspect of the sac (Fig. 24-4B). The sac then is encircled by blunt dissection with a hemostat. In large hernias, which tend to flare out at the fundus, it is easier to carry out the dissection close to the neck of the sac. Once encircled, the sac is incised on its caudad aspect (see Fig. 24-4C). Because abdominal contents adhere to the fundus of the sac, such an incision avoids inadvertent damage to them. Once the sac has been entered and the contents reduced, the incision is carried around to the cephalad aspect of the sac (see Fig. 24-4D). The cut edges of the sac then are held up to permit abdominal contents to fall back into the peritoneal cavity while horizontal mattress sutures are placed at the edges of the fascial defect, using nonabsorbable material of appropriate size (see Fig. 24-4E). We make no attempt to separate peritoneum from fascia and do not "double-breast" the repair. Occasionally, umbilical vessels may require ligation. It usually is easier to obtain a tension-free repair in the transverse direction. If the defect is larger vertically or there is an associated supraumbilical defect, a lon-

gitudinal closure is more appropriate. The redundant sac is excised. Electrocautery is useful in obtaining hemostasis (see Fig. 24-4E). A small button of the fundus of the sac is left attached to the inner surface of the cicatrix and is tacked down to the area of the fascial repair with one nonabsorbable suture (see Fig. 24-4F). After meticulous hemostasis has been ensured, subcutaneous tissues are approximated with interrupted absorbable sutures and a subcuticular skin closure is carried out, also with absorbable sutures (see Fig. 24-4G). A compression dressing is left in place for 4 to 7 days. I place cotton balls soaked in alcohol over the umbilicus and retain them in place with an Elastoplast bandage. Once the alcohol evaporates, the cotton ball dries in the shape of the umbilicus and maintains firm, uniform pressure.

Other techniques of managing the sac include that of Miller, who dissects the entire sac and inverts it into the abdominal cavity without opening it,[54] and that of Benjamin and coworkers,[5] who dissects the sac from the umbilicus, twists it, and then suture ligates it at the fascia before excising its redundant portion. In both these techniques, the sac and fascia are repaired separately. Complications of umbilical herniorrhaphy are extremely uncommon if meticulous hemostasis is carried out. The patient should be observed for the formation of a seroma or hematoma and the development of secondary infection. Recurrence is possible if large defects are closed under tension, or if an as-

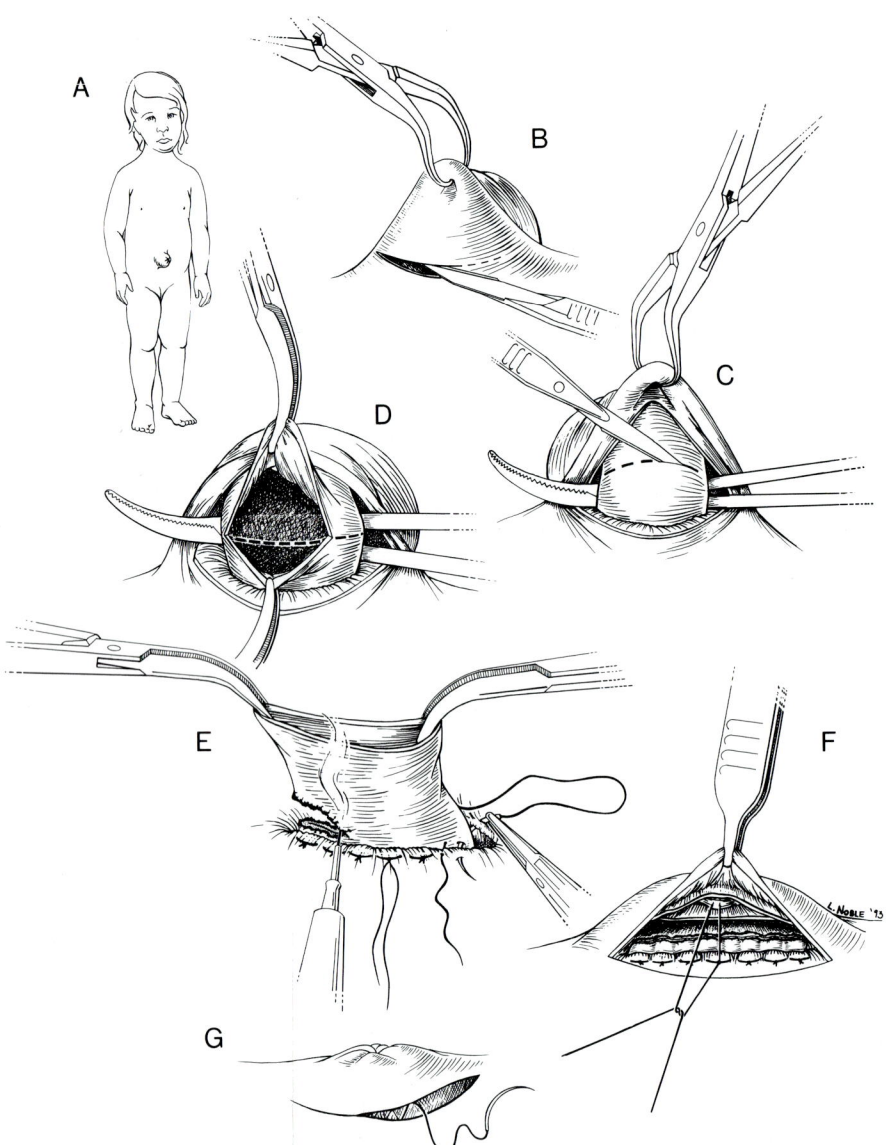

Figure 24-4. (*A*) The typical infantile umbilical hernia. (*B*) The hernia is held at the cicatrix with a towel clip and is elevated. A subumbilical "smile" incision is made in a skin fold. (*C*) The hernia sac is encircled completely by a clamp and is being opened on its caudal aspect. (*D*) The sac is entered and the contents are reduced. The cephalad aspect of the sac then is incised. (*E*) After the fascial defect is repaired with horizontal mattress sutures, the redundant part of the sac is excised using electrocautery. (*F*) The button of sac left on the undersurface of the umbilicus is tacked down to the repaired fascia. (*G*) The subcutaneous tissues are repaired with interrupted sutures of chronic catgut and the skin is closed with a running subcuticular suture of chronic catgut.

sociated paraumbilical hernia is overlooked. We follow Ravitch's[50] suggestion that the undersurface of the linea alba be palpated through the umbilical defect to identify any coexisting paraumbilical hernias.

Concern regarding redundancy of periumbilical skin always exists in large umbilical hernias (see Fig. 24-1). If it is tacked down properly and pressure is applied to prevent the formation of a hematoma, this skin will shrink down to a normal appearance over time. On rare occasions, it may be worthwhile to excise the redundant skin. Various techniques have been described to reconstruct an umbilicus under such circumstances.[15,29,51] I have found the technique described by Jona[34] to be the most satisfactory. This consists of raising a flap based either superiorly or

inferiorly. The flap is about 2.5 cm long and 2.5 cm wide at its distal end. The base is about 1 cm wider than the tip. The flap is sutured into a tube with absorbable sutures so that the epidermis is on the inside. The tube is closed at its tip, which is sutured to the fascia to create a skin-lined pit. I agree with Jona that "it will now collect lint, sand and dirt and should be able to hold a 5 carat Jewel"!

Acquired Umbilical Hernia

Patients with acute abdominal distention (eg, intestinal obstruction) often have a partially unfolded umbilicus. If the intraabdominal pressure persists, the

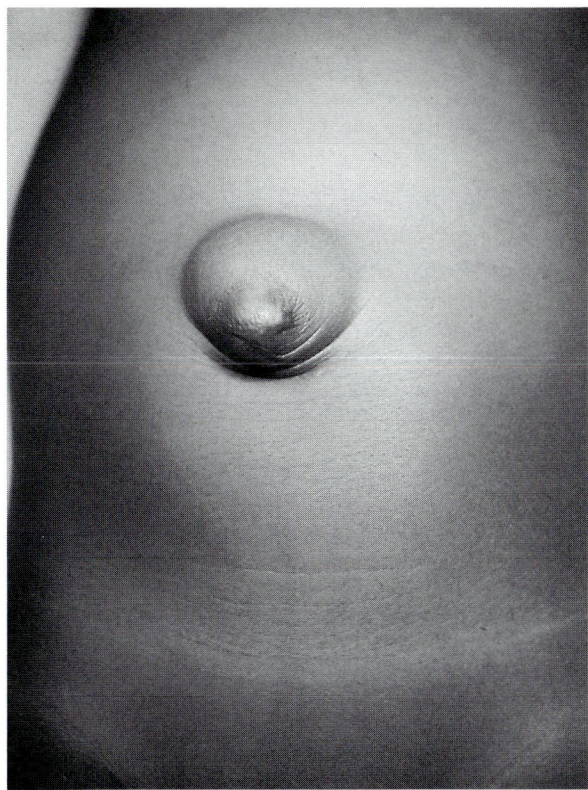

Figure 24-5. Paraumbilical (supraumbilical) hernia in a child. Note that the lower half of the fundus is covered by the cicatrix, whereas the upper half is covered by supraumbilical skin. This is in contrast to Figure 24-6.

umbilical cicatrix gives way, resulting in an acquired umbilical hernia. Acquired hernias may be noted in patients who have ascites resulting from cirrhosis, congestive heart failure, or nephrosis.[55] Patients undergoing peritoneal dialysis also have a higher incidence of umbilical hernias.[56,58] Patients with serious underlying problems generally should not undergo operation unless the hernia incarcerates or becomes extremely large and the overlying skin is thinned down to such an extent that spontaneous rupture is possible.

Paraumbilical Hernia

Paraumbilical hernias occur in all age groups. These lesions are the result of defects in the linea alba and the umbilical fascia, which is a direct extension of the transversalis fascia.[2] They generally are seen in the supraumbilical linea alba, but can occur below the umbilicus. They may occur in association with umbilical hernias and can be multiple when associated with diastasis recti. Paraumbilical hernias do not resolve spontaneously. These patients may have intermittent

abdominal pain (possibly caused by dragging on the fat and peritoneum of the falciform ligament), incarceration, inflammation, or gangrene of the contents (which can occur if the pedicle twists on itself or is gripped tightly at the aponeurosis).

Diagnosis

Supraumbilical hernias must be differentiated from umbilical hernias. In the supraumbilical hernia, about half the fundus of the sac is covered by the umbilicus and the remainder is covered by the skin of the abdomen immediately above the umbilicus (Fig. 24-5). This is in contrast to the umbilical hernia, in which the protrusion is directly under the umbilicus with a circumferentially symmetric bulge (Fig. 24-6). In addition, there is no collar of fibrous tissue at the neck. On occasion, small paraumbilical hernias may be difficult to identify. In such cases, the patient should stand erect and the physician should draw the pulp of the index finger along the linea alba from the xiphoid to the umbilicus and search for a small, palpable nodule, often tender, that indicates the site of herniation.

Operative Technique

Because these hernias do not resolve spontaneously and have a high incidence of incarceration and strangulation, surgical repair always is indicated. In patients with a small paraumbilical hernia separated from the umbilicus, it is advisable to use a skin marker to localize the lesion with the patient erect because it can be extremely difficult to identify once the patient is anesthetized and relaxed. For solitary lesions separated from the umbilicus, a transverse incision directly

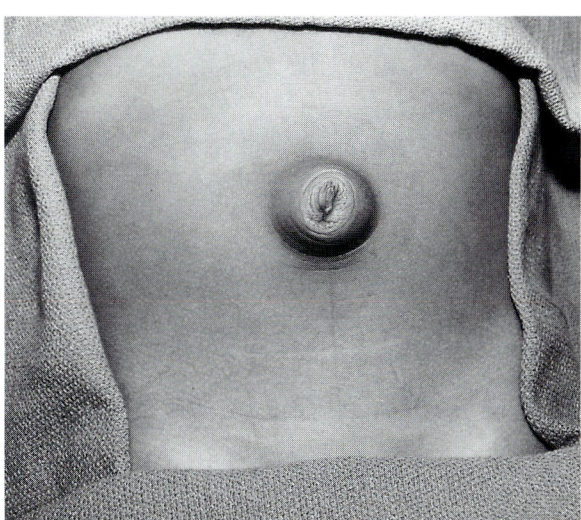

Figure 24-6. A typical umbilical hernia in a child, with the cicatrix in the center of the protrusion and symmetric swelling circumferentially.

over the hernia provides the best exposure. The incision is carried down to the protruding fat, and the linea alba on all sides is dissected out. If the fat is viable, it is reduced into the abdominal cavity and the defect is closed either transversely or vertically, depending on the defect. In patients with strangulated or infected fat, it is best to amputate the herniated preperitoneal fat. In patients with a paraumbilical hernia associated with an umbilical hernia, the incision can be made in the same fashion as for an infantile umbilical hernia except that it is made on the cephalad aspect of the umbilicus. In such cases, a vertical fascial closure generally provides the best results. In patients with multiple fascial defects, the entire linea alba may have to be repaired up to the xiphoid.

Umbilical Hernia in Adults

It is generally believed that umbilical hernias in adults do not represent persistence of infantile hernias, even though Morgan,[44] Haller,[27] and their associates, based on their experience at Johns Hopkins Hospital, have suggested prophylactic repair of umbilical hernias in children to prevent incarceration in adults. Jackson and Moglen,[30] in a retrospective review of adults with umbilical hernias, found that only 10.9% recalled having hernias from childhood. In a series of 71 women, Sibley and coworkers[55] noted that only 2 had recurrence of an umbilical hernia during pregnancy. In both cases, the hernia resolved completely after delivery. One of the women had a recurrence with each of her three pregnancies. None of the 82 men followed up by Sibley and coworkers[55] had a recurrence of their umbilical hernia. In contrast to the infantile hernia, which is a direct hernia, umbilical hernias in adults are indirect herniations through an umbilical canal that is bordered by umbilical fascia posteriorly, the linea alba anteriorly, and the medial edges of the two rectus sheaths on each side.[7,60] Therefore, these hernias tend to incarcerate and strangulate, and do not resolve spontaneously. Askar[2] believes that they actually are paraumbilical hernias that occur just above and to the left of the umbilicus. The incidence of incarceration of umbilical hernias in adults is 14 times that in children. In addition, there is high associated morbidity and mortality. More than 90% of these patients are women, and almost all are obese and multiparous. In this patient population, umbilical hernias incarcerate half as often as do inguinal hernias and three times more often than do femoral hernias.[44] Although Morgan and colleagues[44] report a predominance of black patients, Jackson and Moglen[30] found no racial differ-

ence in incidence. Umbilical hernias in adults also are common in cirrhotic patients with ascites; Chapman and associates[12] have reported an incidence of 24%. It appears that a persistent increase in intraabdominal pressure exerted against a thinned-out umbilical ring and fascia is the cause of herniation in both the cirrhotic patient with ascites and the obese multipara. Umbilical hernias may rupture spontaneously in cirrhotic patients with ascites.[9,25] Unless ascites is controlled before the hernia is repaired[36] or a peritoneovenous shunt is placed at the time of herniorrhaphy, these patients have a high morbidity and mortality, and the hernia tends to recur.[4,9,37] During preoperative care, it must be kept in mind that the hernia may incarcerate as the ring narrows down with successful medical treatment[4,36] or on placement of a peritoneovenous shunt.[19] In a retrospective study, Pescovitz[47] has demonstrated that cirrhotic patients can be operated on without an increase in variceal bleeding. This study contradicts a previous report indicating that umbilical herniorrhaphy interrupts periumbilical portosystemic venous collaterals and increases the likelihood of variceal bleeding by inducing acute portal hypertension.[3]

Diagnosis

The diagnosis of umbilical hernia in adults usually is obvious (Fig. 24-7). In large hernias, complete reduction often is unsuccessful because omentum becomes adherent to the sac. As the hernia enlarges, it becomes oval and has a tendency to sag downward. Patients may complain of a local, dragging pain because of the weight of the lesion. Gastrointestinal symptoms are common, and probably result from traction on the stomach or transverse colon. Attacks of intermittent colicky pain may be caused by subacute intestinal obstruction. In long-standing cases, maceration of adjacent skin surfaces by the panniculus can be noted.

Operative Technique

Nonoperative therapy with a truss is uniformly unsuccessful because these hernias are loculated and often only partially reducible. Furthermore, the hernial orifice lies deep inside fat and cannot be reached by the pad on the truss.[2] In elective cases, it is important to identify the underlying associated pathology and to try and improve the general status of the patient before undertaking surgical correction. These patients often have incarcerated hernias, however, and prolonged preoperative therapy is not possible.

These high-risk adult patients generally are operated on using regional or local anesthesia. In smaller adult umbilical hernias, a subumbilical inci-

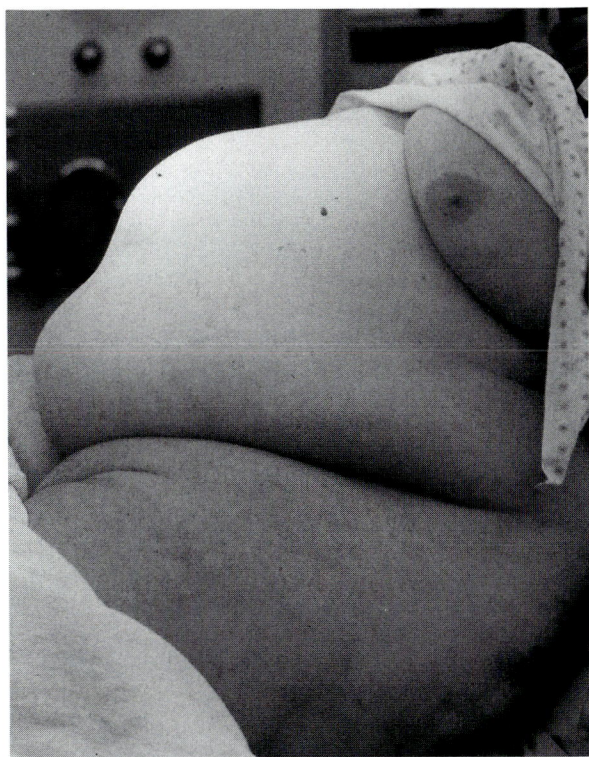

Figure 24-7. An extremely obese, multiparous middle-aged woman with a large incarcerated adult type of umbilical hernia. The fatty panniculus hangs down to the pubis. She had to be anesthetized in the upright position because she was unable to breathe when supine. Strangulated cecum was found in the hernia. Postoperatively, the patient required prolonged ventilatory support, tracheostomy, and a 3-week intensive care unit stay. She finally recovered and was discharged home after 6 weeks in the hospital.

sion can be used, but large hernias, and particularly incarcerated hernias, often require a large incision. Dissection is carried through the subcutaneous fat down to the aponeurotic layer above, below, and on the sides of the sac. The entire mass of skin, fat, and hernia is elevated while the neck of the sac is incised, because adhesions of the omentum or underlying bowel are more likely at the fundus. The incarcerated contents must be evaluated and treated as required. Richter hernias occur occasionally and must be sought carefully. After the contents are dealt with, the sac is repaired and edge-to-edge closure is carried out in either the transverse or the vertical direction, whichever is appropriate. The classic vest-over-pants operation[41,42] generally has been discarded since Farris and coworkers[24] demonstrated that the bursting strength of the wound did not improve by imbrication and actually was impaired to a degree that was pro-

portional to the amount of overlapping and tension. Metheny[43] discussed Farris' paper and indicated that he noted no adhesions between the smooth, peritoneum-covered upper fascial flap and the lower one in a patient on whom he operated for recurrent umbilical hernia 40 years after the original procedure.

The overlying umbilical skin usually should not be excised unless it is macerated or infected. In such cases, a new umbilicus could be created.[24] Askar[2] warns against this, however, because it has been his experience that recurrences occur at the point on the linea alba where the umbilicus is created. To achieve closure without stress in larger hernias, the anterior and posterior rectus sheaths may be incised laterally. On occasion, strips of fascia lata or a prosthetic mesh may be required to obtain tension-free closure.[2] Repair is carried out with nonabsorbable sutures of appropriate size. If the possibility of infection is high, a synthetic, long-lasting but absorbable material may be a better choice. Furthermore, if wound sepsis is feared, the subcutaneous fat and skin should be left open and plans made for delayed primary closure.

Complications include the development of seromas, hematomas, and infections. In addition to local problems, these patients often have respiratory and cardiovascular complications and may require prolonged hospitalization. Recurrence of these hernias appears to be extremely uncommon.[49]

REFERENCES

1. Angel-Lord G. Infantile umbilical hernia. To strap or not to strap. Med J Aust 1971;1:83.
2. Askar OM. Aponeurotic hernias. Recent observations upon paraumbilical and epigastric hernias. Surg Clin North Am 1984;64:315.
3. Baron HC. Umbilical hernia secondary to cirrhosis of the liver. Complications of surgical correction. N Engl J Med 1960;263:824.
4. Belghiti J, Desgrandchamps F, Farges O, Fekete F. Herniorrhaphy and concomitant peritoneovenous shunting in cirrhotic patients with umbilical hernia. World J Surg 1990;14:242.
5. Benjamin B, Vinocur CD, Wagner CW, Weintraub WH. A closed technique for umbilical hernia repair. Surg Gynecol Obstet 1987;164:473.
6. Bergsma D, ed. Birth defects compendium, ed 2. New York, Alan R Liss Inc, 1979.
7. Blumberg NA. Infantile umbilical hernia. Surg Gynecol Obstet 1980;150:187.
8. Buckley DJ, Pemberton PJ. Rupture (evisceration) of an umbilical hernia. (Letter) Med J Aust 1988; 149:715.
9. Bunt TJ, Mohr JD. Ruptured umbilical hernia in cir-

rhotic patients: management with peritoneovenous shunting and herniorrhaphy. South Med J 1985; 78:755.

10. Cameron BH. Two cases of primary bacterial peritonitis presenting with a tender hernia. Aust N Z J Surg 1991;61:794.

11. Channa A, ulHasan N. Opsite-strapping for the treatment of infantile umbilical hernia. J Pak Med Assoc 1984;34:306.

12. Chapman CB, Snell AM, Rowntree L. Decompensated portal cirrhosis: report of one hundred and twelve cases. N Engl J Med 1931;97:237.

13. Chatterjee H, Bhat SM. Incarcerated umbilical hernia in children. J Indian Med Assoc 1986;84:238.

14. Cohen IP. Umbilical hernias and anterior fontanelle size in Jamaican children. West Indian Med J 1989; 38:91.

15. Cone JB, Golladay ES. Purse-string skin closure of umbilical hernia repair. J Pediatr Surg 1983;18:297.

16. Crump EP. Umbilical hernia. I. Occurrence of the infantile type in Negro infants and children. J Pediatr 1952;40:214.

17. Cullen TS. Embryology, anatomy and diseases of the umbilicus together with diseases of the urachus. Philadelphia, WB Saunders, 1916:1.

18. Doraiswamy NV, AlBadr MSK, Issa MA. Obstructed umbilical hernias in childhood in Kuwait—Richter—and other types. Z Kinderchir 1981;32:301.

19. Eisenstadt S. Symptomatic umbilical hernias after peritoneovenous shunts. Arch Surg 1979;114:1443.

20. Ellis H. The umbilical hernia of Queen Caroline. Contemporary Surgery 1980;17:83.

21. Emory JL. Infant deaths associated with tight umbilical binders. Proc R Soc Med 1967;60:10.

22. Evans AG. The comparative incidence of umbilical hernias in colored and white infants. J Natl Med Assoc 1941;33:158.

23. Farris JM. Umbilical hernia. In: Nyhus LM, Harkins HN, eds. Hernia. Philadelphia, JB Lippincott, 1964: 315.

24. Farris JM, Smith GK, Beattie AS. Umbilical hernia: an inquiry into the principle of imbrication and a note on the preservation of the umbilical dimple. Am J Surg 1959;98:236.

25. Fisher J, Calkins WG. Spontaneous umbilical hernia rupture: a report of three cases. Am J Gastroenterol 1978;69:689.

26. Hall DE, Roberts KB, Charney E. Umbilical hernia: what happens after age 5 years? J Pediatr 1981; 98:415.

27. Haller JA, Morgan WW Jr, Stumbaugh S, White JJ. Repair of umbilical hernias in childhood to prevent adult incarceration. Am Surg 1971;37:245.

28. Heifetz CJ, Bilsel ZT, Gaus WW. Observations on the disappearance of umbilical hernias of infancy and childhood. Surg Gynecol Obstet 1963;116:469.

29. Itoh Y, Arai K. Umbilical reconstruction using a cone-shaped flap. Ann Plast Surg 1992;28:335.

30. Jackson OJ, Moglen LH. Umbilical hernia: a retrospective study. Calif Med 1970;113:8.

31. James T. Umbilical hernia in Xhosa infants and children. J Royal Soc Med 1982;75:537.

32. Jeans PL, Wright JE. Strangulated umbilical hernia in infancy. Aust Paediatr J 1984;20:75.

33. Jelliffe DB. The racial incidence of umbilical hernia. J Trop Med Hyg 1954;57:270.

34. Jona JZ. Reconstruction of a lost umbilicus. In: Raffensperger JG, ed. Swenson's pediatric surgery, ed 4. New York, Appleton-Century-Crofts, 1980:175.

35. Lassaletta L, Fonkalsrud EW, Tovar JA, Dudgeon D, Asch MJ. The management of umbilical hernias in infancy and childhood. J Pediatr Surg 1975;10:405.

36. Lemmer JH, Strodel WE, Eckhauser FE. Umbilical hernia incarceration: a complication of medical therapy of ascites. Am J Gastroenterol 1983;78:295.

37. Leonetti JP, Aranha GV, Wilkinson WA, Stanley M, Greenlee HB. Umbilical herniorrhaphy in cirrhotic patients. Arch Surg 1984;119:442.

38. Mack NK. The incidence of umbilical herniae in Africans. East Afr Med J 1945;22:369.

39. Mahorner H. Umbilical and midline ventral herniae. Ann Surg 1940;111:979.

40. Mares AJ, Siplovich L. Obliterated umbilical artery abscess simulating a strangulated umbilical hernia: a late complication of neonatal umbilical artery catheterization. Isr J Med Sci 1984;20:1197.

41. Mayo WJ. Remarks on the radical cure of hernia. Ann Surg 1899;29:51.

42. Mayo WJ. An operation for the radical cure of umbilical hernia. Ann Surg 1901;34:276.

43. Metheny D. Discussion of Farris JM, Smith GK, Beattie AS. Umbilical hernia: an inquiry into the principle of imbrication and a note on the preservation of the umbilical dimple. Am J Surg 1959;98:236.

44. Morgan WW, White JJ, Stumbaugh S, Haller JA Jr. Prophylactic umbilical hernia repair in childhood to prevent adult incarceration. Surg Clin North Am 1970;50:839.

45. Olch PD, Harkins HN. Historical survey of treatment of inguinal hernia. In: Nyhus LM, Harkins HN, eds. Hernia. Philadelphia, JB Lippincott, 1964:1.

46. Orda R, Nathan H. Surgical anatomy of the umbilical structures. Int Surg 1973;58:458.

47. Pescovitz MD. Umbilical hernia repair in patients with cirrhosis. No evidence for increased incidence of variceal bleeding. Ann Surg 1984;199:325.

48. Pilling GP IV. Umbilical hernia. In: Nyhus LM, Condon RE, eds. Hernia, ed 2. Philadelphia, JB Lippincott, 1978:362.

49. Pollak R, Nyhus LM. Epigastric, umbilical and ventral hernias. In: Cameron JL, ed. Current surgical therapy 1984–1985. Philadelphia, BC Decker, 1984:284.

50. Ravitch MM. Umbilical hernia in a child: in repair of hernias. Chicago, Year Book Medical Publishers, 1969:148.

51. Reyna TM, Hollis HW Jr, Smith SB. Surgical management of proboscoid herniae. J Pediatr Surg 1987; 22:911.

52. Rudran V, Jones R. Strangulated umbilical hernia in a child. (Letter) Br J Gen Pract 1992;42:440.

53. Sharaki M, Abdel-Kader M. Umbilical deposits from internal malignancy (the Sister Joseph's nodules). Br Assoc Surg Oncol 1981;7:351.

54. Shaw A. Umbilical hernia. In: Welch KJ, Randolph JG, Ravitch MM, O'Neill JA Jr, Rowe MI, eds. Pediatric surgery, ed 4. Chicago, Year Book Medical Publishers, 1986:735.

55. Sibley WL III, Lynn HB, Harris LE. A 25-year study of infantile umbilical hernia. Surgery 1964;55:462.

56. Tank ES, Hatch DA. Hernias complicating chronic ambulatory peritoneal dialysis in children. J Pediatr Surg 1986;21:41.

57. Vohr BR, Rosenfield AG, Oh W. Umbilical hernia in the low-birth-weight infant (less than 1500 gm). J Pediatr 1977;90:807.

58. von Lilien T, Salusky IB, Yap HK, Fonkalsrud EW, Fine RN. Hernias: a frequent complication in children treated with continuous peritoneal dialysis. Am J Kidney Dis 1987;10:356.

59. Walker SH. The natural history of umbilical hernia. A six-year follow-up of 314 negro children with this defect. Clin Pediatr (Phila) 1967;6:29.

60. Woods GE. Some observations on umbilical hernia in infants. Arch Dis Child 1953;28:450.

Editor's Comment

I was pleased that Radhakrishnan quoted Olch from the first edition of our monograph. When Peter D. Olch worked with Professor Henry N. Harkins on this history presentation, Olch was a junior surgical resident in our program at the University of Washington, Seattle. Shortly thereafter, Peter Olch entered a training program in pathology. Completing same, he then found his true calling, that is, the history of medicine. He became the Deputy Chief, History of Medicine Division, National Library of Medicine, National Institutes of Health, Bethesda, Maryland. Peter Olch will be remembered for his many contributions to our knowledge of medical history, but the most important was his study of William S. Halsted and his lifelong battle against drug addiction. Olch's review of this tale reads like a modern-day novel (Anesthesiology 1975; 42:479). Sadly, Peter D. Olch died of head and neck cancer in the early 1990s.

L.M.N.

Hernia, Fourth Edition, edited
by Lloyd M. Nyhus and Robert E. Condon.
J.B. Lippincott Company, Philadelphia © 1995.

Chapter 25

Epigastric Hernia

Arnold P. Robin

The anatomic feature common to all external hernias is a defect in the aponeurotic–fascial layer that lines the abdominal cavity. Hernias of the anterior abdominal wall aponeurosis that are located in the midline are referred to collectively as hernias of the linea alba. With the exception of umbilical hernias, the most common location of a midline fascial defect is between the xiphoid process and the umbilicus. These upper abdominal midline fascial defects are termed *epigastric hernias.*

HISTORICAL PERSPECTIVE

A review of the historical aspects of epigastric hernia reveals an evolution of the understanding of the anatomic–functional relations of the anterior abdominal wall.[11,19,25] The development of the current clinical approach to this entity also can be traced. Since the first clear-cut description in the mid-18th century by LeDran, the approach to this lesion has reflected the contemporary understanding of the pathophysiology of midline abdominal wall defects.

Arnauld de Villeneuve described an epigastric hernia in 1285, but it was not until 1743 that De-Garengeot first ascribed vague abdominal symptoms to this condition. In 1744, based on his finding of commonly noted gastric symptoms, Gunz promoted the concept that the stomach always was contained in the hernia sac, and thus referred to the lesion as a gastrocele. This concept was discounted by Richter 40 years later. The term *epigastric hernia* was introduced by Leveille in 1812. Detailed anatomic descriptions were provided by Bernitz in 1848 and Cruveilhier in 1849.

The first successful operation on this hernia was reported by Maunior in 1802. Until Terrier's[35] report in 1886, however, the procedure was shunned because of the frequent complication of peritonitis. In the ensuing years, with the advent and acceptance of aseptic technique, repair became more common. In 1887, Luecke[23] described two patients in whom repair of epigastric hernia was followed by the disappearance of chronic gastric symptoms. Perhaps undue en-

thusiasm later was attached to the operation; epigastric symptoms stemming from the intraabdominal disease often were overlooked or attributed incorrectly to the hernia. Numerous reports followed of epigastric hernia and coexisting intraabdominal disease. Capelle[7] reported on 31 instances of repair of epigastric hernias. Four patients later died of gastric carcinoma, 12 continued to have gastric symptoms, and 6 had a recurrence of the hernia. After these reports, the concept of an association between epigastric hernia and intraabdominal disease was touted.[11] Lewisohn[21] recommended that any patient with an epigastric hernia and associated gastrointestinal complaints undergo thorough abdominal exploration at the time of hernia repair.

In the early 20th century, many investigators alleged that traction on the stomach exerted by incarcerated omentum either caused or impaired healing of gastric ulcers.[15,34] Meyer and Ivy[26] simulated this situation experimentally in 14 dogs. Although anatomic deformities of the greater curvature were demonstrated, there were no ulcers. Later reports reflect the currently accepted approach.[8,18,24,29,31,36] In patients with epigastric hernias, the presence of gastrointestinal symptoms should prompt a thorough diagnostic evaluation. Epigastric hernia is an important clinical entity, however, that in and of itself may produce a variety of symptoms.

DEMOGRAPHICS

The actual incidence of epigastric hernia is difficult to determine. Many hernias produce no symptoms, and thus go undiagnosed. Autopsy studies indicate a prevalence of 0.5% to 10% in the general population. These hernias seldom are seen in infants and children. There is a male predominance, with a male:female ratio of at least 3:1. The diagnosis usually is made in the third through fifth decades, and congenital epigastric hernias are rare. The lesion is found with extraordinary frequency among the sepoys of India.[19]

Epigastric hernias account for 0.5% to 5% of all hernias operated on. Iason[19] quotes figures from a multicenter statistical study in which epigastric hernia repairs accounted for 0.7% of all hernia operations. Lindenstein[22] reported the surgical treatment of 850 hernias, of which 13 were epigastric. Of 816 hernias operated on over a 9-year period, Peters and Nesselrode[31] reported 28 epigastric hernias. Elechi,[9] reporting his experience in Nigeria, noted 8 (3.4%) epigastric hernias among 238 hernias repaired. The same author, reporting only strangulated abdominal wall hernias, found 3 of 53 (5.7%) to be epigastric.[10] Reports from the armed services show a somewhat higher proportion, perhaps because of the skewed population or the more frequent routine examination of young men who do not have symptoms. Heydorn and Velanovich[17] reported the United States Army experience with 36,250 hernia repairs over a 5-year period. It is unfortunate, and perhaps testimony to the status afforded this hernia, that epigastric hernias are lumped with other ventral hernias.

ANATOMY AND PATHOLOGY

The linea alba is the midline raphe formed by the junction of the rectus sheaths. It extends from the xiphoid process to the symphysis pubis. Superficial to the linea alba lie only skin and subcutaneous adipose tissue. Deep to the linea alba in the epigastric region is found transversalis fascia, preperitoneal fat, fat of the falciform ligament, and peritoneum. The rectus muscles diverge as they proceed superiorly to insert on the fifth, sixth, and seventh ribs, and on the costal cartilage. Although the linea alba is narrow below the umbilicus, it may be as much as 2.5 cm wide above it. This anatomic feature may account for the rarity of midline hernias below the umbilicus. Several paired neurovascular bundles traverse the linea alba on each side of the midline.

Askar[1] reported a detailed anatomic study of the anterior abdominal wall in 40 cadavers and 25 adult patients undergoing elective abdominal operations. He stressed the microscopic anatomy of the abdominal wall aponeuroses, and the structural–functional and biomechanical relations. Under the dissecting microscope, the anterior abdominal wall aponeuroses are seen to be fine tendinous fibers invested in loose areolar tissue and arranged as interwoven sheets (Fig. 25-1). This arrangement results in a triple-layer crisscross pattern in the anterior and posterior rectus sheaths, and contributes to the anatomic–functional linkage of the muscles of the anterior abdominal wall that allows them to work in concert (Figs. 25-2 and 25-3).

These tendinous fibers do not stop in the midline, but merely decussate, creating an intricate interwoven pattern and linking all layers of the abdominal wall with those of the opposite side. The midline zone generally is obvious to the operating surgeon, and appears whitish, hence the name *linea alba*. Above the umbilicus, the decussation may appear as a single line in the midline (30%) or, more commonly (70%), as a triple decussation pattern (Figs. 25-4 and 25-5). Below the umbilicus, a single line of decussation always is seen. A detailed description of this work also has been published by Askar.[3]

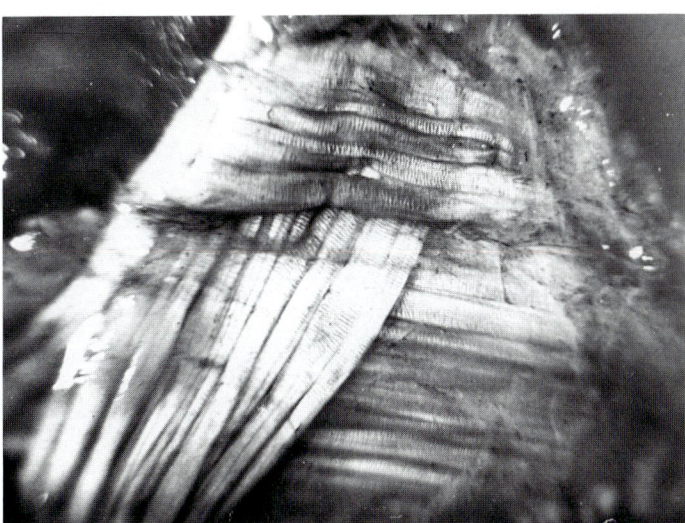

Figure 25-1. Anterior rectus sheath seen under the dissecting microscope. Note fine tendinous fibers arranged as interwoven sheets. (Askar OM. Surgical anatomy of the aponeurotic expansions of the anterior abdominal wall. Ann R Coll Surg Engl 1977;59:313)

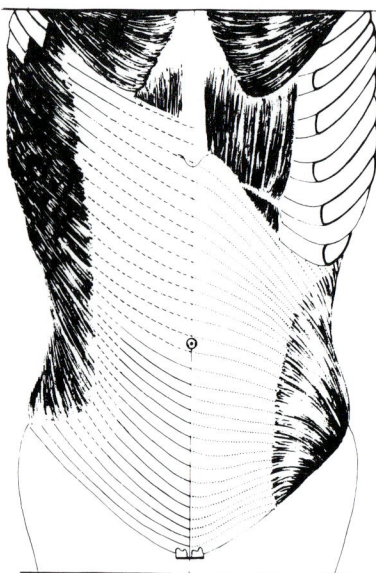

Figure 25-2. Digastric pattern between the external oblique aponeurosis (*right*) and the anterior lamina of the internal oblique aponeurosis (*left*). (Askar O. Surgical anatomy of the aponeurotic expansions of the anterior abdominal wall. Ann R Coll Surg Engl 1977;59:313–321)

Fascial defects may vary in diameter from a few millimeters to several centimeters. Smaller ones often are incarcerated, whereas larger ones usually are readily reducible. Most commonly, a preperitoneal mass of fat attached to the peritoneum by a pedicle is

herniated. The other variety is a true hernia with a peritoneal sac. Peters and Nesselrode,[31] Pollack,[32] and Wilkinson[36] found a sac to be present in 17 of 28, 26 of 45, and 2 of 16 cases, respectively. The sac usually contains omentum, with intestinal contents being rare and only occasional reports of strangulation. In about 20% of patients, multiple fascial defects are present.

ETIOLOGY AND PATHOGENESIS

Epigastric hernia generally is considered to be an acquired lesion, probably related to excessive strain on the anterior abdominal wall aponeuroses. Because of the anatomic features of the defect, however, some authors, such as Pollack,[32] favor a congenital origin. Moschowitz[27] emphasized the importance of blood vessels perforating the linea alba and prolongation of the transversalis fascia at this point. He expressed the opinion that preperitoneal fat enclosed in the falciform ligament would insinuate itself into the fascial foramen created by the vessel, enlarge it, and result in epigastric hernia. This explanation accounted for the uniform absence of a peritoneal sac and the consistent presence of a distinct vessel in his experience. Numerous authors[32,36] have challenged this theory, however, and only rarely have isolated vessels accompanying the hernial mass.

Askar[2,3] applied his studies of the anatomy and function of the anterior abdominal wall to the problem, and emphasized the importance of the pattern

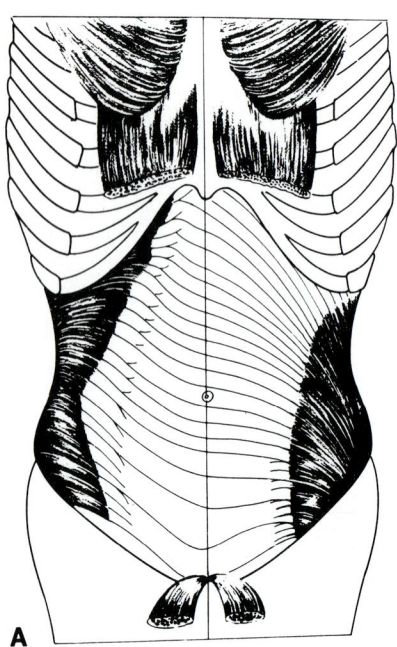

A

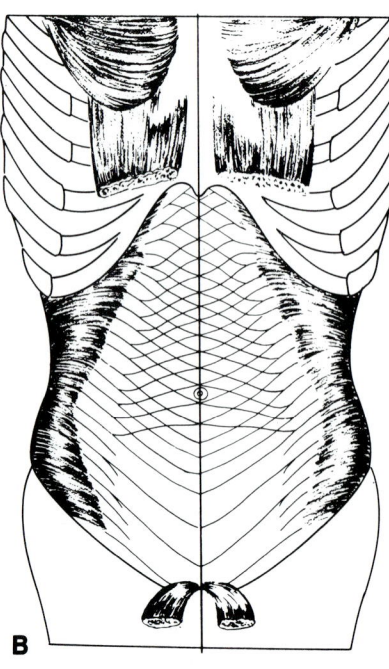

B

Figure 25-3. (*A*) Digastric pattern between the transversus (*right*) and the posterior lamina of the internal oblique aponeurosis (*left*). (*B*) Digastric pattern between the two transversi. (Askar O. Surgical anatomy of the aponeurotic expansions of the anterior abdominal wall. Ann R Coll Surg Engl 1977;59:313–321)

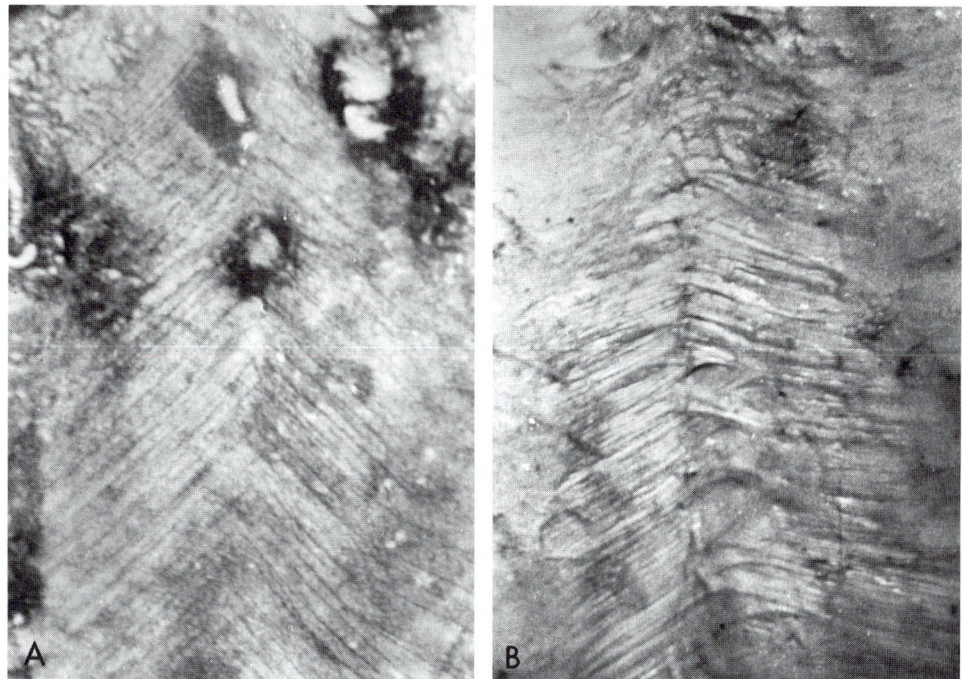

Figure 25-4. (*A*) Single and (*B*) triple pattern of decussation of the internal oblique aponeurosis seen in a midline epigastric incision. (Askar O. Surgical anatomy of the aponeurotic expansions of the anterior abdominal wall. Ann R Coll Surg Engl 1977;59:313–321)

of aponeurotic decussation in the pathogenesis of epigastric hernia. He observed epigastric hernias exclusively in patients who had a single midline pattern of decussation (see Figs. 25-4 and 25-5). The pathogenesis of epigastric hernia also can be related to the

structural–functional relations of the anterior abdominal wall. The midline aponeurotic area may be divided functionally into an upper abdominal "parachute" area, allowing respiratory motion, and a lower "belly support" area, divided by the lowest tendi-

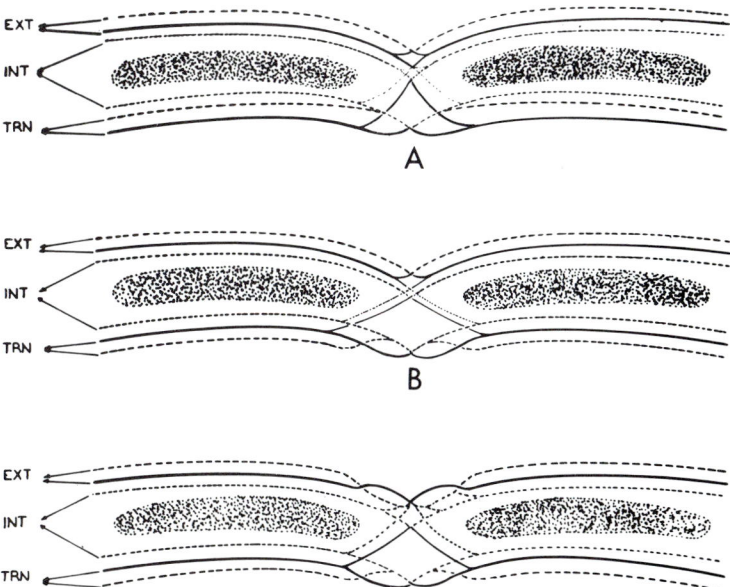

Figure 25-5. (*A*) Single anterior and single posterior lines of decussation (30%). (*B*) Single anterior and triple posterior lines of decussation (10%). (*C*) Triple anterior and triple posterior lines of decussation (60%). Ext, external oblique; int, internal oblique; trn, transversus. (Askar O. Surgical anatomy of the aponeurotic expansions of the anterior abdominal wall. Ann R Coll Surg Engl 1977;59:313–321)

nous intersection. The tendinous fibers are situated obliquely in the aponeurotic sheets, allowing for changes in the shape of the abdominal wall such as would be required during respiration. The midline can change only in length and breadth, however, with an increase in one necessitating a decrease in the other. During abdominal distention, the linea alba must increase in both dimensions. The resultant tearing of fibers or widening of spaces between fibers may play a role in the development of epigastric hernia.

Askar's studies also demonstrated that fibers originating from the diaphragm traverse the upper midline aponeurosis posteriorly and join with fibers of the posterior rectus sheath and middle tendinous intersection. They attach to the linea alba at a site midway between the xiphoid and the umbilicus. These fibers may coordinate respiratory movements of the diaphragm and upper abdomen. Uncoordinated, vigorous, synchronous contraction of the diaphragm and upper abdomen may occur during events such as straining and coughing. The force caused by upward traction on the diaphragm and lateral traction on the tendinous intersection would be maximal at this point of attachment midway between the xiphoid and the umbilicus, the most common site of epigastric herniation.

CLINICAL PRESENTATION

Seventy-five percent of epigastric hernias cause no symptoms. A small subcutaneous mass may be noted by the patient or discovered by the physician during routine examination. Smaller hernias, even when they are not incarcerated, often cause more symptoms than do larger ones. Hernias that give rise to complaints may produce variable and inconstant symptoms, seemingly unrelated to the hernia. Such complaints include epigastric pain that is dull, burning, or colicky and sometimes radiates to the lower abdomen, back, or chest; this occasionally is associated with abdominal distention, dyspepsia, nausea, and vomiting. Typical of epigastric hernia is epigastric pain on exertion. The pain often is exacerbated by bending or standing and relieved by reclining in the supine or prone position.

Incarceration is common, especially in smaller hernias. Friedenwald and Morrison[11] reported only 37 of 65 hernias to be reducible, but strangulation is unusual. Strangulation of preperitoneal fat or omentum results in localized pain and tenderness. Incarceration and strangulation of intraabdominal viscera are extremely rare, and symptoms depend on the incarcerated organ.[6,13,14,16,20,33]

DIAGNOSIS

The diagnosis usually is confirmed on physical examination by the presence of a midline mass. Performing the examination with the patient standing or in tangential light may be helpful. Palpation of the mass occasionally is difficult, especially in obese patients. A local area of tenderness in the linea alba usually is present, however, even in nonincarcerated hernias. This finding, combined with typical symptoms, should prompt surgical exploration for a nonpalpable or occult epigastric hernia.[5,28]

The diagnosis of hernia can be confirmed as the mass becomes more prominent when the patient strains, coughs, or raises the head in the supine position. Despite these maneuvers, differentiating this condition from subcutaneous tumors may be difficult and occasionally must be done at the time of exploration. The characteristic findings of abdominal wall hernias on ultrasound and computerized tomographic (CT) examination have been described by Yeh and coworkers.[37] These modalities may prove useful in the occasional hernia that escapes clinical diagnosis. Yeh and coworkers describe the demonstration of a muscular defect in the abdominal wall. Intestine in the sac may be detected by the demonstration of peristalsis on real-time ultrasonography or by the delineation of contrast medium or air in the loop of intestine on CT scan. Exaggeration of the lesion with straining and reducibility with pressure offer further confirmation.

TREATMENT

In the discussion of the paper by Friedenwald and Morrison,[11] Gilbride stated that "these gentlemen have conferred a dignity and importance on epigastric hernia that it does not deserve." Perhaps this statement should not be interpreted literally; that is, the variety of symptoms described earlier never should be attributed to epigastric hernia. Instead, it should be remembered that, in patients who have vague epigastric symptoms, intraabdominal disease should not be discarded in favor of a more obvious diagnosis. In light of modern diagnostic technology, there is little to recommend routine abdominal exploration in cases of epigastric hernia. In patients with vague or atypical complaints, however, a full battery of diagnostic studies should be undertaken.

Epigastric hernias are unusual in children. In a series of patients aged 2 to 7 years with asymptomatic epigastric or periumbilical hernias, most of the hernias resolved spontaneously with time.[30] Therefore, expectant management has been recommended in young children. The decision for surgical intervention depends on the type and severity of symptoms. In adults, operative intervention is considered the only acceptable therapy.

Numerous techniques have been used for repair of the fascial defect. In most instances, a small hernia traversed by preperitoneal fat is encountered. After the fat is resected in most defects less than 2.5 cm in diameter, simple suture closure suffices. The orientation of the suture closure is a matter of controversy. Although some surgeons claim that a transverse closure is more sound, others favor a vertical closure because of the frequency of multiple defects and of recurrence adjacent to the transverse hernioplasty.[24] Still other surgeons prefer an oblique orientation of the sutures, claiming it to be more anatomic.[2] For these small defects, more elaborate procedures that violate normal surrounding fascia probably are unnecessary and meddlesome.

For larger hernias, some have advocated enlarging the defect transversely and performing a vest-over-pants repair, as in the Mayo repair of umbilical hernias. This technique only seems to create undue tension, and most defects amenable to this repair also are amenable to simple suture repair. Berman[4] advocated a technique of repair in which the rectus sheath is opened anteriorly, on one side, near the line of fusion. The contralateral posterior rectus sheath is incised near its line of fusion, thus creating a short anterior and long posterior fascial flap on one side and the reverse on the other side. The vertical defect is closed in three layers, using imbricated mattress sutures for the fascial flaps and approximating the rectus muscles in the midline as a middle layer.

Askar[2] described a method of dealing with larger defects (> 2.5 cm in diameter) based on studies of the anatomy and biomechanics of the anterior abdominal wall. He advocated separate closure of the peritoneum followed by bridging of the gap with strips of autograft fascia lata (Fig. 25-6). Using the strips, an interwoven mesh is created that is oriented obliquely in line with the native aponeurotic fibers. The strips then are woven into the aponeurotic fibers at the circumference of the defect and fixed in place with nonabsorbable suture material. If synthetic mesh is used, the fibers should be oriented obliquely in a similar manner in line with the native aponeurotic fibers.

The surgeon's choice of technique may be a matter of individual preference, but should be guided by the following general principles (Figs. 25-7 through 25-9):

1. Wide exposure of the linea alba. The skin and subcutaneous tissue should be divided from xiphoid to umbilicus so that multiple defects are not overlooked.

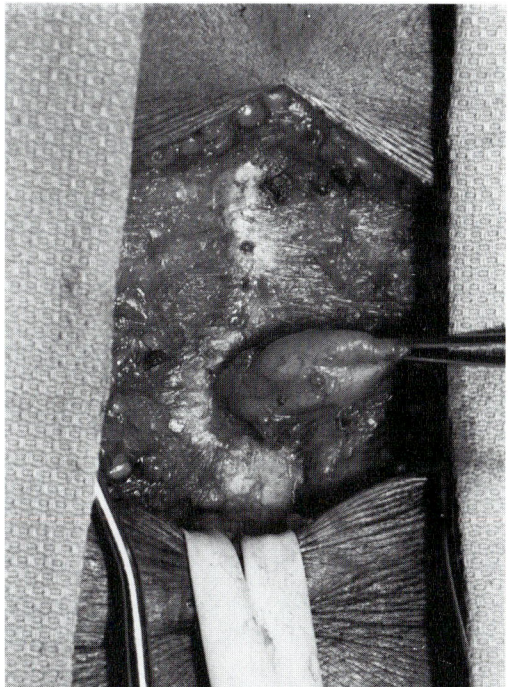

Figure 25-7. The linea alba has been exposed from xiphoid to umbilicus. Preperitoneal fat can be seen exiting from the fascial defect about 3 cm above the umbilicus. A Penrose drain encircles an associated umbilical hernia.

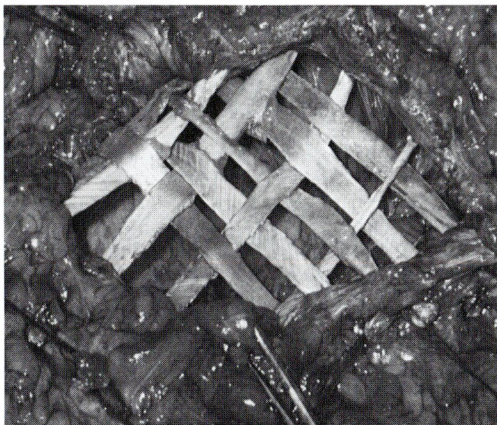

Figure 25-6. Fascial darning technique forming an obliquely oriented crisscross interwoven mesh. (Askar OM. A new concept of the aetiology and surgical repair of paraumbilical and epigastric hernias. Ann R Coll Surg Engl 1978;60:42)

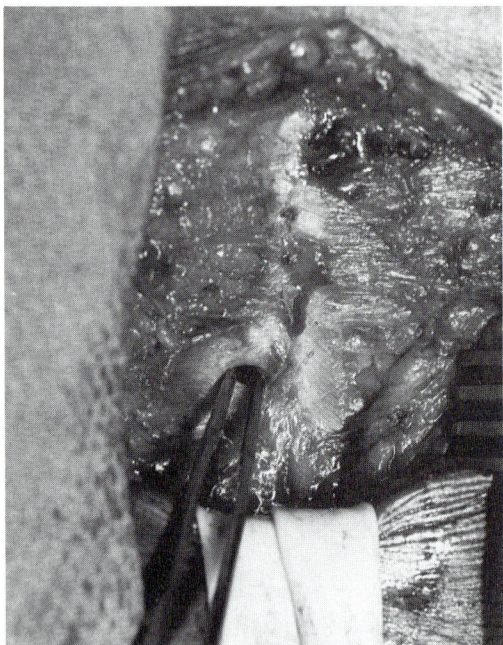

Figure 25-8. The fat has been excised, exposing a small fascial defect. The edges are exposed adequately and do not require acute débridement.

2. The hernia should be exposed by sharp dissection and débridement if necessary.
3. Preparation of the defect for closure. After excision of the sac or preperitoneal fat, it is not essential that the peritoneum be closed as a separate layer, or at all.
4. Anatomic repair without tension.

RESULTS

Most complications of epigastric hernia repair are not unique to this operation. They are the usual complications associated with an abdominal incision or anesthesia, and their rate should be low. Local wound infection is especially worrisome, because it greatly increases the probability of recurrence.

Reported recurrence rates generally are higher than with primary repair of other common hernias. Glenn and McBride[12] reported two recurrences among 14 patients with adequate follow-up. Askar[3] reported preliminary results of a 7% recurrence rate among the first 150 patients in whom the fascia lata darning technique was used for large epigastric or paraumbilical hernias. McCaughan[24] reported a 9.4% recurrence rate among 64 patients with adequate follow-up study.

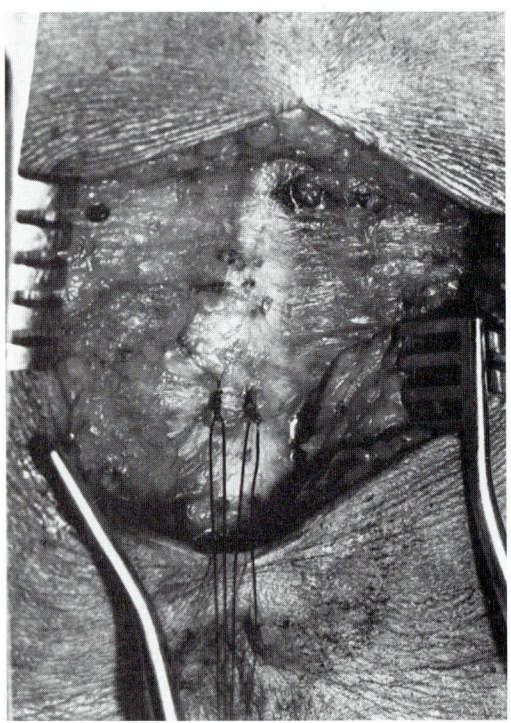

Figure 25-9. The defect has been closed with simple sutures oriented transversely. Vertical closure could have been chosen in this situation because of the proximity to the umbilical hernia.

Obesity and infection have been identified as risk factors leading to a high recurrence rate. In perhaps 50% of patients, however, the recurrence actually represents the persistence of a second hernia or area of weakness that was overlooked at the initial procedure. This last point emphasizes the importance of wide exposure and careful inspection of the entire supraumbilical linea alba.

REFERENCES

1. Askar OM. Surgical anatomy of the aponeurotic expansions of the anterior abdominal wall. Ann R Coll Surg Engl 1977;59:313.
2. Askar OM. A new concept of the aetiology and surgical repair of paraumbilical and epigastric hernias. Ann R Coll Surg Engl 1978;60:42.
3. Askar OM. Aponeurotic hernias: Recent observations upon paraumbilical and epigastric hernias. Surg Clin North Am 1984;64:315.
4. Berman EF. Epigastric hernia: an improved method of repair. Am J Surg 1945;68:84.
5. Brown RN. Nonpalpable epigastric hernias. Arch Surg 1960;81:87.
6. Bryk D. Gastric involvement in abdominal wall hernias. Gastrointest Radiol 1984;9:311.

7. Capelle. Dauerresultate mach operationen der hernia epigastrica. Beitr Klin Chir 1909;63:264.
8. Catanzaro FP. Epigastric hernia simulating gastrointestinal tract disease. USAF Med J 1955;6:1360.
9. Elechi EN. External abdominal wall hernias: experience with elective and emergency repairs in Nigeria. Br J Surg 1987;74:834.
10. Elechi EN, Etawo SU. Strangulated external abdominal wall hernia: experience with 53 cases in Port Harcourt, Nigeria. J Natl Med Assoc 1988;80:788.
11. Friedenwald J, Morrison JH. Epigastric hernia: a consideration of its importance in the diagnosis of gastrointestinal disease. JAMA 1926;87:1466.
12. Glenn F, McBride AF. The surgical treatment of five hundred herniae. Ann Surg 1936;104:1024.
13. Goldman G, Rafael AJ, Hanock K. Acute acalculous cholecystitis due to an incarcerated epigastric hernia. Postgrad Med J 1985;61:1017.
14. Gupta AS, Bothra VC, Gupta RK. Strangulation of the liver in epigastric hernia. Am J Surg 1968;115:843.
15. Hall JN. Epigastric hernia in the soldier. JAMA 1919;73:171.
16. Harison CS. A case of strangulated epigastric hernia. S Afr Med J 1965;39:679.
17. Heydorn WH, Velanovich V. A five-year U.S. Army experience with 36,250 abdominal hernia repairs. Am Surg 1990;56:596.
18. Hinton JW. Abdominal pain due to epigastric hernia. Am J Med Sci 1925;170:748.
19. Iason AH. Hernia. Philadelphia, Blakiston, 1941.
20. Lemonick D, Widmann WD. Epigastric hernia with intestinal obstruction: an unusual complication of a transmesenteric hernia. Arch Surg 1985;120:1390.
21. Lewisohn R. The importance of a thorough exploration of the intra-abdominal organs in operations for epigastric hernia. Surg Gynecol Obstet 1921;32:546.
22. Lindenstein. Zur lehre von der hernia epigastric. Beitr Klin Chir 1908;57:293.
23. Luecke. Operative beseitigung von sog. Fetternien wegen gastralgie. Zentralbl Chir 1887;14:68.
24. McCaughan JJ. Epigastric hernia. Results obtained by surgery. AMA Arch Surg 1956;73:972.
25. McCaughan JJ. Epigastric hernia. In: Nyhus LM, Condon RE, eds. Hernia, ed 2. Philadelphia, JB Lippincott, 1978:369–374.
26. Meyer J, Ivy AC. Studies on gastric and duodenal ulcer: the relation of epigastric hernia to gastric ulcer—a clinical and experimental study. J Lab Clin Med 1922;8:37.
27. Moschowitz AV. The pathogenesis and treatment of hernia of the linea alba. Surg Gynecol Obstet 1914;18:504.
28. Moschowitz AV. Epigastric hernia without swelling. Ann Surg 1917;66:79.
29. Pemberton JJ, Curry FS. The symptomatology of epigastric hernia. An analysis of 296 cases. Minn Med 1936;19:109.
30. Pentney BH. Small ventral hernias in children. Practitioner 1960;184:779.
31. Peters GR, Nesselrode CC. Epigastric hernia: a factor in upper abdominal diagnosis. J Kansas Med Soc 1945;46:289.
32. Pollack LH. Epigastric hernia. Am J Surg 1936;34:376.
33. Serour F. Gastric involvement in an epigastric hernia. (Letter) AJR 1989;152:893.
34. Soper HW. A case of concomitant epigastric hernia and gastric ulcer. N Y Med J 1910;92:259.
35. Terrier F. Hernias epigastriques et ad-umbilicales. Rev Chir 1886;6:985.
36. Wilkinson WR. Epigastric hernia. W V Med J 1949;45:328.
37. Yeh H-C, Lehr-Janus C, Cohen BA, Rabinowitz JG. Ultrasonography and CT of abdominal and inguinal hernias. J Clin Ultrasound 1984;12:479.

Editor's Comment

Professor Omar M. Askar, chairman of the department of surgery at Cairo University in Egypt, has added important anatomic information to the problem of epigastric hernia. His thesis has been presented to the Royal College of Surgeons of England.

My approach to the treatment of epigastric hernia follows that described by Robin. An operation offers the only chance for permanent cure of these defects. I prefer to expose the hernia through a generous midline incision from the xiphoid process to the umbilicus. This allows for an uninterrupted view of the entire linea alba and of associated defects not felt on examination. The hernia and its contents are dissected from the surrounding subcutaneous tissues and fascia to expose the margins of the fascial defect. The superior edge of the ring is incised and then grasped with a Kocher clamp to elevate the anterior abdominal wall and facilitate exposure of the hernial contents and a sac should it exist.

After the hernia is dissected free, a finger is inserted and searches superiorly and inferiorly to define any further weakness that may not be easily visible. If other defects are found, the incision in the linea alba should be extended to incorporate them so that a more complete repair can be accomplished without fear of a late recurrence. Preperitoneal fat usually is excised. If a sac exists, it is opened and any involved viscus is reduced. If evidence from the preoperative evaluation suggests an underlying abnormality, formal exploration of the abdominal cavity is carried out. This maneuver usually is unnecessary and meddlesome when not warranted. The peritoneum is left open, and the formal repair is begun. For an effective closure, it is essential to have at least 2 cm of fascia cleared on each side of the linea alba before suture placement. This is done with nonabsorbable sutures of 0 polypropylene or fine stainless-steel wire. Sutures may be placed in a simple manner, the left margin stitched to the right margin of the linea alba, ensuring at least 1.5-cm bites on both sides separated by about 1 cm. Careful, secure suture tying is essential. Rarely should any subcutaneous drain be placed before the skin is closed. Recurrence is unusual.

In the emergency setting, when compromise of the intestine is suspected, the operative approach is the same, attention to the viability of the remaining intestine being of prime importance. When indicated, the wound should be allowed to heal by delayed primary closure or secondary intention.

L.M.N.

Hernia, Fourth Edition, edited
by Lloyd M. Nyhus and Robert E. Condon.
J.B. Lippincott Company, Philadelphia © 1995.

Chapter 26

Spigelian Hernia

Leif Spangen

Spigelian hernias are rare and generally difficult to diagnose because of their often intramural location and vague and nonspecific symptoms. With the introduction of ultrasonographic scanning (US) and computed tomography (CT), diagnosis has become easier and the number of proven spigelian hernias has increased considerably during the last 15 years.

HISTORICAL REVIEW

Adriaan van den Spiegel[48] (1578–1625) was born in Brussels and studied first in Leiden and later in Padua, where he subsequently held the chair of anatomy and surgery. He did not diagnose spigelian hernia, but was the first to describe the semilunar line; therefore, it also is known as the linea semilunaris Spigeli or the linea Spigeli (Adrianus Spigelius being the Latin form of his name). Spontaneous rupture along the semilunar line first was described by Henry-Francois Le Dran[23] in 1742, but Josef T. Klinkosch[20] was the first to refer to this condition as hernia in the linea semilunaris. More than 350 articles on spigelian hernia have been published, but most authors report only a few cases of their own. Some of the larger series are listed in Table 26-1. All the published reports of spigelian hernia at various points in time are provided in Table 26-2.

REVIEW OF THE LITERATURE

Nine hundred and seventy-nine cases of spigelian hernia treated surgically have been reported so far (see Table 26-2). The age of the patient was provided in 632 cases, the gender in 748, and the location of the hernia in 711. Most spigelian hernias are diagnosed in patients between 40 and 70 years of age. The mean age in the compiled material was 51 years. There were 435 women and 313 men, with mean ages of 50 and 51.5 years, respectively. Three hundred and seventy-six hernias were located on the right side and 335 on the left; there were 32 bilateral hernias. In 6 patients, there was more than one hernia on the same side. Most of the hernias were located below the umbilicus; only 32 were found above this point. Operations for spigelian hernia were performed on patients of all ages, from 6 days to 94 years. Thirty children younger than 16 years (19 boys and 11 girls) were operated on for spigelian hernia. Incarceration at the time of the operation was seen in 138 of 509 reported hernias (27.3%).

DEFINITIONS

The semilunar (spigelian) line (Figs. 26-1 through 26-3) forms and marks the transition from muscle to aponeurosis in the transversus abdominis muscle of the abdomen.[48] It is a lateral convex line between the costal arch and the pubic tubercle. The part of the aponeurosis that lies between the semilunar line and the lateral edge of the rectus muscle often is called the spigelian fascia or zone.

Spigelian aponeurosis is a more accurate anatomic designation, and is the term used here. In Anglo-Saxon literature, the semilunar line often is designated mistakenly as the more medially situated lateral edge of the rectus abdominis muscle. Protrusion of a peritoneal sac, an organ, or preperitoneal fat from its normal position through a congenital or acquired defect in the spigelian aponeurosis is referred to as hernia Spigeli or spigelian hernia. Hernias that penetrate the aponeurosis more medially and protrude into the rectus sheath are referred to as intravaginal hernias (see Fig. 26-2).

Hernias that have arisen within the spigelian aponeurosis after either surgery or direct trauma should not be considered spigelian hernias, but have been referred to as such by several authors. The term *spigelian hernia* usually refers to defects that are located above the inferior epigastric vessels. Hernias that penetrate the spigelian aponeurosis within the Hesselbach triangle (ie, caudal and medial to the inferior epigastric vessels) are called low spigelian hernias (see Fig. 26-3). A spigelian hernia usually is located between the different muscle layers of the abdominal wall and, therefore, is called interparietal, interstitial,

Table 26-1. Large Series of Spigelian Hernias

Author	Year	No. of Hernias
Spangen	1984	45*
Stuckej et al.	1973	43†
Houlihan	1976	31‡
Persson et al.	1975	19
Ponka	1980	19§
Guivarc'h et al.	1988,1989	16
Gullmo	1980,1984	13
Lindholm and Hulin	1969	12
Kienzle and Staemmler	1978	12
Stirnemann	1982	12

*Includes 12 low spigelian hernias.
†Compilation of all spigelian hernias from a single department from 1951 to 1971.
‡Compilation of all spigelian hernias from a single department from 1963 to 1971.
§Includes 2 low spigelian hernias.

intermuscular, intramuscular, or intramural (see Fig. 26-2). In this location, a small hernia is especially difficult to detect by palpation and often is referred to as occult or masked.

The spigelian hernia belt (Fig. 26-4) is a transverse belt lying 0 to 6 cm cranial to the interspinal plane (ie, the horizontal plane through both anterior superior iliac spines). The spigelian aponeurosis is widest here (on average, about 2 cm), and my own observations indicate that 85% to 90% of spigelian hernias arise in this location.[45]

TOPOGRAPHIC ANATOMY

It is difficult to distinguish the internal oblique muscle from the transversus abdominis muscle as natural layers, especially distal to the umbilical plane. The internal oblique muscle ventral to the spigelian aponeurosis may consist of either muscle belly or aponeurosis. When the muscle is aponeurotic, its fibers may be strongly adherent to and contribute to the strength of the spigelian aponeurosis. If the internal oblique

Table 26-2. Total Number of Published Reports of Spigelian Hernia at Different Points in Time

No. of Patients	Year	Author(s)
21	1890	Macready
42	1910	Stuehmer
60	1923	Sandelin
116	1942	River
192	1960	Harless and Hirsch
295	1974	Weiss et al.
554	1976	Spangen
979	1993	Spangen

muscle consists of muscle fibers, the spigelian aponeurosis is not as strongly reinforced.

Below the umbilicus, there are considerable structural variations in both muscle and aponeurotic tissue within both the internal oblique and transversus abdominis muscles. Both present finger-like bands and varying numbers of slit-like gaps.[54] The fibers of the two muscles run almost parallel here, so that the gaps in the muscles may coincide. In such situations, the fibers can be separated more easily, creating a risk of herniation. Above the umbilicus, the fibers cross one another at angles, making herniation less likely.

Above the semicircular line (the line of Douglas), the aponeurosis of the transversus abdominis muscle divides into two layers, which blend with the anterior and posterior lamellae of the rectus sheath.[30] This division occurs within the spigelian aponeurosis, which therefore consists of two lamellae. The dorsal lamella becomes thinner as it approaches the semicircular line. The medial part of the spigelian aponeurosis is weakest within the last few centimeters above the line of Douglas, and this probably is one of the most important reasons that most spigelian hernias are located in the vicinity of this line. Caudal to the line, all fibers from the transversus aponeurosis run to the anterior lamella of the rectus sheath, and the spigelian aponeurosis consists of a single layer again.

The location and appearance of the semicircular line vary widely. The most lateral point of the line is located on average 2 cm cranial to the interspinal plane (ie, within the spigelian hernia belt).[45]

Spigelian hernia is rare in the most cranial part of the abdomen. The muscle belly of the transversus abdominis muscle here reaches to and behind the lateral edge of the rectus muscle. The semilunar line lies dorsal to the rectus muscle and there is accordingly no spigelian aponeurosis in this area (see Figs. 26-1 and 26-4). As a result, herniation through the transversus aponeurosis at this level is intravaginal (see Fig. 26-2). This is another reason why so few spigelian hernias have been found above the umbilicus.

The external oblique muscle, which is the most stable structure in the anterolateral part of the abdominal wall, is aponeurotic ventral to the spigelian aponeurosis throughout its length and prevents the hernia from entering the subcutaneous tissue, which explains why the hernial sac was located subcutaneously in only 18 reported cases. In most instances, the hernia is located between the musculoaponeurotic layers of the anterior abdominal wall.

The internal oblique muscle consists of muscle fibers ventral to the spigelian fascia more often in patients with spigelian hernia than in others (see Fig. 26-2). The width of the spigelian aponeurosis in patients with a hernia does not differ from that in other people.[45] A hernia usually penetrates both the transversus

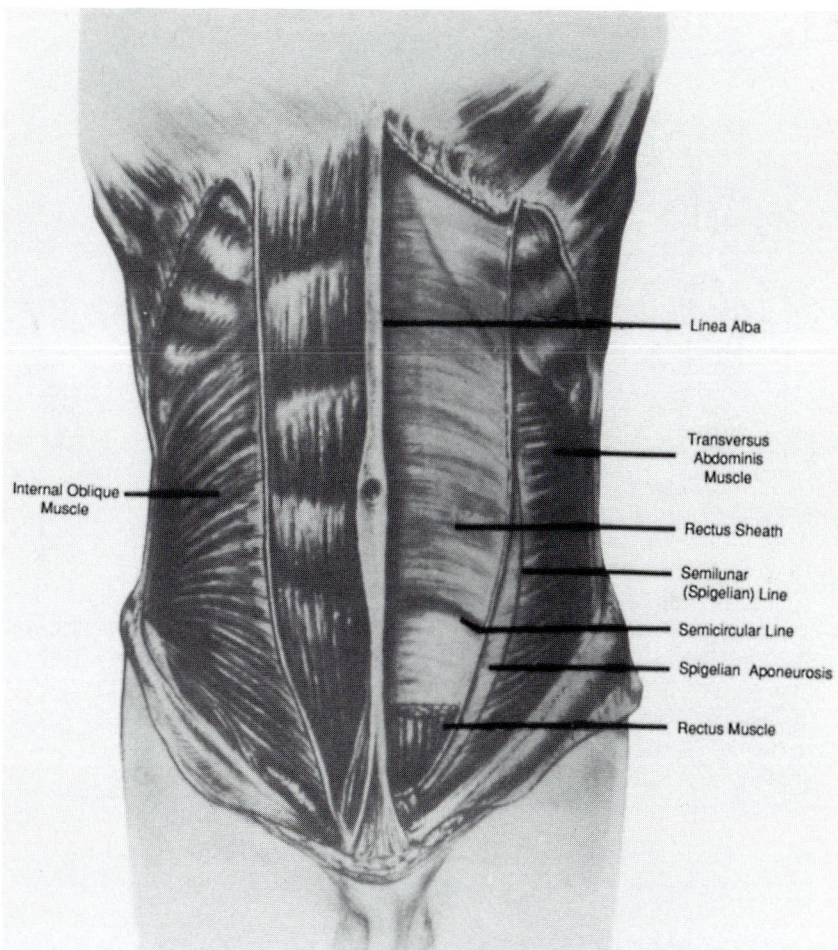

Figure 26-1. Ventral view of the abdominal wall showing the topographic anatomy. To the right, the external oblique muscle and the ventral lamella of the rectus sheath are cut away. To the left, the internal oblique and rectus abdominis muscles are removed. (Reproduced with permission of Acta Chirurgica Scandinavica. From Spangen L. Spigelian hernia. Acta Chir Scand Suppl 1976; 462:7)

abdominis and internal oblique muscles (see Fig. 26-2). The layer between the two oblique muscles is loose and normally acts as a glide layer. The hernial sac can expand easily in this space and, therefore, adopts the typical T- or mushroom-shaped appearance. The hernia expands laterally where more space is present, usually toward the anterior superior iliac spine and the groin. The medial progress of a spigelian hernia is arrested by the fusion of the external oblique aponeurosis with the deeper layers to form the rectus sheath. Occasionally, however, the hernia may protrude intravaginally. It is unusual for the hernia to extend between the transversus abdominis and internal oblique muscles (see Fig. 26-2). This is possible if the internal oblique muscle consists of muscle fibers that are elevated by a small hernia (see Fig. 26-2). When the hernia grows, it probably dissects the muscle fibers so that the sac penetrates the glide layer between the two oblique muscles. The hernial orifice usually is oval, although some are more triangular or round, and the edges are well defined and rigid. Most hernias

are small, the diameter of the orifice usually ranging from 0.5 to 2.0 cm. In hernias of this size, the orifice generally is limited to the spigelian aponeurosis. Orifices with a diameter of 6 to 8 cm have been reported.

ETIOLOGY

Congenital spigelian hernias have been reported, but the lesion is acquired in most cases. The musculoaponeurotic structure within and ventral to the spigelian aponeurosis generally is considered to be the most important contributing factor. The spigelian aponeurosis is one of the congenital weak areas in the ventral abdominal wall. Other predisposing factors are the same as for other types of hernia (eg, those resulting in increased intraabdominal pressure). Spigelian hernia has been observed in patients treated with continuous ambulatory peritoneal dialysis (CAPD). Increased intraabdominal pressure, in combination with weakened connective tissue, is an important factor in

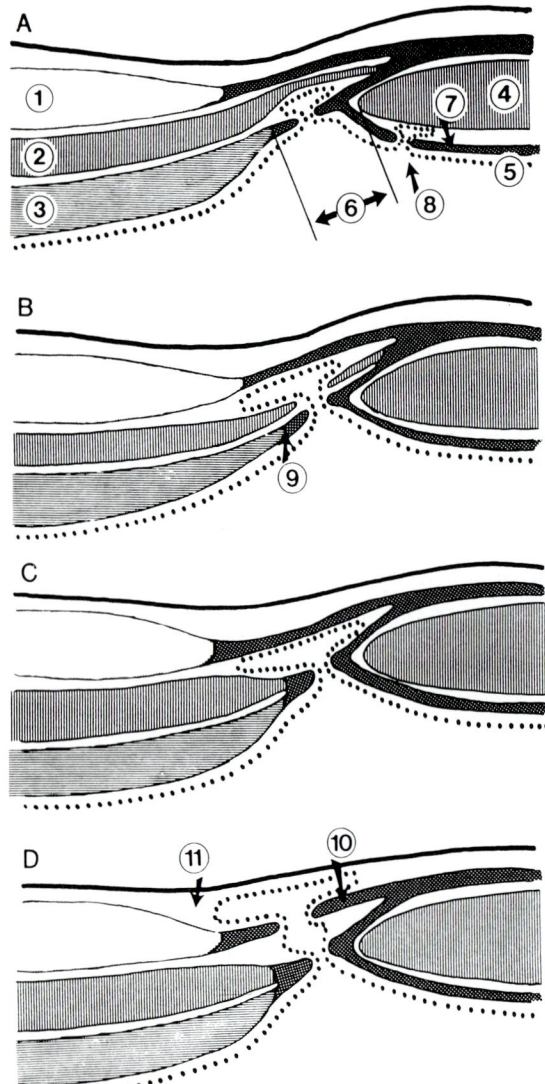

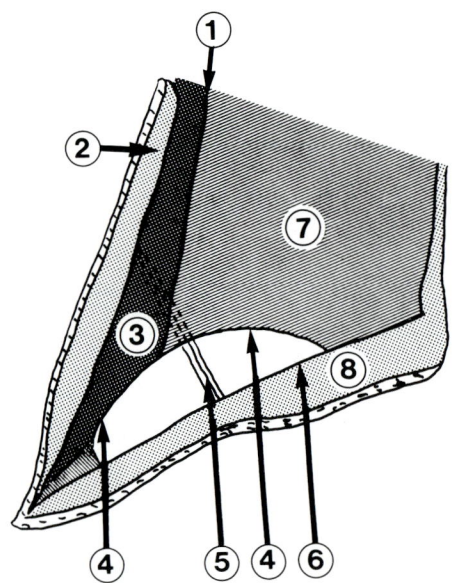

Figure 26-3. Schematic presentation of the anatomy in the Hesselbach triangle. 1, semilunar line; 2, internal oblique muscle; 3, spigelian aponeurosis; 4, arch of transversus abdominis aponeurosis; 5, inferior epigastric vessels; 6, inguinal ligament; 7, transversus abdominis muscle; 8, external oblique aponeurosis.

Figure 26-2. (*A through D*) Schematic cross section of ventral abdominal wall cranial to the semicircular line, indicating the possible location of the hernial sac in spigelian hernias. 1, external oblique muscle; 2, internal oblique muscle; 3, transversus abdominis muscle; 4, rectus abdominis muscle; 5, peritoneum; 6, spigelian aponeurosis; 7, dorsal lamella of the rectus sheath; 8, intravaginal hernia; 9, semilunar line (linea Spigeli); 10, external oblique aponeurosis; 11, subcutaneous tissue.

of the abdominal wall muscles also may contribute. Fat apparently can force its way between the fibers of the spigelian aponeurosis, paving the way for herniation.[21,38] A spigelian hernia may consist of preperitoneal fat alone, and the fact that the hernial sac always

the relatively high incidence of herniation in patients undergoing CAPD. In the upright position, the intraabdominal pressure is greatest in the lower part of the abdomen. This means that the pressure on the abdominal wall is greatest below the navel, which could be another reason spigelian hernias occur most often in this region. Aging and weight loss generally are regarded as important causative factors. Paralysis

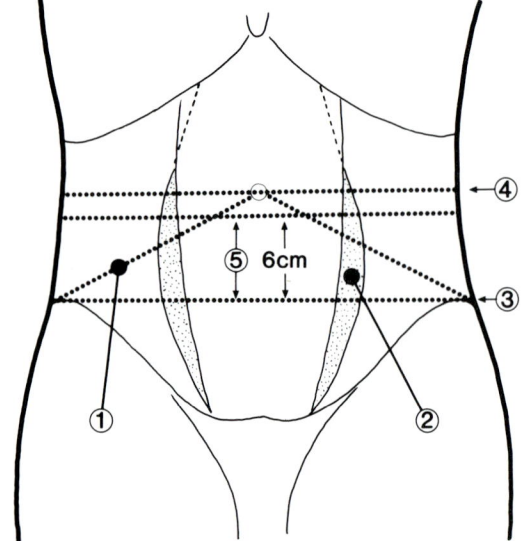

Figure 26-4. Location of spigelian hernia belt in relation to the umbilical plane, the interspinal plane, and the line of Monro. 1, line of Monro; 2, spigelian aponeurosis; 3, interspinal plane; 4, umbilical plane; 5, spigelian hernia belt.

is surrounded by prolapsing preperitoneal fat, being thickest at the top (prehernial lipoma), supports this theory.

It previously was believed that neurovascular openings in the spigelian aponeurosis may become enlarged, permitting herniation.[5] If such were the case, the neurovascular bundle should run beside the hernial sac through the hernial orifice. Such findings have been reported, but this now is considered to be of minor importance. Spigelian hernia is associated with a high rate of incarceration, which probably can be explained by the combination of a small hernial opening with rigid edges and the fact that the hernia often is diagnosed only when symptoms consistent with incarceration are apparent.

DIAGNOSIS

Symptoms

A spigelian hernia in its earliest form often is simply a protrusion of preperitoneal fat through the spigelian aponeurosis—a condition similar to fatty herniation of the linea alba. The hernia also can be part of an extraperitoneal organ, but a peritoneal sac is found in most cases. If the peritoneal sac has content, it usually is greater omentum, small intestine, or part of the colon. Other organs are found in the sac less often

(Table 26-3). Richter-type hernias also have been reported. The symptoms vary considerably, probably because so many different organs can be included in the hernia, resulting in diagnostic confusion. A decisive factor is whether the hernia is repositioned.

The symptoms that cause a patient to consult a physician usually are abdominal pain, a mass in the anterior abdominal wall, or signs of incarceration with or without intestinal obstruction. The pain varies in type, severity, and location, and depends on the content of the hernia. Abdominal pain of uncharacteristic type, not typical of a hernia, is common. Pain often can be provoked or aggravated by maneuvers that increase intraabdominal pressure and is relieved by rest. Intense pain occurs if the hernia is incarcerated, and if intestine is present in the hernial sac at the same time, symptoms of intestinal obstruction may ensue. If the patient has observed local swelling along the semilunar line, a spigelian hernia should be suspected.

Physical Examination

If the hernia produces a palpable mass along the spigelian aponeurosis, the diagnosis generally is easy to make, provided the possibility of this hernia is considered. If the contents of the abdominal wall resistance can be repositioned in the abdominal cavity, a spige-

Table 26-3. Uncommon Contents Found in the Sacs of Spigelian Hernias

Author	Year	Content of Sac	No. of Hernias
Belluzzi	1957	Stomach	1
Kirchberger	1867	Gallbladder	1
Durst et al.	1977	Gallbladder	1
Orokhovskii and Dudnichenko	1989	Strangulated gallbladder with perforation	1
Massabuau et al.	1933	Meckel diverticulum	1
Chalier	1948	Strangulated appendix	1
Ferrand et al.	1956	Strangulated appendix	1
Blikra	1959	Strangulated appendix	1
Hibbard and Schumann	1962	Strangulated appendix	1
Spangen	1976	Strangulated appendix	1
Jain et al.	1977	Strangulated appendix	1
Le Joliff et al.	1985	Strangulated appendix	1
Nauta et al.	1986	Crohn appendicitis	1
Nadjafl and Maurer	1967	Appendix epiploica	1
Biaggi et al.	1977	Appendix epiploica	1
Cullen	1911	Ovary	1
Mathews	1923	Ovary	1
Lamb	1962	Endometriosis in the sac	1
Louw and Lauritzen	1981	Leiomyoma of the uterus	1
Schoofs	1895	Testicle	1
Gravier et al.	1978	Testicle	1
Podkanenev et al.	1986	Testicle	1
Scotte et al.	1991	Urinary bladder	1

lian hernia is highly probable. The same applies if the hernia appears when the patient is upright and repositions spontaneously when the patient lies down, or if it appears when the patient strains or lifts heavy loads. The clinical diagnosis of a palpable hernia is complicated by the fact that the defect often continues to grow laterally and caudally between the two oblique muscles. The palpable mass, therefore, is most prominent lateral to the spigelian aponeurosis.

Patients who complain of pain but have no visible or palpable lump present the greatest difficulty in diagnosis. This condition exists when the hernial sac content is repositioned at the time of examination, or when a small interparietal hernia cannot be detected on palpation.

The hernial orifice, which usually is 0.5 to 2.0 cm in diameter, seldom can be detected by palpation because it is masked by the skin, the subcutaneous fat, and the usually intact external aponeurosis.

The hernial orifice can be palpated through the external aponeurosis in some cases if the patient is examined with a tense abdominal wall. Physical examination should be carried out while the patient alternately tenses and relaxes the abdominal muscles. When the abdominal muscles are tensed, all patients with spigelian hernias have a distinct tender point over the hernial orifice in the spigelian aponeurosis. On palpation, the hernia is pressed against the hernial ring, which is well defined and firm during a Valsalva maneuver. This brings about an afferent flow from the pain and stretch receptors that are present in abundance in the parietal layer of the peritoneum and the preperitoneal fat, and explains the distinct tenderness over the hernial orifice. In small, nonrepositioned but nonpalpable hernias, the explanation for the distinct tenderness on palpation is similar. This finding is not pathognomonic of spigelian hernia, but offers a useful method for screening: patients without distinct tenderness in the spigelian aponeurosis on palpation do not have spigelian hernia, whereas those with positive findings may have. Local tenderness may be the only sign of the hernia.

Sometimes, pinprick and tactile hyperesthesia of the abdominal wall just medial to the hernial orifice can be demonstrated. This is caused by mechanical irritation of the medial sensory branch of the corresponding intercostal nerve.

Diagnostic Procedures

Diagnostic procedures in spigelian hernia are aimed primarily at demonstrating a hernial orifice or sac and obtaining information regarding any sac contents.

Roentgenography

Only a few spigelian hernias have been diagnosed correctly by conventional roentgenographic examination. A prerequisite is that the hernial sac has an intramural or subcutaneous location and that it contains intestine filled with gas or, after a barium meal, intestine filled with contrast medium. The extraabdominal sac then can be visualized in tangential projections. If it contains a portion of large intestine, the sac can be demonstrated after a barium enema.

If the sac is empty, plain abdominal roentgenograms and contrast studies usually are not conclusive. Herniography with positive contrast medium may be attempted, but the diagnostic accuracy of this procedure is low and it carries some complications.[12,13] It has proven difficult to demonstrate small and even

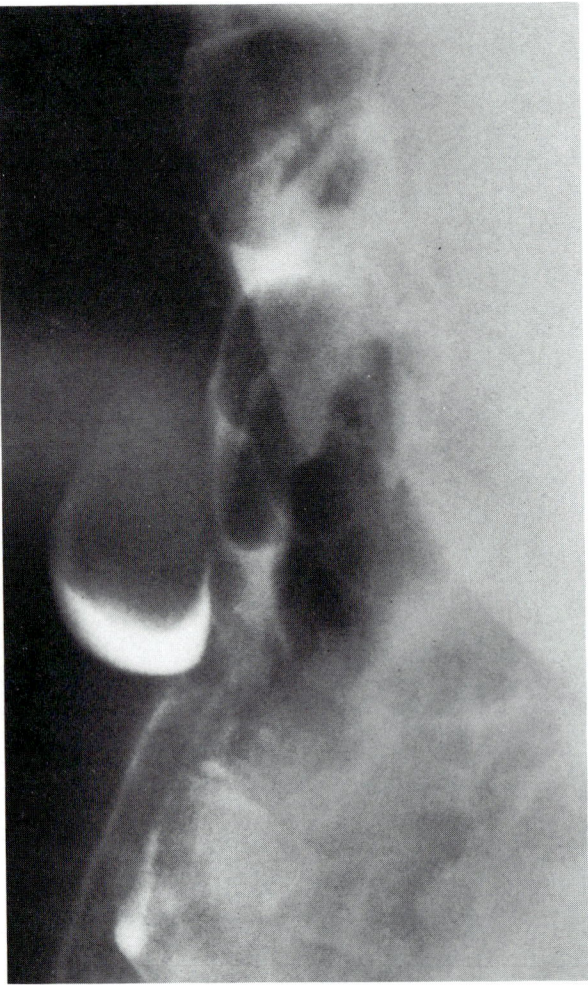

Figure 26-5. Spigelian hernia diagnosed by herniography. Horizontal supine oblique (45 degrees) position; anteroposterior projection.

medium-sized hernial sacs by herniography. Large hernias usually can be detected (Fig. 26-5), but the diagnosis of such lesions frequently is clear after the physical examination.

The hernial orifice cannot be demonstrated by a roentgenographic examination apart from herniography to facilitate the diagnosis of spigelian hernia. No satisfactory roentgenographic method is available for the diagnosis of spigelian hernias not found on physical examination.

Ultrasonic Scanning

Ultrasonic scanning is a valuable diagnostic tool in both palpable and nonpalpable spigelian hernias.[33,44,45,53] It is rapid, accurate, noninvasive, and easy to perform, and the abdominal wall layers can be delineated clearly. The diagnosis is based on demonstration of a hernial orifice in the spigelian aponeurosis, on an interparietally located hernial sac, and on sac content in the form of intestine or omentum. Scanning is begun with parasagittal sweeps, starting at the lateral aspect of the rectus muscle and continuing laterally. The examination is completed with transverse scans and, if necessary, scans in several other planes. The transducer is maintained perpendicular to the abdominal wall at all times. The sweeps are made bilaterally to obtain comparative views.

In the scans (Fig. 26-6), echogenic stripes can be seen below the subcutaneous fat, running almost parallel to the outline of the skin. The deepest stripe represents preperitoneal fat and parietal peritoneum. The other stripes represent muscle and aponeurotic layers of the ventral abdominal wall. The hernial orifice is visualized as a defect in the echo line from the aponeurosis. Usually, there also is an interruption in the stripe representing the preperitoneal fat and peritoneum (see Fig. 26-6). In repositioned hernias, the defect also causes a stronger than normal echo from underlying intestine in contact with the hernial orifice. The visualization of a hernial orifice and the interparietal location of the hernial sac (with preperitoneal fat) establish the diagnosis even in the absence of herniated loops of intestine.

Preperitoneal fat and omentum are highly echogenic, more so than the adjacent subcutaneous fat. Patients with spigelian hernias always have a distinct tenderness over the hernial orifice on palpation. US makes it possible to determine with certainty whether there is a defect in the spigelian aponeurosis.

Computed Tomography

Computed tomography is able to delineate clearly the abdominal wall layers and provides a good alternative method for evaluating the anterior abdominal wall. CT provides information about the hernial orifice, the sac, and the sac contents (Fig. 26-7).

Scanning must include the abdominal wall defect (see Fig. 26-7). If it does not, omental fat in the hernia may be misinterpreted as an abdominal wall lipoma.[43]

Only cross sectional scans can be performed with CT, and the distance between them must be short to demonstrate a hernial orifice.

US and CT probably are equally effective in demonstrating the hernial orifice, but CT may provide

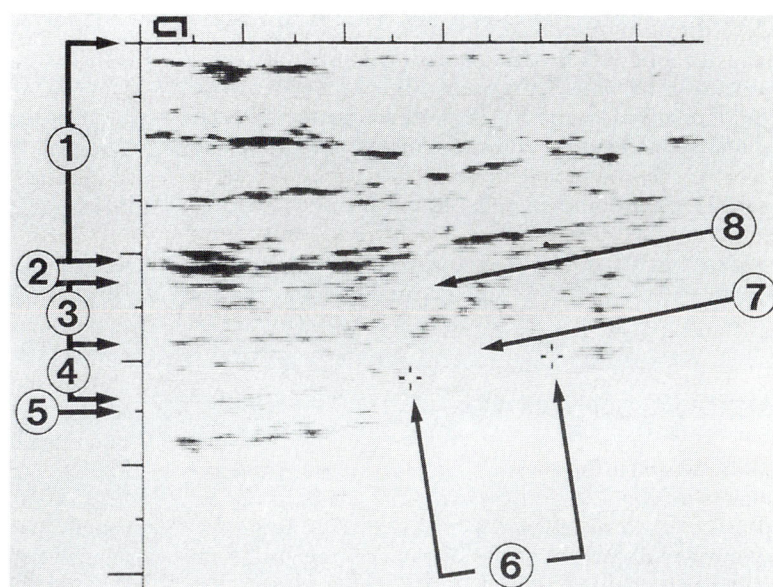

Figure 26-6. Ultrasonographic examination of a patient with a nonpalpable spigelian hernia. A longitudinal section of the left abdominal wall reveals a defect in the preperitoneal fat line and in the line from the internal oblique and transversus abdominis aponeuroses. 1, subcutaneous tissue; 2, external oblique aponeurosis; 3, internal oblique and transversus abdominis aponeuroses; 4, preperitoneal fat; 5, parietal peritoneum; 6, hernial orifice (diameter, 14.7 mm); 7, spigelian hernia containing intestine; 8, prolapsing preperitoneal fat.

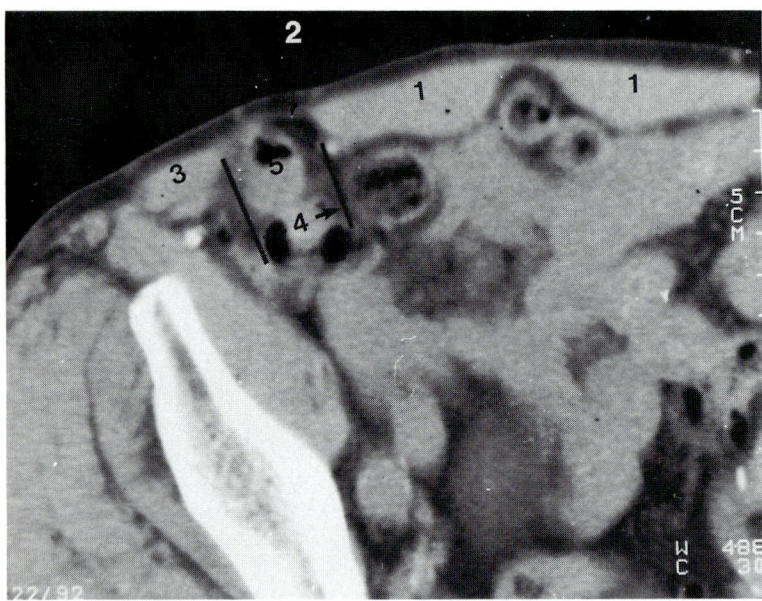

Figure 26-7. CT examination of ventral abdominal wall demonstrating a spigelian hernia on the right side. 1, rectus abdominis muscle; 2, external oblique aponeurosis; 3, lateral abdominal muscles; 4, hernial orifice (2.6 cm); 5, hernial sac containing intestine.

more information regarding hernial sac contents. To identify bowel loops, Yeh and colleagues[53] recommend the routine use of contrast medium in CT scanning of the abdominal wall when hernia is suspected. Bowel loops then are identified more clearly and bowel gas is delineated better. Peristaltic movement of herniated bowel loops also may be demonstrated. US is easier to perform and considerably cheaper than CT, so it seems reasonable to perform US first and supplement it with CT if additional information is required.

US and CT may prove helpful to the surgeon by demonstrating the precise location and extent of the musculoaponeurotic defect. The examinations also provide information regarding the thickness of the abdominal musculature. By performing the tests in connection with the Valsalva maneuver, the contractility of the abdominal muscles and possible muscle paresis (pseudohernia) also can be assessed. As a result, US and CT examination help to identify those patients in whom a synthetic prosthesis may be indicated.

SURGICAL EXPLORATION

Many spigelian hernias are clinically elusive and remain undiagnosed until an exploratory laparotomy is performed to investigate pain of unclear origin or symptoms of incarceration with or without intestinal obstruction.

DIFFERENTIAL DIAGNOSIS

Because a spigelian hernia can cause many different symptoms, the condition can be mistaken for both intraabdominal diseases and other lesions in the abdominal wall.

Most spigelian hernias lie beneath an intact musculoaponeurotic layer. As a result, they often are impalpable or indistinctly felt and may be mistaken for masses within the abdominal cavity. A mass in the abdominal wall found on physical examination may have many causes other than hernia. Besides surgical exploration, US and CT scanning are considered to be the diagnostic methods of choice for the evaluation of masses in the abdominal wall. Lipomas often are tender on palpation and may be located between the muscles in the abdominal wall, making them difficult to distinguish clinically from a spigelian hernia. A lipoma is easy to demonstrate, however, by both US and CT. In addition, there is no defect in the echo line from the aponeurosis. An intravaginal hernia (see Fig. 26-2A), which also may be combined with a spigelian hernia, is difficult to distinguish clinically from a spigelian hernia, and the diagnosis almost always is made at the time of operation. If no acute, tender abdominal wall tumors are found in this area, the possibility of a hematoma or an abscess must be considered. Both hematomas and seromas can be diagnosed by US. If an abscess is present, gas often can be demonstrated with US. In such instances, it is difficult to distinguish between an abscess and an incarcerated hernia containing intestinal gas. A correct diagnosis can be obtained by CT or surgical exploration. An abscess caused by an enteric fistula also may have a small detectable defect in the musculoaponeurotic layer.

Lesions other than hernia can cause tenderness in the spigelian aponeurosis on palpation. With the exception of hernias in the Hesselbach triangle (so-called low spigelian hernias), spigelian hernias are uncommon below the interspinal plane (see Fig. 26-4). If the only sign of hernia is tenderness in the spigelian aponeurosis between the interspinal plane and the deep inguinal ring, an indirect inguinal hernia should be suspected. Patients with symptomatic indirect inguinal hernias may exhibit tenderness in the spigelian aponeurosis several centimeters above the internal inguinal ring.[46] In women, indirect inguinal hernias often emerge high up laterally in the groin and, therefore, may simulate a spigelian hernia. If inguinal or even femoral or obturator hernia is suspected, herniography with positive contrast medium may be diagnostic.[12]

In patients without a palpable hernia or hernial orifice, but with a tender point in the spigelian aponeurosis and uncharacteristic abdominal pain, gastrointestinal and genitourinary disorders must be differentiated from spigelian hernias. A hernia in such patients may not cause symptoms.

In more than 50% of my own patients with proven spigelian hernia, initial neuralgic pain, most often experienced as a well-defined hyperesthetic area in the skin supplied by the medial branch of the corresponding intercostal nerve, can be found.[45] These nerve branches pass through the spigelian aponeurosis and then the anterior lamella of the rectus sheath about one fingerbreadth more medially. Pressure placed on the nerve by the hernia probably causes the symptoms. These sensory nerve branches also can be activated by forceful contraction of the muscles in the abdominal wall. This seems to occur more easily if the patient's weight changes rapidly or if the patient is in poor physical condition. The tenderness on physical examination then is most intense over the neurovascular hiatus in the anterior lamella of the rectus sheath (ie, one fingerbreadth medial to the spigelian aponeurosis). The pain disappears if a local anesthetic is injected toward the nerve opening in the aponeurosis. If a spigelian hernia is present, there also is a tender point over the hernial orifice in the spigelian aponeurosis. Myotendinitis at the transition between muscle and aponeurosis in the external oblique muscle or in tendinous intersections in the rectus abdominis muscle can be differentiated from a hernia by electromyography.

The occurrence of paresis in the abdominal wall musculature (pseudohernia) can be demonstrated with the aid of US and CT.

If a hernial orifice in the spigelian aponeurosis cannot be visualized with US, it is unlikely that one is present, although false-negative US results are obtained occasionally. Some conditions produce false-positive results on US; the posterior lamella of the rectus sheath ends at the semicircular line and a false-positive result may be registered if the line is distinct. A localized weakness within an abdominal wall muscle or aponeurosis in the vicinity of the spigelian aponeurosis, or a focal hypertrophy of the rectus muscle may simulate a hernia clinically. US and CT are helpful in clarifying the diagnosis in such cases. If intestine or an organ is adherent to the spigelian aponeurosis, the criteria for a hernial orifice may be present on US. The spigelian aponeurosis and the connective tissue in the adhesion have about the same acoustic impedance, so a distinct interface cannot be visualized. Defects in the aponeurosis that are of no clinical relevance also sometimes can be found on US or CT.

SURGICAL TREATMENT

Spigelian hernia should be treated surgically. The use of different types of incisions for palpable and nonpalpable hernias should be considered. In palpable hernias, a gridiron incision is excellent. After the external aponeurosis is split, it usually is easy to locate the hernia (Fig. 26-8). The simplest form of hernioplasty generally is sufficient. As a rule, the hernial orifice is so small that the repair will be free of tension and a relaxing incision need not be used.

If a gridiron incision is used, a short incision also should be made in the anterior lamella of the rectus sheath. This provides better exposure of the spigelian aponeurosis and adjacent parts of the posterior lamella of the rectus sheath, reducing the risk of an undetected intravaginal hernial offshoot. Defects in the posterior lamella of the rectus sheath are common and should be closed. A gridiron incision also may be used in patients without a palpable hernia or hernial orifice if US or CT has shown that the hernial sac lies between the two oblique muscles. The hernial sac then is visible when the external aponeurosis is split.

If no palpable hernia or hernial orifice is detected preoperatively but US or CT findings are consistent with a spigelian hernia, a preperitoneal dissection through a paramedian incision provides good exposure (Fig. 26-9). The paramedian incision is made through the ventral lamella of the rectus sheath, and the rectus muscle is retracted laterally so that the pos-

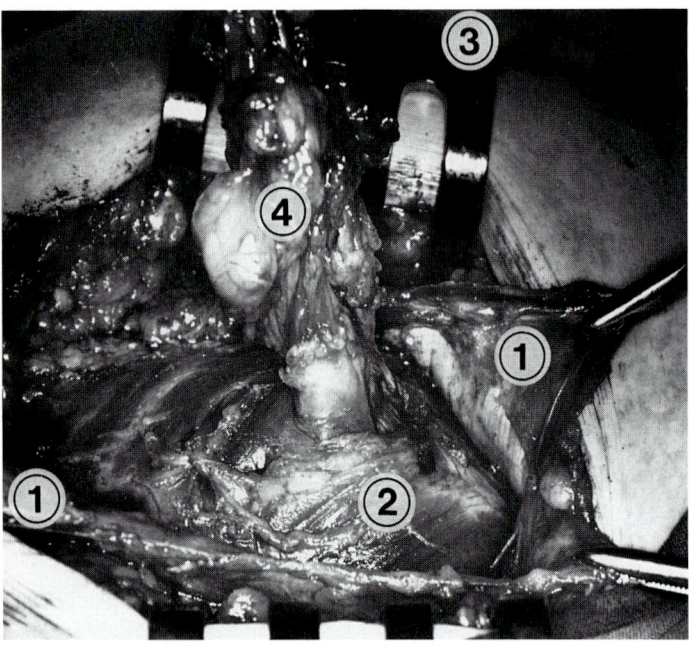

Figure 26-8. A typical spigelian hernia shown through a gridiron incision. The orifice measured 1.5 × 1.0 cm and the sac was 5 cm long and surrounded by preperitoneal fat. 1, external oblique aponeurosis; 2, internal oblique aponeurosis; 3, umbilicus; 4, hernial sac enclosed in preperitoneal fat.

terior lamella can be split longitudinally. Preperitoneal dissection then is carried out down to the spigelian aponeurosis. This enables easy inspection of a large part of the spigelian aponeurosis and the posterior lamella of the rectus sheath. The hernial orifice and additional aponeurotic defects can be exposed without difficulty and closed without cutting muscles and aponeuroses ventral to the spigelian aponeurosis.

If the internal oblique muscle is intact over the hernia, it may be difficult to locate the hernial orifice through a gridiron incision. Identifying the orifice through this incision also may be challenging in the absence of a peritoneal sac in an intubated and relaxed patient, because the orifice usually is small. An aponeurotic defect can be detected more easily on palpation from the peritoneal side. A paramedian approach facilitates hernioplasty and permits preperitoneal exploration and treatment of other abdominal wall hernias. A preperitoneal approach is highly suitable for exploratory laparotomy, which is recommended in patients with preoperative US or CT findings consistent with a spigelian hernia who have no palpable hernia or hernial orifice on physical examination. These patients, who seek medical advice because of pain, may have a quiescent spigelian hernia detected in the course of the investigation. Therefore, the peritoneum always should be opened to identify any other or additional causes of the patient's symptoms. A vertical incision also is a good alternative in patients with intestinal obstruction.

RESULTS

The results of operations for spigelian hernia are excellent, and the risk of recurrence is low. Only six cases of recurrence have been reported. Prosthetic material usually is not used in the repair of spigelian hernia, but may be necessary if the hernial orifice is large or the abdominal musculature/aponeurosis is thin or atrophic because of nerve injury. Other possible indications for the use of prosthetic material in the hernia repair are the presence of several concomitant defects in the spigelian aponeurosis and recurrent herniation.

LOW SPIGELIAN HERNIA

The spigelian aponeurosis also is located caudal and medial to the inferior epigastric vessels in the Hesselbach triangle. Therefore, both direct inguinal hernias and low spigelian hernias may occur within the triangle. Different names have been given to these lower spigelian hernias (eg, parainguinal hernias, hernias through the conjoined tendon, and direct inguinal hernias). This probably explains why so few cases of low spigelian hernia have been reported. As in other spigelian hernias, the hernial orifice is small and localized to a well-defined aponeurotic plane. The low spigelian hernia usually consists of preperitoneal fat alone, but also may involve the bladder. If there is a hernial sac, it typically contains omentum or intestine.

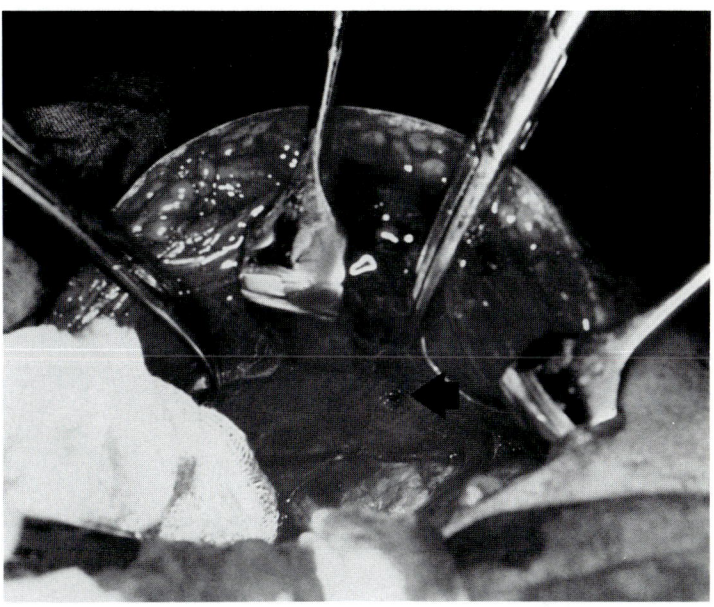

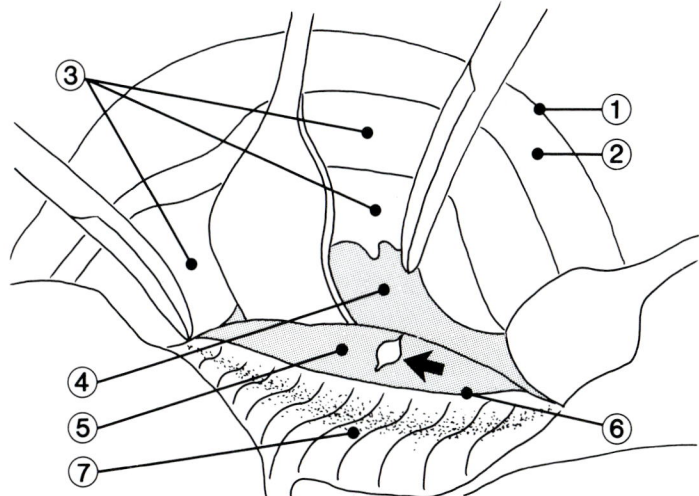

Figure 26-9. Spigelian hernia exposed by preperitoneal dissection 1, skin; 2, subcutaneous fat; 3, rectus abdominis muscle; 4, dorsal lamella of rectus sheath; 5, spigelian aponeurosis; 6, semilunar line; 7, peritoneum. The arrow marks the hernial orifice, which measured 0.4 × 0.3 cm. The hernia consisted of preperitoneal fat only.

Low spigelian hernia is difficult to demonstrate preoperatively, and the diagnosis often is established at the time of surgery for inguinal hernia. It is easier to treat than is a direct inguinal hernia, and the risk of recurrence is lower.

REFERENCES

1. Belluzzi V. Observazioni cliniche. Ernia di Spigelio strozzata contenente lo stomaco. Policlinico Sez Prat 1957;36:1151.
2. Biaggi J, Kuepfer K, Stirnemann H. Die Spiegelische Hernie. Schweiz Med Wochenschr 1977;107:119.
3. Blikra G. Hernia Spigelii T. Norske Laegeforen. 1959;79:1124.
4. Chalier A. Etranglement de l'appendice dans une hernie de la ligne semilunaire de Spigel. Soc Chir Lyon 1948;43:455.
5. Cooper A. The anatomy and surgical treatment of crural and umbilical hernia, part II. London, T Cox, T Bensley, 1807:58–61.
6. Cullen TS, Brödel M. Lesions of the rectus abdominis muscle simulating an acute intraabdominal condition. Bull Johns Hopk Hosp 1937;61:295.
7. Durst J, Mueller G, Muench B. Inkarzeration des Gallenblasenfundus in den linea semilunaris Spigheli. Med Welt 1977;28:490.
8. Ferrand J, Pegullo J, Destaing F, Debaille R. Les her-

nies du sillon latéral de l'abdomen. Presse Med 1956;64:2055.

9. Gravier L, Bernstein D, RuBane CF. Lateral ventral (Spigelian) hernias in infants and children. Surgery 1978;83:288.

10. Guivarc'h M. Traitment chirurgical des hernies anterio-láterales dites de Spiegel. Presse Med 1989; 18:177.

11. Guivarc'h M, Fonteny R, Boche O, Roullet-Audy JC. Hernies ventrales antéro-laterales dites de Spiegel. 16 cas et revue de la litterature. Chirurgie 1988;114: 572.

12. Gullmo Å. Herniography. The diagnosis of hernia in the groin and incompetence of the pouch of Douglas and pelvic floor. Acta Radiol Scand Suppl 1980;361.

13. Gullmo Å, Bromeé A, Smedberg S. Herniography. Surg Clin North Am 1984;64:229.

14. Harless MS, Hirsch JE. Spigelian or spontaneous lateral ventral hernia. Am J Surg 1960;100:515.

15. Hibbard LT, Schumann WR. The spigelian hernia in gynecology. Am J Obstet Gynecol 1962;83:1439.

16. Houlihan TJ. A review of spigelian hernias. Am J Surg 1976;131:734.

17. Jain KM, Hastings OH, Kunz VP, Lazaro FJ. Spigelian hernia. Am Surg 1977;43:596.

18. Kienzle HF, Staemmler S. Die Spieghel-Hernie und ihre Behandlung. Fortschr Med 1978;96:876.

19. Kirchberger J. Ein Fall von herzförmiger Leber, mit ihrem rechten Rande eingebetteter Niere, im Vereine mit einer seltenen Art von Hernia epigastrica lateralis. Wien Klin Wochenschr 1867:996.

20. Klinkosch JT. Divisionem Herniarum Novamgue Herniae Ventralis Speciem Proponit. Dissertationum Medicorum 1764:184.

21. Koljubakin SL. Hernia linea Spigelii. Arch Klin Chir 1925;136:739.

22. Lamb WK. Discussion of Hibbard IF, Schumann WR. The spigelian hernia in gynecology. Am J Obstet Gynecol 1962;83:1445.

23. Le Dran HF. Traité des operations de chirurgi. Paris, 1742:142.

24. Le Joliff L, Letoquart JP, Focaud X, Langella B, Mambrini A. Les hernies Ventrales latérales ou de la ligne de Spiegel. J Chir (Paris) 1985;122:409.

25. Lindholm Å, Hulin E. Hernia Spigelii—ett vanligt förekommande bråck? Nord Med 1969;39:1225.

26. Louw P, Lauritzen JB. Hernia Spigelii fremkaldt af uterusfibrom. Ugeskr Laeger 1981;143:1222.

27. Macready J. Rarer forms of ventral hernia. Lancet 1890;2:963.

28. Massabuau MM, Guibal A, Cabanac. Deux cas de hernies ventrales latérales spontanées étranglées. Presence du divverticule de Meckel dans une de ces hernies. Arch Soc Med Biol Montpellier 1933;14:340.

29. Mathews FS. Hernia through the conjoined tendon. Ann Surg 1923;78:300.

30. McVay CB, Anson BJ. Composition of the rectus sheath. Anat Rec 1940;77:213.

31. Nadjafl A, Maurer W. Die Spiegelsche Hernie. Schweiz Med Wochenschr 1967;97:1070.

32. Nauta RJ, Heres FK, Walsh DB. Crohn's appendicitis in an incarcerated spigelian hernia. Dis Colon Rectum 1986;29:659.

33. Nelson RI, Renigers SA, Nyhus LM, et al. Ultrasonography of the abdominal wall in the diagnosis of spigelian hernia. Am Surg 1980;46:373.

34. Orokhovskii VI, Dudnichenko AS. Incarceration of spigelian hernia with perforation of the gallbladder. Chirurgija (Mosk) 1989;7:136.

35. Persson PH, Grennert L, Jögi P, Pallin B. Diagnos och operativ teknik vid hernia Spigelii. Acta Soc Med Suecanae 1975;84:213.

36. Podkanenev VV, et al. Incarceration of spigelian hernia in a child. Klin Khir 1986;6:72.

37. Ponka JL. Spigelian hernias. In: Joseph K, Ponka MD, eds. Hernias of the abdominal wall. Philadelphia, WB Saunders, 1980:478–486.

38. Read RC. Spigelian hernia. In: Nyhus LM, Condon RE, eds. Hernia, ed 2. Philadelphia, JB Lippincott, 1978:375–382.

39. River LP. Spigelian hernia. Ann Surg 1942;116:405.

40. Sandelin T. Om bråck i linea semilunaris Spigelii. Finska Läkarsällsk. Handlingar 1923;64:268.

41. Schoofs. Un cas de hernie ventrale du testicule. Arch Med Belges 1895:229.

42. Scotte M, Majerus B, Sibert L, Teniere P. Incarcération vésicale dans une hernie de Spiegel. J Chir (Paris) 1991;128:74.

43. Shenouda NF, Hyams BB, Rosenbloom MB. Evaluation of spigelian hernia by CT. J Comput Assist Tomogr 1990;14:777.

44. Spangen L. Ultrasound as a diagnostic aid in ventral abdominal hernia. J Clin Ultrasound 1975;3:211.

45. Spangen L. Spigelian hernia. Acta Chir Scand Suppl 1976;462.

46. Spangen L. Spigelian hernia. Surg Clin North Am 1984;64:351.

47. Spangen L. Spigelian hernia. In: Nyhus LM, Condon RE, eds. Hernia, ed 3. Philadelphia, JB Lippincott, 1989:369–379.

48. Spiegel A. Opera Quae Extant Omnia. Amsterdam, John Bloew, 1645:103.

49. Stirnemann H. Die Spigelische Hernie: Verpasst? Selten? Verlegenheitsdiagnose? Der Chirurg 1982;53: 314.

50. Stuckej AL, Lutjko GD, Tivarovskij VI. Hernias of the Spigeli line. Tsitologiia 1973;15:10.

51. Stuehmer A. Ueber die Hernien der Bauchwand seitlich der Mittellinie unter besonderer Beruecksichtigung der Hernien der linea semilunaris (Spigelii). Bruns Beitr Klin Chir 1910;66:113.

52. Weiss Y, Lernau OZ, Nissan S. Spigelian hernia. Ann Surg 1974;180:836.

53. Yeh HC, Lehr-Janus C, Cohen BA, Rabinowitz JG. Ultrasonography and CT of abdominal and inguinal hernias. JCU 1984;12:479.

54. Zimmerman LM, Anson BJ, Morgan EH, McVay CB. Ventral hernia due to normal banding of the abdominal muscles. Surg Gynecol Obstet 1944;78:535.

Hernia, Fourth Edition, edited
by Lloyd M. Nyhus and Robert E. Condon.
J.B. Lippincott Company, Philadelphia © 1995.

Chapter 27

Interparietal Hernia

Barry Altman

*A typical strangulated interstitial hernia shows signs of acute obstruction, a mass is present
above Poupart's ligament, and the testis on the same side as the lump is absent.*

T.J. Noonan, 1950

DEFINITION

An interparietal hernia is one in which the hernial sac
lies between the layers of the abdominal wall.

HISTORY

In 1661, Thomas Bartholin[4] described the case of a
30-year-old man who had had a tumor of the left
groin for 15 years. After a dose of purging medicine
"from an empiric," the tumor had grown from the size
of a duck's egg to exceed the size of an adult human
head. Bartholin remarked on the fact that it had
grown upward toward the spleen, and that he was unable to find any previous record of a bubonocele's
having done such a thing. This probably is the first
record of an interstitial hernia.

The next report was in 1790, when Petit[34] described a patient he had seen in 1779. Hernu[21] in
1802 described a hernia lying in front of the bladder,
in which the sac shared a common opening with a
scrotal hernia.

In 1814, Hesselbach[22] reported a hernia between
the internal and external oblique muscles. Sir Astley
Cooper[10] already had performed the first successful
repair of a strangulated hernia in this situation in
1812; however, he did not record it until 1827.

The designation *interstitial* first was used by
Goyrand[19] in 1836 to describe a hernia between the
layers of the muscles of the abdominal wall.

Parise[33] in 1851 described inguinal-intrailiac and
inguinal-antevesical hernias. By 1876, Krönlein[24] had
collected and analyzed 23 cases, described the anatomy, discussed the etiology, and given them the name
properitoneal.* The inguinosuperficial type really was

---
*The editors prefer the term *preperitoneal;* although it is etymologically incorrect, it has the advantage of clinical acceptance and conveys the intended meaning clearly (see Chap. 2).

defined for the first time as a variety of interstitial hernia by Küster in 1887.[25]

There were further additions to the literature on
the subject, including a comprehensive study by
Göbell[18] in 1900. By 1931, Lower and Hicken[28] were
able to collect 590 reports of interparietal hernias of
all types, including two patients of their own. Etawo
and Elechi[16] added six more patients to the ever-grow-
ing list.

CLASSIFICATION

Clinical

Macready[29] divided interstitial hernias into those with
and without ventral swelling. This can be a useful division from the clinical point of view, because the former may be diagnosed without undue difficulty, but
the latter are unlikely to be recognized in the absence
of swelling.

Anatomic

The current anatomic classification (Fig. 27-1) is
based on the one used by Fuld.[17]

Preperitoneal
In preperitoneal interparietal hernias, the sac passes
between the peritoneum and the transversalis fascia.
These lesions may be subdivided into inguinopreper-
itoneal, cruropreperitoneal, and simple peritoneal,
depending on whether the sac is associated with an
inguinal or a femoral hernia, or with neither. Depend-

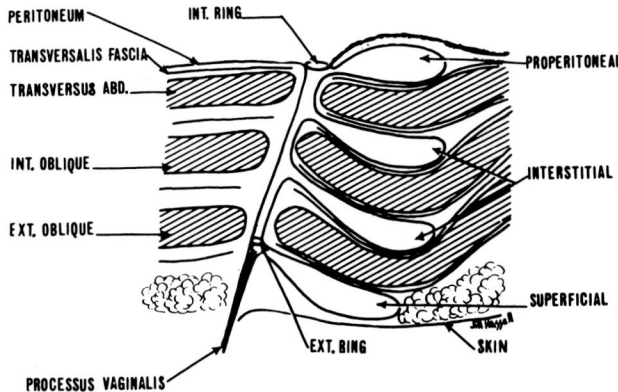

Figure 27-1. Composite diagram of the three principal types of interparietal hernias; monolocular sacs.

ing on the direction in which the sac expands, they may be designated further as follows:

Anterior Iliac. The most common type is anterior iliac, in which the sac lies above and medial to the internal inguinal ring and enlarges upward and outward toward the anterior superior iliac spine.

Inguinoiliac. In inguinoiliac hernias, the sac passes backward to lie in the iliac fossa.

Inguinovesical. The sac passes medially and downward in inguinovesical interparietal hernias, lying in front of or alongside the bladder.

Pelvic or Obturator. The sac of pelvic or obturator hernias passes downward and lies between the peritoneum and the pelvic wall in the region of the obturator foramen.

Inguinocrural. In inguinocrural hernias, the sac passes downward behind the inguinal ligament, lying in the region of the femoral ring.[39]

In addition, Halstead[20] described a preperitoneal hernia in which the sac lay above and medial to the internal ring.

Inguinointerstitial. The sac of an inguinointerstitial hernia may pass between the transversalis fascia and the transversus abdominis muscle, between the transversus abdominis and internal oblique muscles, or between the internal oblique and external oblique muscles. Although the sac usually lies in a clearly defined plane between muscle layers, it may pass between the fibers of the internal oblique.[19,28] The sac usually passes upward and laterally toward the anterior superior iliac spine. It may pass in other directions, however; I have seen a hernia in which the sac

passed upward and medially and presented through the linea semilunaris as a spigelian hernia.[2]

Inguinosuperficial. In inguinosuperficial hernias, the sac passes through the external ring and lies superficial to the external oblique aponeurosis between it and the skin. The sac then usually passes upward and laterally toward the anterior superior iliac spine, but also may pass upward toward the umbilicus or downward over the inguinal ligament to lie over the femoral canal.

Both this superficial inguinocrural hernia and the inguinocrural preperitoneal varieties must be distinguished from the type of sac that passes down the inguinal canal and then beneath the inguinal ligament to enter the femoral canal by way of the femoral ring. This is the true inguinofemoral hernia.

Moynihan[31] insisted that a bilocular sac was essential to the production of an interparietal hernia; Halstead[20] agreed. One loculus lay in the inguinal canal as an inguinal hernia, and the other loculus lay interparietally (Fig. 27-2). Moynihan actually defined an interstitial hernia in these terms, but there have been many examples in the literature of monolocular sacs occurring alone and monolocular sacs occurring independent of a concurrent inguinal hernia. These probably are not as common as the bilocular variety, and this may account for the mistaken impression given by earlier authorities. A report also has been made of two preperitoneal sacs occurring in the absence of an inguinal sac, one extending upward and outward, and the other downward and inward.[23]

The sac may or may not pass through the internal inguinal ring. If it does not, then it may penetrate the fibers of the transversus abdominis and internal oblique muscles to gain its final position. If the sac does pass through the internal inguinal ring, it may share a common opening with an inguinal hernial sac;

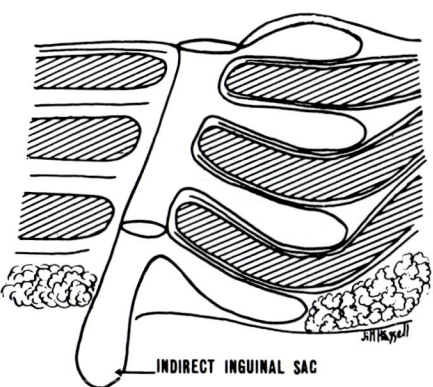

INDIRECT INGUINAL SAC

Figure 27-2. Composite diagram of the three principal types of interparietal hernias; bilocular sacs in association with a patent indirect inguinal sac.

this is the usual situation. It may pass through the internal ring, however, in the absence of a true inguinal sac. Less often, an interparietal sac and an inguinal sac may pass through the internal ring together, yet be entirely unconnected.

ETIOLOGY

Numerous theories have been propounded to explain the occurrence of interparietal hernias. The more logical ones are discussed under the headings of Mechanical Causes and Congenital Causes.

Mechanical Causes

Anatomic Considerations
Eppinger[15] arbitrarily divided the inguinal canal into three parts. The first or innermost part extends from the internal ring to the point where the infundibuliform fascia pierces the transversus muscle. In this part, the transversalis fascia is attached firmly to muscle, but is connected only loosely to the peritoneum.

The second or middle part is surrounded by the internal and external oblique muscles and is reinforced firmly. The third or anterior segment is the space between the internal oblique muscle and the external ring. Here, the internal and external oblique muscles are attached loosely.

Thus, the first and third parts of the inguinal canal are weak areas in which herniation can occur. In the first part, a hernia is preperitoneal, and in the third part, it is interstitial. Hernia does not occur in the second part.

Factors That Cause Obstruction
Factors that obstruct the "normal descent" of an inguinal hernia to the scrotum or its reduction into the peritoneal cavity include narrowing of the abdominal inguinal rings and a constricted sac neck.

Narrowing of the abdominal inguinal rings may come about at the external ring as a result of adhesion formation from an ill-fitting truss (which Halstead thought to be the chief cause), or it may be related to congenital obstruction of the inguinal canal by (1) an incompletely descended testis in the canal, (2) hydrocele of the canal of Nuck,[9] (3) a fallopian tube and ovary,[14] (4) absence of the external ring,[1] or (5) reduction of the contents of an inguinal sac by taxis in the presence of an obstruction at its neck. If the narrowing is at the internal ring, this may force the contents out of the canal into a preperitoneal or an interstitial sac. If the external ring is narrowed, then the contents may enter a superficial sac.

This aspect has been discussed extensively, and it generally has been concluded that the transfer of the contents of an inguinal sac to a preperitoneal one accounts for the condition known as *reduction en masse.* Moynihan found that all specimens of reduction en masse that he examined in hospital museums were of preperitoneal hernias, in which the "reduced" sac always lay outside the peritoneal cavity. It was pointed out by Halstead that it is virtually impossible to reduce an inguinal sac complete with its contents because of the firm attachment of the sac to other structures passing through the canal, but that attempts to reduce an inguinal hernia easily could move the contents from the inguinal sac to a preformed interparietal sac (Figs. 27-3 and 27-4). The truth of this was demonstrated by Corner.[11] It also has been postulated that the interparietal sac is formed as a diverticulum from a previously "normal" inguinal sac by repeated attempts at reduction against an obstructed or narrowed internal ring. It is the consensus that this is not so, and that the sac is preformed.

Congenital Causes

Maldescent of the Testis
The association of an ectopic or incompletely descended testis was mentioned in the early literature. Macready[29] gave the incidence in 129 cases of interparietal hernia as follows: in 73.4%, there was some abnormality of the testis, and in 67.1%, the testis was retained completely or had descended only partially. In some superficial hernias, the testis lies superficial to the external oblique aponeurosis. A scrotum that not only is empty, but is underdeveloped on the side

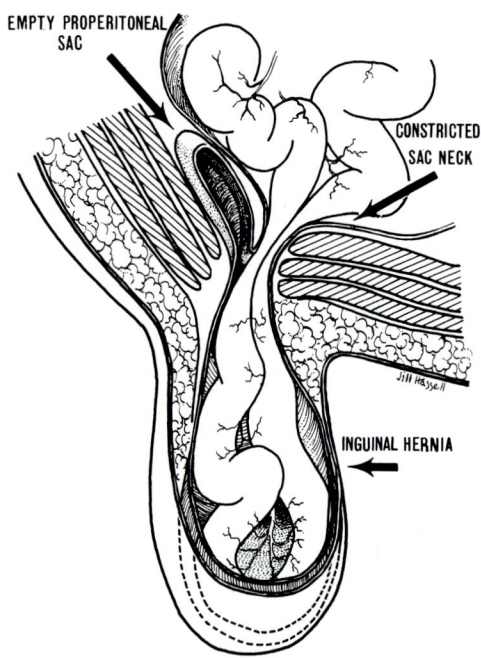

Figure 27-3. Bilocular preperitoneal hernia. The constriction at the neck is above the common opening of the two sacs. Attempted reduction could cause the situation shown in Figure 27-4.

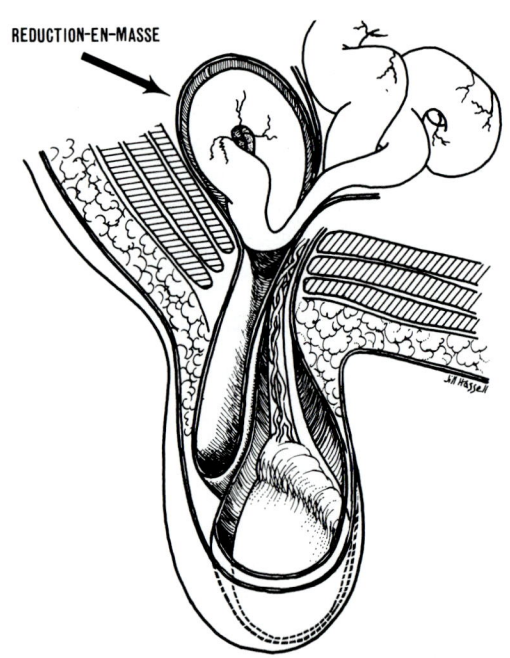

Figure 27-4. Reduction en masse. The constriction above the common opening has prevented reduction of the contents of the inguinal sac into the peritoneal cavity. They have entered the preperitoneal sac, but the intestine still is strangulated.

of the interparietal hernia may be associated with a testicular abnormality. It is implied that the hernial sac follows an ectopic testis and its gubernaculum to its final position.

The interstitial sac, however, may not follow the maldescended or incompletely descended testis. Masih and colleagues[30] described bilateral interstitial hernias in a newborn infant. At 5 days of age, he had huge lower abdominal swellings. The scrotum was empty and underdeveloped. The right testis could be palpated at the apex of the mass on that side. The left testis was palpable at the external ring (Fig. 27-5).

At operation, both masses were found to be interstitial hernias lying between the internal and external oblique muscles. The one on the right was a monolocular sac with the testis adherent to the apex of the interstitial sac. The external ring was tight and poorly formed. On the left side, there was a bilocular sac. The testis lay at the apex of the *inguinal* sac at the apparently normal external ring.

Lambrecht[26] reported two cases in infants; both hernias were on the right side. In one of the infants, who was 8 months of age, the testis could not be palpated.

There appears to be a relationship between the incidence of testicular abnormalities and interparietal hernia, but this cannot be the explanation in all cases.

To cite Macready again, of 457 patients with a hernia in conjunction with anomalies of the testis, only 23 had interstitial hernia. In addition, many patients, including the one originally described by Bartholin,[4] had a normally placed testis, and some other explanation is necessary both for these cases and for cases occurring in women. The relatively small and tight external ring in women may explain the latter.

Congenital Pouches

Rokitansky[36] described the finding of small pouches or diverticula of peritoneum in the region of the internal inguinal ring. Moynihan[31] described similar fossae in fetuses, reporting an incidence of 22%. Similar findings in adults were obtained by Coughlin.[12] It appears that these pouches could form the beginnings of a preperitoneal hernia and, thus, would explain the occurrence of a sac that has no connection with an inguinal hernia.

Although Moynihan supported this idea, he denied that this alone was the cause, and insisted that there always must be a connection with an inguinal sac. He envisaged a small pouch enlarging until its neck merged with that of a concurrent inguinal sac, thus producing an opening from the peritoneal cavity that is common to both of them.

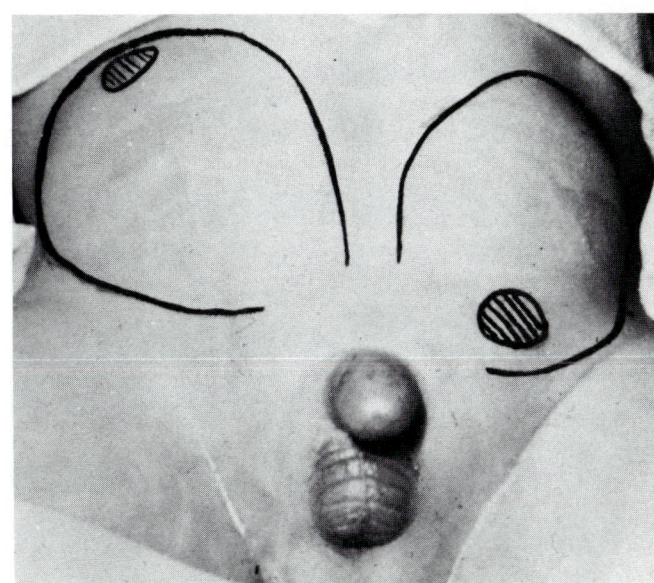

Figure 27-5. Bilateral interstitial hernia in a 5-day-old infant. The extent of the bilateral abdominal masses and the position of the testes are demonstrated clearly. Note the empty and underdeveloped scrotum. (Masih B, et al. Surgery 1971; 69:577.)

Other Congenital Anomalies

Other congenital abnormalities, such as absence of the cremaster muscle, absence of the external abdominal ring, a superimposed abdominal ring, and a dislocated internal ring, in which the internal ring is misplaced congenitally upward and outward, have been suggested.[38]

The theory of association with testicular anomalies is the best supported and has in its favor the higher incidence of interparietal hernia on the right side as compared with the left, there being on the right side a greater percentage of abnormalities associated with delayed descent of the testis and delayed closing of the processus vaginalis.

Russell[37] suggested that all hernias are congenital, and that interparietal hernias are explained by the processus vaginalis becoming caught up between the layers of the abdominal muscles.

On the whole, the etiology of interparietal hernias appears to be multifactorial. Barling[3] believed that all interparietal hernias should be considered congenital, and that mechanical factors, when they occur, are secondary to the congenital defect. This view probably is the most satisfactory given the current state of our knowledge.

INCIDENCE

The incidence of preperitoneal hernia is difficult to assess because many cases probably remain undiagnosed. The interstitial and superficial types, because of the presence of a palpable mass, are more likely to be diagnosed correctly; even so, assessment of incidence is unlikely to be accurate.

The relative incidence, as taken from the literature, remains as given by Lower and Hicken:[28] preperitoneal, 20%; interstitial, 60%; superficial, 20%.

Reports of the absolute incidence vary between authors. The figures for preperitoneal hernia deviate considerably, being given as 1 in 5000 hernias (0.02%) by Bull and Coley[7] and as 0.31% of all hernias in his clinic by Biasini.[6] There also is a wide range of figures for interstitial hernias, from 42 of 50,000 hernias (0.08%)[27] to 6 of 482 hernias (1.2%).[32] The only fact that emerges from a study of incidence is that it depends on recognition of the condition by the surgeon. The impression is that preperitoneal hernias occur much more commonly than do the interstitial or superficial types, but because of difficulty in diagnosis, they have been recognized and reported less often.

There is a distinctly higher incidence in men than in women, perhaps associated with a higher incidence of congenital abnormalities in the inguinal region in men. The male:female ratio of the hernias is reported to be 3.5:1 to 4:1 for the preperitoneal and interstitial types, and 10:1 to 14:1 for the superficial types. Five of the six hernias reported by Etawo and Elechi[16] were in women.

The hernias occur earlier in men than in women. They have been reported from birth to 74 years in men, with a maximum incidence at 30 to 40 years. In women, the greatest proportion are seen at 50 to 60 years.

DIAGNOSIS

Making the correct diagnosis depends first on awareness of the condition on the part of the surgeon. This may sound trite, but as pointed out by Beigler and O'Brien,[5] the diagnosis seldom is made because clinicians become accustomed to classifying hernias in the inguinal region as direct or indirect and do not recognize other types because they are unaware of their existence.

It may be difficult or even impossible to make a correct diagnosis before operation, and in most of the cases reported in the literature, the diagnosis has been made only at laparotomy or autopsy.

In 90% of cases, the patient has intestinal obstruction. This may be accompanied by pain in the suprainguinal region. If the hernial contents are strangulated at the neck of a preperitoneal sac, however, there may be no symptoms referable to the inguinal region.

The presence of a mass makes a correct diagnosis more likely, but a mass occurs only in the interstitial and superficial types. If there is a palpable lump, it is most likely to be felt above and lateral to the internal inguinal ring.[8,32,35]

I saw a 58-year-old man with a 1-year-old recurrence of a right inguinal hernia originally repaired 27 years earlier. He complained of a rapid increase in size and of pain in the right lower quadrant and back. A mass measuring 12×10 cm was present that extended upward and laterally to the anterior superior iliac spine with a cough impulse. It was completely reducible downward and medially. At operation, a well-formed sac containing small intestine was found lying between the external and internal oblique muscles. There was much scarring from the previous repair medial to the internal ring.

It is probable that the recurrence was directed upward and laterally, similar to an interstitial hernia, because of the scarring in the canal. The interstitial sac may have been overlooked at the first repair.

If no mass is palpable, computed tomography of the lower abdominal wall should be considered (see Chap. 26). In a patient with intestinal obstruction, the following criteria may indicate a strangulated interparietal hernia:

1. A long-standing inguinal hernia, especially if there has been a recent prolonged attempt to reduce it with apparent success after a great deal of initial difficulty
2. Abnormal position of the testis with or without an underdeveloped scrotum on that side
3. Pain in the suprainguinal region that is worse on standing and relieved by lying down

Suprainguinal pain may be the only symptom of a nonstrangulated hernia or of one that contains only a knuckle of intestine (Richter hernia) or omentum, but interstitial and superficial hernias also may produce a small mass that appears on standing and disappears on lying down.

The most common presentation, therefore, is colicky pain and absolute constipation, vomiting, and abdominal distention, sometimes with a mass above the inguinal ligament and an abnormally placed testis.

Dass and Wood[13] reported a case of strangulation in an unrecognized interstitial hernia immediately after repair of a large inguinal hernia in an 86-year-old man.

TREATMENT

Initial treatment most commonly consists of urgent operation to relieve intestinal obstruction.

The surgical approach to undiagnosed hernias is abdominal, with exploration revealing a loop of intestine disappearing into a hernial sac, and a mass in the region of the posterior aspect of the inguinal canal. The neck of the sac is divided, the loop of intestine is freed, the neck of the sac is ligated, and the sac is pulled inside out and excised.

In the presence of a mass, a combined inguinal and abdominal approach probably is best, and the recommended incision is made parallel to, but higher than that normally used for herniorrhaphy.[3] This provides better exposure of the site of obstruction. After the intestine is inspected and dealt with as in routine strangulation, the interparietal sac may be excised and its neck closed in the usual manner.

An abnormally placed testis may present a problem. If it is considered desirable and technically possible, the testis may be brought down to the scrotum, but it probably should be removed. Removing the testis not only enables a sound repair to be made, but also prevents the occurrences to which abnormally placed testes are prone—trauma, malignant change, and inflammation. The surgeon then may proceed with routine repair.

As a prophylactic measure during herniorrhaphy in the inguinal and femoral regions, it always is wise to open the sac, examine it, and palpate it carefully for loculi. This is facilitated by free exposure of the entire inguinal canal. By placing traction on the dissected sac, any loculi can be pulled down and the sac can be closed proximally.

Similarly, when an apparently straightforward strangulated inguinal or femoral hernia is repaired, it is advisable to expose the neck of the sac completely to avoid overlooking a preperitoneal sac containing strangulated intestine. If such a sac is missed, the symptoms of intestinal obstruction persist after apparent reduction of the hernia. In the presence of such symptoms, reoperation and a search for a preperitoneal sac are essential.

With regard to conservative treatment of inguinal hernia, it should be pointed out that a truss never should be prescribed if the testis on the side of the hernia is abnormally placed.

The reported mortality for preperitoneal hernia is much higher than for more easily diagnosed varieties of hernia, but should be no greater than for any other type of intestinal strangulation.

REFERENCES

1. Abu-Dalu K, Muggia M, Schiller M. Congenital inguinal hernia—an unusual manifestation. Z Kinderchir 1981;34:290.
2. Altman B. Interstitial presenting as spigelian hernia. Br J Surg 1960;48:60.
3. Barling EV. Interparietal hernia. Aust N Z J Surg 1956;26:32.
4. Bartholin T. Historiarum Anatomicarum et Medicarum Rarorium Cent v, Hist 51. Hafniae, 1661:117.
5. Beigler SK, O'Brien H. Interstitial hernia. Wis Med J 1928;27:407.
6. Biasini A. Contribution to the study of strangulated inguinoproperitoneal hernia. Int Abstr Surg 1949; 88:338.
7. Bull WT, Coley WB. Observations on the mechanical and operative treatment of hernia at the Hospital for Ruptured and Crippled of New York. Ann Surg 1893;17:527.
8. Carpanelli JB. Hernias intersticiales complicadas. Rev Asoc Med Argent 1955;69:384.
9. Coley WB. Inguinal hernia in the female. Ann Surg 1909;50:609.
10. Cooper AP. The anatomy and surgical treatment of abdominal hernia, ed 2. London, Longman, 1827.
11. Corner EM. A case of strangulated hernia, first in one, and then in the second sac (a hernia en bissac) of an inguinal hernia. Med Press Circ ns 1912;94:213.
12. Coughlin WT. Anatomical and pathological observations on the formation of hernia at Hesselbach's triangle. St Louis Cour Med 1905;33:336.
13. Dass T, Wood EF. Accidental strangulation of interstitial hernia following inguinal herniorrhaphy. Arch Surg 1968;96:949.
14. De Garmo WB. Abdominal hernia, its diagnosis and treatment. Philadelphia, JB Lippincott, 1907.
15. Eppinger H. Beiträge zur Pathologischen Anatomie der Hernien in der Leistengegend. Int Beitr z Wiss Med Festschr R Virchow 1891;2:357.
16. Etawo US, Elechi EN. Interparietal hernias: analysis of six cases with literature review. Br J Clin Pract 1987;41:1068.
17. Fuld JE. Interparietal inguinal hernia. Int J Surg 1921;34:132.
18. Göbell R. Ueber interparietale Leistenbrche. Dtsch Z Chir 1900;56:1.
19. Goyrand G. De la hernie inguino-interstitielle. Mem Acad R Med 1836;5:14.
20. Halstead AE. Inguino-properitoneal hernia; inguinointerstitial hernia: report of cases. Ann Surg 1906; 43:704.
21. Hernu C. Observation sur un étranglement intérier d'une portion d'intestin. Rec Period Soc Med Sédillot 1802;11:291.
22. Hesselbach FC. Neueste Anatomisch-Pathologische Untersuchungen über den Ursprung und das Fortschreiten der Leisten—und Schenkelbrüche. Würzburg, Stahel, 1814.
23. Howlett EH. A case of properitoneal hernia. Q Med J 1902;10:336.
24. Krönlein RU. Herniologische Beobachtungen aus der v. Langenbeck'schen Klinik. Arch Klin Chir 1876;19:408.
25. Küster E. Beiträge zur Lehre von den Hernien. Arch Klin Chir 1887;34:202.
26. Lambrecht W. Die interstitielle Liestenhernie des Säuglings. Chirurg 1983;54:541.
27. Langton J. The association of inguinal hernia with descent of the testis. Lancet 1900;2:1857.
28. Lower WE, Hicken NF. Interparietal hernias. Ann Surg 1931;94:1070.
29. Macready JFCH. A treatise on ruptures. London, C Griffin, 1893.
30. Masih B, Swamy S, Altman B. Bilateral interstitial hernia in the newborn infant. Surgery 1971;69:577.
31. Moynihan BGA. The anatomy and pathology of the rarer forms of hernia. Lancet 1900;1:513.
32. Noonan TJ. Interstitial inguinal hernia. Lancet 1950; 2:849.
33. Parise J. Mémoire sur deux variétés nouvelles de hernies. Mem Soc Chir Paris 1851;2:399.
34. Petit JL. Traité des maladies chirurgicales, et des opérations qui leur conviennent, vol 2. Paris, Méquignon l'aîné, 1790:217.
35. Rampini OA, Garbini JJ. Un caso de hernia intersticial. Sem Med (B Air) 1957;3:896.
36. Rokitansky C. A manual of pathological anatomy, vol 2. London, Sydenham Society, 1849.
37. Russell RH. Inguinal herniae: their varieties, mode of origin, and classification. Br J Surg 1922;9:502.
38. Schmidt M. Zur Aufrechterhaltung meiner Erklärung fr die Genese der Hernia inguino-interstitialis und Hernia inguino-properitonealis. Arch Klin Chir 1891;41:292.
39. Zimmerman LM, Anson BJ. Anatomy and surgery of hernia. Baltimore, Williams & Wilkins, 1953.

Hernia, Fourth Edition, edited
by Lloyd M. Nyhus and Robert E. Condon.
J.B. Lippincott Company, Philadelphia © 1995.

Chapter 28

Supravesical Hernia

*Panagiotis N. Skandalakis, Lee J. Skandalakis, Stephen W. Gray,
and John E. Skandalakis*

Because of mankind's erect posture, the anterior abdominal wall is the site of a variety of hernias. Most of these defects protrude through the abdominal wall to form obvious, palpable swellings in the groin. From a beginning in one area, the supravesical fossa, a hernia may take either of two paths. It may appear externally as a direct inguinal or a femoral hernia, or, more accurately, an external supravesical hernia. Much less commonly, such a hernia remains within the abdomen, passing into spaces around the bladder as an internal supravesical hernia (Fig. 28-1). Both rare and invisible, these internal hernias are pathologic curiosities and diagnostic challenges.

HISTORY

Sir Astley Cooper[9] illustrated the first recognizable external supravesical hernia in 1804. Ten years later, Ring[26] described the first authentic internal supravesical hernia. In 1940, Warvi and Orr[32] reviewed the literature and found 38 acceptable cases of internal supravesical hernia, including 1 treated by them. They also reproduced Cooper's illustration of an external supravesical hernia. Keynes,[19] in the first edition of this book, found 41 acceptable and 10 probable cases. In 1970, Adler[1] considered a hernia he treated to be the 58th such case in the world literature. The hernia treated by us became the 59th case of internal supravesical hernia.[29] Two more cases were reported by Guivarc'h and Fallouh[14] in 1977. Ten years later, Ekberg and Kullenberg[12] reported hernial sacs protruding from the supravesical fossa in 5 patients in a series of 19 patients with direct diverticular inguinal hernia (DDIH). An unusual type of supravesical small-bowel hernia associated with herniation of the bladder through a traumatic diastasis of the pubic symphysis was reported by Jacques and colleagues.[17] Chou and coworkers[8] found a supravesical hernia that had caused the bowel obstruction they were investigating. Köksoy and associates identified 64 cases of internal supravesical hernia in the world literature, including

1 of their own (Köksoy F, Soybir G, Yalçin O, Aker UY, Köse H, unpublished data, 1993).

Despite these reports, it is not feasible to tabulate all reported cases because of the confusion in terminology. Warvi and Orr[32] listed 22 terms used to describe the 38 hernias they reviewed. They complained that the term *supravesical hernia* was not in medical dictionaries; this remains true 53 years later! They politely refrained from observing that, for more than a century, the subject of these hernias had been avoided rather than neglected.

Much of the difficulty lies in the failure of patient reports to describe the path taken by the hernial sac. In far too many reports, the origin of the hernia in the supravesical fossa is clear, but the subsequent path of the hernia is obscure. Reduction of the hernia and repair of the hernial ring often have been accomplished without the exploration necessary to understand the anatomic relationship of the hernial sac.

ANATOMY OF THE ANTERIOR ABDOMINAL WALL AND SUPRAVESICAL FOSSA

The posterior surface of the anterior abdominal wall contains three shallow fossae on each side of the midline, which is marked by the obliterated urachus extending from the umbilicus to the dome of the bladder (see Fig. 28-1). From lateral to medial, these fossae are as follows:

Lateral fossa—Lateral to the interior epigastric artery. Location of the internal inguinal ring. Site of indirect inguinal hernia.
Medial fossa—Between the inferior epigastric artery and the lateral umbilical ligament (obliterated umbilical artery). Site of direct inguinal hernia.
Supravesical fossa—Between the lateral umbilical ligament and the middle umbilical ligament (obliterated urachus). Site of supravesical hernia.

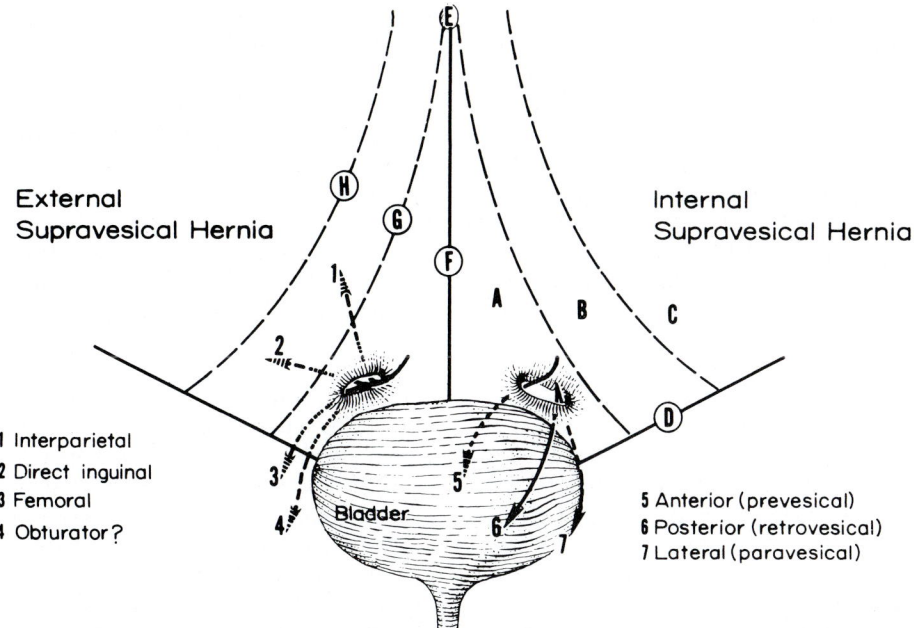

External
Supravesical Hernia

Internal
Supravesical Hernia

1 Interparietal
2 Direct inguinal
3 Femoral
4 Obturator?

Bladder

5 Anterior (prevesical)
6 Posterior (retrovesical)
7 Lateral (paravesical)

Figure 28-1. The bladder and anterior abdominal wall viewed posteriorly. Possible pathways of external supravesical hernias are shown on the left and those of internal supravesical hernias are shown on the right. A, supravesical fossa with mouth of supravesical hernia; B, medial fossa; C, lateral fossa; D, inguinal ligament; E, umbilicus; F, middle umbilical ligament (obliterated urachus); G, lateral umbilical ligament (obliterated umbilical artery); H, inferior (deep) epigastric artery.

The supravesical fossa partially overlies the modern conception of the Hesselbach triangle (Fig. 28-2), so that the lateral umbilical ligament lies within it. Thus, a hernia through either the medial or the supravesical fossa is a direct inguinal hernia. From another point of view, it can be said that a direct hernia may be either an "inguinal direct" (in the medial fossa) or a "supravesical" (in the supravesical fossa) hernia.

The lateral umbilical ligament is not always constant. In about 10% of the population, the terminal portion of the aponeurosis of the internal oblique muscle and the transversus abdominis muscle form the "conjoined tendon." This "tendon" lies close to the

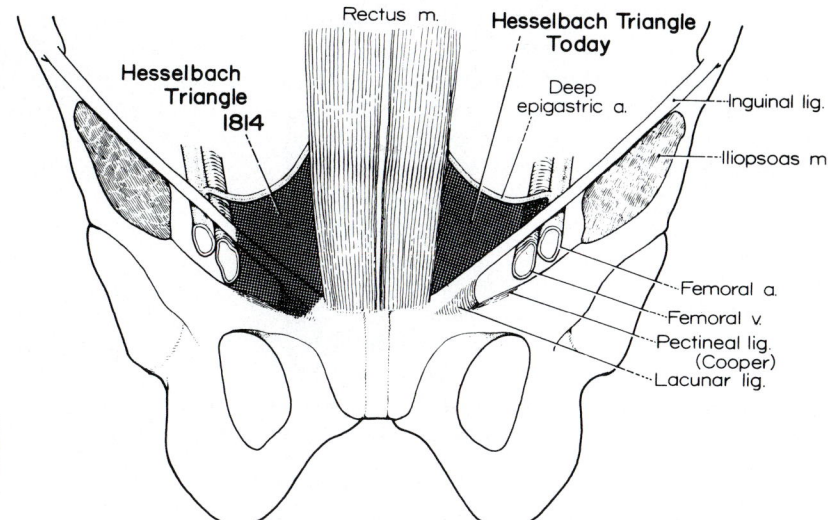

Rectus m.

Hesselbach Triangle
1814

Hesselbach Triangle
Today

Deep
epigastric a.

Inguinal lig.
Iliopsoas m.
Femoral a.
Femoral v.
Pectineal lig.
(Cooper)
Lacunar lig.

Figure 28-2. Hesselbach triangle as originally described (*left*) and as accepted today (*right*). It may be seen that part of the supravesical fossa lies within the triangle.

lateral umbilical ligament. In most patients, the tendon is absent, and we believe that the lateral border of the rectus sheath is the best landmark for recognition of a supravesical hernia (Fig. 28-3). This border always is present, whereas the "conjoined tendon" is not.

The floor of the supravesical fossa is formed by a portion of the endopelvic fascia. If the bladder is empty, the proximal half of the fossa is formed by the transversalis fascia, and the distal half by the vesical fascia, which may be considered to be a part of either the endopelvic fascia or the transversalis fascia. Somewhere between the umbilicus and the semicircularis line of Douglas, the upward continuation of the vesical fascia gradually becomes united with the transversalis fascia.

We agree with Keynes[19] that the lower limit of the supravesical fossa should be the transverse fold of the bladder. This fold is more marked in some individuals than in others, but to go beyond it would expand unnecessarily the concept of the fossa.

Thus, for the surgeon, the lateral limit of the supravesical fossa is poorly defined, whereas for the anatomist, the upper and lower limits seem equally poorly demarcated.

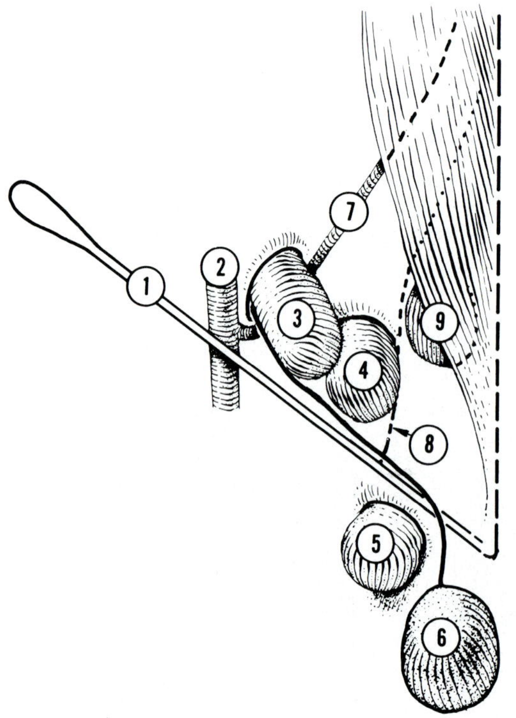

EXTERNAL SUPRAVESICAL HERNIA

An external supravesical hernia forms as a result of failure of the integrity of the aponeurosis of the transversus abdominis muscle and the transversalis fascia, both of which insert into the pectineal ligament (of Cooper). Any defect in the wall of the supravesical fossa permits first a bulge and later a true hernial sac. In relation to the myopectineal orifice of Fruchaud (Fig. 28-4), this defect should be located most medially.[31] The sac usually remains above the pelvis and forms a direct or a femoral hernia.

Perhaps as many as half of all direct inguinal hernias originate in the supravesical fossa.[7] Such hernias may emerge through the lower part of the semilunar zone (spigelian or pararectal hernias) or lateral to the rectus muscle (median or lateral direct hernias). The opening of the hernia may be large enough to extend laterally beyond the lateral umbilical ligament and into part of the triangle of Hesselbach. Keynes[19] observed that hernia from the supravesical fossa to the obturator canal is possible, although it has not been described.

Figure 28-3. Four types of groin hernia and some of the important landmarks. 1, inguinal ligament; 2, femoral artery; 3, indirect hernial sac; 4, direct hernial sac; 5, femoral sac; 6, testis; 7, inferior epigastric artery; 8, lateral umbilical ligament; 9, external supravesical sac emerging from beneath the rectus abdominis muscle. (Rowe JS Jr, et al. Am Surg 1973; 39:269.)

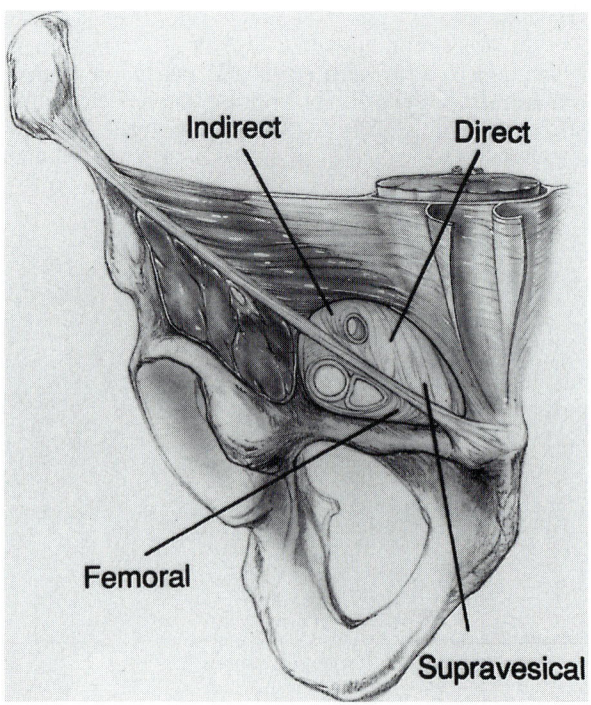

Figure 28-4. Posterior view of Fruchaud myopectineal orifice. (Modified from Wantz GE. Atlas of hernia surgery. New York, Raven Press, 1991.)

Not surprisingly, these hernias frequently coexist with other hernias in this region. The specimen illustrated in Cooper's report of 1804 shows six hernial openings in the abdominal wall; two were in the supravesical fossae. We described a patient who had external supravesical, direct, indirect, and femoral hernias on each side of his body[27] (see Fig. 28-3). We also saw a patient with indirect, direct, interstitial, and external supravesical hernias, all on the same side.[29] Remarkably, there was no hernia on the other side.

External supravesical hernias cause no special symptoms and present no particular diagnostic problems. An external swelling always is present and palpable; repair is as usual for inguinal hernias.

External supravesical hernias are common, comprising about half of all direct groin hernias.[7] Direct hernias account for about 7.5% of all hernias.[33]

Ekberg and Kullenberg[12] classify external supravesical hernias, among other direct inguinal hernias, as DDIHs because of their characteristically narrow neck. They estimate the frequency of DDIH to be about 1% of all hernias in men; these lesions are extremely rare in women.

Diagnosis

The diagnosis of external supravesical hernias is easy if the surgeon remembers the existence of such an entity. In the differential diagnosis of inguinal hernia, any swelling at the medial edge of the triangle of Hesselbach or at the lateral edge of the rectus abdominis muscle should be considered to be a supravesical hernia. If the hernia follows the femoral or obturator route, its diagnosis is difficult but academic. To the inattentive surgeon, an external supravesical hernia is a rarity, but to the thoughtful surgeon who remembers the anatomy of the region, this hernia is not rare.

Treatment

The treatment of external supravesical hernias is surgical. The procedure of choice and the approach used depend on the anatomic location of the swelling; they are the same as for any groin hernia above or below the inguinal ligament.

INTERNAL SUPRAVESICAL HERNIA

There is considerable confusion in the classification of internal supravesical hernias. By definition, they all start in the supravesical fossa, but their subsequent course varies. The terms *prevesical*, *paravesical*, and *retrovesical* have been used by Keynes,[19] Adler,[1] and others. Burton[6] used the terms *prevesical*, *supravesical*, and *paravesical*. He excluded the retrovesical hernias. These terms are readily understood, but they are awkward in combination with the collective term *supravesical*. We have proposed the following classification of internal supravesical hernias based on whether their course is in front of, beside, or behind the bladder[29] (Fig. 28-5):

1. Anterior supravesical hernia
   a. Retropubic supravesical hernia
   b. Invaginating supravesical hernia

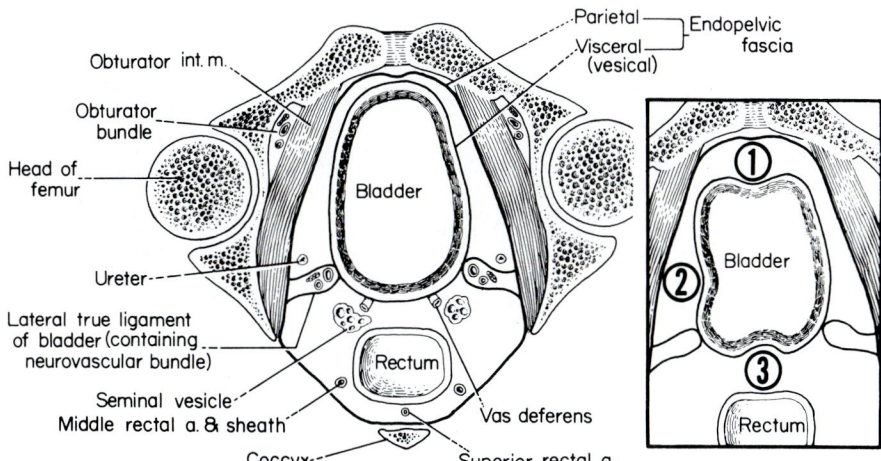

Figure 28-5. Highly diagrammatic section of the body at the level of the acetabulum showing some of the landmarks of the spaces around the bladder. (*Inset*) 1, location of sac in anterior internal supravesical hernia; 2, location of sac in lateral internal supravesical hernia; 3, location of sac in posterior internal supravesical hernia.

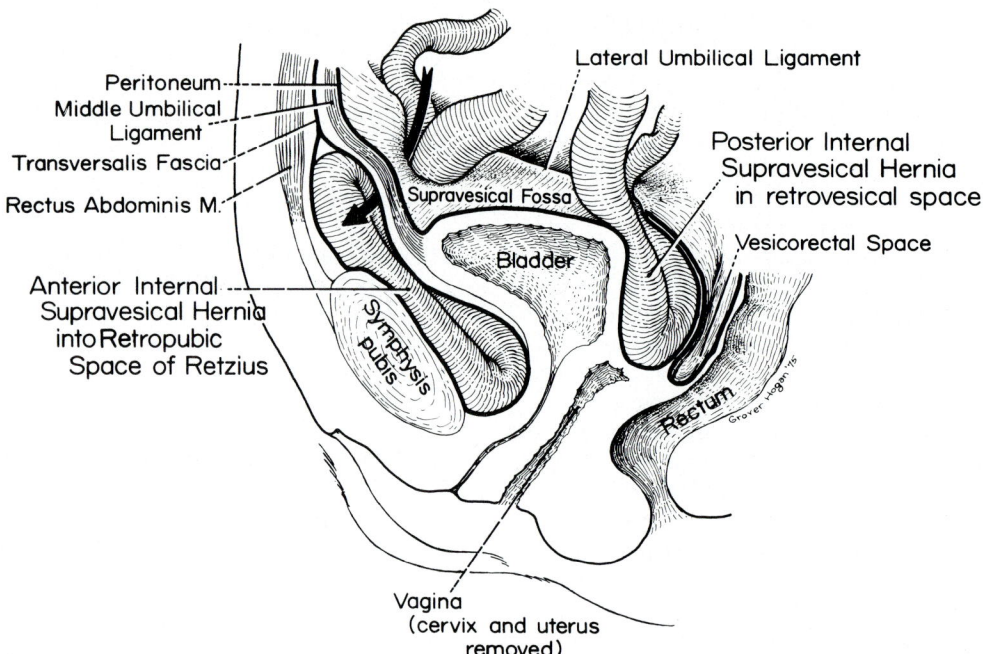

Figure 28-6. Comparison of anterior and posterior internal supravesical hernias. Most are of the anterior type. The posterior hernia is illustrated in a patient who previously had undergone a hysterectomy. (Skandalakis JE, et al. Internal and external supravesical hernia. Am Surg 1976; 42:142–146.)

2. Right or left lateral supravesical hernia
3. Posterior supravesical hernia

Types 1b and 3 are extremely rare.

The anterior retropubic and the lateral hernias pass into the retropubic space of Retzius behind the pubis and in front of the bladder (Fig. 28-6). The in-

vaginating type (1b) pushes in the anterior bladder wall rather than descending behind the pubis (Fig. 28-7). This type has been called *intravesical*,[1] but this term is misleading, because the hernia does not enter the bladder.

The posterior hernias pass into the retrovesical space between the bladder and the rectum in men, or

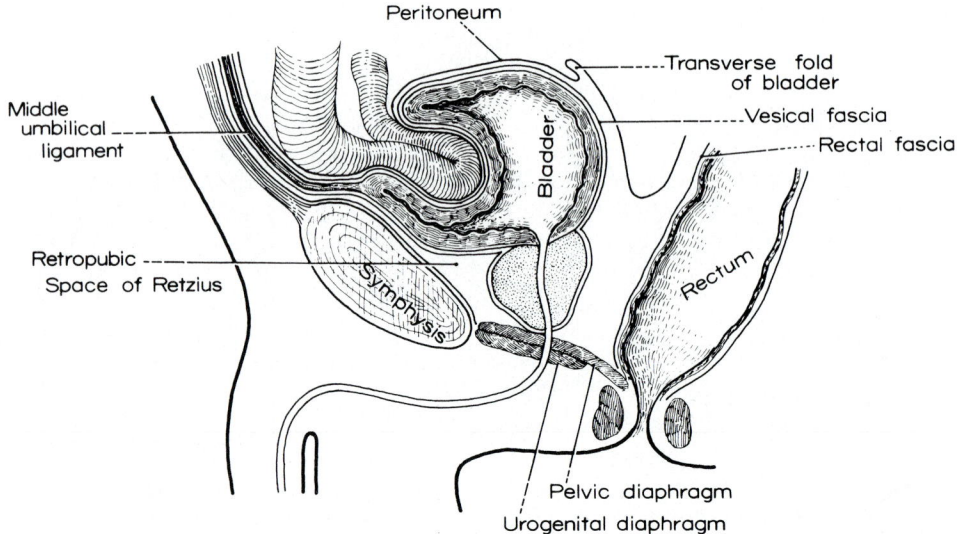

Figure 28-7. Invaginating type of anterior internal supravesical hernia.

between the bladder and the uterus in women. They form a definite, but small group of supravesical hernias (see Fig. 28-6).

In practice, only well-developed anterior and lateral hernias, accurately described by the surgeon, can be classified. A hernia may be reduced and the sac ligated without examination of the pathway the sac has taken. In many cases, the sac is small and the hernia has not descended completely. Anterior retropubic and lateral supravesical hernias are especially difficult to differentiate in the early stages of their development. Attempts at precise classification of many cases in the literature are futile.

Knowledge of the surgical anatomy of the supravesical fossa and the spaces around the bladder is essential to a clear understanding of these hernias. Figure 28-5 shows the bladder and the spaces into which herniation may occur.

Review of Surgical Anatomy

Retropubic Space (Prevesical Space; Space of Retzius)

Boundaries. The retropubic space is situated in front and to the sides of the urinary bladder. Its boundaries are as follows:

Anterior—Symphysis pubis
Lateral—Pubic bone; fascia of internal obturator muscle; superior fascia of levator ani muscle; lateral puboprostatic ligament
Medial—Inferior lateral surface of bladder
Superior—Peritoneum bridging the upper surface of the bladder and the lateral pelvic wall
Posterior—Vascular stalk of the hypogastric artery and vein with its sheath, which reach the posterolateral border of the bladder
Inferior—Puboprostatic or pubovesical ligaments; reflection of the superior fascia of the levator ani muscle to the urinary bladder

The space potentially extends upward and laterally in the anterior abdominal wall to form a triangular space between the lateral umbilical ligaments. The upper limits of the space depend on the level at which the transversalis fascia and the vesical fascia fuse with each other (Figs. 28-8 and 28-9). Thus, the retropubic space is not the small "cave of Retzius" described in some books, but "an extensive bursa-like cleft in the areolar tissue at the sides and front of the bladder that allows the bladder to fill and empty without hindrance."[2]

With the foregoing in mind, this large triangular anatomic area can be summarized as follows: the apex of the triangle is at the umbilicus, the sides are formed by the two lateral umbilical ligaments, and the base is formed by the puboprostatic or pubovesical ligaments.

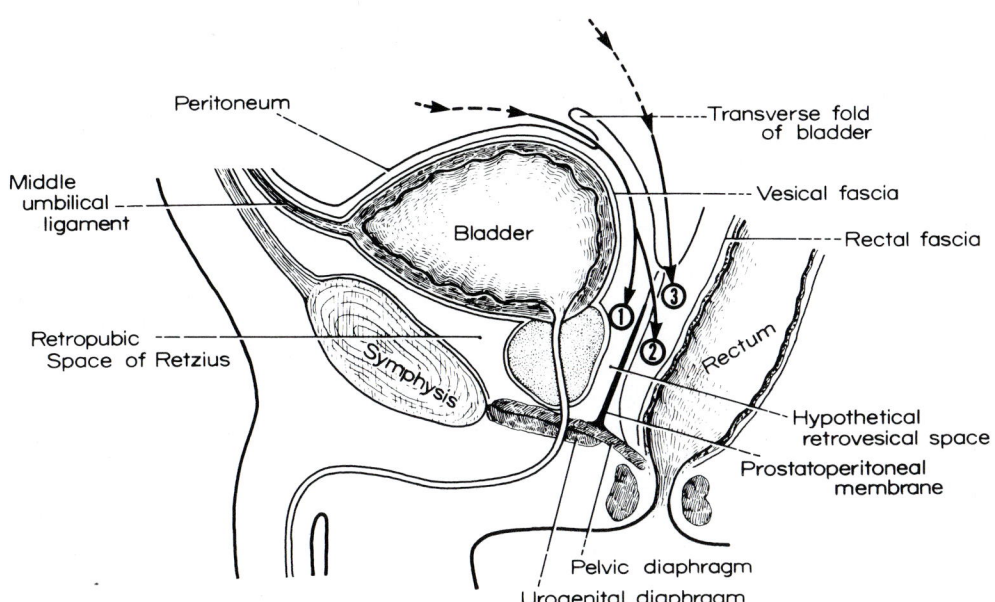

Figure 28-8. Three possible pathways of posterior internal supravesical hernias in men. 1, path of true retrovesical hernia; 2, path of retrovesical hernia; 3, path of hernia through rectovesical pouch.

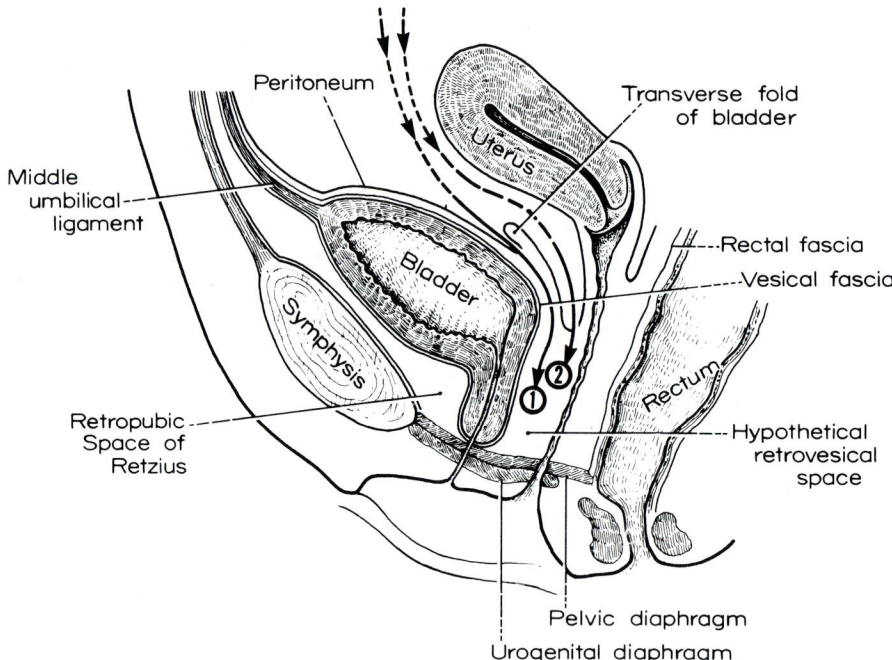

Figure 28-9. Two possible pathways of posterior internal supravesical hernias in women. 1, path of true rectovesical hernia; 2, path of hernia through the vesicovaginal pouch.

Space of Bogros

Boundaries. The French anatomist Bogros (1823) originally described a triangular space (Fig. 28-10) with the following boundaries:

Lateral—Iliac fascia
Anterior—Transversalis fascia
Medial—Parietal peritoneum

The space of Bogros is a lateral extension of the retropubic space of Retzius and may be explored by incising the transversalis fascia from the internal ring to the pubic crest.[3]

Stoppa (personal communication, 1992) believes this cleavable interparietal/peritoneal space to be the lower prolongation of the great posterior paraurinary space. Hureau and colleagues[15,16] consider the posterior paraurinary area to be comprised of (1) the fat of Gerota anteriorly, and (2) a cellular space posteriorly that most likely incorporates the space of Bogros in the internal iliac fossa.

Fat and other connective tissue, either thick or thin, lie within the space between the peritoneum and the transversalis fascia. Fibrous bands are present, and lipomas similar to those in the spermatic cord are found occasionally. The preperitoneal space is exposed by the reflection of parietal peritoneum toward the iliac fossa before it reaches the pubic bone.

Peritoneum. In both men and women, the peritoneum covers the superior surface of the bladder and passes to the posterior surface of the anterior body wall and the lateral pelvic wall. On each side of the bladder, the lateral peritoneum lines the paravesical fossa.

Posteriorly, the peritoneum in men passes to the rectum, forming the rectovesical fossa. In women, it passes to the uterus, forming the uterovesical fossa. Across the upper surface of the bladder is a peritoneal fold, the transverse fold of the bladder, which is the posteroinferior limit of the supravesical fossa. In emaciated male cadavers, this fold can be seen bridging both right and left deep inguinal rings after crossing the lateral umbilical ligaments.

Fasciae. The transversalis fascia envelops the abdominal cavity from the lower surface of the respiratory diaphragm down to the formation of the endopelvic fascia with its subdivisions. It should be remembered that the femoral ring and sheath are part of this fascia, and that it inserts on the pubis and on the pectineal (Cooper) ligament.

The term *transversalis fascia* once was used to identify only the deep fascia covering the internal surface of the transverse abdominis muscle. Today, the term refers to the entire connective tissue sheet lining the musculature of the abdominal cavity. Specific

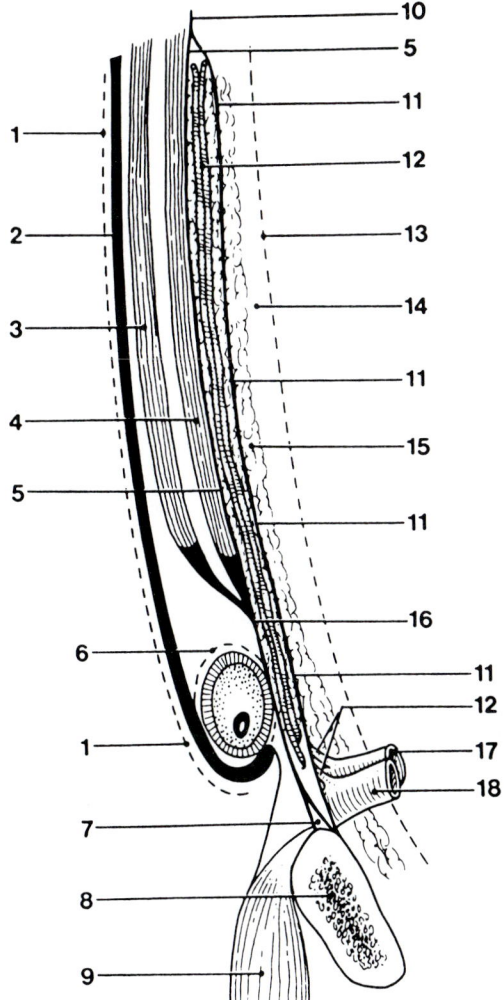

Figure 28-10. The space of Bogros. 1, innominate fascia; 2, external oblique aponeurosis; 3, internal oblique muscle; 4, transversus abdominis muscle; 5, transversalis fascia anterior; 6, external spermatic fascia; 7, Cooper ligament; 8, pubic bone; 9, pectineus muscle; 10, transversalis fascia; 11, transversalis fascia; 12, vessels; 13, peritoneum; 14, home (space) of the prosthesis, space of Bogros; 15, preperitoneal fat; 16, transversus abdominis aponeurosis and anterior lamina of transversalis fascia; 17, femoral artery; 18, femoral vein. (Skandalakis JE, et al. Embryologic and anatomic basis of inguinal herniorrhaphy. Surg Clin North Am 1993; 73:799–836.)

areas of this fascial layer are identified by the muscles they cover, such as "iliacus" or "psoas" fascia.

The composition of the transversalis fascia varies. It is thin and closely adherent in the portion covering the transversus abdominis aponeurosis. It is thick and discrete in other areas.[9] Although it is a weak layer that is useless for hernia repair when used alone, it serves this function well when it is fused with the transversus abdominis aponeurosis.

Cooper's posterior lamina of transversalis fascia is a tissue paper–like membrane covering the preperitoneal fat at the inguinal area (Fig. 28-11). Challenging the popular view of a monolaminar transversalis fascia, Read[25] supports Astley Cooper's observation[9a] that this anatomic feature is bilaminar in nature. Read identifies a posterior lamina deep to the epigastric vasculature attached to the pubic ramus.

The umbilical vesical fascia is an upward continuation of the vesical fascia; it envelops the lateral and middle umbilical ligaments.

The umbilical prevesical fascia is a thin, ill-defined fascia between the umbilical vesical fascia and the transversalis fascia. We believe that these last two fasciae are of no importance to the surgeon, who needs to be concerned only with the retropubic space of Retzius.

The pelvic or endopelvic fascia is the downward continuation of the abdominal fascia. For ease of description, it may be divided arbitrarily into parietal, diaphragmatic, and visceral portions. The parietal portion covers the lateral pelvic wall and its two muscles, the piriformis and the obturator internus. The diaphragmatic portion forms the superior and inferior layers of the pelvic diaphragm (coccygeus and levator ani muscles), as well as the superior layer of the urogenital diaphragm. The inferior layer is not part of the endopelvic fascia. The visceral portion is a reflection of the superficial layer of the pelvic diaphragm to the bladder, rectum, prostate, and vagina.

The bladder and rectum are separated by four layers of visceral fascia: vesical fascia, fascia of seminal vesicles and ductus deferens (two layers), and rectal fascia.

Ligaments of the Bladder. The nine true ligaments of the bladder are special thickened areas of the endopelvic fascia. They are the urachus (median umbilical ligament) in the midline and four paired ligaments; the lateral true ligaments of the bladder, which envelop the vessels and nerves from the lateral pelvic wall to the base of the bladder; the obliterated umbilical (hypogastric) arteries; and the medial and lateral puboprostatic ligaments in men, and the medial and lateral pubovesical ligaments in women.

The seven false ligaments are folds of peritoneum. They are the superior ligament (median umbilical fold) in the midline, covering the urachus, and three paired folds; the lateral superior ligaments (medial umbilical folds) following the obliterated umbilical arteries; the posterior false ligaments (sacrogenital folds) of the retrovesical pouch; and the lateral false ligaments from the lateral bladder wall to the lateral pelvic wall.

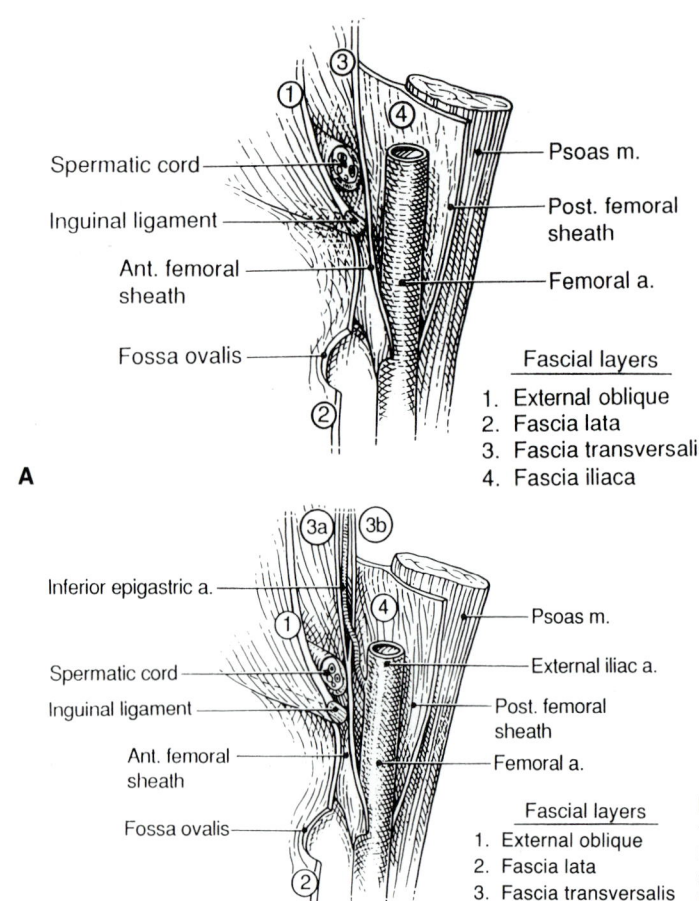

Fascial layers

1. External oblique
2. Fascia lata
3. Fascia transversalis
4. Fascia iliaca

A

Fascial layers

1. External oblique
2. Fascia lata
3. Fascia transversalis
   a. Anterior lamina
   b. Posterior lamina
4. Fascia iliaca

B

Figure 28-11. (*A*) Highly diagrammatic drawing of the transversalis fascia and femoral sheath (old concept). (*B*) Highly diagrammatic drawing of the transversalis fascia and femoral sheath (new concept), emphasizing the bilaminar nature of the transversalis fascia in the inguinal area. (Skandalakis JE, et al. Embryologic and anatomic basis of inguinal herniorrhaphy. Surg Clin North Am 1993; 73:799–836.)

Retrovesical Space

Boundaries in Men. The boundaries of the retrovesical space are as follows:

Anterior—Posterior surface of the bladder with vesical fascia; the lateral true ligament of the bladder
Superior—Peritoneum
Posterior—Anterior surface of the rectum with rectal fascia
Inferior—Rectourethralis ligament; pelvic diaphragm
Contents—Seminal vesicles and ductus deferens

The anterior and posterior boundaries of the space through which a retrovesical hernia passes may differ from those just described. Both the vesical fascia and the rectal fascia are loose connective tissue. Between them lies a stronger fascia (Denonvilliers),

the posterior part of the prostatic fascia or, more accurately, the anterior layer of the prostatoperitoneal membrane. Thus, the true retrovesical space lies between the vesical fascia and the anterior layer of the prostatoperitoneal membrane in men (see Fig. 28-8).

The hernial sac, starting at the bottom of the transverse fold of the bladder (posterior boundary of the supravesical fossa), passes between the vesical fascia and the peritoneum. It then may take either of the two following paths:

1. If the sac follows the bladder wall downward toward the seminal vesicles, its posterior boundary is the anterior layer of the prostatoperitoneal membrane, as shown by path 1 in Figure 28-8. This membrane is attenuated close to the peritoneum, but becomes stronger as it descends toward the prostate. It is here that the surgical/anatomic confusion arises.

2. If the sac travels more posteriorly through the upper, more attenuated part of this membrane, then the posterior boundary becomes the rectal wall because the rectal fascia is too loose to form a barrier. The prostatoperitoneal membrane forms the anterior boundary in this situation, as seen in path 2 of Figure 28-8. If the sac travels still deeper, it is questionable whether the hernia remains a retrovesical hernia or becomes a hernia into the rectovesical pouch. We consider such a rectovesical hernia with an intact pelvic floor to be surgically, if not anatomically, a retrovesical hernia.

If the sac originates in the rectovesical pouch, it passes into the same space, between the prostatoperitoneal membrane and the wall of the rectum (path 3, see Fig. 28-8). Although in the strict sense, its origin is outside the supravesical fossa, the final position of the sac is the same and the distinction is academic. Thus, a hernial sac in the rectovesical space may have its mouth (a) at the bottom of the transverse fold of the bladder, or (b) at the bottom of the rectovesical pouch.

In either situation, the end of the sac lies on the intact pelvic floor. If there is a defect in this floor through which the sac passes, it becomes a perineal hernia.

Boundaries in Women. In women, the situation is confused by the controversy over the existence of the so-called pubocervical ligament, pubocervical fascia, or vesicovaginal septum. We believe that a discussion of this structure is outside the scope of this chapter. The boundaries of the rectovesical space are as follows:

Anterior—Posterior surface of the bladder with vesical fascia; the true lateral ligament of the bladder
Superior—Peritoneum
Posterior—Anterior surface of the vagina with anterior vaginal fascia or the pubocervical ligament
Inferior—Reflection of the posterior vesical fascia and anterior vaginal fascia; pelvic and urogenital diaphragms or the pubocervical ligament; pelvic and urogenital diaphragms

As in men, the retrovesical space may be reached by a hernia starting in the bottom of the transverse fold of the bladder (path 1, see Fig. 28-9) or in the bottom of the vesicovaginal pouch (path 2, see Fig. 28-9).

Incidence

More than 60 cases of internal supravesical hernia were reported in the world literature to 1985. Eight years later, no more than 75 appeared in the literature.

No definite figures can be compiled for the relative frequency of the different types. By far the most common are the anterior retropubic hernias into the space of Retzius. Mauer,[20] analyzing 46 cases in the literature, considered 90% to be anterior. Only 3 confirmed cases of the invaginating type appear to have been reported.[4,5,34] Equally rare are the posterior hernias.[13,23,29]

Men are far more subject to internal supravesical hernias than are women, by a ratio of 5.7:1. More than half of all cases in both sexes occur in the sixth to seventh decade of life. Table 28-1 shows the distribution of 60 patients whose age and sex were known. The youngest patient was a boy 7 years of age;[18] the oldest patients were in their 70s.

Right and left supravesical fossae appear to be affected equally. Mauer[20] observed that this hernia has been reported in France more frequently than in Germany or Anglo-Saxon countries. Guivarc'h and Fallouh[14] referred to no fewer than 18 cases in the French literature over 25 years.

Etiology

To understand the etiology of supravesical hernia, three questions need to be answered:

1. Why does the sac form?
2. Why does it form more often in men?
3. Why are some supravesical hernias external, whereas others remain internal?

Table 28-1. Age and Sex in 60 Cases of Internal Supravesical Hernia

Age Groups (y)	Male	Female	Total
0–9	1	—	1
10–19	—	—	—
20–29	7	1	8
30–39	4	—	4
40–49	5	2	7
50–59	13	1	14
60–69	18	4	22
70–79	3	1	4
80–89	—	—	—
Total	51	9	60

Abnormally deep abdominal fossae produced by abnormally high peritoneal folds over the obliterated urachus and umbilical arteries were the first cause to be suggested. Although variation does exist, such deeper fossae have not been observed in patients with supravesical hernias. Differences in the anatomy of the male and female bladders have been discounted as a cause of male predisposition.[19]

Only the first question can be answered, and only in part. We know that the development of groin hernias depends on the loss of integrity of the transversus abdominis aponeurosis and the transversalis fascia (ie, a defective posterior wall of the inguinal canal). Defects of these structures encourage herniation through any of the anterior abdominal fossae. Keynes[19] suggested that supravesical hernias may result from the presence of other associated hernias by stretching of the peritoneum. More probably, the multiple hernias all are the result of weakness of the muscle and its aponeurosis, and of fascia of the lower abdominal wall.

Symptoms

Symptoms usually are those of acute obstruction of the small intestine, often associated with symptoms of bladder compression. If only the omentum is incarcerated, pain without obstruction may be the only symptom.[14] Remission of attacks may occur after spontaneous reduction of the hernia.[24] Empty hernial sacs have been found at operation.[24,32] Three patients have had asymptomatic hernias found incidentally. Two hernias were found in the course of repair of inguinal hernias[10,20] and one during cystoscopy for urinary problems.[4]

Diagnosis

A supravesical hernia always should be considered in instances of internal pelvic hernia. The diagnosis is not easy to make. There may be no symptoms, or symptoms may be urinary, consisting of frequency or dysuria, or intestinal, consisting of signs of partial or complete obstruction, or incarceration or strangulation.

Intestinal symptoms usually dominate. Urinary symptoms are present in about 30% of patients,[1] but they may be overlooked or considered irrelevant. Suprapubic tenderness may be present early in an acute attack. Intraabdominal contrast medium has been used successfully to identify internal supravesical hernias.[11]

Chou and coworkers[8] used retrograde air insufflation and magnetic resonance imaging to evaluate bowel obstruction in their series of nine patients. The transition zone of the case with supravesical hernia was shown clearly on the coronal image. The diagnosis was made at the time of operation.

Treatment

Conservative treatment is useless; immediate surgical intervention is indicated. The procedure used must be determined in the operating room, according to the anatomic location of the hernia, the contents of the sac, and the viability of the incarcerated loops of intestine.

Unless an unequivocal diagnosis of anterior internal supravesical hernia can be made, an extraperitoneal approach is without merit. A low paramedian incision usually is best. Reduction of the hernia generally is easy, but the ring occasionally must be incised. The posterior margin should be incised upward.[28] The sac almost always is found to contain ileum. The reduced intestine must be examined for viability, and resection and anastomosis performed when necessary.[30] Resection was required in 6 of the 40 cases reviewed by Mauer.[20]

The sac should be closed with polyglycolic acid sutures, especially if there is strangulation and obvious contamination. To avoid future complications, the defect (which usually is 1 to 2 cm in diameter, but sometimes is larger) should be closed after removal of the sac. We have seen no accounts of recurrence of an internal supravesical hernia.

Supravesical hernias and other hernias of the anterior abdominal wall may be associated with pelvic fractures. It is important, therefore, to take care in the diagnosis of hernias in such cases. Jacques and associates[17] note that a preperitoneal approach through a lower abdominal transverse incision provides the best exposure to both groins and the supravesical and prevesical areas. Findings on exploration indicate the required treatment.

Mortality

Before 1957, 6 patients died before surgical treatment could be undertaken. Among 40 patients operated on, 7 died (17.5%). Since 1957, no patient appears to have died as a result of surgical treatment of an internal supravesical hernia.

ACKNOWLEDGMENT

This project was supported by a grant from George St. Stefanakis in memory of his son Stephanos.

REFERENCES

1. Adler GG. Die Hernia supravesicalis. Bruns' Beitr Klin Chir 1970;218:225.
2. Basmajian JV. Grant's method of anatomy, ed 8. Baltimore, Williams & Wilkins, 1971.
3. Bendavid R. The space of Bogros and the deep inguinal venous circulation. Surg Gynecol Obstet 1992;174:355.
4. Blum V. Die Hernia intravesicalis. Wien Klin Wochenschr 1904;17:209.
5. Bräutigam H. Ein Fall von Dnndarmeinklemmung in die Harnblase und deren operative Behandlung. Zentralbl Chir 1944;71:939.
6. Burton CC. Hernias of the supravesical, inguinal, and lateral pelvis fossae: their diagnosis, classification, and relationship. Int Abstr Surg 1950;91:1.
7. Chandler SB. Studies on the inguinal region. II. The anatomy of the inguinal (Hesselbach) triangle. Ann Surg 1946;124:156.
8. Chou CK, Liu GC, Chen LT, Jaw TS. The use of MRI in bowel obstruction. Abdom Imaging 1993;18:131.
9. Cooper A. The anatomy and surgical treatment of inguinal and congenital hernia. London, Longman, 1804.
9a. Cooper AP. The anatomy and surgical treatment of crural and umbilical hernia. London, Longman, 1807.
10. Dall'Acque U. Osservazioni anatomo-patologiche e cliniche sulle ernie. Clin Chir 1907;15:301.
11. Ekberg O. The herniographic appearance of direct inguinal hernias in adults. Br J Radiol 1981;54:496.
12. Ekberg O, Kullenberg K. Direct diverticular inguinal hernia. Acta Radiol 1988;29:57.
13. Finsterer H. Hernia supravesicalis interna incarcerata. Med Klin 1937;33:295.
14. Guivarc'h M, Fallouh H. La hernie supravésicale; a propos de 2 observations. Chirurgie 1977;103:241.
15. Hureau J, Agossou-Voyeme AK, Germain M, Pradel J. Les Espaces Interpariétopéritonéaux Postérieurs ou Espaces Rétropéritonéaux: Anatomie topographique normale. J Radiol 1991;72:101.
16. Hureau J, Pradel J, Agossou-Voyeme AK, Germain M. Les Espaces Interpariétopéritonéaux Postérieurs ou Espaces Rétropéritonéaux: Anatomie tomodensitométrique pathologique. J Radiol 1991;72:205.
17. Jacques LF, Gloviczki P, Patterson DE, Sarr MG. Successful repair of an unusual hernia associated with traumatic pubic diastasis. Mayo Clin Proc 1988;63:492.
18. Johannsen AC. Herniae supravesicales internae. Ugeskr Laeger 1965;127:285.
19. Keynes WM. Supravesical hernia. In: Nyhus LM, Harkins HN, eds. Hernia. Philadelphia, JB Lippincott, 1964.
20. Mauer A. Hernie interne supra-vésicale; contribution à l'étude des hernies internes. Paris, Lang, 1962.
21. McVay CB. Surgical anatomy, ed 6. Philadelphia, WB Saunders Co, 1989.
22. Nathan H. Internal hernia. J Int Coll Surg 1960;34:563.
23. Olivier C, Blondeau P. La hernie interne supravésicale. Presse Med 1951;59:1552.
24. Olivier C, DiMaria G, Mahé F. Une autre observation de hernie supravésicale éntranglée. Mém Acad Chir 1966;92:476.
25. Read RC. Cooper's posterior lamina of transversalis fascia. Surg Gynecol Obstet 1992;174:426.
26. Ring J. A case of internal inguinal hernia. Lond Med Reposit 1814;2:204.
27. Rowe JS Jr, Skandalakis JE, Gray SW. Multiple bilateral inguinal hernias. Am Surg 1973;39:269.
28. Skandalakis JE, Gray SW, Akin JT Jr. The surgical anatomy of hernia rings. Surg Clin North Am 1974;54:1227.
29. Skandalakis JE, Gray SW, Burns WB, Sangmalee U, Sorg JL. Internal and external supravesical hernia. Am Surg 1976;42:142.
30. Tretbar LL, Gustafson GE. Internal supravesical hernia. Am J Surg 1968;116:907.
31. Wantz GE. Atlas of hernia surgery. New York, Raven Press, 1991.
32. Warvi WN, Orr TG. Internal supravesical hernias. Surgery 1940;8:312.
33. Watson LF. Hernia, ed 3. St Louis, CV Mosby, 1948.
34. Zeilinger H. Hernia vesicalis incarcerata. Wien Klin Wochenschr 1949;61:284.

Hernia, Fourth Edition, edited
by Lloyd M. Nyhus and Robert E. Condon.
J.B. Lippincott Company, Philadelphia © 1995.

Chapter 29

Lumbar Hernia

W. Peter Geis and George T. Hodakowski

Lumbar hernias are relatively rare, with only 250 to 300 cases having been reported in the literature. Each hernia represents a type of anatomic parietal wall defect in the lumbar region of the torso, and descriptions vary widely in size, anatomic location, and contents. The lumbar region is a broad anatomic area bordered superiorly by the 12th rib, inferiorly by the iliac crest, medially by the erector spinae muscle group, and laterally by the posterior border of the external oblique muscle as it extends from the 12th rib to the crest of the ilium. Abdominal wall defects in the lumbar region have been referred to as *Petit hernia, Grynfeltt hernia, hernia dorsalis, costoiliac hernia of Larrey,* and *suprailiac hernia of Huguier.* Two specific areas of anatomic weakness have been described within this region. Petit[24] described the anatomic boundaries of the inferior lumbar triangle, while Grynfeltt[9] and Lesshaft[18] independently described an anatomic superior lumbar triangle. Lumbar hernias have been classified as congenital or acquired; spontaneous or posttraumatic; and postoperative incisional. Descriptions of surgical repair of these hernias have addressed the location, size, and cause of the defect. Small defects have been repaired by simple approximation techniques, whereas larger defects have been repaired using fascial flaps, autologous fascial strips, and foreign-body mesh.

HISTORICAL ASPECTS

The first suggestion of the existence of a lumbar hernia defect is attributed to Barbette.[1] Budgen[5] described the first congenital hernia, but did not know that the protrusion was a hernia. Ravaton[27] surgically reduced a strangulated lumbar hernia in a pregnant woman. In 1783, Petit[24] described the anatomic boundaries of the inferior lumbar triangle and reported a case of a patient who had a strangulated hernia through this anatomic location. Goodman and Speese,[8] in reviewing the historical aspects of lumbar hernia in 1916, emphasized that Jeannel[15] clearly identified that the descriptions of the early cases of Ravaton, Budgen, and others were all hernia defects

in the inferior lumbar triangle. It was unclear to Jeannel why the inferior lumbar triangle became identified with Petit's name because Petit described the anatomic defect at a later date than the other authors.

Until 1866, when Grynfeltt[9] described the boundaries of the superior lumbar triangle, all lumbar hernias were thought to emanate from the inferior triangle of Petit. Further, Watson believes that hernias of the superior lumbar triangle were often confused with ventral hernias. Independently, Lesshaft[18] described the same anatomic landmarks as Grynfeltt and called this triangle the *superior lumbar triangle.*

Once these anatomic defects became commonly recognized, reports of series of lumbar hernias began to appear in the literature. In a review of the literature, Goodman and Speese[8] continued to emphasize the inferior lumbar triangle. Swartz[29,30] emphasized that, before 1920, most authors thought that most lumbar hernias presented through the Petit inferior lumbar triangle. In 1923, Ravdin[28] presented the opinion that most lumbar hernias were actually represented by superior lumbar triangle defects (Grynfeltt-Lesshaft). Ravdin, however, excluded traumatic and postoperative incisional hernias from his assessment. Virgillio,[34] in his comprehensive review of the subject, reconfirmed that the superior lumbar triangle represented the most common location of lumbar hernia defects. More recent series (including the series of Watson,[36] Thorek,[32] and Swartz[30]) continue to substantiate the most common site to be through the superior lumbar triangle.

SYMPTOMS AND DIAGNOSIS

Reducible Hernia

The most common finding suggesting lumbar hernia is a flank protrusion usually discovered by the patient. The bulge may be small or large, with the larger hernias passing laterally (Figs. 29-1, *bottom,* and 29-2, *bottom*) along the abdominal wall and presenting with a flank bulge. Postoperative incisional hernias in the lumbar region may be as large as 25 cm in diameter

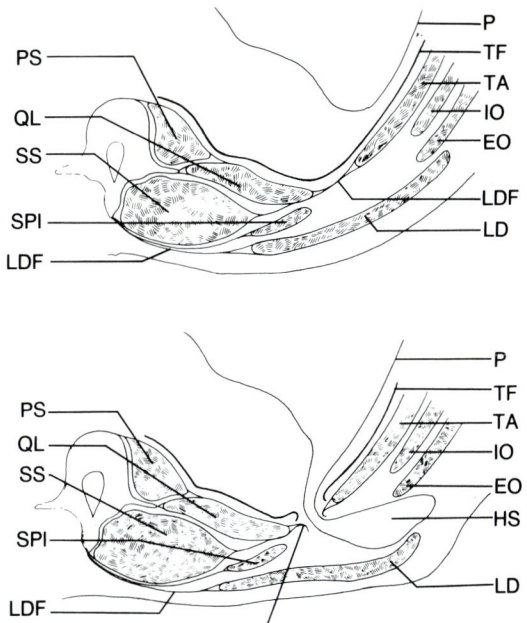

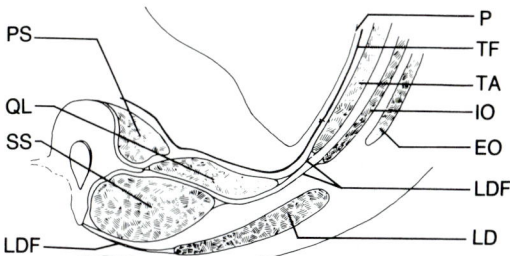

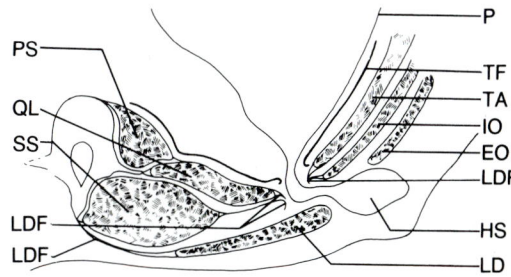

Figure 29-1. Superior lumbar triangle: cross section at point A (Fig. 29-3). *Top,* normal anatomy. *Bottom,* hernia. PS, psoas muscle; QL, quadratus lumborum muscle; SS, sacrospinalis muscle; SPI, serratus posterior inferior muscle; LDF, lumbodorsal fascia; P, peritoneum; TF, transversalis fascia; TA, transversus abdominis muscle; IO, internal oblique muscle; EO, external oblique muscle; LD, latissimus dorsi muscle; HS, hernial sac.

Figure 29-2. Inferior lumbar triangle: cross section at point B (Fig. 29-4). *Top,* normal anatomy. *Bottom,* hernia. PS, psoas muscle; QL, quadratus lumborum muscle; SS, sacrospinalis muscle; LDF, lumbodorsal fascia; P, peritoneum; TF, transversalis fascia; TA, transversus abdominis muscle; IO, internal oblique muscle; EO, external oblique muscle; LD, latissimus dorsi muscle; HS, hernial sac.

and distort the symmetry of the patient's torso. The size and shape of the hernias are variable depending on the posture of the patient. When the patient is in the erect position, the hernia tends to become tense and larger. Coughing produces an impulse and, on percussion, the hernia is tympanic. Congenital hernias, noted at birth or soon thereafter, tend to be large soft masses that increase in size when the child cries. If the hernia is reducible, the protrusion recedes or entirely disappears when the patient is placed in the supine position.

No subjective symptoms are pathognomonic of lumbar hernia. The patient often complains of a dragging sensation, which disappears when the hernia is reduced. Some patients complain of fatigue on exertion or pain and tenderness to palpation. Swartz[29,30] pointed out that palpation of the hernia often results in referred pain along the sciatic nerve distribution, the thigh, or testes. Some authors think that nonspecific referred pain to the anterior and lower portions of the abdomen may occur when the contents of the hernia include viscera, mesentery, or omentum. Others attribute back pain to herniation of adipose tissue in the lumbar area.[13] Ponka,[25] however,

cautions that a thorough musculoskeletal evaluation should be performed before attributing back pain to a lumbar hernia.

Incarcerated Hernia

The lumbar hernias that are most difficult to diagnose are those that are irreducible or strangulated. Watson[36] notes that strangulation in lumbar hernias is unlikely because of the large size of the lumbar hernia defect and broad neck of the sac. In his review of 186 cases of lumbar hernia, strangulation was present in only 8%. Watson notes, however, that spontaneously occurring lumbar hernias are more frequently strangulated than other varieties; his series indicates an 18% incidence of strangulation in spontaneous lumbar hernias. Goodman and Speese[8] noted a 24% occurrence of incarceration in spontaneous lumbar hernias. The most common cause of strangulation in these series was either constriction of the neck of the sac or the occurrence of a volvulus.

The contents of a lumbar hernia may include small or large intestine, mesentery, omentum, the appendix, the cecum, the stomach, ovary, spleen, or rarely, the kidney.[32] Symptoms are most severe when intestinal obstruction occurs. Cramping abdominal pain, vomiting, and distention associated with a tender, nonreducible mass in the lumbar area suggest the diagnosis of an incarcerated lumbar hernia producing intestinal obstruction. Incarceration not involving the gastrointestinal tract is more difficult to diagnose because the tender mass in the lumbar area does not transmit an impulse on straining or coughing and the symptoms of intestinal obstruction are absent.

DIFFERENTIAL DIAGNOSIS

Hernias in the lumbar region are rare. Most nodular masses in the lumbar region prove not to be lumbar hernias. The differential diagnosis of tumefaction in the lumbar area should include: lipoma; soft tissue tumor, including fibroma, rhabdomyoma, or sarcoma; hematoma; abscess; renal tumors; muscular hernia; pannicular lumbosacroiliac hernia; and panniculitis.

Lipoma: The diagnosis of lipoma is easily differentiated from a lumbar hernia. The tumor is slow to grow and is usually mobile and definitively free from the underlying fascia and muscle. It is nontender and does not reduce on recumbency.

Soft tissue tumors: Tumors of the muscle or fascia are not freely movable on physical examination; however, they tend not to be tender and are not reducible. These tumors are firm, and they tend to move with contraction of the muscle group. They may not be easily differentiated from a deep lipoma until operative exploration. Swartz[29] thinks that these tumors are often confused with incarcerated lumbar hernias.

Hematoma: Hematomas should be considered when an antecedent history of trauma is present. There is often tenderness and ecchymosis in the area, but hematomas are not reducible. Athletes and patients receiving anticoagulant medications are likely candidates for flank hematomas.

Abscess: Abscesses of the retroperitoneal space or of the lumbar abdominal wall are invariably associated with focal tenderness, local edema, and occasionally cellulitis. Chills, fever, and leukocytosis strongly suggest the diagnosis. An antecedent history of trauma may indicate an infected hematoma. Perinephric abscesses occasionally protrude into the lumbar region. In the past, Pott disease frequently presented in the weakened area of Petit triangle. The associated tuberculous abscesses were "cold," not especially painful, and often not associated with chills and fever. Abscesses do not reduce in response to local pressure or recumbency and are not tympanic. Radiographic assessment of bone disease should be entertained if the diagnosis of abscess is considered. Contrast-enhanced computed tomography is helpful to delineate the extent of the abscess and the organs involved.

Renal tumors: Both solid and cystic renal tumors, as well as hydronephrosis, may project posteriorly and mimic a lumbar hernia mass. These lesions are not reducible, not tympanic, and usually painless.

Muscle hernia: Muscle hernias are extremely rare. They represent herniation through the overlying lumbodorsal fascia. With relaxation of the muscle, they disappear, leaving no palpable hernia defect in the abdominal wall.

Pannicular lumbosacroiliac hernia: These lesions are herniation of subfascial fat through defects in the lumbodorsal fascia, either in the lumbosacral region or the sacroiliac region. Those in the superior portion of this region mimic incarcerated lumbar hernias but do not contain a hernia sac. They have been described by Herz[13] and have been implicated as the cause of low back pain. The physical findings are a painful, nonreducible nodule in the lumbosacral or sacroiliac region. They often represent trigger points for referred pain to the sciatic region, thigh, or genitalia because they emanate through the fascia near cutaneous branches of lumbosacral nerves. The diagnosis of pannicular lumbosacral hernia may be confirmed by the infiltration of local anesthetic into the region. Alleviation of local and referred pain confirms the diagnosis. These lesions are easily resolved by local exploration, excision of the fatty nodule, and repair of the fascia.

Panniculitis: Panniculitis is a rare inflammatory process that involves multiple areas of subcutaneous fat. It is usually associated with rheumatic manifestations and often is part of a symptom complex of relapsing nodular panniculitis or Weber-Christian disease. Most often, there is a history of repeated episodes of small, tender nonsuppurative fatty nodules reoccurring in multiple locations.

ANATOMIC CONSIDERATIONS

The lumbar region is bordered by the 12th rib superiorly, the erector spinae muscle medially, the crest of the iliac bone inferiorly, and the posterior border of the external oblique muscle laterally. It contains a number of weak points in the parietal wall of the torso through which protrusions or hernias may occur. The two most recognized anatomic weak areas are the superior lumbar triangle (Fig. 29-3) and the inferior lumbar triangle (Fig. 29-4). Less frequently described are smaller irregular openings in the muscles and aponeuroses. These include buttonhole openings in the lumbodorsal fascia secondary to trauma or maldevelopment, described by Thorek,[32] as well as the normally occurring exit sites for the cutaneous branches of the posterior lumbar nerves, originally described by Braun.[4] Further, each of the lumbar triangles has a specific weak point. The superior lumbar triangle exhibits a subcostal weakness in the fascia between the 12th rib and the lumbocostal ligament of Henle. The inferior lumbar triangle has a thin fascial weakness near its apex, described as the *Hartmann fissure*. In addition to the spontaneously occurring areas of vulnerability, surgical incisions, penetrating flank and lumbar trauma, blunt torso trauma, and retroperitoneal abscesses occasionally result in iatrogenic defects that cause diffuse and often large hernia defects.

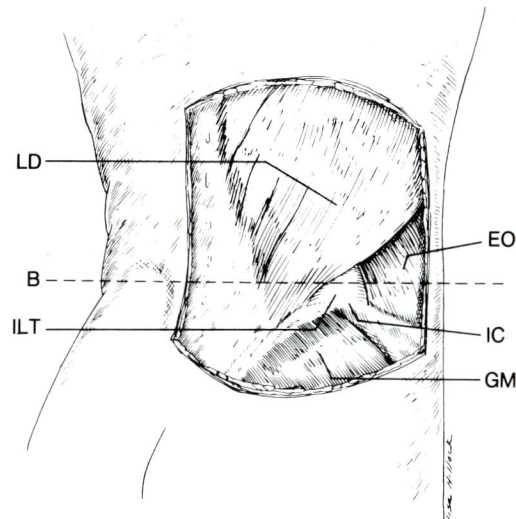

Figure 29-4. Right posterior oblique view: inferior lumbar triangle. LD, latissimus dorsi muscle; EO, external oblique muscle; IC, iliac crest; GM, gluteus maximus muscle and fascia; ILT, inferior lumbar triangle; B, cross-section level for Figure 29-4.

Superior Lumbar Triangle

The superior triangle of Grynfeltt-Lesshaft is larger and more constant than the inferior triangle and probably represents the most common site for protrusion of a spontaneous lumbar hernia. The boundaries of the space are represented in Figure 29-3. It is an inverted triangle, with its base formed by the inferior margin of the 12th rib along with the inferior border of the serratus posterior inferior muscle; the medial border of the triangle is the lateral edge of the quadratus lumborum muscle, which parallels the erector spinae muscle group; the lateral margin is the posterior free border of the internal oblique muscle. These anatomic boundaries are best remembered by referring to the triangle as the *lumbocostal abdominal space.*

The roof of the superior lumbar triangle is formed by the latissimus dorsi muscle (see Fig. 29-1). Hume[14] describes that in some cases the hernia lies beneath the latissimus dorsi muscle, lifting the muscle but not escaping it; however, occasionally the hernia tracts anteriorly beneath the latissimus dorsi to emanate as a protuberance in the anterolateral subchondral region of the abdomen.

The floor of the superior lumbar triangle is formed by the transversalis fascia along with the aponeurosis of the transversus abdominis muscle (see Fig. 29-1, *top*). The posterior extension of the aponeurosis of the transversus muscle splits into three layers, which become the lumbodorsal fascia encompassing

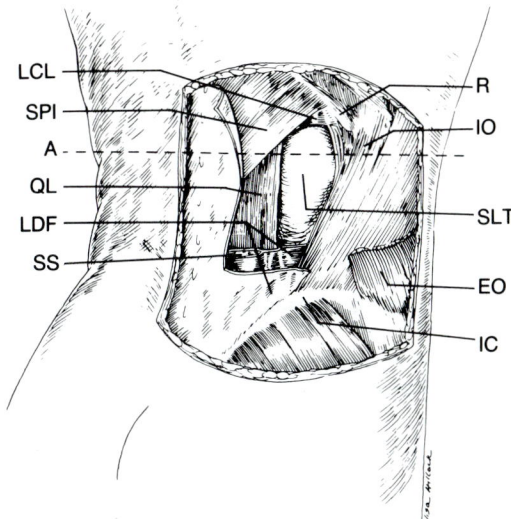

Figure 29-3. Right posterior oblique view: superior lumbar triangle. R, 12th rib; IO, internal oblique muscle; SLT, superior lumbar triangle; EO, external oblique muscle; IC, iliac crest; LCL, lumbocostal ligament; SPI, serratus posterior inferior muscle; QL, quadratus lumborum muscle; LDF, lumbodorsal fascia; SS, sacrospinalis muscle; A, cross-section level for Figure 29-3.

the quadratus lumborum and sacrospinalis muscle group. There are no muscle groups that prevent the protrusion of a hernia in this area, except for the roof of the triangle (latissimus dorsi), which has no fascial attachment laterally and inferiorly.

The fascial floor is dense and of multiple layers posteriorly and medially but is a single layer and comparatively weak laterally as it becomes the aponeurosis of the transversus muscle. Three additional weak points are described and summarized by Swartz.[29,30] The areas are all in the superior aspect of the triangle. Immediately beneath the 12th rib, the fascia is not covered by the external oblique; the fascia is perforated in this area by the 12th dorsal intercostal neurovascular bundle; and immediately adjacent is a weak space between the inferior border of the 12th rib and the lumbocostal ligament of Henle.

The size and shape of the superior triangle are extremely variable; it may take a quadrilateral, deltoid, trapezoid, or polyhedral shape.[36] The shape and size of the triangle alter the degree of weakness and the potential for a superior lumbar hernia. Other factors that alter vulnerability include the length and angle of the 12th rib, the size and shape of the quadratus lumborum and serratus posterior inferior muscles, the variable insertion of the latissimus dorsi on the 11th and 12th ribs, the union of the posterior fibers of the latissimus dorsi with the external oblique, the variable insertion of the fibers of external oblique muscle along the 12th rib, and whether the internal oblique muscle is muscular or aponeurotic at its insertion along the 12th rib. A tall, slim person with acute angulated lower ribs has a smaller superior lumbar space than a short, round-chested person with horizontal ribs,in whom the superior triangle becomes broad and larger.

Inferior Lumbar Triangle

The inferior lumbar triangle described by Petit (see Fig. 29-4) is an upright triangle and is less consistent in its size and shape than the superior lumbar triangle. The space has been described as the lumboiliac abdominal space. The crest of the iliac bone forms the base of the triangle and is a rigid structure. The lateral border of the triangle is the posterior free margin of the external oblique muscle. The medial border is the lateral free border of the latissimus dorsi muscle. The inferior lumbar triangle is found in significantly greater percentages of adults than children. Lesshaft[18] found the area to be present in 77% of adult cadavers and only 25% of infants. Goodman and Speese[8] found the space present in 63% of tall and muscular patients. The overlapping of the latissimus dorsi on the external oblique muscle narrows the defect. Light[20]

emphasized that women with wider pelvises exhibit lateral displacement of the origin of the external oblique muscle as well as more medial position of latissimus dorsi muscle, creating a wider base to the triangle. Goodman and Speese[8] found the base of the triangle to range from essential nonexistence to a maximum of 6 cm in width; the height of the triangle in their subjects ranged from 1 to 8 cm. Swartz[30] reminds us that the border of the latissimus dorsi and external oblique muscle may be contiguous, obliterating the potential hernia space.

The floor of the inferior lumbar triangle is composed of lumbodorsal fascia, which is contiguous with the aponeuroses of the internal oblique and transversus abdominis muscles (see Fig. 29-2). Watson[36] observed that the internal oblique muscle is wholly tendinous. However, attenuated and frayed internal oblique muscle may also be a cause of herniation in this region. Most authors agree that a weak point (Hartmann fissure) is present at the apex of the inferior lumbar triangle. Swartz[29] compares the inferior triangle favorably with the superior triangle by noting that the inferior triangle exhibits no nerves or blood vessels that pierce its floor and no musculature forming the roof of the latter triangle. In contrast, Light[20] describes the iliohypogastric and ilioinguinal nerves to pierce the deep layer of lumbodorsal fascia as they proceed between the transversus abdominis and internal oblique muscles. He also implicates the small apertures that occur in the lumbodorsal fascia for exit of the cutaneous branches of the last three lumbar nerves as potential weak points for herniation.

Diffuse Lumbar Hernias

Diffuse lumbar hernias are among the largest and most grotesque-appearing hernias described. They are most often iatrogenic, occurring at the site of prior surgical incisions. The most frequent operations associated with lumbar hernia are kidney procedures performed through flank incisions. The anatomic layers are often obliterated secondary to the prior surgical procedure. The superior lumbar triangle is usually incorporated as a portion of the hernia defect because of its location with relation to surgical incisions for renal and adrenal surgical exposures.

Diffuse hernias may also be associated with previous trauma and occasionally with large congenital defects. The margins of the diffuse lumbar hernia may exceed the margins of the anatomic lumbar space when the anterior border invades the lateral margin of the rectus sheath. The inferior margin (iliac crest) and the superior margins (12th rib) are immobile structures. When these bony structures comprise the margins of a diffuse lumbar hernia ring, there exists a technical dilemma in providing an adequate repair. Swartz,[29] in his review of the causes of diffuse and large lumbar hernias, describes avulsive defects in the iliac bone secondary to traumatic fractures and gunshot injuries. Herniation through a defect in the iliac crest after the use of the ala of the ilium as a donor site to harvest bone was reported. The common anatomic factor is a large full-thickness bony defect along the wing of the iliac crest.

CLASSIFICATION OF LUMBAR HERNIAS

It is not possible to provide a simple classification for lumbar hernias. A few reasonably inclusive attempts have been made at classification. These include using criteria for: (1) site of protrusion, (2) cause, and (3) contents of the hernia. Each of these classifications is useful, and each provides additional information regarding the expected natural history of the hernia, the proper assessment, and the diagnostic and therapeutic options.

Classification of lumbar hernias based on site of protrusion is useful for describing physical findings during preoperative assessment. The three anatomic sites of protrusion are described in Table 29-1. Synonyms for hernias of the superior lumbar triangle and for the inferior lumbar triangle are also listed in Table 29-1. *Diffuse lumbar hernias* are those that have become enlarged to the degree that they encompass most of the lumbar space and are not confined to either the superior or inferior triangular areas. They are often posttraumatic or postoperative incisional hernias. Congenital hernias may also occur as diffuse lumbar defects. Further, hernias that protrude through the superior or inferior triangles may be secondary to trauma, or they may occur spontaneously. Congenital hernias may protrude from each of the anatomic lo-

cations described; however, they usually occur in the superior triangle.

Thorek[32] proposed a classification based on contents of the hernia to include the presence or absence of a peritoneal hernia sac. His description includes a discussion of the various structures that may be encountered within the hernia at the time of surgical exploration. The classification is useful to describe the intraoperative findings that may be encountered as well as helpful in determining the ideal operative procedure. Thorek described three categories: (1) lumbar hernias containing no peritoneum (no sac), termed *extraperitoneal;* (2) hernias in which the peritoneum was adherent to a viscus or followed the viscus through the hernia ring, termed *paraperitoneal* (these are actually sliding hernias by their description); and (3) hernias in which the peritoneum completely surrounds the contents of the hernia, providing a complete sac in all dimensions of the hernia, termed *intraperitoneal.*

Ponka[25] described a useful classification for lumbar hernias based on etiologic factors. His two major categories are *congenital* and *acquired.* Acquired hernias are subdivided into *spontaneously occurring* hernias and *traumatically induced* hernias. Hernias caused by trauma are further divided into those that follow operative trauma (*incisional* hernias) and nonsurgically induced traumatic hernias.

Swartz[29] proposed a similar classification based on cause. He suggested that all lumbar hernias that occur in infants or children who have obvious defects of the musculoskeletal system in the lumbar region be classified as *congenital* hernias. Using these criteria, about 20% of all reported lumbar hernias are of congenital origin. All lumbar hernias that are not defined as congenital hernias are *acquired* hernias. These are subdivided into *primary* and *secondary* lumbar hernias. Primary acquired lumbar hernias are those that occur

Table 29-1. Classification of Lumbar Hernias

Site of Protrusion	Synonyms
Superior lumbar triangle hernia	Grynfeltt hernia
	Lesshaft hernia
	Superior hernia of Grynfeltt-Lesshaft
	Lumbocostal abdominal hernia
	Costoiliac hernia of Larrey
Inferior lumbar triangle hernia	Petit lumbar hernia
	Hernia of Petit triangle
	Suprailiac hernia of Huguier
	Lumboiliac abdominal hernia
Diffuse lumbar hernia	Incisional lumbar hernia
	Postoperative lumbar hernia
	Flank incisional hernia
	Traumatic lumbar hernia

spontaneously and are not due to trauma, infection in the lumbar region, or previous surgical intervention. This group represents about 55% of reported cases. Predisposing factors include excessive weight loss and pulmonary disease such as bronchitis or emphysema, and they have a predilection for the elderly patient. It has been suggested that the spontaneous hernias may be associated with strenuous physical labor.

The remaining group of acquired hernias are secondary lumbar hernias. They exhibit a definite causal relation to trauma, abscess in the lumbar region, or prior surgical procedures. This category represents about 25% of all lumbar hernias. Traumatic lumbar hernias may be secondary to direct penetrating trauma, as occurred in the case described by Kretschmer[17] in which a patient was gored by a bull. Crush injuries are also responsible for the development of lumbar hernias. Another mechanism in which trauma disrupts integrity of the lumbar area is fracture of the crest of the iliac bone. Operative disruption of the iliac crest has also resulted in the development of secondary lumbar hernias. Postoperative incisional lumbar hernias results in large hernias that are often difficult to repair. Kretschmer[17] reported on 11 patients who developed such hernias after various operations on the kidney. In the past, Watson described Pott disease or caries of the vertebrae as the most frequent cause of secondary acquired lumbar hernias. Infection of the pelvic bones or ribs, liver abscess, and contamination of retroperitoneal hematomas are all infectious processes that have disrupted the integrity of the transversalis fascia or lumbodorsal fascia, resulting in lumbar hernias.

TREATMENT

Lumbar hernias rarely result in strangulation, and therefore the prognosis for most patients is good. However, these hernias gradually increase in size and become symptomatic as well as cosmetically displeasing to the patient. As the hernia becomes larger, a corrective surgical procedure becomes increasingly more difficult and complicated. For these reasons, most lumbar hernias should undergo operative repair at the time of discovery. Some authors recommend delay in operative correction of congenital lumbar hernias until the child is at least 6 months of age. At this interval, the anatomic structures are better developed and more easily defined for surgical correction. If, however, the child undergoes progressive increase in the intensity of symptoms or the physical findings suggest the danger of incarceration or strangulation, then the surgical procedure should not be delayed.

Preoperative Preparation

Before the operative procedure, the surgeon should know the relation between the colon, the urinary tract, and the hernia sac contents. Preoperative barium enema and intravenous pyelogram radiographs should be performed. Some authors also recommend contrast studies of the upper gastrointestinal tract because the small bowel is occasionally included in the hernia contents. Radiographic assessment of the lumbar vertebrae and iliac bone is essential to appraise bony defects in the lumbar spine and ilium. Newer diagnostic modalities such as contrast-enhanced computed tomography may provide the best single study to assess the position of the gastrointestinal tract and urinary tract with relation to the hernia and its contents.[12] It is prudent to prepare the bowel bacteriologically and mechanically before the operative procedure. Patients who have extremely large hernia defects or who are obese should undergo a weight reduction program before operative intervention.

Positioning the Patient in the Operating Room

If the hernia is a small focal protuberance emanating from the inferior lumbar triangle, the oblique position is often adequate. In most circumstances, however, lateral positioning of the patient provides the best access to all the structures requiring exposure. The upper thigh and leg should be extended over the lower leg. The lower hip and knee are flexed to 45 degrees, and the kidney elevator is raised. These maneuvers increase the vertical distance from the 12th rib to the iliac crest and enhance operative delineation of structures. Sterile preparation of the skin and draping of the operative field should include the entire upper thigh, the ipsilateral buttocks, and the gluteal area. Exposure of the thigh may be required for use of fascia lata grafts, and access to the gluteal area provides for rotation of a fascial flap from the gluteus muscles to the lumbar area. Before the surgical procedure, the surgeon should be familiar with the various techniques using fascial strips, flaps, free-sheet grafts, and foreign-body mesh in the repair of lumbar hernias.

Incision

Various authors have described the use of vertical, transverse, or oblique incisions. The vertical incision provides adequate exposure for small hernias in the inferior lumbar triangle of Petit and provides easy access to the gluteal fascia. We prefer the oblique incision described by Ponka in which the skin incision conforms to the neurovascular and dermatome distribution. This incision provides the best exposure of underlying structures in all directions; it is directed from beneath the 12th rib posteriorly in oblique fashion over the apex of the hernia to the anterior portion of the iliac crest (see the diagrammatic sketch inserts in Figs. 29-5 and 29-6).

Exploration: The Sac

The hernia and its contents are never adherent to the skin. The hernia is frequently covered by subcutaneous fat, muscle, and attenuated lumbodorsal and transversalis fascia. These relations are depicted on diagrammatic sketches in Figures 29-1, *bottom*, and 29-2, *bottom*.

During exploration, the hernia mass is carefully separated from surrounding fatty tissue, and a diligent search is made for a sac. Preperitoneal fat adjacent to the hernia sac should be carefully inspected because it may represent mesocolon with associated colonic blood supply, which must not be inadvertently injured. The presence of a paraperitoneal sliding hernia component to the hernia should be treated by inversion and plication of the sliding component, avoiding the viscera and its blood supply. When a sac is present, as either a true peritoneal hernia or a component of a paraperitoneal sliding hernia, the sac should be opened and its contents identified. Inspec-

tion of the interior of the sac also provides the opportunity to evaluate the anatomy of a sliding component and to identify a multiloculated sac. The most common contents of the lumbar hernia sac are intestine (large and small), omentum, preperitoneal fat, mesentery, appendix, cecum, stomach, ovary, spleen, and rarely, kidney.

The presence of a true complete peritoneal hernia sac is uncommon; when present, the sac should be ligated and excised if possible. When the base of the sac is too broad for simple ligation, the sac may be inverted or imbricated, and plicated with interrupted sutures. The goal of hernia repair is to eliminate the protruding defect and to construct an elastic and firm parietal abdominal wall that will withstand the stress of everyday life.

Reconstruction

Reconstruction is the challenging aspect of lumbar hernia surgery. The location and size of the abdominal wall defect influence the operating surgeon's choice of repair. A wide variety of techniques have been described for repair of lumbar hernias. These descriptions have evolved to accommodate the variations in size, location, content, and causes of lumbar hernias that have been encountered by various authors. Ponka[25] described a selective approach to reconstruction. A strong overlapping aponeurotic reconstruction using the patient's intrinsic fascia provides the most functional lateral abdominal wall repair when these tissues are available. Fascia strips,

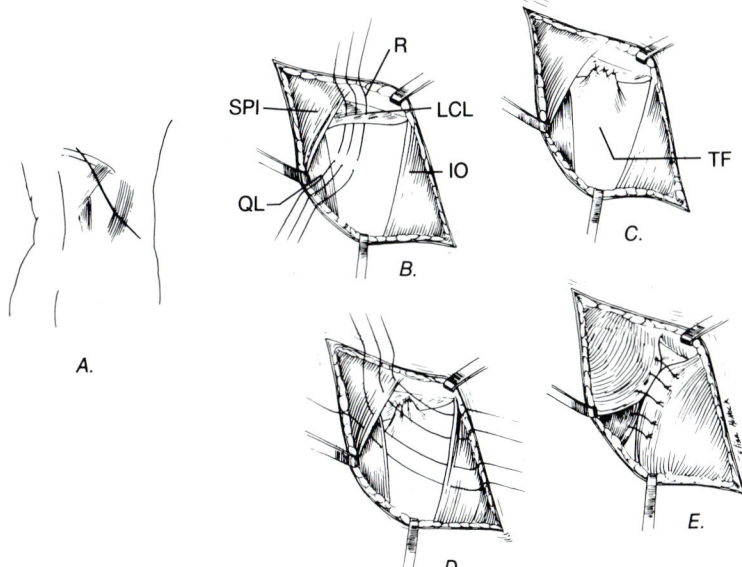

Figure 29-5. (*A* through *E*) Repair of hernia of the superior lumbar triangle. SPI, serratus posterior inferior muscle; QL, quadratus lumborum muscle; R, 12th rib; LCL, lumbocostal ligament; IO, internal oblique muscle; TF, transversalis fasia.

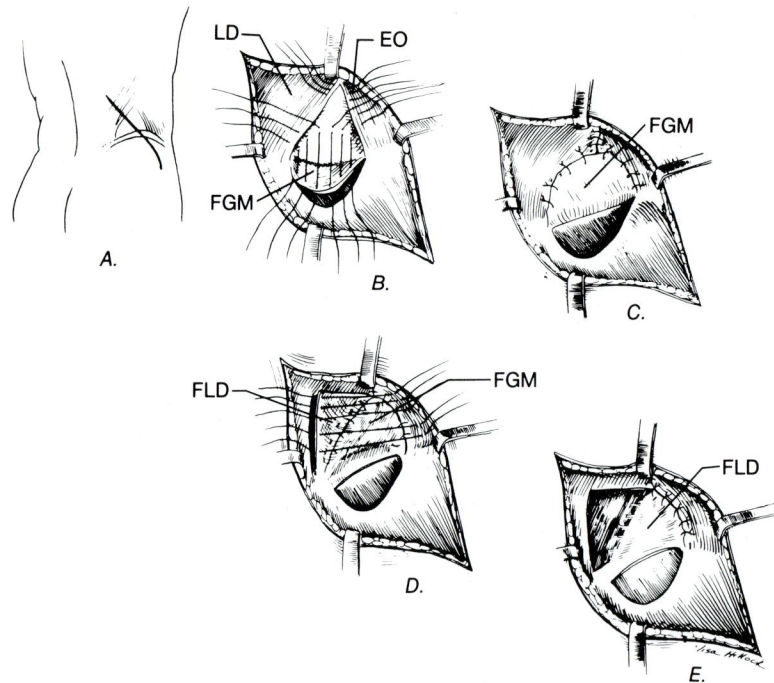

Figure 29-6. (*A* through *E*) Repair of hernia of the inferior lumbar triangle. LD, latissimus dorsi muscle; FGM, fascia of gluteus maximus muscle; EO, external oblique muscle; FLD, fascia of latissimus dorsi muscle.

flaps, free grafts, and foreign mesh should be reserved for circumstances in which the defect is not comfortably repaired with intrinsic tissues. Most lumbar hernias are of moderate or small size, and the surrounding anatomic structures are identifiable by the operating surgeon.

The following discussion describes each surgical approach and the appropriate application.

Simple Closure

Small or moderate-size hernias occurring in the superior or inferior lumbar triangles are securely repaired by approximating the transversalis fascia along with the fascia of the transversus abdominis muscle (see Figs. 29-5 and 29-6). Interrupted, heavy, nonabsorbable sutures are preferred. Reinforcement of the repair is occasionally required. When the hernia occurs in the inferior lumbar triangle, approximation of the fascia of the free edge of the external oblique muscle to the fascia of the latissimus dorsi muscle provides a strong second layer (see Fig. 29-6A).

When the hernia occurs in the superior lumbar triangle, particular attention should be paid to the use of the simple two-layer closure. Approximation of the transversalis fascia to the lumbocostal ligament and the periosteum along the undersurface of the 12th rib is important (see Fig. 29-5). A strong second layer is provided by approximation of the free edge of the fascia of the internal oblique muscle anteriorly with the free edge of the fascia of the serratus posterior inferior muscle and quadratus lumborum muscle posteriorly. Interrupted, heavy, nonabsorbable sutures are used.

Use of Fascial Rotation Flaps and Free Grafts

In moderate-size or large hernias, the addition of one or more layers for reinforcement is necessary. The classic technique was described in 1907 by Dowd.[6] This procedure is outlined in Figure 29-6 and is most useful for larger defects involving the inferior lumbar triangle. After the approximation of the transversalis fascia and fascia of the transversus abdominis muscle layers, the superior portion of the defect is reinforced by approximating the fascia of the free edge of the latissimus dorsi muscle to the free edge of the fascia of the external oblique muscle using interrupted, nonabsorbable sutures. A generous flap of fascia and aponeurosis from the gluteus maximus muscle is elevated and rotated to cover the inferior portion of the defect. The edges of the gluteus maximus fascial flap are sutured to the underlying lumbodorsal fascia and transversalis fascia; the sutures are returned through the edge of the latissimus dorsi fascia posteriorly and through the fascia of the external oblique anteriorly. Finally, Dowd developed an aponeurotic flap using the anterior fascia of the latissimus dorsi. He rotated the flap onto the inferior portion of the defect and over the gluteus fascial flap to reinforce the repair. The free edge of the latissimus flap is sutured by interrupted, nonabsorbable sutures to the fascia of the external oblique anteriorly.

The principles of Dowd's repair are best used when a primary closure cannot be accomplished without undue tension and when a large defect is present in the inferior lumbar triangle. It is also helpful if there is no intrinsic fascia at the base of the inferior triangle along the iliac crest. Many modifications of this technique have been appropriately described. For example, we have split half the aponeurosis of the latissimus dorsi to provide extra fascia for closure of the inferior defect. Another technique is to overlap flaps of transversalis fascia similar to a "vest-over-pants" repair as the first layer. Dowd reinforced the repair using a flap of fascia rotated from the gluteus maximus region. The imbrication of the transversalis fascia has been an important contribution to the successful repair of these hernias and was reemphasized and pictorially described by Watson.[36]

Probably the first use of free fascial grafts to reinforce lumbar hernia repairs was described by Ravdin in 1923.[28] His description identifies a large traumatic hernia of the superior lumbar triangle that required reinforcement due to its size. After closure of the transversalis fascia layer, Ravdin used a free fascia lata graft, which he sutured to the undersurface of the 12th rib to include the lumbocostal ligament. The graft was transfixed laterally to the transversus abdominis and internal oblique aponeuroses and medially to the fascia of the quadratus lumborum. Figure 29-5 provides the anatomic relations. The latissimus dorsi muscle was reapproximated over the surface of the repair. The entire area was reinforced with a second free fascial graft anchored to the latissimus dorsi fascia and to the posterior fascia of the external oblique muscle. Interrupted nonabsorbable sutures were used.

Dowd's descriptions of repair of large defects of the inferior triangle and Ravdin's of repair of large defects of the superior triangle provide the surgeon with the opportunity to modify these techniques to use foreign-body mesh and fascial implants. Historically, Koontz[16] used cutis grafts in large defects. Thorek[32] described the use of tantalum. Hafner and colleagues[10] in 1963 reinforced large defects of the inferior lumbar triangle using Marlex mesh. Tantalum gauze tends to fragment with time after implantation.

Repair With Fascial Strips

Another approach to lumbar hernias of moderate size is to approximate and repair the defect with fascia lata strips. Swartz[29,30] described and diagrammed the technique in detail. The fascial strips are used as large running retention sutures. The free fascial strips are interwoven through adjacent musculofascial structures, the fascia of the latissimus dorsi and external oblique muscles, the transversalis fascia, and the lumbodorsal fascia. The fascial strips are 1 to 1.5 cm wide.

The rationale for use of fascial strips is that they represent living sutures possessing elasticity. In addition, they are not brittle and provide great tensile strength. The strips are obtained from the fascia lata from each thigh, with the strongest fascia obtained from the middle and dorsal portion of the fascia lata.

Repair of Bony Defects

When a portion of the iliac bone has been removed or injured after trauma, the technique of closure must be modified to include repair of the bony defect. In 1949, Lewin and Bradley[19] used the iliopsoas muscle as a pedicle graft partially to replace lost soft tissue mass and the bony defect along the internal aspect of the iliac bone. Pyrtek and Kelly[26] emphasized the importance of closing both the internal opening and the external portion of the bony defect. They repaired two large defects with a double-layer free graft technique using fascia lata and tantalum mesh.

When bone is removed from the iliac crest as a donor site, the defect should be repaired at the time of bone grafting. Small defects may be repaired by a simple two-layer closure. The iliopsoas or iliacus muscle may be used to close the inner aspect; the outer opening may be repaired by a flap of fascia from the gluteus maximus muscle (ala[6]). Occasionally, larger defects require mesh. Pictorial descriptions of repair of bony defects are provided by Swartz.[29] Newer forms of mesh (Mersilene, Marlex, Gore-Tex) are more resilient, are more resistant to decay, and have more tensile strength than previous materials.[2] Most of the wounds require closed-system suction drainage because extensive mobilization of tissue is necessary in all but the smallest of lumbar hernias.

PATIENT CASES: PERSONAL EXPERIENCE

We have reviewed our experience with lumbar hernias during the past 10 years. There have been six patients (four males and two females) ranging in age from 42 to 75 years. All hernias were acquired (Table 29-2). In three patients, the hernia was primary (spontaneous), with two of these being left-sided and one a right-sided lumbar hernia. Two hernia defects occurred in the superior lumbar triangle, and one occurred through the inferior lumbar triangle of Petit. Hernia size varied from 4 to 7 cm in diameter. Two patients had an operative repair of their hernias; the third patient refused surgery. A true peritoneal sac was present in one patient, whose barium enema radiograph delineated the presence of descending colon within the hernia sac (Fig. 29-7). At operative exploration, the hernia and colon contents exhibited a sliding component, and the hernia was designated a

Table 29-2.   A Series of Lumbar Hernias

Sex	Age (y)	Symptoms	Causation	Location	Contents	Duration	Size (cm)	Repair
Female	65	Flank bulge	Primary	Right superior triangle	Colon, no sac	6 mo	7	Closure
Female	75	Flank pain, asymmetry	Primary	Left superior triangle	Not operated on	2 y	5	Not operated on
Male	67	Obstipation, distention, mass	Primary	Left inferior triangle	Descending colon, sac, sliding hernia	3 y	6	Closure
Male	62	Flank pain, flank bulge	Secondary— abscess	Left superior triangle	Retroperitoneal soft tissue, no sac	15 y	12	Closure vest-over-pants
Male	42	Flank bulge, pain	Secondary— incisional	Left superior triangle and diffuse	Colon, no sac	5 y	25	Marlex mesh
Male	51	Bilateral flank pain, bulge, and obstipation	Secondary— trauma and incision	Bilateral superior triangle and diffuse	Colon, kidney, no sac	18 mo	10	Closure

paraperitoneal lumbar hernia (Thorek classification) through the left inferior lumbar triangle. These lumbar hernias were repaired by simple closure of healthy fascia using interrupted nonabsorbable sutures. Simple closure was accomplished after identifying the limited size of the hernia defect, the presence of healthy fascia at the edge, and the lack of abdominal wall tension.

Three of the patients had secondary lumbar hernias. The causative factors were variable. One hernia was an incisional lumbar hernia that followed a right nephrectomy surgical incision. This defect was about 25 cm in its largest diameter and included the superior lumbar triangle. A second patient had bilateral superior lumbar triangle hernias secondary to large posterior bilateral subcostal surgical drainage inci-

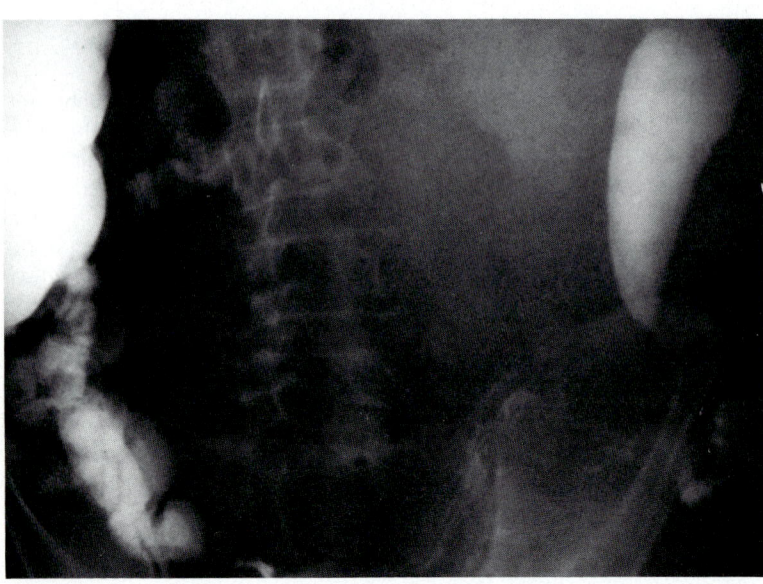

Figure 29-7.   Barium enema showing descending colon as contents of hernia of left inferior lumbar triangle.

sions for blunt torso trauma involving pancreatic and hepatic injuries. The third hernia was a large, 12-cm, left-sided lumbar hernia through the superior lumbar triangle. It occurred after a retroperitoneal abscess of the right lobe of the liver. None of these hernias had a true peritoneal sac, and each contained retroperitoneal structures (extraperitoneal). The large incisional hernia was repaired using two layers of Marlex mesh. The bilateral drain site hernias were repaired by simple closure of the fascia with interrupted sutures. The hernia that occurred secondary to a retroperitoneal abscess was closed by a vest-over-pants repair of the fascia. All patients recovered without morbidity.

REFERENCES

1. Barbette P. Opera chirurgico-anatomica. Lugduni, Gelder, 1672:26.
2. Blasi A, Tufodandria G, Di Cesare F. Uso della rete di Polipropilene nel trattamento dell'ernia di Grynfeltt: descrizione di un caso clinico. Chir Gastroenterol 1993;27:141.
3. Bonner CD, Kasdon SC. Herniation of fat through the lumbodorsal fascia as a cause of low-back pain. N Engl J Med 1954;251:1102.
4. Braun H. Die Hernia lumbalis. Langenbecks Arch Klin Chir 1879;24:201.
5. Budgen J. A remarkable conformation of the urinary parts. Philos Trans R Soc Lond 1728;36(410):138.
6. Dowd CN. Congenital lumbar hernia at the triangle of Petit. Ann Surg 1907;45:245.
7. Florer RE, Kiriluk L. Petit's triangle hernia, incarcerated. Am Surg 1971;37:527.
8. Goodman EH, Speese J. Lumbar hernia. Ann Surg 1916;63:548.
9. Grynfeltt J. Quelques mots sur la hernie lombaire. Montpellier Med 1866;16:323.
10. Hafner CD, Wylie JH, Brush BE. Petit's lumbar hernia: repair with Marlex mesh. Arch Surg 1963;86:180.
11. Hartmann HJ. Die Bauchelltaschen in der Umgebung des Blinddarms. Tubingen, ID,1 1870.
12. Hasaniya NW, Lee Y-TM, Crandall DB. Spontaneous inferior lumbar hernia of Petit: ACT assisted diagnosis. Contemp Surg 1993;43:363.
13. Herz R. Herniation of fascial fat and low back pain. JAMA 1945;128:921.
14. Hume GH. Case of strangulated lumbar hernia. Br Med J 1889;2:73.
15. Jeannel M. La hernie lombaire. Arch Prov Chir Paris 1902;11:389, 521, 649, 713, 1279; 1903;12:91, 159, 281.
16. Koontz AR. An operation for massive incisional lumbar hernia. Surg Gynecol Obstet 1955;101:119.
17. Kretschmer HL. Lumbar hernia of the kidney. J Urol 1951;65:944.
18. Lesshaft P. Lumbalgegren in anatomisch—Chirurgischer Himsicht. Anat Physiol Wissensch Med 1870:264.
19. Lewin ML, Bradley ET. Traumatic iliac hernia with extensive soft tissue loss. Surgery 1949;26:601.
20. Light HG. Hernia of the inferior lumbar space. Arch Surg 1983;118:1077.
21. Lotem M. Lumbar hernia at an iliac bone graft donor site. Clin Orthop 1971;80:130.
22. Marmisse G. Hernie ventrale. Gaz D Hop 1862;35:170.
23. Orcutt TW. Hernia of the superior lumbar triangle. Ann Surg 1971;173:294.
24. Petit JL. Traite des maladies chirurgicales, et des operations qui leur conviennent. Paris, TF Didot, 1774;2:256–258.
25. Ponka JL. Lumbar hernias. In: Ponka JL, ed. Hernias of the abdominal wall. Philadelphia, WB Saunders, 1980:465–478.
26. Pyrtek LH, Kelly CC. Management of hernia through large iliac bone defects. Ann Surg 1960;152:998.
27. Ravaton H. Traite des plaies d'armes a feu. 1750:277.
28. Ravdin IS. Lumbar hernia through Grynfelt (sic) and Lesgaft's (sic) triangle. Surg Clin North Am 1923;3:267.
29. Swartz WT. Lumbar hernia. In: Nyhus LM, Condon RE, eds. Hernia. Philadelphia, JB Lippincott, 1978:409–425.
30. Swartz WT. Lumbar hernias. J Ky Med Assoc 1954;52:673.
31. Thorek M. Lumbar hernia. J Int Coll Surg 1950;14:367.
32. Thorek M. Modern surgical technic. Philadelphia, JB Lippincott, 1950.
33. Tibaudin HA. Lumbar fat hernias as the cause of reflex lumbo-sciaticas. Prensa Med Argent 1959;46:773.
34. Virgillio F. Lumbar hernia. Arch Ital Chir 1925;14:337.
35. Wang J. Lumbar hernia simulating an adrenal pseudotumor: a CT diagnosis. J Formosan Med Assoc 1983;82:795.
36. Watson LE. Hernia, ed 3. St Louis, CV Mosby, 1948:443–455.

Editor's Comment

Jean Louis Petit was born in Paris in 1674. He was a remarkable person, both as a child and as an adult (Surgery 1963;53:699). An unusual circumstance of his childhood was destined to influence his entire life and career. A celebrated anatomist, Alexis Littre (of Littre hernia fame), occupied apartments in the same building in which the Petit family lived. At that time, Littre maintained a dissecting amphitheater and conducted courses in anatomy. A strong attachment developed between Littre and Petit early in the child's life. By the time Jean Louis was 7 years of age, he was a regular and fascinated visitor at Littre's dissections and demonstrations and, even at this early age, was allowed to perform some of the dissections himself. Thus, he learned anatomy as a child of today learns the alphabet. By the time he was 12 years of age, Petit was so adept that he became Littre's demonstrator and was placed in charge of the anatomic amphitheater. Petit was very short, and it was necessary for him to stand on a chair to be seen during the demonstrations.

Petit's remarkable association with Littre continued for 10 years. At the age of 16 years, at Littre's insistence, Petit was sent to study under Castel, the most celebrated surgeon of the day, with whom Petit remained for 2 years.

A prolific writer, Petit contributed information to the fields of general surgery (breast, gallbladder, hernia, aneurysm), orthopedic surgery (fractures, ruptures of the Achilles tendon), and neurosurgery (trephination, coma, cerebral abscess). When the Academy of Surgery of France was founded in 1731 by King Louis XV, Petit was named the first director.

L.M.N.

Hernia, Fourth Edition, edited
by Lloyd M. Nyhus and Robert E. Condon.
J.B. Lippincott Company, Philadelphia © 1995.

Chapter 30

Obturator Hernia

*Lee J. Skandalakis, Panagiotis N. Skandalakis, Stephen W. Gray,
and John E. Skandalakis*

*It remains, now, for us to speak of a hernia so little known that it has not even seemed
possible to many anatomists: It is that which occurs through the oval (obturator) foramen.*
de Garengeot, 1743

*The last case . . . rests its principal practical importance upon the presence of a peculiar
and diagnostic symptom, the spasmodic pain down the limb, which may, in other cases, lead
to its detection, and which has not, that I am aware of, been before noticed.*
John Howship, 1840

Never externally visible, and rarely palpable, hernia through the obturator canal is usually unsuspected and hence undiagnosed before an exploratory operation.

The hernia tends to affect thin, frail women well past middle age. Intestinal obstruction of unknown origin is the usual preoperative diagnosis. There has been little improvement in diagnosis over the last 45 years, although the operative mortality has markedly declined.

Anatomically, obturator hernia, together with inguinal and femoral hernias, belongs to the anterior group of pelvic hernias (Fig. 30-1). In frequency, it belongs to the posterior group of uncommon to rare pelvic hernias (Fig. 30-2). Few surgeons see many in a normal practice.

HISTORY

René Jacques Croissant de Garengeot, in 1743,[21] described a patient in whom he had manually reduced an obturator hernia 10 years earlier. He was able to diagnose the hernia because he remembered a report of two similar hernias read "about 20 or 21 years ago" before the Royal Academy of Surgeons of Paris. This report, in 1722 or 1723, was by Roland Arnaud de Ronsil and is the earliest known description of an obturator hernia. De Garengeot also mentioned six other early instances.

Nyhus[49] pointed out in 1964 that almost all the early reports were published in France. It could well have been called the *French hernia*. Some early terms

used for obturator hernia were *hernie par le trou ovalaire, hernia foramina ovalis,* and *thyroideal hernia.* According to Nyhus (see Editor's Comment), Guillaume Dupuytren (1777–1835) was among the first to write about obturator hernia.

Sporadic reports of this unusual hernia appeared over the next 100 years. In 1848, Hilton[33] may have been the first to attempt surgical repair. He incised the abdomen of a patient under chloroform anesthesia and reduced an unsuspected obturator hernia, but the patient did not live. The first successful operation on record was performed in 1851 by Henry Obre.[50] He used an extraperitoneal approach to a previously diagnosed obturator hernia. The hernia was reduced, and the 55-year-old woman recovered.

John Howship,[35] in his book published in 1840 (Fig. 30-3, *left*), described the pain in the medial aspect of the thigh characteristic of pressure by a hernia on the obturator nerve. Independently described by Moritz Heinrich Romberg[58] in Germany in Dieffenbach's *Operative Chirurgie*, published in 1848 (see Fig. 30-3, *right*), this pain, pathognomonic of obturator hernia, is now called the *Howship-Romberg sign.*

During the remainder of the century, the anatomy of the obturator region became well understood, as shown by two beautiful museum specimens in the Royal College of Surgeons, illustrated by Wakeley.[72] One was made in 1842 (Fig. 30-4).

Horine[34] estimated that there were 258 instances in the literature by 1924. Watson[75] in 1948 found 442 instances, which he reviewed. By 1960, Rogers[56] was able to collect 463, to which he added 12 of his own. We reviewed 50 reports in the English-language literature from 1946 through 1970.[25]

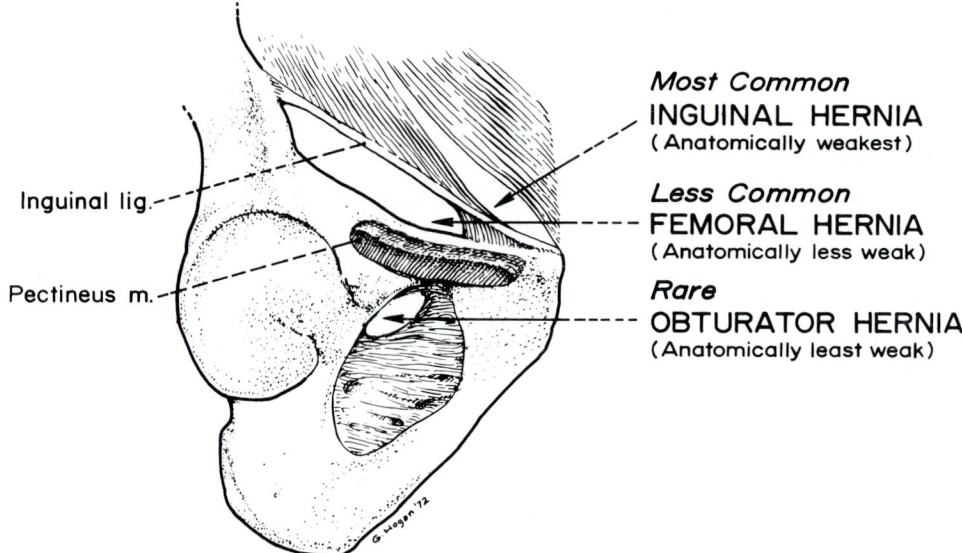

Figure 30-1. Lateral view of the right side of the pelvis and a portion of the abdominal wall showing the relation between the sites of inguinal, femoral, and obturator hernias.

ANATOMIC CONSIDERATIONS

The Obturator Region

The obturator or adductor region lies in the medial portion of the upper third of the thigh between the extensor and flexor muscle groups. The region includes the obturator canal and the origins of the adductor muscles from the margins of the obturator foramen and the obturator membrane.

The region as defined by Anson and McVay[5] is bounded medially by the pubic arch, the perineum, and the gracilis muscle; laterally by the hip joint and the shaft of the femur; superiorly by the horizontal ramus of the pubis; and inferiorly by the insertion of the adductor magnus on the adductor tubercle of the femur.

The Obturator Foramen

The obturator foramen is the largest foramen in the body and is formed by rami of the ischium and pubis. It lies on the anterolateral pelvic wall, inferior to the

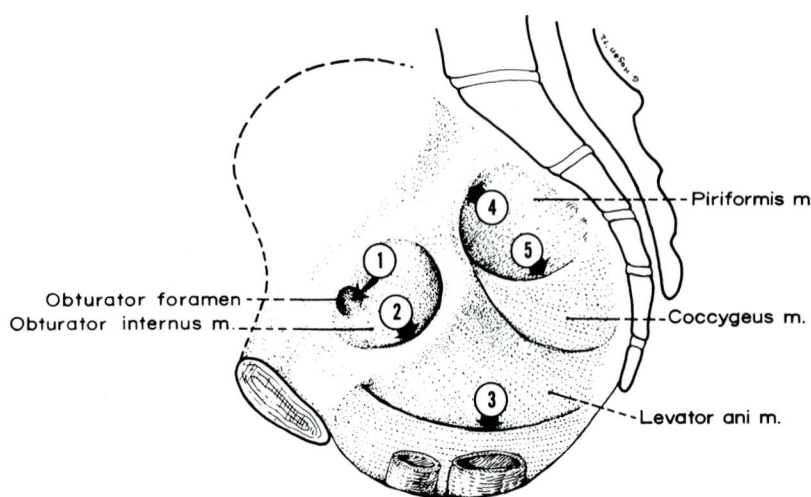

Figure 30-2. Medial wall of the left side of the pelvis showing sites of internal pelvic hernias: (1) obturator hernia; (2) ischiorectal hernia; (3) perineal hernia; (4) suprapiriformis muscle; (5) infrapiriformis muscle.

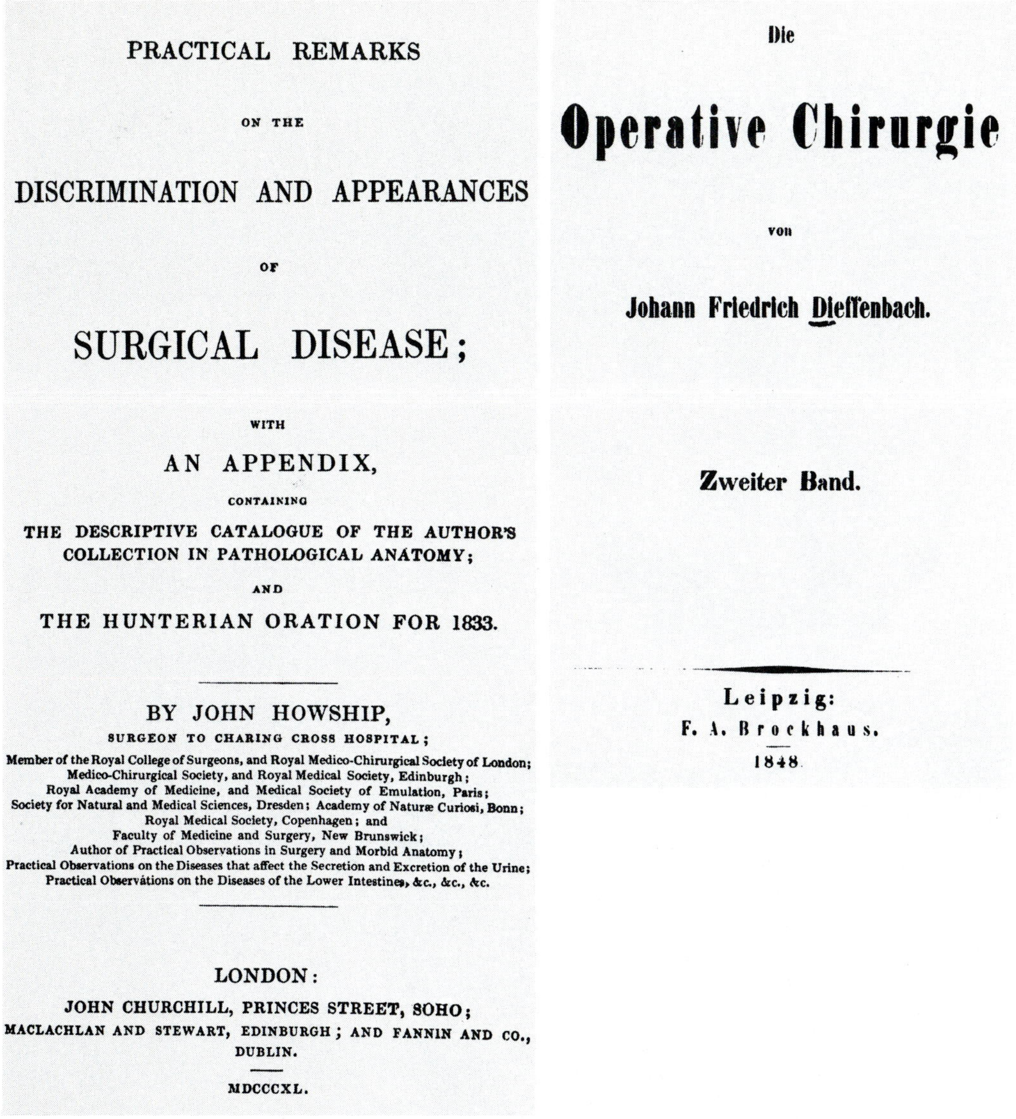

PRACTICAL REMARKS

ON THE

DISCRIMINATION AND APPEARANCES

OF

SURGICAL DISEASE;

WITH

AN APPENDIX,

CONTAINING

THE DESCRIPTIVE CATALOGUE OF THE AUTHOR'S
COLLECTION IN PATHOLOGICAL ANATOMY;

AND

THE HUNTERIAN ORATION FOR 1833.

BY JOHN HOWSHIP,

SURGEON TO CHARING CROSS HOSPITAL;

Member of the Royal College of Surgeons, and Royal Medico-Chirurgical Society of London;
Medico-Chirurgical Society, and Royal Medical Society, Edinburgh;
Royal Academy of Medicine, and Medical Society of Emulation, Paris;
Society for Natural and Medical Sciences, Dresden; Academy of Naturæ Curiosi, Bonn;
Royal Medical Society, Copenhagen; and
Faculty of Medicine and Surgery, New Brunswick;
Author of Practical Observations in Surgery and Morbid Anatomy;
Practical Observations on the Diseases that affect the Secretion and Excretion of the Urine;
Practical Observations on the Diseases of the Lower Intestines, &c., &c., &c.

LONDON:

JOHN CHURCHILL, PRINCES STREET, SOHO;

MACLACHLAN AND STEWART, EDINBURGH; AND FANNIN AND CO.,
DUBLIN.

MDCCCXL.

Die

Operative Chirurgie

VON

Johann Friedrich Dieffenbach.

Zweiter Band.

Leipzig:
F. A. Brockhaus.
1848.

Figure 30-3. (*Left*) Title page of Howship's book in which he described the typical pain of obturator hernia. (*Right*) Title page of Dieffenbach's work on surgery, which contains a description by Moritz H. Romberg of the pain produced by compression of the obturator nerve but no reference to Howship's earlier work.

acetabulum. All but a small area of this huge foramen is closed by the obturator membrane, fibers of which are continuous with the periosteum of the enclosing bones and with the tendinous attachments of the internal and external obturator muscles.

Embryologically, the foramen and its membrane represent an area of potential bone formation that never proceeds to completion. In this sense, the obturator foramen is a lacuna, and the obturator canal is the true foramen.

The Obturator Canal and Its Contents

The obturator canal is a tunnel 2 to 3 cm long that begins in the pelvis at the defect in the obturator membrane and passes obliquely downward to end outside the pelvis in the obturator region of the thigh. It is bounded superiorly and laterally by the wall of the obturator groove of the pubic bone and inferiorly by the free edge of the obturator membrane and the internal and external obturator muscles. Through

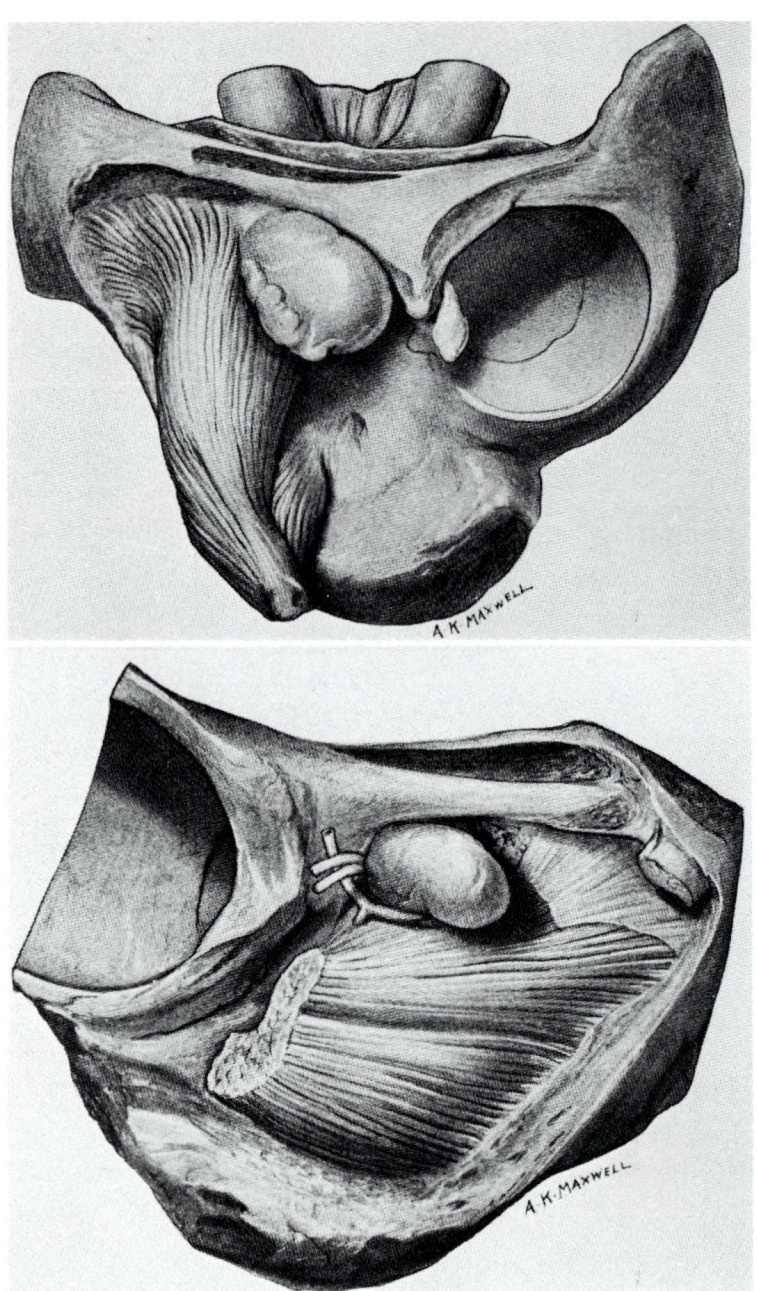

Figure 30-4. Specimens of obturator hernia from the Royal College of Surgeons Museum. The upper specimen dates from 1842. (Wakeley, CPG. Obturator hernia: its aetiology, incidence, and treatment, with two personal operative cases. Br J Surg 1939; 26: 515)

this canal pass the obturator nerve, artery, and vein and the fat body of the obturator canal. Some surgeons consider this last entity to be pathologic. We, however, have found it present in all our dissections. From 0.2 to 0.5 cm in size, we consider this a nice cushion for the obturator nerve and by all means not a pathologic entity. The relations of these structures to one another and to other structures within the pelvis may be seen in Figures 30-5 and 30-6.

The obturator nerve usually enters the obturator canal superior to the artery and vein. Immediately on emerging from the canal, it divides into anterior and posterior divisions. The anterior division emerges between the adductor longus and adductor brevis muscles, while the posterior division emerges between the adductor brevis and adductor magnus muscles. Figure 30-7 shows the muscles innervated by the two divisions. There are afferent fibers from the hip joint

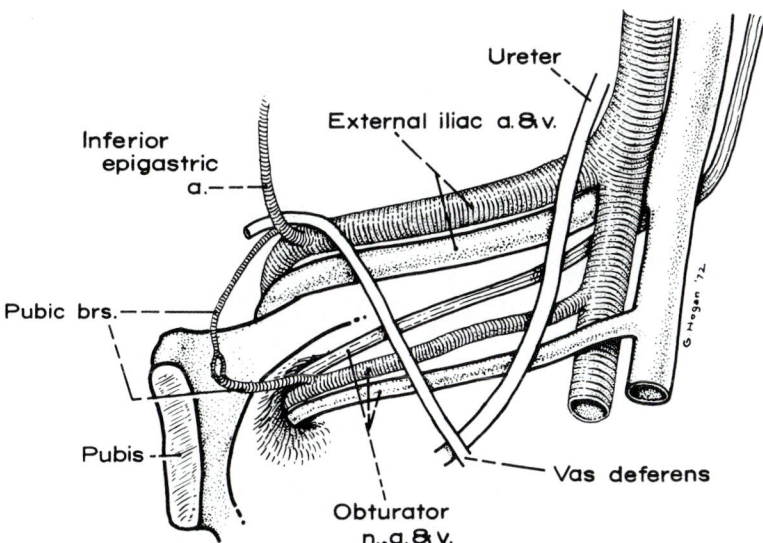

Figure 30-5. Medial wall of the male pelvis showing the structures traversing the obturator canal and their relations to the ureter, ductus deferens, and iliac vessels. (Gray SW, Skandalakis JE, Soria RE, Rowe JS Jr. Strangulated obstructor hernia. Surgery 1974; 75: 20)

and the knee joint as well as from the skin of the medial surface of the thigh.

The obturator artery also divides on emerging from the canal. The medial and lateral branches anastomose to form a ring around the foramen (Fig. 30-8). From this ring, twigs pass to the adductor muscles.

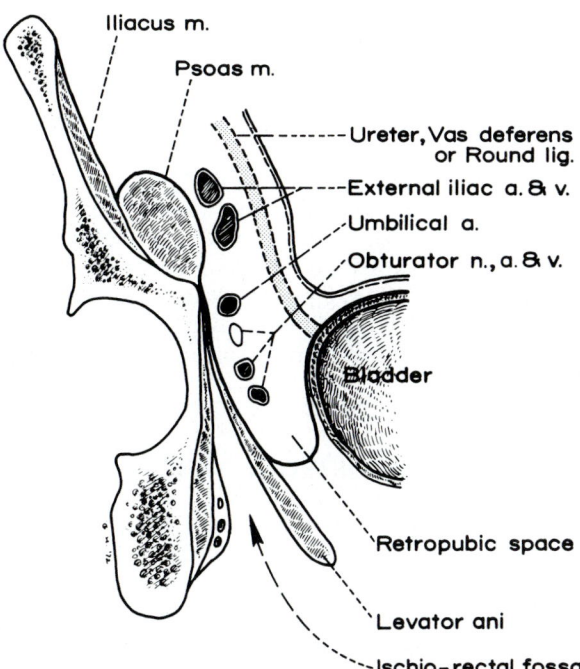

Figure 30-6. Diagrammatic coronal section of the lateral wall of the male pelvis showing the relations of the obturator nerve and vessels to other pelvic structures. (Gray SW, Skandalakis JE, Soria RE, Rowe JS Jr. Strangulated obstructor hernia. Surgery 1974; 75:20)

FORMATION OF OBTURATOR HERNIA

First Stage (Prehernia)

An obturator hernia begins with the entrance of preperitoneal connective tissue and fat into the pelvic orifice of the obturator canal (Fig. 30-9A and B). Such "pilot tags" with no internal dimpling of the peritoneum are common. Anson and colleagues[4] found six examples among 360 body halves dissected. Singer and associates[64] found nine such tags among 14 female cadavers and seven among 30 male cadavers. One example has been found in a living patient.[56] The frequency of pilot tags in cadavers and the rarity of actual obturator hernias in patients suggest that most instances do not progress beyond the asymptomatic prehernia stage.

Second Stage

The second stage (see Fig. 30-9C) begins with the appearance of a dimple in the peritoneum over the internal opening of the obturator canal and progresses to the invagination of a peritoneal sac, which, at first, may remain empty. The sac may follow the anterior or the posterior division of the obturator nerve (Fig. 30-10). The vessels lie lateral to the sac in about half of patients and medial, anterior, or posterior in the remainder.

Third Stage

The third stage begins with the onset of symptoms produced by entrance of an organ, usually the ileum,

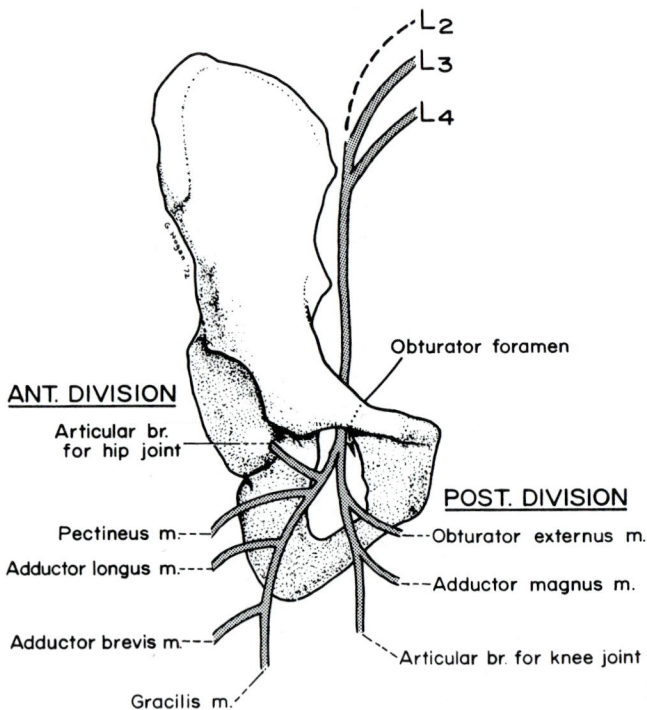

Figure 30-7. The course and distribution of the right obturator nerve.

into the sac (see Fig. 30-9*D*). At first, the herniation is transitory and reduces spontaneously. In a few instances, indications of herniation were present before operation, but the sac, at operation, was empty.[47] Occasionally, there may be areas of scarring on the ileum, indicating repeated herniation and reduction.[69]

Later in the third stage, the herniated knuckle of ileum may fail to reduce spontaneously. If only a portion of the ileal circumference is incarcerated (Richter hernia), the obstruction may be partial or complete (see Fig. 30-9*D*). If an entire loop enters the sac, obstruction is complete (see Fig. 30-9*E*). Adhesions are not common, and the hernia usually can be reduced by traction, although exceptions have been reported.[37,53] If necessary, the ring should be incised at the lower margin. There is always the danger that necrosis of the incarcerated loop may result in preoperative perforation or in tearing during forcible reduction.

ANALYSIS OF REPORTED INSTANCES

Watson found 442 instances of obturator hernia in the literature up to 1946.[75] Since 1946, at least 109 instances of obturator hernia have been reported in the English-language literature. Of these, 41 were from Asian or African hospitals.[2,8,12,40,42,43,65] The largest single series is the 20 hernias reported by Martin and Welch[43] from Thailand.

Little is known of the incidence of this hernia. Rogers[56] stated that there were 12 instances of obtur-

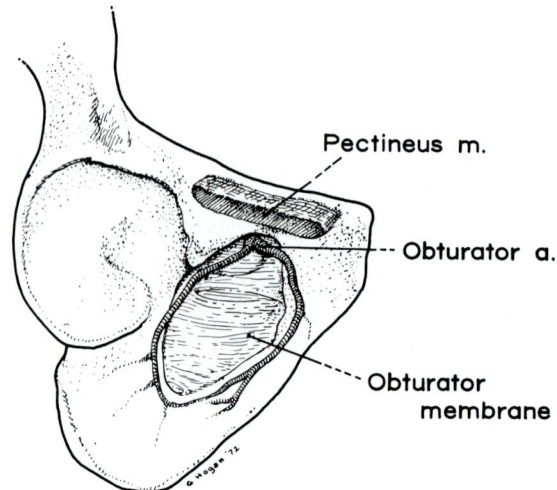

Figure 30-8. The obturator artery divides into a medial and a lateral branch as it emerges from the obturator canal. These branches anastomose distally to form an arterial ring around the obturator foramen.

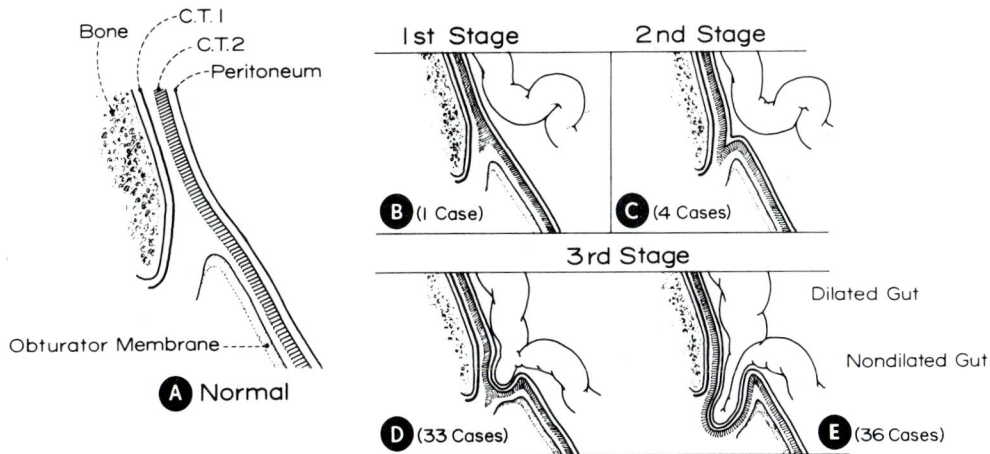

Figure 30-9. The genesis of obturator hernia. (*A*) Section through the obturator canal; pubic bone (*above*) and obturator membrane (*below*) form the boundaries. (*B*) First stage: "pilot tag" of preperitoneal connective tissue in obturator canal. (*C*) Second stage: peritoneal invagination beginning. (*D*) Third stage: partial incarceration (Richter) of an ileal loop. (*E*) Third stage: complete herniation of ileal loop. C.T. 1, periosteal layer; C.T. 2, preperitoneal connective tissue. (Gray SW, Skandalakis JE, Soria RE, Rowe JS Jr. Strangulated obstructor hernia. Surgery 1974; 75:20)

ator hernia among 3000 mechanical intestinal obstructions treated over 22 years at the Los Angeles County General Hospital. Kozlowski and Beal[39] found three hernias in 8 years at Northwestern Memorial Hospital, Chicago. Manning[42] found 4 obturator hernias among 539 hernia operations in 1 year (1964) in a Nigerian hospital. This is an abnormally high incidence, not usual in Nigeria or elsewhere. Bjork and colleagues[9] reported 11 cases of obturator hernia, which represented 0.073% of all (15,098) hernias re-

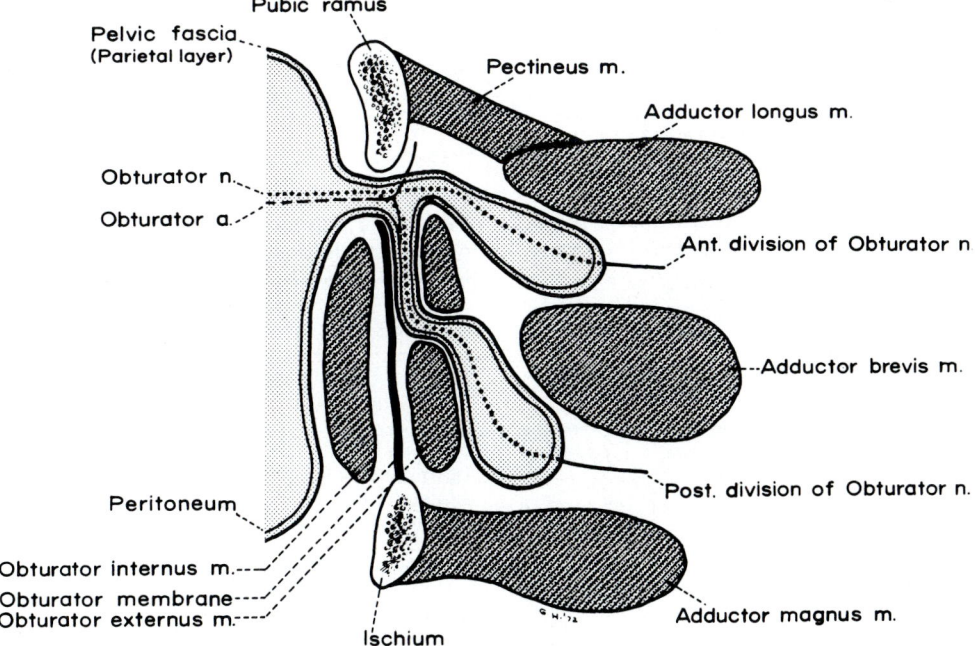

Figure 30-10. Diagrammatic longitudinal section of the upper thigh showing potential pathways of obturator hernia. The hernial sac may follow either the anterior or the posterior division of the obturator nerve. (Gray SW, Skandalakis JE, Soria RE, Rowe JS Jr. Strangulated obstructor hernia. Surgery 1974; 75:20)

paired at the Mayo Clinic. Persson and colleagues[54] found 15 patients (11 women and 4 men) with obturator hernias among 850 patients undergoing herniography for the investigation of groin pain. Five patients underwent surgical exploration, but the presence of a hernial sac was confirmed in only two. These latter two patients continued to exhibit symptoms even after the hernias were repaired. It is easy to see why the word *elusive* has been used to described the diagnosis of obturator hernia.[55,70,77]

Sex, Age, and Side Affected

Only 14 of the 99 hernias occurred in men (Table 30-1). The sex ratio of 1:6.1 is close to that in Watson's[75] older data, for which the ratio was 1:5.3. Singer and colleagues[64] believed that the more vertical direction of the obturator canal in men reduces the predisposition to hernia. The modal group of women were in the eighth decade of life; men appeared to be affected at a slightly younger age. The youngest patient was 30 years of age, the oldest, 93 years of age. The 37 patients from Asian and African hospitals were about 10 years younger than the 62 white patients.

In men, the left side is more often affected than the right; in women, hernia is more frequent on the right side (Table 30-2). Among 31 patients described as emaciated or who had marked weight loss, more lesions were on the left than among patients not so described. Thirty-one patients were described as emaciated, very thin, or frail; only one was described as obese.

Bilateral hernias were reported in two patients. In one, the hernia on the right side occurred 8 weeks after successful reduction of a hernia on the left side.[29] In the second patient, herniated ileum on the right was associated with an empty sac on the left. A third patient had two operations for obturator hernia

Table 30-1. Sex and Age at Operation of 143 Patients With Obturator Hernia

Age (y)	Male	Female
0–9	0	0
10–19	0	0
20–29	0	1
30–39	3	3
40–49	0	7
50–59	2	13
60–69	6	24
70–79	6	40
80–89	1	29
90–99	0	9

Table 30-2. Sex and Side Affected in 141 Patients With Obturator Hernia

Side Affected	Male	Female	Total
Left	10	43	53
Right	8	76	84
Both	0	4	4
Not stated	0	3	3

8 years apart, but it was not known whether the second hernia was a recurrence of the first or was on the contralateral side. Concurrent femoral and obturator hernias have been reported.[74]

Contents of the Hernial Sac

The hernial sac in most instances contained small intestine, usually ileum. In slightly more than half of these hernias, the incarceration was partial (Richter type). Omentum, uterine tubes, urinary bladder, and appendix have been found in a few patients.

Peculiar cases of obturator hernia have been presented by Ng Lung Kit and Collins.[48] A leiomyoma originating from the broad ligament was found within the obturator canal, producing obturator hernia.

In four patients only an empty sac was found.[36,47,56] In two of these patients, the empty sac was asymptomatic; it was found incidentally to elective repair of femoral hernias.[56] Table 30-3 lists the hernial sac contents encountered in 73 patients.

Table 30-3. Contents of Hernial Sac in 122 Instances of Obturator Hernia

Contents	No. of Instances
Ileum	69
"Small intestine"	22
"Small bowel"	5
Jejunum	5
Descending colon	1
Appendix	2 (1)*
Sigmoid epiploicae	1
Bladder	1
Omentum	1 (1)*
Uterine tube	(1)*
None	16
Pilot tag only, no sac	1
TOTAL	124

*In addition to ileum

Symptoms and Signs of Obturator Hernia

Symptoms of obturator hernia are acute, becoming progressively severe, and are relieved only by reduction of the hernia (Table 30-4). Twenty-eight patients had a history of previous attacks, each relieved spontaneously until the last one. The longest such history was 10 years.

Obstruction

Signs and symptoms of partial or complete intestinal obstruction were the presenting complaint in 70 of 79 hernias.

Hip and Knee Pain (Howship-Romberg Sign)

Forty-seven patients experienced pain extending down the inner surface of the thigh to the knee and sometimes lower, occasionally radiating to the hip joint. Flexion of the thigh usually relieves this pain; extension, adduction, or medial rotation exacerbates it. This is the Howship-Romberg sign. The pain results from compression by the hernia of the obturator nerve where it passes through the canal; it especially affects the cutaneous branch of the anterior division (Fig. 30-11). The nerve contains motor as well as sensory fibers, and adductor weakness could probably be shown if pain from the sensory fibers did not mask it. Both sensory loss and motor weakness have been demonstrated after section of the obturator nerve.

The sign is not constant; 38 of 79 patients denied feeling such pain (see Table 30-4). Thus, its absence is not important. Its presence, however, is an indication of pressure on the obturator nerve. If a tumor of one of the pelvic organs is ruled out, the pressure can only be attributed to herniation into the obturator canal. The physician must not overlook the importance of medial thigh pain in elderly patients with numerous rheumatic pains.

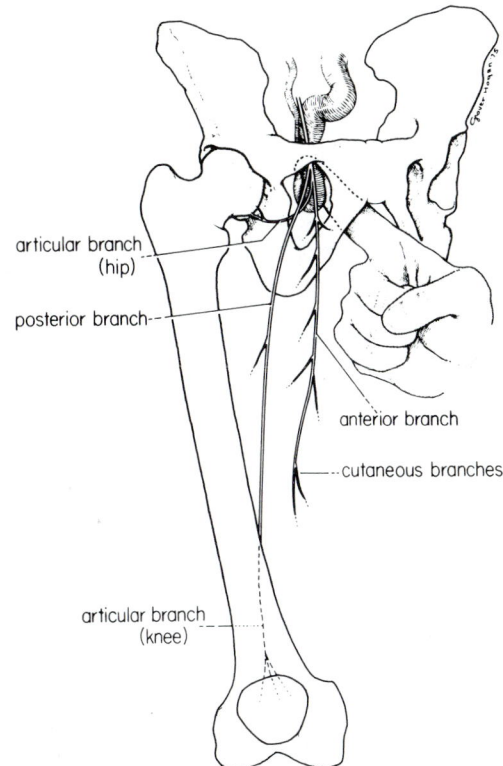

Figure 30-11. Pain results from compression of the obturator nerve by the hernia (Howship-Romberg sign). Either or both divisions may be affected. Palpation of rectum or vagina may help to confirm suspicion of obturator hernia.

The degree and extent of the pain are not important. Extreme pain was experienced by a patient with a spontaneously reducing hernia; at operation, the sac was empty.[47]

Palpable Mass

A hernial mass was palpated in only 15 patients. The optimal position for palpation is with the patient supine, with the thigh flexed, abducted, and rotated outward. Rectal and especially vaginal palpation may help in locating the mass. Tenderness or pain over the tumor suggests strangulation of the hernia.

Previous Attacks

In 28 of 79 patients, there was a history of previous attacks of acute obstruction and subsequent remission. These indicated transient herniation followed by spontaneous reduction. In 12 patients, the attacks occurred within the 6 months preceding operation; in 9, they were within 3 years; and in 7, attacks were experienced from 4 to 10 years earlier.

Table 30-4. Signs and Symptoms Accompanying 118 Instances of Obturator Hernia

Sign or Symptom	No. of Instances	Percentage
Obstruction	88*	74.6
Howship-Romberg sign	49†	41.5
Emaciation or weight loss	42	35.6
History of previous attacks	33	28.0
Palpable mass	19	16.1
Incidental finding (no symptoms)	8	6.8

*Not including 5 equivocal
†Not including 3 equivocal

Associated Diseases

Other coexisting hernias are not uncommon. In one patient, the omentum was strangulated in an inguinal hernia; in another, the same structure was strangulated in a femoral hernia. The ileum was incarcerated in the obturator hernia in both patients.

One patient presented with subcutaneous emphysema of the lateral aspect of the thigh.[37] There was no mass, and there were no symptoms of obstruction; the Howship-Romberg sign was present, and an obturator hernia was correctly diagnosed. A partially incarcerated loop of descending colon had perforated, allowing gas to escape into the tissue spaces of the thigh with formation of an abscess. The colon was repaired and the sinus tract drained. Gaunt and colleagues[22] reported a case of a strangulated hernia in which the associated pain was attributed to a total hip replacement.

Diagnosis

The four signs of obturator hernia are, in order of frequency, intestinal obstruction, the Howship-Romberg sign, a history of previous attacks, and a palpable mass (see Table 30-4). They cannot be called a syndrome or a constellation in any sense. The most frequent combination (obstruction plus Howship-Romberg sign) was present in less than half of patients; in only 3 of the 77 patients who described symptoms were all four signs present.[15,40]

The diagnosis of complete or partial intestinal obstruction is obvious in most instances. The nature of the obstruction is usually in doubt.

Obturator hernia was correctly diagnosed in 24 of 76 patients in whom intestinal obstruction was reported and in 1 patient with incarcerated urinary bladder.[44] In 22 of these patients, the Howship-Romberg sign was the only finding consistently present in addition to the intestinal obstruction. One hernia was correctly diagnosed by roentgenography,[79] and another was correctly diagnosed after recurrence of a previously reduced obturator hernia.[8] In 18 patients in whom obstruction was not correctly diagnosed, the sign was present but did not lead to a correct diagnosis. In some patients, the presence of the sign was remembered only after an operation revealed the hernia.

Roentgenography contributed to the correct diagnosis in four patients, and computed tomography revealed the hernia in one.[45] Since that time, several authors[18] have advocated the use of computed tomography examination. Visualization of the site of obstruction is sometimes possible when the hernia is of

the Richter type, which only partially obstructs the intestinal canal. Glicklich and Eliasoph[24] found that pain in the thigh elicited during the course of a barium enema examination suggested the diagnosis of an incarcerated obturator hernia.

In no instance did a palpable mass alone suggest the diagnosis of obturator hernia. In 8 of the 15 patients in whom a mass was palpated, the correct diagnosis was not made. We believe that many more hernias could be palpated if the suspicion was in the examiner's mind. In a few instances, the presence of a palpable femoral hernia completely masked the coexisting obturator hernia.

Herniography, ultrasonography, and laparoscopy should be added to the diagnostic armamentarium of the surgeon. Herniography has been used successfully by Persson and colleagues,[54] Carriquiry and Piñeyro,[10] and Hall and colleagues.[28]

The Howship-Romberg sign must be considered pathognomonic of obturator hernia. In its absence, correct diagnosis is improbable; in its presence, an obturator hernia should be immediately suspected.

TREATMENT

An ileal loop herniated into the obturator canal may reduce spontaneously, ending a short episode of pain and partial obstruction. At operation, an empty sac is found. If the loop becomes strangulated, surgical intervention is necessary. Treated early, the healthy intestinal loop requires only reduction. If surgical treatment is delayed, gangrene begins, and the strangulated loop must be resected with anastomosis of the healthy intestine. Still longer delay results in rupture of the strangulated loop and onset of peritonitis. Olivier and Noyez[51] consider that delayed treatment is the most important single factor in the mortality of the disease. Resection of some small intestine was found to be necessary in 49 of the 79 collected reports (Table 30-5).

Surgical Approach

A variety of approaches to obturator hernias have been suggested. The important ones are described here.

Abdominal Approach
Through a lower midline incision with the patient in the Trendelenburg position, the pelvis can be inspected. If the hernia has reached the third stage (see Fig. 30-9D and E), the pathologic state is obvious. If the hernia is in the second stage (see Fig. 30-9C) and

Table 30-5. Summary of Treatment in 101 Instances of Obturator Hernia

Treatment	No Repair of Defect Stated	Defect Only Closed	Sac Only Excised	Defect Closed, Sac Excised	Total
Spontaneous reduction before operation				1	1
Reduction only	8	27	6	5	46
Reduction and resection with anastomosis	13	11	3	11	38
Irreducible; resection with anastomosis		2	1	8	11
No operation	2				2
Potential hernia only		3			3
TOTAL	23 (22.8%)	43 (42.6%)	10 (9.9%)	25 (24.8%)	101 (100%)

incarceration is not present, the surgeon should inspect and palpate the obturator area. If there is no dimple in the peritoneum and if the finger does not feel any defect just under the ischiopubic area at the obturator membrane, the surgeon must decide either to dissect for possible herniation of preperitoneal fat, the first stage in the formation of an obturator hernia (see Fig. 30-9B), or to discontinue the operation.

If the intestine is strangulated and the ring cannot be stretched with the finger, the surgeon should remember that the vessels and nerve lie lateral to the sac in half of patients and medial, anterior, or posterior in the remainder. Because the relation of the sac to the vessels and nerves is variable, the ring should be incised at the lower margin. The intestine should be inspected thoroughly to determine whether resection and end-to-end anastomosis are necessary.

Retropubic Approach

A retropubic or retroperitoneal approach was advocated by Cheatle,[11] Henry,[31] and Soothill.[66] Nyhus[49] and Rogers[57] pointed out the advantages of this approach in patients in whom a correct diagnosis was made before operation.

Because of the rarity of the problem, no one author has adequate experience to advocate resoundingly any single surgical approach. We refer the reader to the surgicoanatomic work of Nyhus and Condon elsewhere in this book and to our own book,[65a] *Hernia: Surgical Anatomy and Technique.*

Obturator Approach

If there is a palpable mass in the obturator area, the thigh should be flexed and abducted and a generous incision made just above the mass. The first structure encountered is fascia lata, which should be divided. This division exposes two muscles, the adductor longus medially and the pectineus laterally. These muscles should be drawn back to expose the hernial sac. The principles governing treatment of strangulated femoral hernia should be applied. Closing the defect is not easy. Inversion of the sac and use of the pectineus muscle by suturing it to the periosteum have been advised.

Inguinal Approach

Milligan[46] and Shackelford[62] described an extraperitoneal approach as in inguinal hernia.

Laparoscopic Approach

The possible use of laparoscopy for the surgical treatment of groin hernias was conceived about 15 years ago. Since its conception, this approach has been subjected to clinical trial and proved successful. Although originally directed to the management of indirect inguinal hernias, this technique has since included treatment of obturator hernia.

Combinations

A combination of the abdominal approach and one of the others is at times advisable.

Selection of the Surgical Approach

Shackelford[62] suggested four advantages to the abdominal approach: (1) it establishes the diagnosis; (2) it is the best way to expose the obturator ring; (3) it is the least dangerous to obturator vessels; and (4) it permits intestinal resection when necessary.

The first advantage becomes important when we remember that in the present series, 52 of 79 hernias were not diagnosed as obturator hernias. The fourth advantage gains importance by the fact that in 35 patients, resection of a portion of the intestine was necessary.

The retropubic approach and the obturator and inguinal approaches avoid entering the abdominal cavity. They give good results if it can be ascertained that the obstruction is actually caused by an obturator hernia and the incarcerated structures do not require resection. Because these two aspects of the lesion are the least predictable, the surgeon who uses these procedures may be forced to make a second incision and approach the site of the obstruction through the abdominal wall. The surgeon should be prepared for this possibility before starting to operate.

Repair of the Defect

As in other hernias, after reduction of the contents, the sac should be inverted and ligated and the redundant portion excised. The stump, sutured to the margins of the obturator opening, closes the defect. More effective closure of the defect may be obtained by the use of a flap of autogenous fascia, prepared ox fascia, tantalum mesh, or a polytetrafluoroethylene (Teflon)

Table 30-6. Summary of Methods Used for Closure*

Author	Method
Short (1923)[63]	Plug of rib cartilage
Horine (1927)[34]	Suture sac to peritoneum after inverting apex of sac through defect
Grey-Turner (1938)[26]	Evert sac and ligate base
Wakely (1939)[72]	Ligate sac, then suture strip from innermost fibers of pectineus muscle to periosteum of obturator canal
Throckmorton (1950)[69]	Patch of tantalum gauze
Pender (1950)[52]	Plug of tantalum gauze placed through thigh incision
Rothman (1951)[60]	Patch of peritoneum 1 × 1.5 in
Stone and McLanahan (1954)[68]	Osteoperiosteal flap turned back from inner pubic bone over opening
Harper and Holt (1956)[30]	Close peritoneum over opening from below upward, incorporating base of sac
Gilfillan (1958)[23]	Evert and ligate sac; fill defect with plug of free omentum
Rogers (1960)[56]	Patch of PTFE cloth
Hanley and Hanna (1970)[29]	Fundus of uterus or broad ligament
Larrieu and DeMarco (1976)[41]	Marlex mesh
Arbman (1984)[7]	Bladder wall
Angstman et al (1986)[3]	Obturator foramen was not closed
Gumbs et al (1986)[27]	Close obturator canal with three 1-0 silk sutures
Hershman et al (1986)[32]	Closed with silk or nylon suture
Ng Lung Kit and Collins (1986)[48]	Plug the canal with pectineus muscle
Wadler and Rose (1987)[71]	Suture pectineal muscle to the periosteum of the obturator canal
Bjork et al (1988)[9]	Local obturator fascia for closure of the canal
Carriquiry and Piñeyro (1988)[10]	Place polypropylene mesh beneath pubis and both obturator formina
Young et al (1988)[78]	Either a pursestring suture or interrupted sutures
Rizk and Deshmukh (1990)[55]	Close with size 1-0 polyglycolic acid suture material
Yip et al (1993)[77]	Closure of the defect with interrupted nonabsorbable sutures; with or without sac invagination and with or without sac excision

*Several reports could not be included in this summary because their authors failed to describe the procedure used for repair. We believe it is imperative that future authors provide greater detail on the technique of repair of this rare entity.
PTFE, polytetrafluoroethylene (Teflon)
(Modified from Rogers FA. Strangulated obturator hernia. In: Nyhus LM, Harkins HN, eds. Hernia. Philadelphia, JB Lippincott, 1964)

patch. Rogers[57] summarized the use of these and other materials for closing the obturator defect. Table 30-6 is from Rogers with additions.

Among the 79 patients operated on, repair of the defect was not mentioned for 22 (see Table 30-5). In some of these patients, repair may have been undertaken without being described; in many, we believe no repair was done. This deviation from the usual principles of hernial repair occurs because of the advanced age and acute illness of the patients afflicted with obturator hernia. Despite this high percentage of unclosed defects, there was only one confirmed recurrence that required reoperation.[8] In one other patient, subsequent attacks suggested recurrence,[59] but they could have been produced by a contralateral obturator hernia. A third patient had been operated on 8 years earlier for obturator hernia,[29] but whether on the same or the opposite side was not known. The evidence does not support Shackelford's[62] statement that there is a 10% recurrence rate.

MORTALITY

Among the 98 patients undergoing an operation, there were 13 deaths. The immediate cause of death was reported in seven—four died of acute cardiovascular disease, two of these having wound infection as well; two died of peritonitis only; and another had a fatal pulmonary embolism. The cause of death in the rest was unspecified. One patient died of rupture of a strangulated jejunal loop before an operation could be performed.[25]

The overall mortality for 98 instances was 13.27%. Among 62 white patients, it was 8.97%. Among 31 Asian and 5 African patients, the mortality was 22.2%.

The mortality has declined markedly since Watson reported 48% in 1948.[75] In view of the advanced age of most of the patients and the small number of correct preoperative diagnoses, the operative mortality must be considered to be low.

SUMMARY

From a review of the reported instances of obturator hernia, especially those since 1946, the following generalizations can be made:

1. Obturator hernia chiefly affects women in the seventh and eighth decades of life; it is more frequent on the right side than on the left.
2. Most obturator hernias contain small intestine, usually a knuckle of ileum; obstruction is often partial.
3. Pain in the medial aspect of the thigh, sometimes radiating to hip and knee joints (Howship-Romberg sign), is the only distinguishing symptom. It is not always present or, if present, may be overlooked. A palpable mass is detected only occasionally.
4. A history of previous episodes of acute obstruction followed by remission is common. Strangulation eventually occurs, and surgical intervention is the only effective treatment.
5. We believe an abdominal approach is the treatment of choice unless the diagnosis is certain and incarceration has been brief. Closure of the defect is as necessary in obturator hernia as it is in other types of hernia.

ACKNOWLEDGMENT

This project was supported by a grant from George St. Stefanakis in memory of his son Stephanos.

REFERENCES

*1. Adams HH, Smith DC. Obturator hernia: report of successful operative case. JAMA 1948;137:948.
*2. Ang HB. Obturator hernia. Aust N Z J Surg 1970;40:86.
*3. Angstman KB, Myers JW, Olson RT. Obturator hernia: a rare cause of intestinal obstruction. J Fam Pract 1986;23:370.
4. Anson BJ, McCormick LJ, Cleveland HC. Anatomy of hernial regions: obturator hernia and general considerations. Surg Gynecol Obstet 1950;90:31.
5. Anson BJ, McVay CB. Surgical anatomy, vol 2. Philadelphia, WB Saunders, 1971:1123.
6. Anson BJ, McVay CB. Strangulated obturator hernia with acute gangrenous appendix. Br Med J 1969;1:230.
7. Arbman G. Strangulated obturator hernia: a simple method for closure. Acta Chir Scand 1984;150:337.
*8. Archampong EQ. Preoperative diagnosis of strangulated obturator hernia. Postgrad Med J 1968; 44:140.
*9. Bjork KJ, Mucha P Jr, Cahill DR. Obturator hernia. Surg Gynecol Surg 1988;167:217.
*10. Carriquiry LA, Piñeyro A. Pre-operative diagnosis of nonstrangulated obturator hernia: the contribution of herniography. Br J Surg 1988;75:785.
11. Cheatle GL. An operation for the radical cure of inguinal and femoral hernia. Br Med J 1920;2:68.
*12. Ch'iu HH. Strangulated obturator hernia: report of a case. Chin Med J 1957;75:328.
*13. Craig RDP. Strangulated obturator hernia: a report of 4 cases. Br J Surg 1962;49:426.

*Contains patient reports used for the tables in this chapter

*14. Cubillo E. Obturator hernia diagnosed by computed tomography. AJR 1983;140:735.

*15. Desmond AM, Huter F. Strangulated obturator hernia. Br J Surg 1948;35:318.

*16. Donald JW, Donald JG. Strangulated obturator hernia. South Med J 1968;61:772.

*17. Dwyer WA. Obturator hernia: report of three cases. J Med Soc NJ 1968;63:451.

*18. Fakim A, Walker MA, Byrne DJ, Forrester JC. Recurrent strangulated obturator hernia. Ann Chir Gynaecol 1991;80:317.

19. Franklin RH. Obturator hernia. Lancet 1938;1:721.

*20. Frederick WC, Krant J, Olymbitis JT, Protos AA. Strangulated obturator hernia. NY State J Med 1972;72:1745.

21. de Garengeot RJC. Memoire sur plusieurs hernies singulieres. Mem Acad R Chir Paris 1743;1:699.

*22. Gaunt ME, Tan SG, Dias J. Strangulated obturator hernia masquerading as pain from a total hip replacement. J Bone Joint Surg 1992;74B:782.

23. Gilfillan RR. Obturator hernia. Can J Surg 1958; 1:366.

*24. Glicklich M, Eliasoph J. Incarcerated obturator hernia: case diagnosed at barium enema fluoroscopy. Radiology 1989;172:51.

25. Gray SW, Skandalakis JE, Soria RE, Rowe JS Jr. Strangulated obstructor hernia. Surgery 1974;75: 20.

26. Grey-Turner G. Cited by Franklin RH. Obturator hernia. Lancet 1938;1:721.

*27. Gumbs MA, Pandya GS, Kim YH. Obturator hernia. NY State J Med 1986;86:150.

*28. Hall C, Hall PN, Wingate JP, Neoptolemos JP. Evaluation of herniography in the diagnosis of an occult abdominal wall hernia in symptomatic adults. Br J Surg 1990;77:902.

*29. Hanley JA, Hanna BKB. Obturator hernia: a report of three cases with strangulation occurring twice in two patients. J Ir Med Assoc 1970;63:396.

*30. Harper JR, Holt JH. Obturator hernia. Am J Surg 1956;92:562.

31. Henry AK. Operation for femoral hernia by a midline, extraperitoneal approach. Lancet 1936;1:531.

*32. Hershman MJ, Reilly DT, Swift RI. Strangulated obturator hernia: delayed diagnosis is still the rule. J R Coll Surg Edinburgh 1986;31:282.

33. Hilton J. Case of obturator hernia, with symptoms of intestinal obstruction within the abdomen, to relieve which the abdomen was opened. Lancet 1848;2:103.

34. Horine CF. Obturator hernia. Ann Surg 1927; 86:776.

35. Howship J. Practical remarks on the discrimination and appearances of surgical disease. London, John Churchill, 1840.

*36. Joseph WL, Kipen CS, Longmire WP Jr. Obturator hernia as a cause of acute intestinal obstruction. Am J Surg 1968;115:301.

*37. Kapur BML, Shah DK. Strangulated obturator hernia presenting as subcutaneous emphysema of the thigh. Can J Surg 1969;12:233.

*38. Korvald E, Myhre HO. Hernia obturatoria: report of 2 cases. J Oslo City Hosp 1970;20:121.

39. Kozlowski JM, Beal JM. Obturator hernia: an elusive diagnosis. Arch Surg 1977;112:1001.

*40. Kwong KH, Ong GB. Obturator hernia. Br J Surg 1966;53:23.

*41. Larrieu AJ, DeMarco SJ. Obturator hernia: report of a case and brief review of its status. Am Surg 1976;42:273.

*42. Manning PC. Incidence and management of obturator hernia. West Afr Med J 1966;15:223.

*43. Martin NC, Welch TP. Obturator hernia. Br J Surg 1974;61:547.

44. McCarthy MC. Obturator hernia of urinary bladder. Urology 1976;7:312.

45. Meziane MA, Fishman EK, Siegelman SS. Computed tomographic diagnosis of obturator foramen hernia. Gastrointest Radiol 1983;8:375.

46. Milligan ETC. The inguinal route for the radical cure of obturator hernia. Br Med J 1919;2:134.

*47. Nathan H. Differential diagnosis of obturator and ileocecal hernia. Proc Rudolph Virchow Med Soc City NY 1971;28:152.

*48. Ng Lung Kit HK, Collins REC. Leiomyoma of the broad ligament in an obturator hernia presenting as a lump in the groin. J R Soc Med 1986;79:174.

49. Nyhus LM. Editorial comment. In: Nyhus LM, Harkins HN, eds. Hernia. Philadelphia, JB Lippincott, 1964.

50. Obre H. Case of obturator or thyroidal hernia successfully relieved by operation. Lancet 1851;2:8.

51. Olivier J, Noyez D. Hernia obturatoria: Casuistiek an vergelijikende dissertatie. Acta Chir Belg 1973; 72:116.

*52. Pender BWT. Recurrent obstruction of obturator hernia. Br Med J 1950;2:1038.

*53. Pernworth P. Obturator hernia: report of operation for irreducible incarceration. Am J Surg 1946;71: 539.

*54. Persson NH, Bergqvist D, Ekberg O. Obturator hernia: clinical significance of radiologic diagnosis. Acta Chir Scand 1987;153:361.

*55. Rizk TA, Deshmukh N. Obturator hernia: a difficult diagnosis. South Med J 1990;83:709.

*56. Rogers FA. Strangulated obturator hernia. Surgery 1960;48:394.

57. Rogers FA. Strangulated obturator hernia. In: Nyhus LM, Harkins HN, eds. Hernia. Philadelphia, JB Lippincott, 1964.

58. Romberg MH. Die Operation des singeklemmten Bruches des eirunden Loches: Operatio herniae foraminis ovalis incarceratae. In: Dieffenbach JF, ed. Die Operative Chirurgie, vol 2. Leipzig, FA Brockhaus, 1848.

*59. Rose TF. Obturator hernia: some difficulties in preoperative diagnosis illustrated by two cases with unusual features. Med J Aust 1954;1:13.

*60. Rothman M. The repair of obturator hernia with peritoneal graft. NY State J Med 1951;51:186.

*61. Rowe EB, Bynum GA. Obturator hernia. Am J Surg 1952;18:770.

62. Shackelford RT. Surgery of the alimentary tract. Philadelphia, WB Saunders, 1955:2369.
63. Short AR. The treatment of strangulated obturator hernia. Br Med J 1923;1:718.
64. Singer R, Leary PM, Hofmeyer NG. Obturator hernia. S Afr Med J 1955;29:73.
65. Sinha SN, DeCosta AE. Obturator hernia. Aust N Z J Surg 1983;53:349.
65a. Skandalakis JE, Gray SW, Mansberger AR Jr., Colborn GL, Skandalakis LJ. Hernia: surgical anatomy and technique. New York, McGraw-Hill, 1989.
66. Soothill EF. Obturator hernia. Guys Hosp Rep 1954;103:43.
*67. Srivastava KP, Racela IG, Rohl JJ. Strangulated hernia of the obturator canal as a cause of acute abdomen. Int Surg 1972;57:566.
68. Stone H, McLanahan S. Obturator hernia. In: Lewis DD, ed. Practice of surgery, vol 7. Hagerstown, MD, WF Prior, 1954:68.
*69. Throckmorton TD. Repair of obturator hernia with a tantalum gauze implant. Surgery 1950;27:888.
*70. Tiwary AK, Tie MLH, Lynch G. Obturator hernia: an elusive diagnosis. J R Soc Med 1992;85:180.
*71. Wadler D, Rose RH. Obturator hernias. NY State J Med 1987;87:414.
72. Wakeley CPG. Obturator hernia: its aetiology, incidence, and treatment, with two personal operative cases. Br J Surg 1939;26:515.
*73. Waterfall MC. Recovery from strangulated obturator hernia. Br Med J 1950;1:585.
74. Watkins RM, Leach RD, Elis H. Bilateral obturator herniae and associated femoral hernia. Postgrad Med J 1981;57:466.
75. Watson LF. Hernia, ed 3. St Louis, CV Mosby, 1948:457.
*76. Yanover RR, Podolsky WG, Marks CR. Obturator hernia. NY State J Med 1950;50:2317.
*77. Yip AWC, AnChong AK, Lam KH. Obturator hernia: a continuing diagnostic challenge. Surgery 1993;113:266.
*78. Young A, Hudson DA, Krige JEJ. Strangulated obturator hernia: can mortality be reduced? South Med J 1988;81:1117.
*79. Zausner J, Dumont AE, Ring SM. Obturator hernia. Am J Roentgenol Radium Ther Nucl Med 1972;115:408.

Editor's Comment

Our colleagues have comprehensively covered this subject. In their summary statement, the transabdominal approach for repair is suggested when the diagnosis is uncertain. I concur. If the diagnosis is certain, the obturator foramen is easily approached by the posterior or preperitoneal method. This statement holds as well for the incarcerated or strangulated hernia and is the approach of choice for these complicated problems. Because of the rigidity of the foramen walls, a prosthetic plug or patch is usually necessary to cover the defect.

Guillaume Dupuytren (1777–1835), the greatest of the early vascular surgeons, is credited with many historical firsts. Included among his feats are the following. He was the first successfully to excise the lower jaw (1812). He was the first to ligate the external iliac artery (1815) and the subclavian artery (1819). He was the first to describe a fracture of the lower end of the fibula with displacement (1819). He was the first to divide the sternocleidomastoid muscle subcutaneously for torticollis (1822). He gave the first adequate description of the hip (1826). He devised an operation in which he used his enterotome for making an artificial anus (1828). He was the first to describe an abscess of the right iliac fossa (1829). He was the first to classify burns (1832). And he was the first to write a treatise on war wounds (1834).

Although he is probably best known for his work on fascial contracture of the hand, it is appropriate to mention herein that Dupuytren's work, *de la Hernie Obturatrice* (Paris, Pimbet D, 1819), was one of the first on obturator hernia, a subject that had a very *French* beginning.

Moritz Heinrich Romberg (1795–1873) is best known for his description of achondroplasia and facial hemiatrophy or trophoneurosis, yet the sign for obturator hernia (the Howship-Romberg, or Romberg, sign) is essentially the only means by which this hernia may be suspected preoperatively. This Romberg sign must be differentiated from the other attributed to him, the sign for tabes dorsalis, in which a patient cannot maintain equilibrium when standing with feet together and eyes closed.

A recent experience by our colleague, Dr. Jack Bergstein, in managing an elderly woman with poor connective tissues, may be helpful to readers. This woman had bilateral obturator hernias. The associated tissues around the hernia orifice were such that they would not easily hold sutures. Dr. Bergstein solved this problem by using a modified Stoppa repair, deepening the angle of the chevron and the dissection in the pelvis so that it went inferior and posterior to the obturator foramina, and tacking the deepest portions of the prosthesis in place. The patient recovered without incident. So far, the repairs are holding.

L.M.N.

Hernia, Fourth Edition, edited
by Lloyd M. Nyhus and Robert E. Condon.
J.B. Lippincott Company, Philadelphia © 1995.

Chapter 31

Sciatic Hernia

Sidney Black

Sciatic hernia is the protrusion of a pelvic peritoneal sac and its contents through the greater or the lesser sciatic foramen. This condition is also called *sacro-sciatic hernia, gluteal hernia, ischiatic hernia, ischiocele,* and *hernia incisurae ischiadicae.*

HISTORY

Watson,[19] in 1948, credited the first description of sciatic hernia to Verdier (1753). Bréhant and associates,[4] however, stated that Papen, in 1750, was the first to describe sciatic hernia and that hernia included small intestine, colon, and ovary. The third report was by Schreger in 1818.[19] Summers,[17] in 1922, was the first American to report a sciatic hernia. A second was reported by Brodnax in 1924.[5] The latter hernia was asymptomatic and contained a Meckel diverticulum that was found during an autopsy after a death resulting from head wounds. In a review of the world literature, Watson was able to find only 35 reports until 1948.[19] He thus concluded that sciatic hernia is the rarest of all hernias. In 1958, Gaffney and Schanno[7] collected three additional instances and added one of their own, a hernia that was thought to be congenital.

INCIDENCE

It is impossible to determine statistically the incidence of sciatic hernia. Although more than 30,000 herniorrhaphies were performed at the Mayo Clinic in the 30-year period from 1944 to 1974, not one sciatic hernia was reported (Kurland and Jurasic, personal communication, 1975). Thomas,[18] in analyzing the medical records from two private hospitals in Seattle from 1932 to 1962, during which 21,138 herniorrhaphies were performed, and a 15-year period at King County Hospital, during which 1843 hernia records were assessed, did not find even one patient with sciatic hernia.

Sciatic hernia occurs on the right and left sides about equally.

In the 35 reports Watson[19] collected, 4 hernias were in children younger than 1 year of age, but only one was in a patient between 1 and 10 years of age. A case of an 18-month-old boy with congenital sciatic hernia was reported by Attah and colleagues in 1992.[1] Most of the patients were between the ages of 20 and 60 years. Sex incidence appears to be almost equal, although Bréhant and coworkers[4] stated that this hernia occurs more frequently in women because the female pelvis is relatively larger and more horizontal and the sciatic foramina are larger than in men.[6,8]

CONTENTS OF THE SAC

According to Watson,[19] most of the sacs (12 of 22) contained small intestine; the rest of the sacs contained bladder, ovary, fallopian tubes, colon, omentum, and Meckel diverticula. Sacs containing ureter[2,3] and tumor[15] also have been reported.

ETIOLOGY

Sciatic hernia may be congenital or acquired. Monro, in 1811, suggested that sciatic hernia might be caused by a congenital defect.[19] This congenital defect could be abnormal development of the piriformis muscle or pelvic bones. Relaxation of muscles, severe strain, traction, erosion of muscle caused by tumors in the gluteal area, severe constipation, and accidents have been incriminated as factors in acquired sciatic hernia.

ANATOMY

The anatomy of the region is complex and compact and contains many important arteries, veins, and nerves. The bony structures involved are the posterolateral wall of the pelvis—the sacrum, ischium, and ilium (innominate bone). These are held together by strong ligaments, especially the anterior and posterior sacroiliac ligaments that bind the sacrum and ilium together. These bones form the greater and lesser sciatic notches. The sacrotuberous ligament converts the greater sciatic notch into the greater sciatic foramen. This ligament is a broad band stretching from the free part of the side of the sacrum and coccyx to the medial part of the ischial tuberosity (Figs. 31-1 and 31-2).

The lesser sciatic notch lies between the ischial spine and tuberosity (and the sacrotuberous ligament) and is converted into the lesser sciatic foramen by the sacrospinous ligament. This ligament lies between the sacrotuberous ligament posteriorly and the coccygeus muscle (tail wagger) anteriorly and extends from the side and dorsum of the free parts of the sacrum and coccyx to the ischial spine.

The greater sciatic foramen is called the *porta*, or door, to the gluteal region[9] because all vessels and nerves pass through it to enter the gluteal region. This foramen is filled mostly by the piriformis muscle, a lateral rotator and abductor of the thigh. This pear-shaped muscle takes its origin from the three bars of bone that separate the four anterior sacral foramina and pars lateralis and extends laterally to insert on the medial part of the greater trochanter. The fascia covering this muscle is areolar and weak. The pirifor-

mis muscle converts this foramen into a suprapiriformis area and an infrapiriformis area. Above the piriformis muscle, the superior gluteal artery, vein, and nerve are present. These are located at the medial part as they emerge, and then they extend laterally to innervate the gluteus medius and minimus and the tensor fasciae latae muscles (all important gait stabilizers). Below the piriformis muscle, the inferior gluteal vessels and nerve that supply the gluteus maximus, the sciatic muscle nerve, the nerve to the quadratus femoris muscle, the posterior femoral cutaneous nerve, the nerve to the obturator internus muscle, and the internal pudendal vessels and nerve are present. The sciatic nerve leaves the pelvis below the piriformis muscle near the ischial border of the greater sciatic notch and at the infragluteal fold is about midway between the ischial tuberosity and the greater trochanter.

The lesser sciatic foramen is a small slit bounded by the sacrospinous ligament above, the sacrotuberous ligament below, the tendon on the obturator internus muscle, and the two gemelli laterally. It occurs where the two ligaments cross medially. This lesser foramen transmits the internal pudendal vessels and nerve back into the pelvis and also the nerves to

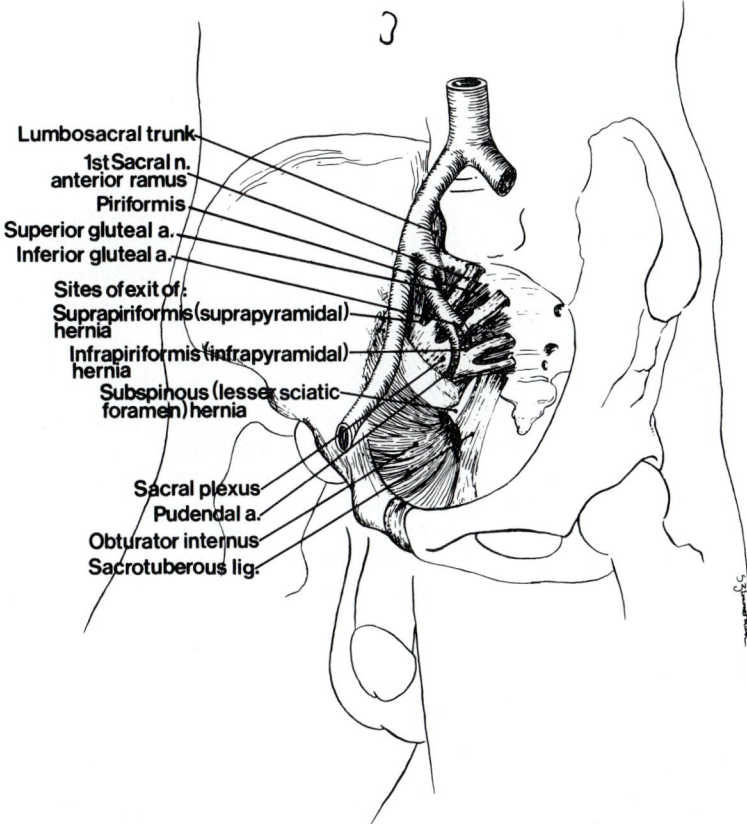

Figure 31-1. Surgical anatomy from within the pelvis, showing the relation of vessels and nerve roots to the sites of exit of the three varieties of sciatic hernia.

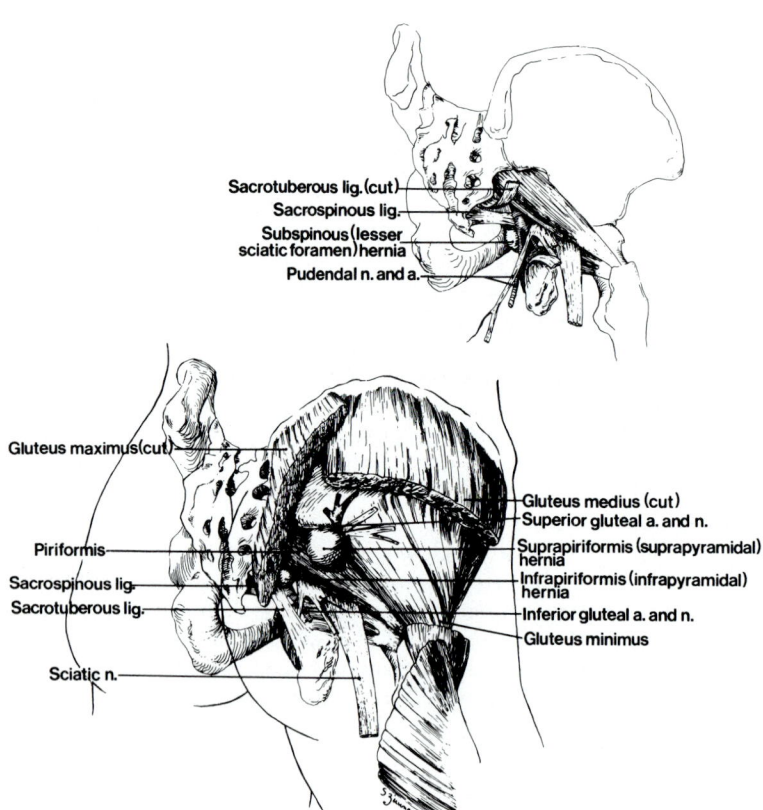

Sacrotuberous lig.(cut)
Sacrospinous lig.
Subspinous(lesser sciatic foramen)hernia
Pudendal n. and a.

Gluteus maximus(cut)

Gluteus medius (cut)
Superior gluteal a. and n.
Suprapiriformis (suprapyramidal) hernia
Infrapiriformis (infrapyramidal) hernia
Inferior gluteal a. and n.
Gluteus minimus

Piriformis
Sacrospinous lig.
Sacrotuberous lig.

Sciatic n.

Figure 31-2. Anatomy of sciatic hernia from the gluteal approach. The sciatic nerve and inferior gluteal and pudendal (internal) vessels and nerves cross over the obturator internus and gemellus muscles.

the obturator internus and the quadratus femoris muscles.

Classification

Sciatic hernias have been classified into three types, according to where they exit from the pelvis. Those that exit through the greater sciatic foramen have also been classified according to their relation to the piriformis muscle. The most common sciatic hernia exits above the piriformis muscle and has been termed *suprapyramidal hernia*. The second most frequent type exits below the piriformis muscle and has been termed *infrapyramidal hernia*. The least common exits through the lesser sciatic foramen and has been termed *subspinous, lesser sciatic,* or *spinous tuberous hernia.*

This classification is descriptive, but use of the terms suprapyramidal and infrapyramidal is anatomically confusing. The pyramidalis (flame-shaped) muscle is an anterior abdominal wall muscle that lies at the lower part of the rectus abdominis muscle. Bréhant and colleagues[4] consistently referred to the piriformis muscle as the pyramidalis muscle, an error in terminology. Watson[19] referred to the piriformis

muscle but spelled it "pyriformis," as did Brodnax.[5] To avoid confusion and to be anatomically descriptive, the classifications for sciatic hernia through the greater foramen should be changed from suprapyramidalis and infrapyramidalis to *suprapiriformis* and *infrapiriformis;* these terms are used in this chapter.

Surgical Anatomy

In women, the abdominal opening of the sac is posterior to the broad ligament just above the uterosacral ligament. In men, the internal opening is in a corresponding place in the posterior lateral pelvis between the rectum and bladder. In the pelvis, the sac of a suprapiriformis hernia lies in front of the piriformis muscle, some of the roots of the sciatic nerve, and the superior gluteal vessels and nerve.

In the suprapiriformis variety, as the sac leaves the pelvis, it is posterior and to the outer side of the superior gluteal vessels and nerve. It is bounded above by the iliac bone and sacroiliac ligament and below by the piriformis muscle.

In the infrapiriformis variety, the sac leaves the pelvis on the inner or medial side of the sciatic nerve, inferior gluteal vessels and nerve, and pudendal vessels and nerve. This is bounded superiorly by the piriformis muscle, inferiorly by the sacrospinous ligament, and posteriorly by the sacrotuberous ligament.

In the subspinous variety, the sac leaves the pelvis medial to the internal pudendal vessels and nerve and the sciatic nerve and is bounded superiorly by the sacrospinous ligament and posteriorly by the sacrotuberous ligament.

The sac may be small and completely covered by the gluteus maximus muscle. As it enlarges, it spreads through the loose areolar tissue to present itself below the gluteus maximus muscle. It has been reported to have attained the size of a man's head.[19]

SYMPTOMS AND DIAGNOSIS

The symptoms of sciatic hernia can be misleading, obscure, and variable, depending on the factors associated with hernia in general and with the structures involved specifically. In some patients, there may be no symptoms, the hernia being discovered accidentally during laparotomy performed for other reasons.

If the hernia is small, there may be only a slight swelling over the gluteal area. As it becomes larger, it may present in the gluteal or infragluteal area as a reducible mass that is aggravated by standing, straining, and coughing and relieved by lying down. The patient may feel gas movements, and bowel sounds may be heard in the mass.

The hernia may be incarcerated but not obstructed. If obstruction of the intestine occurs, the symptoms of small or large intestinal obstruction, or both, dominate; for example, the patient has cramping abdominal pains, distention, possibly nausea and vomiting, and increased bowel sounds. If it can be felt in the gluteal area, the mass is tense and probably irreducible.

If strangulation occurs, there are additional abdominal symptoms such as muscle guarding, tenderness, and decreased bowel sounds. The gluteal mass is tense and tender, and the patient probably has a fever and leukocytosis. Watson[19] found that 8 of 35 hernias were diagnosed at necropsy, and in 6 of these, intestinal obstruction was the cause of death.

Sciatic nerve involvement, both sensory and motor, caused by pressure by the hernia may be the presenting complaint. These may be the symptoms of classic sciatica, with pain radiating down the back of the leg and aggravated by, for example, dorsiflexion and muscle weakness. A patient of Matel's had intermittent painful claudication and muscle weakness for 5 years that was finally relieved by repair of sciatic hernia.[4] Lawson[11] reported a patient with intermittent cramping and right lower-quadrant abdominal pains

radiating down the back of the right leg of 10 years' duration. An emergency operation for acute intestinal obstruction revealed an incarcerated and strangulated "suprapyramidal sciatic hernia" anterior and medial to and pressing on the sciatic nerve.

Urinary disturbance, as reported by Beck and colleagues,[2] may be the only symptom. Beck and associates reported a 66-year-old woman with colicky pains in the left flank and loin and nausea and vomiting as the presenting symptoms. A loop of left ureter was trapped in the suprapiriformis hernial sac, causing hydroureter and hydronephrosis. Beck and coworkers cited Lindblom, who had a similar patient; both patients were treated successfully. Bohnert[3] reported an infant who, in addition to hydrocephalus and other congenital malformations, had bilateral ureteral herniations into the right and left sciatic foramina.

The sacral and gluteal areas should be examined routinely in all patients with intestinal obstruction, sciatic nerve syndromes, and urinary disturbances to rule out sciatic hernia as the possible cause. An increased number of sciatic hernias would probably be recognized, treated, and reported if this were done.

The diagnosis, when in doubt, can be aided by abdominal roentgenograms, including flat-plate and upright films, and, if necessary and permissible, barium roentgenographic studies to help determine if any intestine is in the sac. Barium meal and small intestinal studies should not be done if there are any symptoms of intestinal obstruction. Intravenous pyelography helps to determine if the ureter or bladder is involved.

If the gluteal mass is not reducible and there is not impulse on straining, the differential diagnosis should include lipoma or another benign tumor,[18] cyst, abscess, especially cold or tuberculous, aneurysm of the gluteal or iliac artery, and malignant tumor. I saw a 55-year-old woman with a gluteal mass that could also be felt on rectal examination; the mass was found at operation to have a malignant neurilemoma of the sacral plexus. The tumor had herniated through the greater sciatic notch and had invaded the peritoneum. The patient was treated by hemipelvectomy.

TREATMENT

The treatment of sciatic hernia is surgical, and the operation should be done soon after the diagnosis has been made and the patient has been adequately evaluated and prepared. There are two approaches—transabdominal and transgluteal. Although both approaches must sometimes be used,[15] there are specific indications for each.

Transabdominal Approach

The transabdominal approach is mandatory when there is evidence of intestinal obstruction or strangulation. It is also indicated when the diagnosis is certain and there are additional abdominal or pelvic procedures to be performed. This approach has been advocated by Watson[19] and others because from within the abdomen it is easier to see the relations between the hernial sac and important vessels and nerves. It is also easier to reduce the incarcerated contents, evaluate the viability of the intestine or other viscera contained in the sac, resect the intestine if necessary, and repair the hernial defect with less chance of nerve and vessel damage.

The preferred technique is to have the patient in a slight Trendelenburg position. The peritoneal cavity is entered through a low midline or right or left paramedian incision, depending on the side of the hernia. After the abdomen is explored and the extent and location of the obstruction and the viscera involved are assessed, the rest of the viscera are packed out of the pelvis. The viscera are followed to the internal

opening of the hernial sac, and the relation of the sac to the surrounding vessels and nerves is determined (Fig. 31-3A).

If the incarcerated intestine cannot be gradually withdrawn with gentle traction, the ring of constriction should be gently dilated with the finger or a blunt instrument such as a knife handle. Sometimes, pressure from below on the bulge in the gluteal area, in addition to traction from above, may be successful in reducing the hernia, as suggested by Watson.[19] If this maneuver is unsuccessful, the ring can be cut after the location of the vessels and nerves is assessed so as not to damage them. This cutting of the ring and piriformis muscle is done under direct vision. As the surgeon remembers, sees, and feels that the sac in the suprapiriformis variety exits laterally to the superior gluteal vessels and nerve, he or she should incise the neck of the sac and piriformis muscle away from these structures, that is, posteriorly, laterally, and inferiorly, as recommended by Skandalakis and colleagues.[16] Multiple small radial incisions can be made, the finger or instrument inserted, and the ring stretched (see Fig. 31-3B). In the rarer infrapiriformis variety, the sac ex-

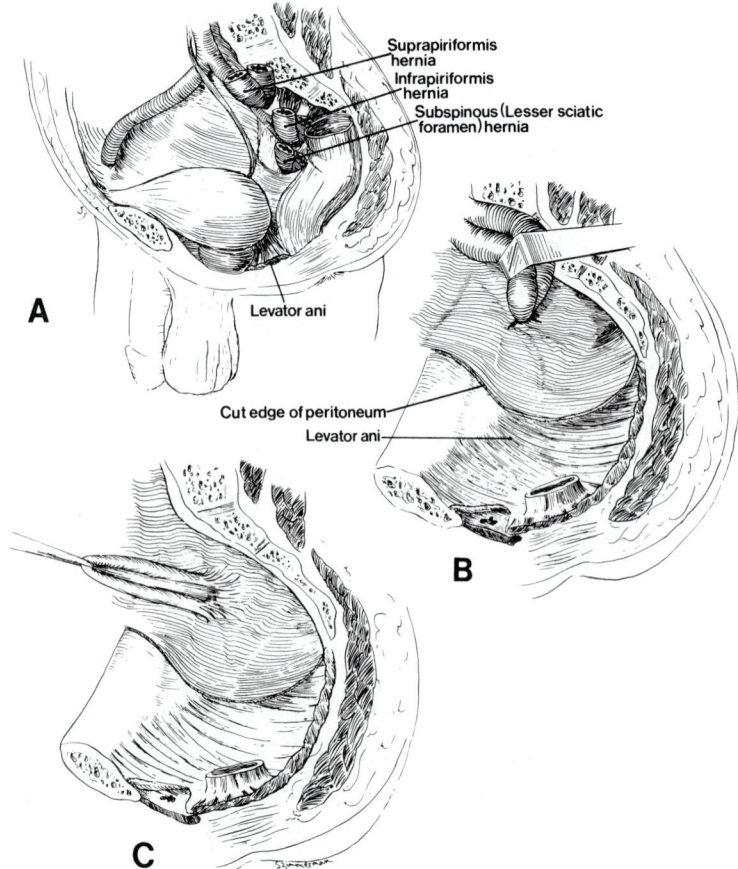

Figure 31-3. Transabdominal view of sciatic hernias. (A) Determining relation of hernial sac to surrounding vessels and nerves. (B) Trapped intestine retracted; neck of sac incised. (C) Peritoneal sac inverted.

its medially to the vessels and nerves, and therefore the neck of the sac and the piriformis muscle should be incised in a medial or superior direction or a medial and superior direction. In subspinous hernias, the neck of the sac should also be incised medially, and the obturator internus may be incised.[16] After the contents of the sac have been reduced and treated as indicated, the sac is pulled out from the sciatic foramen (see Fig. 31-3C).

Before ligation of the sac or reperitonealization of the area, the repair should be performed (Fig. 31-4A). Watson[19] described turning up a flap of fascia from the piriformis muscle and suturing it to the area of the anterior sacroiliac ligament or fascia and periosteum of the iliac bone. The fascia of the piriformis muscle is usually too thin and areolar to be used, however, so it is probably advisable to use fascia lata or prosthetic material such as polyester fiber mesh (Mersilene) or stainless steel wire mesh (Surgaloy; see Fig. 31-4B). Mesh is especially necessary when the sciatic

opening is large as a result of congenital deficiency or atrophy of the piriformis muscle. Sadek and associates[15] used stainless steel wire mesh successfully to repair the large defect caused by a neurofibroma.

If the opening is small, a few interrupted nonabsorbable sutures can be used to close the opening by suturing the piriformis muscle with its fascia to the periosteum of the iliac bone.

Another method described by Watson[19] for repair of a smaller hernial defect is to fold the sac on itself, suture it, and use it as a wad to close off the opening (see Fig. 31-4A). This wad technique using peritoneum was questioned by Nyhus.[13,14] The technique, however, has merit because of its ease of performance and safety. Rather than peritoneum, a sheet of polypropylene monofilament mesh (Marlex) can be rolled into a snug wad and used to partially fill the area and plug the opening after the technique advocated by Lichtenstein and Shore[12] for the treatment of femoral and recurrent inguinal hernia.

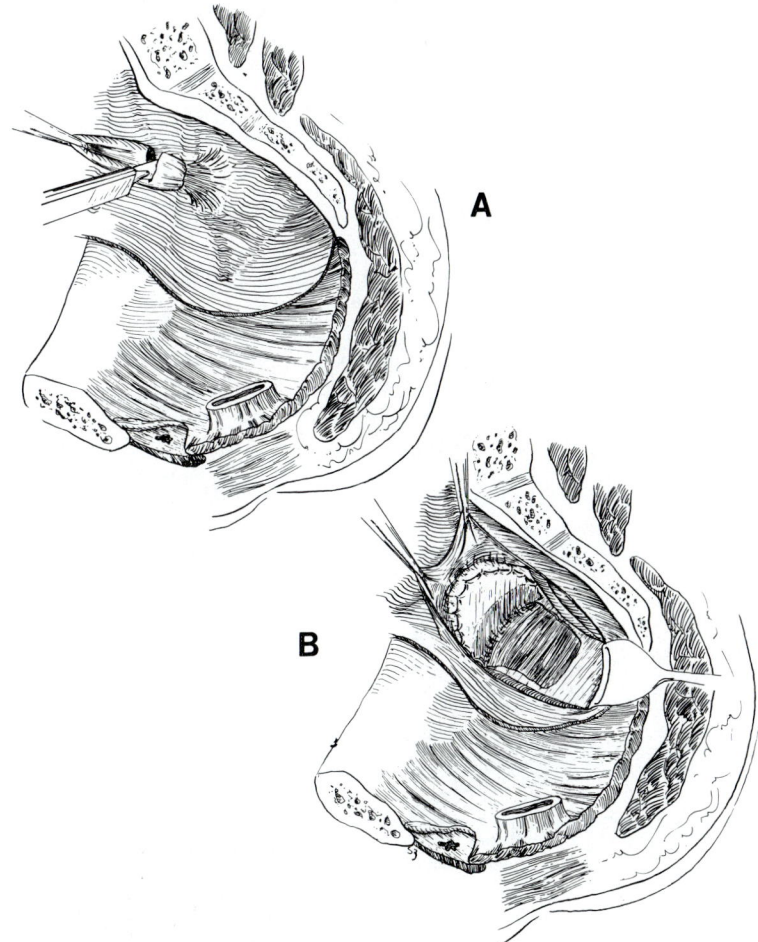

Figure 31-4.   Transabdominal repair of sciatic hernia. (A) Neck of sac ligated; excess sac excised or plicated and used as a plug. (B) Alternative method: Peritoneum, hypogastric vessels and sacral plexus retracted; flap of fascia from piriformis muscle or polyester (Mersilene) mesh gauze sutured to fibrous tissue over ilium to close defect and reperitonealize the area.

Transgluteal Approach

The transgluteal approach may be used when the diagnosis is certain and the contents of the hernial sac are reducible. It is also indicated when the gluteal area is to be explored to ascertain the nature of a mass beneath the gluteus maximus muscle.

The patient is placed in the prone position with the involved side higher than the opposite one and the thigh free to be moved. The locations of the posterior superior iliac spine, tip of the coccyx, top of the greater trochanter, and ischial tuberosity are marked on the skin. The incision is made from the posterior edge of the greater trochanter and should cross the hernial mass. At the level of the middle of the incision, the gluteus maximus muscle is incised and separated in the direction of its fibers. This is at the level of the *key line*, defined by Grant[9] as the "line joining the midpoint between the posterior superior iliac spine to the tip of the coccyx to the top of the greater trochanter." This key line is at the lower border of the piriformis muscle. The gluteus maximus muscle is adequately retracted, beginning at the greater trochanter, and because it is the only muscle that crosses the greater trochanter, the cleavage plane is easy to follow

(Fig. 31-5A). To help slacken the gluteus maximus muscle, the thigh is extended and laterally rotated, which is the action of this muscle. The piriformis muscle, the superior and inferior gluteal vessels and nerves, and the sciatic nerve and other structures are identified. The sac is gently freed from the adjacent muscles, vessels, and nerves and opened. The contents are identified, and viability is ascertained before the contents are returned to the peritoneal cavity. If an intestinal resection is required, an abdominal approach is also necessary.

If the hernia is incarcerated, the constricting ring should be treated in the manner described in the transabdominal approach. In suprapiriformis hernias, the stretching and cutting of the constriction should be made in the adjacent piriformis muscle in a downward and outward direction (see Fig. 31-5B). In infrapiriformis and lesser sciatic foraminal hernias, these incisions are made in an upward and inward direction to avoid nerve and vessel injuries. After the contents are reduced and the neck of the sac is ligated, the excess sac may be excised or used with the piriformis as part of the repair (see Fig. 31-5C). Fascial flaps, fascia lata, and polyester fiber mesh (Mersilene) can be used to bridge the gap between the piriformis mus-

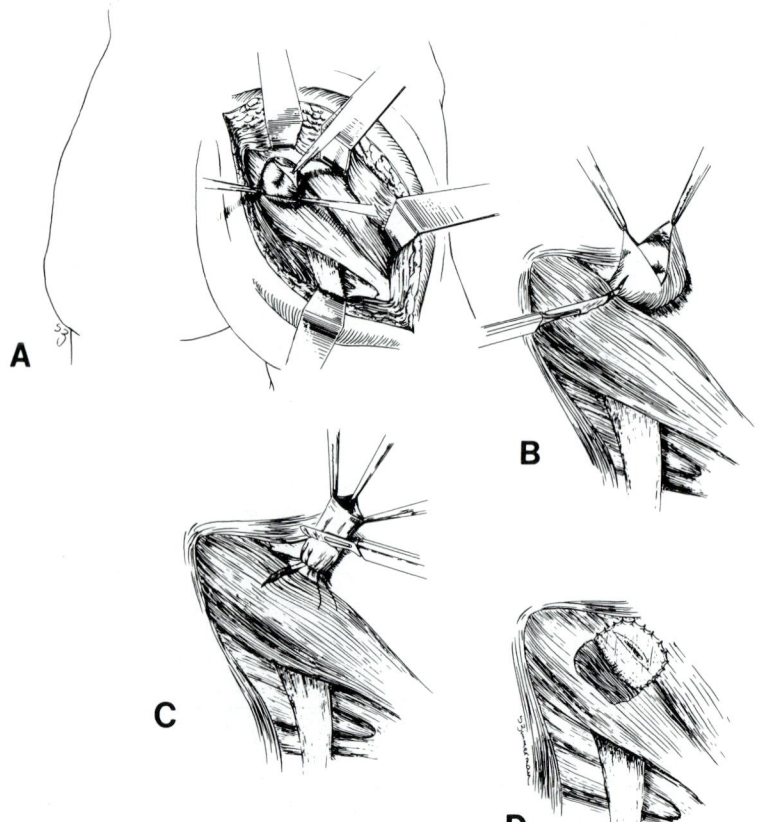

A

B

C

D

Figure 31-5. Transgluteal repair of sciatic hernia. (*A*) Gluteus maximus separated. (*B*) Sac opened; ring around neck of sac incised to reduce contents. (*C*) Neck of sac ligated; excess sac excised. (*D*) Flap of fascia from piriformis muscle or polyester mesh gauze used to close defect.

cle and iliac bone or between the piriformis muscle and ischial bone (see Fig. 31-5*D*).

The hernial defect can be closed by suture of the piriformis muscle to the gluteus maximus and medius muscles, as described by Gaffney and Schanno in 1958.[7] Those authors stated that at no time during the operation was the sciatic nerve seen in their patient, a 5-month-old girl. Henegar and coworkers[10] described a new technique with which they repaired a suprapiriformis hernia in a 22-month-old boy. It consisted of mobilizing the gluteus maximus muscle by transecting it near its insertion and visualizing the sciatic nerve and superior and inferior gluteal vessels. Exact treatment of the sac is not mentioned, but the authors stated:

> Since the right ureter and caecum are in this region it was considered unwise to try to invert the sac blindly. The pyriformis muscle was then approximated to the gluteus medius by means of interrupted No. 60 cotton sutures leaving room enough only for the superior gluteal vessels and nerve to come through. The gluteus maximus muscle was then sutured at its insertion.

The girl was followed for 1 year and the boy for 6 months. Both periods are obviously too short to evaluate the efficacy of the repairs.

Most surgeons reporting on sciatic hernias favor an abdominal approach, but occasionally the gluteal approach is the one of choice. A combined operation, such as that reported by Sadek and associates[15] to repair the hernia and then remove a large benign tumor, sometimes is necessary. A combined approach is also necessary if, during exploration through the gluteal approach, gangrenous intestine is encountered.

REFERENCES

1. Attah M, Jibril JA, Yakubu A, Kalayi GD, Nmadu PT. Congenital sciatic hernia. J Pediatr Surg 1992;27:1603.
2. Beck WC, Baurys W, Brochu J, Morton WA. Herniation of the ureter into the sciatic foramen ("curlicue ureter"). JAMA 1952;149:441.
3. Bohnert WW. Ureteral sciatic hernias: case report of infant with bilateral ureteral herniation into the sciatic foramina. J Urol 1971;106:142.
4. Bréhant J, Pinet F, Leca A, Garchon G. Hernie ischiatique. Mem Acad Chir 1960;86:937.
5. Brodnax JW. Sciatic hernia: report of a case of herniation of Meckel's diverticulum through the greater sciatic foramen. JAMA 1924;82:440.
6. Cali RL, Pitsch RM, Blatchford GJ, Thorson A, Christensen MA. Rare pelvic floor hernias: report of a case and review of the literature. Dis Colon Rectum 1992;35:604.
7. Gaffney LB, Schanno J. Sciatic hernia: a case of congenital occurrence. Am J Surg 1958;95:974.
8. Ghahremani GG, Michael AS. Sciatic hernia with incarcerated ileum: CT and radiographic diagnosis. Gastrointest Radiol 1991;16:120.
9. Grant JCB. A method of anatomy, ed 6. Baltimore, Williams & Wilkins, 1958.
10. Henegar GC, Hudson CB, Jensen GL. Sciatic notch hernia: report of a case, description, new operative approach. Arch Surg 1952;64:399.
11. Lawson R. Sciatic hernia. Can Med Assoc J 1948;59:265.
12. Lichtenstein IL, Shore JM. Simplified repair of recurrent and femoral hernias by a plug technique. Presented at Clinical Congress, American College of Surgeons, Miami Beach, October 1974.
13. Nyhus LM. Editorial comment, chap 43. In: Nyhus LM, Harkins HN, eds. Hernia. Philadelphia, JB Lippincott, 1964.
14. Nyhus LM. Editorial comment, chap 26. In: Nyhus LM, Condon RE, eds. Hernia, ed 2. Philadelphia, JB Lippincott, 1978.
15. Sadek HM, Kiss DR, Vasconcelos E. Sciatic hernia caused by a neurofibroma: surgical repair with a stainless steel wire mesh. Int Surg 1970;54:135.
16. Skandalakis JE, Gray SW, Akin JT. Surgical anatomy of hernial rings. Surg Clin North Am 1974;54:1227.
17. Summers JE. Sciatic hernia. Ann Surg 1922;75:672.
18. Thomas GF. Sciatic hernia. In: Nyhus LM, Harkins HN, eds. Hernia. Philadelphia, JB Lippincott, 1964:650.
19. Watson LF. Hernia, ed 3. St Louis, CV Mosby, 1948:476.

Editor's Comment

Sidney Black is the Chicago counterpart of Charles Griffith of Seattle (see Chap. 5). Both clinical surgeons have had a long and in-depth interest in gross anatomy. Dr. Black has taught surgical anatomy to medical students for 32 years. Thus, when he advises a change in nomenclature (ie, *suprapiriformis hernia* instead of *suprapyramidalis hernia*) to assist in our understanding, we should carefully review his points.

I note that Dr. Black has credited Summers (1922) rather than Brodnax (1924), who was given this honor in the first edition of *Hernia*, with reporting the first sciatic hernia in America. I suppose that we must continue to remember Brodnax because his first description was that of a patient with a sciatic hernia containing a Meckel diverticulum. After all, Littre managed to gain the status of immortality on the basis of the slim observation of two examples of Meckel diverticulum in inguinal hernial sacs.

I note that the wad technique has been given new vitality. In the first edition of *Hernia,* I commented that the suggestion of suturing wadded peritoneum as a pad to the sciatic defect was open to question. It was reminiscent of the suggestion made by Sir G. Lenthal Cheatle (Br Med J 1921;2:1025) that coiled autogenous saphenous vein be used to plug the femoral canal in the repair of a femoral hernia. I added that it would seem appropriate to rely on one of the newer prosthetic materials rather than on either wadded peritoneum or thin piriformis fascia. I recognized in 1974 that the wad technique has been promulgated for more common types of hernias. I continue to believe that there must be a better way.

(Dr. Black is a founding member of the American Association of Clinical Anatomists. Surgeons interested in the relation of human gross anatomy to operative procedures should seek membership in the young but vital organization.)

L.M.N.

Perineal Hernias

Part Five

Hernia, Fourth Edition, edited
by Lloyd M. Nyhus and Robert E. Condon.
J.B. Lippincott Company, Philadelphia © 1995.

Chapter 32

Perineal Hernia
Russell K. Pearl

Perineal hernias are among the most uncommon hernias encountered in surgical practice. These unusual hernias may be difficult to recognize clinically and can be classified into two types—primary and secondary. Primary perineal hernias result from congenital or acquired defects between the muscles and fascia that form the pelvic floor and are exceedingly rare. Secondary perineal hernias are true incisional hernias that occur infrequently after pelvic exenteration, abdominoperineal resection of the rectum, or perineal prostatectomy. Proper management of perineal hernias depends on an understanding of their cause and natural history as well as familiarity with the wide array of surgical techniques used to repair these uncommon hernias.

PRIMARY PERINEAL HERNIA

Primary perineal hernias have been recognized since de Garengeot's original description of this condition in 1736. In the second edition of *Hernia* (1978),[11] Koontz discussed a total of 92 patients with primary perineal hernias from an extensive review of the literature, which included a patient report that he had written in 1951. The total number of patients reported is still less than 100.

Primary hernias of the perineum occur most commonly in patients between 40 and 60 years of age and develop five times more frequently in women than in men.[11] The female predominance of this entity is probably related to the broader pelvis in women and the attenuation and weakening of the pelvic floor during pregnancy and childbirth. Other factors that contribute to the formation of primary perineal hernias include chronic ascites, obesity, and recurrent infection of the pelvic floor.

The two types of primary perineal hernia, anterior and posterior, depend on the relation of the hernia to the superficial transverse perineal muscles[17] (Fig. 32-1). In an anterior perineal hernia, the defect is through the urogenital diaphragm bounded by a triangular space formed by the bulbocavernosus muscle medially, the ischiocavernosus muscle laterally, and the superficial transverse perineal muscle posteriorly. If the hernial sac emerges between the ischiopubic bone and the vagina, the hernia may present as a labial mass, which has sometimes been referred to as a *pudendal hernia.* Anterior perineal hernias are said never to occur in men.

The muscular defect of a posterior perineal hernia is posterior to the superficial transverse perineal muscle through the levator ani muscle or between the levator ani and coccygeus muscles. If the levator ani muscle is not anchored to the obturator fascia, a potential space known as the hiatus of Schwalbe develops.

The hernial sac of a primary perineal hernia may contain intestine, bladder, or omentum, depending on the location of the defect. Strangulation of the contents of the hernial sac does not occur frequently because the neck of the sac is usually wide and encircled by relatively elastic tissues.

The symptoms of perineal hernia are not pronounced and are ordinarily confined to complaints of a perineal, labial, or gluteal mass that may cause discomfort to the patient while sitting. If a portion of the bladder is within the hernial sac, the patient may describe difficulty with urination.

The most important physical sign is the presence of a soft perineal mass, which is usually reducible. The direction of reduction, together with a palpable defect in the pelvic floor, helps to differentiate a primary perineal hernia from a sciatic hernia, which emerges posteriorly through the greater or lesser sacrosciatic foramen yet may also present as a mass along the inferior margin of the gluteus maximus muscle. Many other causes of perineal masses may be mistaken for primary perineal hernias. These include various types of soft tissue tumors, hematomas, cysts, and abscesses, all of which are generally irreducible. The clinician should exclude the diagnosis of rectocele, cystocele, and rectal prolapse by careful physical examination. In addition, plain roentgenograms of the pelvis and barium enema examination, especially postevacuation roentgenograms, may help to confirm the presence of a perineal hernia.[18]

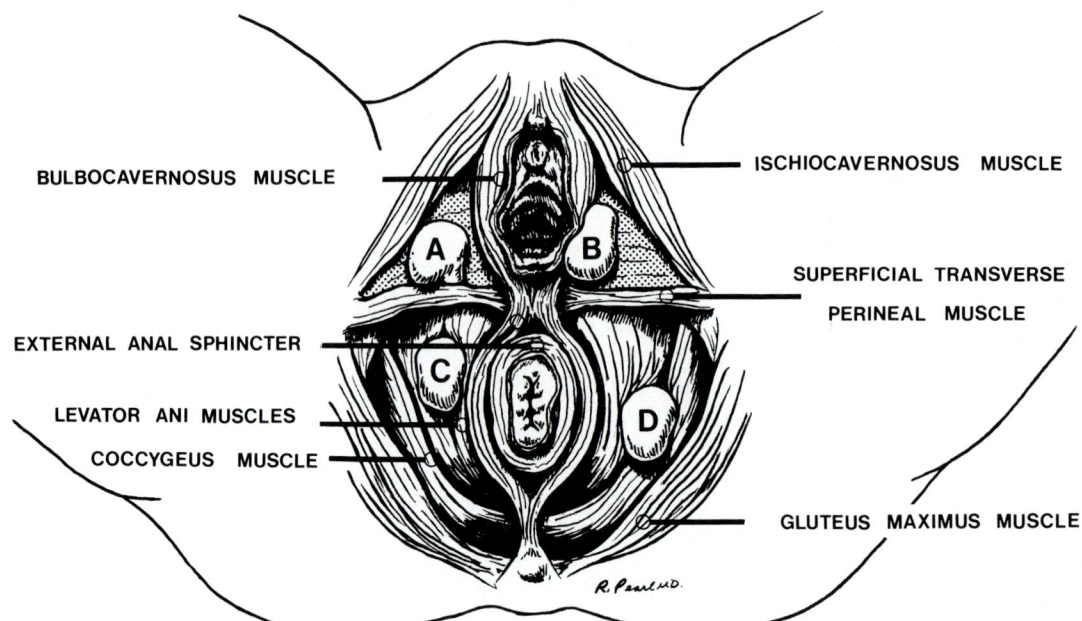

Figure 32-1. Anatomy of the perineum demonstrating primary perineal hernias. (*A*) Anterior perineal hernia emerging through the urogenital diaphragm (*shaded*). (*B*) Anterior perineal hernia bulging into the posterior part of the labia (pudendal hernia). (*C*) Posterior perineal hernia emerging through the levator ani muscle. (*D*) Posterior perineal hernia emerging between the levator ani and coccygeus muscles.

Two newer imaging techniques have been reported to aid in the diagnosis of perineal hernia. Computed tomography of the lower pelvis may demonstrate herniated loops of bowel and associated mesenteric vessels residing in the ischiorectal fossa.[5] Also, dynamic proctography may help pinpoint the location of a defect in the pelvic floor as well as delineate other causes of outlet obstruction, such as rectocele and internal rectal prolapse.[13]

Repair of primary perineal hernias using the abdominal, perineal, and combined abdominoperineal routes has been reported. The consensus appears to be that the abdominal approach is preferable because the contents of the sac can be reduced more directly, minimizing the risk of injury to the intestine or bladder, and a securer closure of the defect can be carried out. Because most of these pelvic floor defects are small, primary closure with nonabsorbable suture material can ordinarily be successfully accomplished. In situations in which the defect is large or cannot be closed satisfactorily without undue tension, nonabsorbable synthetic mesh such as polypropylene (Marlex) can be used. Perhaps the only time the combined approach is advantageous is in the rare instance in which a pouch of skin and subcutaneous tissue into which a large hernia protrudes remains and needs to be excised.

Defects in the pelvic floor can be developmental in origin, but these events are exceedingly uncommon. Prenatal perforation of the extraperitoneal part of the rectum associated with a pararectal defect in the levator ani muscles and extravasation of meconium into the buttock has been reported, presenting as a discolored, gas-filled gluteal swelling at birth.[6] These infants were successfully treated with diverting colostomies and drainage of the collection of meconium. Although no specific repair of the levator ani muscles was attempted, the defects closed spontaneously.

SECONDARY PERINEAL HERNIA

The development of a perineal hernia after the removal of pelvic organs and adjacent portions of the pelvic floor is infrequent. These incisional hernias complicate less than 1% of abdominoperineal resections of the rectum and only about 3% of pelvic exenterations for advanced malignant tumors of the pelvis.[3,14,15] Most of these hernias occur in women, probably because of the width of the female pelvis and the relative frequency of pelvic exenteration for gynecologic cancer. Other factors that may contribute to the formation of secondary perineal hernias in-

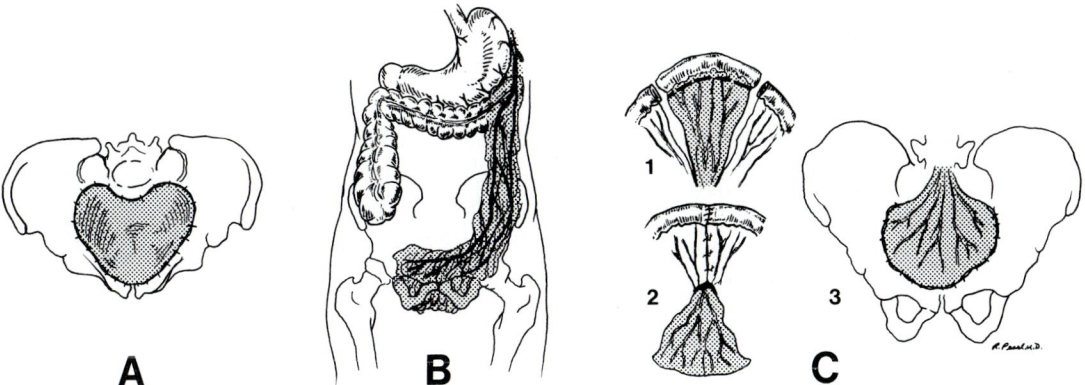

Figure 32-2.   Repair of incisional perineal hernias. (*A*) Polypropylene mesh. (*B*) Omental graft (in this case, based on the left gastroepiploic artery). (*C*) Mesenteric leaf repair of the pelvic floor.

clude removal of the coccyx as part of the operative procedure, postoperative perineal infections, and complications of radiation therapy that may interfere with perineal wound healing. In addition, the potential for a perineal hernia to develop is related to the length of the mesenteric blood vessels and nerves that are the main support of the intestines. If a loop of small intestine cannot reach the perineum, it is unlikely that it will become incarcerated in a perineal hernia.

A secondary perineal hernia usually presents as a palpable perineal mass, which may annoy the patient while sitting. Occasionally, the skin overlying the her-

nia may become ulcerated, and in extreme instances, frank evisceration may develop, prompting emergency surgical correction. Most of these hernias present within a year of an operation.

Many ingenious methods have been proposed for repairing incisional perineal hernias (Figs. 32-2 and 32-3). In addition to primary suture of the defect or reinforcement of the defect with free fascial grafts or synthetic mesh, several types of tissue grafts and myocutaneous flaps have been described to help reconstruct the pelvic floor.[1,4,16]

Among the tissue grafts reported to be useful in separating the abdominal contents from the pelvic de-

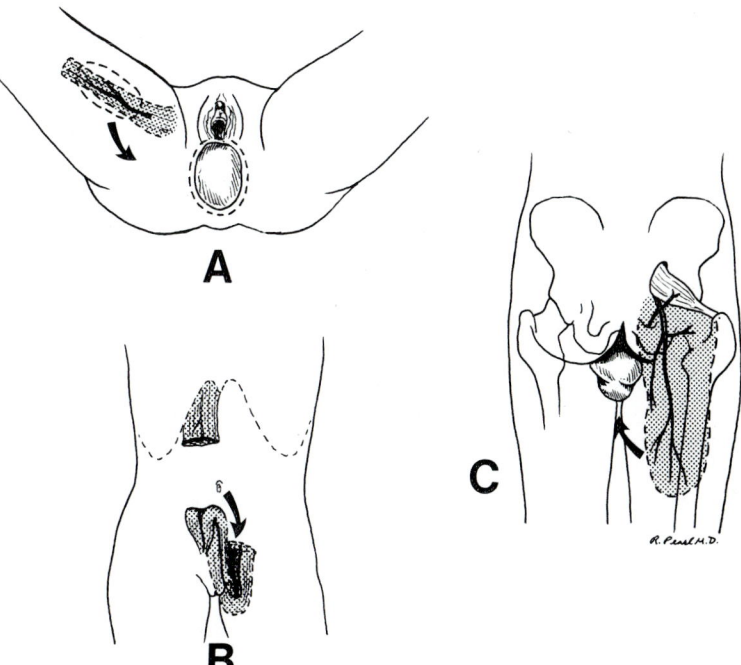

Figure 32-3.   Myocutaneous flaps for the repair of defects of the pelvic floor. (*A*) Gracilis myocutaneous flap. (*B*) Rectus abdominis muscle flap. (*C*) Gluteal thigh flap.

fect are the creation of an omental carpet and the interposition of a mesenteric leaf. By mobilizing the greater omentum from the transverse colon, a well-vascularized apron of omentum can be placed over a synthetic mesh repair of the defect to help reperitonealize the pelvic floor and provide pelvic support to the intestines. In the mesenteric leaf repair, a segment of small intestinal mesentery is interposed as a peritoneum-covered pelvic lid by suturing the edges of the leaf to the margins of the true pelvis.

Myocutaneous flaps are particularly useful for the reconstruction of large, chronically inflamed, or heavily irradiated defects.[12] They offer the advantage of providing a large quantity of strong, healthy tissue to fill the defect without major functional or esthetic loss to the patient.

The gracilis myocutaneous flap has been useful in this regard.[2] The gracilis muscle originates from the medial lower half of the pubic body and the upper half of the inferior pubic arch, and it inserts on the medial surface of the upper portion of the tibia. Its blood supply is usually from branches of the deep femoral artery, which enter the muscle in its upper third. The nerve supply is derived from the anterior branch of the obturator nerve. The graft can be rotated up into the perineum by detaching it at its insertion and suturing it in place to obliterate the defect.

The gluteal thigh flap is a versatile myocutaneous graft developed for closure of large wounds of the perineal and postsacral regions.[9] This flap includes the inferior portion of the gluteus maximus muscle and the direct cutaneous territory of the inferior gluteal artery to the posterior thigh.

A novel approach to reconstructing the pelvic floor is detaching the rectus abdominis muscle superiorly but retaining its attachment at the symphysis pubis, basing its blood supply on the inferior epigastric vessels.[8] The rectus muscle is then placed in the depth of the pelvic defect and sutured to the pelvic walls to form a strong, well-vascularized muscular sling; then the abdominal incision is closed.

The technique for repairing a perineal hernia should be tailored to each patient. In general, the best operation is one that is simple, yet effective. For example, a small, clean perineal hernia surrounded by relatively healthy tissue can be repaired with a piece of polypropylene mesh sutured in place during a laparotomy. In contrast, a large, chronically infected or heavily irradiated field of tissue surrounding an incisional perineal hernia mandates the use of a well-vascularized myocutaneous flap.

REFERENCES

1. Alexander JC, Beazley RM, Chretien PB. Mesenteric leaf repair of pelvic defects following exenterative operations. Ann Surg 1975;182:767.
2. Bell JG, Weiser EF, Metz P, Hoskins WJ. Gracilis muscle repair of perineal hernia following pelvic exenteration. Obstet Gynecol 1980;56:377
3. Brotschi E, Noe JM, Silen W. Perineal hernias after proctectomy. Am J Surg 1985;149:301.
4. Buchsbaum HJ, White AS. Omental sling for management of the pelvic floor following exenteration. Am J Obstet Gynecol 1973;117:407.
5. Cali RL, Pitsch RM, Blatchford GJ, Thorson A, Christensen MA. Rare pelvic floor hernias: report of a case and review of the literature. Dis Colon Rectum 1992;35:604.
6. Davies MRQ, Cywes S, Rode H. Prenatal perforation of the extraperitoneal part of the rectum, associated with a developmental defect of the pelvic floor. Z Kinderchir 1984;39:271.
7. De Garengeot RJC. Sur plusieurs hernies singulieres. Mem Acad R Chir Paris 1743;1:699.
8. Giampapa V, Keller A, Shaw WW, Colen SR. Pelvic floor reconstruction using the rectus abdominis muscle flap. Ann Plast Surg 1984;13:56.
9. Hurwitz DJ, Walton RL. Closure of chronic wounds of the perineal and sacral regions using the gluteal thigh flap. Ann Plast Surg 1982;8:375.
10. Koontz AR. Perineal hernia: report of a case with many associated muscular and fascial defects. Ann Surg 1951;133:255.
11. Koontz AR. Perineal hernia. In: Nyhus LM, Condon RE, eds. Hernia, ed 2. Philadelphia, JB Lippincott, 1978:453.
12. Leuchter RS, Lagasse LD, Hacker NF, Berek JS. Management of postexenteration perineal hernias by myocutaneous axial flaps. Gynecol Oncol 1982;14:15.
13. Lubat E, Gordon RB, Birnbaum BA, Megibow AJ. CT diagnosis of posterior perineal hernia. AJR 1990;154:761.
14. McMullin ND, Johnson WR, Polglase AL, Hughes ESR. Post-proctectomy perineal hernia: case report and discussion. Aust N Z J Surg 1985;55:69.
15. Rutledge RN, Smith JP, Wharton JT, O'Quinn AG. Pelvic exenteration: an analysis of 296 patients. Am J Obstet Gynecol 1977;129:881.
16. Sarr MG, Stewart JR, Cameron JC. Combined abdominoperineal approach to repair of postoperative perineal hernia. Dis Colon Rectum 1982;25:597.
17. Skandalakis JE, Gray SW, Akin JT. The surgical anatomy of hernial rings. Surg Clin North Am 1974;54:1227.
18. Trackler RT, Koehler PR. The radiographic findings in posterior perineal hernia. Radiology 1968;91:950.

Hernia, Fourth Edition, edited
by Lloyd M. Nyhus and Robert E. Condon.
J.B. Lippincott Company, Philadelphia © 1995.

Chapter 33

Prolapse of the Rectum

David A. Appel and Gordon L. Telford

Prolapse of the rectum, or procidentia, is the descent of the full thickness of the rectum through the anal orifice. This prolapse initially occurs only while the patient is straining at stool and is easily reduced after defecation. Subsequently, the rectum may prolapse at rest and be difficult to reduce manually. After prolonged periods of prolapse, incarceration and strangulation may occur in severe cases.

The condition most frequently confused with rectal prolapse is partial-thickness, or mucosal, prolapse. On physical examination, with rectal prolapse, there are concentric or circular folds of mucosa, with the lumen of the rectum often being slightly posteriorly placed. Simple mucosal prolapse is characterized by radial folds of mucosa with a central lumen (Fig. 33-1). Anorectal tumors may prolapse through the anal orifice and be confused with procidentia.[7] Perineal hernias without prolapse (enterocele) must also be differentiated from true prolapse because their treatment, as in all other entities encompassed by the differential diagnoses, is different.

EPIDEMIOLOGY

Procidentia is believed to be a relatively rare disease, although accurate figures on its incidence are not available. Substantial series of patients have been reported from Western industrialized countries and from developing nations indicating that procidentia is not likely a disease associated with affluence and the consumption of refined food products like hemorrhoids, colorectal cancer, and diverticular disease.

Rectal prolapse has been found to be rare in men older than 45 years of age and women younger than 20 years of age.[19] Most patients who require an operation are elderly women. Forty to 50% of these women are nulliparous; therefore, birth trauma is ruled out as a cause of rectal prolapse. The association of psychiatric disorders is frequently observed with this disease, but an etiologic relation was not documented in a well-designed epidemiologic study.

Another condition causally associated with rectal prolapse is pelvic neuropathy, including tabes dorsalis, multiple sclerosis, and pelvic trauma. Patients with dysenteric infections also have been noted to develop rectal prolapse.[4] Patients with chronic constipation who have to strain excessively to defecate appear to also have an increased incidence of rectal prolapse. There is one group that practices, as a religious rite, excessive straining with an empty rectum as if to have a bowel movement; these people frequently have prolapse.[4]

In older people, excessive straining at stool appears to be the common denominator. This sort of behavior is seen frequently in patients with severe psychoneuroses who reside in mental institutions and in patients with dysenteric infections. As a rule, rectal prolapse spontaneously resolves in children when they begin walking normally. Therefore, nonoperative management is appropriate initially.

CAUSES

Although the precise cause of rectal prolapse is not known and has been debated in the medical literature since the early 1900s, there are many theories. A thorough discussion of the subject was published by Moschowitz in 1912.[13] He stated that all abdominal wall hernias, of which rectal prolapse was an example, were believed to occur at the points of exit from the abdominal cavity of the viscera and blood vessels. Moschowitz did not believe that hernias were caused by persistence of a congenital sac; he believed that the sac developed at a weak point in the fascia. Herniation occurred, in his model, secondary to increased intraabdominal pressure. Moschowitz believed, therefore, that procidentia originates as a hernia in the pouch of Douglas. Because of adherence of the peritoneal reflection to the rectum and the relative fixation of the anus, the hernia presents as an intussusception through the anal canal. This intussusception would explain the posteriorly placed orifice that is

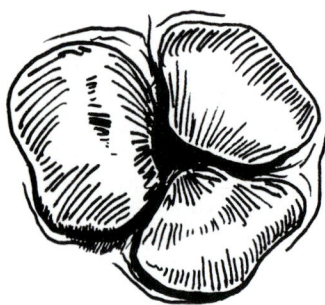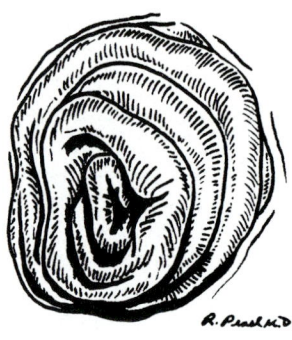

Figure 33-1. (*Left*) Radial folds of mucosa with prolapse of internal hemorrhoids. (*Right*) Concentric circular folds with procidentia.

seen in prolapse and the occasional presence of the small intestine in the sac. Based on this theory, Moschowitz's therapy was directed toward plication of the transversalis fascia anterior to the rectum through a series of pursestring sutures placed in the fascia to close the defect. Because recurrence rates after the Moschowitz operation were as a high as 48%, this operation was abandoned.

Because the Moschowitz operation failed to achieve satisfactory results and did not lead to the development of more efficacious treatments, other causative theories were developed. Rectal prolapse looks like an intussusception. Cineroentgenographic defecograms by Theuerkauf and associates[18] demonstrated intussusception of the rectosigmoid as the patient strained at stool. This intussusception could be either congenital or acquired. Cineroentgenographic studies by Broden and Snellman[5] located the leading edge of the intussusception 6 to 8 cm from the anal verge, whereas Theuerkauf and coworkers[18] believed that it was higher, at the pelvic brim, 15 to 18 cm from the anal verge.

With the etiologic concept of intussusception came changes in treatment that generally have been more successful than steps taken to repair the hypothesized sliding perineal hernia. Yet there are features of procidentia that are not typical of intussusception seen elsewhere in the gastrointestinal tract in adults. First, the leading edge of the intussusception is not a tumor, diverticulum, suture line, or fixation of a point, as in a stoma. Second, the mechanism of intussusception elsewhere is inherent in the normal motility of the intestine. Small intestinal intussusception occurs as the pathologic leading edge is propelled by the antegrade motility of the intestine.

The causative mechanisms involved in procidentia appear to be both a sliding perineal hernia and an intussusception of the colon. Therefore, in selecting a procedure to correct procidentia, fixation or resection directed toward preventing intussusception generally is the most effective means of therapy.

PRESENTATION AND ASSOCIATED CONDITIONS

The most important presenting sign in these patients is the prolapse of the rectum. Most patients also complain of other difficulties in managing their bowel habits—chronic constipation, fecal incontinence, or both. In one series, 64% of patients also complained of straining, urgency, and frequency. Another condition commonly associated with rectal prolapse is proctitis cystica profunda.[17] Symptoms of this condition are generally the same as those of solitary rectal ulcer, including bleeding, mucous discharge, tenesmus, and constipation. These erythematous lesions of the rectum on biopsy show cystic glandular structures deep to the mucosa in the submucosa and muscularis. Care must be taken in interpreting biopsies of these lesions because casual inspection may result in an incorrect diagnosis of invasive carcinoma. The lesions are usually located anteriorly, and 15 to 28 patients with proctitis cystica profunda were found by Stuart[17] to have prolapse of the rectum. In patients with solitary rectal ulcer and in those with proctitis cystica profunda, surgical treatment of the prolapse results in healing of the inflammatory lesions.

The association of solitary rectal ulcer and proctitis cystica profunda with procidentia is so strong that the presence of these lesions anteriorly in the rectum led Ihre[8] to describe patients with solitary rectal ulcer and proctitis cystica profunda but without clinically evident prolapse as having internal procidentia. However, surgical treatment of prolapse in patients with solitary rectal ulcer and proctitis cystica profunda without prolapse has not resulted in healing of these lesions.[3,9]

Occasionally, patients with lower gastrointestinal bleeding secondary to procidentia, who do not have prolapse at rest, are unaware of their prolapse. In these patients, the bleeding occurs only while the rectum is prolapsed, and repair of the prolapse stops subsequent episodes of bleeding.

The diagnosis of procidentia in a patient whose rectum is prolapsed at rest or who can prolapse the rectum with a simple Valsalva maneuver is no problem. In other patients in whom prolapse is suspected because of rectal ulcer, proctitis cystica profunda, occult bleeding, or a history of prolapse with straining, the best means of demonstrating the prolapse is to give the patient an enema, have the patient strain, and examine the patient while he or she is on the toilet or in the squatting position. It is absolutely necessary that the prolapse be seen by the operating surgeon before operative intervention not only to establish the diagnosis but also to rule out simple mucosal prolapse and to help plan the operative procedure.

CONSEQUENCES OF PROLAPSE

The consequences of prolapse of the rectum include development of an abnormally deep anterior peritoneal reflection, diastasis of the levator muscles with pelvic floor weakening, patulous anal sphincters with incontinence, elongation of the mesorectum with loss of the anorectal angle, and extensive redundancy of the sigmoid colon (Fig. 33-2). Each of these consequences was once believed to be a causative factor of procidentia. Now all are believed generally to occur secondary to the prolapse.[19] Complications arising from the anatomic abnormalities occurring with prolapse include fecal incontinence, incarceration or even strangulation of the prolapse, and bleeding. Few operations that have been developed for the treatment of prolapse are directed toward correction of all these anatomic abnormalities. One operation that does correct all the abnormalities is presented later.

TREATMENT

Most children have spontaneous resolution of their prolapse as they grow older, and expectant treatment suffices. For children with troublesome mucosal prolapse and occasionally for children with full-thickness prolapse, submucosal injection of a sclerosing solution such as sodium tetradecyl sulfate or sodium morrhuate is effective. Care must be taken not to inject excessive sclerosing agent because anal stenosis may result. Surgical procedures are almost never needed for children with rectal prolapse.

In adults, the treatment of rectal prolapse is surgical. These operations are done through the abdomen or the perineum. Abdominal procedures include sigmoidectomy, with or without rectal fixation, and sacral rectopexy, known as the Ripstein or Wells procedure. Perineal procedures include perineal rectosigmoidectomy with or without levator repair, as described by Altemeier and colleagues,[1] and sacral fixation of the rectum with postanal repair, as described by Prasad and associates.[15] Anal circlage using a variety of synthetic or autogenous materials and sclerotherapy of the anal mucosa are used under certain circumstances. Less frequently used procedures include anterior fixation of the sigmoid colon or the rectum, rectal mucosal stripping with muscular reefing, cul-de-sac closure, transabdominal anterior levator repair, posterior sacral exposure with fixation, and combined abdominoperineal resection of the rectum and anus.

Abdominal Sigmoidectomy With Rectal Fixation

Abdominal sigmoidectomy with rectal fixation is becoming increasingly popular in the treatment of rectal

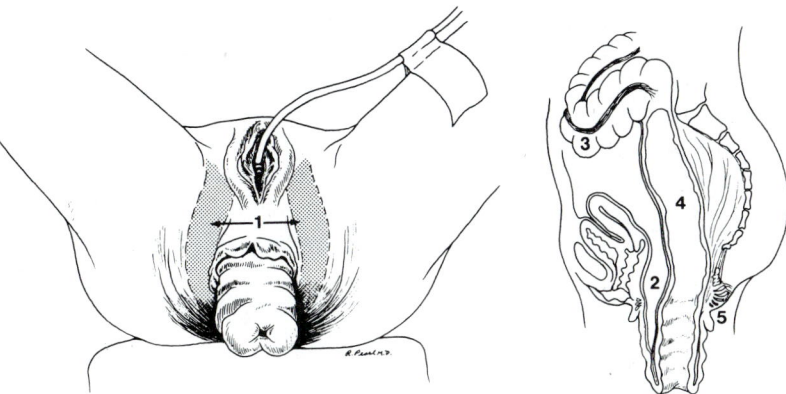

Figure 33-2. Anatomic features of severe rectal prolapse. (1) Diastasis of levator ani muscles. (2) Deep pouch of Douglas. (3) Redundant sigmoid colon. (4) Straightening of the rectum (long rectal mesentery, lack of fixation of rectum to sacrum). (5) Patulous anus (lax internal and external sphincters).

prolapse.[19] The technique involves resection of the redundant sigmoid colon with anastomosis to the rectum just below the pelvic brim (Fig. 33-3). Preceding sigmoidectomy, there should be full mobilization and fixation of the rectum to the sacrum. Through a lower midline incision, the rectum is mobilized by first incising the peritoneum on either side of the rectum down to the peritoneal reflection. Posterior mobilization in the presacral space is performed down to the level of the levator muscles. The lateral pelvic stalks and inferior mesenteric vessels are carefully preserved. After mobilization, cephalad traction is placed on the rectum, and rectal fixation or a rectopexy is performed. Rectopexy may be performed by suturing the rectum to the presacral fascia or by using prosthetic mesh to attach the rectum to the sacrum. Details are presented later.

The rationale for this procedure is that fixation of the rectum prevents intussusception and procidentia, while resection of redundant sigmoid improves bowel function and also prevents intussusception. In 102 patients reported by Watts and colleagues,[19] there were only two recurrences, and 56% of patients reported improvement in bowel function. Madoff and colleagues[11] reviewed 47 patients at the University of Minnesota who underwent colon resection and suture rectopexy for treatment of procidentia. There were only three recurrences (6.3%). Of the 20 patients that presented with constipation, 10 were improved after operation (50%). Of the 21 patients who presented with incontinence, 8 (38%) improved. Although the numbers are small, the data indicate that this procedure improves preoperative constipation.

In a prospective study, McKee and colleagues[12] compared abdominal rectopexy with and without sigmoidectomy. One group underwent rectopexy alone, while the other underwent rectopexy with sigmoidectomy. There was significant improvement in patients with constipation who underwent sigmoidectomy in addition to rectopexy. This was demonstrated both clinically and on the basis of colonic transit studies. Four of the five incontinent patients in the rectopexy-alone group reported improvement, whereas there was no change in the other group. These data appear to indicate that sigmoidectomy is useful in managing constipation and that the constipating effects of rectopexy may improve patients with incontinence.

Sacral Rectopexy

Sacral rectopexy involves fixation of the mobilized rectum to the presacral fascia using synthetic material or autogenous fascia. The original procedure, as described by Ripstein, involved the use of autogenous fascia lata to attach the rectum to the sacrum. To avoid a leg incision, prosthetic materials have replaced the use of autogenous fascia. A variety of synthetic materials have been used, including polytetrafluoroethylene, polypropylene (Marlex), and polyvinyl alcohol (Ivalon). The original procedure has been modified because Ripstein used a 360-degree wrap of the rectum, which can result partial obstruction and severe constipation (Fig. 33-4). A partial wrap as described by Wells is recommended.[20]

A standard lower midline abdominal incision is made and the rectum mobilized by incising the lateral peritoneal reflections on either side of the rectum down to the peritoneal reflection and connecting these incisions anteriorly. Blunt dissection is used to enter the presacral space posterior to the rectum. Mobilization continues inferiorly to the level of the leva-

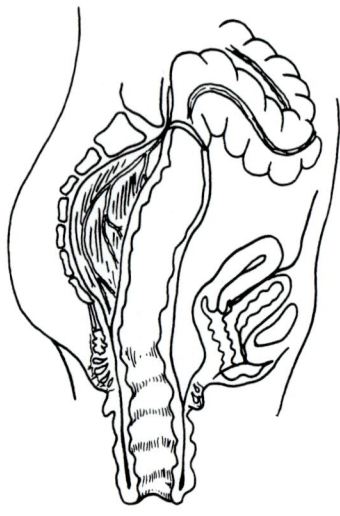
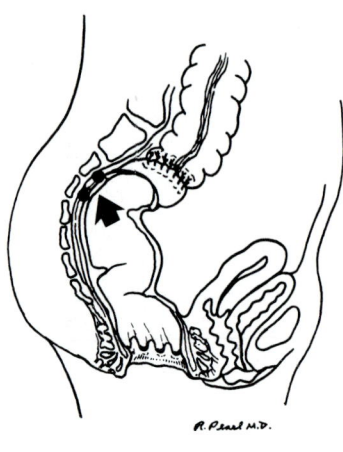

R. Pearl M.D.

Figure 33-3. Abdominal sigmoidectomy with rectal fixation. (*Left*) Prolapsed rectum, showing loss of sacralization and redundancy of the sigmoid colon. (*Right*) Redundant sigmoid colon resected. The rectum is sutured to the presacral fascia (*arrow*).

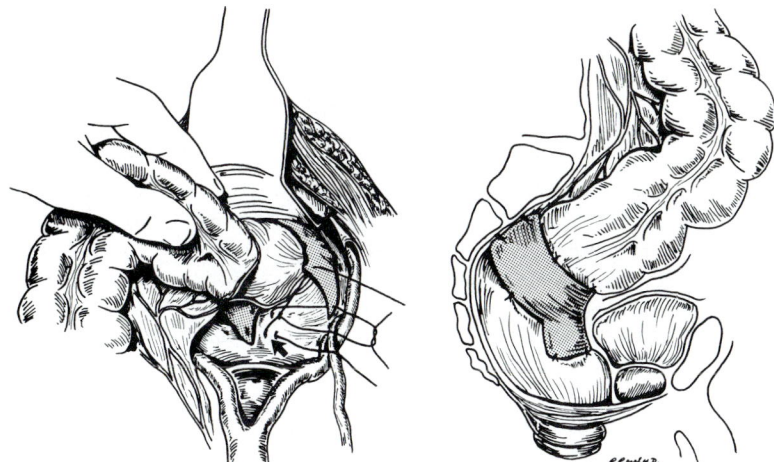

Figure 33-4. Ripstein rectopexy. (*Left*) After full mobilization of the rectum, a strip of synthetic mesh is wrapped around the rectum, and both ends of the mesh are sutured to the presacral fascia. (*Right*) Lateral view showing seromuscular tacking sutures to the anterior and lateral rectal walls.

tors. Bleeding is minimized by using blunt dissections and staying superficial to the presacral fascia. Care is taken to preserve the superior hemorrhoidal artery.

Once rectal mobilization is accomplished and hemostasis obtained, four or five nonabsorbable double-armed sutures are placed in the presacral fascia in the midline. These should be placed as low as possible in the pelvis. A 5 × 15 cm piece of prosthetic material is then cut. The sutures in the presacral fascia are placed through the middle of the prosthetic material, which is oriented transversely, and then tied securely (Fig. 33-5). The rectum is drawn up out of the pelvis as far as possible, and the prosthetic material is sutured to the anterolateral walls of the rectum with a series of interrupted seromuscular sutures. The peritoneum is then closed over the repair.

In a large series published by Gordon and Hoexter[6] of 1111 operations performed by 102 members of the American Society of Colon and Rectal Sur-

geons using the traditional 360-degree wrap, complications occurred in 16.5% of patients, and the recurrence rate was 2.3%. Complications included bleeding (2.6%), abscess (1.5%), stricture (1.8%), and fecal impaction (6.7%). Bleeding occurs most often when a presacral vein is pierced during presacral fixation. Frantic attempts at coagulation and suture ligature are often unsuccessful and may lead to more severe bleeding. Often, tying of the offending suture is all that is necessary. Troublesome bleeding that is unresponsive to conservative measures may be treated by the judicious use of sterile thumbtacks, as described by Nivatvongs and Fang.[14]

The polyvinyl alcohol sponge rectopexy was initially described by Wells. It is probably the most frequently used procedure in Great Britain.

Historically, the most frequently seen complication of the Ripstein procedure has been fecal impaction caused by the obstruction resulting from the re-

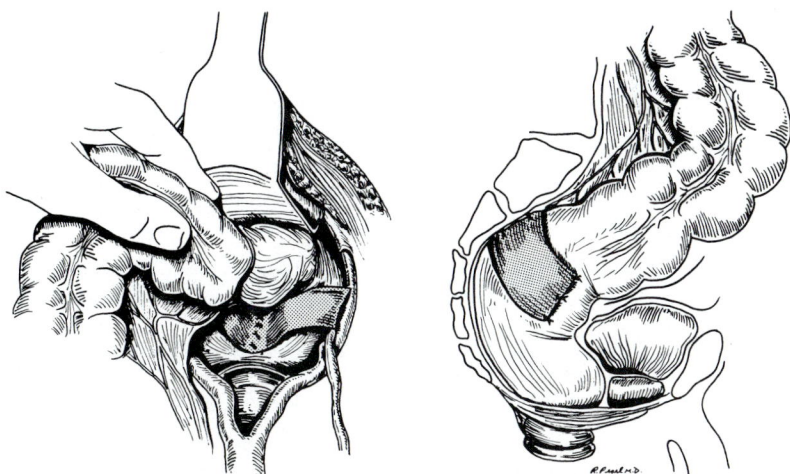

Figure 33-5. Wells rectopexy. (*Left*) After full mobilization of the rectum, a strip of synthetic material is sutured to the presacral fascia. After the rectum is drawn out of the pelvis, the ends of the synthetic material are sutured to the anterolateral walls of the rectum. (*Right*) Lateral view of the completed posterolateral wrap. Notice the gap in the wrap anteriorly.

active fibrosis surrounding the synthetic material. Roberts and colleagues[16] reported an incidence of 7.4%, which is comparable to the 6.7% reported by Gordon and Hoexter.[6] In the original Ripstein procedure, the wrap was complete anteriorly (360 degrees). The modified procedure described by Wells uses a posterolateral wrap of the mobilized rectum. The anterior wall is not encircled, making partial obstruction and fecal impaction less likely.

A laparoscopic modification of this procedure was described by Berman.[2] Thumbtacks are used to fix the synthetic material to the sacrum, and staples are used to attach the rectum to the prosthetic material.

Perineal Rectosigmoidectomy

Perineal rectosigmoidectomy with and without posterior rectopexy and postanal levator repair has traditionally been reserved for the elderly or debilitated patient who cannot tolerate an abdominal procedure. It is intended to correct both the pathologic anatomy of the prolapse and to restore fecal continence. The procedure may be performed under local or regional anesthesia. A minimum of 5 cm of prolapse is required.

After routine preoperative preparation of the colon, a 1:200,000 solution of epinephrine is injected circumferentially deep to the submucosa of the prolapsed segment about 1.5 cm proximal to the dentate line, when the anastomosis will be hand sewn, or 2.5 cm proximal if a stapling device will be used (Fig. 33-6A). This provides adequate length for anastomosis yet prevents postoperative protrusion. A full-thickness transverse incision is made through the prolapsed segment anteriorly and carried posteriorly, taking care to securely ligate all bleeding vessels (see Fig. 33-6B). Stay sutures of 2-0 polyglycolic acid (Vicryl) are placed in the four corners of the rectal remnant as the incision is carried posteriorly. The mesentery of the prolapsed segment is divided close to the bowel wall because these vessels may retract into the abdomen once divided. With the mesentery divided, the prolapse may be completely unfolded. Traction is applied to the segment to achieve adequate resection of the redundant rectosigmoid (see Fig. 33-6C).

Sacral rectopexy is performed at this time. The prolapsed segment is elevated anteriorly to expose the presacral space. A series of interrupted nonabsorbable sutures are used to fix the sigmoid colon to the presacral fascia above the levators (Fig. 33-7). The levator ani muscles are approximated posteriorly using 2-0 nylon suture. The rectosigmoid is then brought down to expose the levator diaphragm anteriorly. A levatoroplasty is then completed by approximating the two arms of the puborectalis muscle with a series of nonabsorbable sutures. This step accomplishes reinforcement of the attenuated pelvic diaphragm (Fig. 33-8).

The anterior wall of the redundant rectosigmoid is then incised longitudinally at the point of anastomosis. The anterior half of the bowel is divided, and anastomosis is undertaken using a series of interrupted 3-0 Vicryl sutures (Fig. 33-9). The bowel is

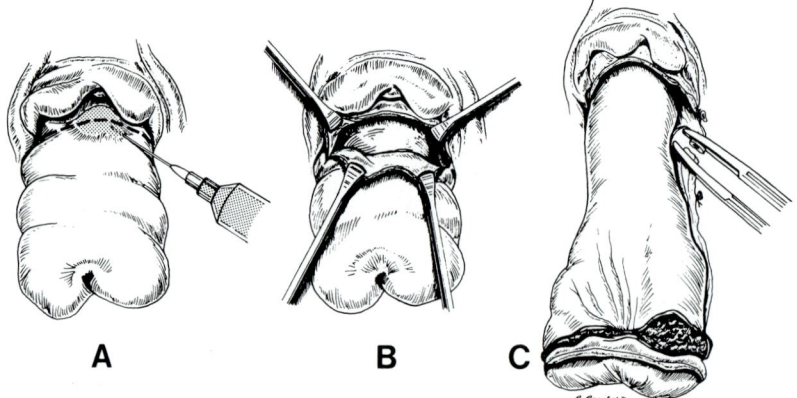

A **B** **C**

Figure 33-6. Perineal proctectomy with posterior rectopexy and postanal levator repair. (*A*) After the full extent of the prolapse is reproduced by applying gentle traction on the rectal wall, a dilute epinephrine solution (1:200,000) is injected into the outer layer of the prolapsed rectal wall to minimize bleeding. (*B*) A circular incision is made through the full thickness of the outer layer of the prolapsed segment just proximal to the everted dentate line. The incision should enter the deep cul-de-sac anteriorly and is best accomplished with electrocautery. Allis clamps are applied to the divided edges of the rectum. (*C*) The rectal prolapse is completely unfolded. The mesenteric vessels are carefully ligated close to the intestinal wall.

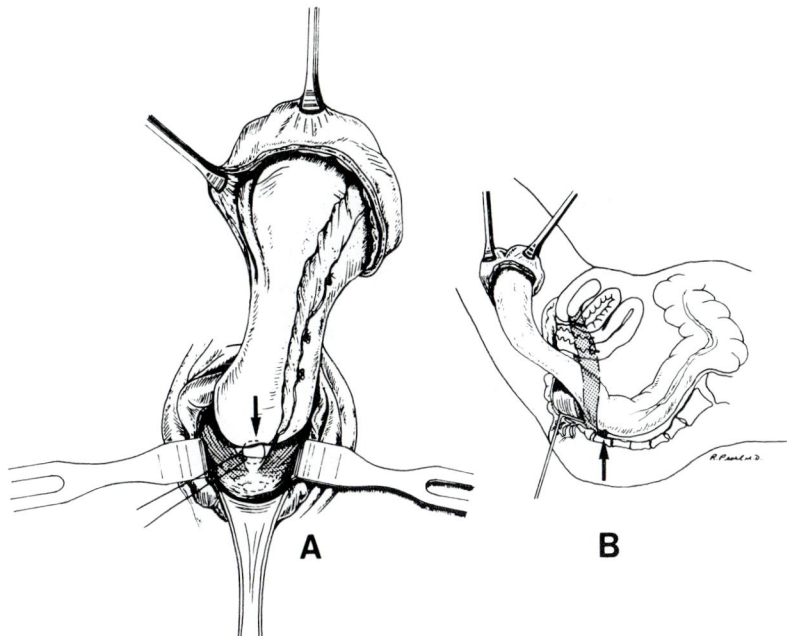

Figure 33-7. Perineal proctectomy (*continued*). (*A*) After the full extent of the prolapse is unfolded, it is elevated anteriorly to expose the presacral space. A posterior rectopexy is performed (*arrow*) by approximating the seromuscular layers of the intestinal wall to the precoccygeal fascia above the levator ani muscles with 2-0 silk sutures. (*B*) Lateral view showing the completed posterior rectopexy (*arrow*). Note that the fixation is above the levator ani muscles (*shaded area*).

then fully transected, carefully dividing mesenteric vessels, and the posterior half of the anastomosis is completed. The sutures are full thickness and approximate sigmoid colon to rectum just above the dentate line. Once completed, the anastomosis retracts into the anal canal (Fig. 33-10). When a stapler is used, pursestring sutures of 2-0 Prolene are placed in the transected ends of the bowel. The circular stapler is inserted into the proximal sigmoid colon, and the

proximal pursestring is tied. The device is partially advanced through the anus and the distal pursestring secured. Firing the instrument completes the anastomosis.

The procedure has been shown to be effective and well tolerated by most patients. Williams and colleagues[21] reported a series of 104 patients treated by this method. The recurrence rate was 10%, most of which occurred after 30 months of follow-up. Com-

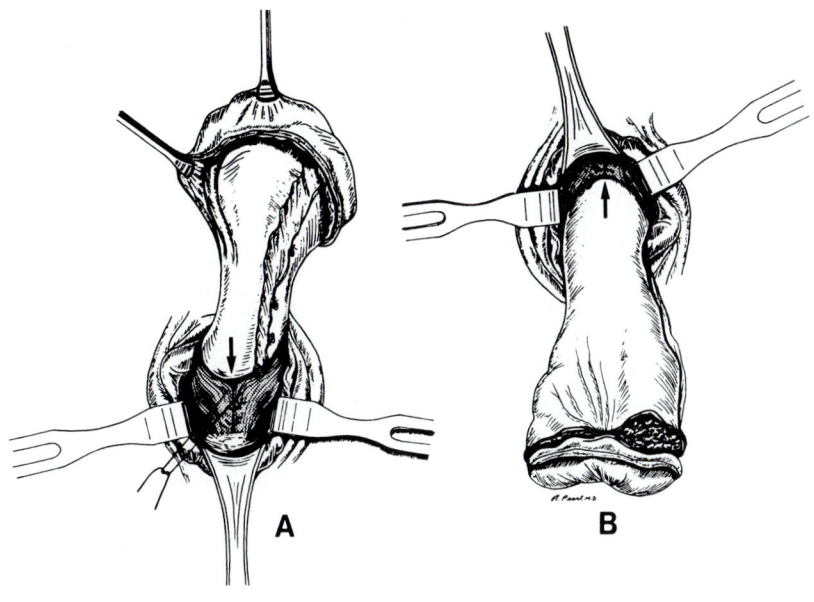

Figure 33-8. Perineal proctectomy (*continued*). (*A*) The levator ani muscles are approximated posteriorly (*arrow*) with four 2-0 polypropylene sutures. This posterior levator repair pushes the intestine anteriorly to help recreate the anorectal angle. (*B*) One or two 2-0 polypropylene sutures are used to approximate the levator muscles anterior to the rectum to reinforce the pelvic floor.

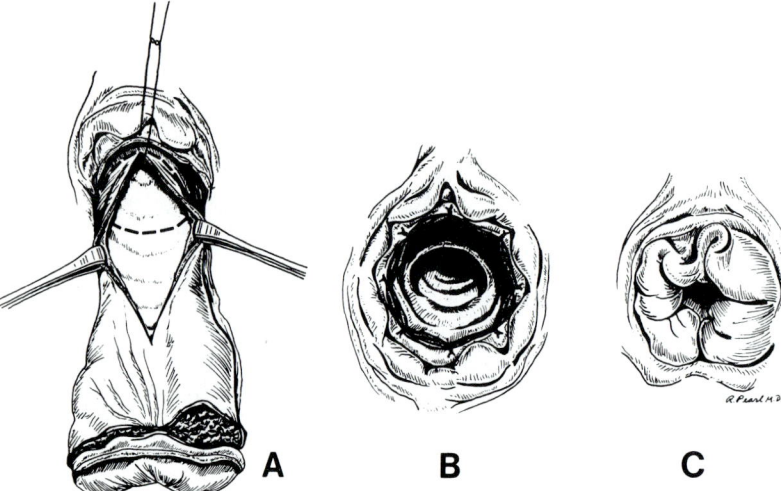

Figure 33-9. Perineal proctectomy (*continued*). (*A*) The anterior wall of the unfolded prolapse is divided longitudinally up to the level of the proposed anastomosis and sutured to the dentate line with interrupted 3-0 polyglycolic acid sutures. The remainder of the prolapse is amputated and sutured to the dentate line in a circumferential manner (*dotted line*). (*B*) Completed anastomosis. (*C*) Appearance of the anus after the suture line is reduced.

plications developed in 12% and were relatively minor. No deaths occurred, and the median hospital stay was only 4 days.

Anal Circlage

Anal circlage involves encirclement of the anus with a foreign material to narrow the anal orifice and prevent external prolapse. In the classic operation described by Thiersch, silver wire was placed in the perianal space. The use of wire has been abandoned because of complications such as breakage and ulcerations. Other materials, such as nylon, Mersilene, Dacron, polypropylene mesh (Marlex), Teflon, fascia lata, silicone rubber, and Silastic have been used.

Of all the procedures for rectal prolapse, anal circlage does the least to treat the disease. It only hides the procidentia and converts external prolapse into internal prolapse. For this reason, it is usually reserved for high-risk patients who are too ill to tolerate abdominal procedures or perineal resection.

Anal circlage is usually done under local or regional anesthesia with the patient in the lithotomy position.[10] Radial incisions are made in the left-posterior and right-anterior quadrant of the perianal area and carried 2 to 3 cm deep into the ischiorectal fat (Fig. 33-11). With a curved hemostat, a tunnel is developed at the deepest extent of the incision, passing beneath the superficial external sphincter and circumferentially around the anal canal. A 1.5-cm–wide segment of nonabsorbable material is then passed through the

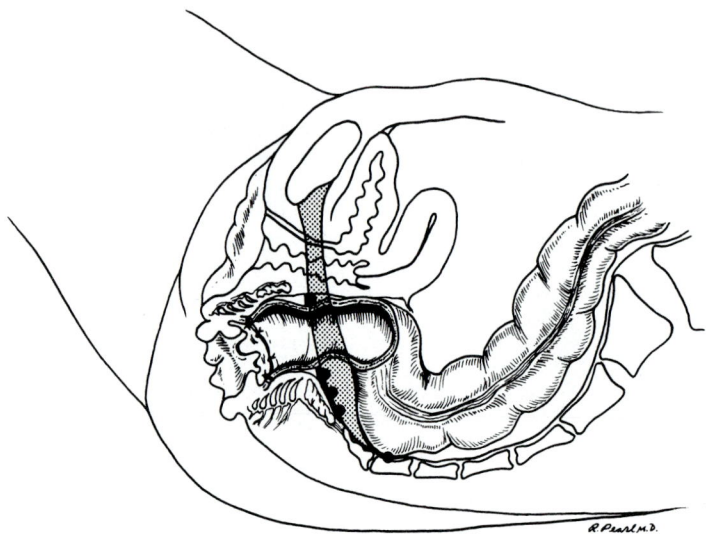

Figure 33-10. Perineal proctectomy (*continued*). Summary of the repair, illustrating the posterior rectopexy and postanal levator repair (*black dots*). Notice how the anorectal angle has been reestablished.

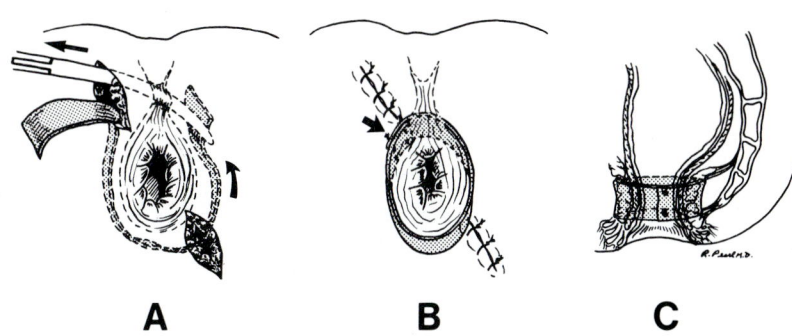

Figure 33-11. Anal circlage procedure. (*A*) Superficial and deep portions of the external sphincter are encircled with a strip of synthetic material tunneled through left posterior and right anterior skin incisions. (*B*) Anal circlage completed. The ends of the strip are either sutured or stapled to each other (*arrow*). (*C*) Lateral view showing position of the band. Note how it passes through the deep postanal space.

tunnel on both sides of the anus. The ends are brought out through the left-posterior incision and sutured together to narrow the anal orifice so that it snugly admits the distal interphalangeal joint of the surgeon's finger. The incisions are then closed. After operation, the patient is given a stool softener.

PREOPERATIVE AND POSTOPERATIVE CARE

All patients having procedures for procidentia must have mechanical and antimicrobial bowel preparation before operation. Patients with incarcerated prolapse must be operated on urgently after resuscitation to avoid the septic risks of strangulation. Stool softeners should be given in the postoperative period. Such medication may be needed for the patient's lifetime after rectopexy or anal circlage.

SURGICAL CHOICE

More than 130 operations have been described for the treatment of rectal prolapse. Described in this chapter are the principles of the most widely performed procedures for procidentia. Abdominal sigmoidectomy with rectal fixation is a relatively simple procedure to perform, and recurrence rates are about 5% to 6%. It has the advantage of simultaneously treating both prolapse and constipation. Fears about anastomotic leakage and pelvic sepsis in the presence of a foreign body when Marlex or other artificial material is used for fixation have generally been unfounded. The procedure is well suited to younger, low-risk patients.

Sacral fixation is ideally suited to the patient with prolapse who does not have significant redundancy of the sigmoid colon. Patients with preoperative incontinence may also benefit from this procedure because the constipating effects of rectopexy may protect against incontinence. The Wells rectopexy is preferred because the rectum remains free anteriorly, and the risk of postoperative fecal impaction is minimized.

For the elderly, high-risk patient with significant prolapse or incarcerated prolapse, the perineal rectosigmoidectomy is the procedure of choice. It is easy to perform and can be done under local or regional anesthesia. Recurrence rates are acceptable, and morbidity is minimal. Well-controlled studies are required to determine whether this procedure may someday become the preferred therapy for all patients with procidentia.

Anal circlage should rarely be done. Inevitably, some patients want the least invasive procedure or are too ill to tolerate even perineal resection under regional anesthesia. The use of silver wire should be avoided, and synthetic suture material or mesh should be used to encircle the anal canal.

REFERENCES

1. Altemeier WA, Culbertson WR, Schwengert C, Hunt J. Nineteen years' experience with the one-stage perineal repair of rectal prolapse. Ann Surg 1971;173: 993.
2. Berman IR. Sutureless laparoscopic rectopexy for procidentia. Dis Colon Rectum 1992;35:689.
3. Biehl AG, Ray JE, Gathright JB. Repair of rectal prolapse: experience with the Ripstein sling. South Med J 1978;71:923.
4. Boutsis C, Ellis H. The Ivalon sponge-wrap operation for rectal prolapse. Dis Colon Rectum 1974;17:21.
5. Broden B, Snellman B. Procidentia of the rectum studied with cineradiography: a contribution to the discussion of causative mechanisms. Dis Colon Rectum 1968;71:330.
6. Gordon PH, Hoexter B. Complications of the Ripstein procedure. Dis Colon Rectum 1978;28:277.
7. Greenwald ML, Banerjel SR, Cherry DA, Walters DL. Perineal resection for colorectoanal intussusception. Contemp Surg 1993;43:81.
8. Ihre T. Studies of anal function in continent and incontinent patients. Scand J Gastroenterol 1974;9 (Suppl):25.
9. Keighley MRB, Shouler P. Clinical and manometric features of the solitary rectal ulcer syndrome. Dis Colon Rectum 1984;27:507.

10. Labow S, Rubin RJ, Hoexter B, Salvati EP. Perineal repair of rectal procidentia with an elastic fabric sling. Dis Colon Rectum 1980;23:467.
11. Madoff RV, Williams JG, Wong WD, Rothenberger DA, Goldberg SM. Long-term functional results of colon resection and rectopexy for overt rectal prolapse. Am J Gastroenterol 1992;87:101.
12. McKee RF, Lauder JC, Poon FW, Aitchison MA, Finley IG. A prospective randomized study of abdominal rectopexy with and without sigmoidectomy in rectal prolapse. Surg Gynecol Obstet 1992;174:145.
13. Moschowitz AV. The pathogenesis, anatomy and cure of prolapse of the rectum. Surg Gynecol Obstet 1912;15:7.
14. Nivatvongs S, Fang DT. The use of thumbtacks to stop massive presacral hemorrhage. Dis Colon Rectum 1986;29:589.
15. Prasad ML, Pearl RK, Abcarian H, et al. Perineal proctectomy, posterior rectopexy and post-anal levator repair for the treatment of rectal prolapse. Dis Colon Rectum 1986;29:547.
16. Roberts PL, Schoetz DJ, Coller JA, Veidenheimer MC. Ripstein Procedure—Lahey clinic experience: 1963–1985. Arch Surg 1988;123:554.
17. Stuart M. Proctitis cystica profunda: incidence etiology and treatment. Dis Colon Rectum 1984;27:153.
18. Theuerkauf FJ, Beahrs OH, Hill JR. Rectal prolapse, causation and treatment. Ann Surg 1970;171:819.
19. Watts JD, Rothenberger DA, Buls JG, et al. The management of procidentia, 30 years' experience. Dis Colon Rectum 1985;28:96.
20. Wells C. Rectal prolapse. Nurs Times 1971;67:345.
21. Williams JG, Rothenberger DA, Madoff RD, Goldberg SM. Treatment of rectal prolapse in the elderly by perineal rectosigmoidectomy. Dis Colon Rectum 1992;35:830.

Editor's Comment

Rectal prolapse combines pathophysiologic features of both a levator diaphragm hernia and an intussusception of the rectosigmoid. Drs. Appel and Telford have described the best procedure in use today, an operation that combines rectopexy and resection.

All surgeons with any experience in the management of rectal prolapse would agree that rectopexy is an essential feature of successful correction. The Ripstein approach, as pointed out by the authors, which involved the placement of a prosthesis for rectopexy across the anterior aspect of the rectum, fails because of the associated complication of obstruction. The original approach advocated by Wells, but now modified to use Marlex mesh instead of Ivalon, in which the prosthesis is placed on the posterior aspect of the rectum and is noncircumferential, achieves a satisfactory rectopexy. I have become convinced over the last decade that resection of redundant sigmoid improves the results and is an important feature of the operation.

Appel and Telford do not mention closure of the hernia orifice in the pelvic diaphragm, which is a regular feature of rectal prolapse. I believe the hernia deserves repair. After thorough mobilization of the rectum and rectosigmoid from the sacrum and pelvic diaphragm, the rectum is pushed anteriorly, and the levator diaphragm is closed posterior to it with interrupted sutures. The rectum is then laid in the reconstructed hollow of the pelvis and the point for rectopexy fixed in the midportion of the sacrum. Then, a judgment can be made about resection of the redundant colon so that a comfortable anastomosis will lie just distal to the pelvic brim.

My experience with cerclage is not different from that cited by these authors: it is associated with a high incidence of complications and does not do anything to correct the fundamental problem. In my experience, the Altemeier operation also fails. I think it does so because the extent of resection, rectopexy to the sacrum, and reconstruction of the pelvic diaphragm are all less satisfactory than with a transabdominal approach. With modern anesthetic techniques, the former concern about a transabdominal approach in an elderly patient is no longer applicable, and I believe the Altemeier approach should be relegated to the group of procedures of only historical interest.

R.E.C.

Intraabdominal Hernias

Part Six

Hernia, Fourth Edition, edited
by Lloyd M. Nyhus and Robert E. Condon.
J.B. Lippincott Company, Philadelphia © 1995.

Chapter 34

Mesenteric Hernia

Alex M. Stone, Yves Janin, and Leslie Wise

Internal hernias are protrusions into pouches or openings in the visceral peritoneum, in contrast to hernias through defects in the retaining walls of the abdomen. Transmesenteric hernias are intraperitoneal hernias that *have no sac* and consist of the protrusion of a loop of intestine through an aperture in the mesentery. As with other hernias, mesenteric hernias may lead to intestinal obstruction, strangulation, and, subsequently, gangrene of varying lengths of intestine. Internal hernias may also occur through defects in the omentum and the broad ligament, and, similar to mesenteric hernias, *have no sac*. In a collected series of 11,270 patients with acute intestinal obstruction,[13,31] 94 patients (0.8%) had internal hernias. This incidence appears to vary in different patient populations; White[71] reported that the incidence of internal hernias as a cause of acute intestinal obstruction in Africans was 13%.

Mesenteric hernias may be of congenital origin, accounting for most reports in the medical literature on this subject, or they may be postsurgical (iatrogenic) in origin. In addition, mesenteric hernias may arise after traumatic injuries.

HISTORY

Rokitansky,[53] in 1836, reported the first incidence of transmesenteric hernia, an autopsy finding in which the cecum alone herniated through a hole near the ileocolic angle. The first instance found at autopsy of herniation through the transverse mesocolon was reported by Loebl in 1844.[46] Turel,[69] in 1932, was the first to describe a herniation through a defect in the sigmoid mesocolon.

Holes in the mesentery were not infrequently described by the early anatomists and pathologists. Mitchell[47] stated that these defects were seen in about 1 of every 400 cadavers. He found three ileocecal mesenteric defects in 1000 necropsies and a fourth cadaver, with an ileocecal mesenteric defect closed by a membrane, devoid of fat. None of these defects contributed to the cause of death. Watson[70] found an opening in the mesentery of the ileocecal region in 3 of 1600 autopsies, and Meade[45] cited Whitnal and Simpson as having found two, in the examination of 50 cadavers.

The first reports of successful operative treatment of patients with mesenteric hernias were by Marsh,[41] in 1888, and Ackerman,[1] in 1902. One hundred fifty patients with idiopathic hernias through defects of the mesentery of the small intestine and mesocolon were collected from the English and European literature and reviewed.[30]

In 1878, Le Moyne,[38] in his thesis, recognized the existence of an unusual form of intestinal obstruction in which there was an aperture in the ileocecal mesentery through which the intestine herniated. In 1883, Coats,[12] in his *A Manual of Pathology*, first postulated that the defect in the mesentery was congenital. The most important characteristic of ileocecal mesenteric defects was noted by Le Moyne,[38] who observed that the margin of the mesenteric defect was thickened and contained one of the arterial branches destined to the terminal ileum. Eight years later, Treves,[68] lecturing at the Royal College of Surgeons in England, described the characteristics of these mesenteric defects: "The holes were round; they were situated in the mesentery of the terminal part of the ileum; their margins were distinct, being often thickened and opaque, and around a part of the margin it was not uncommon to find one of the terminal branches of the superior mesenteric artery." Treves observed an area of the ileal mesentery of a well-rounded or oval shape in the fetus that was circumscribed by the anastomosis of the ileocolic branch of the superior mesenteric artery with the last of the intestinal arteries. At the autopsy of a 52-year-old man, Treves reported that the serous membrane that formed this area was thin, clear, and atrophied to a cribriform structure, pierced by about 20 holes. He noted that this area was remarkable insofar as it had no fat and no visible blood vessels, even in injected specimens, and was never occupied by any mesenteric glands. This area subsequently has been named *Treves field* (Fig. 34-1).

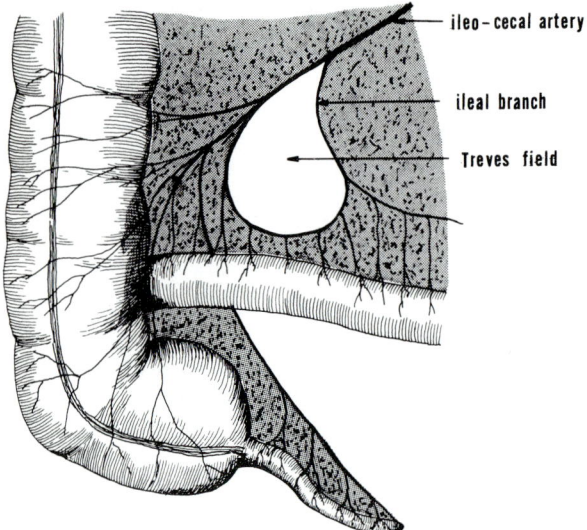

ileo-cecal artery

ileal branch

Treves field

Figure 34-1. Congenital mesenteric defect in the ileocolic mesentery (Treves field).

PATHOGENESIS

Three etiologic hypotheses have been proposed for idiopathic (congenital) holes in the mesentery. Federschmidt[21] stated that the defects represented a partial regression of the dorsal mesentery in the human being. Menegaux[46] postulated that fenestration occurred during the developmental enlargement of an inadequately vascularized area. Dolton[20] added that "the ileocecal mesentery, due to the descent of the cecum, undergoes considerable and rapid lengthening in fetal life." Multiple mesenteric fenestrations, as reported in the ileocecal area by Treves,[67] Long,[39] and Gatewood,[24] along the mesenteric border of the small intestine are common in the mesentery of the goose, possibly lending some support to the hypothesis of Federschmidt as outlined earlier. Judd[33] and Kiebel and Mall[35] believed that because the greater part of the gut is displaced from the abdominal cavity into the umbilical cord in fetal life, considerable pressure may cause the colon to continue along the path of least resistance and gradually force its way through the delicate structure of the mesentery. Macklin[40] postulated that when two epithelial layers are apposed with a deficient intervening supporting stroma of connective tissue, coalescence inevitably takes place, with the development of a space or defect.

Acquired mesenteric hernia has a completely different cause. Most of these defects occur after surgical resection of the small intestine or of the colon. If the mesenteric defect created by the bowel resection is not surgically repaired, or if the repair is inadequate or does not properly heal, a mesenteric hernia is the end

result. The incidence of this problem is unknown because only a small fraction of the patients with acquired mesenteric hernias come to surgical attention. In addition, it is not an anatomic finding that routinely would be noted in autopsy studies. Furthermore, a small mesenteric hernia is more likely to result in symptoms (partial or complete intestinal obstruction) than a large hernia, which is usually asymptomatic. There is also a more unusual variety of mesenteric hernia secondary to trauma. Penetrating stab wounds are the most common etiologic factor.

For all types of mesenteric hernias, symptoms result because of intestinal obstruction. A pressure differential cannot exist within the abdominal cavity. The intestine finds its way into the defect by virtue of peristaltic movement and the natural property of the intestine to occupy the entire peritoneal cavity. Among 139 patients with idiopathic mesenteric hernias, 24 patients (17%) had a history of intermittent episodes of crampy abdominal pain. This suggests that the mesenteric defect had been present throughout the life of the patient and that a loop of intestine had intermittently herniated through this defect, followed by spontaneous reduction. The final acute episode is most probably caused by the development of distention in a loop of intestine that has accidentally prolapsed through the mesenteric defect (unlike external hernias whereby a pressure differential exists across the defect). This results in a gas-trap mechanism,[16] which draws loops of intestine through the aperture until incarceration occurs. This gas-trap mechanism was demonstrated experimentally by Gatch and associates.[23] As peristalsis continues and increases, various lengths of intestine extrude through the defect. Thus, the size of the hole does not limit the size of the prolapsed intestine. This was shown by Brown[9] and MacLean,[24] who reported herniation of the entire small intestine through a small mesenteric defect.

The rapid onset of intestinal gangrene in a large number of patients is precipitated by the anatomic characteristics of these hernias. They have no limiting sac (as in external hernias), and because most of the defects are small (2–3 cm) with long portions of intestine passing through, it is not difficult to imagine how a considerable amount of tissue may occupy these small defects, quickly resulting in ischemia and gangrene. The pressure of the herniated intestine and its thickened mesentery compresses the vessels in the free margins of the mesenteric defect and may be responsible for ischemic changes in the loop forming the margin of the defect. This explains how it is possible for the loop of bowel forming the margin of the defect to be found to be gangrenous, whereas the herniated intestine may be completely viable. In addition to the packing of tissues through the defect, with resulting strangulation, there is no limitation to the occurrence of volvulus, either of the herniated loop or a redundant loop forming the margin of the defect (ie, sigmoid colon[71]).

Another cause of gangrene in a portion of the intestine that did not herniate was reported by Cullen,[14] who described a patient with a herniation of a loop of sigmoid colon through a defect in the mesentery of the ascending colon. This patient had gangrene of more than 5 ft of nonherniated terminal ileum. This gangrene was explained on the basis of compression of the terminal ileum by the taut mesentery of the distended sigmoid mesocolon.

Causes of obstruction can be found other than compression of the herniated loops of intestine that occupy the mesenteric defect or comprise its borders. Pye-Smith[50] reported on a patient in whom a Meckel diverticulum passed through a defect in the mesentery of that part of the intestine from which it arose (distal ileum) and, after encircling the intestine, became attached by its tip to the mesentery above the defect and produced obstruction. McWharter[44] described a patient in whom the lower end of the omentum was bifid, and both ends, after encircling the jejunum, fused through the opening in the mesentery of the upper part of the jejunum and caused obstruction.

INCIDENCE AND LOCATION

No sex or age predominance has been demonstrated for congenital mesenteric hernia. The ages of the patients at presentation ranged from the moment of birth[65] to 88 years of age.[63] Seventy-one percent of the reported mesenteric hernias occurred through defects in the mesentery of the small intestine.[30] Ileocecal defects[52] accounted for 54% of these instances and 39% of the entire group of mesenteric defects. However, the site of the defect in the mesentery of the small intestine was not specified in one fourth of the patients. Mesocolic defects were responsible for 26% of the instances reported. Defects in the transverse mesocolon were the most common defects (59%).

In addition, several investigators[10,37,46,48,51,55,61,62] reported the incidental finding of a defect in the transverse mesocolon in patients who were operated on for peptic ulcer disease. The small intestine herniated into the lesser sac through a defect in the gastrocolic omentum in three patients,[11,13,48] and in two of them,[11,48] it reemerged through an aperture in the gastrohepatic ligament.

Two instances of herniation through a defect in the mesentery of a Meckel diverticulum were reported, one by Dickenson[19] and the other by Dalinka and associates.[17] Rooney and colleagues[54] reported the only instance of herniation through a defect in the mesoappendix.

Ileocolic defects, the most common cause of congenital mesenteric hernias, are circular or oval and lie in the area of the mesentery between the ileocolic trunk and the last ileal branch of the superior mesenteric artery (see Fig. 34-1). The defect does not usually reach the mesenteric border of the ileum and is separated from the base of the mesentery by a firm edge. Most of the defects are 2 to 3 cm in diameter. The smallest was 1.6 cm in diameter.[15] The largest, which was found in an African, measured 30 by 40 cm and ran from one end of the mesentery to the other.[56] Although these defects are usually single, Gatewood[24] described a patient with an ileocecal mesenteric hernia who had multiple small and large defects along the mesentery of the small intestine. The ileocolic artery may be absent and replaced by a strongly developed right colic artery, as reported by Hommes.[29] In such an instance, the right colic artery anastomoses with an enlarged terminal intestinal vessel, named the *arteria ilei magna* by Hommes. Transverse mesocolic defects are most frequently bounded by the vascular arch formed by the middle and left colic vessels. Defects of the sigmoid mesocolon are usually circular and lie in its lower lead immediately above the superior rectal vessels.

Among the 150 patients reviewed, the small intestine herniated in 130 patients (87%), whereas the colon herniated in 14 patients (9%). The cecum and the sigmoid colon accounted each for 43% of these instances. There were two herniations of a Meckel diverticulum. Pye-Smith[50] reported on a patient with a herniation of a Meckel diverticulum through an opening in the mesentery of the intestine from which it arose, and Dickenson[19] described a herniation of a Meckel diverticulum through a hole in the base of its own mesentery. Sohn,[57] Nikisin,[47f] and Kagan[34] each reported on patients with herniation of the stomach through a defect of the transverse mesocolon. Six patients had herniation of more than one part of the gastrointestinal tract, and for seven patients, the herniated viscus was not mentioned. The length of the herniated small intestine varied from a short loop to the entire small intestine from the ligament of Treitz to the ileocecal valve.[24]

COMPLICATIONS

Vascular Compromise

In mesenteric herniation, vascular compromise of the intestine in the form of strangulation or gangrene may supervene extremely rapidly. The shortest duration of symptoms, with gangrene found at operation, was 6 hours, as reported by Williamson.[72] Vascular compromise occurred in 59% of the patients. Vascular compromise of the small intestine occurred in 52.5% of the patients with a mesenteric hernia and 62.5% of the patients with a herniated loop of small intestine. Vascular compromise of the colon occurred in 6% of the patients with a mesenteric hernia and in 36% of the patients with a herniated loop of colon.

Volvulus

Volvulus of the gastrointestinal tract was found in 17% of the patients, and it was associated with strangulation or gangrene in 83% of them. Volvulus of the small intestine occurred in one sixth of the patients with a herniated loop of small intestine, and it was accompanied by strangulation or gangrene in 79% of them. The volvulus may not affect the herniated segment but instead may involve that portion of the intestine through the mesentery of which the herniation has taken place. White[71] reported on two patients with herniation of the ileum through a defect in the sigmoid mesocolon who had a secondary volvulus and gangrene of the sigmoid colon. Sohn[57] described an instance of herniation of the stomach with a concomitant 180 degrees of volvulus and gangrene in a patient with a defect of the transverse mesocolon.

Constrictions of the herniated intestine were described in two patients.[26,45] Staab[60] reported on a patient with herniation of the small intestine through an ileocecal mesenteric defect and four constrictions of the small intestine, two of which were close together near the cecum and two others that were also close together and about 5 ft from the first pair.

Herniation through an ileocecal mesenteric defect may be found incidentally during appendectomy.[19,24] The tip of a noninflamed appendix[36] or a gangrenous appendix[19] may be found to be adherent to the herniated loop of small intestine. Also, Meckel diverticulitis was found in a patient who underwent exploration for intestinal obstruction secondary to incarceration of the small intestine through a mesenteric defect.[27]

ASSOCIATED ANOMALIES OF THE GASTROINTESTINAL TRACT

Associated anomalies of the gastrointestinal tract have been reported in patients with mesenteric hernias. In adults, these include incomplete rotation or malrotation of the colon,[43,47d,54] and of the sigmoid mesocolon associated with herniation through the mesosigmoid,[6] and Ivemark syndrome.[54] Murphy[47e] found that among 11 infants with herniation of the small intestine through a mesenteric defect, 10 had associated anomalies. Seven infants had multiple anomalies. The

most frequent anomaly of the gastrointestinal tract reported in infants with a mesenteric hernia was small intestinal atresia, which was found in half of infants. Among these infants, ileal atresia was the most common type, accounting for two thirds of the instances. Two infants had associated cystic fibrosis. Three infants had incomplete rotation of the colon; one infant had intestinal duplication; and one other was found to have Hirschsprung disease. A mesenteric hernia was also reported in an infant with erythroblastosis fetalis.[42]

SIGNS AND SYMPTOMS

The most common symptom was pain, which was sudden in onset and severe in more than half of patients. The pain is most frequently located in the epigastrium and the periumbilical area. Vomiting was the next most common symptom, and constipation occurred in about one fourth of patients. Infants usually presented with persistent vomiting and abdominal distention.[3,8,42,47b,59,74]

Twenty-seven patients (18%) had a history of intermittent attacks of severe abdominal pain, occasionally associated with vomiting and constipation, which subsided spontaneously. The incidence would probably have been much higher but for the fact that in a number of reports, no mention was made of the history of the patient. Thirteen patients had a single previous attack, 11 days[64] to 13 years[22] before the final episode. Eleven patients had numerous previous attacks. Three patients had vague abdominal complaints for several years. Four patients had more unusual histories. Odermatt,[47g] in 1926, reported on a patient with a 3-year history of abdominal distress, vomiting, and weight loss, who was thought to have a carcinoma of the intestine and who died of a gangrenous hernia of the transverse mesocolon. Atherton[4] reported on a patient with an 8-year history of recurrent attacks of abdominal pain, which increased in frequency, became stronger, and lasted longer as the final attack approached. Cullen,[14] in 1936, reported on a patient with a history of abdominal pain relieved by vomiting and sometimes precipitated by strenuous exercise. Moulay and associates[47c] described a patient with mesenteric herniation and gangrene of four fifths of the small intestine and all of the sigmoid colon who had a 2-year history of postprandial periumbilical pain, nausea, abdominal distention, and constipation lasting for 2 to 3 days and then subsiding spontaneously. All these reported case histories imply intermittent incarceration of the mesenteric hernia with spontaneous reduction before the attack that brought the patient to medical attention.

Seven patients had a history of trauma occurring from 4 years to just before the onset of symptoms. In four patients, the symptoms were reported to have started during strenuous activity, such as chopping wood,[47a] cranking a car,[18] pitching forward on the ground,[58] and straining during a bowel movement.[41] Whether the trauma initiated incarceration of a congenital mesenteric hernia or whether the trauma bears some etiologic responsibility as a cause of the hernia can only be speculated from these reports.

On physical examination, these patients inevitably appeared to be severely ill. In every instance, there was abdominal tenderness, which was most frequently right-sided but was occasionally diffuse, accompanied by varying degrees of distention and peristaltic patterning. Peristalsis was obstructive in character in most patients, but, with the onset of intestinal gangrene, auscultation revealed a silent abdomen. A shock-like state was often associated with necrosis of the incarcerated intestine. A palpable abdominal mass was present in 11 patients (7%). Of these, eight patients had gangrene, and one had volvulus of the herniated intestine. The mass was usually sausage-shaped and tympanitic, with a succussion splash elicited in some of the patients. An abdominal mass does not always represent herniated intestines. This is illustrated by the report of Heaney and Simpson,[28] who reported on a patient who presented with two abdominal masses located in the left and right upper quadrants, respectively, both with visible peristalsis. These represented the halves of the stomach compressed by the small intestine that had herniated through the transverse mesocolon into the lesser sac and then through the gastrohepatic omentum. In infants, hemorrhagic discoloration of the skin of the abdominal wall may be noted in the presence of gangrene and perforation of the intestine.[3]

LABORATORY FINDINGS

The laboratory findings are essentially those of acute intestinal obstruction with leukocytosis and varying degrees of hemoconcentration. Strangulation and gangrene occur more rapidly than changes in the laboratory findings, accounting for the fact that the severity of the physical signs, in almost every reported instance, outstripped the severity of the laboratory changes. Roentgenography has been universally of little use in providing clues as to the cause of the intestinal obstruction.

PREOPERATIVE DIAGNOSIS

The most common diagnosis preoperatively was that of intestinal obstruction, in 70% of the patients. In 7% of the patients, a preoperative diagnosis of acute ap-

pendicitis was made. Only three instances of transmesenteric herniation were diagnosed preoperatively as internal hernias. Baty[7] and Johnson[32] each diagnosed an internal hernia from clinical information, and Mueller[47d] diagnosed a transverse mesocolic herniation with the use of a barium enema.

Herniation and incarceration through a mesenteric defect may follow an unrelated condition, and this results in a delay in diagnosis. Barnett[5] reported on a patient with an incarcerated mesenteric hernia, who, together with his friends, had abdominal cramps and vomiting after a beer party and who was at first diagnosed as having gastritis.

An acute intestinal obstruction with strangulation in the absence of an external hernia and with no history of previous surgical procedures must always suggest the possibility of an internal hernia, especially if the patient has a history of chronic intermittent abdominal distress and if a palpable abdominal mass is found on examination. In the case of acquired mesenteric hernia, there is little way to make a definitive preoperative diagnosis over the far more common strangulated intestinal obstruction due to adhesions. The distinction is moot, however, because the pathology is usually obvious at the time of laparotomy.

SURGICAL MANAGEMENT

An incarcerated internal hernia rapidly produces strangulation and gangrene. An early operation, in theory, should decrease the necessity for resection of the intestine, thus lowering the mortality. The importance of severe abdominal pain and vomiting, with other signs of intestinal obstruction, should be recognized early and should lead to early laparotomy. Procrastination can only lead to worsening of the general condition of the patient and further loss of viability of the intestine. Thirteen of the 150 patients collected from the literature by Janin and colleagues[30] were not operated on, and they all died. The mesenteric hernia was completely missed at the first operation in two patients[4,25] and was found but not repaired in a third patient.[49] Although two of these patients were later reoperated on, and the hernias were reduced, all three patients died. Treatment depends on the viability of the intestine. If the herniated loops are gangrenous, resection is necessary, with or without primary anastomosis. If the intestine is viable, reduction of the incarcerated intestine with repair of the defect, using interrupted nonabsorbable sutures, is recommended.[30,73] This was the most common procedure reported, having been performed in 55% of the 150 patients reviewed.[30] It was also associated with the lowest mortality, 20%. Twenty-five percent of the patients had a resection of the small intestine with an end-to-end anastomosis. A Mickulicz resection of the small intestine was performed in 5% of the patients. Each procedure resulted in a mortality of about 30%. One patient had a resection of the colon with colostomy and lived. Three patients had a resection of segments of both small intestine and colon, and all lived. The youngest patient to survive a Mickulicz resection of the small intestine for a transmesenteric hernia with gangrene and perforation of the small intestine was a 2.5-hour-old infant.[65] Note that mortality rates and results reviewed in this overview should be viewed with some skepticism because the reports reviewed span more than 150 years of surgical literature. Mortality rates of patients seen at the time of this writing should be considerably lower.

If a mesenteric defect is discovered during laparotomy for an unrelated problem, it is imperative that it be closed. This is illustrated by Meade's[45] report of a patient who was found at appendectomy to have a defect in the ileocecal mesentery that was not closed. The patient had signs and symptoms of intestinal obstruction 7 days after operation and was found to have 6 feet of gangrenous intestine secondary to herniation through the mesenteric defect.

POSTOPERATIVE COMPLICATIONS

Five early complications were seen after operation. Fecal fistulas developed in two patients who had undergone resection of gangrenous ileum with or without ileocolostomy.[16,71] A pelvic abscess followed resection of gangrenous ileum and ileocolostomy.[16] In one patient, multiple fistulas of the small intestine developed secondary to the ligature of a bleeding vessel in the edge of the mesenteric defect,[71] and in another patient, an abscess of the lesser sac formed after reduction of a hernia of the transverse mesocolon.[55] Both these patients died. The mortality associated with acute intestinal obstruction secondary to mesenteric hernias was 33%, more than double the mortality of acute intestinal obstruction from all causes.

REFERENCES

1. Ackerman J II. Intra-abdominal hernia through an orifice in the transverse mesocolon. Nord Med Ark 1902;2:1.
2. Agarwai SL, Singh RPA. A review of intestinal obstruction. Int Surg 1966;46:113.
3. Arnheim E, Razin E. Mesenteric hernias in infancy and childhood. J Mt Sinai Hosp NY 1961;28:543.
4. Atherton AB. Case of strangulation of a loop of ileum through a hole in the mesentery with a Meckel's diverticulum attached. Br Med J 1897;2:975.
5. Barnett SW. Hernia of the jejunum through an aperture in the mesentery of the small intestine. J Iowa State Med Soc 1934;24:202.
6. Barone CA. Obstrucao intestinal em adulto por hernia transmesenterica de megasigmoide. Hospital (Rio de Jan) 1969;75:115.
7. Baty JA. Internal strangulation through an aperture in the mesentery. Br Med J 1938;1:671.
8. Blandy JP. Neonatal intestinal obstruction from a congenital hole in the mesentery. Br J Surg 1960;48:133.
9. Brown HP Jr. Intra-peritoneal hernia of the ileum through a rent in the mesentery. Ann Surg 1920;72:516.
10. Caire A. Un cas de hernie trans-mesocolique. Bull Mem Soc Chir Marseille 1939;4:418.
11. Cattophadhyay TK, Sarathy VV, Iyer KS. Internal herniation through gastrocolic and gastrohepatic omenta. Jpn J Surg 1982;12:453.
12. Coats J. A manual of pathology. Philadelphia, Henry C Lea, 1883:577.
13. Corberi O, Crespi G, Deho E, et al. Le ernie interne addominali: prezentazione di 10 casi trattadi. Minerva Chir 1980;35:1685.
14. Cullen TS. Intestinal obstruction due to a hole in the mesentery of the ascending colon. JAMA 1936;106:895.
15. Cutler GD. Mesenteric defects as a cause of intestinal obstruction. Boston Med Surg J 1925;192:305.
16. Cutler GD, Scott WH Jr. Trans-mesenteric hernia. Surg Gynecol Obstet 1944;79:509.
17. Dalinka MK, Wunder JF, Wolfe RD. Internal hernia through the mesentery of a Meckel's diverticulum. Radiology 1970;95:39.
18. Deaver JB. Acute abdomen. Surg Gynecol Obstet 1920;30:30.
19. Dickenson GK. Holes in the mesentery with herniation of the intestine. JAMA 1907;48:1267.
20. Dolton EG. Mesenteric defects. Br J Surg 1944;31:275.
21. Federschmidt F. Die praformierten lucken im mesenterialen gewebe: Ihre genese und die in ihrem gefolge auftretenden krankenhaften veranderungen. Disch Z Chir 1920;158:205.
22. Frazier CH. Acute intestinal obstruction of unusual origin: operation, recovery. Philadelphia Med J 1899;3:174.
23. Gatch WD, Trusler HM, Ayers KD. Effects of gaseous distention on obstructed bowel: incarceration of intestine by gas traps. Arch Surg 1927;14:1215.
24. Gatewood J. Intra-peritoneal hernias through mesenteric defects. West J Surg 1934;42:191.
25. Godard II, Smith P. Les hernies de l'arriere carite des epiplons: a propos de quelques varietes complexes. Rev Chir 1929;67:265.
26. Gross RE. The surgery of infancy and childhood. Philadelphia, WB Saunders, 1953:445.
27. Hamaker WD. A unique case of bowel obstruction. JAMA 1914;62:204.
28. Heaney FS, Simpson GCE. Two cases of hernia

through the transverse mesocolon. Br J Surg 1925;13:387.

29. Hommes JH. Darmverschluss durch einklemmung in meseneriallucken. Zentralbl Chir 1930;57:862.

30. Janin Y, Stone AM, Wise L. Mesenteric hernia. Surg Gynecol Obstet 1980;150:747.

31. Janin Y, Stone AM, Wise L. Intestinal obstruction during pregnancy. Unpublished collected series, 1986.

32. Johnson RJ. Internal hernia. Arch Surg 1950; 60:1171.

33. Judd JR. Mesenteric defects with special reference to their etiology and report of rare case of colonic obstruction. Surg Gynecol Obstet 1929;48:264.

34. Kagan M. Ein fall von ileus bei innerer einklemmong des magens und dunndarms in einer mesokolonlucke. Zentralbl Chir 1928;55:1995.

35. Kiebel F, Mall FP. Human embryology, vol 2. Philadelphia, JB Lippincott, 1912:32.

36. King ESJ. Intestinal herniation through a mesenteric hiatus. Br J Surg 1935;22:504.

37. Lefene C. Un cas de hernie transmesocolique. Bull Mem Soc Nat Chir 1927;53:790.

38. Le Moyne JM. Contribution a l'etude de l'occlusion intestinale. Thesis No. 457, Paris, A Parent, 1878.

39. Long ER. Acute intestinal obstruction in newborn infants from hernia of lower ileum through congenital mesenteric opening. Trans Chicago Pathol Soc 1927;12:333.

40. Macklin CC. Alveolar pore in the lungs of man and other mammals. Anat Rec 1935;61(Suppl):33.

41. Marsh H. Case of intestinal obstruction treated by laparotomy: recovery, remarks. Br Med J 1888; 1:1157.

42. May SC, Brintnall ES. Strangulated transmesenteric hernia in an erythroblastic newborn. Surgery 1953;33:312.

43. Mayo CW, Stalker IK, Miller JM. Intra-abdominal hernia: review of 39 cases in which treatment was surgical. Ann Surg 1941;114:875.

44. McWharter CI. Ends of omentum fused through opening in mesentery producing acute intestinal obstruction: chronic symptoms since childhood; resection of omentum with relief. Surg Clin North Am 1928;8:535.

45. Meade HS. Hernias through the mesentery of the ileo-cecal junction. Ir J Med Sci 1942;6:103.

46. Menegaux G. Les hernies dites trans-mesocolique: mesocolon transverse. J Chir 1934;43:321.

47. Mitchell IJ. Strangulated internal hernia through a mesenteric hole. Ann Surg 1899;30:505.

47a. Mock CJ, Mock HE Jr. Strangulated internal hernia associated with trauma. Arch Surg 1958;77:881.

47b. Moore TC. Trans-mesenteric hernia in infancy. Surgery 1957;41:438.

47c. Moulay T, Moulay A, Mathqual A. Une cause rare d'occlusion intestinale aigue: hernie transmenterique du grele et de l'anse sigmoide. Lyon Chir 1971;67:465.

47d. Mueller EC. Congenital internal hernia. Am J Surg 1959;97;201.

47e. Murphy AD. Internal hernias in infancy and childhood. Surgery 1964;55:311.

47f. Nikisin F. A case of trans-mesocolic herniation of the small bowel. Cas Lek Cesk 1927;66:429.

47g. Odermatt W: Die hernien der bursa omentalis. Schweiz Med Wochenschr 1926;56:459.

48. Pfanner W, Staunig K. Ueber die netzbeutel-hernien und ihre bezeilhungen zum ulcus ventriculi: Zugleich ein beitrag zur rontgendiagnostik derselben. Bruns Beitr Klin Chir 1921;121:376.

49. Pringle J II. Hernia across the lesser sac of the peritoneum. Glasgow Med 1919;4:129.

50. Pye-Smith RJ. Acute intestinal obstruction caused by a fish-fin lodging above a Meckel's diverticulum. Lancet 1889;1:472.

51. Reinhardt AD. Hernia mesocolica media and hernia bursae omentalis mesocolica. Beitr Pathol Anat 1916;63:649.

52. Rivkind AI, Shiloni E, Muggia-Sullam M, et al. Paracecal hernia: a cause of intestinal obstruction. Dis Colon Rectum 1986;29:752.

53. Rokitansky C. Uber innerer darmeinschnurungen. Med Jahrb Osterr Staates 1836;19:632.

54. Rooney JA, Carroll JP, Keeley JL. Internal hernias due to defects in the meso-appendix and mesentery of small bowel, and probable Ivemark syndrome. Ann Surg 1963;157:254.

55. Schumacher ED. Die hernien der bursa omentalis mit abnormen eintrittspforten: Die transhaesio intestini. Beitr Klin Chir 1910;66:507.

56. Sharma BD, Bhargava KS, Galviya UL. Transmesenteric hernia. Arch Surg 1968;96:306.

57. Sohn A. Zur kasuistik des darmverschlusses infloge innerer einklemmung in einer mesenteriallucke und uber den volvulus des sanduhrmagens. Dtsch Z Chir 1921;167:124.

58. Speidel FW. An interesting case. Louisville Med Month 1895;2:479.

59. Spencer R. Intestinal obstruction in the newborn associated with faulty development of the midgut and its mesentery. Surg Gynecol Obstet 1952;95:568.

60. Staab EC. Eight cases of abdominal surgery. St Thomas's Hosp Rep Lond 1891;21:169.

61. Steindl H. Transhaesio intestini tennis supra-gastrica. Wien Klin Wochenschr 1920;15:327.

62. Stocker-Dreyer V. Uber lucken im mesocolon transversum: correspondence. Blatt Schweiz Aertze 1919;49:1985.

63. Strenger G. Intestinal obstruction due to mesenteric hiatus. Am J Surg 1949;78:129.

64. Taneja OP, Eggleston FC. Factors influencing morbidity and mortality in acute intestinal obstruction. Indian J Surg 1962;24:755.

65. Tow A, Hurwitt ES, Wolf JA. Meconium peritonitis due to incarcerated mesenteric hernia. Am J Dis Child 1954;87:192.

66. Treves F. Surgical applied anatomy. Philadelphia, Henry C Lea, 1883:298.

67. Treves F. The anatomy of the intestine, anus, and peritoneum in man. Br Med J 1885;1:470.

68. Treves F. Hunterian lectures, 1885. The anatomy of

the intestinal canal and peritoneum in man. London, HK Lewis, 1885:28.

69. Turel SJ. Mesenteric holes or rents as a cause of intestinal obstruction. Int J Surg 1932;45:462.
70. Watson LR. Hernia. St Louis, CV Mosby, 1938:420.
71. White A. Mesenteric hernia and double volvulus in the African in Rhodesia. J R Coll Surg Edinburgh 1962;7:138.
72. Williamson JCFL. Internal hernia through congenital aperture in mesentery: strangulation. Br J Surg 1933;20:684.
73. Yip AWC, Tan KK, Choi TK. Mesenteric hernias through defects of the mesosigmoid. Aust N Z J Surg 1990;60:396.
74. Zimmerman LM, Laufman H. Intra-abdominal hernias due to developmental and rotational anomalies. Ann Surg 1953;138:82.

Editor's Comment

A number of peculiar internal hernias evolve, including paraduodenal and paracecal hernias, hernias of the intersigmoid fossae and foramen of Winslow, defects in the small intestinal and colonic mesenteries, and omental holes. Pritchard and Price-Thomas (Dis Colon Rectum 1986;29:657) reported for the first time the interposition of transverse colon in the subphrenic space, but in that instance, the colon passed posterior to the liver. This is in contrast to Chilaiditi syndrome, in which the intestine passes anterior to the liver to reach the right anterior subphrenic space. The syndrome occurs more readily if the liver is small or atrophic, the intestine is unduly mobile, the thoracic cage is wide (emphysema), the diaphragm exhibits eventration or a hernial defect, or the abdominothoracic pressure gradient is increased. In most patients, Chilaiditi syndrome is an incidental roentgenographic finding, and the patients have no symptoms. Contrariwise, in the patients presented by Pritchard and Price-Thomas, the colon passed posterior to the liver and became incarcerated in the subphrenic space with subsequent progression to obstruction and strangulation.

L.M.N.

Hernia, Fourth Edition, edited
by Lloyd M. Nyhus and Robert E. Condon.
J.B. Lippincott Company, Philadelphia © 1995.

Chapter 35

Retroanastomotic Hernia

Joseph M. Vitello and Robb H. Rutledge

Retroanastomotic hernias are uncommon, often difficult to diagnose, and, most important, frequently preventable. This acquired, internal hernia causes no more than 0.6% to 5.8% of all cases of intestinal obstruction. Failure to diagnose and properly treat this condition may result in significant morbidity and mortality. The original description of a retroanastomotic hernia occurred as a complication of a gastrojejunostomy, although herniation of bowel theoretically may occur behind any anastomosis. Herniation may involve an afferent or efferent loop, or occur regardless of the type of anastomosis or the direction of the intestinal segment. Once awareness exists regarding the potential for retroanastomotic herniation, simple maneuvers to prevent this iatrogenic problem are easy to undertake.

HISTORICAL ACCOUNT

In 1897, Bunddee[3] described the death of a patient with a retroanastomotic hernia that occurred 2 weeks after a gastroenterostomy for malignant gastric outlet obstruction. Bunddee's recommendation was to obliterate the retroanastomotic space with omentum, and this still represents a viable option to prevent herniation. Petersen[20] reported two similar fatal occurrences in 1900. His advice was to close all gaps and construct the afferent loop as short as possible. Because of his excellent, well-illustrated report, he generally is given credit for describing this condition. The first afferent loop retroanastomotic hernia was reported by Kelling[12] in 1900 and by Weber[23] in 1901. In all these early accounts, the pathologic findings were discovered at the autopsy table! W.J. Mayo in 1902 described the first successful preoperative diagnosis and surgical correction of a retroanastomotic hernia in a patient who had undergone a gastroenterostomy for peptic ulcer disease. Although Mayo succeeded in correcting the problem, he failed to elucidate the important principle of closing the site of the hernia. It was Gray[8] in 1904 who emphasized the critical factor in preventing a retroanastomotic hernia: closure of the retroanastomotic space at the original operation.

This simple, yet occasionally overlooked principle is the key to preventing retroanastomotic hernias. The topic has been reviewed by many authors, including Newsom and Kukora,[18] and Rutledge.[21]

RETROANASTOMOTIC SPACES

After any gastrojejunal anastomosis, potential retroanastomotic spaces are created. The boundaries of these spaces have limited elasticity and, therefore, represent theoretic hernial rings. The spaces are similar whether the operation is a simple gastroenterostomy or a gastric resection with gastrojejunostomy. When an antecolic gastrojejunostomy is performed, one large space is created (Fig. 35-1). It is bounded anteriorly by the afferent jejunal segment, the gastroenterostomy, and the gastric remnant; superiorly by the peritoneal reflections of the gastric remnant; posteriorly by the posterior peritoneum, transverse colon, mesocolon, and omentum; and inferiorly by the ligament of Treitz. These theoretic spaces that may be formed frequently become obliterated with adhesions or adherent viscera. For example, the gastric remnant and transverse colon often are densely adherent, predisposing to an anterior abdominal wall. This adherence explains in part why this type of hernia does not occur more frequently. If a gastric bypass or anterior gastroenterostomy is performed without resection, the boundaries of the hernial space are similar except that the gastroenterostomy becomes the roof of the space and the distal stomach wall forms the posterior margin. A few well-placed sutures will ensure adhesion and permanent obliteration of these theoretic spaces, thereby protecting against future herniation.

When a retrocolic anastomosis is performed, two potential spaces are formed (Fig. 35-2). Because of these spaces and the fact that revision of this anastomosis is difficult, antecolic anastomoses are preferred. The more important lower space is bounded anteriorly by the afferent jejunal loop and the gastric remnant, superiorly by the transverse mesocolon, posteriorly by the parietal peritoneum, and inferiorly by

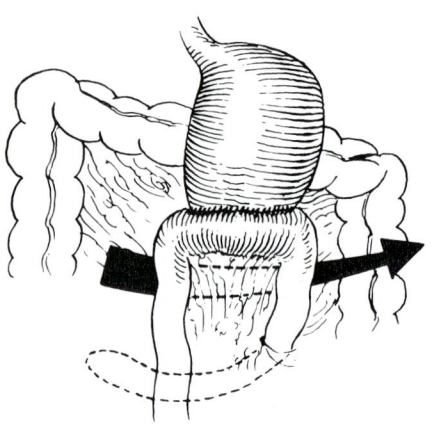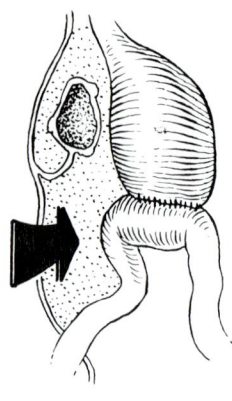

Figure 35-1. Retroanastomotic space after an antecolic anastomosis. (*Left*) Front view. (*Right*) Lateral view.

the ligament of Treitz. There exists a theoretic upper space above the mesocolon; however, no herniation in this area has been reported. The gastrojejunocolic fistula occurs after a retrocolic gastrojejunal anastomosis.

TYPES OF HERNIAS

Retroanastomotic hernias may involve the afferent loop, the efferent loop, or both. Since the development and widespread success of pharmacologic therapy for peptic ulcer disease, the use of surgical intervention for ulcers has declined significantly. As fewer and fewer gastric resections have been performed for ulcer disease, the overall incidence of retroanastomotic herniation has decreased. Highly selective vagotomy is being used increasingly as the procedure of choice for the surgical treatment of peptic ulcer disease, and this should reduce the incidence of retroanastomotic hernia even further.

Afferent loop hernias usually occur after an antecolic anastomosis because the longer afferent segment associated with this procedure may slip back into the retroanastomotic space (Fig. 35-3). Nearly all

afferent loop hernias occur in a right-to-left direction and in cases in which the afferent limb is anastomosed to the lesser curve of the stomach (antiperistaltic). In most patients, the ligament of Treitz is identified to the left of the midline. If the afferent loop is positioned along the lesser curvature of the stomach, the loop must be longer, twisted about 135 degrees, and slightly folded on itself. Markowitz[14] correctly points out that, with this configuration, the surgeon not only creates a hernial ring, but actually places a loop of intestine within it. If the ligament of Treitz happens to be closer to the midline, the afferent limb may come straight up to the lesser curvature. Efferent loop hernias are about three times more common than afferent loop hernias. This is related directly to the surgeon's conscious attempt to keep the afferent limb as short as possible. Efferent loop herniation is equally common after antecolic and retrocolic gastroenterostomy. It does not seem to matter whether the afferent loop is sutured to the lesser or the greater curve of the stomach (Fig. 35-4). About 75% of the hernias occur in a right-to-left direction. It is postulated that the high position of the gastrojejunostomy in the left upper quadrant and the fact that the bulk of small intes-

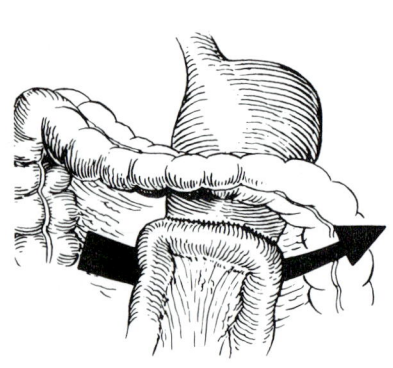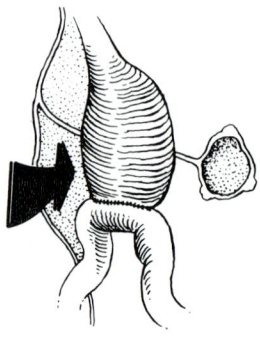

Figure 35-2. Retroanastomotic spaces after a retrocolic anastomosis. (*Left*) Front view. (*Right*) Lateral view.

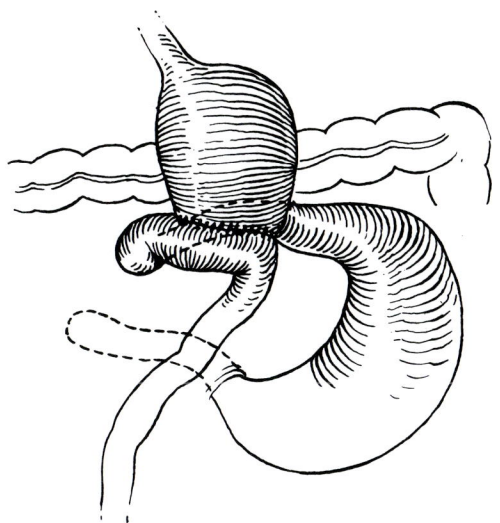

Figure 35-3. Afferent-loop hernia.

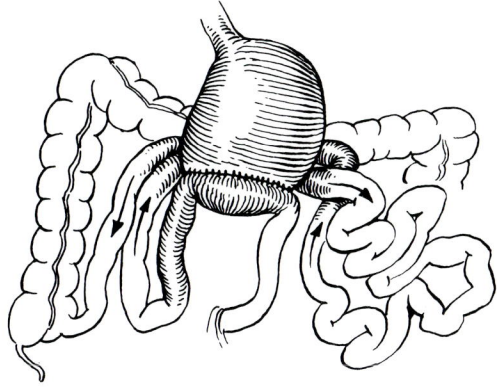

Figure 35-4. Efferent-loop hernia.

tine tends to end up primarily on the right side of the abdomen facilitates the development of a retroanastomotic hernia.[2] This assumption implies that the loops of small bowel remain without adhesions and float freely, which usually is not the case. Actually, a strong case could be made for the formation of small-bowel adhesions in the presence of this type of anastomosis to prevent future herniation. If a hernia does occur, it typically involves a large segment of the distal

small intestine. Rarely, a mobile cecum and right colon may herniate through the retroanastomotic space. Large efferent loop hernias may obstruct the afferent loop, so that some patients may have combined afferent and efferent loop obstruction.

Rarely, a retroanastomotic hernia may contain only omentum. This may result in few symptoms unless there is torsion or infarction of the omental segment or the omentum directly obstructs either the afferent or efferent loop.

Although the classic historical account of these hernias involved a gastroenterostomy, other types of reconstruction after gastric surgery are not immune

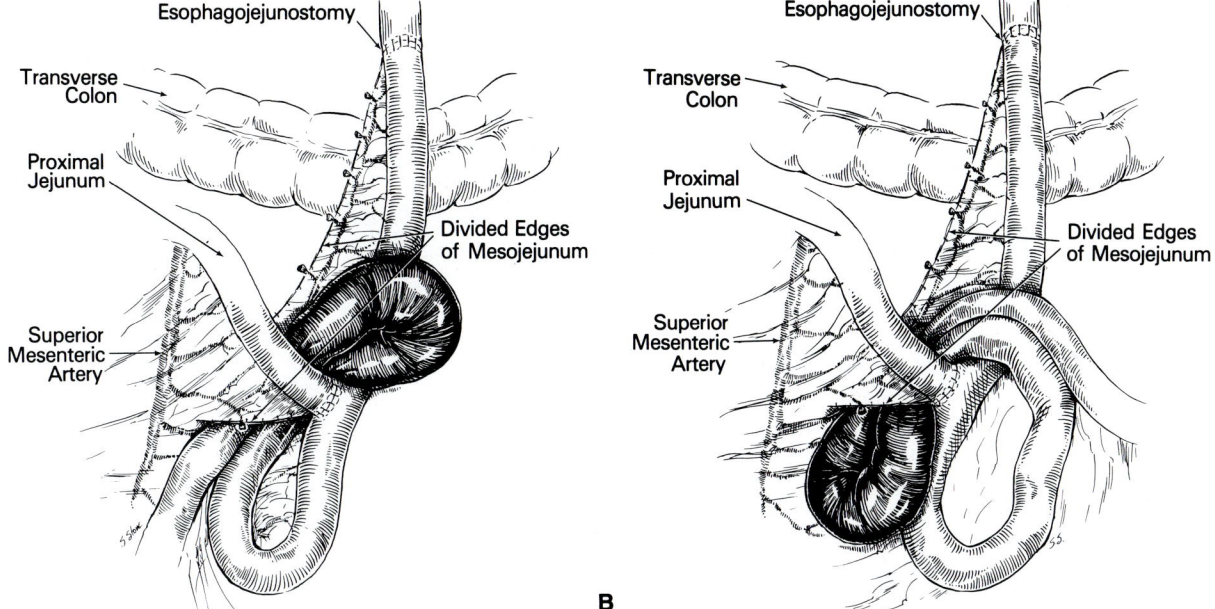

Figure 35-5. Herniation and strangulation of small bowel after a total gastrectomy with Roux-en-Y reconstruction. (*A*) Clockwise rotation. (*B*) Counterclockwise rotation. (Newsom BD, Kukora JS. Congenital and acquired internal hernias: unusual causes of small bowel obstruction. Am J Surg 1986; 152:281)

to this complication. Newsom and Kukora[18] reported the passage of the entire small bowel behind the defunctionalized limb of a Roux-en-Y esophagojejunostomy after a total gastrectomy (Fig. 35-5). These same authors described another hernia associated with a Roux-en-Y anastomosis several years after a pancreaticojejunostomy for chronic pancreatitis.

CLINICAL FEATURES

Internal abdominal herniation rarely is diagnosed accurately before surgery. About 25% of retroanastomotic hernias manifest within the first postoperative month, often while the patient remains hospitalized from the original operation. Another 25% present within the first year, and the remainder are noted any time thereafter.[2]

Patients with an afferent loop hernia usually complain of constant upper abdominal pain. This is in contrast to the typical adhesive small-bowel obstruction, which tends to cause cramping pain. Vomiting usually is a prominent, yet nonspecific finding. The vomiting may be nonbilious and proceed to retching. Physical examination of the abdomen generally does not reveal distention. Bowel sounds may be preserved until late in the course of the disease and typically are not hyperactive or dominated by borborygmi. Mild to moderate tenderness and guarding are noted in the upper abdomen. The presence of peritoneal signs usually signifies ischemia or the occurrence of gangrenous changes in the involved bowel segment. The absence of tachycardia, marked leukocytosis, or peritoneal signs does not exclude gangrenous bowel. It is because of this latter fact that there is a delay between the onset of symptoms and operative intervention in many patients.

Patients with an efferent loop hernia are more likely to have the classic findings associated with bowel obstruction. Colicky, generalized abdominal pain associated with bilious vomiting is typical. Abdominal distention may be more prominent, depending on the length of small bowel involved in the hernia. Diffuse, poorly localized abdominal tenderness and guarding are noted unless the involved segment of intestine has gone on to infarction. If infarction has occurred, the patient may be in shock and have the characteristic findings of an acute abdomen. Again, absence of these findings does not exclude vascular compromise of the involved intestinal segment. If the hernia occurs while the patient remains hospitalized from the original operation, the findings are confusing and delay in diagnosis is the norm. A high index of suspicion must be maintained to achieve a timely diagnosis and avert disaster and mortality. As general surgeons grow more comfortable with both diagnostic and therapeu-

tic laparoscopy, this technique should be considered in patients who have abdominal pain soon after surgery, when many retroanastomotic hernias occur.

Because postoperative pancreatitis is a well-described complication of all gastric and upper abdominal operations, elevated amylase levels often are ascribed to the pancreas. Intestinal obstruction, however, including that caused by afferent or efferent loop retroanastomotic hernias, can mimic postoperative pancreatitis and result in markedly elevated serum amylase levels.[6,17] Failure to recognize this fact can delay diagnosis. Olson and colleagues[19] showed that the hyperamylasemia associated with acute afferent loop obstruction is caused by duodenal hypertension with resultant backpressure into the pancreatic ducts. McGowan and Wills[16] studied 12 patients with Billroth II gastrectomies and elevated amylase levels. In 11 patients, the hyperamylasemia was caused by an afferent loop obstruction. Amylase elevation is not specific for pancreatitis;[22] in the presence of a recent gastroenterostomy, retroanastomotic hernia should be included in the differential diagnosis of upper abdominal pain and hyperamylasemia. Radiographic examination of the patient with a retroanastomotic hernia may be helpful, but is not always diagnostic. With an afferent loop obstruction, radiographs may disclose a distended gastric remnant and a mass in the

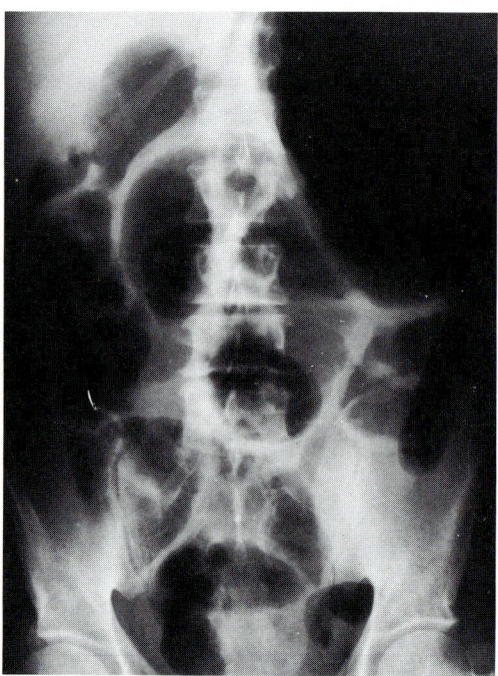

Figure 35-6. Plain radiograph of a patient with an efferent retroanastomotic hernia producing a simultaneous afferent-loop obstruction 3 months after a gastric resection. Massive dilation of the stomach and small intestine is shown.

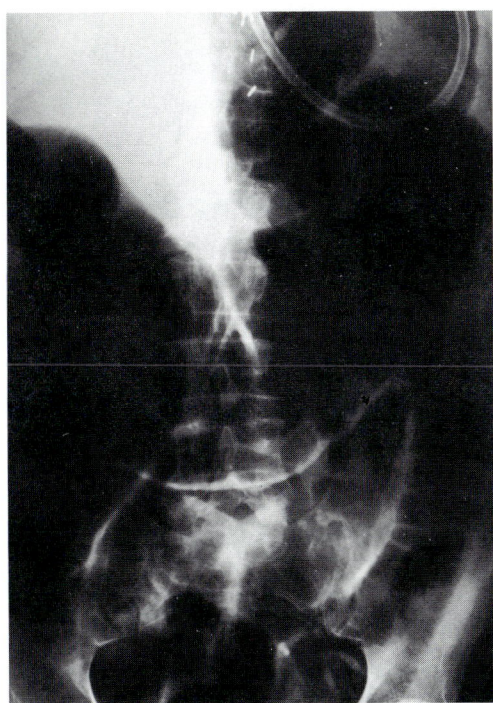

Figure 35-7. Plain radiograph of a patient with a massive efferent retroanastomotic hernia 2 weeks after a gastric resection with an antecolic anastomosis. The film demonstrates marked dilation of the small intestine and right colon.

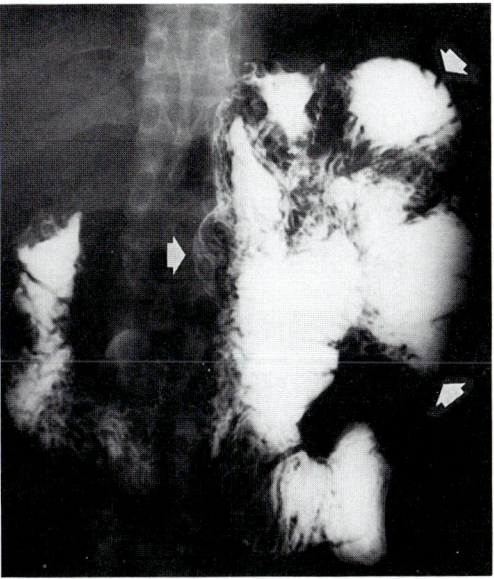

Figure 35-8. Efferent-loop retroanastomotic hernia. Herniated loops form an encapsulated group in the left upper abdomen (*arrows*). An afferent loop with a duodenal diverticulum also is visualized. (Ghahremani GG, Meyers MA. Iatrogenic abdominal hernias. In: Meyers MA, Ghahremani GG, eds. Iatrogenic gastrointestinal complications. New York, Springer-Verlag, 1981)

left upper quadrant. In an efferent loop hernia, the initial films may be normal, only to evolve into a clearly evident mechanical small-intestinal obstruction (Fig. 35-6). If the patient has had a previous antecolic anastomosis, the cecum and right colon may be markedly distended, suggesting a primary colon obstruction (Fig. 35-7). Rarely, a barium contrast upper gastrointestinal study is needed to make the diagnosis (Fig. 35-8). Afferent loop obstruction is more difficult to detect. It may be identified when a computed tomogram of the abdomen performed in search of a cause for abdominal pain reveals a distended, fluid-filled afferent loop (Fig. 35-9). Radionuclide scans

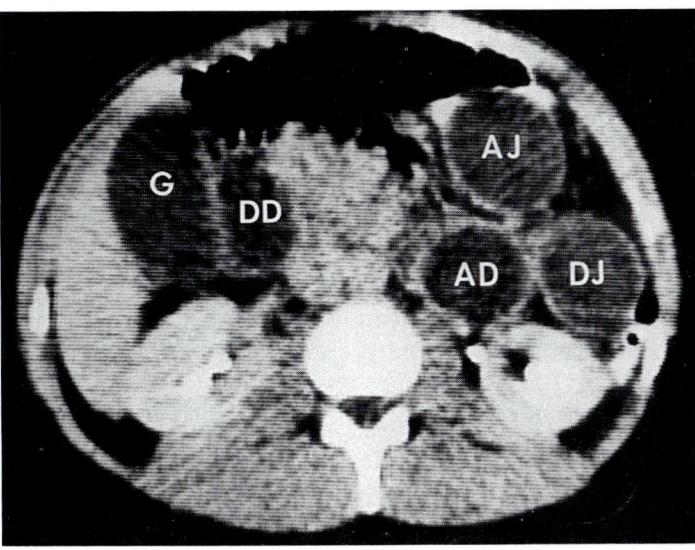

Figure 35-9. The CT appearance of an obstructed afferent loop is highly characteristic, presenting as a constellation of peripancreatic cystic masses of nearly equal diameter. This midabdominal CT scan shows a distended gallbladder (G), descending duodenum (DD), ascending duodenum (AD), descending jejunum (DJ), and ascending jejunum (AJ), all on a long afferent loop. (Gale ME, Gerzof SG, Kiser LC, et al. CT appearance of afferent loop obstruction. AJR 1982; 138:1085)

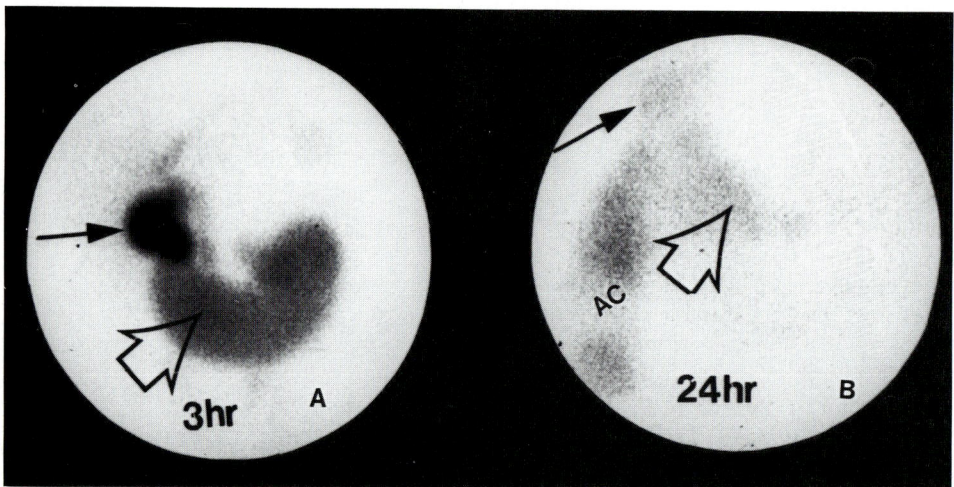

Figure 35-10. 99mTc-PIPIDA scan in a patient with an obstructed afferent loop. Three- (*A*) and 24-hour (*B*) delayed views show residual activity in the gallbladder (*arrow*) and duodenum (*open arrow*). AC, ascending colon. (Rao K, Gooneratne N, Asokan S, et al. Afferent loop obstruction documented with hepatobiliary imaging. Gastrointest Radiol 1983; 8:345)

also can be used to reveal afferent loop obstruction (Fig. 35-10). Isotopic agents excreted by the biliary tree enter the duodenum and may demonstrate an obstructed afferent loop.[7]

Although most cases of retroanastomotic hernia occur as acute obstruction soon after the original operation, about 10% occur as vague, chronic abdominal pain representing intermittent partial obstruction. These symptoms may persist unchanged for many years until the hernia is corrected, or they may progress to a complete closed-loop obstruction necessitating emergent operation.

SURGICAL THERAPY

Prevention is the primary therapy for retroanastomotic hernia. Most of these lesions can be prevented if the surgeon remembers to obliterate the potential hernial orifice. Despite meticulous surgical technique, however, a retroanastomotic hernia may occur and require intervention.

PROPHYLAXIS

If an antecolic gastrojejunostomy is chosen for reconstruction after a gastric resection, the afferent loop should be kept as short as possible. This may be facilitated by the resection of some omentum. The anastomosis should be performed so that the loop lies comfortably (ie, the jejunal loop should not be forced into a position that is dogmatic for the surgeon). Often, the afferent loop seems to lie nicely adjacent to the greater curvature of the stomach because it comes straight up from the ligament of Treitz without angulation or excess length. If the ligament of Treitz is more medial in location, the afferent limbs lie more comfortably and are sutured more easily along the lesser curve of the stomach. In this circumstance, the retroanastomotic space may be closed by suturing the jejunal mesentery to the transverse mesocolon. Adequate space must be allowed for the transverse colon, but this can be accomplished and the possibility of retroanastomotic hernia still be virtually eliminated.

If a retrocolic gastrojejunostomy is performed, the lower hernial space can be closed by suturing the mesentery of the afferent loop to the posterior parietal peritoneum, as advocated by Cannon and Weeks.[4] If the ligament of Treitz and the fourth portion of the duodenum are mobilized, the afferent loop can be made extremely short, so there is essentially no hernial space. Dunphy[5] described the performance of a "no-loop" retrocolic anastomosis by mobilizing the ligament of Treitz and closing the mesocolic defect below the afferent loop. The upper posterior space normally does not need to be closed, but careful suturing of the mesocolic aperture to the gastric remnant is essential in any anastomosis. Addison[1] reported the occurrence of hernias through the transverse mesocolon when this was not done. If these simple maneuvers are used, the incidence of retroanastomotic hernia can be minimized. Newsom and Kukora[18] reported that in only one of six cases of retroanastomotic hernia was specific mention made in the operative note of an attempt to close an offending defect during the original operation. This highlights the importance of closing at the end of each operation all potential hernial spaces that may have been created.

TREATMENT OF EXISTING HERNIAS

As with any hernia, after the diagnosis is secured, a retroanastomotic hernia should be reduced and the defect closed to prevent recurrence. Recalling that most of these hernias occur in a right-to-left direction may simplify the operation. Nonviable or questionably viable intestine should be resected and appropriate reanastomoses performed. The duodenal stump should be inspected, especially if the original operation was recent. If there is any question regarding the integrity of the duodenal suture or staple line, a tube duodenostomy should be placed to help avert the catastrophic events of duodenal stump blowout.

When an afferent loop hernia is reduced, the surgical options to prevent recurrence include (1) shortening of the long afferent limb, (2) anastomosis to the efferent limb, (3) conversion to a Henle type of reconstruction, or (4) change to a Roux-en-Y or Roux-19 anastomosis.[10]

When an efferent loop hernia is reduced, the intestine is less likely to be damaged if it is pushed or "milked" out, as with reduction of an intussusception. Pulling the intestine out may create a tear and result in leakage of obstructed intestinal contents into the peritoneal cavity, placing the patient at risk for an intraabdominal abscess. Decompression of distended bowel may be required to accomplish the reduction, especially if the intestinal loop has been obstructed for a long time. Takedown of the gastrojejunostomy and resection of a segment of chronically obstructed bowel sometimes are necessary to achieve a successful outcome.

OTHER RETROANASTOMOTIC HERNIAS

Iatrogenic retroanastomotic hernias can occur after operations on areas other than the stomach, although historically these are the most common. The principles of therapy remain the same. Prevention is paramount, but once the hernia has occurred, prompt diagnosis and treatment are necessary to avoid morbidity and mortality.

COLOSTOMY

If a sigmoid colostomy is fashioned, a potential hernial space will exist between the colon and the lateral abdominal wall. Internal hernias have occurred through this aperture (Fig. 35-11). This complication

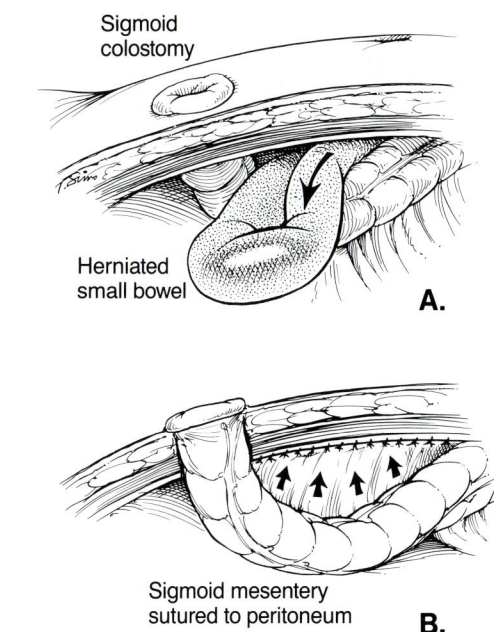

Figure 35-11. (*A*) Small intestine herniated through an unclosed mesenteric defect with a transperitoneal colostomy. (*B*) Closure of the mesenteric defect to prevent a hernia.

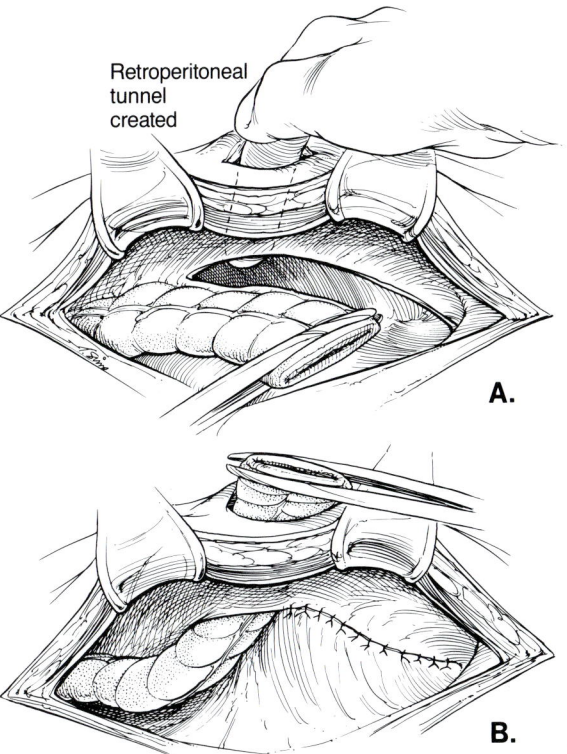

Figure 35-12. Steps in the construction of a retroperitoneal sigmoid colostomy. (*A*) Creation of the tunnel. (*B*) The colostomy in position.

can be prevented by closing the defect between the colonic mesentery and the lateral peritoneal reflection. If this attempt fails, a hernia still may result. Another method of avoiding this complication is to bring the colostomy out in a retroperitoneal path to the abdominal wall. This technique, which often is used in patients with ascites to minimize fluid leak, avoids a potential hernia space (Fig. 35-12). Fixation of the colon where it becomes retroperitoneal remains necessary because a loop of small bowel may slip posteriorly. The high prevalence of small-bowel adhesions probably contributes to the low incidence of this type of hernia.

The operation for an existing hernia involves reduction of the hernia contents, resection of any intestine if necessary, and closure of any defect. Generally, the colostomy can be left unchanged unless a large parastomal hernia is coexistent.

The creation of an ileostomy, a urinary-ileal conduit, or virtually any stoma can result in a potential hernia space. In the case of the ileum, hernia formation can be minimized by suturing the mesentery to the anterior peritoneum, starting at the falciform ligament and continuing to the point of peritoneal exit.

BYPASSED SMALL INTESTINE

Because the jejunoileal bypass for the treatment of morbid obesity no longer is performed, most surgeons will not encounter a retroanastomotic hernia related to this procedure. Although many of these operations have been reversed because of a multitude of complications, there still are patients with intact bypasses who are at risk for the development of an internal hernia.[9] With the Scott modification of the jejunoileal bypass, the distal end of the excluded bowel routinely was sutured to either the cecum, the transverse colon, or the sigmoid. In each case, a potential hernia space was created that would allow a retroanastomotic hernia to form unless the mesenteric defect was closed (Fig. 35-13). A patient with this problem may be seen with the findings of an acute abdomen. Plain abdominal radiographs and contrast-enhanced upper gastrointestinal studies are not helpful because the obstructed intestine is not in continuity with the rest of the digestive tract. Computed tomography can be useful in demonstrating the distended, fluid-filled loops of the bypassed bowel segment. Diagnosing a retroanastomotic hernia in this setting requires a keen awareness of the condition.

Several treatment options are available. The surgeon may be able to reduce the hernia and close the defect. Alternatively, some bypassed intestine may require resection, or the ileocolostomy may have to be disassembled and the distal end brought out as a mucous fistula. Rarely, the entire bypassed segment requires resection.

VASCULAR GRAFTS

Although it no longer is a routine practice, a femoral-femoral bypass graft may be placed in the retropubic position through the space of Retzius to avoid external compression. The graft inadvertently may enter the peritoneal cavity during placement and tunneling, or erode into the coelom at a later date. By either mechanism, the intraperitoneal portion of the graft forms an unsuspected hernial ring (Fig. 35-14). A

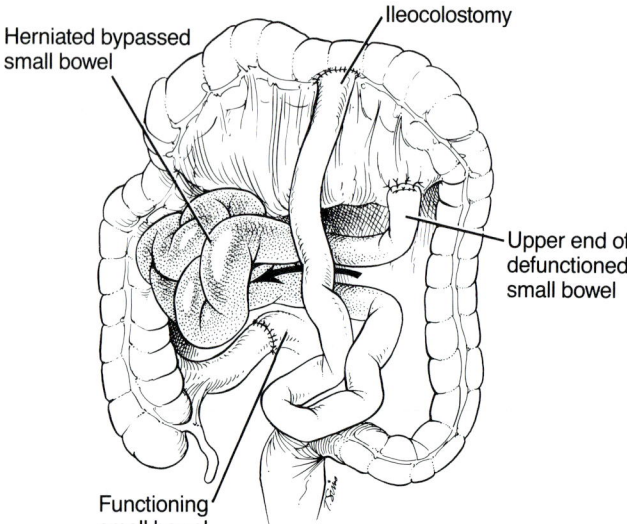

Figure 35-13. Retroanastomotic hernia of a bypassed small intestine after a Scott type of jejunoileal bypass.

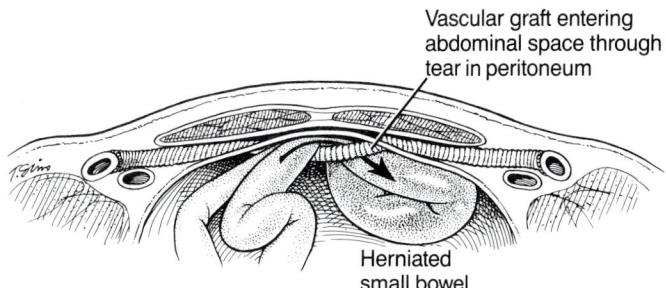

Figure 35-14. Herniated small intestine around an inadvertent intraperitoneal portion of a femoral-femoral bypass graft.

loop of intestine herniating anterior to the graft will result in bowel obstruction.[11] The same potential exists for other intraperitoneal grafts, such as an aortic-superior mesenteric artery bypass or a standard aortic bifurcation graft with a redundant limb that erodes the posterior peritoneum. Confronted with such a situation, the surgeon should reduce the hernia, resect the intestine if indicated, and return the vascular graft to an extraperitoneal position. The graft itself usually is not infected, but the surgeon must use good judgment and clinical correlation with the patient's condition and presentation to make this determination.

PARATRANSPLANT HERNIAS

Kyriakides and coworkers[13] reported three cases of internal hernia through a defect overlying a renal allograft. A small, unrecognized rent in the peritoneum

made during the transplant procedure is the most likely predisposing cause of such a hernia. The small intestine herniates through this tear and comes to lie over the extraperitoneal transplant (Fig. 35-15).

Although the clinical features often resemble those of small-intestinal obstruction from other causes, the diagnosis may be confused with a rejection episode. Because the immune systems are suppressed in transplant recipients and peritonitis has a high mortality rate in this patient population, this retroanastomotic hernia represents a surgical emergency.

CONCLUSIONS

Retroanastomotic hernias are rare and potentially preventable. With the decline in elective gastric surgery, the frequency of these hernias associated with gastroenterostomy is decreasing. Retroanastomotic hernias can occur around colostomies, ileostomies, bypassed small intestine, vascular grafts, and renal transplants. Prompt diagnosis, often based on a high index of suspicion, and expeditious surgical intervention are essential to minimize the morbidity and mortality related to these iatrogenic intraabdominal hernias.

REFERENCES

1. Addison NV. Herniation through the transverse mesocolon following partial gastrectomy. Br J Surg 1960;47:381.
2. Bastable JRG, Huddy PE. Retroanastomotic hernia. Br J Surg 1960;48:183.
3. Bunddee. Demonstration eines falles von Achsendrehung des Dunndarms und des Zugehorigen Mesenteriums. Dtsch Med Wochenschr 1897;23:146.
4. Cannon JA, Weeks WH. Complications of the internal ring left unclosed in gastroenterostomy. Ann Surg 1953;138:772.
5. Dunphy JE. A method of handling the jejunal loop in gastrectomy with a posterior anastomosis. Surg Gynecol Obstet 1960;110:109.
6. Everett WG, Sampson D. Afferent loop obstruction mimicking acute pancreatitis. Br J Surg 1969;56:843.

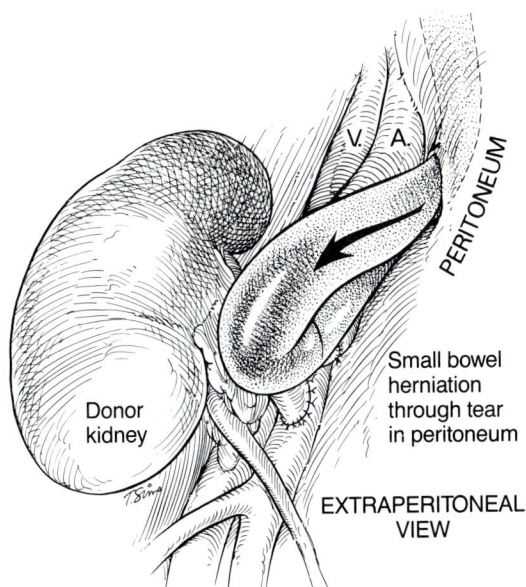

Figure 35-15. Paratransplant hernia. Small intestine herniating through a peritoneal tear made during extraperitoneal renal transplantation.

7. Ghahremani GG. Internal abdominal hernias. Surg Clin North Am 1984;64:393.

8. Gray HMW. A cause of intestinal obstruction after gastroenterostomy. Lancet 1904;2:256.

9. Harmon JW, Aliapoulas M, Braasch JW. The excluded small bowel segment. Arch Surg 1976;111:953.

10. Herrington JL. The afferent loop syndrome. Am Surg 1968;34:321.

11. Jordan FT, Schurz JW, Hoshal VL Jr. Internal hernia and gangrenous intestine: a rare complication of a femoral-femoral bypass graft. Am Surg 1984;50:290.

12. Kelling G. Studien zur Chirurgie des Magens. Arch Klin Chir 1900;62:1.

13. Kyriakides GK, Simmons RL, Buis J, Najarian JS. Paratransplant hernia. Am J Surg 1978;136:629.

14. Markowitz AM. Internal hernia after gastrojejunostomy. Surgery 1961;49:185.

15. Mayo WJ. Complications following gastroenterostomy. Ann Surg 1902;36:231.

16. McGowan GK, Wills MR. Diagnostic value of plasma amylase especially after gastrectomy. BMJ 1964;1:160.

17. McMaster P, Wijetunge DB. Postgastrectomy afferent loop obstruction due to efferent loop herniation simulating acute pancreatitis. Br J Surg 1976;63:526.

18. Newsom BD, Kukora JS. Congenital and acquired internal hernias: unusual causes of small bowel obstruction. Am J Surg 1986;152:279.

19. Olson C, Hinshaw DB, Carter R. Serum amylase levels in experimental intestinal obstruction with special references to the acute afferent loop syndrome. Surg Gynecol Obstet 1960;110:66.

20. Petersen W. Ueber Darmverschlingung nach der Gastroenterostomie. Arch Klin Chir 1900;62:94.

21. Rutledge RH. Retroanastomotic hernias after gastrojejunal anastomoses. Ann Surg 1973;177:547.

22. Salt WB, Schenker S. Amylase—its clinical significance: a review of the literature. Medicine (Baltimore) 1976;55:269.

23. Weber W. Ueber Misserfolge nach Gastroenterostomie wegen Stenose und ihre Verhutung. Beitr Klin Chir 1901;31:240.

Editor's Comment

Further reading may be found in the writings of Herrington and Sawyers (eg, Herrington JL, Sawyers JL. Remedial operations. In: Wastell C, Donahue PE, Nyhus LM, eds. Surgery of the esophagus, stomach and small intestine, ed 5. Boston, Little, Brown, 1995).

L.M.N.

Hernia, Fourth Edition, edited
by Lloyd M. Nyhus and Robert E. Condon.
J.B. Lippincott Company, Philadelphia © 1995.

Chapter 36

Paraduodenal Hernia
Robert A. Brigham

In my opinion this disease is a congenital anomaly in the development of the peritoneum.
Edmund Andrews, 1923

An internal hernia, according to Zimmerman and Laufman,[13] is a defect in peritoneal development within the normal boundaries of the intact endoabdominal fascia. It may be preperitoneal, endoperitoneal, retroperitoneal, or foraminal. The nomenclature associated with further classification of internal hernias is, at best, confusing. This is partially because of the rarity of this type of hernia and misunderstanding of its pathogenesis. About one half of all internal hernias are paraduodenal hernias. Cogswell and Thomas[3] stated that a paraduodenal hernia is a condition in which most or all of the small intestine is incarcerated behind the folds of the mesocolon, making its entrance in the area of the duodenojejunal junction. Paraduodenal hernias are formed by anomalies of gut rotation and reduction, and may result in intestinal obstruction. More than 1800 patients with paraduodenal hernia have been described, with most of the knowledge concerning this entity derived from isolated patient reports.[6] The clinical importance of knowledge of this lesion lies in the considerable increase in morbidity and mortality that result from delay in its diagnosis. A clear understanding of the anatomy and pathogenesis of paraduodenal hernias aids in the prompt recognition and proper surgical treatment of the condition.

NORMAL GUT ROTATION AND REDUCTION

The primitive gut forms during the fourth week of embryonic life and is divided into the foregut, the midgut, and the hindgut. The midgut, supplied by the superior mesenteric artery, has as its derivatives the small intestine, cecum, appendix, ascending colon, and proximal transverse colon. The midgut initially is suspended by a dorsal mesentery, which rapidly elongates. Because of the limited space within the abdominal cavity, the midgut intestinal loop migrates through the umbilical cord into the extraembryonic coelom as it elongates. The midgut loop has two limbs: (1) a cephalic or prearterial limb, which forms most of the small intestine; and (2) a caudal or postarterial limb, which forms the terminal ileum and right half of the colon. The junction of the two limbs is demarcated by the attachment of the yolk stalk. At this stage in development, the midgut loop rotates 90 degrees counterclockwise in relation to the dorsal mesenteric attachment and axis of the superior mesenteric artery.

Growth and differentiation continue until the 10th week, when the abdominal cavity has enlarged enough to allow the midgut to return to the abdomen. The prearterial segment returns first and passes behind the superior mesenteric artery. As the midgut continues to return, it undergoes a further 180-degree counterclockwise rotation, resulting in the prearterial segment being situated to the left of the superior mesenteric artery and the postarterial segment to the right of and ventral to the artery. After total intestinal reduction, the proximal portion of the colon lengthens, displacing the cecum and appendix to the right lower quadrant.

As the final positions are assumed, the anatomic relations of the prearterial and postarterial segments to the superior mesenteric artery are apparent. Knowledge of these relations provides the basis for proper surgical treatment of a paraduodenal hernia. Fixation of the right midgut occurs last, with fusion of the ascending colonic mesentery to the posterior abdominal wall. The previous small-intestinal rotation results in a line of attachment of the mesentery of the jejunum and ileum from the duodenojejunal junction downward to the ileocecal junction. Numerous reviews have been published concerning anomalies of gut rotation. For an excellent review of the developmental anatomy, the article by Gray and associates[5] is recommended.

PATHOGENESIS OF PARADUODENAL HERNIA

Credit for the first description of a paraduodenal hernia is given to Neubauer in 1786. He attributed the formation of these hernias to a defect in peritoneal development. This precipitated numerous arguments regarding the pathogenesis of paraduodenal hernias and became the subject of extensive anatomic investigation. Treitz and Waldeyer, nearly 100 years later, painstakingly described numerous folds and fossae through which intestine could herniate, resulting in what they referred to as a hernia retroperitonealis. Several other authors added to the growing confusion and terminology surrounding the pathogenesis of a paraduodenal hernia. By the turn of the 20th century, two theories emerged as the most popular explanations for the formation of this entity.

In 1899, Moynihan described nine different fossae in the vicinity of the duodenum. His explanation for their occurrence was based on a process he referred to as physiologic adhesions. Moynihan proposed that the fossae were fusion folds that originated in fetal life. He believed that, during normal rotation of the gut, portions of the common dorsal mesentery adhered to and then fused with the posterior abdominal wall, forming peritoneal folds and a subsequent fossa. The formation of these fossae is variable and their terminology confusing. Most investigators believe that only five of these are of clinical importance. Moynihan[10] proposed that a hernia was acquired by gradual enlargement of an existing fossa. The fossa of Landzert was implicated as the etiologic source for a left paraduodenal hernia and the mesentericoparietal fossa, or fossa of Waldeyer, as the opening for a right paraduodenal hernia.

Acceptance of Moynihan's theory remained until 1923, when Andrews[1] offered a more plausible explanation for the formation of a paraduodenal hernia. He did not dispute the existence of the fossae described by Moynihan, but questioned the mechanism by which the fossa could expand to accommodate nearly all the small intestine. Andrews believed that no differential pressures developed within the peritoneal cavity that could account for this phenomenon. In addition, the content of a paraduodenal hernia consistently was small intestine, with omentum uniformly absent. For these reasons, Andrews proposed that paraduodenal hernias form as a consequence of a congenital anomaly in the development of the peritoneum, with imprisonment of the small intestine beneath the developing colon. As a result, he believed that the term *duodenal hernia* was a misnomer. Although there have been equally enthusiastic proponents for both theories, most surgeons today agree with Andrews.

CLINICAL PRESENTATION AND DIAGNOSIS

Paraduodenal hernias represent the major subclassification and account for 53% of all internal hernias. Although internal hernias are responsible for only 1% of all cases of intestinal obstruction, 50% of patients with paraduodenal hernias have intestinal obstruction. Therefore, general surgeons need to be familiar with and understand this entity. These hernias are encountered in men three times more often than in women, but their exact incidence is unknown.[7] Anatomically, paraduodenal hernias are classified as either right or left, with the left variety occurring about three times more often than the right.

Clinically, patients most commonly have recurrent, ill-defined episodes of abdominal pain, often progressing to partial or complete intestinal obstruction. Actual strangulation of a closed loop of intestine may develop rapidly, with its corresponding increase in morbidity and mortality. The chronic digestive complaints of these patients frequently are attributed to gallbladder disease because the pain often occurs after meals. At times, a patient may describe relief of the pain on assumption of the recumbent position. The results of a physical examination are relatively nonspecific unless the hernia is large enough to produce an abdominal mass. Abdominal distention is a variable finding.

The diagnosis of paraduodenal hernia may be entertained if a patient has these ill-defined complaints that are not clearly typical of any particular symptom complex. A definitive preoperative diagnosis can be made by a well-performed upper gastrointestinal series with small-intestinal follow-through. The first person to visualize an intraabdominal hernia roentgenologically was Kummer.[8] His original description remains the standard today: "There is total absence of small intestine in the true pelvis in the upright position; the small intestine is confined in a smooth, sharply circumscribed mass." Taylor[12] further refined this description by stating that there was a "bunched up appearance of small gut, as if it were contained in a bag." The clumping of intestinal coils that is characteristic of a paraduodenal hernia is seen in Figure 36-1. Exner[4] established criteria for differentiating right and left paraduodenal hernias. Barium studies demonstrate a circumscribed ovoid mass of intestinal loops to the left of the midline in a left paraduodenal hernia or to the right in a right paraduodenal hernia. Despite manipulation by the radiologist, the intestinal coils cannot be displaced. There is an absence of small

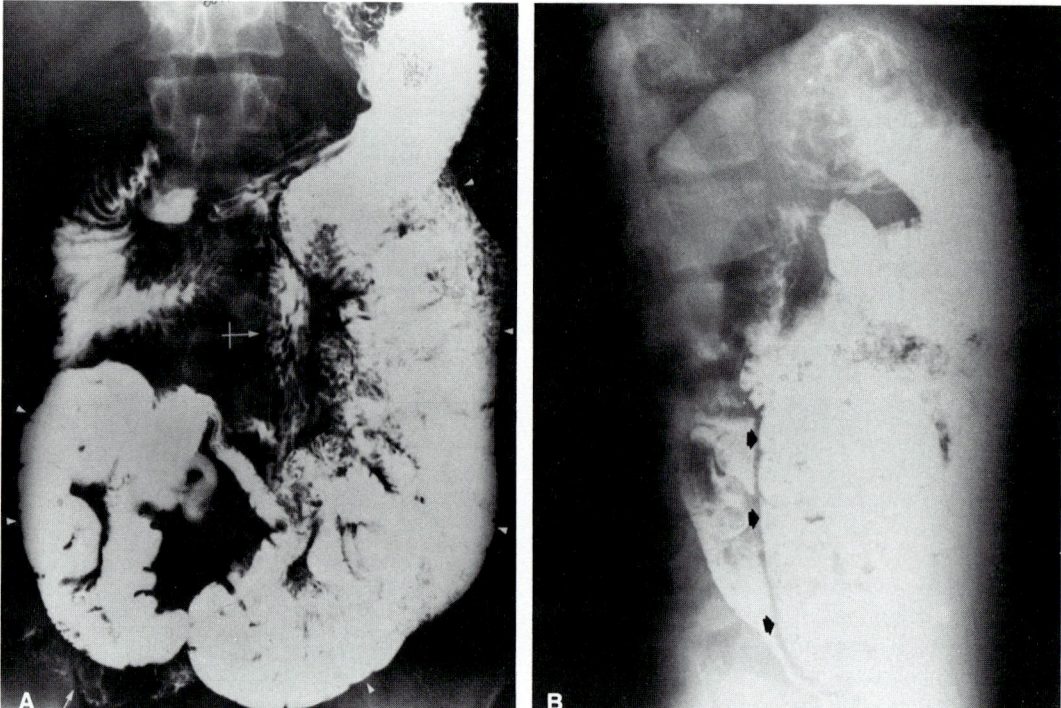

Figure 36-1. (*A*) Upper gastrointestinal series 60 minutes after ingestion of barium. There is a smooth contour to the slightly dilated small intestine in the hernial sac (*arrowheads*). Entrance loop (*crossed arrow*) and short segment of ileum outside sac (*arrow*) are seen. (*B*) Lateral view of upper gastrointestinal series. Arrows mark the classic finding of small intestine posterior to anterior borders of the vertebrae. (Brigham RA, Fallon WF, Saunders JR, et al. Paraduodenal hernia: diagnosis and surgical management. Surgery 1984; 96:498)

intestine in the pelvis except when a greater amount of the terminal ileum is outside the hernial sac. A loss of intestinal motility may be visualized with moderate intestinal dilation.

Another method of diagnosing paraduodenal hernia is based not on visualization of the herniated intestine, but on the disturbances in normal anatomy of the mesenteric vasculature. Meyers[9] noted that, in both right and left paraduodenal hernias, there was reversed looping of the jejunal artery branches of the superior mesenteric artery. He and others[14] advocated the use of selective mesenteric angiography in the evaluation of a suspected paraduodenal hernia. Computed tomography is effective in the preoperative diagnosis of this entity.[11]

Although some patients have complete obstruction and their condition is not diagnosed until laparotomy, many paraduodenal hernias can be detected by these properly performed studies. Preoperative identification of this abnormality allows the surgeon to plan a safe, corrective surgical procedure.

TREATMENT

Whether the hernia is encountered as an incidental finding at laparotomy or is identified adequately before surgery, safe operative therapy requires a thorough understanding of the difference in anatomy between the right and left varieties. The basic principle to be followed is reduction of the hernia and repair of the defect by either closure or wide opening of the hernial orifice. Initial exploration often reveals the classic empty abdomen sign, with only a segment of ileum present in the abdominal cavity and the remainder of the small intestine encased in the hernial sac.

Right Paraduodenal Hernia

An understanding of the anatomic characteristics of a right paraduodenal hernia depends on knowledge of the underlying congenital abnormality. The abnormality occurs when the prearterial portion of the mid-

gut loop is in a nonrotated position. Despite this configuration, the postarterial segment continues to rotate into its normal position. This rotation results in trapping of the prearterial segment in a sac. The relationship of the vascular structures to this sac is extremely important. A fold of mesentery raised by the superior mesenteric artery and ileocolic artery is in intimate association with the neck of the sac (Fig. 36-2). The mesentery of the ascending colon and part of the transverse colon compose the anterior wall. The hernial orifice lies just to the right of midline and is directed to the left, where the afferent and efferent loops of the small intestine can be identified entering and leaving the sac. The duodenum marks the superior border of the hernia and the lumbar spine marks its posterior border.

Knowing the intimate association of the superior mesenteric and ileocolic vessels with the neck of the sac makes the proper technique for surgical correction more obvious. Any attempt to open the sac near its orifice must be avoided because this uniformly results in damage to branches of the superior mesenteric artery and probable compromise of the intestine. The surgical approach to right paraduodenal hernia described by Bartlett and colleagues[2] is recommended. In this approach, the prearterial and postarterial segments of the intestine are replaced in the position they normally would occupy at the end of the

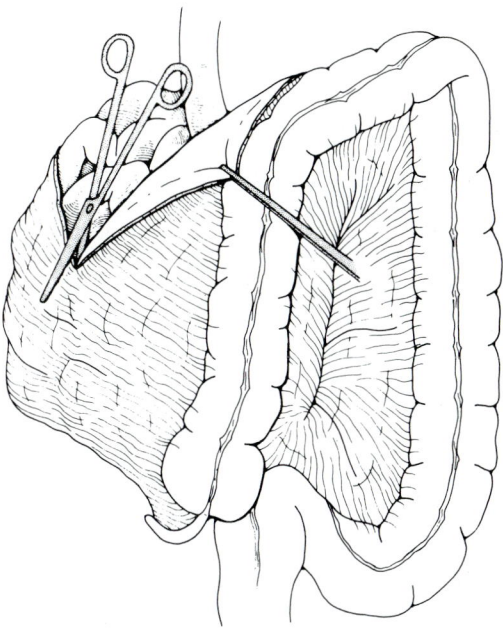

Figure 36-3. Repair of right paraduodenal hernia. Division of the lateral attachments of the ascending colon, transferring it to the left side and allowing reduction of the small intestine. (Brigham RA, Fallon WF, Saunders JR, et al. Paraduodenal hernia: diagnosis and surgical management. Surgery 1984; 96:498)

first stage of rotation, with the duodenum, jejunum, and most of the ileum to the right of midline, and the terminal ileum, cecum, and colon to the left of midline. This procedure effectively eliminates the small hernial orifice and allows for safe reduction of the herniated intestine. It is accomplished by dividing the lateral attachments of the ascending colon (Fig. 36-3) and transferring it to the left side of the abdomen. The hernial sac thus becomes part of the general abdominal cavity.

Left Paraduodenal Hernia

Although it is not as easily explained as a right paraduodenal hernia, the formation of a left paraduodenal hernia follows a similar pattern. This hernia also involves an anomaly of gut rotation and reduction. The prearterial segment of the midgut rotates in the normal pattern. This rotation results in passage of the gut behind and to the left of the superior mesenteric artery (Fig. 36-4). At that point, it enters into the fossa of Landzert, an unsupported area of the descending mesocolon. The intestine then is trapped under the developing mesocolon as the descending colon seeks its normal attachment. The normal attachments of the cecum likewise develop, and the

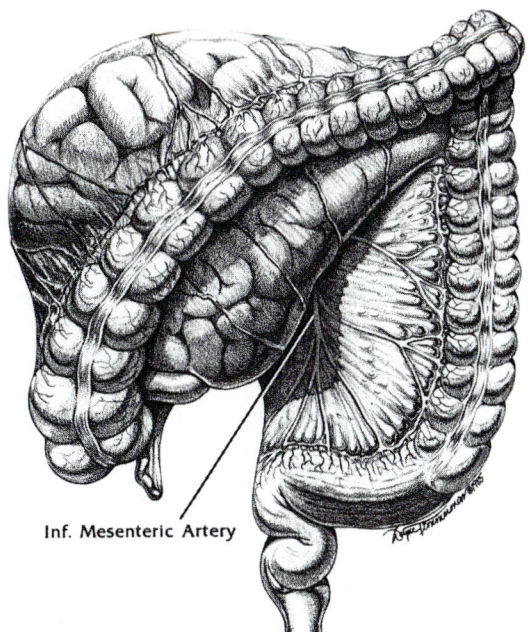

Inf. Mesenteric Artery

Figure 36-2. Right paraduodenal hernia. The hernial orifice lies to the right of midline, with the mesentery of the ascending colon forming the anterior wall of the sac. The superior mesenteric and ileocolic arteries are in intimate association with the neck of the sac.

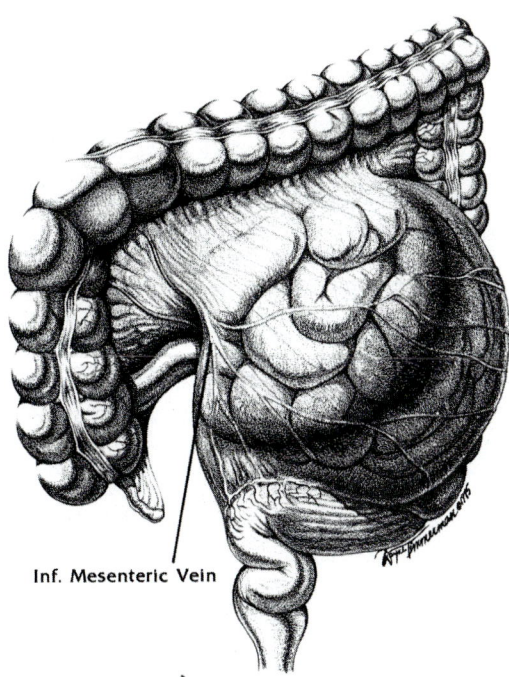

Figure 36-4. Left paraduodenal hernial orifice lies to the left of midline, with the mesentery of the descending colon forming the anterior wall of the sac. The inferior mesenteric vein lies in the lateral margin of the sac.

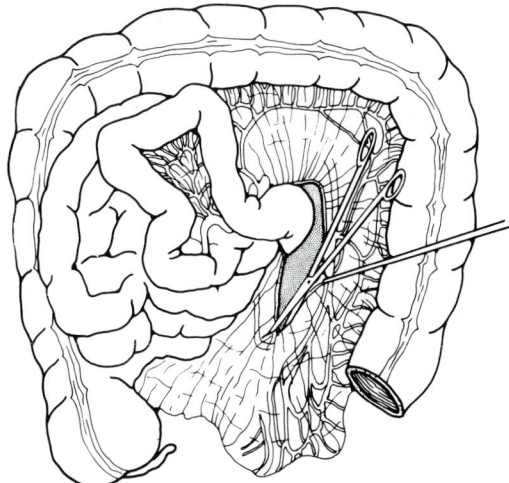

Figure 36-5. Repair of left paraduodenal hernia. Incision of the sac along an avascular plane to the right of the inferior mesenteric plane, allowing reduction of the small intestine. (Brigham RA, Fallon WF, Saunders JR, et al. Paraduodenal hernia: diagnosis and surgical management. Surgery 1984; 96:498)

cecum locates in the right lower quadrant. The inferior mesenteric vein lies in the lateral margin of the sac with the inferior mesenteric artery, and its branches become an integral part of the sac.

This intimate association of the inferior mesenteric vessels with the hernial orifice must be kept in mind during the surgical approach to a left paraduodenal hernia. Extreme care must be taken during attempts at reduction of the herniated intestine to avoid injuring these vessels. Several operative approaches have been advocated to accomplish this task. Although Bartlett[2] indicated that these vessels can be divided without compromising the intestine, preservation of the inferior mesenteric vein and artery whenever possible is recommended, consistent with achieving complete reduction and satisfactory repair of the hernia. This is accomplished best by incising the sac in an avascular plane just to the right of the inferior mesenteric vein, as shown in Figure 36-5. When this incision is made, the intestine is reduced easily and the sac opened widely to the peritoneal cavity. On occasion, the intestine can be reduced manually through the neck of the sac and the defect closed with simple sutures. This reduction is unusual, however, because of the frequent occurrence of scarring and adhesions of the intestine at the sac orifice. Again, if this maneuver is performed, painstaking care must be taken to ensure that the inferior mesenteric vessels are not compromised.

SUMMARY

Although it is a rare cause of intestinal obstruction and abdominal pain, paraduodenal hernia must be considered in the evaluation of patients with atypical abdominal symptoms. The best explanation for the formation of these hernias is a congenital abnormality of gut rotation and reduction resulting in entrapment of the small intestine behind the developing mesocolon. Upper gastrointestinal series with small-intestinal follow-through and computed tomography provide good means of preoperative diagnosis, with selective mesenteric angiography used to define equivocal cases. Once the diagnosis is made, surgical therapy can be carried out if the surgeon possesses a thorough knowledge of the unique anatomy of these hernias. With careful preservation of the mesenteric vessels, the hernia may be reduced safely and the defect closed primarily or the sac opened widely.

REFERENCES

1. Andrews E. Duodenal hernia: a misnomer. Surg Gynecol Obstet 1923;37:740.
2. Bartlett M, Wang C, Williams W. The surgical management of paraduodenal hernia. Ann Surg 1968;168:249.

3. Cogswell H, Thomas C. Right paraduodenal hernia. Ann Surg 1941;114:1035.

4. Exner F. The roentgen diagnosis of right para-duodenal hernia. Am J Roentgenol 1933;29:585.

5. Gray SW, Skandalakis LJ, Rowe Jr JS, Skandalakis JE. Vascular compression of the duodenum. In: Nyhus LM, Baker RJ, eds. Mastery of surgery, ed 2. Boston, Little, Brown & Co, 1992:764.

6. Guillino D, Giordano O, Guillino E. Les hernies internes de l' abdomen: a propos de 14 cas. J Chir (Paris) 1993;130:179.

7. Jones TW. Paraduodenal hernia and hernias of the foramen of Winslow. In: Nyhus LM, Harkins HN, eds. Hernia. Philadelphia, JB Lippincott, 1964.

8. Kummer E. Signes radiologiques de la hernie interne duodenojejunale. J Radiol Electrol 1921;5:362.

9. Meyers M. Paraduodenal hernias. Radiology 1970;95:29.

10. Moynihan GBA. On retroperitoneal hernia. New York, William Wood & Co, 1906.

11. Olazabol A, Guasch I, Casas D. Case report: CT diagnosis of nonobstructive left paraduodenal hernia. Clin Radiol 1992;46:288.

12. Taylor J. X-ray diagnosis of right paraduodenal hernia. Br J Surg 1930;17:639.

13. Zimmerman L, Laufman H. Intraabdominal hernias due to developmental and rotational anomalies. Ann Surg 1953;138:82.

14. Zollinger RM Jr. Congenital mesocolonic or paraduodenal hernias: an embryologic basis for classification and operative repair. In: Nyhus LM, Condon RE, eds. Hernia, ed 2. Philadelphia, JB Lippincott, 1978:488–494.

Hernia, Fourth Edition, edited
by Lloyd M. Nyhus and Robert E. Condon.
J.B. Lippincott Company, Philadelphia © 1995.

Chapter 37

Hernia of the Broad Ligament

Frederick A. Slezak and Thomas M. Schlueter

Hernia of the broad ligament, a protrusion of an intraabdominal viscus through or into a defect of the supporting structures of the uterus, is an uncommon type of internal hernia (Fig. 37-1). Rarely diagnosed preoperatively, these hernias present with acute abdominal symptoms of incarceration and often intestinal strangulation. Primary broad ligament hernias are presumed to involve parauterine defects of congenital, inflammatory, or traumatic origin. Iatrogenic broad ligament defects from uterine suspension procedures or other manipulations of the adnexa with intestinal herniation are secondary (postoperative) broad ligament hernias.

ANATOMY

The broad ligaments of the uterus are formed by layers of peritoneum covering the intestinal and vesical surfaces of the organ. These layers are carried laterally in a tripod fashion to the side walls of the pelvis (Fig. 37-2). The superior extent of the broad ligament contains the fallopian tube. Immediately below the tube, the anterior and posterior peritoneal folds condense to form the relatively avascular mesosalpinx, which is bounded by the fallopian tube superiorly, the uterus medially, the ovary laterally, and the ovarian ligament proper inferiorly. The ligamentum ovarii proprium is a condensation of the posterior leaf of the broad ligament, below which is the broad ligament proper. The anterior leaf of the ligament covers the round ligament of the uterus and forms the mesoligamentum teres. The lateral extent of the broad ligament covers the ovarian vessels, forming the infundibulopelvic ligament, or suspensory ligament of the ovary.

SECONDARY BROAD LIGAMENT HERNIA

Posterior plication of the round ligaments through surgically created defects of the broad ligaments for uterine retroversion was described by both Webster[78] and Baldy.[6] Enlargement of this portion of the medial broad ligament can lead to an internal hiatus (Fig.

37-3). The first case of small-intestinal obstruction through a surgically created defect of the broad ligament from this procedure was reported by Richardson.[68] Hernias through these iatrogenic defects resulting in intestinal obstruction are considered secondary broad ligament hernias.

The popularity of the Webster-Baldy uterine suspension in the early part of the 20th century coincides with numerous reports of intestinal obstruction through medial broad ligament defects. Twenty-nine cases of intestinal herniation after uteropexy have been reported. After Pulrang's[63] summary of this surgical complication in 1944, the frequency of reports has diminished.[41,44,70]

Intestinal obstruction has been described after other types of uterine suspension procedures involving manipulation of the round ligaments without broad ligament defects.[51] In addition, broad ligament defects with intestinal obstruction have occurred after salpingo-oophorectomy.[81]

PRIMARY BROAD LIGAMENT HERNIA

Historical Perspective

In 1861, Quain[64] described the first case of an incarcerated hernia through an aperture of the right broad ligament in a 36-year-old woman at autopsy. Although scattered reports appeared in the foreign literature,[16,24,33,34] Fagge's[25] description of two cases in 1918 renewed interest in this entity.

Seventy-four cases of primary broad ligament hernia have been documented in the world literature, including 47 reported in the English language. Most have appeared as single case reports, with the subject reviewed by Baron,[8] Robert and Margulies-Winaver,[70] and Cleator and Bowden.[19]

Clinical Experience

We have encountered four cases of primary hernia of the broad ligament at Akron City Hospital since 1969.

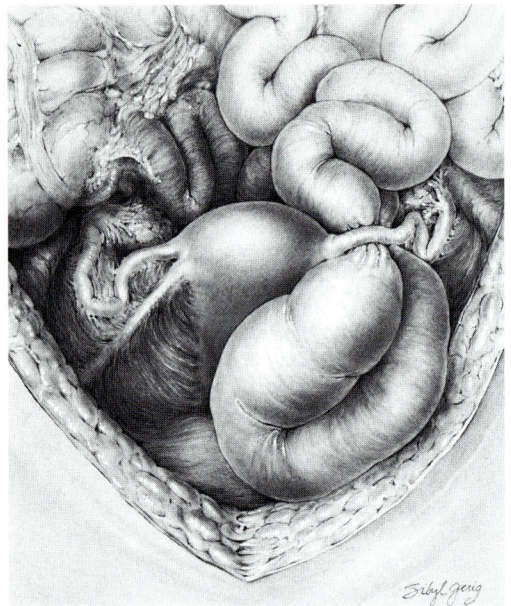

Figure 37-1. Hernia of the broad ligament. Typical appearance with small-intestinal herniation through the left mesosalpinx.

Details of these hernias are summarized in Table 37-1 and are incorporated into this review.

Clinical Features

The typical patient found to have herniation through the broad ligament is a middle-aged woman with small-intestinal obstruction who has been pregnant and has no history of abdominal surgery. The average patient age is 47 years, and the youngest patient ever described was 16 years.[72] The condition occurs most often in the fifth and sixth decades of life.

Incidence

The true incidence of broad ligament hernias is obscure. Hansmann and Morton,[30] in their review of intraabdominal hernias in 1939, found 18 cases of broad ligament hernia in 467 cases of internal hernia, representing about 4%. The authors suggest that an internal hernia in the pelvis of a woman is almost certain to involve the broad ligament. Internal hernias are the cause of about 0.9% (range, 0.5%–3.0%) of all cases of intestinal obstruction.[12] Primary broad ligament hernias comprise less than 7% of all internal hernias and 0.1% of those that cause intestinal obstruction.[38]

Cause

Pelvic infection, congenital defects, and trauma all have been implicated as the cause of primary broad ligament apertures leading to hernia. Infection with destruction of broad ligament tissues and hiatus formation appears unlikely. Quain,[64] Finlaison,[26] and Merscheimer and coworkers[50] report previous pelvic infection as a precursor to the development of broad

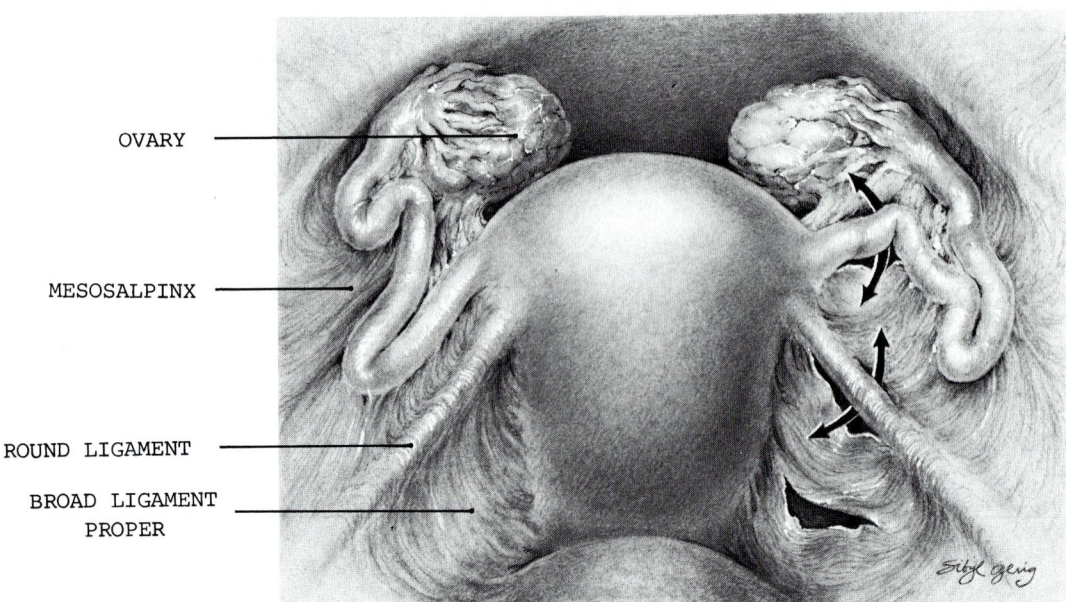

OVARY

MESOSALPINX

ROUND LIGAMENT

BROAD LIGAMENT PROPER

Figure 37-2. Anatomy of the broad ligament and adnexal structures. Common sites of broad ligament defects: broad ligament proper, mesosalpinx, and mesoligamentum teres.

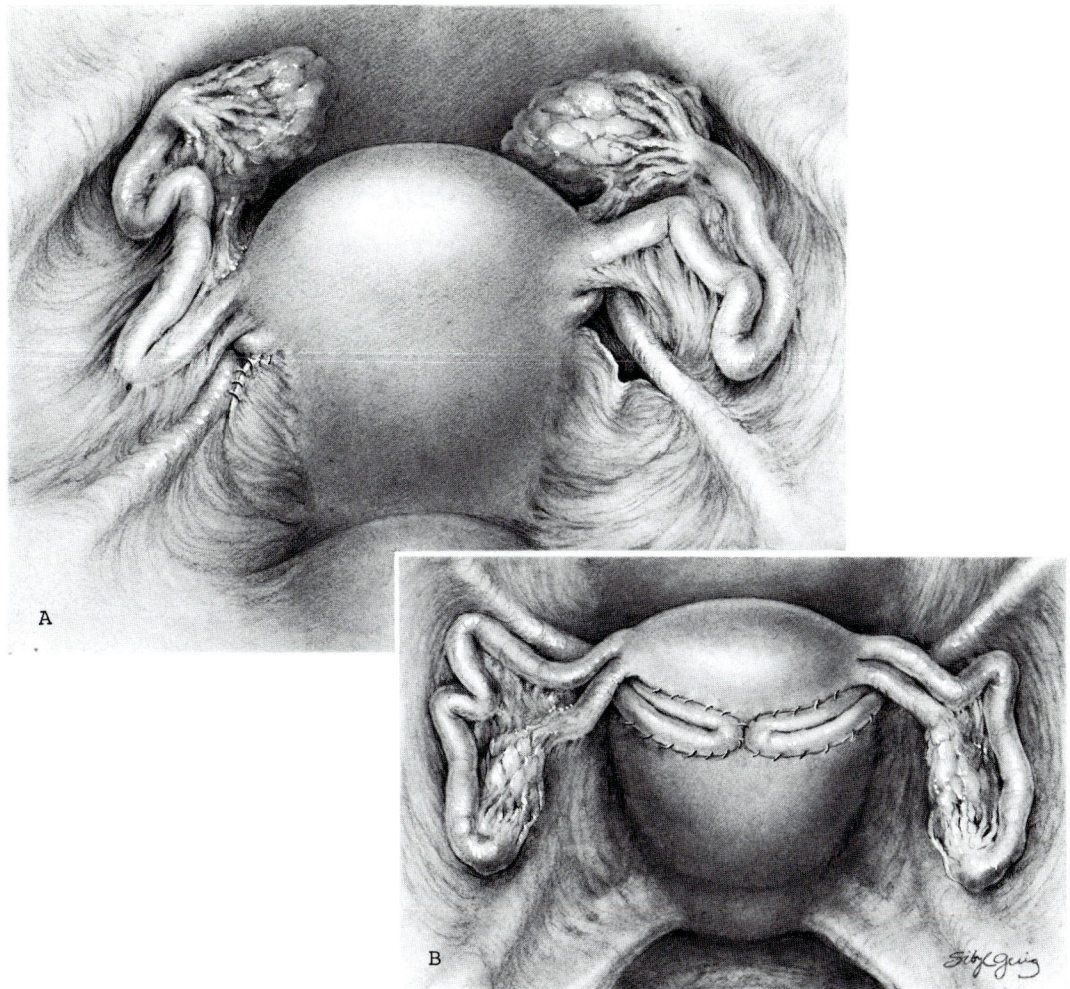

Figure 37-3. Webster-Baldy uterine suspension. (*A*) Anterior view with left parauterine defect. (*B*) Posterior view of round ligament plication.

Table 37-1. Primary Hernias of the Broad Ligament Seen at Akron City Hospital

Patient	Year	Age	Side	Previous Pregnancy	Previous Surgery	Type of Hernia	Structure	Diagnosis	Treatment
I	1969	50	Left	Yes	No	Through broad ligament	Small bowel	Small-bowel obstruction	Closure of defect
II	1969	50	Left	Yes	Yes	Through broad ligament	Small bowel	Small-bowel obstruction	Closure of defect; bowel resection
III	1979	53	Right	Yes	No	Through broad ligament	Small bowel	Appendicitis	Closure of defect
IV	1981	51	Left	Yes	No	Through broad ligament	Ileum	Correct diagnosis by ultrasound	Closure of defect; bowel resection

ligament defects. Biopsy of the fibrous margin of the defect has not assisted in determining the cause.[19]

Defects of the broad ligament without herniation of a viscus, discovered at laparotomy for other conditions, have been reported infrequently.[31,32,35,79] Occasionally included in reviews of broad ligament hernias, these reports suggest that presumed congenital openings in the supporting structures of the uterus are rare.

A congenital origin of parametrial defects has been proposed in 14 cases (19%). Criteria include bilateral defects or nulliparity without a previous pelvic operation or infection. Only eight cases of primary broad ligament hernia are specified definitely as nulliparous, indicating a probable congenital basis for the defect.[4,10,21,25,29,37,72,76] Bilateral defects with unilateral herniation are likely of congenital origin, but have been discovered only in multiparous women.[5,43,57,59] No case of broad ligament herniation in a nulliparous patient with bilateral broad ligament defects has been reported. Occasionally, a congenital cause has been proposed in the absence of the above criteria.[71,74]

The most common cause of broad ligament hernia appears to be trauma associated with a previous pregnancy. Torsion of the gravid uterus may lead to tearing of the uterine supporting structures and subsequent parametrial defects. More than 85% of these hernias have occurred in parous women. In 1955, Allen and Masters[1] described a combination of obstetric laceration of the uterine ligaments and the pelvic congestion syndrome. The authors did not associate these lacerations of the parametrium with broad ligament hernias. Mustier,[53] however, described a patient in whom dyspareunia and dysmenorrhea developed after a traumatic delivery only to disappear during the course of a second pregnancy before the discovery of a nonobstructive broad ligament hernia during a cesarean section. A relationship to both the Masters and Allen syndrome and spontaneous reduction of the hernia during pregnancy was proposed.

Reports of intestinal herniation into the broad ligament occurring during pregnancy have been few. These hernias generally involve the sigmoid colon and the left broad ligament.[14,35,45]

Previous abdominal surgery, exclusive of uterine suspensory procedures, may play a causative role. Manipulation of pelvic structures during laparotomy could produce defects of the broad ligament. Such defects with hernia more accurately are termed secondary broad ligament hernias. Redwine[66] reported a case of small-intestinal herniation through the right broad ligament after electrocoagulation of the same broad ligament for endometriosis.

Anatomic Features

Herniation occurs with equal frequency in the right and left broad ligaments, although defects discovered during pregnancy are left-sided and often involve sigmoid colon. Bilateral defects are uncommon (five cases) and bilateral herniation has not been reported. The direction of the herniating viscus is variable.

Herniation occurs through both layers of the broad ligament in most cases (Table 37-2). Beneath the round ligament (mesoligamentum teres) and through the mesosalpinx are other common sites of defects (see Fig. 37-2). Herniation often occurs into the mesometrium through the posterior leaf. The presence of a hernial sac is unusual and may represent components derived from the remaining intact layers of broad ligament. Therefore, most broad ligament hernias are false hernias.

The herniating viscus is small intestine in more than 90% of cases. Less common structures include sigmoid colon (four cases), ovary (three cases), cecum (two cases), omentum, appendix, and ureter.

Clinical Presentation

Although hernias of the broad ligament have been discovered at laparotomy for other reasons, most present with acute abdominal symptoms. More than 50% of patients manifest findings of small-intestinal obstruction (Table 37-3). Nonobstructive broad ligament hernias apparently are unusual.[21,35,53]

Unless the defect is suspected after previous uteropexy,[2] accurate preoperative diagnosis is distinctly uncommon. Rose[72] arrived at the correct preoperative diagnosis in a 16-year-old nulliparous woman with symptoms of nausea and vomiting found to have right adnexal fullness on pelvic examination. Rabushka[65] correctly diagnosed herniation of the sigmoid colon through the broad ligament by barium enema. Suzuki and coworkers[77] suspected the diagnosis on the basis of pelvic computed tomography. The fourth hernia

Table 37-2. Primary Hernia of the Broad Ligament: Analysis of 78 Cases

Site of Broad Ligament Herniation	No. of Cases
Through the broad ligament	36
Into mesometrium	19
Through mesosalpinx	10
Under round ligament	8
Suspensory ligament of ovary	1
Unspecified	4

Table 37-3. Primary Hernia of the Broad Ligament: Analysis of 78 Cases

Preoperative Diagnosis	No. of Cases
Small-bowel obstruction	39
Ovarian torsion or cyst	8
Appendicitis	7
Acute abdomen	6
Correct diagnosis	4
Autopsy	3
Pelvic pain	2
Ectopic pregnancy	2
Cesarean section	2
Ileocolic fistula	1
Pain	1
Volvulus	1
Adhesions	1
Cholecystitis	1

we saw was suspected clinically and confirmed by pelvic ultrasonography. In general, the clinical signs and symptoms are those of acute intestinal obstruction, with sudden, cramping abdominal pain followed by nausea, vomiting, distention, absence of flatus, accentuated bowel sounds, and abdominal tenderness. Pelvic examination may reveal an adnexal mass. Abdominal roentgenograms may confirm dilated loops of bowel with or without a pelvic mass effect. Occasionally, barium enema or other radiologic studies may lead to a correct diagnosis.

Treatment

Surgical intervention is the optimum treatment, but often is delayed unintentionally until progressive signs of obstruction and bowel infarction are obvious. After reduction of the hernia, the defect is closed primarily with nonabsorbable sutures. On occasion, division of the superior margin of the aperture is satisfactory for both release of the obstruction and treatment; rarely is hysterectomy necessary. Bowel resection is dependent on surgical findings. The opposite broad ligament should be inspected for a similar hiatus.

Morbidity and mortality are related directly to delay in diagnosis and treatment. No recurrences have been reported.

SUMMARY

Hernia of the broad ligament is an unusual internal hernia, representing less than 7% of all internal hernias. Obstetric trauma may be a causative factor in most cases. Secondary herniation through the broad ligament can occur after surgical manipulation of the adnexal structures, especially after uterine suspension procedures. The diagnosis should be considered in a woman with acute intestinal obstruction who has a history of previous uteropexy. A small-bowel obstruction arising in the pelvis of a parous woman who has not had an abdominal operation is likely to involve the broad ligament.

REFERENCES

 1. Allen WM, Masters WH. Traumatic laceration of uterine support. Am J Obstet Gynecol 1955;70:500.
 2. Amadei A. Occlusione intestinale da pregressa isteropessia alla Dartigues. Gior Ital Chir 1946;2:261.
*3. Andren-Sandberg A, Ihse I. False hernia through parametric defects. Acta Chir Scand 1981;147:381.
 4. Arianoff AA, Vielle G, Gose CL, Dewulf E. Obstruction by a hernia of the small gut in an opening of the suspensory ligament. Acta Gastroenterol Belg 1972;35:400.
 5. Armstrong CP, Drummond A. Small bowel obstruction and perforation through a defect in the broad ligament. J R Coll Surg Edinb 1983;28:333.
 6. Baldy P. Retroplacements of the uterus and their treatment. Surg Gynecol Obstet 1903;28:333.
*7. Bard P. Occlusion du grêle dans une brèche péritonéale du Douglas. Lyon Chir 1945;40:216.
 8. Baron A. Defect in the broad ligament and its association with intestinal strangulation. Br J Surg 1948;36:91.
*9. Barr HA. Strangulated hernia of the small intestine through the left broad ligament. South Texas Med Rec 1920;14:5.
10. Bartsch GH. Darmeinklemmung durch Luckenbildung im breiten Mutterband. Zentralbl Chir 1940;67:1714.
*11. Bates GJ, Bennett IC, Furnival CM, Gough IR. A strangulated hernia through the broad ligament causing ureteric obstruction. J R Coll Surg Edinb 1983;28:335.
12. Bertelsen S. Mesenteric hernia. In: Nyhus LM, Condon RE, eds. Hernia, ed 2. Philadelphia, JB Lippincott, 1978:485.
*13. Bolin TE. Internal herniation through the broad ligament. Acta Chir Scand 1987;153:691.
14. Bordenca MJ. Hernia through the broad ligament complicating pregnancy. Obstet Gynecol 1959;13:311.
*15. Bowles HE. Hernia through the broad ligament. Surgery 1939;5:382.
16. Burianek B. Incarceration of a loop of the small intestine between folds of the broad ligament of the right side. Cas Lek Cesk 1914;53:789.

*Patient reports included in tables in this chapter.

*17. Caplan S. Strangulated hernia of the broad ligament. BMJ 1930;1:950.

*18. Cilley R, Poterack K, Lemmer J, Dafoe D. Defects of the broad ligament of the uterus. Am J Gastroenterol 1986;81:389.

19. Cleator IGM, Bowden WM. Bowel herniation through a defect of the broad ligament. Br J Surg 1972;59:151.

*20. Cooper RW. Strangulation of small intestine. Aust N Z J Surg 1931;1:325.

21. Delannoy E, Gautier P, Devambez J. Hernie de l'appendice à travers une brèche du ligament large: découverte opératoire chez une malade atteinte de cancer du corps associée à un fibrome utérin calcifié at a un kyste dermoïde de l'ovaire. Bull Assoc Gynecol Obstet 1950;2:439.

*22. Dornan WE. Hernia into the broad ligament. BMJ 1928;2:528.

*23. Dunn L. Hernia in the broad ligament from the clinical viewpoint. Surg Gynecol Obstet 1926;42:398.

24. Ertl. Darmeinklemmung bewirkt durch einem Spalt des runden Mutterbandes. Allgem Wien Med Zeitung 1864;9:231.

25. Fagge CH. Two cases of strangulated retroperitoneal hernia into pouches of the broad ligament. Br J Surg 1918;5:694.

26. Finlaison FH. Intestinal hernia between folds of the broad ligament. BMJ 1946;1:51.

*27. Füssell K. Rare forms of ileus caused by intestinal strangulation. Zentralbl Chir 1937;64:1288.

*28. Goode TV, Newbern WR. Intestinal obstruction associated with defects in the broad ligaments of the uterus. Am J Surg 1944;65:127.

29. Gray TWA, Baillie DM. Hernia of the ovary and fallopian tube into the broad ligament. Can Med Assoc J 1933;29:647.

30. Hansmann GH, Morton SA. Intra-abdominal hernia. Arch Surg 1939;39:973.

31. Herrmann E. Aus dem Krankenhous der Wiener Kaufmannschaft Recessus Parauterinus. Zentralbl Gynakol 1925;45:63.

32. Hightower CC, Hightower CC Jr. Congenital hernia of the posterior sheath of the broad ligament. Miss Dr 1948;25:391.

33. Holmer. Om Laparotomi eller Enterotomi i Tilfälde af "Ileus." Nord Med 1874;6:1.

34. Honsell B. Ueber Darmeinklemmung in einer Lücke der Mutterbänder. Beitr Klin Chir 1900;29:374.

35. Hunt AB. Fenestrae and pouches in the broad ligament as an actual and potential cause of strangulated intra-abdominal hernia. Surg Gynecol Obstet 1934;58:906.

*36. Janes R. Two cases of intestinal obstruction due to strangulation of a loop of small intestine in an opening of the left broad ligament. Br J Surg 1929;17:333.

37. Johnson GL. Intestinal obstruction secondary to a hiatus in the uterine broad ligament. Mil Med 1965;130:1014.

38. Jones TW. Paraduodenal hernia and hernias of the foramen of Winslow. In: Nyhus LM, Harkins HN, eds. Hernia. Philadelphia, JB Lippincott, 1964:577–578.

*39. Karaharju E, Hakkiluoto A. Strangulation of small intestine in an opening of the broad ligament. Int Surg 1975;60:430.

*40. Koch HC. Ein Fall von Hernia interna in einmen Loch im Ligamentum latum. Der Chirurg 1941;13:23.

*41. Kristiansen FV. Tyndtarmsstrangulation i defekter i parametriet. Ugeskr Laeger 1979;141:3455.

*42. Kyosola K. Simultaneous occurrence of ovarian torsion and gangrenous strangulation through a congenital opening in the mesosalpinx. Ann Chir Gynaecol 1977;66:290.

43. Leahy P, Galvin C. Small bowel obstruction through a defect in the broad ligament. Ir Med J 1984;77:355.

44. Livaudais W Jr, Hartong JM, Otterson WN. Small bowel herniation through a defect in the broad ligament. Am J Obstet Gynecol 1979;133:927.

45. Masmonteil F, Vautier J. Intestinal occlusion during pregnancy; strangulation of sigmoid in breech of broad ligament; case. Bull et Mem Soc d Chir de Paris 1938;30:463.

*46. Massè, Ducassou. Deux nouveaux cas d'entranglement de l'intestin à travers le ligament large. Mem Acad de Chir 1949;75:648.

*47. Masson JC, Atkinson W. Hernias into the broad ligament. Proc Staff Mayo Clin 1933;8:293.

*48. Matheson NM. Unusual cause of intestinal obstruction. J Obstet Gynecol Br Emp 1934;41:410.

*49. Mathieson AJM, Millar WG. Ileovaginal fistula complicating internal hernial strangulation through a broad ligament defect. Br J Surg 1971;58:353.

50. Merscheimer WL, Kazarian KK, Roeder WJ. Internal hernia due to defects in the broad ligament: report of two cases. Rev Surg 1973;30:241.

51. Michael MA. Internal hernia following round ligament suspension. JAMA 1936;107:1293.

*52. Muheim E. Strangulation of the small intestine into the ligamentum latum. Schweiz Med Wochenschr 1960;90:988.

53. Mustier MJ. A propos d'un cas de hernie de l'intestin à travers une brèche du ligament large. Bull Fed Gynecol Obstet Franc 1964;16:377.

*54. Natalini G, Trancanelli V, Gerli P, et al. Ernia interna di un orificio del legamento largo dell'utero. Minerva Chir 1980;35:1359.

*55. Nikolajsen IL, Toft P. Tyndtarmshernie gennem en defekt i ligamentum latum. Ugeskr Laeger 1986;148:1833.

*56. Panek V, Pros JR. Acute intestinal occlusion due to diseases or abnormalities of adnexa. Cas Lek Cesk 1950;89:943.

57. Papas HN. Intestinal obstruction associated with pouches and fenestrae in the broad ligament. Am J Obstet Gynecol 1960;80:172.

*58. Papin M. Hernie étranglée è travers le ligament large. Mem Acad de Chir 1944;70:123.

59. Petereit MF. Internal hernia through a mesosalpinx

defect: a rare cause of distal mechanical small bowel obstruction. S D J Med 1973;26:29.

*60. Pidcock BH. Two cases of intestinal obstruction. BMJ 1924;1:369.

*61. Probst H, Wetzels E. Lückenbildung in der Plica lata. Klin Khir 1952;184:285.

*62. Puhr L. Innere inkarceration auf Grund der Entwicklungsstörungen der Plica Lata. Orv Hetil 1931:16.

63. Pulrang S. Disastrous sequelae to the Webster-Baldy operation. Am J Surg 1944;65:281.

64. Quain. Case of internal strangulation of a large portion of the ileum. Trans Pathol Soc Lond 1861;7:103.

65. Rabushka SE. Colon hernia through a hiatus in the broad ligament. Obstet Gynecol 1968;31:261.

66. Redwine DB. Symptomatic internal hernia of the broad ligament: a complication of electrocoagulation therapy of endometriosis. Obstet Gynecol 1989;73:495.

*67. Reineke ED. Foramen-like defects in the broad ligament of the uterus. Zentralbl Allg Pathol 1937;69:81.

68. Richardson EP. Intestinal obstruction following the Webster-Baldy operation for retroversion. Surg Gynecol Obstet 1920;31:90.

*69. Ritchie AJ, Humphreys WG. Internal herniation of small bowel through a broad ligament defect. Br J Hosp Med 1991;45:109.

70. Robert GH, Margulies-Winaver D. Les hernies de l'intestin à travers les breches du ligament large: contribution à l'étede des hernies internes. Rev Fr Gynecol Obstet 1961;56:283.

71. Rochet, Barrie. Ileus par etranglement du grele au travers d'une brèche du ligament large. Lyon Chir 1979;38:600.

72. Rose D. Congenital bowel invagination into the broad ligament. Obstet Gynecol 1962;21:218.

*73. Sarbu, Pandele. Etranglement de l'intestin a travers le ligament large. Mem Acad Chir 1948;74:434.

74. Shepard VD, Waugh JM. Hernia into suspensory ligament of ovary producing acute intestinal obstruction. Proc Staff Meet Mayo Clin 1942;17:126.

*75. Simstein NL. Internal herniation through a defect in the broad ligament. Am Surg 1987;53:258.

76. Stimson CM. Hernia strangulated through the broad ligament. Am J Obstet Gynecol 1928;15:251.

77. Suzuki M, Takashima T, Funaki H, et al. Radiologic imaging of herniation of the small bowel through a defect in the broad ligament. Gastrointest Radiol 1986;11:102.

78. Webster GA. Principle and practice in surgical treatment of retrodisplacement of the uterus. JAMA 1901;37:913.

79. Williams GA. Arteriovenous aneurysm of the uterus. Am J Obstet Gynecol 1954;67:198.

*80. Zikry A. Intestinal strangulation through defects in the broad ligament. J Egypt Med Assoc 1951;34:670.

81. Zoefgen W. Spätileus durch postoperative Hernienbildung im Ligamentum latum. Deutsch Med Wochenschr 1926;52:450.

General Aids to Repair

Part Seven

Hernia, Fourth Edition, edited
by Lloyd M. Nyhus and Robert E. Condon.
J.B. Lippincott Company, Philadelphia © 1995.

Chapter 38

Anesthesia for Herniorrhaphy

Alon P. Winnie and Richard W. Rosenquist

The selection and delivery of a safe, effective anesthetic for herniorrhaphy is based on several criteria, including the patient's medical condition and preference, the type and location of the defect, the surgical technique to be used for the repair, the anticipated duration of the procedure, whether the surgery is urgent or elective, and whether the operation will be performed on an inpatient or outpatient basis. This chapter reviews the anesthetic options available for herniorrhaphy, with an emphasis on the way in which factors related to the patient, the surgery, and the anesthesia determine the appropriate anesthetic choice for both intraoperative and postoperative pain.

SURGICAL FACTORS

Site of Surgery

The location of a hernia is an important determinant of anesthetic requirements. The repair of a diaphragmatic or umbilical hernia requires profound muscle relaxation, inguinal herniorrhaphy requires much less, and femoral herniorrhaphy requires little or no relaxation. The degree of physiologic dysfunction, and hence the potential for morbidity and mortality, increases with the level of the herniorrhaphy and decreases with the age of the patient. For example, herniorrhaphy carried out below the level of the diaphragm interferes little with ventilatory and cardiocirculatory function in infants or adults, whereas repair of a diaphragmatic hernia can produce severe ventilatory and cardiac impairment in adults, greater impairment in children, and life-threatening ventilatory inadequacy in infants.

Duration of Surgery

The anticipated duration of any surgery can alter the choice of anesthesia. Although regional analgesia can be prolonged almost indefinitely with the use of long-acting agents or continuous techniques, a patient who remains on the operating table for several hours be-

comes uncomfortable in the unanesthetized areas, with resultant restlessness and agitation. This problem can be offset somewhat by the judicious use of analgesics and ataractics; however, excessive doses of these agents produce the central depression and hypoventilation that regional anesthesia is intended to avoid. The skill of the surgeon plays a particularly important role in this respect, because it has been well documented that the likelihood of complications increases concomitantly with the duration of surgery.

PATIENT FACTORS

Physical Status

One of the most important functions of the anesthesiologist is to assess the status of the patient's organ systems and to select an anesthetic that provides the best operative conditions while producing the fewest deleterious effects on organ function. This is the major objective of the preanesthetic visit, during which the chart is reviewed, the patient is examined, additional studies or consultations are requested if necessary, and the anesthetic alternatives are discussed with the patient. In addition to providing the anesthesiologist with critical information about the patient's physical status, the preanesthetic visit also has an important psychological impact on the patient; this visit has been shown to allay apprehension better than any available premedication.

Age

The aging process results in progressive changes in the function of most of the vital organs and in the ability of the body to respond to stress. These anatomic and physiologic changes require alterations in anesthetic technique to accommodate decreased metabolism of injected and inhaled anesthetic agents, and decreased volume of distribution, slower renal excretion, and greater spread of intraspinal local anesthetics.[8] Thus, the induction of both regional and general anesthesia becomes increasingly complex and sometimes hazardous as the age of the patient increases.

Weight

Patient weight is of special concern to the anesthesiologist for several reasons. First, the dosage of virtually all anesthetic agents and adjuncts is based on weight. In addition, morbidly obese patients provide a serious challenge to the anesthesiologist in the administration of general anesthesia, and particularly in the establishment of an airway and maintenance of adequate ventilation. Finally, regional anesthesia techniques are much more difficult to carry out in obese patients because key landmarks are hard to identify and the target of the needle is located much deeper.[1]

Habitus

In addition to anatomic abnormalities, variations in normal body build also can pose a serious threat to the safe implementation of certain anesthetic techniques. Congenital craniofacial anomalies such as the Pierre Robin syndrome present difficult problems of intubation and airway management, as do burn contractures of the neck and face. Subtler and perhaps more treacherous are the airway problems of the pyknic patient, whose short neck, large tongue, and protruding teeth can cause considerable difficulty in establishing and maintaining an airway after reductions of anesthesia, and may provide an insurmountable obstacle to endotracheal intubation. In these circumstances, anesthesia for elective herniorrhaphy should be approached cautiously, because the anesthetic may pose a greater risk to the patient than the surgical procedure for which it is being administered. Regional anesthesia circumvents the entire problem, but may be inappropriate for children and some uncooperative adults.

Respiratory System

The respiratory system is responsible for the uptake of inhaled anesthetics from the anesthetic machine and their delivery to the circulatory system. All anesthetic agents, including narcotics and local anesthetics, have a depressant effect on the respiratory centers. This effect, combined with the mechanical changes in ventilation that result from pain caused by the surgical procedure, make it imperative that the

functional status of the patient's respiratory system be assessed before the type of anesthesia is selected.

As part of this evaluation, a recent history of cough, sputum production, hemoptysis, upper respiratory tract infection, or fever should be sought because these symptoms imply hypersecretion, which may lead to an increased incidence of pulmonary complications.[3,6] A history of asthma or chronic obstructive pulmonary disease also is important, because these disease processes may cause progressive functional impairment and result in pulmonary complications.

For patients with a significant history of pulmonary disease or obvious clinical findings, many bedside tests have been advocated to measure pulmonary function and determine the need for further laboratory tests. In the final analysis, however, arterial blood gases are the most sensitive indicators of pulmonary adequacy and invariably indicate whether additional pulmonary studies are required.

Cardiocirculatory System

The cardiocirculatory system is responsible for the uptake of inhaled anesthetics from the lungs and for the delivery of both inhaled and parenteral anesthetics to the central nervous system. All anesthetic agents, however, including narcotics and local anesthetics, are capable of producing myocardial depression. Therefore, careful assessment of the functional status of the cardiocirculatory system is essential to an appropriate anesthetic choice.

A history of dyspnea, orthopnea, or other signs and symptoms of recent congestive heart failure contraindicate the use of the more cardiac depressant anesthetics until this condition has been treated adequately. A history of hypertension is equally important, because this may cause exaggerated pressor responses to anesthetic maneuvers such as intubation, and because antihypertensive medications can interact with anesthetic agents and result in severe hypotension. A history of recent chest pain or a documented myocardial infarction within the past 6 months represent almost absolute contraindications to elective surgery, because the incidence of repeated infarction and subsequent mortality is increased markedly during the first 6 months after the initial event. After that time, morbidity and mortality decrease progressively until, at the end of 1 year, the incidence of infarction equals that of the general population of the same age.[7,12,20,21] Patients in this category should be monitored carefully throughout the perioperative period because this has been shown to decrease their morbidity and mortality.[16]

Preanesthetic Laboratory Testing

For many years, the use of multiple preoperative screening tests has been advocated. Chest roentgenography, electrocardiography, hemoglobin or hematocrit determination, an SMA 6 or greater profile, a coagulation profile, and a urinalysis are ordered routinely to prevent the case "from being delayed or cancelled." Recent studies have indicated that extensive screening tests carried out in the absence of known or suspected conditions fail to detect occult diseases.[9,18] In the face of increasing pressure to control medical costs, a trend toward little or no routine preoperative screening is developing, although biochemical studies of known or suspected medical problems always are indicated before anesthesia and operation.

Concurrent Drug Use

It is vital that the anesthesiologist be aware of any drugs the patient is taking, including prescription drugs, over-the-counter medications, and illegal substances. The interaction of anesthetic drugs with drugs taken by the patient may preclude the use of certain agents because of increased risks.

Many antihypertensive drugs interfere with the synthesis, storage, release, or reuptake of catecholamines, or block the adrenergic receptors, all of which result in reduced sympathetic tone. It is common practice, however, to treat hypertension with a combination of agents, each of which partially inactivates only one or two of the mechanisms essential for sympathetic responsiveness, minimizing the interference with the body's homeostatic mechanisms.

Patients receiving psychotropic medications such as tricyclic antidepressants and monoamine oxidase inhibitors may have exaggerated responses to the stresses of anesthesia and operation. In the past, it was recommended that these medications be discontinued 2 or more weeks before surgery. Today, patients continue to take these medications and are monitored carefully during operation to ensure rapid, careful blood pressure control if necessary.

Intravenous drug abuse is of concern to the anesthesia provider primarily because of the potential for concurrent diseases such as infection, phlebitis, pulmonary embolism, bacterial endocarditis, hepatitis, and the acquired immunodeficiency syndrome. Because of the risks associated with withdrawal, the simplest approach is to maintain the patient's drug use at the accustomed level and to avoid agonist/antagonists or pure antagonists.

Cocaine, the most widely used of all illicit drugs, carries additional dangers. It prevents presynaptic reuptake of norepinephrine into the nerve endings and can cause hypertension, tachycardia, ventricular arrhythmias, coronary artery spasm, mydriasis, hyperglycemia, and hyperthermia. The life-threatening potential of these conditions is exacerbated by anesthetic agents and the stress of surgery.

Anesthetic History

The anesthetic history of both the patient and the family should be obtained before surgery. A history of unexplained fever that occurred intraoperatively during a previous anesthetic exposure, or of relatives who died unexpectedly during surgery indicates that the patient may be at risk for malignant hyperpyrexia. Malignant hyperpyrexia is a pharmacogenetic disease, which means that the tendency for the syndrome to develop is determined genetically, but that it usually occurs only on exposure to anesthetic agents and adjuncts. Although a full-blown reaction may be triggered spontaneously by anxiety, fear, or surgical stress, it most often is precipitated by halogenated inhaled anesthetics, succinylcholine, or both.

In a typical case, a dose of succinylcholine that ordinarily would cause fasciculations followed by flaccid paralysis results in excessive fasciculations and rigidity rather than relaxation. If the anesthetic is continued in the face of this response, a rapidly progressive fever develops, associated with hypercapnia, hypoxemia, and ventricular dysrhythmias. A full-blown episode was almost uniformly fatal in the past, but earlier recognition and aggressive pharmacologic and physical treatment have reduced the mortality significantly. Nonetheless, if the typical abnormal response to succinylcholine or halogenated anesthetic agents occurs, both the anesthetic and the operation should be discontinued as rapidly as possible.

ANESTHESIA FOR REPAIR OF HERNIA IN ADULTS

Because current practice (and the insurance laws that influence it) calls for uncomplicated herniorrhaphy to be performed on an outpatient basis, the preoperative evaluation and control of concurrent medical problems has become increasingly important. The anesthetic used must interact favorably with the patient's coexisting medical conditions while it facilitates the surgical repair and provides some control of postoperative pain. If the patient is treated at an outpatient facility, complete and rapid recovery from the anesthetic also is essential.

General Anesthesia

General anesthesia offers the advantages of rapid induction, good muscle relaxation, and certainty of action. A detailed discussion of all the techniques of general anesthesia is beyond the scope of this discussion, but the importance of knowledge and skill on the part of the anesthesiologist cannot be overemphasized. A thorough understanding of both the primary pharmacologic effects of the various anesthetic agents and their effects on the patient's medical conditions is essential to safe anesthesia. For optimal results, the decision to use general anesthesia is less important than the selection of the particular anesthetic agent for the individual patient.

Regional Anesthesia

The benefits of regional anesthesia are being recognized increasingly for many types of surgery. For herniorrhaphy, regional anesthesia offers several advantages over general anesthesia. Regional analgesia can be confined to a limited area and need not interfere with the function of other organs. The sensory blockade provided is complete and limits nociassociation and other abnormal reflex mechanisms that may be the cause of alterations in cardiovascular and respiratory function. There is considerably less postoperative nausea, retching, and vomiting after regional anesthesia, and the immediate postoperative period is pain-free. In addition, the use of continuous techniques allows maintenance of the analgesic state well into the recovery period, avoiding the need for systemic narcotics and other drugs that may have adverse respiratory and cardiocirculatory effects. All these factors permit earlier ambulation and resumption of oral feeding, both of which enable earlier discharge from the hospital.

Regional anesthesia does have disadvantages, however. Many of the techniques are more difficult to master than are techniques of general anesthesia, so the incidence of inadequate anesthesia is higher. Complications may result from improper technique or from inappropriate management of physiologic responses to regional anesthesia. The procedures cannot be performed on patients who are unwilling or unable to cooperate, and some patients simply dislike being awake during the surgical procedure. Many patients, however, readily accept regional anesthesia when they are informed that the proper preoperative and intraoperative use of narcotics, sedatives, and tranquilizers allows them to sleep peacefully throughout the entire operation.

To achieve optimal results with regional anesthesia, the physician who performs it must have a thorough knowledge of the nerve supply of the region, the best site for blocking the appropriate nerves, and the perineural relations at the site of the block. He or she also must be expert in the use of various techniques of regional anesthesia, and must be aware of the advantages, disadvantages, and possible complications of each. In addition, the anesthesiologist must have a complete knowledge of the pharmacology of local anesthetic agents in both normal and abnormal physiologic states. Finally, it is essential that the surgeon appreciate the limitations of each regional technique, be willing to wait until analgesia is complete, and handle the deeper tissues carefully, particularly the spermatic cord and the hernia sac. This latter requirement is especially important when the anesthetic is a field block or local infiltration.

There is an increasing body of evidence indicating that the type of anesthesia used affects not only the performance of the surgery itself, but also the amount of postoperative pain that the patient experiences. It appears that regional (or local) anesthesia, especially if it is applied some time before the incision is made, is associated with a significant decrease in postoperative pain. This also is the case if a regional anesthetic or local infiltration is carried out before a general anesthetic. It is postulated that this preemptive analgesia results from the prevention of nociceptive impulses entering the central nervous system during and immediately after surgery, suppressing the formation of the sustained hyperexcitable state in the central nervous system that is thought to be responsible for the maintenance of postoperative pain.[2,4,5,13,22]

Techniques of Regional Anesthesia

Unlike general anesthetic techniques, it is important to consider regional anesthetic techniques in some detail because it may be the surgeon, rather than the anesthesiologist, who provides the anesthesia in many operations. Regional techniques that may be used for the repair of inguinal, femoral, or umbilical hernias include local infiltration, field block, paravertebral block, epidural block, and subarachnoid (spinal) block. Intercostal nerve blocks also may be used, but these are most effective for umbilical or other upper abdominal herniorrhaphies. In selecting a specific technique, it must be remembered that the farther from the central nervous system the local anesthetic is deposited, the greater is the dose of local anesthetic required to produce anesthesia. This fact may limit the choice of anesthetic technique in elderly or debilitated patients.

No operation that entails the use of local anesthetics should be initiated without the availability of equipment, drugs, and trained personnel for imme-

Table 38-1. Cardiopulmonary Resuscitation Equipment for Treatment of Local Anesthetic Toxicity

Agent or Equipment	Use in Resuscitation
Diazepam or thiopental	Control of local anesthetic–induced seizures
Succinylcholine	Control of muscular contractions induced by seizure and facilitation of endotracheal intubation
Anesthesia machine or ambu bag	Provide positive-pressure ventilation with supplemental oxygen
Face mask, oropharyngeal airways, laryngoscopes, endotracheal tubes, stylets	Control of the airway
Suction device	Cleaning any oral secretions or vomit from the airway
Vasopressor drugs: ephedrine, phenylephrine, epinephrine	Support of the blood pressure
Electrocardiogram, blood pressure, O_2 saturation	Monitoring of physiologic parameters

diate cardiovascular and pulmonary resuscitation. These are summarized in Table 38-1.

LOCAL INFILTRATION

The equipment necessary for local infiltration and field block is a 10- or 20-mL Luer-Lok syringe; one 25-gauge, 4-cm needle for intracutaneous injection; and two 22-gauge, 8-cm needles for subcutaneous and deeper infiltration. Fresh, unopened bottles of local anesthetics should be used for the block. If epinephrine is desired, it is preferable to add it to the local anesthetic solution at the time of injection rather than to use a solution that contains epinephrine. Solutions that are premixed with epinephrine by the manufacturer are more costly, but even more important, the decreased pH of the solution that is necessary to preserve the epinephrine slows the onset of the local anesthetic significantly. Although any of the available local anesthetics are suitable, 0.5% lidocaine or 0.5% mepivacaine is used most frequently for local infiltration. Lidocaine provides anesthesia for about 1½ hours and mepivacaine for about 2½ hours. For greater duration, or for prolonged postoperative pain relief, 0.125% or 0.25% bupivacaine often is used, despite its slow onset. An agent that is underused for local infiltration is etidocaine, which has the same duration as bupivacaine but a faster onset of action than lidocaine. In addition, it provides a more profound motor block than does bupivacaine. Regardless of the local anesthetic chosen, if not contraindicated, the addition of epinephrine enhances surgical hemostasis and delays absorption of the local anesthetic, resulting in an increased duration of anesthesia and a decreased risk of systemic toxic reactions. It is extremely important that the epinephrine be measured accurately with a tuberculin syringe, using 0.1 mL of 1:1000 epinephrine for each 20 mL of local anesthetic solution to produce the optimal concentration of 1:200,000.

The most effective technique of local infiltration, first developed by Harvey Cushing, consists of successive infiltration and incision of the various layers of the abdominal wall and direct injection of the ilioinguinal nerve when it is exposed. After the surgical field has been prepared, a series of intracutaneous injections is made with a 22-gauge needle along the course of the contemplated incision (Fig. 38-1A). About 10 mL of the anesthetic solution is injected into the skin, with the needle almost parallel to the skin surface. The right-handed operator should begin the infiltration at the medial end of the incision on the right side and at the lateral end on the left.

Subcutaneous infiltration is carried out next with an 8-cm, 22-gauge needle (see Fig. 38-1B and C), and a total of 10 to 15 mL of solution is injected as the needle is advanced and withdrawn along the line of incision. The point of the needle is guided by the second and third fingers of the operator's left hand placed on the skin of the inguinal region, and it is relatively easy to feel the needle as it is advanced and directed beneath the skin in all but extremely obese patients. Analgesia may by expected within 1 to 2 minutes after infiltration, because small, virtually unprotected nerves are bathed by the injected anesthetic.

After analgesia is complete, the incision is made through the skin down to the aponeurosis of the external oblique muscle (see Fig. 38-1D through F). The edges of the incision are separated gently and infiltration is carried out along the line of the next incision with another 10 mL of the anesthetic solution. After 2 to 3 minutes, the aponeurosis is incised, exposing the spermatic cord and the internal oblique muscles. The ilioinguinal nerve and the inguinal branch of the iliohypogastric nerve (when this is present) are found at the lateral edge of the incision. Two to 3 mL of the anesthetic solution is infiltrated around each of these nerves, with care taken to avoid intraneural injection or traction. If the internal oblique muscle is to be incised to permit better visualization of the internal

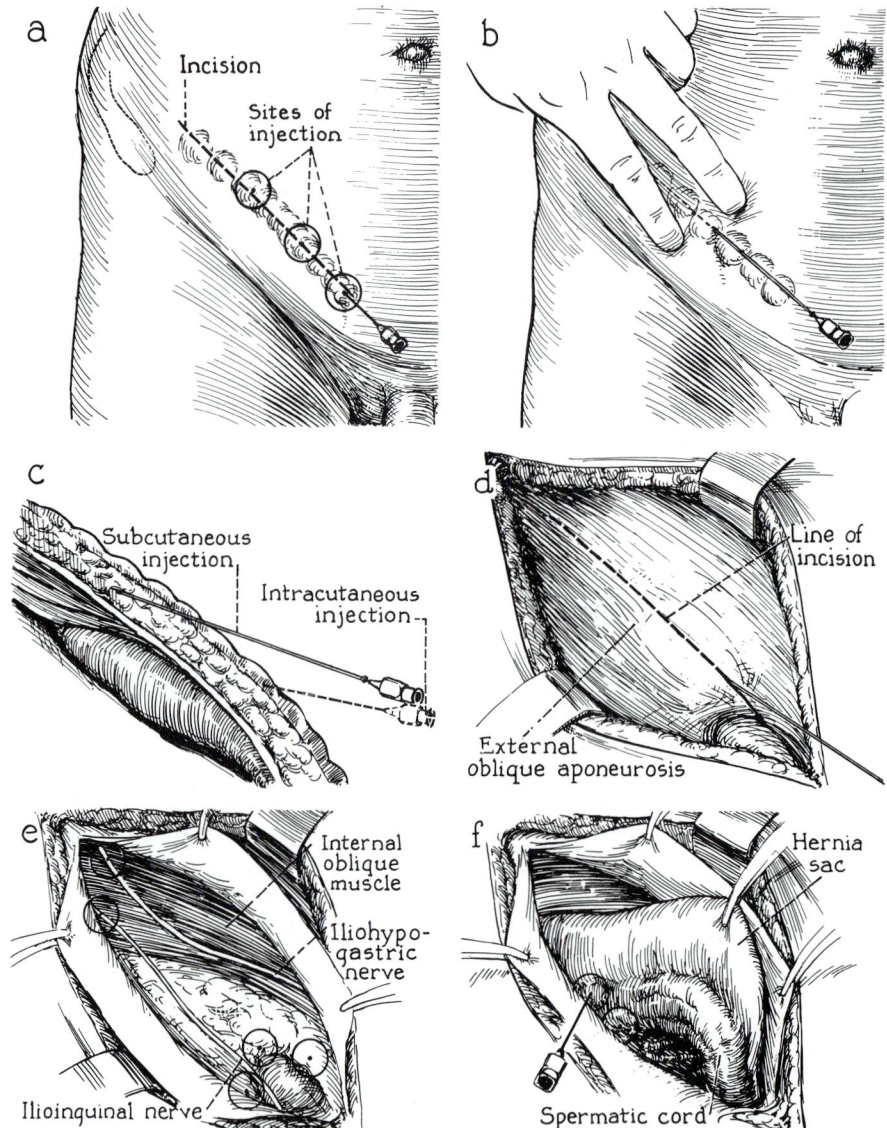

Figure 38-1. Technique of local infiltration of anesthetic solution for inguinal hernia repair. (*a*) A series of intracutaneous injections are made along the proposed line of the incision. (*b*) Subcutaneous injection using an 8-cm, 22-gauge needle guided by the fingers of the left hand. (*c*) Cross section of the injection site showing the relationship between the intracutaneous and subcutaneous injections. (*d*) Injection of the aponeurosis of the external oblique muscle along the line of incision. (*e*) Injection of the ilioinguinal and inguinal branches of the iliohypogastric nerves and the peritoneum of the hernial sac. (*f*) Injection of the spermatic cord.

ring, it first is infiltrated with an additional 8 to 10 mL of anesthetic.

The final step is to inject 5 to 10 mL of local anesthetic into the region of the internal inguinal ring to block the genitofemoral nerve and the sensory fibers of the spermatic plexus. Lidocaine and mepivacaine are recommended because they diffuse into the spermatic cord better than do other agents. No attempt should be made to infiltrate this structure be-

cause injury to the vessels of the cord can result in serious hematomas. If the hernia is irreducible, the edges of the sac are infiltrated carefully, and if intestine or omentum is strangulated, it also must be infiltrated to avoid the severe pain that can result from tension or torsion of strangulated intestine or omentum that has become adherent to the sac.

Although the method described produces surgical analgesia, it provides little or no muscle relaxation. If the operation involves suture of the lacunare (Gimbernat) and pectineale (Cooper) ligaments, these structures should be infiltrated before suturing. It also is advisable to infiltrate over the pillars of the external ring, because branches from the 12th thoracic nerve occasionally reach this point. The technique of infiltration described herein entails the use of less than the maximum dose of anesthetic agent. In infants and children, smaller volumes and decreased concentrations of the drug are needed. In these patients, many surgeons use local infiltration and general anesthesia to provide lighter planes of general anesthesia during the operation and relief of pain afterward.

The only important complication of local infiltration and field block is a systemic toxic reaction, which can be prevented by avoiding intravascular injection and limiting the total dosage to that indicated in Table 38-2. A toxic reaction usually is manifested by twitching or convulsions, cardiovascular collapse, or both, but it generally is preceded by restlessness. Therefore, if a patient becomes restless and irritable during a procedure being performed under infiltration or field block, the anesthetist should administer diazepam or thiopental intravenously in small, incremental doses, as well as oxygen by mask, to avert the development of an overt convulsion. Because they can interfere with adequate ventilation and consequently produce asphyxia and hypertension, convulsions should be terminated by the intravenous injection of diazepam or thiopental and by ventilation with 100% oxygen. If this does not terminate the convulsion, succinylcholine should be administered by the anesthetist so that ventilation can be controlled and intubation accomplished if necessary. If a reaction is accompanied by hypotension or bradycardia, appropriate doses of vasopressors or anticholinergic agents should be injected intravenously.

Field Block

Field block anesthesia for the repair of inguinal hernia has been popular among surgeons for more than 80 years. It offers several advantages over local infiltration. The anesthesia does not distort the surgical field, and blockage of ilioinguinal, iliohypogastric, and lower thoracic nerves results in better muscle relaxation. Although surgeons can perform field block alone, many find it expeditious to have the anesthesiologist carry out the procedure before the operation.

The disadvantages of the technique include a higher failure rate than is encountered with local infiltration and the need for a larger amount of local anesthetic. In addition, if the technique is carried out as originally described, the inguinal canal must be infiltrated blindly through the skin, which can result in injury to the spermatic cord.

The technique of field block is depicted in Figure 38-2. The operator usually stands on the side to be injected. An intracutaneous wheal is raised just above the anterior superior iliac spine, and an 8-cm, 22-gauge needle is inserted through the wheal and advanced carefully, penetrating the fascia and aponeurosis of the external oblique muscle. Thirty to 40 mL of local anesthetic agent is injected between this aponeurosis and the internal oblique muscle along the lateral half of the line connecting the anterior superior iliac spine and the umbilicus. This anesthetizes the iliohypogastric and ilioinguinal nerves, as well as branches of the 11th and 12th thoracic nerves.

Next, an intracutaneous wheal is raised just above the pubic tubercle, and several 5- to 10-mL injections are made along the horizontal ramus of the pubis on each side of the spermatic cord, with great care taken to avoid puncturing the femoral vein. This can be prevented by palpating the femoral artery with the left

Table 38-2. Doses of Local Anesthetic Agents Commonly Used for Regional Techniques

Agent	Local Infiltration and Field Block (%)	Intercostal and Paravertebral Block (%)	Epidural Block (%)	Maximum Dose* (mg/kg)
Procaine (Novocain)	0.5	1–2	1–2	10–15
2-Chloroprocaine (Nesacaine)	0.5	1–2	2–3	10–15
Lidocaine (Xylocaine)	0.5	1	1–2	5–7[+]
Mepivacaine (Carbocaine, Polocaine)	0.5	1	1–2	5–7
Prilocaine (Citanest)	0.5	1–3	1–3	10[‡]
Bupivacaine (Marcaine, Sensorcaine)	0.25	0.25–0.50	0.25–0.75	3–4
Etidocaine (Duranest)	0.25	0.5–1.0	1.0–1.5	3–5
Tetracaine (Pontocaine)	0.1	0.1–0.2		0.2–0.5

*Maximum doses for healthy young adults. Minimal doses necessary should be used in all instances, but in cachectic, aged patients and seriously ill patients, the maximum limits should be decreased.
[+]When using the upper dosage limits, epinephrine 1:200,000 should be added to minimize blood levels.
[‡]If the dosage exceeds 600 mg, methemoglobinemia may become clinically evident.

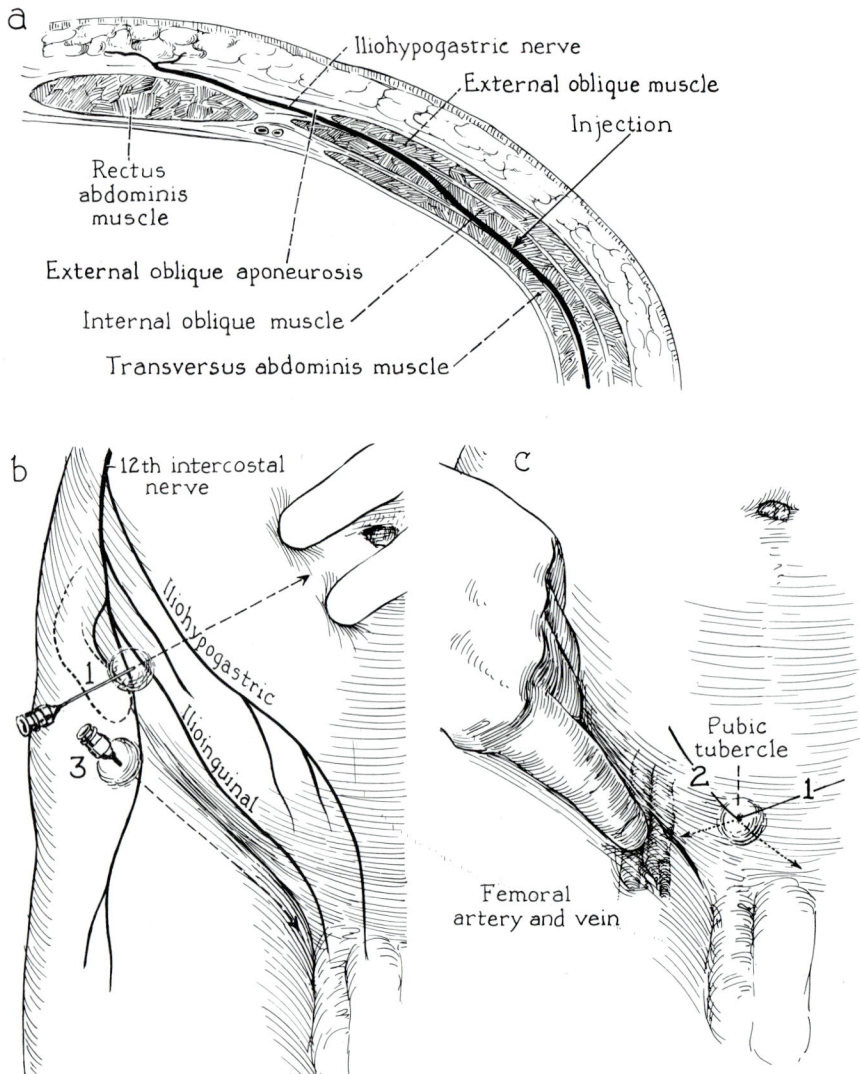

Figure 38-2. Technique of field block of inguinal region. (*a*) Schematic cross-section of the abdominal wall showing the relation of the iliohypogastric nerve to the muscle and fascial layers. Note that, in the lateral aspect of the abdominal wall, the nerve lies deep to or runs in the substance of the internal oblique muscle. (*b*) Site and direction of injections for (1 and 2) blocking the iliohypogastric and ilioinguinal nerves, and (3) the external femoral cutaneous and femoral branches of the genitofemoral nerves. (*c*) Injections along the ramus of the pubis on each side of the spermatic cord, with care taken to avoid the femoral vessels.

forefinger below the inguinal ligament at the level of the femoral ring and keeping the point of the needle at least 2 cm from the artery. Additional 5- to 10-mL injections are made along the horizontal ramus of the pubis to a point 3 to 4 cm beyond the midline (see Fig. 38-2*C*).

At this point, 10 to 20 mL is infiltrated subcutaneously just below the inguinal ligament from the anterior superior iliac spine to the medial aspect of the thigh (see Fig. 38-2), to block the overlapping branches of the external femoral cutaneous and genitofemoral nerves, which may supply the skin and other tissues of the inguinal region.

Although older techniques of inguinal field block involved percutaneous infiltration of the inguinal canal to anesthetize the spermatic cord, the genitofemoral nerve, and the peritoneum of the internal inguinal ring, this may lacerate the delicate vessels of the spermatic cord, causing trauma and hemorrhage. It is safer for the surgeon to infiltrate the region of the inguinal ring under direct vision.

Subarachnoid Block

The technique of spinal anesthesia for inguinal herniorrhaphy is well known and does not warrant detailed discussion here. The excellent results obtained with this procedure in innumerable patients during the past 90 years attest to its usefulness. Spinal anesthesia is simple to carry out and almost always effective. It produces rapid analgesia and any degree of muscle relaxation required. The technique entails the use of only small amounts of local anesthetics, and virtually eliminates any risk of a systemic toxic reaction.

The major disadvantage of spinal anesthesia is the possibility of hypotension caused by the production of sympathetic blockade. The incidence of hypotension can be minimized by "preloading" the patient with several hundred milliliters of lactated Ringer solution just before administration of the anesthetic (the actual volume administered depends on the patient's cardiocirculatory status). Nonetheless, serious hypotension may occur in the best of hands, especially in patients with arteriosclerosis or hypovolemia, even if they are treated with fluids and vasopressors. Spinal headache occurs in 2% to 10% of patients, but can be reduced considerably by the use of appropriate needles. A summary of the technique of subarachnoid block is contained in Table 38-3. We prefer to use a hyperbaric solution and seek a level of anesthesia up to the 9th or 10th thoracic dermatome, but it must be emphasized that this level is adequate for inguinal herniorrhaphy only if the surgeon is gentle and avoids traction on the spermatic cord and

surrounding viscera, because a level of T5 is required to provide complete anesthesia of the abdominal viscera.

Epidural Block

Segmental epidural block is one of the best techniques of anesthesia for the repair of an inguinal hernia.

Although the single-shot technique can be used, the continuous catheter technique is preferable because it provides better control of the extent, duration, and intensity of analgesia, and allows postoperative analgesia with all of its benefits. A total of 10 to 12 mL of local anesthetic usually produces analgesia from the 9th or 10th thoracic to the 3rd or 4th lumbar dermatomes. This procedure is performed more easily, more quickly, and with less discomfort to the patient than is local infiltration, field block, or paravertebral block, and it provides more certain analgesia. Furthermore, because of the larger volumes of local anesthetic solution required to carry out the latter technique in obese patients or those who have a large, incarcerated hernia, segmental epidural block reduces the possibility of a systemic toxic reaction. A test dose of local anesthetic (2–3 mL) with epinephrine 1:200,000 always should be administered before the full dose is given. The rapid development of numbness and tingling or motor block of the legs indicates accidental subarachnoid (spinal) injection, whereas a transient increase in the pulse rate on the electrocardiogram indicates intravascular injection.

Headache associated with lumbar puncture does not occur after epidural block unless the dura has been perforated, and the risk of neurologic sequelae is theoretically less than that of subarachnoid anesthesia. Unless a subarachnoid or epidural block extends

Table 38-3. Doses of Anesthetic Agents for Spinal Anesthesia for Inguinal Herniorrhaphy (Administered in the Lateral Position)

Agent (as injected)	Average Dose (mg)	Volume of Solution (mL)	Duration of Effect (min)	Specific Gravity Compared to CSF (Baricity)
Tetracaine (0.5% in dextrose 5%)	8–10	1.6–2.0	90–180*	Hyperbaric
Tetracaine (0.5% in CSF)	8–10	1.6–2.0	90–180*	Isobaric
Procaine (5% in dextrose 5%)	100–125	2.0–2.5	45–60*	Hyperbaric
Procaine (5% in CSF)	100–125	2.0–2.5	45–60*	Isobaric
Lidocaine (5% in dextrose 7.5%)	75–100	1.5–2.0	60–90*	Hyperbaric
Bupivacaine (0.75% in dextrose 8.5%)	10–15	1.4–2.0	90–110	Hyperbaric
Bupivacaine (0.5%)	15–20	3.0–4.0	90–110	Isobaric

*Duration may be increased by an average of 50% by adding epinephrine 1:10,000.
CSF, cerebrospinal fluid.

far above the 10th thoracic segment, the degree of hypotension caused by sympathetic blockade is mild, but the magnitude is the same with either technique. An additional advantage of continuous epidural block is the fact that the catheter may be left in place to provide postoperative analgesia. Although this analgesia has been provided in the past with intermittent injections of local anesthetics, more recently small (3- to 5-mg) doses of morphine have been injected into the epidural catheter, providing as much as 24 hours of pain relief without the anesthesia and motor block caused by local anesthetics. The epidural administration of morphine after operation requires close surveillance of the patient, because rare cases of delayed respiratory depression have been described. The incidence of this complication can be minimized by using a combination of dilute local anesthetics and narcotics.

Complications of epidural block include accidental injection of the therapeutic dose into the subarachnoid space and a systemic toxic reaction from an intravascular injection. Both problems can be avoided by the routine use of a test dose with epinephrine, as described earlier. Treatment of a total spinal block consists of artificial ventilation with 100% oxygen and support of the circulation with appropriate fluid or vasopressor therapy. If a toxic reaction progresses to overt convulsions, it usually can be terminated by hyperventilation with oxygen and the intravenous administration of diazepam in 0.1- to 0.2-mg/kg increments or thiopental in 25-to 50-mg increments.

Caudal Anesthesia

Caudal anesthesia may be used in place of lumbar epidural or subarachnoid block for inguinal hernia repair. It rarely is used in adults (although it can be), but is an excellent method in children and infants. To achieve anesthesia in adults, a 1½-inch, 21- or 22-gauge needle is inserted through the sacrococcygeal ligament and 25 to 30 mL of local anesthetic is injected, depending on the size of the patient. The volume may be reduced to 15 to 20 mL by using a 3½-inch spinal needle and advancing it several inches into the caudal canal, but this carries a greater risk of intravascular and even subarachnoid injection. As with lumbar epidural block, a continuous technique may be used to provide better control of the extent, duration, and intensity of analgesia. Whichever technique is used, as with epidural block, injection of the total volume of local anesthetic should be preceded by a test dose of 3 mL with epinephrine to ensure that the catheter or needle is not in the subarachnoid space or in a blood vessel. Such a caudal block should produce

analgesia extending from T9 or T10 to S5. In infants and children, a small injection into the caudal canal with a 25-gauge needle can be used to provide surgical anesthesia, but the injection more often is made at the end of a procedure performed under general anesthesia to provide prolonged postoperative pain relief.

Paravertebral Block

If segmental analgesia and muscle relaxation are desired, and there is a contraindication to subarachnoid, epidural, or caudal anesthesia, paravertebral block of T10-12, L1, and L2 can be performed. The technique is difficult and unpleasant for the patient because it requires multiple "needle sticks" and paresthesias. Figure 38-3 indicates the important landmarks for the

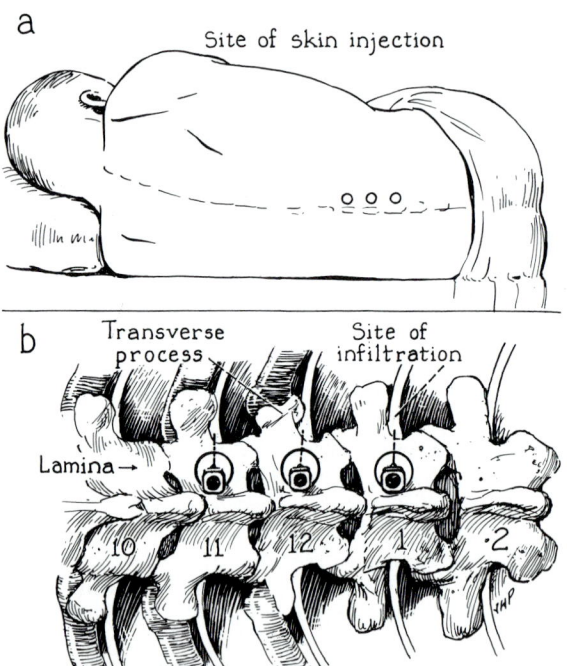

Figure 38-3. Technique of paravertebral—lower thoracic—somatic nerve block. (*a*) Position of the patient for block on the right side. Note that the skin wheal is formed 1.5 cm lateral to the tip of the spinous process of the vertebra. (*b*) The needle is advanced through the skin wheal perpendicular to the skin until the lateral edge of the lamina is contacted. The needle then is withdrawn until its point is in the subcutaneous tissue, the skin is moved laterally about 0.5 cm, and the needle is advanced again in a sagittal plane until it slips just lateral to the lamina and engages the transverse ligaments. Carefully advancing the needle with constant pressure on the syringe results in a sudden loss of resistance to injection as the needle passes through the transverse ligaments into the paravertebral region in the vicinity of the nerve. Five milliliters of anesthetic solution then is injected in the vicinity of the nerves.

block. After a paresthesia has been elicited at each level (indicating contact with the nerve), 5 mL of local anesthetic is injected to block each nerve. Because anesthesia is restricted to one side and fewer vasomotor segments are involved, this technique produces less hypotension than does epidural, subarachnoid, or caudal block. However, because accurate placement of the needle at each of the five nerve roots is essential for optimal anesthesia, the chances of incomplete anesthesia are greater with this technique.

Regional Anesthesia for Femoral Hernia

Repair of femoral hernias may be performed using local infiltration, paravertebral block of the 1st through 3rd lumbar nerves, subarachnoid or caudal block extending to the 1st lumbar dermatome, or segmental epidural block involving the 12th thoracic to the 3rd lumbar spinal dermatomes. The neuroanatomy of the region is such that field block is not practical.

Regional Anesthesia for Umbilical and Ventral Hernias

Repair of an umbilical hernia may be performed with the same anesthetic techniques used for inguinal and femoral hernias, except that the level of the analgesia needs to be higher. In addition, bilateral blocks of the 7th through 10th intercostal nerves may be used. Because intercostal blocks do not produce vasomotor blockade, there is little or no risk of the hypotension that often accompanies subarachnoid, epidural, and caudal blocks. Carried out correctly, the technique produces complete anesthesia of the abdominal wall, including the parietal peritoneum, and results in relaxation of the abdominal muscles. The primary disadvantage of this technique is that it does not interrupt visceral afferent fibers, and manipulation of herniated intestine or omentum may provoke discomfort if the physician is not extremely careful and gentle.

ANESTHESIA FOR INGUINAL HERNIA REPAIR IN CHILDREN

Because a large proportion of pediatric patients who are operated on for inguinal hernia repair are younger than 3 years, this group must be given special consideration. Successful management of anesthesia in these patients requires careful attention to detail, a

knowledge of the pharmacologic and anatomic differences between children and adults, and equipment designed specifically for the size of the patient. The physiologic responses of infants and children to stress are qualitatively similar to those of adults, but infants and children require quantitatively less stress to produce a response.

Preoperative Preparation

During the preoperative visit to the pediatric patient, the anesthesiologist should attempt to gain the confidence and friendship of the child and the parents by exhibiting consideration, sympathy, understanding, and, most important, tactful honesty. Even though the patient's parents are an integral part of the preoperative visit, unless the patient is very young, the anesthesiologist should address the patient so that the child does not feel manipulated. Because the rapport thus gained may be of little value if the child cannot recognize the anesthesiologist, the preoperative visit should be made wearing operating room attire. Children younger than 6 years do not understand or remember descriptions of anesthetic methods; therefore, we do not discuss anesthesia except in the broadest sense. Induction methods may be discussed with older children, and they may indicate a preference for a given technique. Once agreement has been reached, the anesthesiologist should follow through with the agreed-on plan if at all possible.

Preanesthetic medication should complement the psychological preparation of the patient and not substitute for it. Many pediatric hospitals provide a preanesthetic or induction room where the atmosphere is quiet and resembles that of a child's bedroom, and sympathetic, understanding personnel are present to reassure the patient. In addition, in many institutions, a parent is encouraged to hold and comfort the child during the induction of anesthesia to minimize the stress of the surgical experience.

Complications of Inguinal Hernia in Children

Incarceration of hernial contents occurs more often in children younger than 1 year than in older children. Resection of the intestine because of strangulation rarely is necessary in children, apparently because of the extreme reversibility of circulatory disturbances of the intestine in this age group. Extravasation of blood and serum into a segment of strangulated intestine can deplete the blood volume significantly and reduce the ability of the patient to withstand the stresses imposed by anesthesia and surgery. Appropriate fluid therapy is critical in these young patients. Indwelling intravenous plastic catheters should be placed percutaneously if possible, and surgical venous cutdown should be carried out to allow adequate fluid replacement if necessary. It is current surgical practice to explore the contralateral inguinal region when one hernia is repaired in a child. Because most elective pediatric hernia repairs are uncomplicated, the contralateral exploration does not prolong anesthesia appreciably and morbidity is not increased. Because the patient's condition could deteriorate unexpectedly under anesthesia and contraindicate exploration of the contralateral inguinal region, the obvious hernia always should be repaired first.

Every attempt should be made to induce anesthesia quickly and smoothly. The attention of the child must be held by the anesthesiologist and all external stimuli excluded until the patient is anesthetized completely. In younger children and infants, induction is accomplished best with the parents present. Sleep may be induced by the open administration of nitrous oxide, halothane, enflurane (Ethrane), or isoflurane; by the rectal administration of barbiturates with ultrashort action; by the intramuscular administration of ketamine; and by the intravenous administration of barbiturates, ketamine, etomidate, midazolam, propofol, or narcotics in appropriate doses. After induction, the anesthetic management differs little from that in adults.

Regional anesthesia often is neglected in pediatric patients. Children who are old enough to understand the procedure tolerate regional techniques as well as (and in many cases better than) adults, provided the anesthetist takes the time to establish rapport. If the child is too young, small doses of ketamine administered intramuscularly create a permissive state that allows the use of regional techniques that otherwise would be impossible. For herniorrhaphy of almost any type, caudal anesthesia is a useful technique. A 25-gauge, $\frac{5}{8}$-inch needle, or a 20-gauge, $1\frac{1}{4}$-inch intravenous catheter is inserted easily through the sacrococcygeal ligament. By varying the amount of drug administered, anesthesia appropriate for any level of hernia can be obtained. There also has been a recent resurgence in the popularity of spinal anesthesia for pediatric herniorrhaphy. Most anesthetists who prefer regional anesthesia in children administer a light general anesthetic to reduce emotional stress during the operation. Even when a general anesthetic has been used as the primary anesthetic for a herniorrhaphy, some pediatric anesthetists administer a caudal anesthetic at the end of the procedure to provide prolonged postoperative pain relief.[17]

ANESTHESIA FOR OUTPATIENT HERNIORRHAPHY

For many decades, inguinal herniorrhaphy has been carried out in infants and young children on an outpatient basis, because these patients can be carried home in the arms of their parents. Inguinal herniorrhaphy in ambulatory adults, which is becoming increasingly more common because of economic pressures, is not new either. Harvey Cushing described hernia repair under cocaine infiltration half a century ago, and since that time, many repairs have been performed on outpatients using local anesthesia. The renewed interest in ambulatory herniorrhaphy in adults is a result of the cost savings inherent in avoiding hospitalization. Ambulatory surgical centers have evolved within hospitals and freestanding surgical centers have become common. The resultant economic benefits, the availability of improved anesthetic techniques, and professional encouragement have resulted in increasing acceptance by both patients and surgeons. Studies comparing the cost of herniorrhaphy performed as an outpatient versus an inpatient procedure at the same hospital have shown significant savings associated with ambulatory herniorrhaphy.[15]

The anesthetic techniques and agents used for outpatient herniorrhaphy play a major role in surgical success, more so than with inpatient procedures. General anesthesia is feasible, but requires the most prolonged postoperative recovery and is associated with a much higher incidence of nausea and vomiting. A short-acting regional anesthetic by itself or combined with the injection of a long-acting local anesthetic allows early return of motor and bladder function, avoiding the urinary retention and immobilization that may be associated with the use of long-acting regional blocks.[19] A mounting body of evidence indicates that infiltration of the surgical site before incision provides immediate postoperative pain relief and decreases the degree of postoperative pain after the local anesthetic has worn off. This also may be accomplished with the use of cryoanalgesia (whereby the ilioinguinal nerve is frozen during herniorrhaphy) to provide several days of postoperative pain relief. In the absence of postoperative pain, patients recover and return to full function more quickly than when traditional forms of anesthesia and postoperative analgesia were used. Perhaps most important is the fact that several comparative studies have found no difference in postoperative complications between patients undergoing outpatient and inpatient herniorrhaphy. Because hernia recurrence rates after ambulatory herniorrhaphy also are comparable to or better than those after inpatient procedures, there appears to be no surgical disadvantage to performing hernia repair on an outpatient basis.[11,14,19,23]

REFERENCES

1. Buckley FP, Robinson NB, Simonowitz DA, Dellinger EP. Anaesthesia in the morbidly obese. A comparison of anesthetic and analgesic regimes for upper abdominal surgery. Anaesthesiology 1983;38:840.
2. Bugedo GJ, Carcamo CR, Mertens RA, Dagnino JA, Munoz HR. Preoperative percutaneous ilioinguinal and iliohypogastric nerve block with 0.5% bupivacaine for post-herniorrhaphy pain management in adults. Reg Anesth 1990;15:130.
3. Cohen MM, Cameron CB. Should you cancel the operation when a child has an upper respiratory tract infection? Anesth Analg 1991;72:282.
4. Cousins MJ. Acute pain and the injury response: immediate and prolonged effects. Reg Anesth 1989;14:162.
5. Ejlersen E, Andersen HB, Eliasen K, Mogensen T. A comparison between preincisional and postincisional lidocaine infiltration and postoperative pain. Anesth Analg 1992;74:495.
6. Empey DW, Laitinen LA, Jacobs L, Gold WM, Nadel JA. Mechanisms of bronchial hyperreactivity in normal subjects after upper respiratory tract infections. Am Rev Respir Dis 1976;113:131.
7. Goldman L, Caldera DL, Nussbaum SR, et al. Multifactorial index of cardiac risk in noncardiac surgical procedures. N Engl J Med 1977;297:845.
8. Hilgenberg JB. Inhalation and intravenous drugs in the elderly patient. Seminars in Anesthesia 1986;5:44.
9. Kaplan EB, Sheiner LB, Boeckmann AJ, Roizen MF. The usefulness of preoperative laboratory screening. JAMA 1985;253:3576.
10. Kitz DS, Lecky JH, Slusarz-Ladden C, Conahan TJ. Inpatient vs day surgery—difference in resource use, patient volume and anesthesia reimbursement. Anesth Analg 1987;66:597.
11. Kornhall S, Olsson AM. Ambulatory inguinal hernia repair compared with short-stay surgery. Am J Surg 1976;132:32.
12. Mangano DT, Browner W, SPI Research Group. Prediction of cardiac morbidity and mortality in patients undergoing noncardiac surgery. N Engl J Med 1990;323:1781.
13. McQuay HJ, Carroll D, Moore RA. Postoperative orthopaedic pain—the effect of opiate premedication and local anesthetic blocks. Pain 1988;33:291.
14. Morris D, Ward AW, Handyside AJ. Early discharge after hernia repair. Lancet 1968;1:681.
15. Pineault R, Contandriopoulos A-P. Randomized clinical trial of one day surgery—patient satisfaction, clinical outcomes, and costs. Med Care 1985;23:171.
16. Rao TK, Jacobs KH, El-Etr AA. Reinfarction following anesthesia in patients with myocardial infarction. Anesthesiology 1983;59:499.
17. Rice LJ, Hannallah RS. Local and regional anesthesia. Motoyama E, Davis PJ, eds. Smith's anesthesia for infants and children. St Louis, CV Mosby Company, 1990:393–426.
18. Roizen MF. Preoperative evaluation. In: Miller RD, ed. Anesthesia, ed 3. New York, Churchill Livingstone, 1990:743.
19. Ryan JA, Adye BA, Jolly PC, Mulroy MF II. Outpatient inguinal herniorrhaphy with both regional and local anesthesia. Am J Surg 1984;148:313.
20. Steen PA, Tinker JH, Tarhan S. Myocardial reinfarction after anesthesia and surgery. JAMA 1978;239:2546.
21. Tarhan S, Moffitt E, Taylor WF, Giuliani ER. Myocardial infarction after general anesthesia. JAMA 1972;220:1451.
22. Tverskoy M, Cozacov C, Ayache M, Bradley EL Jr, Kissin I. Postoperative pain after inguinal herniorrhaphy with different types of anesthesia. Anesth Analg 1990;70:29.
23. Young DA. Comparison of local, spinal, and general anesthesia for inguinal herniorrhaphy. Am J Surg 1987;153:560.

Special Comment

Use of Local Anesthesia to Expose and Repair a Recurrent Inguinal Hernia by the Posterior Approach

James A. Bulen and Sam Maywood

The posterior approach to the groin described by Henry and popularized by Nyhus, Condon, and Wantz is an effective method for repairing a recurrent inguinal hernia. In previous descriptions, this surgery required a general, spinal, or epidural anesthetic to provide adequate pain relief and muscle relaxation. Because of coexistent medical problems, such as cardiopulmonary disease, some patients are serious anesthetic risks. We have found that these individuals can be cared for easily and effectively by using local anesthesia supported by an anesthesiologist who is experienced in managed anesthesia care.[1,2]

I have become familiar with the posterior approach to the groin and have performed many primary inguinal hernia repairs using local anesthesia. Combining the posterior approach with local anesthesia has allowed me to repair recurrent inguinal hernias easily in an outpatient setting. Patients experience about as much stress as they would during a primary repair. Fourteen patients have been operated on using this technique, with no morbidity. Although this is a small series, it suggests that the outpatient setting can be used for recurrent inguinal hernia repair with gratifying results. I recommend this to patients and surgeons who enjoy the use of outpatient facilities.

Anesthesiologist Dr. Sam Maywood describes his technique:

> *After careful preoperative assessment and placement of monitors, the patient is initially treated with intravenous midazolam (Versed) citrate 1–3 mg and a narcotic, my usual choice being fentanyl citrate 25–75 μcg. The dosage varies with the age, size, condition of the patient and any underlying systemic illness. Oxygen is administered by mask or nasal cannula before the induction. When the surgeon is ready to give the local, a short acting barbiturate like methohexital (Brevital) sodium or propofol (Diprivan) is given through the intravenous line. This provides sufficient amnesia for two to three minutes while the surgeon injects the initial dose of local anesthetic into the surgical site. The airway is maintained with simple chin support, and the majority of patients rarely desaturate, nor experience any significant change in their cardiovascular or pulmonary status. The patient is then allowed to awaken slowly. Careful attention and communication are provided from then on to assure comfort. Occasionally a patient may feel some pain or pressure; the surgeon administers more local anesthesia, and I may give more Brevital or Diprivan. Our technique has been extremely successful. The local anesthesia eliminates postoperative pain for six to twelve hours. The patients are usually quite awake and can be discharged home quickly and safely. A 60 mg. injection of ketorolac (Toradol) tromethamine is often given intramuscularly, while in the recovery room, to help decrease their postoperative discomfort.*

When the anesthesiologist approves, local anesthesia consisting of 20 mL of equal parts 1% lidocaine hydrochloride (Xylocaine) and 0.25% bupivacaine hydrochloride without epinephrine (Marcaine) is injected. Ten-milliliter syringes and 2-inch, 25-gauge needles are used. This solution is injected in about equal parts into the subcutaneous tissue of the planned incision site and deep to the external oblique muscle, especially where the ilioinguinal, iliohypogastric, and genitofemoral nerves enter the operative field. The nurse then shaves and prepares the patient, and the operative field is draped and set up. This delay allows time for the local anesthetic to become effective. An incision is made about 1½ fingerbreadths superior to the pubis or through the old scar, as appropriate. Dissection continues to the level of the external oblique and landmarks are checked again. The external oblique is divided superior and medial to the previous suture line. The anterior rectus sheath is divided, the rectus is retracted medially, and the muscle fibers of the internal oblique and transversus muscles are separated. The internal inguinal ring, triangle of Hesselbach, femoral ring, areas behind the pubis and rectus, and preperitoneal tissue superior and medial to the incision are exposed. During the dissection, an additional 10 to 35 mL of the anesthetic mix is injected in small increments, as indicated by the patient. This amount of local anesthetic is safe.[3] The patient may be awake or dozing, but can respond to questions and cough on request. The hernia defects are defined and these findings are coordinated with the preoperative description. A large piece of mesh is inserted. The hernia openings themselves usually are not repaired, but 1 to 3 sutures may be placed to triangulate and hold the mesh in place. The mesh is not trimmed unless absolutely necessary, removing only the minimum so that it does not wrinkle. Enough mesh is used to extend widely beyond all defects and suture lines. During the procedure, the wound is irrigated with antibiotic solution, supplementing the preoperative intravenous antibiotics. At the time of closure, an additional 10 mL of 0.5% bupivacaine is injected into the wound in a distribution similar to the initial injection.

The anesthesiologist observes the surgeon's progress and monitors the patient throughout the procedure. The analgesia is coordinated so that the patient is alert during the wound closure. The patient discusses the operation as the bandage is being applied and usually expresses surprise that the surgery is completed and was a painless experience. Patients typically remain in the recovery room for 45 to 90 minutes, and are released after they have voided, ambulated, and taken fluids.

REFERENCES

1. Amado WJ. Local anesthesia. Surg Clin North Am 1993;73:436.
2. Mann M. Local anesthesia with MAC. In: Bulen JA, Bridgman C, eds. The hernia solution, a comprehensive guide to patient care. Escondido, CA, Advanced Health Press, 1992:161–162.
3. Ritchie J, Murdock, Greene NM. Pharmacological basis of therapeutics, Goodman and Gilman, 8th edition. Pergamon Press, 1990:321–324.

Editor's Comment

Bulen and Bridgman (The hernia solution: myths, facts, answers. Escondido, CA, Advanced Health Press, 1992) have produced an authoritative guide for patients with a variety of hernial problems. Patients are concerned and wish to have a source to study that speaks to the details of the cause of hernia, its treatment, and the results of hernia operations. Bulen and Bridgman have given us such a source of information.

L.M.N.

Hernia, Fourth Edition, edited
by Lloyd M. Nyhus and Robert E. Condon.
J.B. Lippincott Company, Philadelphia © 1995.

Chapter 39

Pneumoperitoneum in Giant Hernia

Edward E. Mason

Pneumoperitoneum is an old procedure that was used for the treatment of pulmonary tuberculosis because it elevated the diaphragm and helped to collapse areas of cavitation in the lung. Occasionally, pneumoperitoneum was used in the radiologic study of intraabdominal organs or to outline a communication between the abdomen and a suspected diaphragmatic hernia in situations that now would be studied by imaging with computerized tomography, ultrasound, or magnetic resonance. It was obvious from radiographic studies of the abdomen of patients receiving long-term treatment of pulmonary tuberculosis with pneumoperitoneum that large increases in intraabdominal space occurred. Before 1940, no one made the connection between this observation and the use of pneumoperitoneum to reestablish abdominal space in patients with giant hernia.

I was provided the opportunity as a medical student to see patients with tuberculosis while working in a state tuberculosis sanitarium and for several years in a veterans hospital, at the time that streptomycin first was used experimentally in national cooperative protocols, and I reported the first such study in patients with intestinal tuberculosis.[13] I was prepared by this experience to be receptive to a new use for this old treatment when, in 1951, an Argentine surgeon, George Reales, described to me the use of pneumoperitoneum to prepare patients with giant hernia for operation.

Reales had been watching the repair of a large abdominal wall defect by Owen H. Wangensteen at the University of Minnesota, while I was assisting. Wangensteen used a pedicled fascia lata graft to fill in the defect. It was a long and complicated procedure. After the operation, Reales mentioned to me that they had a simpler way to treat giant hernias in Argentina, and he described Moreno's use of pneumoperitoneum. When I returned to the University of Iowa to practice surgery in 1953, I began looking for patients with "inoperable hernias" and subsequently reported an experience with nine patients.[9]

There were references in the surgical literature of the first half of the 20th century to the loss of abdominal domain in patients with large hernias. This ter-

minology was designed to focus attention on the risk of suddenly reducing viscera from a large hernia into an abdomen of inadequate capacity. The concept of progressive pneumoperitoneum to prepare a space for herniated viscera seems obvious today. There was considerable delay, however, between the first papers describing the technique and its widespread use. Now, with the frequent use of insufflation in laparoscopic surgery, there may be an increased use of pneumoperitoneum in the preparation for repair of giant hernia.

Incarceration and adhesions may prevent reduction of a hernia. In giant hernias, loss of the right of abdominal domain may cause incarceration. Before 1940, patients were prepared for repair of giant hernia using purges and tubes to empty the gastrointestinal tract. Surgeons knew that there often was a need for more abdominal room, but they did not have an effective way of creating the needed space before Moreno's work. The mortality rate was high because of increased intraabdominal pressure, elevation of the diaphragm, interference with ventilation, and impairment of venous return through the vena cava. The answer, 50 years ago, was to declare large hernias inoperable, a solution that relieved the surgeon but not the patient. Most patients with inoperable hernias underwent a series of unsuccessful repairs, which supported the conclusion that they were inoperable. On October 7, 1940, Ivan Goñi Moreno reported his use of pneumoperitoneum for the reestablishment of abdominal room for the contents of giant hernia to his colleagues in Argentina, and subsequently to surgeons in North America.[4]

PATHOPHYSIOLOGY OF THE ABDOMINAL WALL

In early embryogenesis, the intestines develop outside the body. As they are reduced into the abdomen, a cavity develops to accommodate them. At any time in life that abdominal contents again leave the abdomen, the process is reversed and the abdominal cavity decreases in size. Enlargement occurs gradually, in response to a need, by stretching of the abdominal wall, as is illustrated by the increase in abdominal volume that occurs during pregnancy or in a patient with ascites. Less obvious is the shrinkage of the abdominal space that occurs during the development of a giant hernia. The abdominal wall is a muscular organ that exerts a low-grade pressure on its contents. If there is an attached sac of peritoneum and skin, viscera are pushed out into this diverticulum.

It takes time for a hernia to become so large as to be irreducible, and inoperable. It also takes time to restore operability by stretching the abdominal space. There is a certain degree of tolerance to more rapid changes in intraabdominal volume that is evident from our ability to ingest a large meal.

The average normal intraabdominal pressure is 8 cm H_2O.[2] A pressure of 1 cm H_2O is equivalent to a pressure of 1 mmHg. In the standing position, the pressure is about 20 cm H_2O in the lower abdomen and less than 8 cm H_2O near the diaphragm. Coughing, vomiting, or straining elevates the pressure to as high as 80 cm H_2O. In experimental animals, elevation of the abdominal pressure to 30 mmHg stops urine flow. Radiologists apply pressure to the abdomen during intravenous pyelography to stop the flow of urine and to provide a more concentrated dye in the kidneys and upper collecting system.

In 1931, Overholt[14] conducted a study to determine what effect the injection of air into the abdominal cavity would have on intraabdominal pressure in dogs. He found that the first 100 mL of air was accompanied by a rise in pressure of 8 cm H_2O. A significant amount of additional air then could be introduced with no further rise in pressure until a critical volume finally was reached. At that point, the intraabdominal pressure rose with each successive injection of air. Moreno used a manometer to monitor pressures during pneumoperitoneum and reported that the highest pressures obtained were 30 to 40 cm H_2O.

INDICATIONS

Loss of abdominal domain is the major reason for using pneumoperitoneum, not the presence of a large defect in the abdominal wall. The ideal candidate is a patient with a relatively small defect but a large sac of herniated viscera that have not been reduced for so long that the abdominal cavity no longer has a place for these organs. There is no certain way to determine loss of domicile. The risk associated with a sudden increase in intraabdominal pressure is so great that peritoneum should be used if there is any question about operability because of the large size of the hernia: better "air" than "err." Pneumoperitoneum, therefore, can be considered diagnostic as well as therapeutic be-

cause the air allows the surgeon to increase intraabdominal contents gradually while observing the reaction of an awake and alert patient.

Most of the giant hernias prepared with pneumoperitoneum have been incisional, but the method also works well with scrotal hernias.[1] Mansuy and Hager[8] described a patient with large bilateral scrotal hernias who was prepared in this manner. Whelan and Eaker[20] used pneumoperitoneum for the secondary repair in two babies with omphalocele. Spratt[18] reported the use of pneumoperitoneum for congenital omphalocele in a 10½-month-old child, and Steichen[19] did so in an 8-month-old child.

Contraindications to the use of pneumoperitoneum are those that would make the patient a poor candidate for hernia repair even after completion of the pneumoperitoneum. Old age is more often a reason for using the method than not. In a patient with limited cardiopulmonary reserve, tolerance to daily 500-mL injections of air may be the best way to determine candidacy for such treatment and for hernia repair.

DECISION TREES

Major decisions regarding treatment must be made at two points in the care of a patient with giant hernia: (1) when the patient first is encountered and operability of the hernia is under consideration; and (2) in the operating room, after all adhesions have been lysed, any compromised bowel has been removed, injured bowel has been repaired, and it is time to close the fascial defect (Fig. 39-1).

Decisions that must be made before surgery include those regarding (1) the presence or absence of urgent problems that may require an early operation, such as strangulated bowel or bowel obstruction; (2) what to do about obesity that is so severe as to prevent or compromise the success of hernia repair; and (3) loss of abdominal domain. Moreno's first patient had a bowel obstruction when first seen, but the pneumoperitoneum relieved this by compressing the contents of the hernia sac and reducing the hernia. It is a testimony to the confidence of Moreno in his own logic that he solved both the problem of incarceration and the need for additional abdominal space in his first patient. He also addressed the problem of existing heart disease. The patient tolerated gradual increases in abdominal pressure. If the hernia had been reduced urgently without this preparation, the patient's heart may not have withstood the changes in circulation that would have occurred.

A severely obese patient was admitted to the University of Iowa Hospitals and Clinics (UIHC) with bowel obstruction from incarceration of a giant her-

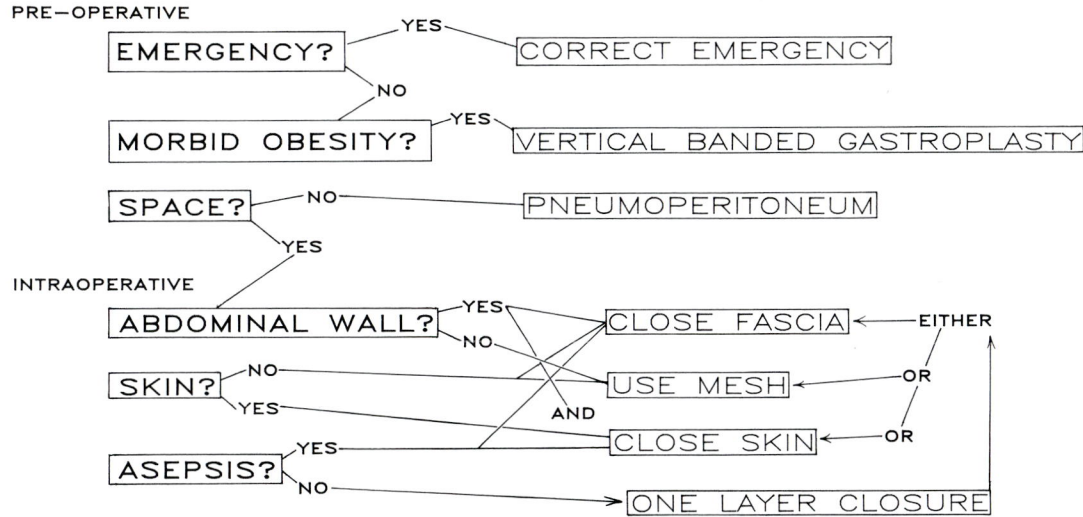

Figure 39-1. Giant hernia decision tree.

nia. As with Moreno's patient, the bowel obstruction was relieved by pneumoperitoneum. When adequate stretching had been performed, a vertical banded gastroplasty (VBG) was done at the same time as the hernia repair. The patient lost 90 lb in 4 months and the repair remained secure. Another patient treated with pneumoperitoneum at UIHC also illustrates some of the long-range planning that is required during various stages of the care of these patients. The patient weighed 253 lb and had obstruction and vomiting. She had a hernia that extended down to the middle of her thighs. A large, hot, red mass had developed at the most dependent part of the hernia sac and had broken down, leaving a dirty ulcer, the base of which was formed by bowel. Simple elevation of the sac relieved the obstruction and allowed time to improve the patient's general condition. The ulcer and a section of small bowel were removed. The hernia was partially repaired, leaving a smaller fascial defect and closing the hernia sac and skin. Pneumoperitoneum was started within a few days of the emergency operation. Thus, to achieve maximum safety and optimal outcome, decisions may be required during an emergency operation regarding further plans for expansion of the abdomen and staging of operative repair. This patient subsequently regained enough weight to cause a recurrence of her hernia and to require an operation to control her weight.

Decisions are required in the operating room at the time of wound closure that may influence the future course and success of treatment. Operation is undertaken either as an emergency or with the expectation that conditions are optimum under the existing circumstances. Finally, the defect must be closed, with a permanent repair of the hernia if this is safe and feasible, but with less than complete repair if necessary; without foreign material if possible, but with Marlex mesh if required; and with closure of the skin if possible, but with healing of the skin and subcutaneous tissues by secondary intention, skin graft, or delayed closure if indicated.

Emergency Conditions

Fifty years ago, patients with giant hernias presented a dilemma if they had bowel obstruction or an acute abdomen. The hernias reached tremendous size in part because they were considered inoperable and were allowed to remain for years. Then, suddenly, a condition would develop that required a life-saving operation. With our understanding of abdominal pressure and volume relationships today, there is no real contradiction. These patients must undergo operation for the emergency condition, but the hernia still should not be repaired. The hernia sac is opened and the portion that is nonviable is excised, but as much of the sac as possible is preserved so that the sac can be closed without any attempt at repair of the hernia after completion of the emergency procedure.

The lesson learned from these emergency operations is that there is no obligation to repair a hernia just because an emergency operation is required. An operation is performed to correct the urgent condition, but the skin is closed without repair of the fascial defect. Within a few days, pneumoperitoneum is begun.

The skin over a huge and redundant hernia may become edematous and infected, and give the appearance of a strangulated hernia, but actually represent nothing more than an abscess in the wall of the hernia. If it is neglected, such a condition may lead to an ulcer on the bottom of the hernia sac with bowel in the base, but this is not life-threatening. If a strangulated hernia is present, however, incision and drainage of what is mistakenly thought to be an abscess may lead to death, or at least to an intestinal fistula. One patient had a huge hernia with incarcerated transverse colon that had perforated spontaneously, forming an abscess. The abscess then had drained into the colon, and the patient had continued to have bowel movements. If bowel obstruction and signs of peritonitis are absent, localized infection may be the most urgent therapeutic problem. It may be possible to excise an abscess that is well localized. It is crucial that hernia and abscess be differentiated when a mass is detected in an old incision. With cardinal signs of inflammation, and especially with evidence of fluctuation, incision and drainage may be preferable to excision as the initial treatment.

Obesity

Moreno's first experience with pneumoperitoneum was in a 65-year-old patient with heart disease who also was obese. Obese patients in the 1940s were instructed to diet and to return when they had lost weight. Morbidly obese patients usually did not return after such instructions. In the early experience at UIHC, it was apparent that obesity often was a contributing factor to the development of extremely large hernias. In a few of these early patients, after the use of pneumoperitoneum and successful repair of the hernia, continuing or recurrent obesity contributed to recurrence of the hernia.

At the suggestion of Kremen, intestinal bypass was used in two such patients in 1955. In the first case, an end-to-side jejunoileal anastomosis was used but the patient continued to gain weight. Therefore, the second patient was treated by the anastomosis of 18 inches of jejunum to the transverse colon. The patient was dependent on intravenous feeding, and more small bowel had to be moved into the functioning stream. Intestinal bypass was abandoned and a search was begun for another effective therapy for obesity. This led to the introduction of gastric bypass.[12]

Gastric bypass was an analogue of Billroth II gastrectomy that was used for the treatment of peptic ulcer. VBG, which evolved from gastric bypass, is an operation designed specifically for the treatment of morbid obesity and no longer has either the capability of influencing gastric acid secretion or of causing malabsorption.[11] Since November 1980, VBG has re-

mained the operation of choice for morbid obesity at UIHC.

Treatment of morbid obesity takes precedence over elective hernia repair. In most patients, after weight reduction is obtained by VBG, the hernia can be reduced and repaired without pneumoperitoneum. The reduction of intraabdominal (visceral) fat may leave room for the hernia contents. If any doubt exists regarding the adequacy of the abdominal cavity after weight reduction, the patient should be prepared for hernia repair with progressive pneumoperitoneum.

Koontz[6] in 1958 expressed frustration with the morbidly obese and a misunderstanding of them that is widely held. He wrote that most of these patients were excessively fat, that they got that way from "disgusting self indulgence," and that, because they lie about what they eat, they also would lie about adhering to any recommended diet. This widely shared attitude has interfered with the treatment of severe obesity and its complications, including some giant hernias. Morbid obesity now is accepted as a disease that is out of control, and a small meal–sizing upper gastric segment can be provided by an operation that forces these patients to follow a weight-reducing diet, an appropriate form of behavior modification.

VBG has been the operation of choice because it avoids the risks of a bypass operation and, if performed properly, allows most patients to maintain their weight at a satisfactory level. VBG reduces weight through a 100-fold decrease in the capacity for a meal. It also is an antireflux operation if the pouch is measured and the vertical staple line is made parallel to the lesser curvature. Performed improperly, VBG may cause reflux. This results from failure to measure the pouch intraoperatively or to achieve a pouch of uniformly small diameter, with the partition parallel to the lesser curvature. VBG is not an operation that surgeons should undertake occasionally. It requires dedication to the care of the severely obese and experience with the technique. It also requires personal follow-up of patients by the surgeon who performs the operation.

Moreno was under the impression that a large hernia contributed to respiratory insufficiency. Because these patients so often are morbidly obese, it is possible that the obesity contributed to the impaired breathing. If obese hypoventilation is present, the patient must be hospitalized and prescribed a weight-reduction diet with adequate protein and a graduated exercise program as the initial step in an extended, closely monitored, and well-supervised rehabilitation program. VBG can be performed later and the hernia repaired much later. This sequence should not be started on an outpatient basis because the patient cannot cooperate and the situation is too urgent. Ineffectual treatment is the reason these cases become so complicated. Inpatient care is expensive, but necessary. After VBG, outpatient treatment is used until patients reach a steady weight; by that time, pneumoperitoneum may not be needed. The exact sequence of treatment should be tailored to the individual patient.

Moreno believed that pneumoperitoneum reduced edema of the abdominal and hernial contents, and improved circulation in the lower extremities. Again, rapid initial weight loss may be caused by the loss of retained fluid that follows a reduction in caloric intake. If a patient is obese and caloric intake is reduced, one of the first changes that occurs is an unloading of excess body fluid. The heavier is the patient, the greater is the diuresis with early calorie restriction. Dependent edema in large, redundant hernias should be treated by elevation of the affected tissues. This requires bed rest, but the patient should walk at frequent, regular intervals to prevent deep venous thrombosis.

Our medical care system tends to resist the treatment of severely obese patients. Many laypersons and professionals believe that severe obesity can be controlled with diet if the patient will just exert a little willpower. Because of the high cost of hospital care and the real need to hospitalize a patient with severe obesity, hypoventilation, and giant hernia for a prolonged period to reduce weight, expand the abdominal cavity, and improve cardiorespiratory function, more of the surgeon's time may be expended in explaining the treatment plan to third parties than in treating the patient. Giant hernias, like severe obesity, often are the result of misunderstanding and neglect. Effective treatment requires a long-term plan for complete and sustained rehabilitation. More is involved than operative therapy. A change in the patient's way of life may be required.

Adequacy of the Abdominal Cavity

The decision regarding the need for pneumoperitoneum is based on the size of the hernia in relation to the abdominal cavity. Forcing the hernia contents into the body cavity without reestablishing "right of abdominal domain" compresses the vena cava and interferes with venous return, sometimes resulting in acute hypotension (Fig. 39-2).

How can it be determined whether the abdominal cavity has been stretched adequately? Ravitch used a cross-table lateral radiograph taken with the patient supine to determine readiness for operation. He first described this in the preparation of a child with giant

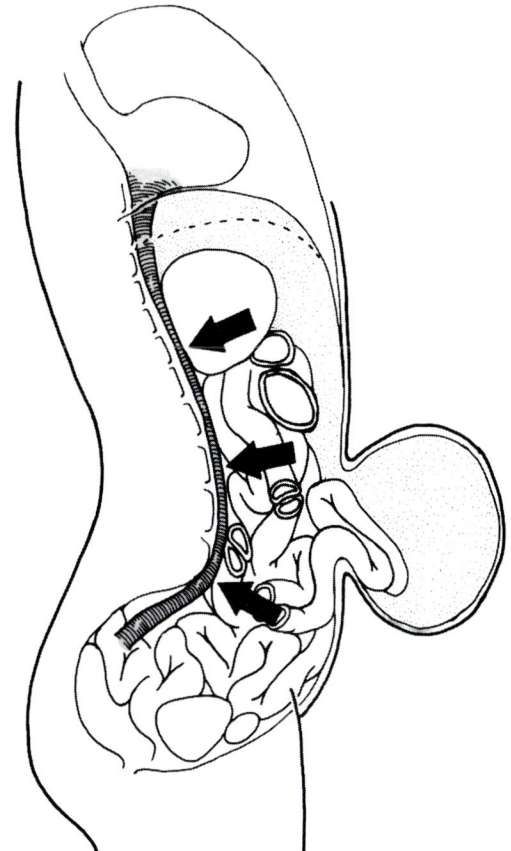

Figure 39-2. Excessive intraabdominal pressure elevates the diaphragm and compresses the vena cava.

eventration after omphalocele, but it also is helpful in determining when an adult is ready for surgery. The exposure should be that of a chest radiograph rather than a huge abdomen because it is the air-filled hernia sac that is of interest, not the abdominal contents. When it appears that the hernia sac is filled with air and the viscera have been reduced so that they provide the appearance of a fluid level at or below the anterior abdominal wall, the defect in the abdominal wall can be closed easily and safely. If extensive adhesions are present between the viscera and the hernia sac, or the fascial ring, the viscera will not drop back into the abdomen. Upright, front and lateral radiographs of the abdomen, showing the diaphragm, are helpful in estimating the relative volumes of the hernia sac and intraabdominal air. Incarcerated, herniated viscera must replace the abdominal air at the time of repair. Often, a hernia that initially is incarcerated reduces during progressive pneumoperitoneum because the air not only expands the hernia sac, but compresses the contents. If the hernia sac contains nothing but air, the progressive pneumoperitoneum has achieved its purpose and the actual repair can proceed.

Intraoperative Decisions

The remainder of the decisions in the decision tree (see Fig. 39-1) relate to closure of the defect. The use of pneumoperitoneum does not guarantee that a complete repair can be accomplished. The abdominal wall and skin must be assessed and the septic status of the wound determined. A huge hernia can be associated with a small fascial defect, and repair of such a lesion is ensured by reestablishment of the abdominal space (Fig. 39-3).

If the neck of the sac is extremely wide, it may not be possible to bring the edges of the defect together, even though there is adequate intraabdominal space. This is more common in the upper abdomen. The edges often can be brought together, however, if all sutures are placed and held up, and adjacent sutures are crossed while each is tied. Prolonged retraction of the wound margins of the upper abdomen may appear to leave too much space for approximation of the fascial edges. An attempt should be made to repair the defect without mesh. It is much safer to close a fascial defect under tension when the viscera are reduced easily than to force such a closure when there is inadequate room.

It is possible to close a wound with too much abdominal wall tension, even though there is adequate abdominal room. The excess tension may not become evident until the patient returns with recurrent herniation around the edge or along both sides of the repair. This may be in the form of multiple small hernias along both sides of the wound where sutures have cut through the abdominal wall in a horizontal direction. Experience and judgment is necessary in determining whether to lay all the sutures and then pull the wound edges together under some tension or to place Marlex mesh as a temporary or permanent gusset in part or all of the defect. The addition of a patch of Marlex mesh over a wound that has been closed under tension may not prevent rows of small, paraincisional hernias from developing as a result of horizontal cutting by sutures that are tied too tightly.

Hernias may develop because of poor tissues in the abdominal wall, and excessive tension in a hernia repair may result in poor tissues. Some patients should be advised preoperatively that several stages may be required to repair their hernia. It is possible to close a defect partially and place a sheet of mesh in what remains, then to remove the mesh later and close the remaining fascial defect. The presence of the mesh provides an opportunity for the adjacent abdominal wall to expand toward the defect and to become functional as an encompassing musculofascial structure.

If there is a history of loss of abdominal wall from excision or infection, the use of prosthetic material in the repair may be required. There are two solutions to this dilemma. One is to repair the hernia partially at a first-stage operation, so that a smaller neck remains, and then simply to close the hernia sac and

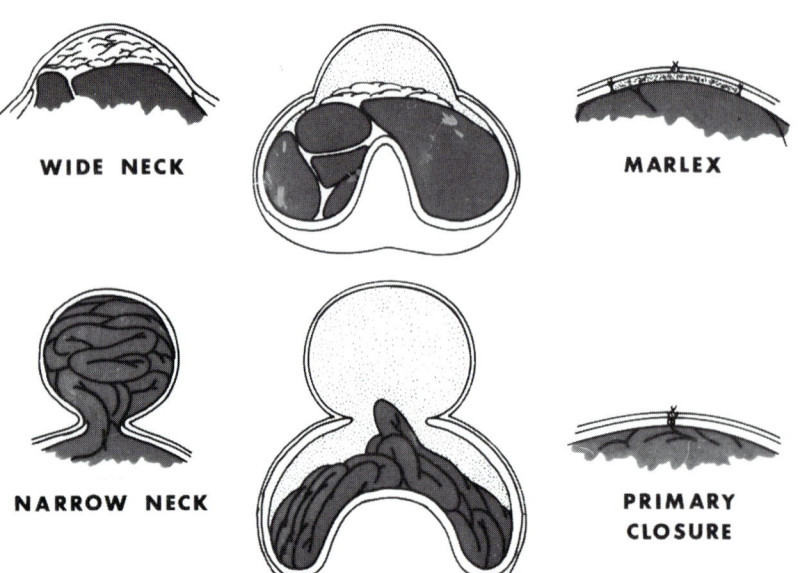

WIDE NECK

NARROW NECK

MARLEX

PRIMARY CLOSURE

Figure 39-3. The failure of pneumoperitoneum to stretch the abdominal wall when the fascial defect is large, and the increase in abdominal volume when the neck of the sac is small but the hernia is large, are depicted.

skin. After the abdominal wall has accommodated to the new demands, the repair is completed as a second-stage procedure. Pneumoperitoneum can be used between stages if necessary.

The other alternative is to cover the fascial defect with a synthetic mesh. If the abdominal wall is inadequate, Marlex mesh may be indicated. If there is contamination from gangrenous bowel or infected or ulcerated skin, it may be necessary to leave the skin open. If the defect is so large as to prevent closure, it may be possible to close part of the defect in the fascia and to close the rest of the area with hernia sac and skin. The skin incision for repair of giant hernia should be made through the hernia sac and skin, so that these tissues remain available until late in the operation. Only after the fascial defect is closed should the skin and sac be removed. If sufficient abdominal wall or skin is not available, the fascial defect can be closed with mesh and the wound left open.

If contamination or sepsis is present, a one-layer closure is indicated to provide both internal and external drainage. The ability of the peritoneal cavity to take care of contamination of the internal surface of a one-layer closure is excellent, and frequent wet dressings are effective in keeping the outer wound clean while granulation tissue forms. Bowel should not be left uncovered in a wound that is healing by contraction of granulation tissue. The contraction of granulation tissue can tear exposed bowel and the opening in the bowel will enlarge progressively as contraction progresses. This is in contrast to bowel fistulas in the depths of a wound, where contraction of scar tissue may close the fistula. It is better to place Marlex mesh in a contaminated wound than to leave bowel exposed and subject to the formation and contraction of granulation tissue. Granulation tissue will form on the surface of bowel and grow into the mesh. The mesh stabilizes the granulating tissue so that it is less likely to contract and tear the bowel.

There may be no way to avoid contact between the bowel and Marlex mesh. This is preferable to leaving bowel in an open wound, however. Adhesions do form between bowel and Marlex mesh if they are in contact. If this occurs, and if further operative treatment is required, timing and nutrition become important in the preservation of bowel integrity during the subsequent operation. Surgery should be delayed until healthy granulation tissue has had time to develop between the bowel and the mesh. This provides the adherent bowel with a thick wall so that dissection from adherent mesh is safe. In a patient with a complicating intestinal fistula that prevents use of the digestive tract, for example, 1 or 2 months of parenteral nutrition may be required to support the production of such tissue. Once the serum albumin has reached a normal concentration and the granulation

tissue has matured, it is possible to dissect between the bowel and the mesh without entering the lumen of the bowel. The mesh may contain "buttonholes," but it can be replaced with a fresh piece. Early attempts to divide adhesions between the bowel and the Marlex mesh may result in further damage to the bowel, additional fistulas, loss of the bowel, and, possibly, the death of the patient. Thus, the success of intraoperative decisions depends on appropriate preoperative preparation and timing of the operation. Preparation may require more than the use of progressive pneumoperitoneum. Marlex mesh used before or during the repair may add to the complexity of the decision tree, but remains a useful adjunct in the treatment of giant hernias, even in contaminated wounds.

TECHNIQUE

The only equipment needed is a large syringe, a stopcock, and a needle that is long enough to reach the peritoneal cavity. To keep the needle in a constant position during manipulation of the syringe, a length of tubing is placed between the stopcock and the needle, and a hemostat is clamped on the shaft of the needle at the level of the skin. A 20-gauge needle is adequate. If a larger needle is used, air is more likely to leak from the needle holes in the peritoneum, especially after repeated refills. The site chosen for injection should be away from the hernia and any scars that may suggest the adherence of bowel. A site near the costal margin in the midclavicular line has a thinner layer of subcutaneous fat than do other areas if the patient is obese. At UIHC, we have used a site in line with the left midclavicular line and just below the costal margin. Moreno recommended the use of a spinal puncture needle inserted at the midpoint of a line running from the anterior superior iliac spine to the umbilicus.

A mercury manometer always is available at the bedside for blood pressure measurement. This device can be connected to the system used for injecting air, and pressure measurements taken and recorded. The initial pressure usually is about 8 mmHg. At the time that the patient is feeling too full to accept more air, the pressure will be higher than 20 mmHg.

The skin and peritoneum are infiltrated with local anesthetic using a small-gauge needle. Aspiration is used to ensure that the needle is not in a vein. Air should enter the peritoneum with almost no resistance. As the abdomen is distended, air usually rises into the hernia sac. If the injection causes pain, the inflation should be stopped until the pain abates. If several attempts to inflate the abdomen cause pain, the injection should be postponed until another time. Injections are continued at daily intervals for several days and then at longer intervals such that the patient always has a full feeling.

Steichen suggested the use of a polyethylene catheter that is made for intravenous use and can be left in place for repeated injections in infants with significant eventration from congenital omphalocele. Raynor and Del Guercio[17] recommend a 5F pigtail catheter threaded over wire. The wire is placed through a needle after proper positioning has been established by the injection of iodized oil (Lipiodol). The pigtail catheter is rigid enough to prevent kinking and is sutured in place. This avoids repeated needle sticks in an infant. Most adults do not mind the use of a new needle with each refill. This approach has the advantage of being less likely to leak air.

Initial injections range from 500 to 4500 mL in adults, and the total amount of air can be as much as 23 L in divided refills over as much as 60 days. Median values at UIHC have been seven injections with a total of 13 L of air given over 4 weeks, but there is great variation. Pingree and Clark recommend refills every 24 hours for only 7 days. Whelan and Eaker used four doses of 150 to 350 mL over 4 days in a 6-year-old child with a ventral hernia that resulted from a first-stage omphalocele repair, and then gave 10 more doses on an outpatient basis over 6 months, with a last dose of 1500 mL. Both the initial and the total amount of air injected are governed in part by the size of the hernia. More air is required for a large hernia because of the larger volume of the hernia and the fact that both the hernia and the abdomen must be distended. If the patient has heart disease, the progressive stretching should be done at a slower rate over a longer period. Air can be removed easily if the pneumoperitoneum proves to be excessive. This is one of the great advantages of the technique over an attempt to reduce and repair a giant hernia without such preparation. Injections are spaced to keep the patient feeling full. If this degree of inflation is not reached and maintained, there may not be adequate space for the hernia contents at the time of repair, even though the injections are continued for several weeks.

Shoulder pain is to be expected when the patient is upright during the first few days. It is caused by stretching of the suspensory ligaments of the liver. Normally, the liver is held against the diaphragm by a vacuum and the suspensory ligaments are not stretched. It is only when air or fluid fills the space between the liver and the diaphragm that the liver is suspended by the suspensory ligaments. The suspensory ligaments are an extension of the capsule of the liver and share the sensitivity to stretching. Referred pain to the shoulder can occur because of chemical irritation, as with acid gastric juice. Air is not irritat-

ing, however, and the pain that is referred from air in the upper abdomen is present more often when the patient is upright because the air rises to a position that allows the liver to leave the diaphragm and stretch the suspensory ligament. If previous operations in the upper abdomen have created adhesions between the liver and the diaphragm, the patient may not complain of shoulder pain in the upright position after the initial pneumoperitoneum. This pain disappears after a few days. It can be severe enough early to raise questions regarding some complication of the pneumoperitoneum. For this reason, we usually begin the treatment in the hospital and continue it on an outpatient basis.

Physicians have voiced concern about all the injected air going into the hernia sac and failing to stretch the abdominal cavity. The skin and hernia sac have a limited capacity, even when they are stretched, and additional air stretches the abdomen. When the first patients were treated at UIHC, we painted the skin with tincture of benzoin and used adhesive tape to support and compress the hernia sac. Such support is indicated if the pneumoperitoneum is begun a few days after completion of an emergency operation and the closure consists of only hernia sac and skin.

It is more comfortable for the patient and perfectly safe to avoid the use of adhesive plaster and allow the hernia sac to distend. The hernia sac will enlarge, but the skin is surprisingly strong, even when it is stretched to its limit. If enough air is used, all areas of the "balloon" eventually enlarge, including the thicker-walled abdominal cavity. Air is much cheaper than adhesive tape. In addition, the skin will be in better condition at the time of operation if no tape blisters are present. If the patient feels more secure with external support, there is a binder made in panels and of a material that allows the Velcro to attach at any point on the outside surface so that it provides maximum conformity and adjustability, does not slide up and down, and is comfortable.*

RISKS

The injection of air into the abdomen poses little risk. Air embolism is a theoretic risk peculiar to pneumoperitoneum. Such a reaction in patients with giant hernia has not been observed at UIHC, and Moreno reported no instances during his experience. Air embolism is uncommon, but those who use peritoneum should take care, especially during the initial intro-

---

*Dale Abdominal Binder, Dale Medical Products, Inc., 7 Cross Street, P.O. Box 1556, Plainsville, MA 02762-0556.

duction of air, to aspirate and ensure that no blood is present in the syringe before beginning the insufflation. The amount of air introduced should be small at first until it is apparent that the patient is tolerating the injection and that the air is going into the peritoneal cavity. Air in the right heart displaces blood so that the heart cannot eject the contents effectively (air is compressible) and sudden circulatory collapse and loss of consciousness ensue. Such a reaction in a patient receiving intraperitoneal air should lead to an immediate presumptive diagnosis of air embolism. The patient should be turned on the right side with the head of the table raised to allow the air to rise and be displaced by blood entering the right ventricle. This should result in the immediate return of cardiac output, consciousness, and blood pressure.

The use of nitrous oxide as an anesthetic agent in a patient with pneumoperitoneum is hazardous.[3,5] To be effective as an anesthetic agent, nitrous oxide requires a high concentration. It is much more soluble in water than is nitrogen. As a result, it moves rapidly through the bloodstream and tissue fluids, and into the air-containing space, until the concentration in the abdominal cavity equals that in the lungs. Nitrogen, which comprises the major gas in the abdominal space, is less soluble in water and therefore moves much less rapidly. As a consequence, soon after a patient begins breathing nitrous oxide, the abdomen contains both the nitrogen that already was present and the rapidly moving, large volume and high concentration of nitrous oxide. The total volume of gas in the abdomen is doubled within 5 or 10 minutes, causing a rapid and marked increase in intraabdominal pressure (see Fig. 39-2) with an intolerable compression of the vena cava and elevation of the diaphragm. An increase in the pulse rate, more rapid respiration, and a fall in blood pressure result; if the increased intraabdominal pressure is not relieved, death soon follows. A rapid incision into the distended hernia sac will relieve the excessive pressure in the abdomen if the surgeon recognizes the problem during the induction of anesthesia. The danger of nitrous oxide in the presence of pneumoperitoneum should be discussed with the anesthesiologist before anesthesia is induced.

Leakage of air from the abdomen into the tissues at the site of puncture of the peritoneum may develop in older patients with weaker tissues. There is no danger to the patient from subcutaneous emphysema. Air that leaks, however, does not distend the abdomen. The pneumoperitoneum becomes ineffective if the leak is large. Puncture of the bowel is unusual, and results in a hole of inconsequential size. The inserted needle should not be moved in such a way as to sweep the point through an arc and thereby lacerate the bowel. If the insufflation is too great at any one time and the patient has respiratory distress, it is a simple matter to remove some of the air. This seldom is required.

RESULTS

The results of pneumoperitoneum are evident when the hernia sac is opened, provided the stretching has been adequate and adhesions do not hold the bowel in the hernia sac. All the bowel usually is within the abdomen. There may be many adhesions that need to be divided. The bowel should be examined before the repair is begun to ensure that no potential sites of obstruction remain or injuries to the bowel have been overlooked. The fascial edges usually are approximated easily. Long-term results of the hernia repair depend on other factors, such as body weight, the absence of wound infection, and the strength of the tissues. There is a period after the air is removed and the defect in the abdominal wall is repaired before the tissues regain their normal tone. This allows the wound to heal without the tension and compression that would exist between tissue and sutures if the wound could have been forced closed without such preparation. Moreno demonstrated the laxity of the abdominal wall by operating on a few patients under local anesthesia, and reported excellent relaxation with no difficulty in maintaining the bowel in the abdomen. In most patients, no foreign material is required beyond the usual sutures. There is none of the concern about circulation and breathing that used to mark the early postoperative course after repair of a giant hernia. Because of the blunt dissection carried out by the air, the hernia usually is reduced, fewer adhesions are present, and the bowel is handled less during the operation. Early resumption of bowel function is the norm.

The recent interest in laparoscopic surgery has made insufflation of the abdomen commonplace, and surgeons may become more receptive to the use of progressive pneumoperitoneum in the preparation for repair of giant hernia. One of the chief advantages of the laparoscopic approach for cholecystectomy and other operations is reduction in the amount of postoperative discomfort. How much does distention of the abdomen by the gas used during a laparoscopic operation, and the subsequent relaxation of abdominal muscles, contribute to patient comfort during the early postoperative period? A study of the course of recovery in patients who begin with laparoscopic operations and then are converted to open procedures may provide an answer to this question. Patients who have giant hernias repaired after progressive pneumoperitoneum have an easy and rapid recovery.

REFERENCES

1. Connolly DP, Perri FR. Giant hernias managed by pneumoperitoneum. JAMA 1969;209:71.
2. Drye JC. Intraperitoneal pressure in the human. Surg Gynecol Obstet 1948;87:472.
3. Eger EI, Saidman LJ. Hazards of N2O anesthesia in bowel obstruction and pneumothorax. Anesthesiology 1965;26:61.
4. Goñi Moreno I. Chronic eventrations and large hernias. Surgery 1947;22:945.
5. Hunter AR. Problems of anesthesia in artificial pneumothorax. Proc Soc Med 1955;48:765.
6. Koontz AR. Hernias that have forfeited the right of domicile: use of pneumoperitoneum as an aid in their operative cure. South Med J 1958;51:165.
7. Kremen AJ, Linner JH, Nelson CH. An experimental evaluation of the nutritional importance of proximal and distal small intestine. Ann Surg 1954;140:439.
8. Mansuy MM Jr, Hager HG. Pneumoperitoneum in preparation for correction of giant hernia. N Engl J Med 1958;258:33.
9. Mason EE. Pneumoperitoneum in the management of giant hernia. Surgery 1956;39:143.
10. Mason EE. Rehabilitation of the ruptured gourmand. The Manitoba Medical Review 1963;43:129.
11. Mason EE. Vertical banded gastroplasty for obesity. Arch Surg 1982;117:701.
12. Mason EE, Ito C. Gastric bypass in obesity. Surg Clin North Am 1967;47:1345.
13. Mason EE, Kridelbaugh WJ, Crouch WH, Ward M. Streptomycin in the treatment of tuberculous enteritis: a report of thirty-three cases. Am J Med Sci 1949;217:28.
14. Overholt RH. Intraperitoneal pressure. Arch Surg 1931;22:691.
15. Pingree JH, Clark JH. Pneumoperitoneum. A neglected procedure for the repair of large abdominal hernias. Arch Surg 1968;96:252.
16. Ravitch MM. Giant omphalocele: second stage repair with the aid of pneumoperitoneum. JAMA 1963;185:122.
17. Raynor RW, Del Guercio LRM. The place for pneumoperitoneum in the repair of massive hernia. World J Surg 1989;13:581.
18. Spratt JS. Artificial pneumoperitoneum, efficacy in enlarging the peritoneal cavity for early closure of congenital omphalocele. Am J Surg 1961;101:375.
19. Steichen FM. A simple method for establishing, maintaining, and regulating surgically induced pneumoperitoneum in preparation for large hernia repairs. Surgery 1965;58:1031.
20. Whelan TP Jr, Eaker AB. Pneumoperitoneum in preparation for second-stage omphalocele repair. Surgery 1962;51:263.

Editor's Comment

The first papers on this subject were by Ivan Goñi Moreno of Argentina. Mason has demonstrated clearly how these original concepts can be translated into day-to-day practice.

In this era of active research and publication, it is almost impossible to think of a new approach. Ivan Goñi Moreno is credited accurately with being among the few who have produced such an approach. The idea is particularly praiseworthy because the technique that Goñi Moreno promulgated in 1940 truly works.

I have had some experience with this method since 1949. I never cease to be amazed at how pneumoperitoneum, properly applied, converts seemingly impossible hernia operations into procedures of almost ludicrous ease.

Goñi Moreno (1905–1976) was born in Paris and reared there in a traditional Argentinian home. He opted for his Argentinian nationality at an early date. Associated with many academic greats, such as Foussay and Finochietto, Goñi Moreno developed an early and lasting interest in teaching. He traveled extensively in Europe, studying under Professors Gasset, Rouviere, and Monod.

Goñi Moreno's first manuscript, published in 1927, was on inguinal hernias. This paper was but a prelude to the work for which he always will be remembered, *Progressive Pneumoperitoneum in the Treatment of Voluminous Eventrations*. Immediately before his death, Goñi Moreno was designated Master in Surgery of the Argentinian Surgical Society, the highest honor of the organization.

Interest in the use of pneumoperitoneum has escalated today because of advances in laparoscopic surgery.

L.M.N.

Hernia, Fourth Edition, edited
by Lloyd M. Nyhus and Robert E. Condon.
J.B. Lippincott Company, Philadelphia © 1995.

Chapter 40

Herniography

Sam G.G. Smedberg

Roentgenographic demonstration of the peritoneal lining of the abdominal cavity using insufflated air as a negative contrast medium, so-called pneumoperitoneum, first was performed in 1914.[2] This technique has been used to demonstrate hernias. Its use never became widespread, however, because of low accuracy.

Positive-contrast peritoneography provides a more detailed view of the peritoneal lining of the abdominal wall, and the peritoneal covering of intraabdominal organs also can be demonstrated. The technique was developed in animal experiments during the 1950s.[2,25] Peritoneal reactions to the water-soluble contrast media were studied. A transient peritoneal inflammatory reaction was seen, but no residual inflammation or scarring. Peritoneography subsequently was applied in patients in the diagnosis of intraabdominal disease,[13] and was refined further by the use of computerized tomographic scanning.[27]

Positive-contrast peritoneography used for the diagnosis of hernias in the inguinofemoral region and the pelvis is called herniography. Herniography first was used for the demonstration of occult contralateral hernias in pediatric patients with unilateral hernias to avoid negative contralateral explorations and to clarify questionable clinical findings.[4] The pediatric use of herniography is not discussed in this chapter. In adult patients, herniography has been performed routinely since the early 1970s.[15,16] Only occasional adult patients were examined with herniography before 1972. Since then, the use of herniography has been increasing, primarily in Europe. Technical aspects, roentgenographic interpretation, clinical use, and indications have been studied further, and herniography has been used as a diagnostic aid in clinical trials.

INDICATIONS

Herniography is indicated primarily in patients with groin pain suggesting primary or recurrent hernia that cannot be verified by clinical examination, and in patients with inconclusive clinical findings. In high-risk patients with manifest hernias, the appearance of

a hernia on the herniographic picture can help the surgeon determine whether to operate and which surgical procedure to use. Finally, herniography is used for scientific purposes as a sensitive and reliable method of diagnosing recurrent hernia in patients operated on in clinical trials.

Patients who have symptoms indicative of a hernia but with no palpable lesion represent a well-known challenge for surgeons. The surgeon must choose either to wait until a clinically manifest hernia develops or to explore the groin surgically and run the risk that no hernia is found. Obscure groin pain and uncertain findings at clinical examination have been the main indications for herniography in most studies.[1,6,8,12,16,19,22,28,32,34,35] The roentgenographic demonstration of a hernia qualifies the patient for surgical treatment, provided other causes of groin symptoms have been ruled out.[26,28]

Preoperative herniography generally is not indicated in patients with palpable hernias. Overlooked hernias at operation are well-known but infrequent causes of recurrence, and should be prevented by more careful surgical exploration rather than by the use of herniography. A randomized study was performed to assess the value of improved preoperative diagnosis.[23] The authors concluded that preoperative herniography in clinically manifest hernias does not influence the surgical treatment of these patients. Preoperative radiologic diagnosis of palpable hernias, however, may be desirable in selected cases (eg, in patients with high operative risks and those who have hernias with atypical clinical features).

The clinical diagnosis of a recurrent hernia sometimes is uncertain. Operative evaluation also is more difficult in the previously operated groin because of scarified and disarranged tissues. Exploratory surgery is discouraged in questionable recurrent cases. Herniography is recommended before surgery is decided on. The use of herniography in manifest recurrent hernias also has been considered justified.[5,21,35] There is an increased risk of overlooking combined defects at the time of operation. In manifest recurrent hernias, however, the use of new operative techniques, such as preperitoneal dissection and implantation of a synthetic graft covering the whole inguinofemoral region, which is being recommended both through open and laparoscopic surgery, prevents the possibility of overlooking combined defects and reduces the need for herniography based on this indication.

In clinical trials, herniography is superior to physical examination for both preoperative and postoperative diagnosis. Recurrences can be found before they become clinically manifest, and follow-up time may be reduced.[31]

TECHNIQUE

A detailed description of the herniographic technique in adult patients has been provided by Gullmo and associates.[16,18] To achieve a good examination, it should be performed on a table that permits fluoroscopy with a tilted tube. The patient should void before the examination to prevent accidental puncture of the bladder and displacement of the peritoneal lining of the inguinal fossae by the distended bladder. No other preparation of the patient is necessary, although the routine use of atropine as premedication has been recommended.[22] With the patient in the supine position, the abdominal wall is punctured under sterile conditions in the lower left quadrant, lateral to the rectus muscle, or in the midline below the umbilicus. The puncture is facilitated by a small incision made in the skin after the induction of local anesthesia. A mandrin-equipped plastic catheter similar to that used for percutaneous cholangiography, or a similar device, is used. A 20- to 22-gauge needle or a Veres needle may be used. The point of the mandrin should be blunted to avoid perforation of the intestine. The catheter is guided into the lesser pelvis and its position tested by the instillation of a few milliliters of saline solution. There should be no resistance to the injection. The table is tilted 25 degrees, with the foot of the table lowered, and 50 to 80 mL of contrast medium is injected, initially under fluoroscopic guidance. A nonionic, low-osmolar, positive-iodine contrast medium such as iohexol (Omnipaque), 240 mg/mL, is used. The patient then is turned to the prone position. As the patient strains and turns from side to side, the contrast medium pools in the inguinal region, the lowest part of the abdominal cavity in this position.

Exposures are made in standard views to demonstrate possible hernias and specify the types of hernias found. Additional exposures may be necessary. Both groins are examined. The inguinal region is visualized best with the tube tilted 25 to 30 degrees caudally. The views obtained are exact anteroposterior views with the streak of the crena ani projected through the symphysis and oblique views with the patient turned about 20 degrees to the right and to the left. Femoral hernias are revealed better with the tube at right angles to the table. For optimal contrast filling of the groins during exposure, the patient is asked to strain repeatedly. A rolled, hard pillow under the abdomen may enhance the filling of the inguinal regions. Hernial contents of the intestine or omentum may obstruct the neck and give falsely normal results. Palpable hernias should be reduced, therefore, to permit filling of contrast medium. Finally, the pouch of Douglas and the pelvic floor are exposed in the standing patient.

INTERPRETATION

The appearance of the peritoneal lining in the groin has no relationship to the muscles and aponeuroses in the region. The herniographic landmarks separating the three inguinal fossae on each side are the median umbilical fold (obliterated urachus) in the midline, the medial umbilical fold (obliterated umbilical artery) separating the supravesical fossa from the medial inguinal fossa, and the lateral umbilical fold (inferior epigastric artery and vein) separating the medial inguinal fossa from the lateral inguinal fossa (Fig. 40-1). The epigastric fold normally is the least prominent fold.

In the normal groin, the inguinal fossae do not reach beyond the rim of the pubic bone in the medial part of the posterior inguinal wall, but the lateral fossa and the lateral part of the medial fossa may cross this border (Fig. 40-2).

Indirect hernias emerge from the lateral fossa, lateral to the epigastric notch. The lateral margin forms a smooth continuation of the lateral lower abdominal wall. Indirect hernias are principally uniform in shape, with an oblique course along the cord or the round ligament within the inguinal canal, and are classified easily according to their width and extension (Fig. 40-3).

Direct hernias vary significantly in shape and size. Most often, the rupture or bulging is located within the medial fossa (lateral direct hernia), but it frequently also can be seen bulging from the suprapubic fossa (medial direct hernia [Fig. 40-4]). Sometimes a double direct hernia is found, with the medial umbilical fold separating the two parts of the hernia (Fig. 40-5). Direct hernias generally are broad-based and dome-shaped, but may appear with a narrow neck on rare occasions.

Broad and deep fossae are caused by an acquired laxity of the posterior inguinal wall without hernial rupture. The diagnostic criteria are not well defined,

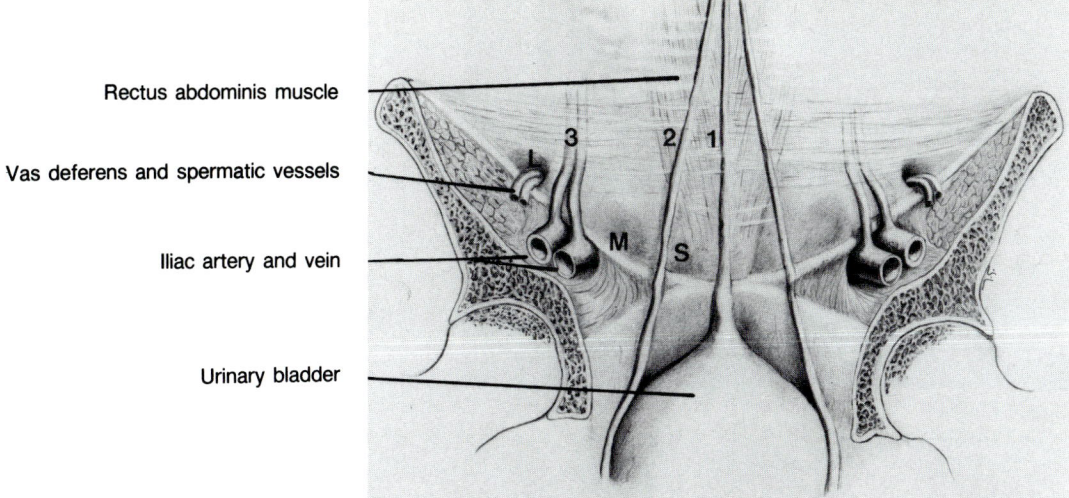

Rectus abdominis muscle

Vas deferens and spermatic vessels

Iliac artery and vein

Urinary bladder

Figure 40-1. The lower anterior abdominal wall seen from behind. 1, median umbilical fold (obliterated urachus); 2, medial umbilical fold (obliterated umbilical artery); 3, lateral umbilical fold (inferior epigastric artery and vein); S, supravesical fossa; M, medial inguinal fossa; L, lateral inguinal fossa.

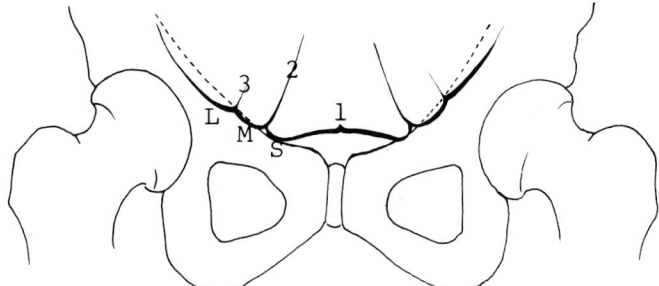

Figure 40-2. Drawing of a normal herniogram. 1, median umbilical fold; 2, medial umbilical fold; 3, lateral umbilical fold; S, supravesical fossa; M, medial inguinal fossa; L, lateral inguinal fossa.

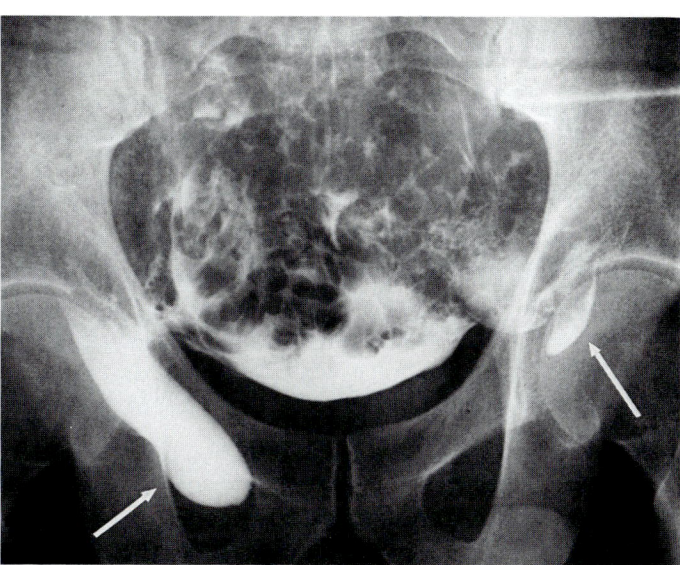

Figure 40-3. Bilateral indirect hernias (*arrows*) in a 40-year-old man. The right-sided hernia, reaching beyond the external inguinal ring, was palpable.

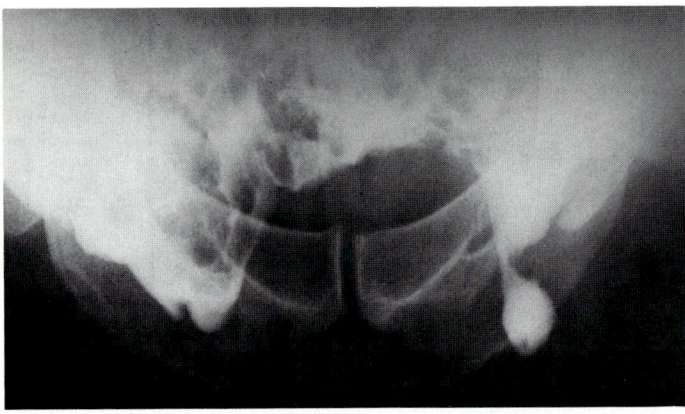

Figure 40-4. A lateral direct hernia and a small indirect hernia on the left side, and a medial direct hernia on the right side, in a 54-year-old man. The left-sided hernia was palpable.

and the diagnosis depends greatly on the experience of the investigator. The inguinal fossae project below the normal position at the rim of the pubic bone, and the medial umbilical fold usually is displaced medially (Fig. 40-6).

Femoral hernias are located more inferiorly and posteriorly than are inguinal hernias. They sometimes are seen while the patient remains in the supine position after the injection of contrast medium, before turning to the prone position. Femoral hernias are directed caudally and are shown best with the tube at right angles to the table. The typical femoral hernia is pear-shaped, with a long, narrow neck corresponding to the passage through the femoral canal, which clearly illustrates the risk of incarceration of femoral hernias (Fig. 40-7). It may be difficult to distinguish this hernia from a lateral direct hernia, particularly in femoral hernias with a broad infundibulum. Oblique views and femoral vein phlebography to rule out compression of the vein by a femoral hernia may be helpful in such cases.[16]

Inguinofemoral hernias are broad, combined defects in the transversalis fascia, resulting in shallow hernias with a direct portion in continuity with a femoral defect (often wide) across the iliopubic tract (see Fig. 40-5C).

Sliding hernias may be difficult to diagnose by herniography. The diagnosis should be suspected when the palpable finding does not correspond to a sac of the same size or shape. Often, only a claw-like peritoneal irregularity is seen in combination with an incomplete delineation of the inguinal fossae (Fig. 40-8). A barium enema can disclose the true nature of the hernia.

Obturator hernias are rare findings, often seen as diverticula localized in the upper, lateral corner of the obturator foramen. They have the same caudal direction as do femoral hernias, but protrude beneath the superior pubic ramus (Fig. 40-9).

Other rare hernias revealed incidentally by herniography include perineal hernias, which are seen as diverticula of the pouch of Douglas, and prevesical hernias, which appear as pouches posterior to the symphysis pubis in the space of Retzius. Pelvic hernias are studied best with the patient in the upright position.

The diagnosis of spigelian hernias requires an examination in specific positions.[16] Hernias sometimes are found corresponding to the site of clinical symptoms. Abnormal findings are rare, however, and ultrasonography may be preferable in these cases.[16,33]

Other hernias of the anterior abdominal wall that can be demonstrated by herniography are umbilical hernias, incisional hernias, and interparietal hernias.

Different types of combined hernias are seen frequently. The interpretation can be difficult, and the use of oblique views is shown in Figure 40-5.

Recurrent hernias are seen as clearly as are primary hernias. The herniographic landmarks may be distorted by the previous repair. Otherwise, the specified diagnoses are made using the same criteria as for primary hernias. Recurrent hernias often have a fibrous, narrow neck (Fig. 40-10). Even in direct recurrent hernias, a narrow neck, indicating risk of incarceration, has been found in almost one third of patients.[29] True recurrent hernias caused by ruptured repairs and hernias that were overlooked during operation or developed afterward may be identified if preoperative herniography is performed.[23,31]

COMPLICATIONS

The overall complication rate after herniography is reported to be 5.8%, which is equal to or lower than the rate in intravenous pyelography.[7] Most complications are minor; major complications are rare. The potential risks relate to puncture of the abdominal

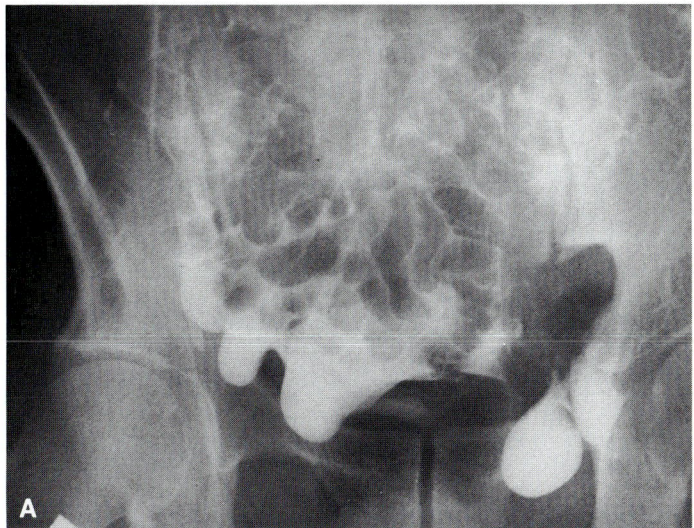

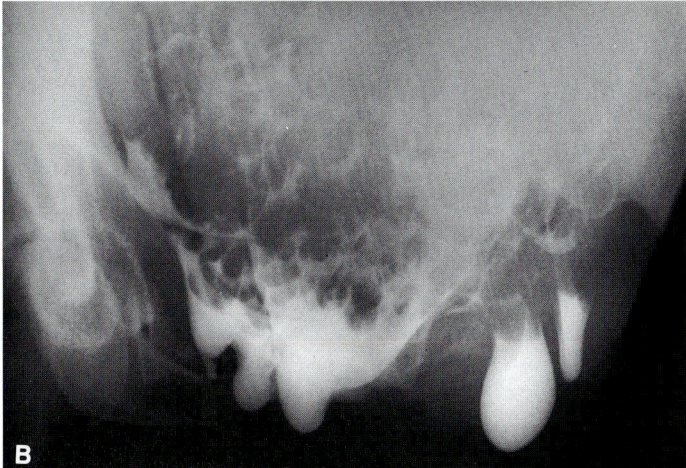

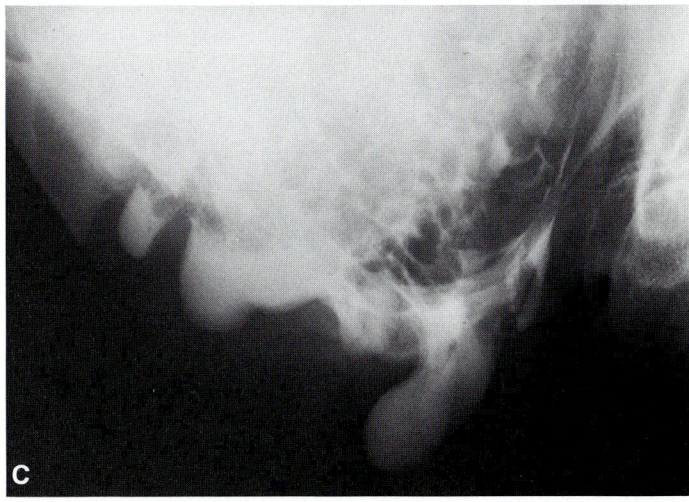

Figure 40-5. A 54-year-old man with a palpable hernia in the left groin. (*A*) An approximate anteroposterior view demonstrating three small hernial sacs on the right side, two direct and one indirect hernias, and two hernial sacs on the left side, difficult to specify anatomically. (*B*) Oblique view with the right side down. The three inguinal fossae on the right side, with their respective hernias, are demonstrated clearly, as are the two hernial sacs on the left side. (*C*) Oblique view with the left side down. On the right side, the lateral direct hernia is directed anteriorly over the inguinal ligament. The medial direct hernia is combined with a broad femoral bulging, pointing caudally, thus constituting an inguinofemoral hernia. On the left side, a small indirect protrusion is seen lateral to the two other sacs, emerging from the medial fossae.

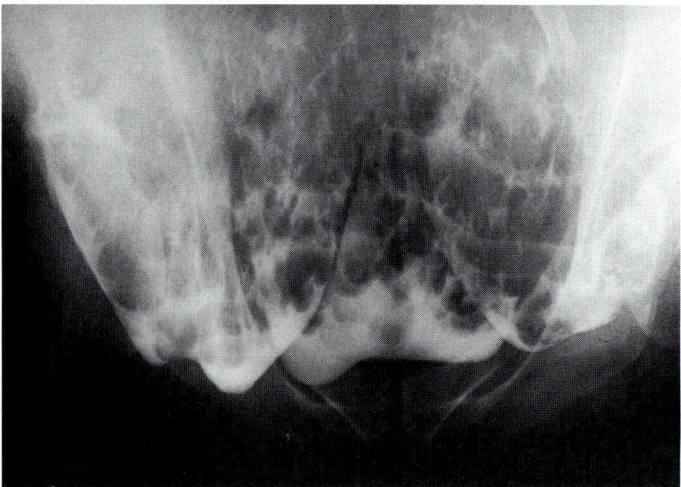

Figure 40-6. A 54-year-old man with broad and deep fossae bilaterally and medial displacement of the medial umbilical folds.

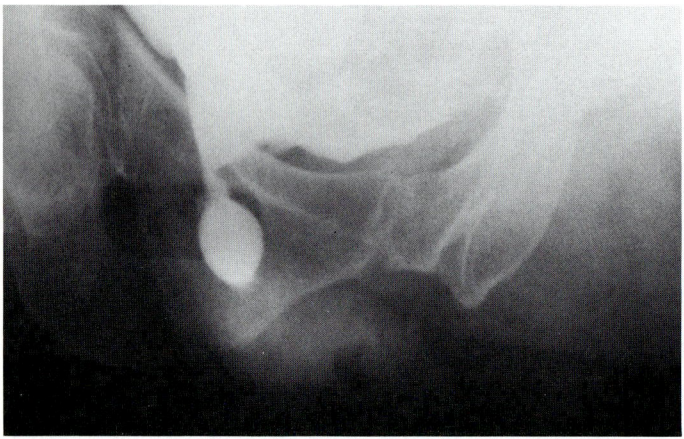

Figure 40-7. A 61-year-old woman with continuous right-sided groin pain but no palpable hernia. Herniography demonstrates a typical femoral hernia, with a long, narrow neck.

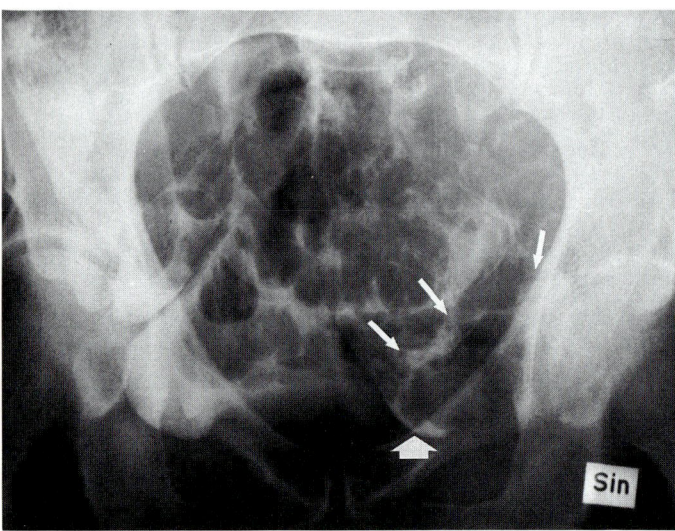

Figure 40-8. A 45-year-old man previously operated on three times on the right side, with left-sided symptoms of a hernia. An incomplete delineation of the posterior wall is seen on the left side (*small arrows*) in addition to a claw-like formation (*large arrow*), indicating a sliding hernia. On the right side, a broad direct recurrent hernia is seen protruding from the suprapubic fossa.

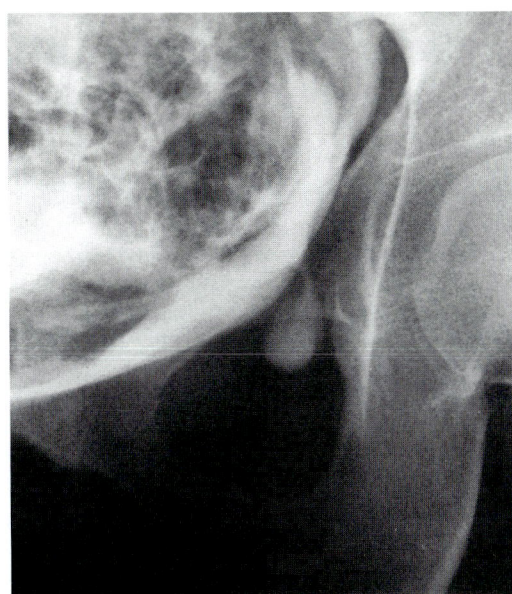

Figure 40-9. An obturator hernia on the left side found incidentally in a 34-year-old woman.

wall, incorrect positioning of the catheter or needle for the injection of contrast medium, and adverse reactions to the contrast medium. The use of nonionic, low-osmolar contrast media has reduced markedly the pain that often accompanied the injection of the contrast media previously used.[10]

During puncture of the abdominal wall, there is a risk of injury to branches of the epigastric vessels. Hematoma and bleeding in the abdominal wall have been described.[7,16] Diagnostic abdominal paracentesis has been used for more than a century, and although intestinal perforation and serosal damage have been reported to occur frequently in emergency situations, there have been few complications related to the puncture itself.[14] Intestinal perforation also has been reported in herniographic examinations, although with a low frequency.[7,16] Intestinal perforation is seen primarily in the early experience of the investigator. Puncturing the right iliac fossa increases the risk of perforation of a mobile cecum. Two cases of severe complications with intramural small-intestinal hematomas and one case of cellulitis of the abdominal wall have been reported, all in pediatric patients.[3,5] The use of a metal needle instead of a catheter probably increases the risk of injection into the intestine.[5] This risk can be reduced by blunting the point of the mandrin. Two decades of herniographic experience at Helsingborg Hospital includes one patient with retroperitoneal bleeding caused by puncture of a tumor,[28] and one patient each with retroperitoneal and intraperitoneal bleeding, probably caused by puncture of mesenteric and omental vessels. Transfusions were given, but surgical exploration was not necessary in any case. Occasional cases of intestinal perforation have been noted. The patients have been treated with antibiotics and there have been no adverse sequelae.

The puncture of the peritoneum and the injection of contrast medium may induce vasovagal reactions. Therefore, premedication with atropine has been recommended.

CLINICAL EXPERIENCE

The use of herniography in adults has been reported comprehensively, mainly by Gullmo and Ekberg.[6,7,9,16–18] Its diagnostic accuracy in detecting hernia has been high, with only exceptional false-positive

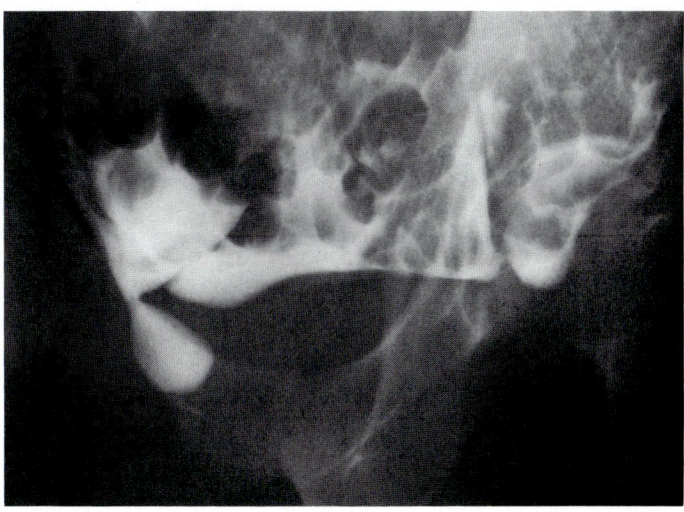

Figure 40-10. A lateral direct recurrent hernia in a 55-year-old man operated on 1 year earlier for a Bassini repair of a direct hernia.

or false-negative findings.[22,23,28,30] The specific diagnosis of the type of hernia is less accurate. If a single hernia is present, the herniographic diagnosis of the type is fairly good, with available figures indicating an accuracy of 78% to 92% compared to operative findings.[23,28] In combined hernias, however, the different diagnostic criteria used in herniography and operation, mainly in regard to direct hernias, make the herniographic diagnosis less accurate. The herniographic diagnosis is based on the appearance of the inguinal wall during straining in the prone position, whereas the operative diagnosis is made with the patient relaxed in the supine position. Herniography appears to be more sensitive in these cases.

According to the published literature, herniography in adult patients is a sensitive, reliable, and safe diagnostic method, capable of demonstrating nonpalpable hernias and clarifying the source of obscure groin pain. Groin pain has become the major and clinically important indication for herniography in adults. Even asymptomatic contralateral hernias have been found frequently, as reported in practically all series. In cases of indirect or femoral hernia, this additional information may be of great value to the patient.

For postoperative follow-up, the diagnosis obtained with herniography also has proved to be more accurate than the clinical diagnosis. In follow-up studies after hernia operations, herniography was performed in patients who had symptoms but no palpable recurrence. The detection of nonpalpable, symptomatic cases of recurrence increased the recurrence rates by about 40% after operations for both primary and recurrent hernias.[29,30] These results were confirmed in a German study.[35] In a clinical trial using postoperative herniography as part of routine postoperative follow-up, additional asymptomatic, nonpalpable recurrences were found.[31] Thus, from a scientific point of view, recurrence rates based only on clinical findings do not have acceptable reliability. Furthermore, we found it possible to determine both the type and the cause of recurrence by comparing preoperative and follow-up herniographic examinations, and correlating the postoperative findings with the operative diagnoses and the repairs performed.[30,31]

In clinical trials, the possibility of improving the clinical diagnosis with herniography facilitates the study of many diagnostic and therapeutic hernia problems. In one study, the clinical consequences of an improved preoperative diagnosis obtained through the routine use of preoperative herniography in manifest hernias was evaluated. Operative judgment and procedures were not found to be altered by preoperative herniography in palpable hernias.[23] In another study, ligation of the resected indirect hernial sac was found not to be necessary.[31] Studies comparing different methods of repair are being performed.

COMMENTS

The high diagnostic accuracy of herniography in detecting hernias is an obvious consequence of the technique itself. Determining the specific type of hernia is more difficult, and accurate interpretation of the study requires significant experience. Clinical examination is unreliable in this respect, however, and herniography is the best method available.[24] Furthermore, herniography clearly demonstrates the size and shape of the hernia and the appearance of the hernial neck, and thus the potential risk of incarceration. Distinguishing between a normal posterior inguinal wall, broad and deep fossae, and a direct hernia is difficult, and there is no clear line of demarcation between these findings. The same diagnostic difficulties also apply to surgical exploration.[20] It should be pointed out that herniographic and operative diagnoses are based on different anatomic structures. The operative evaluation of the posterior inguinal wall, for example, does not include the peritoneal lining.

Herniography plays a major role in two important hernia-related diagnostic problems. The first is the clinical problem of obscure groin pain, including postoperative pain without palpable recurrence. The second is the challenge of defining recurrence and measuring and comparing operative results. The definitions of recurrent hernia used in different series vary significantly, including recurrences noticed by the patient, recurrences causing symptoms that indicate a second operation, recurrences that are operated on, palpable hernias except minor asymptomatic bulging at the pubic tubercle, and any palpable abnormality indicating a recurrent hernia. This complicates the comparison and evaluation of results. Standardized diagnostic criteria for recurrence are just as valuable as is the operative classification of hernias in evaluating the results of surgery. The use of herniography allows clinical materials to be compared, something that previously has been difficult. "A reporting of the true recurrence rate without herniography is no longer conceivable."[35]

Critics of the technique have cited the potential complications caused by direct puncture of the abdominal cavity, the injection of contrast medium, and irradiation of the pelvic region in young patients. It is agreed, however, that herniography may be useful in the treatment of patients with rare, recurrent, and questionable hernias. Furthermore, herniography is of great interest from an academic point of view. It "enhances our understanding of the dynamics of hernia development and the principles of surgical repair."[21]

REFERENCES

1. Berg van den JC, Strijk SP. Groin hernia: role of herniography. Radiology 1992;184:191.
2. Birtzle H. Ist die Peritoneographie als röntgenologische Untersuchungsmetode möglich und brauchbar? Rofo Fortschr Geb Rontgenstr Neuen Bildgeb Verfahr 1961;95:824.
3. Butch JL, Kuhn JP. Intramural hematoma of the small bowel: a possible lethal complication of herniography. Surgery 1978;83:121.
4. Ducharme JC, Bertrand R, Chacar R. Is it possible to diagnose inguinal hernia by x-ray? J Can Assoc Radiol 1967;18:448.
5. Ducharme JC, Guttman FM, Poljicak M. Hematoma of the bowel and cellulitis of the abdominal wall complicating herniography. J Pediatr Surg 1980;15:318.
6. Ekberg O. Inguinal herniography in adults: technique, normal anatomy and diagnostic criteria for hernias. Radiology 1981;138:31.
7. Ekberg O. Complications after herniography in adults. Am J Roentgenol 1983;140:491.
8. Ekberg O, Blomquist P, Olsson S. Positive contrast herniography in adult patients with obscure groin pain. Surgery 1981;89:532.
9. Ekberg O, Kullenberg K. Direct diverticular inguinal hernia. Acta Radiol 1988;29:57.
10. Ekberg O, Nilsson PE. Herniography: comparison of morbidity and image quality after use of high and low osmolality contrast media. Invest Radiol 1986;21:404.
11. Ekberg O, Persson NH, Abrahamsson PA, et al. Longstanding groin pain in athletes. A multidisciplinary approach. Sports Med 1988;6:56.
12. Fenn K, Keller G, Kühn R. Die Peritoneographie zum Nachweiss nicht tastbarer Hernien. Radiologe 1982;22:166.
13. Gelfand DW. Positive contrast peritoneography: the abnormal abdomen. Am J Roentgenol 1973;119:190.
14. Giacobine JW, Siler VE. Evaluation of diagnostic abdominal parasentesis with experimental and clinical studies. Surg Gynecol Obstet 1960;110:676.
15. Gullmo Å. Om herniografi. Swed Soc Med Radiol 1973;2:19.
16. Gullmo Å. Herniography: the diagnosis of hernia in the groin and incompetence of the pouch of Douglas and pelvic floor. Acta Radiol Suppl 1980:361.
17. Gullmo Å. Herniography. World J Surg 1989;13:560.
18. Gullmo Å, Broomé A, Smedberg S. Herniography. Surg Clin North Am 1984;64:229.
19. Hall C, Hall PN, Wingate JP, et al. Evaluation of herniography in the diagnosis of an occult abdominal wall hernia in symptomatic adults. Br J Surg 1990;77:902.
20. Halverson K, McVay CB. Inguinal and femoral hernioplasty: a 22-year study of the author's methods. Arch Surg 1970;101:127.
21. Lancet, editorial. Herniography. Lancet 1980;2:1065.
22. Magnusson J, Gustafson T, Gullstrand P, et al. Herniography: a useful diagnostic method in patients with obscure groin pain. Ann Chir Gynaecol 1984;73:91.
23. Magnusson J, Gustafson T, Gullstrand P, et al. Preoperative herniography in clinically manifest groin hernia: a prospective randomized trial. The Society of University Surgeons, Sixth Tripartite Meeting, Boston, February 1985:168.
24. Ralphs DNL, Brian AJL, Grundy DJ, et al. How accurately can direct and indirect inguinal hernias be distinguished? BMJ 1980;280:1039.
25. Rollino A. Studi sperimentali sulla peritoneografia; la tollerabilita locale e generale all Urografin iniettato nella cavita peritoneale. Minerva Chir 1956;11:234.
26. Roos H, Smedberg S. Symptomatic non-palpable inguinal hernias. Postgrad Gen Surg 1992;4:131.
27. Roub LW, Drayer BP, Orr DP, et al. Computed tomographic positive contrast peritoneography. Radiology 1979;131:699.
28. Smedberg SGG, Broomé AEA, Elmér O, et al. Herniography in the diagnosis of obscure groin pain. Acta Chir Scand 1985;151:663.
29. Smedberg SGG, Broomé AEA, Elmér O, et al. Herniography: a diagnostic tool in groin symptoms following hernial surgery. Acta Chir Scand 1986;152:273.
30. Smedberg SGG, Broomé AEA, Elmér O, et al. Herniography in primary inguinal and femoral hernia: an analysis of 283 operated cases. Contemp Surg 1990;36:48.
31. Smedberg SGG, Broomé AEA, Gullmo Å. Ligation of the hernial sac? Surg Clin North Am 1984;64:299.
32. Smedberg SGG, Broomé AEA, Gullmo Å, et al. Herniography in athletes with groin pain. Am J Surg 1985;149:378.
33. Spangen L. Spigelian hernia. Acta Chir Scand Suppl 1976:462.
34. Verhaar JA, Pot JH. De waarde van de herniografie bij onbegrepen pijn in de lies. Ned Tijdschr Geneeskd 1985;129:359.
35. Wrazidlo von W, Karl E-L, Koch K. Herniendiagnostik durch Peritoneographie. Fortschr Röntgenstr 1989;150:699.

Hernia, Fourth Edition, edited
by Lloyd M. Nyhus and Robert E. Condon.
J.B. Lippincott Company, Philadelphia © 1995.

Chapter 41

Biomaterials in Hernia Repair

Alonzo P. Walker

The use of biocompatible materials in repairing ventral and inguinal hernias is now commonplace. Over the preceding four decades, many such materials have been evaluated in animal models and used in the clinical setting. In developing these biomaterials, which are both synthetic and natural, the goal has been to identify the ideal material that best restores the integrity of the abdominal wall, is lasting and easy to use, does not stimulate excessive foreign-body reaction, becomes incorporated into the surrounding native tissue, and is tolerated well, even in the presence of infection.

The indications for the use of biocompatible materials in abdominal wall hernia repair are as replacement for lost musculofascial tissue when primary approximation cannot be achieved and as reinforcement of a primary repair. These materials also may be used as reinforcement of herniations related to native tissue weakness that results in visceral protrusion and its distressing associated symptoms.[29]

TYPES OF BIOCOMPATIBLE MATERIALS

Various types of biocompatible materials have been developed for use in hernia repair.

The characteristics desired of the ideal material, natural or synthetic, have been described by both Cumberland[4] and Scales.[26] Initially, biomaterials were used primarily for the repair of ventral hernias in which tissue deficits existed. The synthetic materials that have proven most desirable and usable now also are accepted in the repair of primary and recurrent groin hernias.

Natural Biomaterials

The natural biomaterials listed in Table 41-1 are not used routinely in hernia repair. Autogenous fascia lata, the most desirable of these, has proved to be an excellent biomaterial for repairing large incisional and groin hernias.[29] The sheets of fascia lata are used as an onlay to provide reinforcement after the repair of a primary or recurrent inguinal hernia. In the repair of an incisional hernia, the sheets of fascia lata are placed as an onlay using a double layer or as an inlay immediately in the preperitoneal plane.

Clinical experience with porcine dermal collagen for the repair of inguinal or incisional hernias is limited. This material is obtained from porcine corium that has been treated by proteolytic enzyme digestion to remove noncollagenous elements. It then is immersed in glutaraldehyde to delay absorption and reduce antigenicity. Although its successful use has been reported by Sarmah and Holl-Allen,[25] no long-term results are available. Furthermore, this material has been evaluated in only a few patients.

Bovine pericardium has not been evaluated in the clinical setting. Obtained fresh from bovine hearts, it is prepared in a lyophilized (non–cross-linked) and cross-linked form by treatment with glutaraldehyde. In the report by James and colleagues,[11] the glutaraldehyde-prepared grafts showed good incorporation into the abdominal wall muscles and developed a strong, stable fibrous tissue replacement suitable for abdominal wall support. The lyophilized grafts were resorbed, and proved to be unsuitable.

The clinical experience with human dura also is limited, and no reported series of patients has been evaluated over the long term. The dura used for hernia repair is preserved tissue obtained from tissue banks that has been sterilized with radiation. It is reported to be as efficacious as synthetic material.[13] The death of a patient with Creutzfeldt-Jakob disease has been reported after the use of lyophilized irradiated human cadaver dura, however. Contamination of the dura with the Creutzfeldt-Jakob disease agent was found. The use of dura is not recommended because the method of sterilization does not appear to inactivate the Creutzfeldt-Jakob disease agent.[8]

The use of autogenous dermal or whole-skin graft is primarily of historical interest. This material was used mainly in the repair of ventral hernias. Several local problems were associated with its use, but the major complication was inability to maintain the integrity of the abdominal wall. The skin that is used now usually is applied as a component of a musculo-

Table 41-1. Natural Biocompatible Materials in Hernia Repair

Autogenous dermal grafts
Whole skin grafts
Dermal collagen homografts
Porcine dermal collagen
Autogenous fascial heterografts
Lyophilized aortic homografts
Preserved dural homografts
Bovine pericardium

Table 41-2. Nonabsorbable Synthetic Biocompatible Materials in Hernia Repair

Polypropylene mesh (Marlex, Prolene)
Tantalum mesh
Polyester cloth (Dacron)
Nylon cloth (Dacron)
Fiberglass sheeting
Polyester sheeting (Mylar)
Nylon mesh
Synthetic acrylic cloth (Orlon)
Polyvinyl sponge (Ivalon)
Stainless steel mesh
Polytetrafluoroethylene mesh (PTFE) (Teflon; Gore-Tex)
Polytetrafluoroethylene
Polyvinyl cloth (Vinyon-N)
Dacron mesh (Mersilene)
Polypropylene mesh and gelatin film (Gelfilm)
Silicone-velvet composite (Rhodergon velvet)
Dacron-reinforced silicone sheeting (Silastic)
Expanded polytetrafluoroethylene weave (e-PTFE) (Gore-Tex)
Carbon fiber

fasciocutaneous flap. These types of reconstruction have a long history of success,[9] but the tissue is not considered to be a biomaterial and is not addressed further in this chapter.

Carbon Fibers

The use of carbon fibers in the clinical setting for the repair of abdominal wall defects has not been reported. Interest in this biocompatible material was generated by results of clinical studies showing the induction of fibrous tissue proliferation in tendons and ligaments[18] for the repair of full-thickness abdominal wall defects in an animal model.[22] One study, using fabricated carbon-fiber implants, demonstrated significant, high-quality tissue ingrowth when compared to polypropylene mesh. In addition, the implant did not cause the chronic foreign-body inflammatory reaction that occurs with polypropylene mesh. Based on these observations, it is considered useful as a replacement for lost tissue or as a reinforcement for weak tissues in hernia repair.[22]

SYNTHETIC BIOCOMPATIBLE MATERIALS

A large volume of experimental and clinical data is available regarding the use of synthetic materials in hernia repair. These materials are listed in Table 41-2. Since 1952, the impetus has been to develop, evaluate, and use materials that have the ideal qualities set forth independently by Cumberland and Scales. Compared to the materials developed and used until that time, none had better qualities or generated better results than autogenous fascia lata. Autogenous fascia lata produced excellent results in groin and incisional hernias when it was used as free grafts (sheets) and as musculofasciocutaneous flaps in large incisional hernias. Because of the need for an additional operative procedure to obtain fascia lata and the associated patient discomfort, however, the

evaluation of synthetic materials continued. Polypropylene mesh and expanded polytetrafluoroethylene (PTFE) are the synthetic materials used most widely in hernia repair today.

Polypropylene Mesh

The classic experimental and clinical studies reported by Usher and colleagues[32,33] established the use of polypropylene mesh in hernia repair. This material is readily available, strong, and nonabsorbable. It is a monofilament that is inert, porous, thin, and firm but pliable. Polypropylene mesh is not rejected by the body and is able to withstand infection. Microscopically, it induces an intense foreign-body inflammatory reaction; its interstices are infiltrated completely by fibroblasts, with subsequent dense fibrous scar formation.[7]

Inguinal Hernia Repair

In groin hernias, polypropylene mesh was used by Usher and associates[32,33] only for large direct and indirect defects repaired by either the Bassini or the Halsted technique. The routine use of polypropylene in this manner was not accepted. In 1970, Lichtenstein reported early data on hernia repair without disability. He recommended that the repair of both primary direct and recurrent hernias be reinforced with polypropylene mesh to prevent recurrence. Because of the high recurrence rate of groin hernias, the application of polypropylene mesh was prompted by its success in recurrent ventral hernias.[12] Repairing recurrent hernias with prosthetic mesh has become standard practice. Recurrence rates improve markedly when this prosthesis is placed in the preperitoneal space.[23,24] The recurrence rate was 1.7% in the series reported by Nyhus and associates,[24] compared to 19% in other series. Although polypropylene mesh is accepted and used routinely for the repair of recurrent groin hernias, its use in primary repair has met with resistance. This application is increasing slowly, and large series have been reported.[28] The preperitoneal approach for mesh placement is advocated by Stoppa[30] and the anterior approach, termed the *tension-free hernioplasty,* is recommended by Lichtenstein and coworkers.[19,20] The combined results of five different series involving 3019 operations using different approaches for mesh placement yielded a failure rate of only 0.2% and an infection rate of 0.03%.[28] In most of the operations reported in this collected series, the mesh was placed by an anterior approach. This approach avoids tension on suture lines, does not alter normal anatomy, permits a true tension-free hernia repair, and addresses the problem of recurrent hernia directly. Use of the mesh is considered safe. The procedure is simple, rapid, and effective; is considered to be less painful; and allows an earlier return to unrestricted physical activity.[20]

Although the routine use of polypropylene mesh in primary groin hernia repair is not generally accepted, objections may subside with the introduction of the laparoscopic approach. This technique takes advantage of the knowledge gained from using mesh in primary inguinal hernias and placing it by a preperitoneal approach. No long-term series of patients with mesh placed by the laparoscopic approach are available, however. It also is not known whether mesh placed using the laparoscope is as effective as that placed by the anterior or preperitoneal approach.

Incisional Hernia Repair

The use of polypropylene mesh for the repair of primary or recurrent incisional abdominal wall hernias is well established. Since the reports by Usher and colleagues,[32,33] it has been considered the prosthetic material of choice for the repair of these hernias. If a defect is not large and native tissue can be approximated safely, the mesh is placed as an onlay for reinforcement of the repair. If large abdominal wall defects are present, the mesh is used as a replacement for the absent musculoaponeurotic tissue using the method described by Condon.[3] A double layer of the mesh is placed: one as an inlay and the other as an onlay. The bowel, including the stomach, must be protected from the mesh by the omentum or the peritoneum. If both are absent, the hernia sac may be used, with the mesh placed in the preperitoneal space. Because of the intense inflammatory foreign-body reaction caused by polypropylene mesh, direct contact with bowel should be avoided. The bowel may become densely adherent, which can lead to visceral erosion, fistula formation, and other reported complications. In the most recent series of 50 consecutive cases reported by Molloy and colleagues,[21] there were no bowel complications. There were 8 wound infections, all of which responded to appropriate antibiotic therapy. Graft removal was not required. Six patients had wound sinuses that either healed spontaneously or responded to removal of only the involved portion of the graft. The recurrence rate of 8% in this series was similar to that of earlier reported series.

Polytetrafluoroethylene

Polytetrafluoroethylene is a nonabsorbable biomaterial that is used widely as a vascular graft. In the initial evaluation by Usher and Wallace,[34] it demonstrated filmy adhesions to bowel and was separated easily. Microscopically, it did not demonstrate a foreign-body reaction in the tissues and caused little surrounding inflammation. Despite these observations, it was not evaluated further for use in abdominal wall repair until the report by Sher and colleagues.[27] In that study, PTFE with specifications different than that used for vascular prostheses was evaluated. This material had a smaller pore size, was thinner and less porous, and was prepared as flat pieces. The pieces were implanted in the abdominal wall of rats. At the end of a 10-week period, the intraabdominal reaction was considered equal to that caused by polypropylene mesh. In the subcutaneous tissue, the gross appearance did not differ significantly from that of polypropylene mesh. The major difference was noted microscopically; polypropylene caused more fibrous scar tissue formation. These authors stated that a properly formulated PTFE prosthesis is as effective as polypropylene mesh in abdominal hernia repair.

Because of continuing interest in the use of this prosthesis for abdominal wall repair, Lamb and colleagues[14] evaluated a microporous PTFE graft. Their results indicated that there was no difference in collagen accumulation between the PTFE mesh and the polypropylene mesh. No hernias occurred in either group. PTFE produced a slight inflammatory response on the peritoneal surface, but was well incorporated into the surrounding fibrous tissue, with many fibroblasts present. These findings also suggested that a microporous formulation of PTFE would be a satisfactory fascial substitute.

Subsequent reports by Law and Ellis[16] indicated that PTFE caused less dense peritoneal adhesion formation. In addition, Law[15] demonstrated that PTFE retained adequate strength to provide a sound repair, that collagen infiltration occurred, and that the graft–tissue bond became progressively stronger over time.

The initial clinical experience with expanded PTFE was a case report by Hodges-Hamer and Scott.[10] Bauer and colleagues[1] described their experience with 28 patients in whom the material was used as a replacement for large abdominal wall defects. They reported a 10% recurrence rate (3 patients) and a 7% wound infection rate (2 patients). In one of the infected wounds, removal of the prosthesis was necessary because of extensive contamination and lack of response to local therapy. On removal, a large amount of purulent material was present beneath the prosthesis. In the hernias that recurred, the defect was present at the prosthesis–patch interface. All recurrences presented within 9 months of the initial operation. Overall, 23 of the patients did well, with no demonstrated reaction to the PTFE over the mean follow-up period of 22.5 months. These authors reported no complications related to bowel adhesion formation, no prosthesis erosion into bowel, and no fistula formation. The absence of these complications was attributed to the softness of the material and the minimal inflammatory response it elicited.

Van der Lei and colleagues[35] described their experience with 11 patients followed up for a mean of 31.5 months. Overall, the clinical findings were similar to those of Bauer and colleagues.[1] In one patient with a postoperative wound infection, complete graft removal was necessary because of persistent infection and poor response to local wound care and systemic antibiotic therapy. Hernia recurrence also presented at the prosthesis–tissue interface. To address this type of recurrence, these authors recommended that the prosthesis be implanted with a 1- to 2-cm overlap of the musculofascial wound edge.

No long-term or large series of patients have been reported to establish the overall efficiency of expanded PTFE compared to the known results for polypropylene mesh. The early clinical experience suggests that it is a satisfactory material for the replacement of lost tissue and that it prevents the local complications of dense adhesion to bowel, viscera erosion, and fistula formation that occur when polypropylene mesh is placed in direct contact with bowel.

For the repair of large hernia defects that require replacement tissue, we use expanded PTFE and polypropylene mesh in a composite, bilaminar fashion. Expanded PTFE is placed on the peritoneal site of the defect as an inlay and polypropylene mesh is placed as an onlay using the method described by Condon.[3]

This technique does not require dissection of the preperitoneal space for graft placement, and there is no possibility of bowel coming into contact with the expanded PTFE patch. Our use of this composite repair is based on the results of a study we conducted in an animal model.

Expanded Polytetrafluoroethylene in Inguinal Hernia Repair

The use of expanded PTFE in groin and inguinal hernia repair was reported initially by Elliott and Juler.[7] They compared expanded PTFE to polypropylene mesh placed in the groin of rabbits and sutured in place between the transversalis fascia and the peritoneum. At the end of the experiment, both materials were examined grossly and microscopically. They observed that the polypropylene mesh was crumpled, had lost its shape, and had formed a ball of scar tissue with surrounding scar contracture. Histologically, the fibers of the polypropylene mesh were encased in a dense mass of scar tissue. The expanded PTFE maintained its position and shape as it had been implanted. The authors noted an ingrowth of fibroblasts into the interstices of the patch and only a minimal inflammatory reaction and limited distortion of the graft. In addition, they noted the development of a thick "neofascia" around the PTFE similar to that which occurs when PTFE is used as a vascular prosthesis. Based on these observations, they indicated that the material is a satisfactory adjunct in groin hernia repair.

Clinical experience with the expanded PTFE patch was reported by Law and Ellis[17] in a group of patients with recurrent inguinal hernia. The repair was approached anteriorly and sutured in a tension-free manner. The authors reported a complication rate of 15% (eight patients). The predominant problem was seroma formation (five patients), which responded to simple aspiration with no long-term sequelae. There were five cases of recurrence: two femoral hernias, two medial hernias at the pubic tubercle, and one hernia that was referred to as a preperitoneal recurrence. Deysine[6] reported his experience with expanded PTFE in a group of 90 patients, 33 of whom underwent inguinal hernia repair. The repairs were primary in 15 patients and recurrent in 18 patients. He reported no complications or recurrence. Berliner[2] reported his experience in 350 patients who had inguinal hernias repaired with the expanded PTFE patch placed as an inlay. He included patients with both recurrent and primary hernias, although most were primary defects. The failure rate was 1.1% (4 patients). A sinus tract infection developed in 1 patient and ultimately required graft removal. Microscopically, Berliner observed bacterial in-

Table 41-3. Inguinal Hernia Repair With Expanded Polytetrafluoroethylene

Author	Year	No. of Patients	Mean Follow-up (mo)	Percent Recurrence Rate (no. of cases)
Law and Ellis*	1990 (1984–1988)	52	25	10 (5)
Deysine†	1992 (1985–1989)	33	24	0 (0)
Berliner†	1993 (1984–1990)	350	41.8	1.1 (4)

*Recurrent only.
†Primary and recurrent.

filtration throughout the interstices of the graft. Overall, he considered the expanded PTFE patch a satisfactory prosthesis for the repair of primary or recurrent groin hernias, although he indicated that not all groin hernias require the use of prosthetic material. In this report, only 15% of the 2331 inguinal hernias that were repaired during the period of evaluation required a prosthetic patch. The Shouldice repair that Berliner usually performed could not be done in a tension-free manner. Reported series of inguinal hernia repair using expanded PTFE are listed in Table 41-3.

Graft Infections in Expanded Polytetrafluoroethylene

Expanded PTFE appears to be a satisfactory biomaterial for hernia repair; however, experience with this material is not as extensive as with polypropylene mesh. A major concern with the placement of biomaterials is the possibility of graft infection, which is considered to be their most serious local complication. Graft infection does not seem to be a significant problem with expanded PTFE, but when it occurred in the series reviewed, graft removal was necessary. These infections did not respond to local care or systemic antibiotic therapy. In the reported cases of graft infection, *Staphylococcus* was the only bacterial organism identified. The bacteria infiltrate the material deeply and are difficult to eradicate. The presence of bacteria infiltrating the graft was shown well in the material retrieved by Berliner.[2]

The finding of staphylococci is not unexpected, because it is well known that *Staphylococcus aureus* and species of coagulase-negative staphylococci are the bacteria isolated most commonly from biomaterial-associated infections. Because these organisms infiltrate the graft material, effective treatment of the infection usually requires removal of the prosthesis.

Antibiotic wound irrigation has not been shown to be beneficial in preventing graft wound infection. Because the placement of synthetic materials may increase the risk or severity of wound infection, the administration of prophylactic antibiotics is recommended. Unless other patient risk factors are present, an antistaphylococcic agent is appropriate.

Absorbable Synthetic Mesh

Absorbable synthetic mesh (Table 41-4) is an unsatisfactory prosthesis for use as a permanent graft for abdominal wall replacement. Using an animal model, Lamb and colleagues[14] demonstrated that adequate fibrous tissue incorporation did not occur before hydrolysis of implanted polyglactin mesh. After 12 weeks of observation, gross hernias were present in four of the ten animals with this material, compared to none of the animals with expanded PTFE and polypropylene mesh. In a more recent animal study, similar results were obtained. Tyrell and colleagues[31] evaluated both polyglactin and polyglycolic acid mesh compared to polypropylene mesh and expanded PTFE for abdominal wall replacement. By the end of the 10 weeks of observation, all animals with absorbable mesh had ventral hernias, compared to none of those with nonabsorbable mesh. These observations are supported by the clinical findings in a report by Dayton and colleagues.[5] In that study, polyglycolic acid mesh was used to repair contaminated abdominal wall defects. In six of the eight patients in whom the mesh was placed, abdominal wall hernias developed at the site of mesh placement over 18 months of follow-up. Based on these observations and results, absorbable mesh should not be used as a permanent replacement for lost tissue, but may be satisfactory for use in the treatment of contaminated wounds. Once the patient has recovered, a nonabsorbable material (eg, expanded PTFE patch, polypropylene) may be used to repair the defect.

Table 41-4. Absorbable Synthetic Biocompatible Materials in Hernia Repair

Polyglycolic acid mesh (Dexon)
Polydioxanone
Polyglactin mesh (Vicryl)

REFERENCES

1. Bauer JJ, Salky BA, Gelerent IM, et al. Repair of large abdominal wall defects with expanded polytetrafluoroethylene (PTFE). Ann Surg 1987;206:765.
2. Berliner SD. Clinical experience with an inlay expanded polytetrafluoroethylene soft tissue patch as an adjunct in inguinal hernia repair. Surg Gynecol Obstet 1993;176:323.
3. Condon RE. Prosthetic repair of abdominal hernia. In: Nyhus LM, Condon RE, eds. Hernia, ed 3. Philadelphia, JB Lippincott, 1989:559–566.
4. Cumberland VH. A preliminary report on the use of prefabricated nylon weave in the repair of ventral hernia. Med J Aust 1952;1:143.
5. Dayton MT, Buchele BA, Shirazi SS, Hunt LB. Use of an absorbable mesh to repair contaminated abdominal-wall defects. Arch Surg 1986;121:954.
6. Deysine M. Hernia repair with expanded polytetrafluoroethylene. Am J Surg 1992;163:422.
7. Elliott MP, Juler GL. Comparison of Marlex mesh and micron microporous Teflon sheets when used for hernia repair in the experimental animal. Am J Surg 1979;137:342.
8. F.D.A. Drug Bull. Possible association between dura matter graft and CJD. April 1987.
9. Fayman MS, Schein M, Saadia R. Abdominal wall reconstruction after open management of the septic abdomen. S Afr J Surg 1990;28:62.
10. Hodges-Hamer DW, Scott NB. Replacement of an abdominal wall defect using expanded PTFE sheet (GORE-TEX). Surgeon's Workshop 1985;30:65–67.
11. James NL, Warren-Poole LA, Schindhelm K, et al. Comparative evaluation of treated bovine pericardium as a xenograft for hernia repair. Biomaterials 1991;12:801.
12. Kaufman M, Weissberg D, Bider D. Repair of recurrent inguinal hernia with Marlex mesh. Surg Gynecol Obstet 1985;160:505.
13. Klein L, Mericka P, Pinter L. Use of dura mater allografts in operations of abdominal wall hernias. Beitr Orthop Traumatol 1990;37:499.
14. Lamb JP, Vitale T, Kaminski DL. Comparative evaluation of synthetic meshes used for abdominal wall replacement. Surgery 1983;93:643.
15. Law NW. A comparison of polypropylene mesh, expanded polytetrafluoroethylene patch and polyglycolic acid mesh for the repair of experimental abdominal wall defects. Acta Chir Scand 1990;156:759.
16. Law NW, Ellis H. Adhesion formation and peritoneal healing on prosthetic materials. Clinical Materials 1988;3:95.
17. Law NW, Ellis H. Preliminary results for the repair of difficult recurrent inguinal hernias using expanded PTFE patch. Acta Chir Scand 1990;156:609.
18. Lemaire M. Reinforcement of tendons and ligaments with carbon fibers: four years, 1300 cases. Clin Orthop 1985;196:169.
19. Lichtenstein IL, Shulman AG. Ambulatory outpatient hernia surgery. Including a new concept, introducing tension-free repair. Int Surg 1986;71:1.
20. Lichtenstein I, Shulman AG, Amid PK. The tension-free hernioplasty. Am J Surg 1989;157:188.
21. Molloy RG, Moran KT, Waldron RP, et al. Massive incisional hernia: abdominal wall replacement with Marlex mesh. Br J Surg 1991;78:242.
22. Morris DM, Haskins R, Marino AA, et al. Use of carbon fibers for repair of abdominal-wall defects in rats. Surgery 1990;107:627.
23. Nyhus L. The recurrent groin hernia: therapeutic solutions. World J Surg 1989;13:541.
24. Nyhus L, Pollak R, Bombeck T, et al. The preperitoneal approach and prosthetic buttress repair for recurrent hernia. Ann Surg 1988;208:733.
25. Sarmah BD, Holl-Allen RTJ. Porcine dermal collagen repair of incisional herniae. Br J Surg 1984;71:524.
26. Scales JT. Materials for hernia repair. Proc R Soc Med 1953;46:647.
27. Sher W, Pollack D, Paulides CA, Matsumoto T. Repair of abdominal wall defects: Gore-Tex vs. Marlex graft. Am Surg 1980;46:618.
28. Shulman AG, Amid PK, Lichtenstein IL. The safety of mesh repair for primary inguinal hernias: results of 3,019 operations from five diverse surgical sources. Am Surg 1992;58:255.
29. Smith RS. The use of prosthetic materials in the repair of hernias. Surg Clin North Am 1971;51:1387.
30. Stoppa R, Warlaumont CR, Verhaeghe PJ, et al. Prosthetic repair in the treatment of groin hernias. Int Surg 1986;71:154.
31. Tyrell J, Silberman H, Chandrasoma P, et al. Absorbable versus permanent mesh in abdominal operations. Surg Gynecol Obstet 1989;168:227.
32. Usher FC, Fries JG, Ochsner JL, et al. Marlex mesh, a new plastic mesh for replacing tissue defects. I. Experimental studies. Arch Surg 1959;78:131.
33. Usher FC, Fries JG, Ochsner JL, et al. Marlex mesh, a new plastic mesh for replacing tissue defects. II. Clinical studies. Arch Surg 1959;78:138.
34. Usher FC, Wallace SA. Tissue reaction to plastics, a comparison of nylon, Orlon, Dacron, Teflon, and Marlex. Arch Surg 1958;76:997.
35. Van der Lei B, Bleichrodt RP, Simmermacher RKJ, et al. Expanded polytetrafluoroethylene patch for the repair of large abdominal wall defects. Br J Surg 1989;76:803.

Editor's Comment

The two most common prosthetic materials used in hernia repair today are polypropylene mesh (Marlex) and expanded PTFE sheets (Gore-Tex). Each has advantages and disadvantages. The advantages of polypropylene mesh are that it has a long history of use, is a monofilament material, supports the development of a strong layer of scar tissue, and often can be left in situ if it becomes infected, with eventual healing of the wound. Its disadvantages are that it is relatively inelastic and has no intrinsic antibacterial activity.

The advantage of PTFE is that it does not stimulate an intense inflammatory reaction, so the development of peritoneal adhesions is reduced or eliminated when this prosthesis is placed within or comes into contact with the peritoneum. It also is intrinsically strong, although more subject to shear forces than is polypropylene mesh. Because of the lack of adhesion formation, PTFE has a major advantage in forming the internal layer of a two-layer ventral hernia repair. Its primary disadvantages are that it does not lead to the formation of a stable, dense scar. Instead, the prosthesis becomes encased in a layer of connective tissue, with minimal connective tissue ingrowth. PTFE prostheses always can be removed with a minimum amount of sharp dissection. This feature, coupled with the fact that the prosthesis must be removed if it becomes infected, makes it somewhat less desirable than polypropylene mesh for most cases requiring prosthetic repair.

R.E.C.

Diaphragmatic Hernia

Part Eight

Hernia, Fourth Edition, edited
by Lloyd M. Nyhus and Robert E. Condon.
J.B. Lippincott Company, Philadelphia © 1995.

Chapter 42

Paraesophageal Hiatal Hernia

Galen Perdikis and Ronald A. Hinder

Herniation of abdominal contents through the diaphragmatic hiatus has been recognized for many centuries, with the first successful surgical repair performed by Postempski[20] in 1889. Paraesophageal hiatal hernia first was described by Akerlund[1] in 1926, who noted it to be a relatively uncommon type of hiatal hernia.

There are three types of hiatal hernia: (1) sliding hiatal hernia, in which the gastroesophageal junction migrates cephalad through the esophageal hiatus (Fig. 42-1); (2) paraesophageal hernia, in which the fundus herniates into the thorax in association with a normally positioned gastroesophageal junction (Fig. 42-2); and (3) mixed hernia, in which both the gastroesophageal junction and the fundus herniate into the thorax (Fig. 42-3). A paraesophageal hernia tends to enlarge over time and the stomach eventually may become situated entirely within the thorax (Fig. 42-4). The consequences of a sliding hernia are largely physiologic because this type of hernia affects the functional integrity of the gastroesophageal junction and can result in gastroesophageal reflux disease. In contrast, a paraesophageal hernia has less of an effect on the physiology of the gastroesophageal junction, but may lead to catastrophic complications such as gastric volvulus, incarceration, ulceration, perforation, and mediastinitis. A mixed hernia has the characteristics of both types and may behave similar to either.

INCIDENCE

The incidence of paraesophageal hernia is difficult to ascertain. Postlethwait,[21] in a study of 7310 patients with hiatal hernias, reports a prevalence of 14.3% for paraesophageal hernias. This figure seems high and may be the result of the inclusion of combined hernias in the paraesophageal hernia group. Various other series report figures ranging from 3.5%[14] to 33%.[11] Overall, paraesophageal hernias comprise about 5% of all hiatal hernias.[6,11,17] Compared to sliding hernias, paraesophageal hernias tend to occur in older patients. The median age is 61 years for patients with

paraesophageal hernias and 48 years for those with sliding hernias.

PATHOGENESIS

A sliding hiatal hernia appears to develop because of weakening of the phrenoesophageal membrane over time[9] and loss or weakening of the attachment of the gastroesophageal junction to the preaortic fascia and the median arcuate ligament. This allows for movement and, thus, herniation of the junction through the hiatus.

Paraesophageal hernia develops in a different manner. Pearson and colleagues[19] have suggested that a paraesophageal hernia is merely an extension of a sliding hernia, but this view is not accepted by most others.[11,17,18] A widened hiatus anterior to the esophagus, possibly congenital in origin,[15] is a consistent finding in patients with a paraesophageal hernia. Occasionally, the left bundle of the right crus is absent and the defect extends into the left leaf of the diaphragm. This defect tends to have a firm, fibrous rim.[17] It is a lateral defect that may be caused by pressure on the left bundle of the right crus by the stomach, resulting in atrophy and extension of the defect to the left. The gastroesophageal junction remains fixed to the preaortic fascia and the median arcuate ligament. The fundus acts as the leading point and herniates first. The structures that normally would prevent displacement of the stomach, the gastrosplenic and gastrocolic ligaments, are abnormally lax.[17] The greater curvature then is able to roll up into the thorax in front of and to the left of the fixed gastroesophageal junction. Because the stomach is fixed at the gastroesophageal junction, the herniated stomach tends to rotate around its longitudinal axis (organoaxial volvulus [Fig. 42-5]). Rotation may occur around the transverse axis (mesentericoaxial volvulus [Fig. 42-6]), but this is less common.

Occasionally, herniation occurs through a congenital defect in the diaphragm immediately to the left of the hiatus known as the canalis paraesophagalis diaphragmatis.[12] This is termed a *parahiatal hernia* and

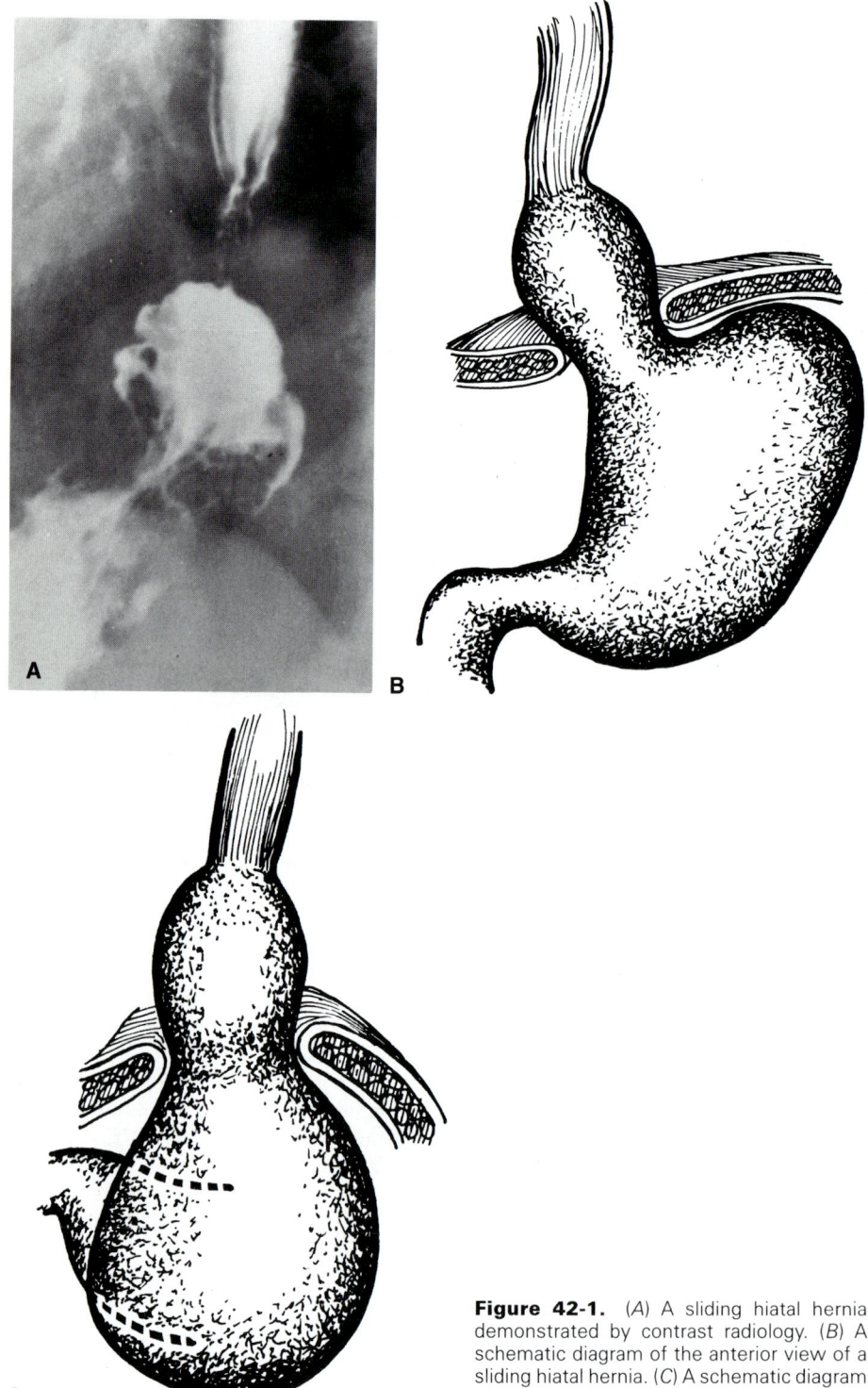

Figure 42-1. (*A*) A sliding hiatal hernia demonstrated by contrast radiology. (*B*) A schematic diagram of the anterior view of a sliding hiatal hernia. (*C*) A schematic diagram of the lateral view of a sliding hiatal hernia.

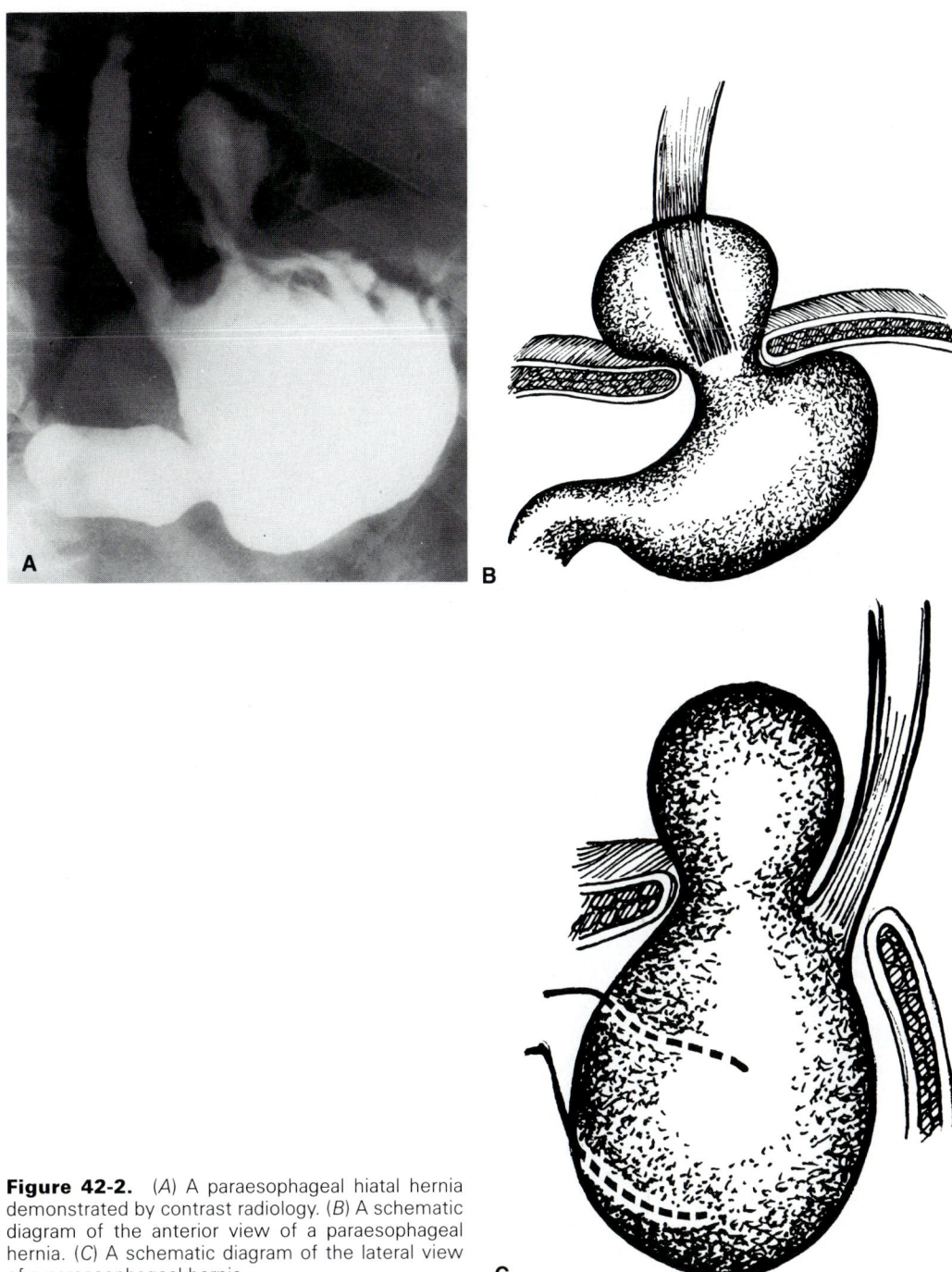

Figure 42-2. (*A*) A paraesophageal hiatal hernia demonstrated by contrast radiology. (*B*) A schematic diagram of the anterior view of a paraesophageal hernia. (*C*) A schematic diagram of the lateral view of a paraesophageal hernia.

is extremely rare. If the strand of diaphragmatic tissue that separates the parahiatal hernia from the true hiatus ruptures, it is impossible to differentiate between a parahiatal and a paraesophageal hernia. A mixed hernia develops when there is an anterior hiatal defect associated with loss of fixation of the gastroesophageal junction.

Special mention should be made of iatrogenic paraesophageal hernias. In a series of 101 patients with paraesophageal hernias, spanning two decades,

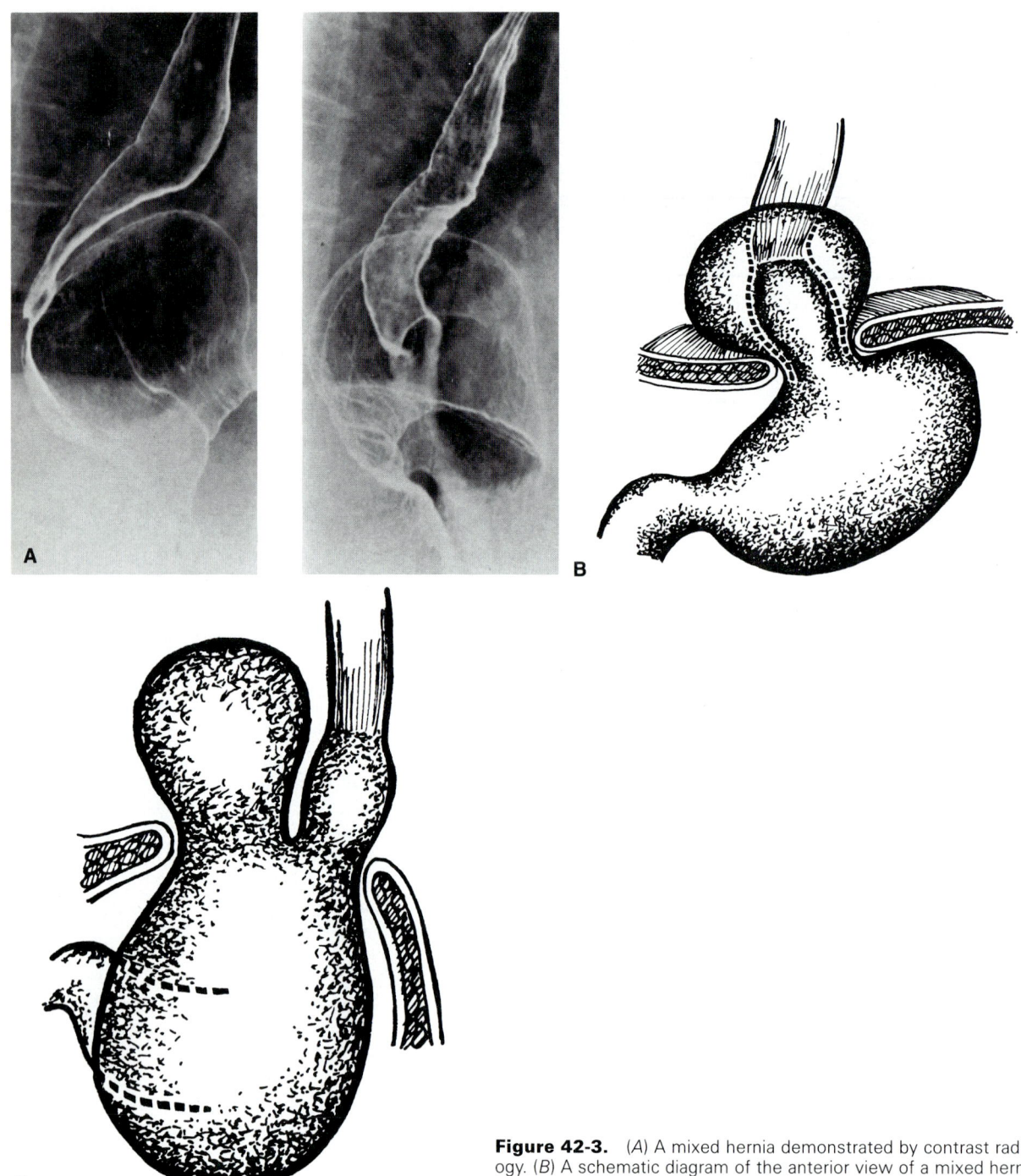

Figure 42-3. (*A*) A mixed hernia demonstrated by contrast radiology. (*B*) A schematic diagram of the anterior view of a mixed hernia. (*C*) A schematic diagram of the lateral view of a mixed hernia.

the defects were identified as being iatrogenic in origin in 13 cases.[24] Ten of these hernias occurred after antireflux procedures. Esophagomyotomy, esophagogastrectomy, and placement of an Angelchik prosthesis accounted for the other 3 cases. The pathogenesis of iatrogenic paraesophageal hernias in this series

was most commonly disruption of the hiatal repair. Other pathogenetic mechanisms included disruption of the phrenoesophageal membrane by operative dissection, postoperative gastric dilation, and failure to recognize esophageal shortening or an existing hiatal defect. A study in children reports the incidence of

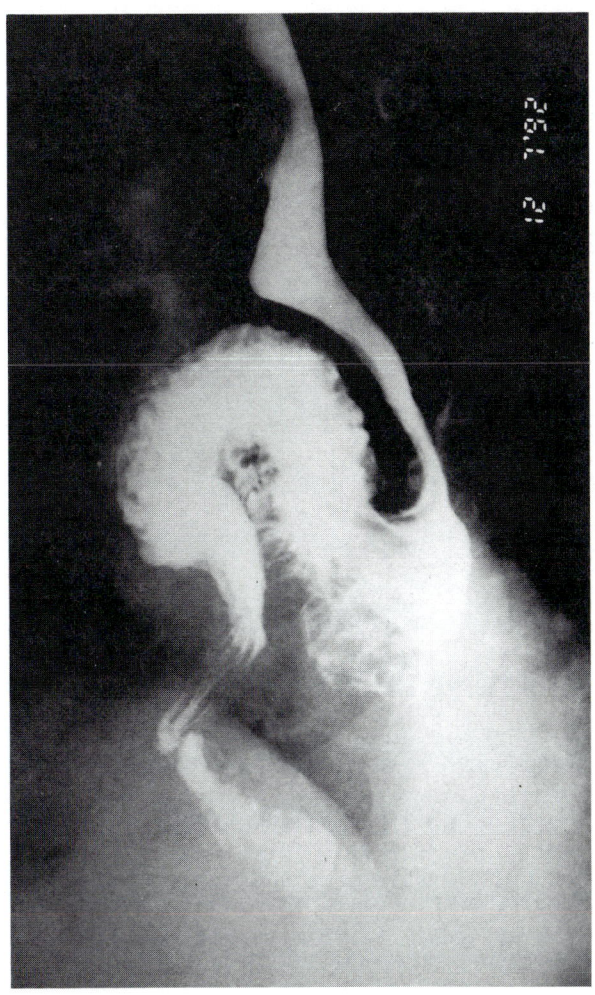

Figure 42-4. A completely intrathoracic stomach is demonstrated in this radiograph. The arrow indicates the diaphragm.

paraesophageal hernia after Nissen fundoplication to be 16.8%;[3] the defect was seen most commonly in patients who did not have a crural repair. It also was concluded that patients younger than 1 year were at highest risk for the development of a paraesophageal hernia after Nissen fundoplication.

CLINICAL PRESENTATION

The symptoms caused by a paraesophageal hernia are mechanical in nature because of the characteristic anatomic defect seen in these patients. Many patients with a paraesophageal hernia have no symptoms and the condition goes undetected until it is noted incidentally on a routine thoracic radiograph. The most common symptom is epigastric or substernal pain;[10]

however, symptoms generally are vague and intermittent, and include postprandial indigestion, substernal fullness, nausea, and, occasionally, retching. Dysphagia also can be a presenting symptom, but seldom is as severe as that associated with a peptic stricture of the esophagus. Obstruction to swallowing is uncommon and, when present, usually is intermittent.[10] The symptoms of postprandial fullness and dysphagia result from compression of the lower esophagus by the cardia and twisting of the gastroesophageal junction as the stomach rotates around either its transverse or its longitudinal axis.[7]

Symptoms of gastroesophageal reflux are relatively uncommon and usually are present only when the lower esophageal sphincter is defective. Occasionally, reflux symptoms may occur in a patient with a normal lower esophageal sphincter. This is possible when obstruction at the level of the diaphragm causes an elevation of pressure in the intrathoracic gastric pouch of sufficient magnitude to overcome the pressure generated by the normal lower esophageal sphincter.

Some patients with a paraesophageal hernia have anemia caused by chronic blood loss. The bleeding usually is associated with vascular engorgement of the portion of the stomach that is situated above the diaphragm, and is caused by venous obstruction at the hiatus that results in a slow ooze from the mucosa. Some patients have a gastric ulcer at the point of constriction and may bleed from this. A recent study reported the incidence of gastric ulceration to be 23% in a series of 34 patients with paraesophageal hernia.[22] Although most patients bleed insidiously, as many as one third may have hematemesis.[26]

Respiratory complications also can result from the presence of a paraesophageal hernia. Dyspnea may occur because of mechanical compression of the lung by a large hernia and pneumonia may result from repeated aspiration.[26] Occasionally, other organs can herniate through the defect. Farrell and coworkers[12] reported a case of colonic obstruction caused by incarceration of the splenic flexure of the colon in a paraesophageal hernia. Another case has been reported in which the entire spleen herniated into the thorax through a paraesophageal hernia.[4]

One fifth of patients with a paraesophageal hernia are seen as a surgical emergency, with excessive bleeding, incarceration, volvulus, strangulation, and perforation. If incarceration of the stomach occurs, the patient's symptoms become more severe and continuous. Gastric volvulus results in increased pain and symptoms of obstruction. If the volvulus compromises the venous and, possibly, the arterial blood supply, necrosis and perforation with resulting sepsis and shock may develop. The mortality rate at this stage of the disease approaches 50%.[13]

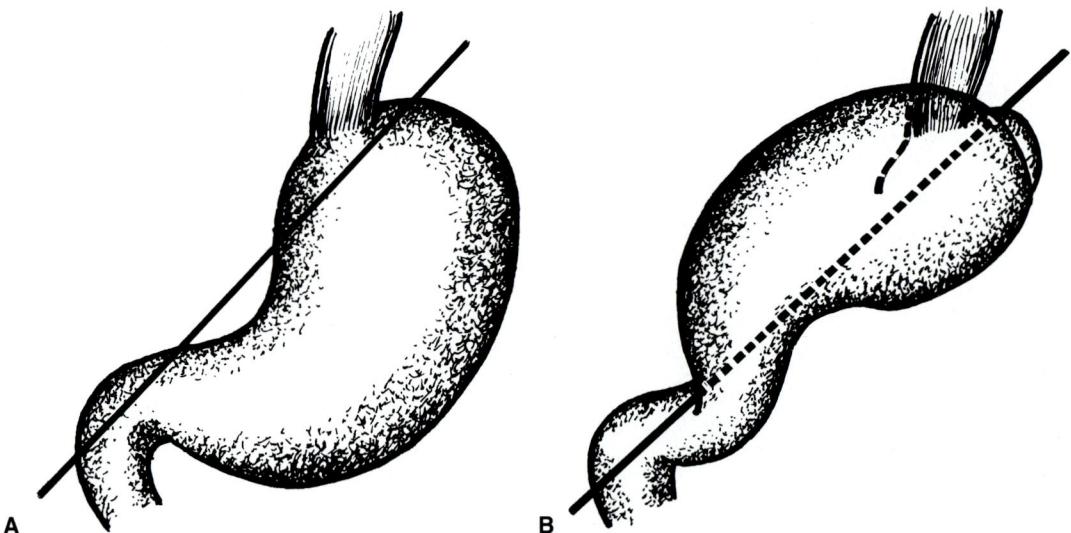

Figure 42-5. Organoaxial volvulus of the stomach. (*A*) Before volvulus. (*B*) After volvulus. The stomach may obstruct at the gastroesophageal junction or in the pyloroduodenal region.

INVESTIGATIONS

An upright radiograph of the thorax often is all that is required to make the diagnosis. A retrocardiac air–fluid level is diagnostic of a paraesophageal hernia or an intrathoracic stomach (Fig. 42-7). Contrast studies almost always are diagnostic of paraesophageal hernia because this lesion is fixed and does not reduce spontaneously as sliding hiatal hernias sometimes do. Flex-

ible esophagogastroscopy allows for a retroflexed view of the gastroesophageal junction. Using this method, a paraesophageal hernia is identified as a separate orifice adjacent to the gastroesophageal junction (Fig. 42-8). Gastric rugal folds are seen to ascend into the hernia. A mixed hernia is diagnosed by noting the presence of a separate gastric pouch or orifice (paraesophageal component) that usually arises halfway up the side of a sliding hiatal hernia (Fig. 42-9). The

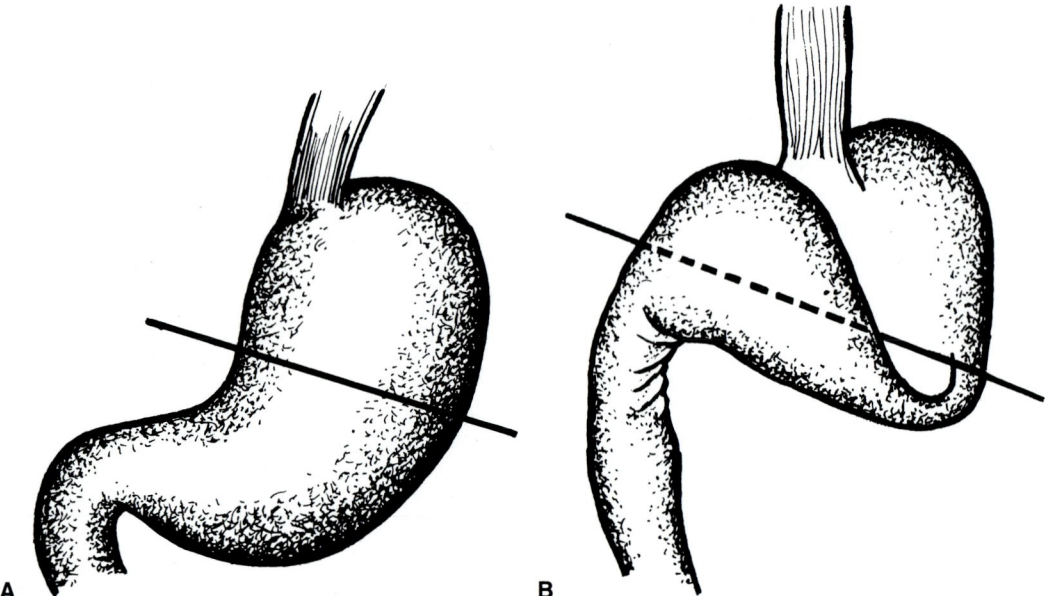

Figure 42-6. Mesentericoaxial volvulus of the stomach. (*A*) Before volvulus. (*B*) After volvulus. The stomach may obstruct in the fixed pyloroantral region.

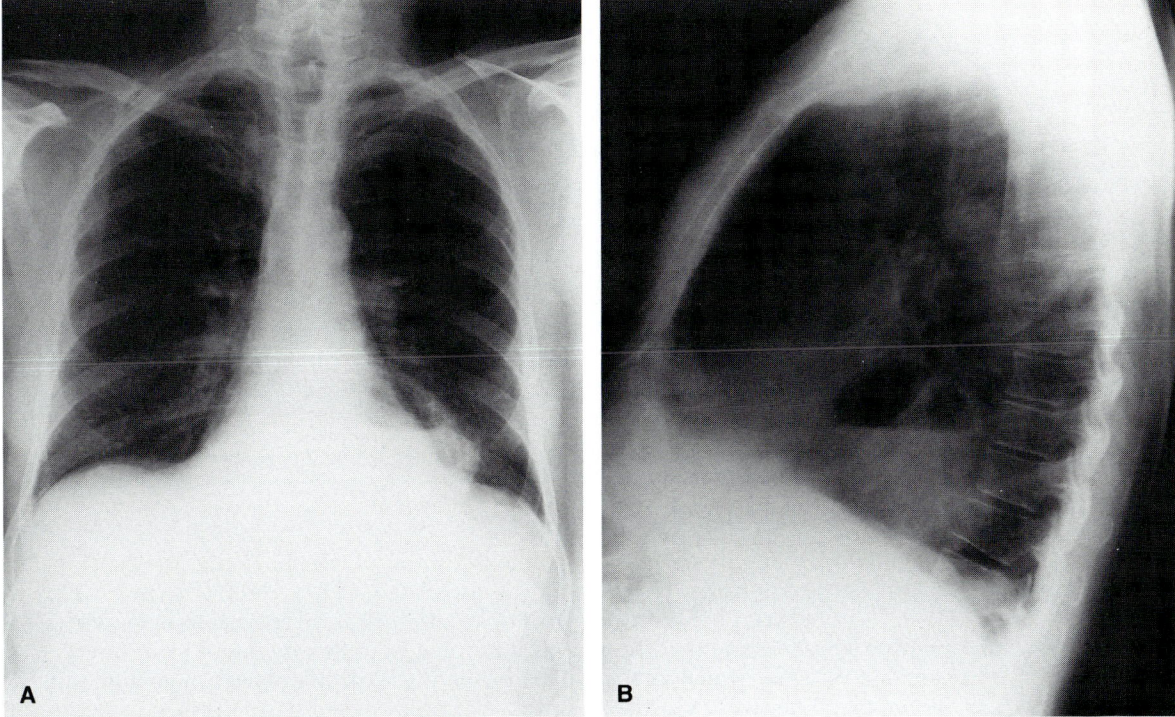

Figure 42-7. Radiograph of a patient with a paraesophageal hernia. The hernia is diagnosed by the presence of a retrocardiac air–fluid level. (*A*) Posteroanterior view. (*B*) Lateral view.

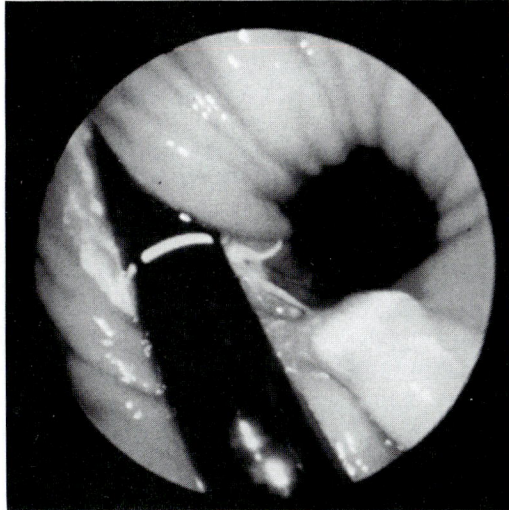

Figure 42-8. A retroflexed endoscopic view of a paraeso-phageal hiatal hernia. Note the separate orifice to the side of the gastroesophageal junction. The gastric rugal folds ascend into the hernia.

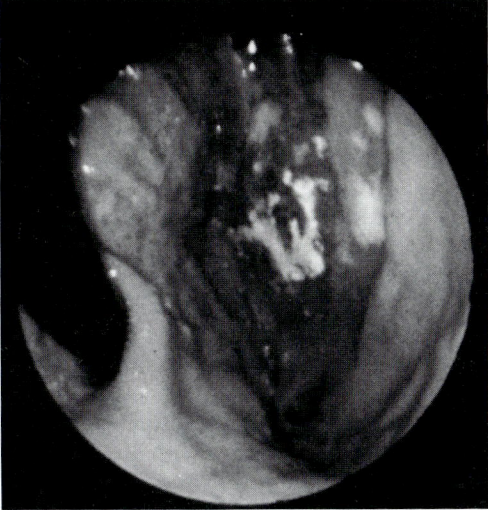

Figure 42-9. A retroflexed endoscopic view of a mixed hia-tal hernia. The paraesophageal hernia begins about halfway up the side of the sliding hiatal hernia, both of which ride high up into the thorax.

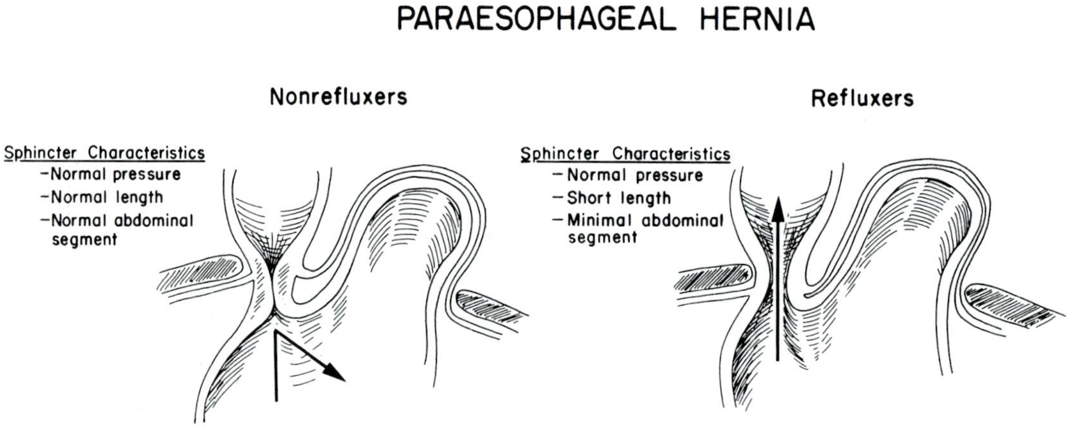

PARAESOPHAGEAL HERNIA

Nonrefluxers   Refluxers

Sphincter Characteristics
 −Normal pressure
 −Normal length
 −Normal abdominal
  segment

Sphincter Characteristics
 −Normal pressure
 −Short length
 −Minimal abdominal
  segment

Figure 42-10. A schematic diagram of the anatomic and manometric differences between patients with paraesophageal hernia with reflux and those without reflux as defined by 24-hour esophageal pH monitoring.

sliding hiatal hernia is diagnosed by identifying gastric rugal folds above the level of the diaphragm. Ideally, there should be at least 2 cm between the crural impression (which is identified by requesting that the patient sniff) and the squamocolumnar junction to make the diagnosis of sliding hiatal hernia.[8] Gastroscopy can be confusing in the presence of a paraesophageal hernia because of distortion of the stomach. It often is impossible to locate and intubate the pylorus at endoscopy.

PATHOPHYSIOLOGY

The gastroesophageal junction is important in preventing gastroesophageal reflux. Several physiologic tests have been developed to study the integrity of the gastroesophageal junction. Ambulatory esophageal pH monitoring provides objective evidence of increased esophageal acid exposure. The integrity of the gastroesophageal junction is dependent on the relationship between the pressure of the lower esophageal sphincter, its overall length, and the length of the portion that is exposed to the positive intraabdominal pressure. A deficiency in any of these characteristics results in incompetence of the lower esophageal sphincter and leads to gastroesophageal reflux, regardless of the presence of a hernia[5,8,26,28] (Fig. 42-10). Stationary manometry allows for accurate assessment of the characteristics of the lower esophageal sphincter (Table 42-1).

A paraesophageal hernia usually does not affect the competence of the lower esophageal sphincter. Occasionally, however, a paraesophageal hernia may lead to shortening of both the overall and the intraab-dominal portion of the sphincter, especially if the lesion is associated with a sliding hernia.[26] This may lead to lower esophageal sphincter incompetence and gastroesophageal reflux disease. Furthermore, loss of fixation of the gastroesophageal junction associated with a sliding or mixed hernia results in poor esophageal body function and may be associated with poor clearance of the refluxed material. This results in increased exposure time of the lower esophagus to acid pH.[8]

THERAPY

The presence of a paraesophageal hernia is an indication for surgical repair. In a report by Skinner and Belsey,[23] 6 of 21 patients who received conservative treatment of a paraesophageal hernia because of minimal symptoms died of the complications of strangulation, perforation, severe hemorrhage, or acute dilation of the herniated stomach. These life-threatening complications often occur without warning, and any patient found to have a paraesophageal hernia should be advised to undergo elective repair. Postlethwait[21]

Table 42-1. The Lower Limit of Normal Values for Manometry of the Lower Esophageal Sphincter

Sphincter Parameter	Lower Limit of Normal
Pressure	6 mmHg
Total length	2 cm
Intraabdominal length	1 cm

(Zaninotto G, DeMeester TR, Schwizer W, et al. The lower esophageal sphincter in health and disease. Am J Surg 1988;155:104)

noted an operative mortality rate of 19% among patients who underwent emergency operation, compared to the mortality rate of less than 1% obtained by Skinner and Belsey with elective repair.[23]

The surgical approach can be divided into five steps:[17]

1. Reduction of the herniated stomach: The stomach is relatively easy to mobilize and reduce. There usually are no adhesions between the stomach and the hernia sac, and the stomach can be reduced with gentle traction. Intubating the stomach with an Ewald tube results in decompression, allowing for easier reduction of the stomach into the abdomen.[17]

2. Herniotomy: The hernia sac always should be excised. This is achieved by incising the sac along the lateral border of the hiatal defect and peeling it away from the soft tissues of the mediastinum. If the sac is not excised, fluid and air can accumulate later and may cause pain and fever.[2]

3. Herniorrhaphy: The hiatal defect is closed with interrupted mattress sutures. Often, the poor quality of the tissue surrounding the defect makes the use of pledgets advisable to help buttress the sutures and achieve a good repair.[17] The repair, especially in the case of a lateral defect, should continue up to and abut on the esophageal wall. If the defect is large, the left and right bundles of the right crus should be approximated in front of the esophagus. The esophagus should not be dissected away from the preaortic fascia.

4. Antireflux procedure: There is no consensus of opinion as to whether an antireflux procedure should be added to the operation. Adding an antireflux procedure significantly lengthens the operative time and increases the amount of dissection necessary around the lower esophagus. This is significant because most of these patients are elderly. In the elective setting, it is sensible to base the decision to add an antireflux procedure on comprehensive preoperative testing. If the patient has evidence of reflux on 24-hour pH testing and an incompetent sphincter on manometry, an antireflux procedure in the form of a fundoplication should be added. We prefer the Nissen fundoplication (Fig. 42-11). If the patient is found to have a competent lower esophageal sphincter, no antireflux procedure is necessary unless a significant amount of dissection around the gastroesophageal junction

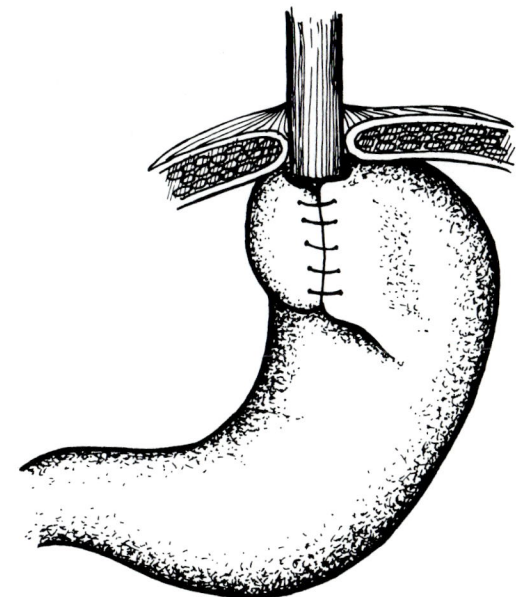

Figure 42-11. A schematic diagram of a Nissen fundoplication.

is required. Often, there is no opportunity to assess the lower esophageal sphincter adequately before surgery. Under these circumstances, a reasonable assessment of the gastroesophageal junction can be obtained by palpating the junction and determining its degree of fixation to the preaortic fascia. If the gastroesophageal junction is well tethered, the sphincter probably is competent and no antireflux procedure is necessary.[17] It is felt that, in this situation, dissection of the gastroesophageal junction may predispose to a "slipped fundoplication" if the crural repair fails. This is particularly likely to occur in elderly patients with a paraesophageal hernia and poor tissue quality.[11,14] If the gastroesophageal junction is mobile, Menguy[17] suggests posterior gastropexy (the Hill procedure) because it is easy to perform, is effective in stabilizing the gastroesophageal junction, and does not require dissection of the preaortic fascia.

5. Gastropexy: Gastropexy usually is not indicated, but should be considered if the stomach is mobile after reduction. It also is used to fix the stomach in its intraabdominal position. Many forms of gastropexy are possible. Ellis and associates,[11] and Wichterman and colleagues[27] suggest the use of a tube gastrostomy. This is performed easily and is effective in preventing gastric volvulus. The tube gas-

trostomy should be placed as high up on the fundus of the stomach as possible to obtain the best results. Menguy[17] prefers a gastropexy done with two rows of sutures attaching most of the greater curvature of the stomach to the underside of the abdominal wall (Fig. 42-12). This method not only prevents gastric volvulus, but also prevents recurrent herniation if the crural repair fails. If the patient is too old to tolerate anesthesia and major surgery, anterior gastropexy alone often is all that is required to prevent the complications of volvulus and can be performed under local anesthesia.

It is possible to approach paraesophageal hernias using the laparoscope. These hernias usually are easy to reduce, making them amenable to the laparoscopic approach. Dissection of the large hernia sac and mobilization of the cardia can be difficult, however, and should not be undertaken laparoscopically until experience has been obtained in the laparoscopic approach to this area. We have used laparoscopy in operating on three patients with paraesophageal hernias, including one patient who had a totally intrathoracic stomach. The repair always was associated with a Nissen fundoplication.

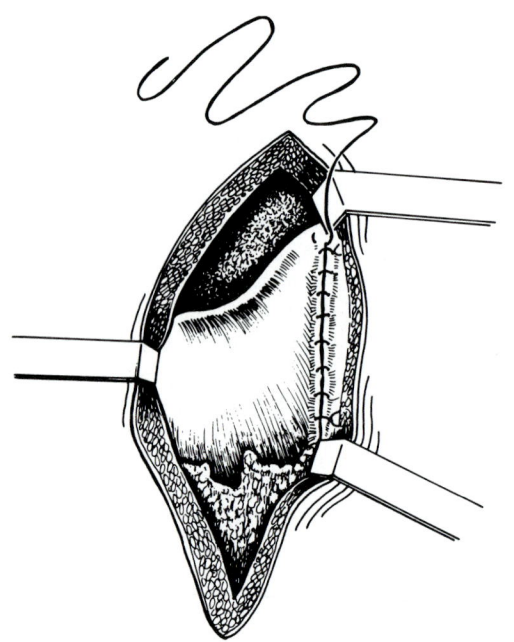

Figure 42-12. The anterior gastropexy illustrated here can be performed as part of the repair of a paraesophageal hernia.

SUMMARY

Paraesophageal hernia results from herniation of the stomach through an enlarged hiatus in association with a fixed gastroesophageal junction. If it is associated with a sliding hiatal hernia, it is known as a mixed hernia. Symptoms usually are vague, but one fifth of these patients have severe life-threatening complications such as incarceration, strangulation, perforation, or excessive hemorrhage. Paraesophageal hernias are diagnosed easily either by the detection of a retrocardiac air–fluid level on thoracic radiography, by contrast radiology, or by esophagogastroscopy. Lower esophageal sphincter incompetence may occur as a result of shortening of the intraabdominal portion of the sphincter. The treatment is surgical. In an elective repair of a paraesophageal hernia, an antireflux procedure should be performed only if physiologic testing reveals gastroesophageal reflux on the basis of an incompetent lower esophageal sphincter. If preoperative testing is not possible, posterior gastropexy (the Hill procedure) is an effective and appropriate antireflux procedure if the gastroesophageal junction appears to be mobile at the time of surgery. Anterior gastropexy prevents recurrent volvulus and may be effective on its own in the treatment of patients who are poor operative candidates.

REFERENCES

1. Akerlund A. Hernia diaphragmatica Hiatus Oesophagei Vom Anatomischen Und Rontgenologischen Gesichtspunkt. Acta Radiol 1926;6:3.
2. Allen B, Tompkins RK, Mulder DG. Repair of large paraesophageal hernia with complete intrathoracic stomach. Am Surg 1991;57:642.
3. Alrabeeah A, Giacomantonio M, Gillis DA. Paraesophageal hernia after Nissen fundoplication: a real complication in pediatric patients. J Pediatr Surg 1988;23:766.
4. Battu P, D'Cruz IA, Holman M, Locksmith JP. Noninvasive imaging of a retrocardiac spleen: unusual component of paraesophageal diaphragmatic hernia. Chest 1992;101:1159.
5. Bombeck TC, Dillard DH, Nyhus LM. Muscular anatomy of the gastroesophageal junction and role of the phrenoesophageal ligament. Ann Surg 1966; 164:643.
6. Chapman JE, Kamath MV, Wilson BW. Combined paraesophageal and sliding hiatal hernia. South Med J 1988;81:1177.
7. Dalgaard JB. Volvulus of the stomach. Acta Chir Scand 1952;103:131.
8. DeMeester TR, Lafontaine E, Joelsson BE, et al. Re-

lationship of a hiatal hernia to the function of the body of the esophagus and the gastroesophageal junction. J Thorac Cardiovasc Surg 1981;82:547.

9. Eliska O. Phreno-oesophageal membrane and its role in the development of hiatal hernia. Acta Anat (Basel) 1973;86:137.

10. Ellis FH Jr. Diaphragmatic hiatal hernias: recognizing and treating the major types. Postgrad Med 1990;88:113.

11. Ellis FH Jr, Crozier RE, Shea JA. Paraesophageal hiatus hernia. Arch Surg 1986;121:416.

12. Farrell B, Gerard PS, Bryk D. Paraesophageal hernia causing colonic obstruction. J Clin Gastroenterol 1991;13:188.

13. Hill LD. Incarcerated paraesophageal hernia: a surgical emergency. Am J Surg 1973;126:286.

14. Hill LD, Tobias JA. Paraesophageal hernia. Arch Surg 1968;96:735.

15. Kleitsch WP. Embryology of congenital diaphragmatic hernia. I. Esophageal hiatus hernia. Arch Surg 1958;76:868.

16. Landreneau RJ, Johnson JA, Marshall JB, et al. Clinical spectrum of paraesophageal herniation. Dig Dis Sci 1992;37:537.

17. Menguy R. Surgical management of large paraesophageal hernia with complete intrathoracic stomach. World J Surg 1988;12:415.

18. Payne WS. In discussion: Wichterman K, Geha AS, Cahow CE, et al. Giant paraesophageal hiatus hernia with intrathoracic stomach and colon: the case for early repair. Surgery 1979;86:497.

19. Pearson FG, Cooper JD, Ilves R, et al. Massive hiatal hernia with incarceration: a report of 53 cases. Ann Thorac Surg 1983;35:45.

20. Postempski P. Nuovo processo operativo per la riduzione cruenta delle ernie diaframmatiche da trauma e per la sutura delle ferite del diaframma. Bull Reale Accad Med Roma 1889;15:191.

21. Postlethwait RW. Surgery of the esophagus. New York, Appleton-Century-Crofts, 1979:195–255.

22. Rakic SR, Pesko P, Dunjic M, Gerzic Z. Healing of gastric ulcer associated with paraesophageal hernia after hernial reduction. Am J Surg 1992;163:443.

23. Skinner DB, Belsey RHR. Surgical management of esophageal reflux and hiatus hernia. Long-term results with 1030 patients. J Thorac Cardiovasc Surg 1967;53:33.

24. Streitz JM, Ellis FH Jr. Iatrogenic paraesophageal hiatus hernia. Ann Thorac Surg 1990;50:446.

25. Treacy PJ, Jamieson GG. An approach to the management of para-oesophageal hiatus hernias. Aust N Z J Surg 1987;57:813.

26. Walther B, DeMeester TR, Lafontaine E, et al. Effect of paraesophageal hernia on sphincter function and its implication on surgical therapy. Am J Surg 1984;147:111.

27. Wichterman K, Geha AS, Cahow CE, et al. Giant paraesophageal hiatus hernia with intrathoracic stomach and colon: the case for early repair. Surgery 1979; 86:498.

28. Zaninotto G, DeMeester TR, Schwizer W, et al. The lower esophageal sphincter in health and disease. Am J Surg 1988;155:104.

Editor's Comment

Perdikis and Hinder have outlined clearly both the diagnostic approach and the major technical steps in the treatment of paraesophageal hiatus hernia. Some points deserve emphasis. One concerns the importance of iatrogenic factors in the etiology of paraesophageal hernia. Children who have had operative correction of reflux esophagitis are reasonably prone to the development of a paraesophageal hernia. Presumably, the reason is excess straining secondary to crying in young infants. Paraesophageal hernias also develop in adults, particularly after esophagectomy for cancer with replacement using a stomach or colon tube. The primary factor seems to be difficulty in securing adequate fixation of the stomach or colon tube completely around the periphery of the diaphragmatic hiatus.

Most patients with spontaneous paraesophageal hernias are elderly. It is not unusual for a surgeon to be consulted in regard to a patient who has a complication of paraesophageal hernia, only to discover that the referring physician has been aware of the hernia's presence for 15 or 20 years and done nothing about it. This therapeutic inertia occurs because most physicians believe that paraesophageal hernias do not lead to significant complications or carry a significant mortality risk. Such an assumption is clearly wrong. Most physicians also believe that surgical repair has a high recurrence rate, a view supported by the results of half a century ago. This assumption is outdated. We have missionary work to do among the physicians. They need to be taught, as indicated by Perdikis and Hinder, that paraesophageal hernia, like any other hernia of the abdominal wall, should be repaired on diagnosis to avoid complications and the risk of mortality. Furthermore, effective operative therapies are available and patients should not be denied the benefits of operative correction of a paraesophageal hernia.

The presence of esophagitis can be a differential diagnostic problem. Most patients with a paraesophageal hernia have at least intermittent obstruction because of partial gastric volvulus within the chest. This results in secondary retention of food in the distal esophagus and consequent inflammation. It is well to recognize that only a few patients with a paraesophageal hernia also have an incompetent lower esphageal sphincter; in most, the apparent esophagitis results from the intermittent obstruction and food retention that accompanies the hernia. Therefore, in most cases, a fundoplication is unnecessary and, in my view, meddlesome. The notion that the fundoplication acts as a big fist and helps to reduce the future risk of recurrence is not well founded.

There are some patients in whom the tissues of the diaphragm adjacent to the enlarged hiatus are of such poor quality that a secure primary repair cannot be constructed. We have used a Marlex prosthesis to reinforce the diaphragm in this situation for some years, with salutary results.

R.E.C.

Hernia, Fourth Edition, edited
by Lloyd M. Nyhus and Robert E. Condon.
J.B. Lippincott Company, Philadelphia © 1995.

Chapter 43

Congenital Diaphragmatic Hernia

Jean-Martin Laberge, David L. Sigalet, and Frank M. Guttman

HISTORY

The first traumatic diaphragmatic hernia was described by the French Army surgeon Ambroise Paré in 1597 and the first congenital diaphragmatic hernia (CDH) was described by Riverius in 1679. One century later, Morgagni described the anterior hernia that now bears his name. In 1848, Bochdalek reported on the posterolateral diaphragmatic foramen. A congenital hernia first was repaired successfully by Heidenhain in 1902, and in 1920, Aue, Heidenhain's assistant, reported a second successful repair. In 1925, Hedblom described 44 children with congenital posterolateral diaphragmatic hernias, 22 of whom lived. Because of a 75% mortality rate within the first month after birth, Hedblom recommended early operation. Philemon E. Truesdale in 1935 reported one of the first American series, successfully repairing 9 of 10 hernias in children aged 17 months to 15 years in his hospital in Fall River, Massachusetts. Ladd and Gross[18] in 1940 presented a series of 16 patients, with 9 survivors. The youngest patient was 40 hours of age at the time of operation. The first survivor operated on before 24 hours of age was described by Gross in 1946. Since that time, the focus of attention has shifted to diaphragmatic hernias that are diagnosed before or immediately at birth.[21] These represent the majority of cases and continue to have a high mortality, although some recent improvement has been gained with the use of extracorporeal membrane oxygenation (ECMO).[19,23,29]

POSTEROLATERAL CONGENITAL DIAPHRAGMATIC HERNIA OF BOCHDALEK

Embryology

During the third to fourth week of gestation, the mesenchyme between the pericardium and the coelomic cavity gives rise to a membranous infolding that extends anteriorly and is known as the septum transversum. It first forms at the cervical level, then moves down to arrive at the lower thoracic level. At this point, it divides the chest and abdominal cavities by fusing with similar infoldings arising posteriorly (the dorsal mesentery) and laterally (the pleuroperitoneal membranes). The last area to close is the site of the Bochdalek hernia, the posterior pleuroperitoneal canal. The left side closes after the right. This separation of the body cavities is complete by 8 to 9 weeks of fetal life. Development of the mesenchyme between the membranes results in the muscular development of the diaphragm. During this same period, the primitive lung buds are developing. The intestinal tract also is growing rapidly into the coelomic cavity and returns to the abdomen during the ninth and tenth weeks of gestation. The classic theory is that the intestines prevent closure of the pleuroperitoneal canal because of their premature return into the abdomen or because of a delay in fusion of the pleuroperitoneal membrane with the rest of the diaphragm. The presence of intestine in the chest then impairs lung development. A large body of experimental work in a fetal lamb model has demonstrated that similar pulmonary hypoplasia and secondary pathophysiologic changes occur after the induction of CDH in the second trimester.[7,13]

This theory is challenged by the fact that large omphaloceles can be associated with CDH.[3] Results of experimental studies in rats and mice have shown that a vitamin A–deficient diet during pregnancy or the administration of a 2,4-dichlorophenyl-p-nitrophenyl ether (nitrophen) can result in a high incidence of CDH in the offspring.[15] In this model, hypoplasia of the lung buds precedes hypoplasia of the posthepatic mesenchymal plate, suggesting that lung hypoplasia may be the primary factor leading to the diaphragmatic defect.[17] Human patients in whom symptoms appear late in childhood, however, have apparently normal lung development.[9]

Anatomy

The most common and severe diaphragmatic hernia of congenital origin is the posterolateral type known as a Bochdalek hernia.

The anatomy of the posterior diaphragmatic defect is variable. It occurs on the left side in 80% to 85% of patients. In less than 10% of cases, a hernial sac is present, usually consisting of a thin mesothelial membrane. The defect itself may be small, or it may be large and involve most of the diaphragm. The posterior rim often appears to be minimal, but usually can be mobilized by unrolling it from the kidney capsule and chest wall. Occasionally, the diaphragm is absent or the defect is bilateral.

On the left side, the abdominal viscera most often found in the chest are the stomach, small intestine, colon, spleen, and left lobe of the liver. Occasionally, the pancreas, kidney, and adrenal gland are included. On the right side, there usually is much less intestine, with the liver blocking the defect. The liver itself may be in the chest. Nonrotation of the intestine usually is associated with the defect.

During intrauterine growth, the presence of the abdominal contents in the chest compresses the ipsilateral lung, which also may affect the contralateral lung because of the mobile mediastinum in the fetus. In babies with symptoms shortly after birth, hypoplasia of both lungs is a constant finding. These lungs have reduced-size bronchi, less bronchial branching (typically, 6–8 generations of bronchi compared with 15 in normal newborns), and decreased alveolar surface area.[4,10] The ipsilateral lung is affected more than the contralateral lung. The pulmonary vasculature also is abnormal, with an increase in the thickness of the arteriolar smooth muscle and extension of this muscularization down to the capillary level of the alveoli. This may impair pulmonary function further by increasing pulmonary artery pressure and resulting in right-to-left shunting.[10,27]

Etiology and Incidence

The cause of CDH is unknown. Vitamin A deficiency and nitrophen ingestion have been shown to contribute to its development in gravid rats. There also are some reports of familial CDH.[14] The incidence of diaphragmatic hernia varies from 1:2000 for all births to 1:4000 to 1:12,500 for live births. Anomalies, especially of the central nervous system, are present in a major proportion of stillborn infants.[25]

Pathophysiology

Before birth, the size of the defect, the volume of herniated viscera, and the duration of compression determine the severity of symptoms and physiologic defects. Babies with acute respiratory distress in the newborn period usually have severe lung hypoplasia and compression after birth from air distention of the intestine (Fig. 43-1A). This results in hypoxia, hypercarbia, and acidosis. In turn, these produce pulmonary vasoconstriction with secondary pulmonary hypertension and a right-to-left shunt. This increases the hypoxemia, leads to metabolic acidosis, and completes the vicious circle of persistent fetal circulation or, more accurately, persistent pulmonary hypertension of the newborn (PPHN).[11] Left untreated, the condition leads to early death. If good intestinal decompression is achieved, correction of the diaphragmatic defect itself does little to affect this process (see Fig. 43-1B through D). Early repair actually may worsen pulmonary compliance.[22,26]

In those patients whose symptoms develop after 24 hours of life, pulmonary hypoplasia is mild and correction of the defect usually is successful.

There is another group of patients with early symptoms who do well initially after repair and then suddenly experience persistent pulmonary hypertension. This is the most characteristic example of the importance of pulmonary vascular reactivity in the outcome of these infants. The factors responsible for ending the "honeymoon" period probably are multiple. The pulmonary vascular bed is hyperactive, possibly because of the abnormal arteriolar muscularization. There also may be a lack of production or early depletion of pulmonary vasodilators. The focus recently has shifted from prostaglandins to nitric oxide, also known as endothelium-derived relaxation factor.[20] Barotrauma also contributes to the pathophysiology. More attention is being given to limiting ventilation pressures in babies with CDH, but the most important index is the transpulmonary pressure gradient, which is defined as airway pressure minus intrapleural pressure. A negative intrapleural pressure (ie, a chest tube on suction) increases the gradient and causes more barotrauma. Excessive ventilation in general results in overdistention of alveoli, interstitial and mediastinal emphysema, possible pneumothorax, and even subcutaneous emphysema. The serious conse-

Figure 43-1. (A) Chest roentgenogram of a newborn infant with a left posterolateral diaphragmatic ▶ hernia. Note distended bowel loops in the left chest, mediastinal shift, and minimal lung volumes. (B and C) Same patient after 2 (B) and 4 (C) days of venoarterial extracorporeal membrane oxygenation. Note progressive improvement in lung volume bilaterally, without repair of the diaphragmatic defect. (D) After repair of the diaphragmatic hernia. Note the absence of a chest tube, and persistent right mediastinal deviation. This could be misinterpreted as being a tension pneumothorax on the left.

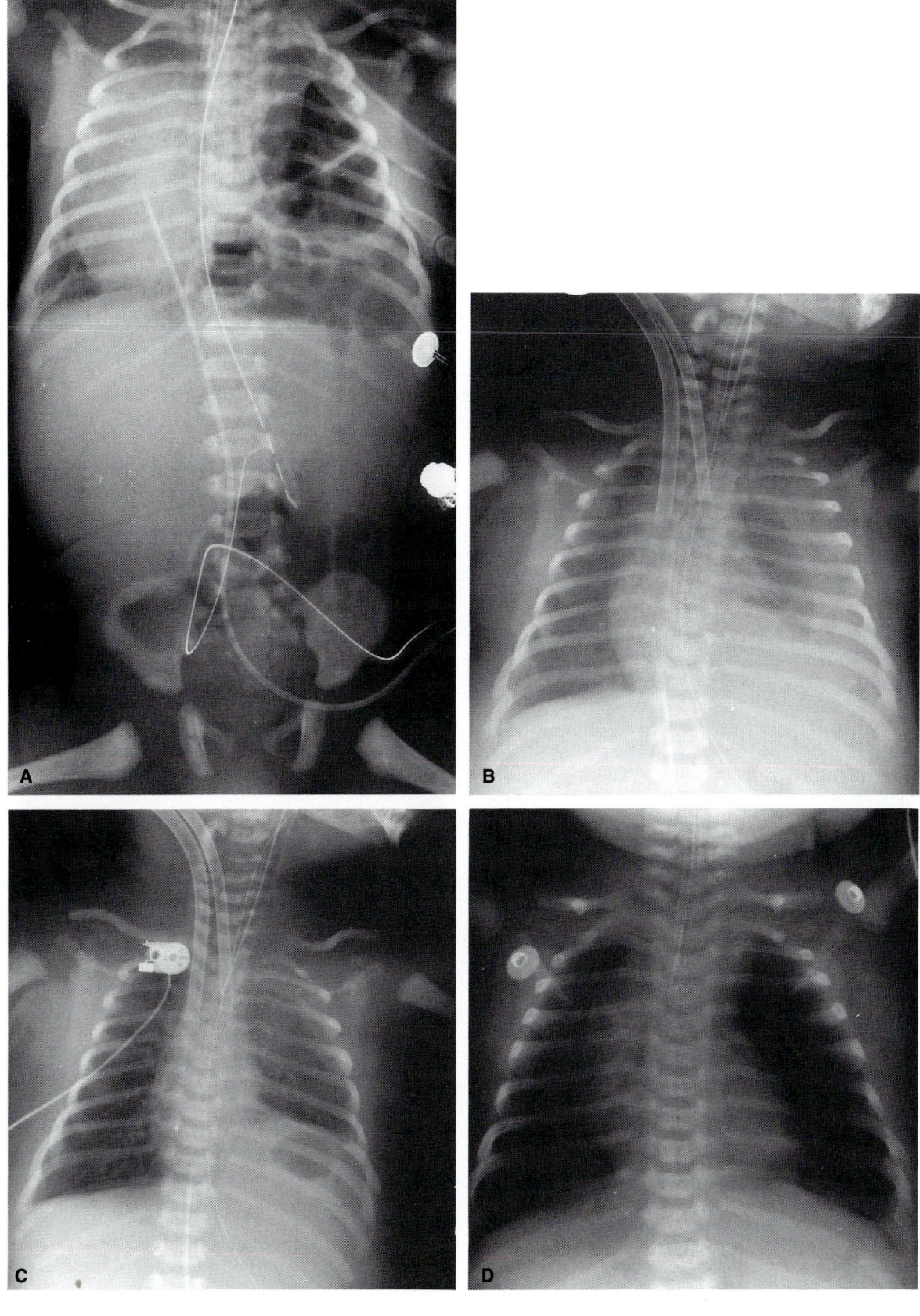

quences of pneumothorax are well known, and the distention of alveoli and interstitial emphysema cause stretching and compression of arterioles and capillaries (air-block syndrome), contributing to the pulmonary hypertension.[8] There also is experimental evidence suggesting a deficiency of surfactant in these patients, adding to the likelihood of barotrauma-induced lung injury.[12]

These pathophysiologic features suggest a variety of alternative therapies, such as direct vasodilation with nitric oxide, alternate ventilator strategies, and ECMO, which are discussed later.

Symptoms and Signs

Before birth, a diaphragmatic hernia may be suggested by the presence of polyhydramnios, or it may be discovered incidentally on ultrasound examination. Sonographic signs include a mediastinal shift and the presence of the gastric bubble in the chest. The condition has been discovered as early as 18 weeks' gestation. In severely affected babies, respiratory distress, cyanosis, and tachypnea are present at birth. The physical signs include absent breath sounds, a scaphoid abdomen, and drawing in of the intercostal muscles. Displacement of heart sounds away from the side of the hernia is a prominent feature, and a misdiagnosis of dextrocardia is common. In patients with mild defects, the symptoms may not appear until after 24 hours of life, a few months of life, or even in later childhood. The diagnosis in the latter patients often is made because of gastrointestinal complications such as partial obstruction. In such patients, physical signs include thoracic bowel sounds on the affected side. Occasionally, the defect may be found incidentally on a chest roentgenogram.

Differential Diagnosis

The diagnosis usually is straightforward. Congenital cystic adenomatoid malformation can mimic loops of intestine in the chest, especially when a tentative diagnosis is made in utero by ultrasound. In newborn infants, a roentgenogram that includes the chest and abdomen confirms the paucity of intestinal loops in the abdomen and a gastric bubble (or preferably a nasogastric tube) in the chest (see Fig. 43-1A). In older infants, staphylococcal pneumonia with pneumatocele has to be considered in the differential diagnosis, but can be excluded by the history and a plain anteroposterior and lateral roentgenogram, occasionally with the help of ultrasound and barium enema. A diaphragmatic eventration can be difficult to differen-

tiate; ultrasound, fluoroscopy, and even pneumoperitoneography may be required.

Preoperative Care

As soon as the diagnosis is suspected, without waiting for roentgenographic confirmation, a nasogastric tube should be passed to decompress the stomach. A distended stomach further impairs ventilation and reduces the venous return to the heart by shifting the mediastinum. Ventilation by mask is contraindicated for the same reasons. If the child has any respiratory distress, endotracheal intubation must be performed early. The most important factor in the initial resuscitation is to avoid high ventilation pressures. It is not necessary to see ample chest movements or hear good air entry to consider the ventilation adequate. Attempts to achieve good chest excursion often lead to pneumothorax, usually on the contralateral side, where the lung is more compliant. Instead, low peak pressures (20–25 cm H_2O) and a high ventilation rate (80–100 breaths per minute) should be achieved, initially by manual ventilation. If a manometer is not available, the physician must have a hand almost "fibrillating" on the bag. Hypercarbia with severe acidosis is the rule, and hyperventilation by hand with an FIO_2 of 1.0 is the safest maneuver to use until blood gas values or transcutaneous oxygen monitoring is available. In our experience, and that of others, retinopathy of prematurity never is seen with CDH.[7]

If a prenatal diagnosis is made, the infant should be delivered at a tertiary-care center. If the baby is born at a hospital where a pediatric surgeon and tertiary neonatal care are not available, arrangements for transfer should be made immediately. The essential steps for transfer of the newborn infant are gastric decompression with an adequate tube (a 10F Replogle tube is ideal), endotracheal intubation with low-pressure and high-frequency ventilation, maintenance of normothermia, establishment of intravenous access, and availability of tube thoracostomy in case of sudden deterioration. The placement of arterial cannulas, monitoring of ventilation by frequent blood gas determinations, and administration of sodium bicarbonate all are useful, but should not delay transfer. Prolonged resuscitation and "stabilization" by inexperienced personnel often result in a pneumothorax and deteriorating condition.

Once the infant is at the tertiary-care center, stabilization measures can be completed. It previously was thought that immediate operation to repair the hernia was the only way to save these infants. It now generally is accepted that reduction of the herniated viscera solves only a small part of the problem, and that operation decreases pulmonary compliance in some cases.[22,26] The child is maintained with intravenous fluids, sedation, paralysis, and continued nasogastric suction. A second roentgenogram that includes the chest and abdomen confirms the diagnosis and the side of the hernia, and identifies a superimposed pneumothorax. Low-pressure, high-frequency ventilation is used to keep blood gas parameters in the range of optimal pulmonary vasodilation ($Po_2 > 100$, $Pco_2 < 40$, and $pH > 7.5$). Monitoring should include preductal and postductal transcutaneous oxygen monitoring or pulse oximetry, as well as an umbilical artery line. A right radial artery line also can be useful to evaluate shunting through the patent ductus arteriosus and oxygenation to the brain. Sodium bicarbonate or tromethamine (if the CO_2 level remains high) are given to correct metabolic acidosis. Other metabolic disturbances, such as hypoglycemia and hypocalcemia, also are avoided. The babies should be kept warm, well-sedated, and paralyzed because cold stress or any external stimulus may augment pulmonary vasospasm. If the child can be stabilized with conventional respirator management for 24 hours, semielective hernia repair can be done at that time. In this type of patient, the risk of late-developing PPHN is low.

If these parameters cannot be achieved with conventional ventilation, more aggressive therapy is indicated. Systemic hypotension often occurs when gas exchange remains poor. This further decreases tissue oxygen delivery, increases the metabolic acidosis, and contributes to pulmonary hypertension. Systemic blood pressure should be supported with dopamine or dobutamine infusion (usually 5–10 µg/kg/min for each). In this setting, high-frequency ventilation (800–1800 breaths per minute) has its proponents, but has had no consistent success. Pharmacologic manipulation of the pulmonary vascular bed has been used with success in some patients, but the individual response varies. Tolazoline, an α-adrenergic antagonist and histaminergic agonist with a direct relaxing effect on arterioles, has been the agent used most widely. Its selectivity for the pulmonary vasculature is minimal, and systemic hypotension usually accompanies its use. Complications such as bleeding can occur, and when a favorable response is elicited, it often is temporary. The overall result is that tolazoline does not improve survival, and its use has been abandoned.

Our approach to the patient who is failing with conventional therapy is to use ECMO support, which gives the hyperreactive pulmonary vascular bed a chance to stabilize (generally, 7–10 days) and allows the lungs to recover from the insult of the original resuscitation without further barotrauma. The indications for ECMO have become standardized. We use an oxygenation index of greater than 40 for 3 hours (oxygenation index = mean airway pressure × F_{IO_2}

× 100/postductal Pao_2). Other indications for ECMO are Pao_2 less than 40 mmHg for 2 hours or severe cardiac dysfunction unresponsive to dopamine and epinephrine. Such infants have less than a 20% chance of survival with conventional therapy.[5] We feel strongly that aggressive attempts at conventional ventilation only increase damage to the hypoplastic lungs and decrease the likelihood of success with ECMO. We use venoarterial ECMO routinely with CDH, because mediastinal shifts make it difficult to maintain adequate flows with venovenous ECMO. The child is maintained with ECMO until weaning trials show adequate pulmonary function, without PPHN. After 12 to 24 hours of stability, the child is weaned off ECMO, and the CDH is repaired after another 24 to 48 hours. During the period of ECMO, the child remains sedated and the lungs are ventilated gently, often with impressive improvements in lung volume and reduction of the herniated viscera (see Fig. 43-1). Because of the fear of recurrent PPHN after surgery, some advocate repair while ECMO is being used. This is associated with increased complications and deaths, however, primarily from bleeding. It also interferes with repair of the associated nonrotation. In our experience, PPHN has not recurred when repair is performed after weaning from ECMO.

If the child cannot be weaned from ECMO after 2 to 3 weeks, we consult with the family and repair the defect on ECMO, with the clear understanding that the ECMO support will be withdrawn if significant improvement does not occur within 4 to 5 days. No reliable predictors of pulmonary hypoplasia incompatible with survival are available for prospective guidance in making the decision to institute ECMO. Recent studies suggest, however, that the functional residual capacity of the lungs in patients with severe hypoplasia can be used as a predictor of survival early in the ECMO course.[1]

Operation

One of the most important elements of the operation is to continue to ventilate the child with high frequency and low pressures. A subcostal incision generally is preferred to a thoracic incision because it facilitates reduction of the viscera into the abdomen and allows lysis of the Ladd bands associated with the nonrotation (Figs. 43-2 through 43-5). Once the hernia is reduced completely and the intestine is eviscerated, a search is made for the hernial sac, which is resected if found. The hypoplastic lung usually can be seen through the diaphragmatic defect. The degree of hypoplasia can be estimated grossly by the size of the lung and the presence or absence of distinct lobes. No

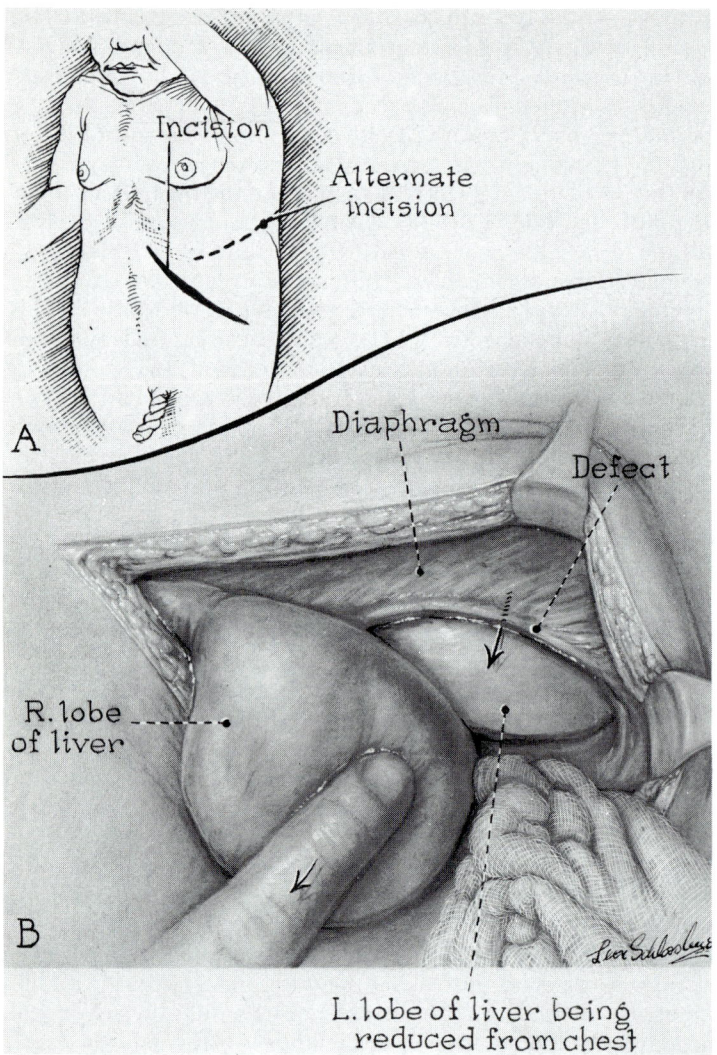

Figure 43-2. (*A* and *B*) The defect as seen at laparotomy. The intestines entering the chest are concealed behind the liver and the pack. The baby is rotated so that a thoracotomy incision may be added if necessary. The entire left lobe of the liver was in the chest.

attempt should be made to expand the lung forcefully.

The posterior edge of the diaphragm is dissected and unrolled if necessary, and the defect is closed with interrupted horizontal mattress sutures of silk or Prolene. If there is moderate tension on the sutures, pledgets should be used.[16] If tension is excessive, a patch should be applied (see Fig. 43-4). We prefer a polytetrafluoroethylene (Gore-Tex) patch. Special attention should be paid to the medial extent of large defects adjacent to the esophagus. This is the usual site for recurrent herniation. If the crus is underdeveloped, multiple small, interrupted sutures in the esophageal wall may be required.

After closure of the diaphragmatic defect, the abdominal cavity is explored and the peritoneal bands overlying the duodenum are divided. We do not be-

lieve that appendectomy should be performed in these patients. The abdominal wall is stretched manually before the abdomen is closed. If the fascia is under too much tension, it should be left open or the defect should be enlarged with polypropylene mesh. The skin then can be undermined and closed with minimal tension. Reoperation for ventral hernia may be avoided by the use of a mesh. In rare cases in which even the skin cannot be closed, a formal silo pouch must be constructed. There is no need for a gastrostomy. A Replogle nasogastric tube provides adequate gastric decompression for as long as necessary.

We prefer not to use a chest tube to drain the ipsilateral thoracic cavity because it may increase the transpleural pressure[8] (Fig. 43-6). If a tube is used, it may be clamped and used to remove or add air to stabilize the mediastinal position. Others leave it

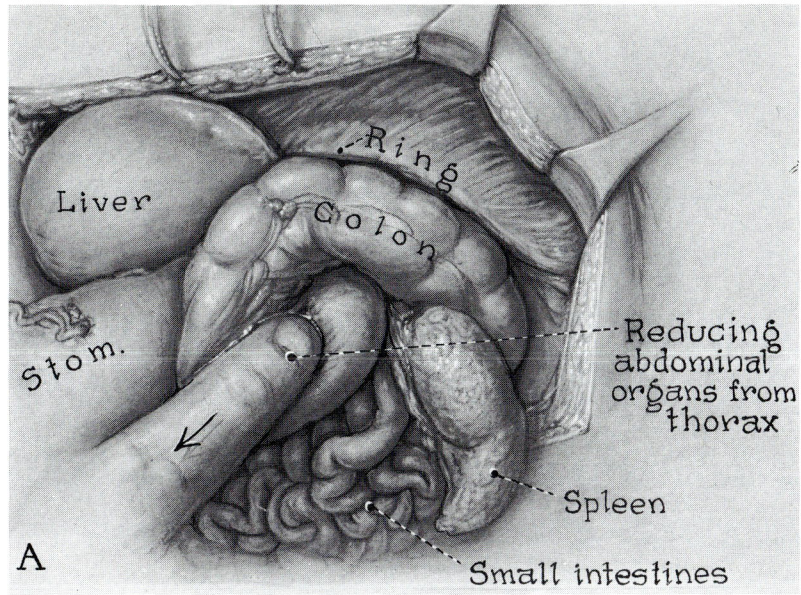

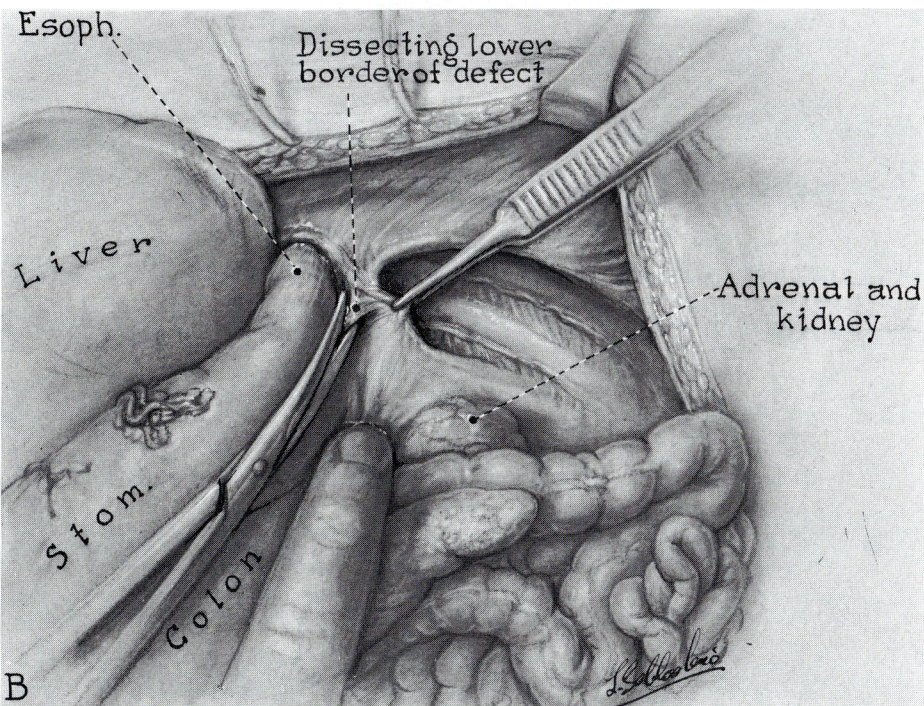

Figure 43-3.   With delivery of the left lobe of the liver and of the intestines, the nature of the defect is disclosed. There is a good strip of diaphragmatic muscle anteriorly and, after removal of the obscuring serosal covering, a clear band of diaphragmatic muscle can be dissected out lateral to the diaphragmatic crura and passing into a thick, rolled edge of diaphragm posteriorly (*A*). This splays out in white fibrous tissue, to disappear at about the posterior axillary line, just as the anterior muscle disappears into the chest wall at about the anterior axillary line, leaving the intervening portion of the circumference of the diaphragm totally defective (*B*).

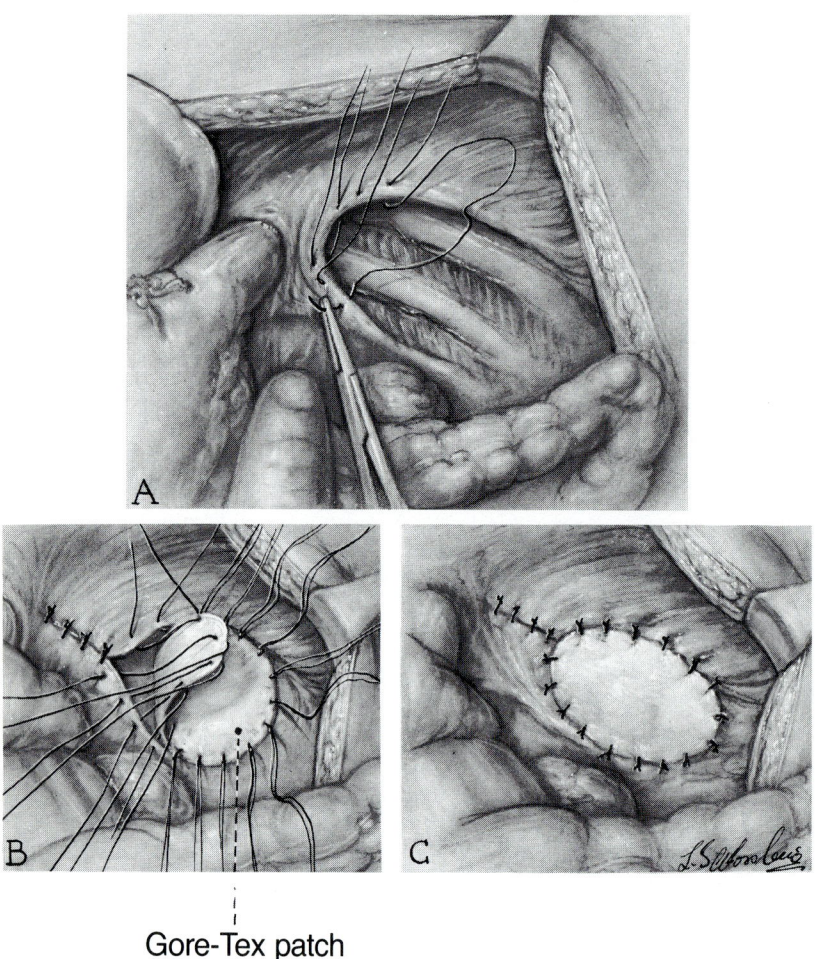

Gore-Tex patch

Figure 43-4. It was possible to approximate the edges of the diaphragmatic defect for about the medial third with permanent sutures (*A*). Excessive tension prevented primary closure. A patch of Gore-Tex was inserted as shown and closed the defect nicely, the lateral sutures being taken through the chest wall (*B* and *C*). In most instances, closure by direct suture is possible.

attached to a plastic bag or to balanced drainage. Placing the tube to suction or an underwater seal definitely is contraindicated.

After operation, even if their condition appears to be improved, these babies should be kept paralyzed on low-pressure, high-frequency ventilation with 100% oxygen.

Postoperative Care

Patients in whom symptoms develop after several hours of life usually can be weaned from the ventilator rapidly and extubated. Because most of these babies do well, this discussion focuses on the infants that are most ill, those in whom symptoms develop in the first hours of life.

A chest roentgenogram is taken immediately after the operation and at 4- to 6-hour intervals during the first 48 hours to detect a contralateral pneumothorax and monitor the mediastinal shift and pulmonary expansion. The chest roentgenogram should be interpreted carefully, because all the roentgenographic signs of an ipsilateral tension pneumothorax will be present: air, a lung that appears collapsed (but actually is hypoplastic and therefore cannot expand), a diaphragm that is flattened after the repair, and a mediastinum that still may be shifted toward the contralateral side (see Fig. 43-6*A*). The contralateral lung usually is less hypoplastic, and it may take a few hours or many days for the mediastinum to shift gradually, helping to fill the ipsilateral chest as the air is absorbed (see Fig. 43-6*B* through *D*). Aspiration of the ipsilateral "pneumothorax" in patients whose condition is stable may have disastrous consequences.

If hypoxia, pulmonary hypertension, and a right-to-left shunt develop postoperatively and are refractory to conventional therapy, ECMO should be reinstituted.

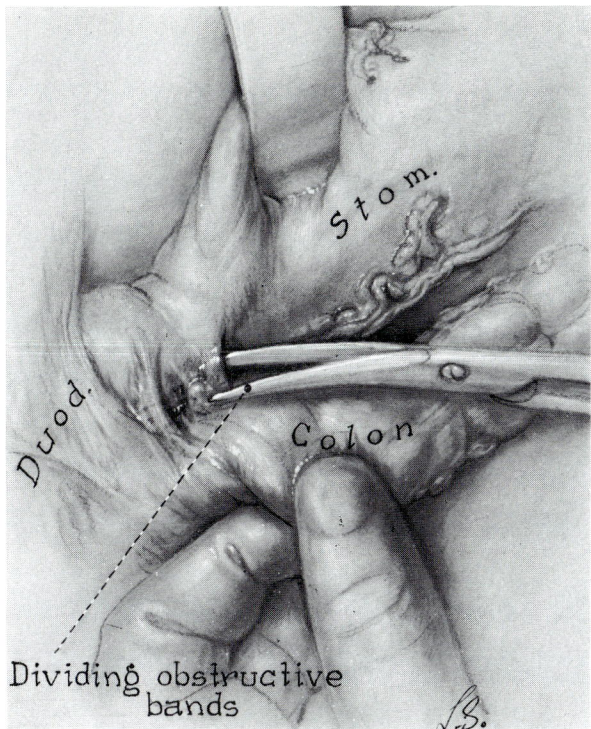

Figure 43-5. As in most children with a hernia this extensive, there was malrotation of the colon with the cecum in the right upper quadrant, complete absence of fixation of the mesentery of the small intestine, and abnormal peritoneal bands from the colon and the cecum crossing over the duodenum. These are shown here being divided in the Ladd maneuver to prevent subsequent duodenal obstruction.

Results

The survival rate in most series is close to 100% for patients whose symptoms develop after 24 hours of life. Long-term follow-up studies show normal lung volumes, with mild, asymptomatic decreases in forced expiratory volume consistent with emphysematous changes.[9] Chest roentgenograms also may be normal, or they may show persistent ipsilateral hypoplasia with contralateral hyperinflation.

In contrast, infants whose symptoms develop within 24 hours after birth have a poorer prognosis; survival rates vary from 40% to 80% when ECMO support is required.[19,29] These infants usually have larger hernial defects requiring a patch, and a high rate of complications such as gastroesophageal reflux (40%), recurrent herniation (up to 50%), and neuromotor delay (30%). The neurologic status of ECMO survivors has been studied intensely. The incidence of deficit and delay is less than that of equivalently ill newborns treated with conventional respirator man-

agement. There is no evidence to suggest that carotid artery ligation is harmful. Although this represents a distinct improvement over the survival rates obtained before the availability of ECMO,[23] there remains a subgroup of patients who cannot be salvaged because of pulmonary hypoplasia.

The true survival rate may be even worse, because many children with CDH die soon after birth, before transportation, and are never included in large series from pediatric surgical centers.[25]

For patients with early symptoms who survive, the long-term outcome is generally good, although many require readmission to the hospital for pneumonia, bronchitis, or other respiratory problems, especially in the first few years of life. The alveolar units of the lung continue to grow in size after birth, and can compensate for some of the hypoplasia. The limits of this compensation are not known.[2] Roentgenographic evidence of definite pulmonary hypoplasia and hyperinflation persist, and pulmonary function tests reveal more marked emphysematous changes and decreased volumes. Longer follow-up is required to assess the outcome in these more severely affected individuals.

Future Developments

Improvement in the outcome of patients with severe CDH has been inconsistent and difficult to achieve over the past 20 years. One major cause of death in CDH remains delay in diagnosis and poor initial resuscitation. From 1980 to 1985, 19 infants with CDH in whom symptoms developed within the first hour of life were transferred to our hospital. Of these, 1 died during transportation and 5 had contralateral pneumothorax before surgery, some with marked subcutaneous emphysema. Four of these 5 babies died. As the use of prenatal ultrasound becomes more common, antenatal diagnosis of CDH with subsequent delivery in a tertiary-care center should improve the survival of some of these infants.

Reduction and closure of the diaphragmatic hernia in utero is physiologically sound and technically feasible, as demonstrated experimentally by the works of Haller and others. Harrison's group has pioneered the use of in utero surgery. Despite impressive technical developments, however, the results of antenatal diaphragmatic hernia repair remain poor.[13] Most of the lethal or severe anomalies associated with CDH (eg, central nervous disorders, trisomy) can be detected in utero by ultrasound and amniocentesis. Even when these associated lethal malformations are excluded, it is difficult to predict which patients have

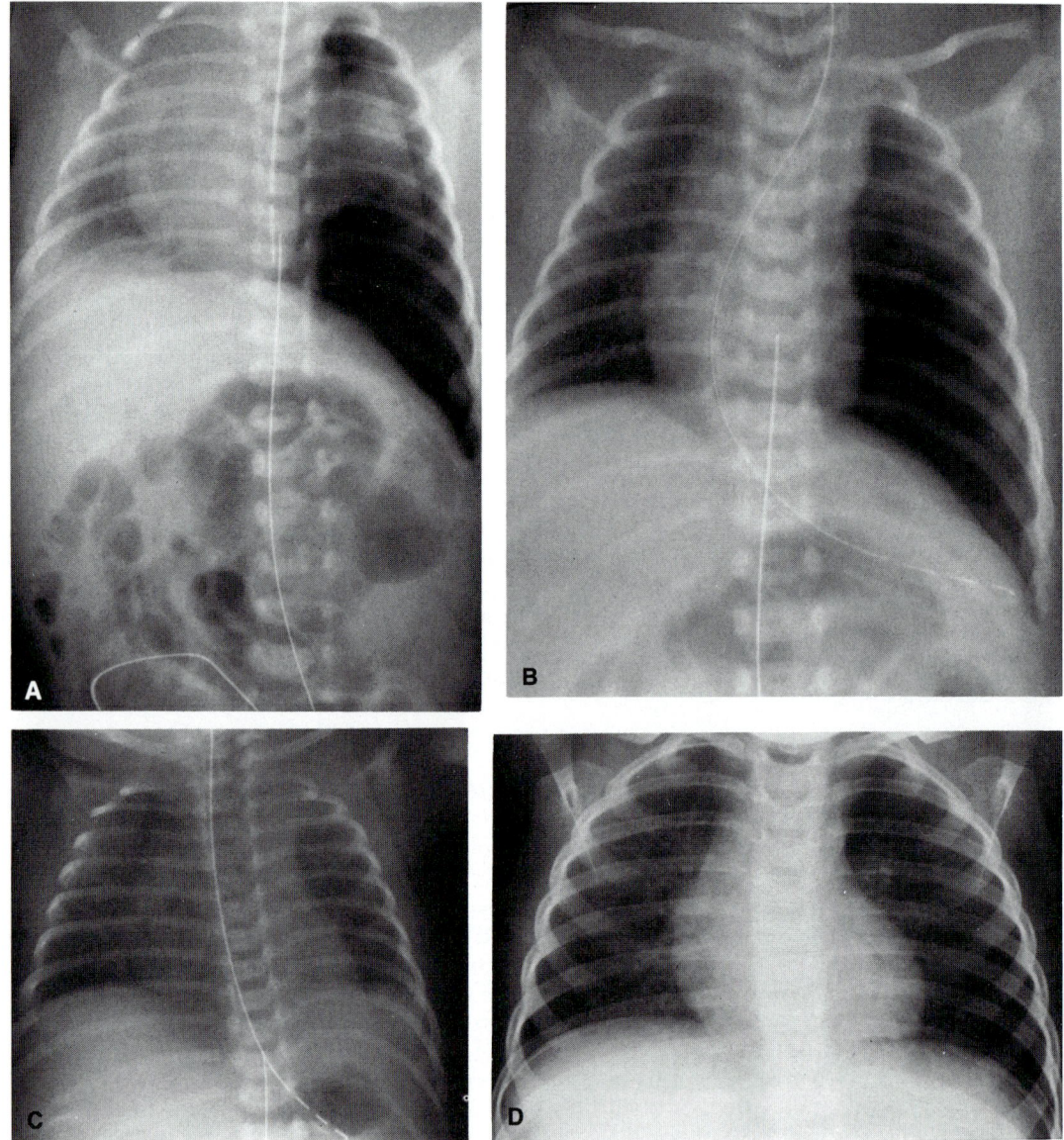

Figure 43-6. (*A*) Twenty-four hours after operation. No intrathoracic drain was used. The mediastinum still is shifted partly to the right, the diaphragm is low, and there is pneumothorax surrounding the hypoplastic left lung. Although all the usual roentgenographic signs of tension pneumothorax are present, aspiration or drainage of the chest is not required and may be dangerous because the child's condition is stable. (*B*) Forty-eight hours later. The lungs are expanding slowly and the mediastinum is returning to the midline. (*C*) One week after operation. The hypoplastic lung does not occupy all the left chest, which is filled by a small effusion. The effusion disappears gradually over time. (*D*) Two years later. The left lung is slightly hyperlucent. The patient has no symptoms.

such severe hypoplasia that survival is doubtful, justifying surgery in utero. This is the subject of an ongoing trial.[13] Our group and other researchers are working to increase pulmonary development in utero, while still others are investigating postnatal lung transplantation.[6]

LATE PRESENTATION

Occasionally, CDH is discovered in older children who have few or no symptoms despite the presence of multiple loops of intestine in the chest on roentgenography. This variation indicates that CDH is a dy-

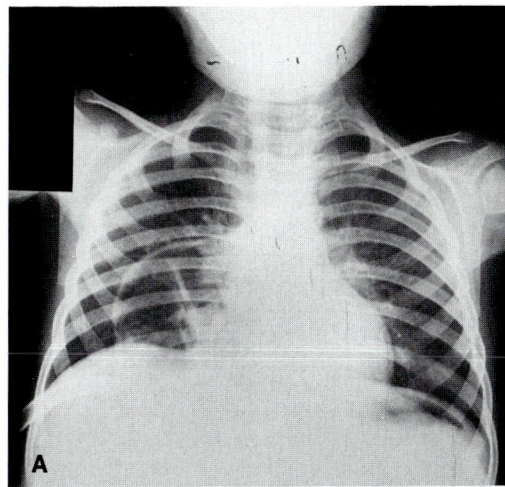

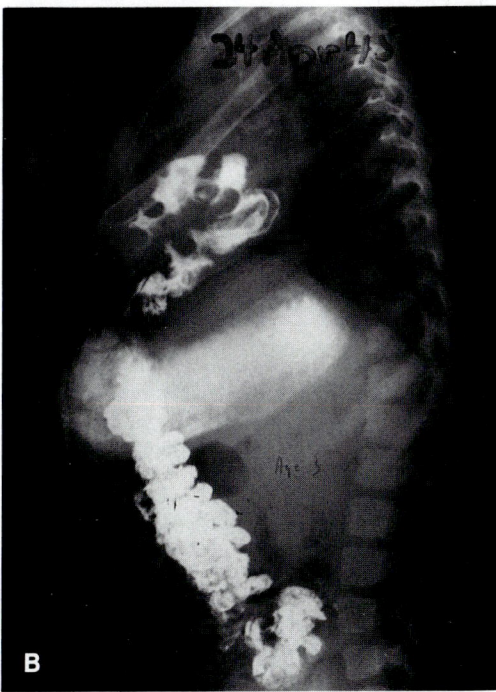

Figure 43-7. Hernia of Morgagni. (*A*) Plain roentgenogram showing an air-filled loop in the chest. (*B*) Barium enema in the same patient, showing the colon passing through the retrosternal defect.

namic process, and that intestine may move in and out of the chest. As a result, the defect is diagnosed by ultrasound in utero in some fetuses but not others, and some newborn infants have severe bilateral pulmonary hypoplasia whereas others do not, all depending on the amount of intestine in the chest and the timing of herniation (before or after birth). Even if a patient has no symptoms, the hernia should be

repaired to avoid the complications of intestinal obstruction, volvulus, or appendicitis in the chest. Gastric volvulus, acute or chronic, also can occur from lack of fixation of the stomach. We usually perform a gastropexy at the time of diaphragmatic hernia repair in this group of patients.

HERNIA OF MORGAGNI

The foramen of Morgagni is a parasternal or retrosternal defect resulting from a failure of fusion between the septum transversum and the sternum or anterior ribs. The defect usually is small and contains a sac with herniated omentum, transverse colon, or, less often, liver, small intestine, or stomach. Although many anterior hernias cause no symptoms and are discovered incidentally on chest roentgenography, infants usually have respiratory distress and cyanosis similar to that seen with Bochdalek hernias.[24]

Associated anomalies such as congenital heart disease are common in these infants and may represent a minor variant of the Cantrell pentalogy. This rare anomaly consists of defects in the abdominal wall (epigastric omphalocele), sternum, pericardium, heart, and anterior diaphragm. Plain roentgenograms usually differentiate hernias through the foramen of Morgagni from other anterior mediastinal masses. Contrast studies of the upper gastrointestinal tract or colon and computerized tomography may be required at times to confirm the diagnosis (Fig. 43-7).

Because of potential incarceration, the hernia should be repaired unless there are contraindications to general anesthesia and laparotomy. An upper abdominal approach is preferred, with reduction of the viscera, excision of the sac, and closure of the defect with interrupted nonabsorbable sutures.

REFERENCES

1. Antunes MJ, Cullen J, Greenspan JS, Wolfsen PJ, Spitzer AR. Assessment of pre-operative lung function in CDH: a predictor of outcome. Abstract 10, 9th Annual Children's National Medical Centre ECMO Symposium, Keystone, CO, February 1993.
2. Beals DA, Schloo BL, Vacanti JP, Reid LM, Wilson JM. Pulmonary growth and remodelling in infants with high-risk congenital diaphragmatic hernia. J Pediatr Surg 1992;27:997.
3. Beardmore HE, Martini M. Omphalocele associated with diaphragmatic hernia. Z Kinderchir Suppl 1968; 5:39.
4. Bohn D, Tamura M, Perrin D, Barker G, Rabinovitch M. Ventilatory predictors of pulmonary hypoplasia in

congenital diaphragmatic hernia, confirmed by morphologic assessment. J Pediatr 1987;111:423.

5. Breaux CW, Rouse TM, Cain WS, Georgeson KE. Improvement in survival of patients with congenital diaphragmatic hernia utilizing a strategy of delayed repair after medical and/or extra corporeal membrane oxygenation stabilization. J Pediatr Surg 1991;26:333.

6. Crombleholme TM, Adzick NS, Hardy K, et al. Pulmonary lobar transplantation in neonatal swine; a model for treatment of congenital diaphragmatic hernia. J Pediatr Surg 1990;25:11.

7. de Lorimier AA. Diaphragmatic hernia In: Ashcraft KW, Holder TM, eds. Pediatric surgery, ed 2. Philadelphia, Saunders, 1993:204–215.

8. de Luca U, Cloutier R, Laberge J-M, et al. Pulmonary barotrauma in congenital diaphragmatic hernia; experimental study in lambs. J Pediatr Surg 1987;22:311.

9. Freyschuss U, Lannergan K, Freneker B. Lung function after repair of congenital diaphragmatic hernia. Acta Paediatr Scand 1984;73:589.

10. Geggel RL, Murphy JD, Langleben D, et al. Congenital diaphragmatic hernia: arterial structural changes and persistent pulmonary hypertension after surgical repair. J Pediatr 1985;107:457.

11. Gersony WM. Neonatal pulmonary hypertension: pathophysiology, classification and etiology. Clin Perinatol 1984;11:517.

12. Glick Pl, Stannard V, Leach EL, et al. Pathophysiology of congenital diaphragmatic hernia II. The fetal lamb CDH model is surfactant deficient. J Pediatr Surg 1992;27:382.

13. Harrison MR, Adzick NS. The fetus as a patient: surgical considerations. Ann Surg 1991;213:279.

14. Hitch DC, Carson JA, Smith EI, et al. Familial congenital diaphragmatic hernia is an autosomal recessive variant. J Pediatr Surg 1989;24:860.

15. Iritani I. Experimental study on embryogenesis of congenital diaphragmatic hernia. Anat Embryol (Berl) 1984;169:133.

16. Kimura K, Tsugawa C, Matsumoto Y, Soper R. Use of pledget in the repair of diaphragmatic anomalies. J Pediatr Surg 1991;26:84.

17. Kluth D, Peterson C, Zimmermann ZH. The developmental anatomy of congenital diaphragmatic hernia. Pediatr Surg Int 1987;2:322.

18. Ladd WE, Gross RE. Congenital diaphragmatic hernia. N Engl J Med 1940;223:917.

19. Lally KP, Paranka MS, Roden J, et al. Congenital diaphragmatic hernia: stabilization and repair on ECMO. Ann Surg 1992;216:569.

20. McQueston JA, Kinsella JP, McMurtry IF, Abman SH. Changes in endothelium-dependent and independent vasodilation during chronic intrauterine pulmonary hypertension in fetal lambs. Abstract 56, 9th Annual Children's National Medical Centre ECMO Symposium, Keystone, CO, February 1993.

21. Molenaar JC, Bos AP, Hazebroek FWJ, Tibboel D. Congenital diaphragmatic hernia, what defect? J Pediatr Surg 1991;26:248.

22. Nakayama DK, Motoyama EK, Tagge EM. Effect of preoperative stabilization on respiratory system compliance and outcome in newborn infants with congenital diaphragmatic hernia. J Pediatr 1991;118:793.

23. Nguyen L, Guttman FM, DeChadarevian JP, et al. The mortality of congenital diaphragmatic hernia: is total pulmonary mass inadequate, no matter what? Ann Surg 1983;198:766.

24. Pokorny WJ, McGill CW, Harberg FJ. Morgagni hernias during infancy: presentation and associated anomalies. J Pediatr Surg 1984;19:394.

25. Puri P, Gorman WA. Natural history of congenital diaphragmatic hernia: implications for management. Pediatr Surg Int 1987;2:327.

26. Sakai H, Tamara M, Hosokura Y, Bryan AC, Barker GA, Bohn DJ. Effect of surgical repair on respiratory mechanisms in congenital diaphragmatic hernia. J Pediatr 1987;111:432.

27. Shochat SJ. Pulmonary vascular pathology in congenital diaphragmatic hernia. Pediatr Surg Int 1987;2:331.

28. Truesdale PE. Diaphragmatic hernia in children with a report of thirteen operative cases. N Engl J Med 1935;213:1159.

29. West KWW, Bengston K, Rescorla FJ, Engle WA, Grosfeld JL. Delayed surgical repair and ECMO improves survival in congenital diaphragmatic hernia. Ann Surg 1992;216:454.

Hernia, Fourth Edition, edited
by Lloyd M. Nyhus and Robert E. Condon.
J.B. Lippincott Company, Philadelphia © 1995.

Chapter 44

Traumatic Diaphragmatic Hernia

John J. Fildes

Both blunt and penetrating injuries to the diaphragm produce a variety of hernias. The abdominal viscera usually herniates through the traumatic defect, but may enter the chest through a congenitally weak portion of the diaphragm. The clinical presentation can be immediate or delayed for several years. Because of the highly variable nature of traumatic diaphragmatic hernia, it is difficult to diagnose and treat. Ideally, all traumatic diaphragmatic hernias should be treated at the time of injury to avoid incarceration and strangulation. If this could be accomplished, the 20% to 60% mortality rate that is associated with obstruction and delayed repair would be reduced to that associated with exploratory laparotomy for trauma.[1]

Efforts have been made to diagnose and treat traumatic diaphragmatic hernias immediately. Liberal use of exploratory laparotomy has been effective, but the rate of unnecessary laparotomy is high.[10] Other diagnostic modalities, such as diagnostic peritoneal lavage, laparoscopy, and thoracoscopy, can reduce the rate of unnecessary laparotomy while providing acceptable accuracy and sensitivity.[9,11,13] As a result, the incidence of delayed traumatic diaphragmatic hernias is decreasing.

Early diagnosis and treatment are necessary to decrease the overall mortality and morbidity of this surgically correctable injury.

ANATOMY AND PHYSIOLOGY

The diaphragm is a large, sheet-like muscle attached to the lower ribs. It forms the boundary between the abdomen and thorax. Because it is not flat, the upper abdomen is inserted into the lower thorax. During exhalation, the diaphragm rises as high as the fourth intercostal space. Therefore, all injuries to the lower thorax carry the risk of injury to the diaphragm and the intraabdominal viscera. These are classified as thoracoabdominal injuries, and they are distributed in the area depicted in Figure 44-1. The upper border of this region is formed by the fourth intercostal space anteriorly and the scapular tips posteriorly. The lower border follows the insertion of the diaphragm along the costal margin anteriorly and the 12th rib posteriorly. Although it is possible for wounds outside this region to produce diaphragmatic injuries, it is much less common.

The diaphragm contains several foramina through which important gastrointestinal and vascular structures pass. These include the esophageal hiatus, the aortic hiatus, and the hiatus of the inferior vena cava. In addition, there are other areas that may be congenitally predisposed to the development of diaphragmatic hernias, such as the foramina of Bochdalek and Morgagni, as well as the pericardial base.

The neurovascular supply to the diaphragm arises primarily from the phrenic nerve and phrenic artery. The reasonably constant anatomic distribution of these structures protects them from injury. Care must be taken to identify these vessels, however, to avoid injuring them during the dissection and repair of diaphragmatic hernias.

The diaphragm is the major muscle of respiration. During contraction, it flattens out. This produces a net negative intrapleural pressure and initiates the inspiratory phase of the ventilatory cycle. During relaxation, the diaphragm rises into the thorax, assisted by the net positive pressure produced in the peritoneum. This produces positive intrapleural pressure and exhalation. Although the diaphragm is assisted by the ability of the intercostal muscles to produce the "bucket handle" movement of the ribs, it can perform 100% of the work required for effective ventilation.

Like cardiac muscle, the diaphragm is never at rest. It functions during both wakefulness and sleep. This property, combined with the presence of positive peritoneal pressure and negative intrathoracic pressure, creates a situation that makes spontaneous healing of diaphragmatic injuries improbable. These factors are most obvious with the development of left-sided traumatic diaphragmatic hernias. Injuries to the right diaphragm are buttressed by the liver. It is not known whether this relationship promotes healing or simply provides a mechanical barrier to enlargement and herniation. Both early and delayed traumatic dia-

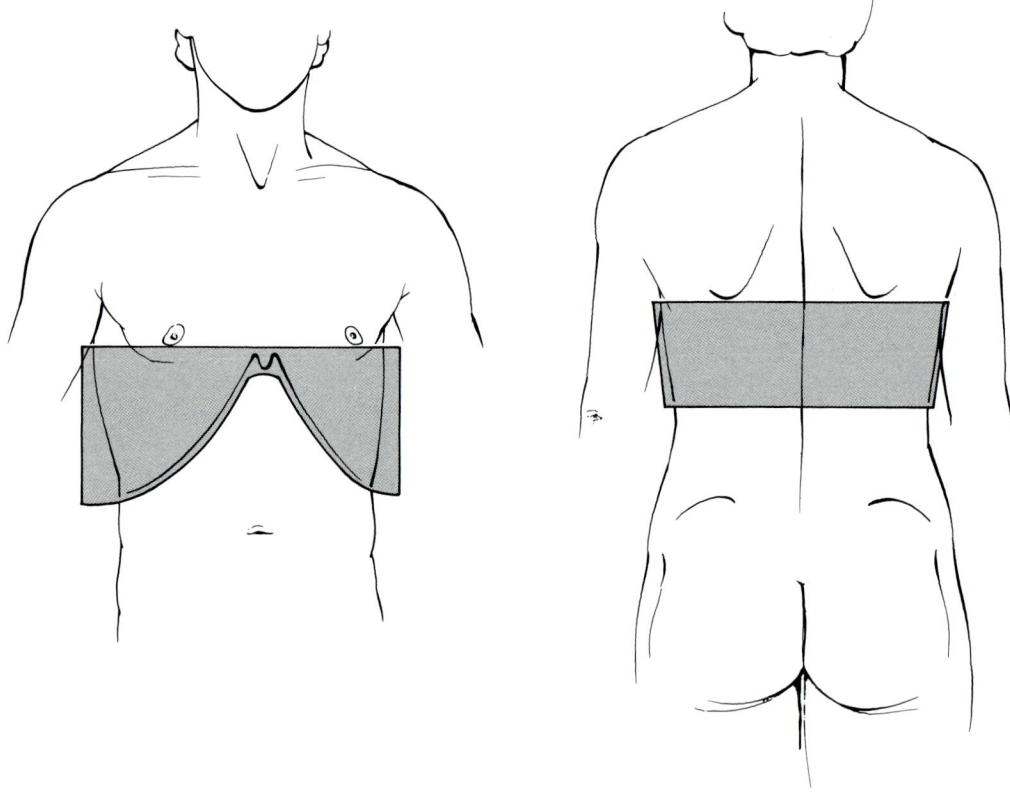

Figure 44-1. The thoracoabdominal region represents the circumferential surface anatomy of the diaphragm. Anteriorly, it extends from the fourth intercostal space to the inferior costal margin. Posteriorly, it extends from the tips of the scapulae to the level of the 12th thoracic vertebra.

phragmatic hernias are less common on the right than on the left, but they are not unusual[2] (Fig. 44-2).

CAUSE

Injuries to the diaphragm can be produced by blunt or penetrating trauma. Although the size and location of these injuries are different, they ultimately are subject to the same pathophysiologic factors.

Blunt injuries characteristically are caused by abdominal trauma that produces an abrupt increase in the intraperitoneal pressure. This causes the diaphragm to tear across the dome. Historically, these injuries were produced by such events as logs striking the abdomen, wagons or vehicles rolling across the abdomen, and horse kicks. More recently, decelerating injuries from motor vehicle crashes and falls are responsible for most diaphragmatic tears. The frequent association of this injury with pelvic fracture has made diaphragmatic evaluation a necessary component of the diagnostic work-up. These tears are more com-

mon on the left than on the right, presumably because the liver acts as a cushion.

Another form of blunt injury is diaphragmatic laceration by bone fragments from lower rib fractures. In patients with multiple rib fractures and flail chest, diaphragmatic lacerations should be suspected and an appropriate diagnostic evaluation conducted.

Still another form of blunt traumatic diaphragmatic hernia occurs when the abdominal viscera is forced through one of the natural foramina of the diaphragm. Patients with preexisting hiatal hernias are at risk when intraperitoneal pressures are elevated abruptly during trauma. Herniations through the aortic and caval hiatus are rare because of their retroperitoneal position and firm investment by the crural fibers.

An important subgroup of traumatic diaphragmatic hernias through preexisting foramina occurs in patients with congenital diaphragmatic abnormalities. Some of these may be hernias that have been present from birth, causing few symptoms and remaining clinically undetected. Others can be present from birth and cause absolutely no symptoms. Still others

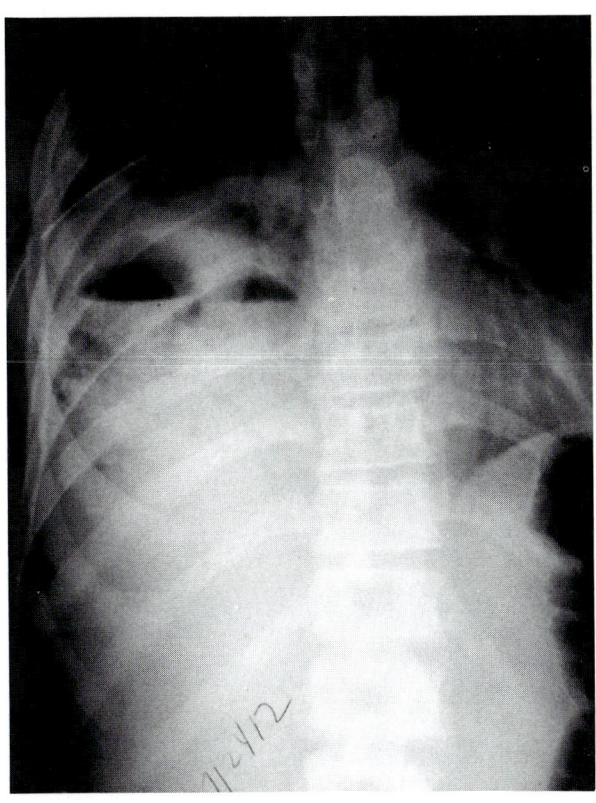

Figure 44-2. This thoracoabdominal roentgenogram demonstrates air–fluid levels above the right diaphragm 4 days after blunt abdominal trauma. Exploratory laparotomy revealed that the colon had herniated through a radial tear in the right diaphragm.

may occur in areas of diaphragmatic weakness that are unable to withstand the pressure produced by abdominal trauma. These include the foramen of Morgagni, the foramen of Bochdalek, and the pericardial base.

Penetrating trauma can produce defects in the left or right diaphragm that are single or multiple. Because most assailants are right-handed and confront their victims face to face, the left diaphragm is injured more commonly. The defects created by stab wounds and gunshot wounds usually are small and often are associated with injuries to the intraabdominal viscera.[5]

DIAGNOSIS

The accurate diagnosis of diaphragmatic injury is a difficult clinical challenge. Historically, most early reports identified traumatic diaphragmatic hernias at postmortem examination. Some described abdominal visceral herniating through lower chest wounds. Oth-

ers related a history of intermittent pain and obstruction combined with the presence of lower bowel sounds in the chest. The mortality of these patients exceeded 80%.[3] The widespread clinical use of chest roentgenography began with the introduction of the high-vacuum hot cathode tube in 1917. Images of traumatic diaphragmatic hernias were obtained and there was a proliferation of reports in the medical literature.[4] By 1924, 283 cases of traumatic diaphragmatic hernia had been reported in the world literature.[8] It was evident from these early reports that traumatic diaphragmatic hernias were diagnosed either at the time of injury or after an interval of days or years. A system of diagnostic classification based on the time of diagnosis (ie, early versus late) continues to be the most useful clinical approach. The major emphasis, however, has shifted away from the identification of late traumatic diaphragmatic hernias and focuses on the diagnosis and treatment of diaphragmatic defects at the time of injury. Table 44-1 lists the diagnostic tests that have been used to identify traumatic diaphragmatic hernias.

Penetrating Diaphragmatic Injury

The early diagnosis of diaphragmatic injuries depends on a high index of suspicion. Patients who sustain penetrating trauma in the thoracoabdominal region (Fig. 44-3) are at highest risk. The diaphragmatic defects usually are small and abdominal viscera seldom herniate through them. Intraabdominal injuries also can be present. Because of the vague clinical signs, ancillary diagnostic tests are required. Mandatory laparotomy has been advocated to prevent

Table 44-1. Diagnostic Methods Described for Traumatic Diaphragmatic Hernia

Most Common
History and physical examination
Chest roentgenogram
Diagnostic peritoneal lavage
Computed tomography
Contrast studies of the stomach and colon
Magnetic resonance imaging
Laparoscopy or thoracoscopy
Laparotomy

Others
Fluoroscopy
Pneumoperitoneum
Sonography
Liver-spleen radionuclide scans
Intraperitoneal contrast

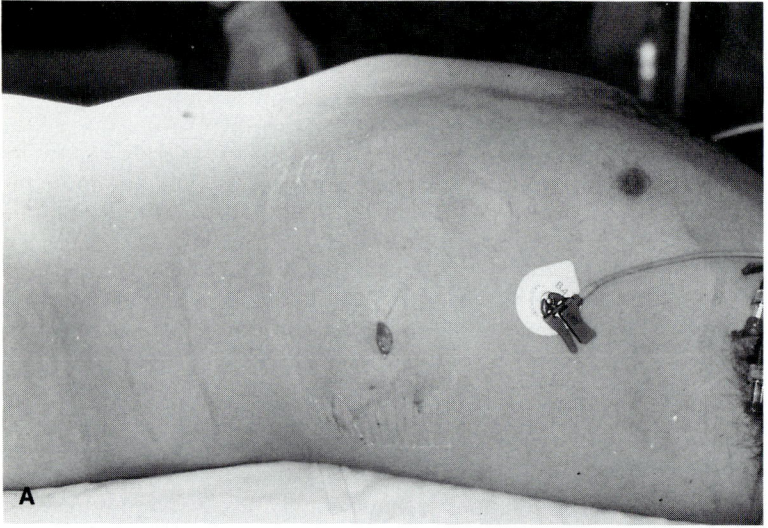

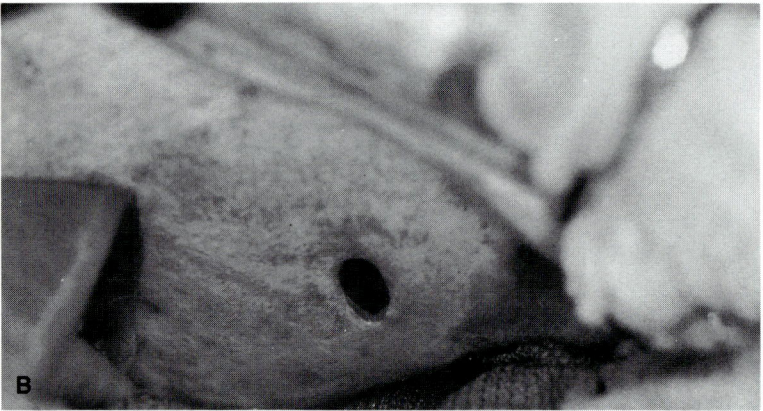

Figure 44-3. (*A*) Stab wound in the left thoracoabdominal area. (*B*) A 2.5-cm laceration of the left diaphragm was identified during laparotomy.

missed diaphragmatic injuries.[10] Although the sensitivity and specificity of this procedure approaches 100%, false-negative results can be obtained if the intraoperative examination of the diaphragm is not conducted carefully and systematically. This usually occurs when life-threatening intraabdominal injuries exist and the search for diaphragmatic defects is abbreviated or overlooked. Diagnostic peritoneal lavage is a useful test. A reduced cell count of 10,000 red blood cells per cubic millimeter has been shown to be 95% sensitive.[11] The overall morbidity and mortality associated with the 1% rate of false-negative results must be weighed against the test's ability to reduce the number of unnecessary laparotomies, with their attendant morbidity. Our experience with this test has been good. Traumatic diaphragmatic hernias rarely are discovered in patients who have undergone diagnostic peritoneal lavage with negative results (using 10,000 red blood cells per cubic millimeter as the positive margin). Laparoscopy is being evaluated for the diagnosis of diaphragmatic injuries after penetrating trauma[9] (Fig. 44-4). The use of 0- and 30-degree laparoscopes combined with the steep reverse Trendelenburg position allows the surgeon to see most of the diaphragm. A reported complication of this procedure is the development of tension pneumothorax during gas insufflation of the peritoneum. The use of lower insufflation pressures in awake patients does not allow complete evaluation of the diaphragm. Missed injuries have been reported with this technique.[14] Gasless laparoscopy using an abdominal lift device, angled laparoscopes, and aggressive gravity retraction of the upper abdominal viscera may avoid these problems (Fig. 44-5). This procedure requires general anesthesia, however, and has not been evaluated thoroughly.

In summary, the diagnosis of a penetrating diaphragmatic injury requires a high index of suspicion. The risk/benefit evaluation of each diagnostic study must weigh the risk of a late traumatic diaphragmatic hernia after a false-negative test result against the benefit of early diaphragmatic repair. The risk of gen-

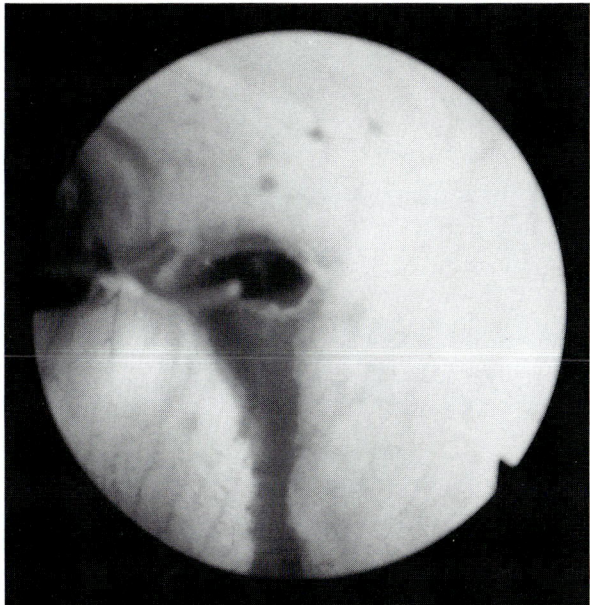

Figure 44-4. Appearance of a penetrating diaphragmatic injury produced in the laboratory. It is viewed through a 10-mm laparoscope 0-degree camera at an insufflation pressure of 12 to 15 mmHg. Note how the defect is maintained open. (Courtesy of Christopher Salvino, MD)

eral anesthesia, negative laparotomy, and procedural complications also must be considered. Our practice is to perform diagnostic peritoneal lavage on all patients with penetrating trauma in the thoracoabdominal region (see Fig. 44-1). A cell count of 10,000 red blood cells per cubic millimeter or the presence of lavage fluid in a chest tube are considered positive results and mandate exploratory laparotomy.

Blunt Diaphragmatic Injury

The early diagnosis of blunt diaphragmatic injuries traditionally has centered on the identification of abdominal viscera above the diaphragm using chest roentgenography (Fig. 44-6). Because blunt injuries produce large radial tears, it is common for herniation to occur at the time of injury. The stomach, colon, and small bowel are the most likely organs to herniate through the defect. On a chest roentgenogram, they are identified by characteristic gas shadows or the presence of a nasogastric tube above the diaphragm. About 20% of blunt diaphragmatic injuries cannot be diagnosed on initial chest roentgenography. If the injury has occurred on the right or left posterior portions of the diaphragm, herniation may be delayed. The most common finding on initial chest roentgenography is elevation and haziness of the diaphragm on the affected side. The costophrenic angle usually is blunted and patients experience respiratory distress. These findings, combined with a high index of suspicion, should prompt diagnostic evaluation. The simplest test is an upright and lateral chest roentgenogram. The lateral view sometimes reveals abdominal viscera above the diaphragm. Upper and lower gastrointestinal studies using contrast medium are performed to delineate the stomach, proximal small bowel, and colon. The use of contrast medium can be combined with computed tomography to identify herniated viscera.[6] Computed tomography, however, has not been uniformly successful in identifying discrete diaphragmatic tears without herniation. This has been most evident in the search for right-sided injuries. Magnetic resonance imaging has been advocated for such cases, because it produces good-quality im-

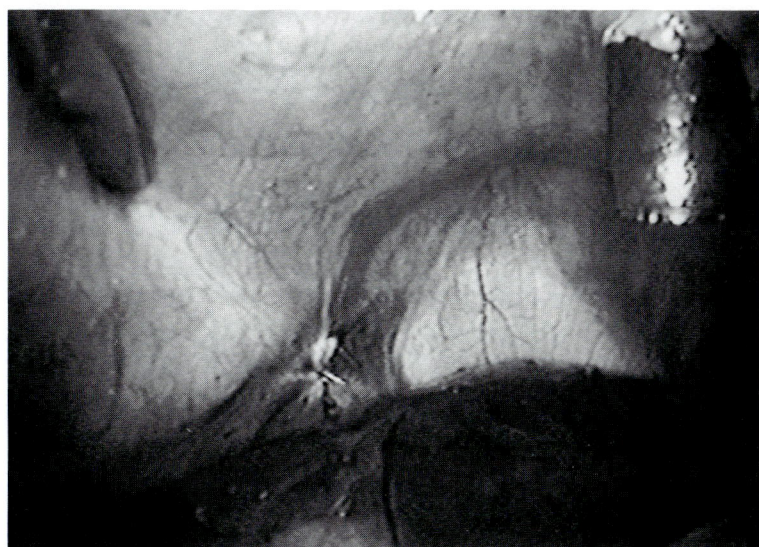

Figure 44-5. Appearance of a penetrating diaphragmatic injury produced in the laboratory. It is viewed through a 10-mm laparoscope 0-degree camera using an abdominal wall lift device to facilitate gasless laparoscopy. Note that the defect has been repaired.

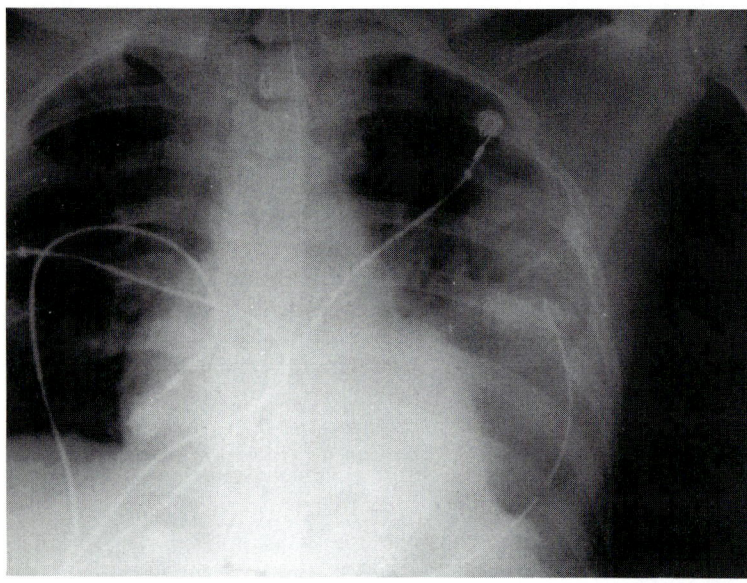

Figure 44-6. The initial chest roentgenogram of a patient who sustained blunt abdominal trauma reveals herniation of the stomach into the left hemithorax. Note the position of the nasogastric tube above the level of the diaphragm.

ages of the diaphragm itself.[12] Clinical experience with this modality is developing.

Late Diaphragmatic Hernia

The diagnosis of late traumatic diaphragmatic hernias requires the identification of abdominal viscera above the diaphragm and a history of penetrating or blunt abdominal trauma. The interval from injury to identification can vary from a few days to several years. Some patients have a history of intermittent gastrointestinal symptoms combined with chest pain. Others may have intestinal obstruction. In still others, strangulation, shock, and respiratory distress develop rapidly. The diagnosis requires awareness of the condition on the part of the surgeon. Initial chest roentgenography is diagnostic in many cases (Fig. 44-7). The presence of intraluminal gas shadows in the chest is pathognomonic. Upper and lower gastrointestinal studies with contrast medium, computed tomography, and magnetic resonance imaging are useful in difficult cases.

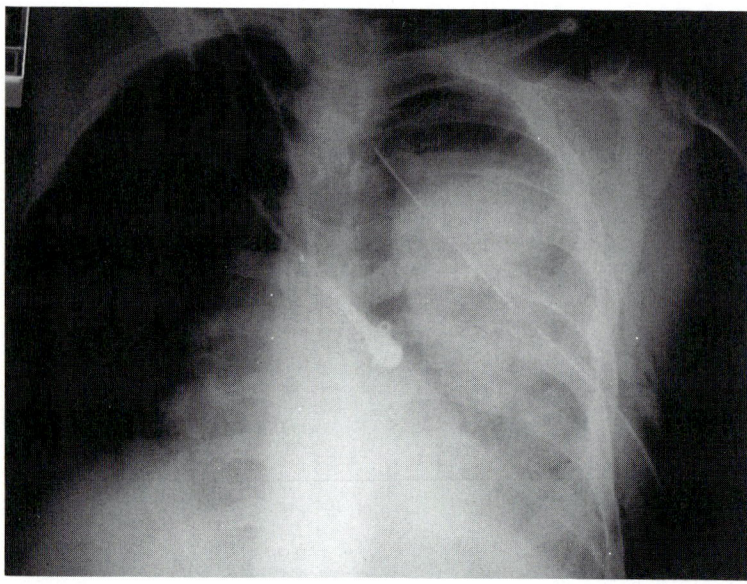

Figure 44-7. Chest roentgenogram showing small bowel herniated into the left hemithorax. The patient sustained a left thoracoabdominal stab wound 1 year before admission.

TREATMENT

Early Diaphragmatic Hernia

Wounds of the diaphragm require surgical repair as soon as they are detected. Operation must be undertaken urgently because herniation and strangulation dramatically increase mortality and morbidity.

For acute injuries, the best approach is through the abdomen. Both blunt and penetrating diaphragmatic trauma are associated with injuries to the intraabdominal viscera. Celiotomy allows the surgeon to assess the intraabdominal contents completely at the time of diaphragmatic repair. Control of gastrointestinal contamination is important to limit pleural contamination. A chest tube is required to reexpand the lung, drain the pleura, and monitor bleeding in the case of concomitant thoracic injury. Repair of the diaphragm is straightforward. Penetrating wounds produce small, well-defined defects, whereas blunt trauma causes large, radial tears. Both injuries can be closed in two layers using nonabsorbable sutures. The interrupted suture technique is preferred, but the use of interlocked running sutures and running horizontal sutures has been described. Because these techniques carry the risk of recurrent hernia formation if the suture breaks or tears through the diaphragm, however, continuous sutures are not recommended.

The stellate diaphragmatic laceration is more difficult to treat. This wound should be closed with interrupted nonabsorbable sutures whenever possible. It sometimes is necessary to use a single-layer technique because of the limited amount of usable tissue. Permanent prosthetic material occasionally is required. If contamination is present, the use of prosthetic material should be delayed. In this case, the abdominal injuries are repaired, the diaphragm is repaired, and prosthetic reconstruction is delayed until the risk of intraabdominal sepsis has passed.

Another type of acute injury occurs when the diaphragm detaches from the posterolateral thoracic wall. If the diaphragm cannot be sutured at its original insertion site, it can be reattached to the intercostal muscles one level above.

Late Diaphragmatic Hernia

The late repair of a traumatic diaphragmatic hernia is approached best through the chest. Because these hernias do not have a true peritoneal sac, adhesions form rapidly between the abdominal viscera and the lung. As a result, hernias diagnosed a few weeks after injury should be repaired using a thoracotomy. All patients should be prepared with gastric and colonic decompression. Gavage is used in unobstructed patients. Perioperative antibiotics must be effective against enteric pathogens and include coverage for empyema or pulmonary infection when present. The first step is to establish adequate exposure. Next, all adhesions must be divided. The diaphragmatic defect may not be identified until this is complete. When the thickened fibrotic ring is found, it may need to be divided in the direction of the muscle fibers to reduce the abdominal viscera. Careful dissection of the defect usually can mobilize enough chronically retracted diaphragm to facilitate primary closure. Prosthetic materials such as Marlex, Prolene, or Gore-Tex can be used to reinforce or bridge defects.

The results of surgical repair of traumatic diaphragmatic hernias are good. Recurrence usually is the result of injuries overlooked during the treatment of acute wounds or of technical problems in the repair of late hernias. The mortality associated with incarceration and strangulation remains high, emphasizing the need for aggressive measures directed toward immediate repair.

REFERENCES

1. Arendrup HC, Arendrup KD. Traumatic diaphragmatic hernia. In: Nyhus LM, Condon RE, eds. Hernia, ed 3. Philadelphia, JB Lippincott, 1989:708.
2. Boulanger BR, Milzman DP, Rosati C, Rodriguez A. A comparison of right and left blunt traumatic diaphragmatic rupture. J Trauma 1993;35:255.
3. Bowditch HI. Diaphragmatic hernia. Buffalo Med J 1883;9:65.
4. Carman RD, Fineman S. Roentgenologic diagnosis of diaphragmatic hernia, with report of seventeen cases. Radiology 1924;3:26.
5. Demetriades D, Kakoyiannis S, Parekh D, Hatzitheofilou C. Penetrating injuries of the diaphragm. Br J Surg 1988;75:824.
6. Demos TC, Solomon C, Posniak HV, Flissak MJ. Computed tomography in traumatic defects of the diaphragm. Clin Imaging 1989;13:62.
7. Girzadas DV, Fligner DJ. Delayed traumatic intrapericardial diaphragmatic hernia associated with cardiac tamponade. Ann Emerg Med 1991;20:1246.
8. Hedblom CA. Diaphragmatic hernia: a study of three hundred and seventy-eight cases in which operation was performed. JAMA 1925;85:947.
9. Invatury RR, Simon RJ, Weksler B, Bayard V, Stahl WM. Laparoscopy in the evaluation of the intrathoracic abdomen after penetrating injury. J Trauma 1992;33:101.

10. Madden MR, Paull DE, Finkelstein JF, et al. Occult diaphragmatic injury from stab wounds to the lower chest and abdomen. J Trauma 1989;29:292.
11. Merlotti GJ, Dillon BC, Lange DA, Robin AP, Barrett JB. Peritoneal lavage in penetrating thoraco-abdominal trauma. J Trauma 1988;28:17.
12. Mirvis SE, Keramati B, Buckman R, Rodriguez A. MR imaging of traumatic diaphragmatic rupture. J Comput Assist Tomogr 1988;12:147.
13. Ochsner MG, Rozycki GS, Lucente F, Wherry DC, Champion HR. Prospective evaluation of thoracoscopy for diagnosing diaphragmatic injury in thoracoabdominal trauma: a preliminary report. J Trauma 1993;34:704.
14. Salvino CK, Esposito TJ, Marshall WJ, Dries DJ, Morris RC, Gamelli RL. The role of diagnostic laparoscopy in the management of trauma patients: a preliminary assessment. J Trauma 1993;34:506.

Medicolegal Aspects of Hernia

Part Nine

Hernia, Fourth Edition, edited
by Lloyd M. Nyhus and Robert E. Condon.
J.B. Lippincott Company, Philadelphia © 1995.

Chapter 45

Medicolegal Aspects of Hernia

Melvin E. Ehrhardt and Raymond Fish

A chapter on the medicolegal problems of herniorrhaphy is useful only if it is of practical value to surgeons and is written in language they understand. For that reason, historical development has been left for others, and there is some concentration on workers' compensation as a clear-cut example of statutory treatment of the subject. The issue of informed consent is important for any surgical procedure, and the topics of personnel relations and responsibilities can be discussed with reference to herniorrhaphy.

This chapter is important because it provides surgeons with tools to practice defensive medicine and, it is hoped, to prevent a medicolegal courtroom encounter. Each day surgeons must make momentous decisions: who should undergo surgical treatment, when should the operation be done, what procedures should be used, and how should the conditions and decisions be explained to a patient and sometimes to parents. Seldom do these decisions require explanation to anyone, much less a lawyer. But when they do have to be explained to a lawyer it is often in the context of justification. A lack of information or misinformation on the part of the surgeon leaves him or her open to attack. An ounce of prevention *is* worth a pound of cure.

The area of medicolegal problems is changing so quickly that the alert practitioner should be reading special publications such as the *Citation* and the *Journal of Legal Medicine* along with other, more familiar medical journals. Basic changes, such as in the legal definition of death and the law's approach to abortion, occur literally overnight, so newspapers and magazines also become vital resource materials. The material presented here includes background information and vocabulary suitable for use in further independent pursuit. Specifically, principles and concepts are discussed with the intent to clarify an often confusing area. Thus, clearly defined legal issues are dealt with only briefly, whereas the broad, gray areas are discussed in some detail.

The overview of principles and concepts of the medicolegal aspects of herniorrhaphy as discussed here is *not* legal advice. That advice comes only from the physician's own attorney, who must be familiar with facts, situations, and individuals. The information in this chapter is designed to alert the reader to problem areas; and even if facts utilized seem similar, nothing here is intended to solve legal questions. State laws vary, and here the laws of Illinois are used as examples.

One of the cardinal principles of the law in all of its manifestations is that legal rights carry corresponding legal duties. The right to earn one's livelihood, in this situation as a surgeon, carries with it the duty to follow the rules that govern the practices of the profession. The chapter is organized in the chronology of the physician–patient relationship, from the time the patient gives consent through the time the physician finds himself or herself in the courtroom. Within that chronology is embedded the rights–duties structure familiar to attorneys and often painfully foreign to physicians.

SURGICAL CONSENT

One of the cardinal rights in the Anglo-American system of law is the right to privacy, a right that courts have interpreted to include a right to care for one's body as one sees fit. It is the right to choose between herbal tea and chemotherapy or to make no choice. The law as it has evolved requires as a general rule that a person demonstrate that he or she has freely exercised this right, as evidenced by a written consent form signed by the patient before a surgical procedure is performed. The essential elements of the form are a specific dated authorization that includes the names of the surgeon and the hospital. Although most state laws do not require the written form on the chart (most hospitals do), the state laws are usually quite specific about what qualifies a person to consent to a surgical procedure. Because these qualifications are the law, the surgeon must know them so that the correct party ultimately signs the form. Illinois statutes, as a typical example, require that a person be 18 years of age to sign his or her own consent form. That general rule is simple enough, but the gray areas, the exceptions, can prove to be quicksand. For example, most state statutes create an exception for life-threatening situations. If a minor is admitted with a strangulated hernia or a traumatic laceration and the parents or legal guardian cannot be contacted, the surgical procedure may be undertaken to correct the life-threatening situation without the required parent–guardian consent. If the situation is not life threatening but the patient cannot sign the consent form and the legal guardian cannot be reached, then next of kin or a spouse can be asked to sign. It is important to point out that each state may have different ages of consent, may have actually defined "life threatening" in specific terms, and may have even defined "next of kin" and "spouse" for consent purposes.

Emancipation by marriage or pregnancy constitutes another exception to the age-of-consent statute. If a person is younger than the defined age designation but married or pregnant, the form may be signed by that person. Despite the exception it is still advisable to have both the parent and the emancipated minor sign. Illinois has additional exceptions to the general rule, but they apply to situations involving birth control, venereal disease treatment, and drug abuse. The obvious social policy values shaping those exceptions are not present in hernia care but are mentioned because exceptions can appear both in logical and illogical places.

Some people, including physicians, often consider the age at which liquor can be legally consumed to be the magic number that fits every situation, including giving medical consent. This rationale is commonly used and commonly wrong, and it can also not be assumed that the person who appears in the office with the minor is the legal guardian for purposes of signing the surgical consent form. Legal custody, usually decided by a court, could, for example, be in an aunt or in a state children's division. Legal custody is the critical factor contained in the authority to sign a consent form, and it must be determined authoritatively.

INFORMED CONSENT

Life would be simple if the surgeon could only slide a sheet of paper across the desk, direct a signature, and whisk the document away or, better yet, send someone else to take care of it. But because a vital right is involved, here as in all other areas of the law the consent must be *informed*. It is an active area of litigation, and the surgeon may safely assume that lawyers will quiz their clients closely on the events surrounding the signing of the form. The courts generally hold the

surgeon responsible for informing the patient of the following:[1]

1. The diagnosis
2. The general nature of the contemplated procedure
3. The risks involved with that procedure
4. The prospects for success
5. The prognosis if the procedure is not performed
6. The alternative methods of treatment, if any

Full disclosure is required so that the patient knows exactly what his or her decision involves. And the decision is the patient's, not the physician's; the patient can disregard all advice and order herbal tea. Dispensing the information is the physician's duty, and for all practical purposes it is not delegable. The courts do not hold nurses liable for explaining the surgical procedure and possible complications but do clearly expect the surgeon to take the time to discuss the operation with the patient. The language used must be understandable by a layperson (*Corn v French*, 289 P2d, 1973 [1955]).

It is suggested that the surgeon who repeatedly performs similar procedures develop a fact sheet containing all the general information that the courts of the jurisdiction expect him or her to have discussed with the patient. The fact sheet can be a general outline in plain English to aid the surgeon in remembering to cover all points. The surgeon can then leave the fact sheet with the patient, dictating for the chart that the operation was discussed with the patient and the fact sheet given to the patient. In attorneys' terms the surgeon has begun to build a record, since documentation is much more readily believed than remembered testimony. The fact sheet with the chart is a convincing indication that the surgeon made an honest effort to see that the patient's consent was informed.

A 1972 decision is an excellent example of the pitfalls of informed consent (*Canterbury v Spence*, 464 F2d 772 [DC Cir 1972]). The patient suffered paralysis after a laminectomy. The surgeon claimed the incidence of postoperative paralysis was 1%. The court of appeals said that full disclosure includes informing the patient of a 1% complication.

Thus, the test for determining whether a particular peril must be divulged is its materiality to the patient's decision: all risks potentially affecting the decision must be unmasked. *And to safeguard the patient's interest in achieving his own determination on treatment, the law must itself set the standard for adequate disclosure. (Canterbury v Spence, p 787) (Emphasis supplied.)*

In a 1981 case a bilateral inguinal hernial repair was followed by permanent bilateral testicular atrophy and total sexual impotence. A jury found that a surgeon had failed to obtain informed consent because the possibility of testicular atrophy had not been explained. The appellate court upheld the decision. In this case (*McKinney v Nash* App 174 Cal Rptr 642), the surgeon testified that, after a bilateral inguinal hernial repair, swelling caused by bleeding occurs in about 4% to 5% of patients. Also, bilateral testicular atrophy can be expected in one tenth of 1% of patients. The surgeon did not inform the patient of any of these risks. The patient testified that he would have declined the operation if he had been informed of such risks.

In the same case the surgeon commented to the patient that the hernial repair would be simple and without problems. It was found that this statement did not satisfy the requirements of an express contract for which the patient could recover for breach of contract. Some courts might consider such a statement a "guarantee," and it is best to be open with patients about risks. If a mentally competent patient refuses an elective operation because of an open discussion of unavoidable risks, it is best not to perform the operation.

In the same case (*McKinney v Nash*) there was some evidence that the patient's general practitioner had administered testosterone and similar hormone injections for weakness and "hot flashes" for a period before the operation. The relevance of these facts to this case is unclear, but the importance of a full medical history before surgical treatment is brought to mind.

A 1972 California Supreme Court case also treats informed consent. Again the controversy arose as a result of a complication of the operation, a ruptured spleen (*Cobbs v Grant*, 103 Cal Rptr 505,502 P2dl). The operation involved was a subtotal gastrectomy, but a ruptured spleen is certainly a possible complication of a diaphragmatic hernial repair. The surgeon in the litigated case had not discussed the possibility that rupture of the spleen could occur during the course of the operation. The plaintiff claimed that either the operation was performed negligently or else a battery had been committed on the patient, since no consent had been given for a splenectomy. The litigation could probably have been avoided by the surgeon if he had obtained a surgical consent that included information about possible complications. It is because the question of informed consent (as opposed to age of consent or capacity to consent) is such an area of active litigation that the surgeon performing herniorrhaphy is well advised to document carefully and completely, on the patient's chart, that the physician has discussed all of the points mentioned previously.

PARTIAL CONSENT

Partial consent refers to the situation in which a patient accepts part of the services offered by the physician but refuses others. The most common situation tested in courts involves the patient's consenting to an operation such as herniorrhaphy but refusing a blood transfusion deemed necessary by the physician (*People v Labrenz*, 41 Ill 618, 104 NE 2d 769 [1952]). Because partial consent is bound up with the right of the patient to refuse cancer treatment and expensive life-sustaining measures, it is a topic alive with practical legal issues and moral implications. It has long been accepted by the American Medical Association that patients have the right to refuse treatment against medical advice, but that position represents complete lack of consent, a step beyond the present, more difficult problem. The greater difficulty involved in partial consent has to do with the legal nature of the physician–patient relationship.

When the relationship is initiated the physician and patient can agree to relate to each other in a certain manner. The physician and the patient essentially form a contract; by virtue of that mutual agreement, each accepts certain responsibilities and obligations with the anticipation that each will perform certain duties.

If a physician and patient can agree to surgical care with restrictions such as no blood transfusions, it is best to put that agreement in writing. There are good reasons for this: the law requires that agreements of more than 1 year be reduced to writing (consider the possible long-term nature of an agreement to perform an operation), and agreements in writing are the best kind of proof in a courtroom. Even a letter from the patient can be sufficient proof of consent to surgical treatment with reservations. One must also document the explanation of the possible consequences of the patient's limited consent. A partial consent relationship is not inadvisable as long as it is documented.

OTHER TYPES OF CONSENT

To round out the issue of consent, two additional situations should be considered: emergency consent and court-ordered consent. The concept of emergency consent arises from the law's presumption that a patient wishes to be given the usual medical treatment even though the patient is unable to communicate that wish. Because the law presumes that a patient would agree that life should continue, the physician, when faced with an unconscious patient or one in a situation so acute that time is the critical factor, should treat and ask questions about consent later (*Cotnam v Wisdon*, 83 Ark 601, 104 SW 164 [1907]).

Court-ordered consent flows from two sources. The ancient doctrine of *parens patriae* delimits the concept that the state has the power to assume legal custody of a minor when the best interests of the minor are involved. A 1972 case in which a court ordered a cleft lip repair after the parents refused the operation is an example (*In re Karvach*, 199 NW2d, 147). The second thrust involves the situation in which the minor requires a surgical procedure or medical care and the legal guardian, for purposes of consent, refuses. The legal structures of many states are organized so that a juvenile court can declare the minor neglected for medical purposes and the care proceeds (Ill Rev Stat ch 37, §701). Specific statutes, rather than a broad legal concept, are typically involved.

Another kind of court-ordered consent usually is of a statutory nature and involves involuntary psychiatric commitment procedures. Because these procedures vary greatly from state to state, the physician who is presented with the involuntarily committed person for herniorrhaphy should determine the legal status in the jurisdiction.

An unusual consent conflict arose in connection with the hernia of an incarcerated patient (*Bowers v County of Essex*, 641 NY S2d 959, Supp [1983]). In this case the patient was advised by his physician that he needed a hernial repair. The patient listed the condition on a medical report form that was filled out when he was admitted to the Essex County Jail. Six months later the patient was taken by the sheriff to another physician who noted the hernia. The physician allegedly stated that such a hernia would usually be operated on, but he refused to operate unless the sheriff authorized the operation. The sheriff did not authorize the operation, and the patient later sued.

In an appellate court decision the Court of Essex County ruled that some operations, such as a bunionectomy, can be delayed but the hernia should have been repaired. The court held that the physician had the responsibility to prescribe and order the required treatment. If the sheriff then refused to produce the patient for the operation, the doctor would have been relieved of further responsibility. In making its decision, the court quoted the landmark case of *Pike v Honsinger* (155 NY 201, 49 NE 760):

> When a physician agrees to treat a patient, he obligates himself to use his best judgment and to use reasonable care in the exercise of his skill and the application of his learning to accomplish the treatment for which he is employed. That his services are rendered gratuitously or at the request of someone other than the patient does not affect the physician's liability.

Another case of a prisoner with a hernia involved a patient whose hernia was diagnosed by the prison physician. The physician recommended surgery within several days and said the patient's condition was serious, even life threatening. The health management organization providing medical services to the prison delayed the surgery for 10 months. During this time the hernia grew larger. Testimony later presented showed that delays in hernia surgery were common in the prison, often lasting more than a year. The prisoner claimed that the delay in surgery constituted cruel and unusual punishment (*Johnson*, 941 F2d 705).

MALPRACTICE

Perhaps the most difficult term to define is the one that physicians hear daily—*malpractice*. Generally, malpractice is a breech of professional duty. The courts have defined that duty in terms of "due care" or "standard of care." The standard-of-care concept simply means that a physician is expected to display that degree of care and skill that other prudent physicians of similar background and training would have displayed in the same situation. Typically, when a malpractice case is tried, other physicians (expert witnesses) with equal training are called to testify concerning the correct treatment under circumstances identical to those involved in the litigation. The standard of care used by the defendant is then at issue.

The patient has a right to expect to receive routine, standard, acknowledged medical care when the patient obtains the services of a physician. He or she has no right to expect miracles. (One way to attempt to avoid some malpractice problems is simply to avoid guaranteeing results.) It is unwise for a surgeon to use the following language: "I will fix your hernia and you will never have any trouble with it again." There is considerable difference between that statement and this: "With your consent, I will repair your hernia; most patients who have a hernia don't have trouble with their hernia again." The differences between these two statements are not too subtle for most patients. A helpful habit surgeons might develop is to use such words as "most patients" and "usually" when talking with patients. The courts have specifically said that promising a patient particular results, or indicating that a particular complication will not occur, operates as a guarantee. In a 1923 California case (*Crawford v Duncan*, 61 Cal App 647, 215, p 753) the radiologist assured the patient that her neck would return to normal color and texture after radiation therapy and that there would be no scar. The patient sued successfully on what the court found to be a cosmetic guarantee. The case is old, but the precedent remains.

Except for the contract situation of guarantee, the plaintiff-patient must prove that the defendant-physician's lack of care caused the patient some harm. If the surgeon performs a hernia operation in a way that deviates from the way that is usual and recommended, the patient must prove that the unusual surgical procedure was the cause of the subsequent injury. If something else caused the injury, or if there were no injury but a good result, the patient would not be compensated by the court. The burden of proving both the injury and the cause rests with the plaintiff-patient. The plaintiff's lawyer must prove with evidence admissible at trial that the proper standard of care was not used by the physician and that the failure caused the plaintiff's injuries. The jury may compensate the plaintiff-patient for all of the medical expenses, for lost time, for pain and suffering incurred, and for future pain and suffering. Malpractice awards have mushroomed, and suits have proliferated to the point that insurers have hiked premium levels to stratospheric heights. Perhaps the most unpredicted medical revolution of the past 15 years was the profession's response to the rates charged for malpractice insurance. In state after state, legislatures have waded into the controversy. None of the solutions has eliminated the whole concept of malpractice, so standards of care are still the rule. The cases, however, have put some limits around actionable conduct.

A physician is also not liable for an honest error of judgment. The law does not demand infallibility of any physician. If he complies with recognized standards a single error will not subject him to liability. In retrospect he may realize that his judgment was wrong, but as long as it was reasonable he is not liable.[2]

Two judicial treatments nicely illustrate the interaction of the concepts of due care and error in judgment.

In a case heard on appeal and decided by the Supreme Court of Montana in 1970 these facts were involved: The surgeon palpated a mass in the inguinal area of an 8-year-old girl. The mother of the child thought that the lump developed after a fall from a bicycle. The general surgeon diagnosed a hernia and recommended surgical treatment, which was performed and which revealed that the lump was a fat pad. The surgeon then obtained a second consent (obtained properly in both instances) and explored the opposite inguinal region, and no hernia was found on the other side. The plaintiff sued for misdiagnosis and unnecessary surgery. In part, the court said:

Testimony at the trial indicated what procedure is followed and what tests are used to diagnose a hernia; that bilateral hernias are common in children; and, that difficulties inherent in examining children will occasionally result in an operation on the wrong side of the child. Two doctors examined the child and both diagnosed the probable existence of a hernia. The only test to determine if the lump was a fat pad or a hernia was to explore it surgically. The fat pad was discovered and Dr. Movius testified that it was unique in his experience of 33 years of practice as a general surgeon.... In the absence of a showing that the defendant acted without ordinary care, diligence or skill, or that he did not make a proper and skillful diagnosis, or that he deviated from established proper medical procedure as practiced in his neighborhood, we must uphold the trial court's directed verdict. (Doerr v Movius, 463 P2d 477, Mont [1970])

The court found for the doctor because the allegations of unnecessary surgery and misdiagnosis could not be proved. The surgeon, the court found, had used due care and had not deviated from standard medical practice, so the surgeon could not be held liable (*Doerr v Movius*, p 479).

The second case (*Engle v Clark*, 346 SW2d 13 Ky [1961]) involved a patient who died of peritoneal hemorrhage 14 hours after repair of an epigastric hernia. The surgeon misdiagnosed the postoperative condition as pulmonary embolus rather than hemorrhage, a misdiagnosis the court found to be well within a reasonable standard of care. The hemorrhage resulted from the slippage of the ligature from the umbilical vein. The plaintiff's contention was that two ligatures should have been used in tying off the vein. The defendant-physician proved the standard of care to be tying off the vein with one ligature. The Kentucky appellate court denied a motion for a new trial, accepting the misdiagnosis and use of one ligature within the ambit of due care for the hernia operation.

Alternative surgical techniques were discussed by the Supreme Court of Delaware in 1961 (*Di Fillipo v Preston*, 173 A 2d 333). The patient lost her voice after a thyroidectomy damaged the recurrent laryngeal nerve. The defendant-surgeon had used the standard surgical procedure, but the plaintiff contended that the Lahey procedure (involving dissection and exposure of the laryngeal nerve) should have been used. The court said:

While Dr. Graubard might well prefer the Lahey technique, at least an equal number of his fellow surgeons throughout the country apparently prefer the so-called standard technique. Since both are recognized as acceptable, it follows that the choice by Dr. Preston of one of two acceptable techniques was not a negligent act on his part. (Di Fillipo v Preston, p 337)

Not all surgeons win lawsuits and appeals, but perhaps no one is more aware of that than today's surgeon.

A bad result, in itself, is not evidence of negligence or malpractice. A lower court dismissed a malpractice case against a surgeon who unintentionally punctured the bladder of a 3-year-old child while repairing a right inguinal hernia and removing a hydrocele. The court of appeal upheld the decision (*Detillier v Groome*, La App 296 So2d 875). It was held that puncture of the bladder was not the result of negligence or improper procedure but rather a complication that is always a threat in a hernioplasty. One judge was uneasy with the decision.

> *I find it difficult to find logic in the explanation of Dr. ——— that it is difficult to distinguish between the bladder and the hydrocele and yet state that the puncture of the bladder occurred in only 2 out of 100 operations. It seems more reasonable that the infrequency of the occurrence suggests a conclusion of negligence when the puncture does occur. However, we cannot substitute our untrained medical evaluation (although it seems reasonable) for the cumulated corroborative opinions of the members of the medical profession. Accordingly, I am compelled to concur (with the opinion that the physician was not negligent). [Parenthetical statements added.]*

In another case a patient's testis atrophied after an operation. The physician had noted swelling of tissues at the time of and after the operation and had made a sufficient opening through the inguinal ring. Still, probably because of postoperative swelling, the testis atrophied. Before trial, the patient died of unrelated causes. The jury found that the physician had provided an opening through the inguinal ring that would be sufficient for normal circulation. The appellate court upheld the decision (*Goodnight v Phillips*, 458 SW2d 196).

Statute of Limitations

There is a technical legal definition of the statute of limitations, but for our purposes it can best be defined as the time during which legal action must be brought on the allegation of a specific act of wrongdoing. It is generally the function of the state legislature to set the statutory period of years for each actionable wrong (civil or criminal act). Typically the figure for malpractice is from 2 to 5 years; however, it is not only the time that is important but also when the court will consider that the statute begins to "run" or "toll."

In some states the statute may not start running in malpractice actions until the damage is discovered or should have been discovered by the patient. In these states, if a hemostat is left in the abdomen during hernial repair, the statute will not begin running on the date of the procedure but on the date it was or should have been discovered.

In one case it was thought that a portion of a patient's vas had been severed during a hernia operation when the patient was 4 months old. This apparently led to sterility, which was discovered after the patient was married. Malpractice action was brought 21 years after the alleged act of negligence. The case was heard in Wisconsin, which at that time had a 3-year statute of limitations applicable to medical malpractice. The discovery rule was not recognized in that state. The Supreme Court of Wisconsin held that

> *This court has recognized that many states have adopted by court decision the "discovery rule," i.e., that the cause of action accrues when the alleged injury is discovered or should have been discovered. We have repeatedly stated that if a change in the statute of limitations was in order, the legislature was the proper body to make that change. (Rod v Farrell, Wis 291 NW2d 568)*

Some courts have interpreted the statutory period as not beginning to run until the patient ends the physician–patient relationship with the defendant-physician. A third formula involves the age of emancipation. In some states if a physician treats a minor the statute does not begin to run until the patient is emancipated or reaches the age of majority. The pediatric surgeon who repairs a hernia in a newborn may be subject to suit 18 or 20 years later, no matter what the formula for adults is for the statutory period.

These relatively long spans of time during which the physician-surgeon is subject to suit have contributed to the malpractice insurance crisis. But sound policy reasons created the statute in the first place. It seems patently unfair that the person who had been carrying around a hemostat should be denied relief because under normal circumstances its presence would not be discovered until long after the operation. It is also not fair that a surgeon face the prospect of suit on the first operation he or she performs until the day he or she dies—hence the limitation.

Contributory Negligence

Malpractice actions are often defended by one of the few legal theories that is almost self-explanatory: *contributory negligence*. The law has long recognized the situation in which the wrongdoing of the plaintiff contributed to the injury. Its application in malpractice results in the defendant's arguing that the plaintiff was at least as negligent as the defendant. The theory of comparative negligence assigns percentages of negligence to patient and physician. Under contributory or comparative negligence the plaintiff-patient will attempt to prove not only the causal relation between the defendant and the injury but also that the plaintiff did not, for example, mislead the physician and did not add to the injuries as a result of his or her own negligence.

ALTERNATIVES TO MALPRACTICE ACTIONS

We have already mentioned legislative involvement in the malpractice field, and some of that involvement now includes examination of new methods of compensating for injuries resulting from medical negligence. The methods are outlined briefly because they may be the law of malpractice in the next few years.

Arbitration Clauses and Panels

Either by legislation or agreement by the parties the dispute between physician and patient would be brought before an arbitrator or a panel. The record would be examined, and both the physician and the patient would be heard. The panel might be empowered to call other witnesses, including experts, before rendering a decision and settlement. The decision might or might not be binding, depending on the legal framework under which arbitration is designed. This solution is essentially an out-of-court settlement made after a courtroom-like investigation.

No-Fault Payment

A new idea in compensating injured parties has come out of the law of automobile accidents. The no-fault insurance concept is premised in the notion that time and money are spent in the almost fruitless search for a wrongdoer. The Anglo-American system is geared to the rather puritanical approach that if there is injury, there is fault, and when there is fault someone must pay. No-fault simply means that everyone insures himself or herself against injuries without regard to who did what bad thing. It is especially appealing in the medical field, since even defending a malpractice action can leave overtones of guilt in the community. There are many permutations of no-fault, including combinations with arbitration.

Limits of Liability

Because some malpractice awards have been astronomical, legislatures have been asked to limit the amount recoverable from a physician. The suggestion is based on the observation that a small error can lead to a huge recovery when future earnings are compensated. It has also been proposed that compensation be based on the amount of negligence proved, not on the amount of damage suffered by the plaintiff. It is equally possible to limit liability by constructing standard tables of recovery so that juries do not award different amounts for identical injuries. (While all of these alternatives are being considered, and perhaps afterward, the physician is bound by the standard of due care, examined by peers and by patients.)

PATIENT ABANDONMENT

As has already been established, the physician–patient relationship is based on a contract, a legal entity that results in rights and duties flowing to both parties. Once the physician undertakes the care of a patient, he or she is bound by a contractual, legally enforceable duty to continue the care of the patient or be chargeable with patient abandonment. Actually the duty continues until the patient receives notice, preferably by registered letter, that the physician is discharging the patient with reasonable time to obtain the services of another physician.[2] Unavailability does not discharge the duty; the physician must provide a substitute who will take calls.

Several cases have delimited the boundaries of patient abandonment. They should be looked at carefully because this issue has clearly become a litigation target.

A 1969 Texas court of appeals case (*Childs v Weiss*, 440 SW2d 104) was faced with these facts: A woman in labor presented herself to a hospital emergency department. The nurse on duty called Dr. Weiss who had never seen the patient, Mrs. Childs, before.

Dr. Weiss, under these circumstances, was under no duty whatsoever to examine or treat Mrs. Childs. When advised by telephone that the lady was in the emergency room, he did what seems to be a reasonable thing and inquired as to the identity of her doctor who had been treating her. Upon being told that the doctor was in Garland, he stated that the patient should call the doctor and find out what should be done. This action on the part of Dr. Weiss seems to be not only reasonable but within the bounds of professional ethics. (Childs v Weiss, p 107)

An hour later Mrs. Childs was delivered of the baby in a car en route to another medical facility. The baby lived 12 hours. Because the court found that medical judgment did not indicate an emergency and because no physician–patient relationship existed, it found that there had been no abandonment of the patient.

Since the 1960s the public has come to expect hospitals to provide care to all who present themselves to emergency departments. Under the federal COBRA anti-dumping legislation (COBRA 42 USC 1395 dd) it is illegal to discharge or transfer patients in labor (and patients who are otherwise unstable) unless (1) the benefits of transfer outweigh the risks or (2) the patient refuses to stay at the hospital.[3] The legal outcome of the Childs case would likely be different in the 1990s. The physician should understand the increasing public expectations related to the right of everyone to have competent, prudent health care.

Issues of patient abandonment were included in a case involving a hernial repair after which the patient suffered pain and lack of sexual function (*Collins v Meeker*, 424 P2d 488 Kan [1967]). The external inguinal ring had been closed too tightly on the spermatic cord, and the patient eventually underwent orchiectomy. The patient sued the referring physician, the surgeon who performed the herniorrhaphy, and the surgeon who explored the herniorrhaphy site. Another surgeon not named in the suit performed the orchiectomy. The surgeon who explored the surgical site found no basis for the patient's complaints and then discharged him from his care, telling him that he was "sick in the head" (a singularly unfortunate way to end any relationship). Aside from the issues of negligence the court responded to the abandonment charge:

> In other words, once initiated, the relationship of physician and patient continues until it is ended by the consent of the parties, revoked by dismissal of the physician, or until his services are no longer needed. A physician has a right to withdraw from a case but if he discontinues his services before the need for them is at an end, he is bound first to give notice to the patient and afford the latter ample opportunity to secure other medical attendance of his own choice. If a physician abandons a case without such notice and opportunity to procure the services of another physician, his conduct may subject him to the consequences and liability resulting from abandonment of the case ... (Collins v Meeker, p 498) (Emphasis supplied.)

The court concluded that the combination of negligence in not discovering the condition causing the injury and the discharge by advising the patient that he was sick in the head constituted adequate grounds for remanding the case to the trial court.

DELEGATION OF RESPONSIBILITIES IN THE HOSPITAL

Just as the art of the surgeon has evolved from the Civil War reliance on whiskey and a cautery poker, so has the role of the hospital evolved from that of a human warehouse. For the purposes of this chapter the most striking evolution has been in the legal relationships between physician and hospital and between physician and other health care professionals and workers. The language itself dramatizes the change.

"Master of the Ship" Theory

The old concept of master of the ship almost speaks for itself: The surgeon was compared to the captain of a seagoing vessel; the surgeon was ultimately responsible for everything that occurred in the operating room. The surgeon was the head of the surgical team, the law said, and therefore responsible for each person's actions. The law, slowly perhaps, came to recognize that there were other professionals who had, in the more complex surgical system, specific responsibilities. For example, the sponge nurse is responsible for the sponge count, and the anesthesiologist makes independent decisions.

> Most states hold the surgeon responsible for all negligence which occurs in the operating room at the time he is performing surgery on the patient. While the negligent persons technically may be employees of the hospital, most courts hold that they are, for purposes of performing surgical procedures "borrowed servants" and are responsible for the total supervision and control of the operating room.[2]

A Colorado case is illustrative. While putting on his gown in the operating room a surgeon told an orderly to turn the anesthetized patient on the patient's side. The surgeon then told the same orderly to strap the patient. While the orderly went to get a strap, the patient fell from the operating table and was injured. During the ensuing lawsuit the surgeon argued that he was not liable for the mishap because operation had not begun. The court replied:

> Thus the point at which the surgeon assumes supervision and direction in the operating room is the crux of the problem, not the time when he begins to operate on the patient. We point out that Dr. Beadles' liability in this action is not predicated upon lack of professional skill. (Beadles v Metayka, 311 P2d 711 [1957])
>
> Under the particular facts in the instant case, the jury was justified in determining that Dr. Beadles had entered the operating room and had assumed command and responsibility by giving direct orders concerning the placing of the

patient in position on the operating table even though he was not actually at the side of the patient at that moment ready to make the first incision. (Beadles v Metayka, p 714)

In another case a physician performed a hernia operation on a patient and was told that the sponge count was correct. The physician did not remember removing all the sponges and questioned the nurses and obtained a radiograph that revealed a sponge still in place after surgery. The patient was still in the recovery room and was returned to surgery. The patient sued. The trial court granted the patient's motion for summary judgment as to liability only. The Court of Appeals of Washington reversed this judgment. The court held that the surgeon complied with the medical standard of care when he relied on the positive assertion of the nurses that all sponges had been retrieved. The court held the hospital liable under the doctrine of respondeat superior. The physician was not vicariously liable for the negligence of nurses under the "master of the ship" doctrine (*Van Hook v Anderson* 824 P2d 509-WA [1992]; The Regan Report on Nursing Law. 32[11], 1992).

Respondeat Superior

Respondeat superior (let the master answer) is also called vicarious liability. It is an ancient method of fixing liability—so ancient that it involved masters and servants. If the servant harmed another, the master was liable. When the implications of the application became clear the defense was made that some actions of servants (employees) were beyond the master's control. Respondeat superior hardened into a formula for attaching liability, one that courts reasoned would spread the cost of injuries. Suffice it to say that the formula is applied by courts in medical situations, as in instances of posttransfusion hepatitis (*Cunningham v MacNeal Memorial Hospital*, 266 NE2d 897 Ill [1970]). In one such case the patient in whom hepatitis developed after a transfusion sued the hospital. The hospital was defended on the theory that all standard procedures had been followed and that no laboratory test existed for detecting hepatitis in blood. After finding that the hospital was not negligent the court went on to find that the transfusion involved a sale, not a service. Because, and only because, it was a sale, a commercial transaction, the hospital was liable vicariously for injury that resulted from the sale. The net effect was to spread the cost for injuries resulting from hepatitis to all consumers. Someone has been injured, the courts reason, and even without negligence the injury still exists and must be compensated.

New Relationships

Trends today find surgeons being held responsible only for those events under their control. Courts are finding others such as hospital administrators, nurses, and other health care workers liable for their own actions, and the standard-of-care concept is being applied to them.

The Darling Case

When drafting the complaint that formally begins a lawsuit, lawyers generally include as defendants anyone connected with the fact situation out of which the lawsuit grew. The lawyer is attempting to ensure that anyone liable for the injury does not escape liability, and the lawyer is gaining access to information that probably would not be available unless the person or entity were a party to the lawsuit. When the lawyer representing an 18-year-old man named Darling sued, he named Charleston (Illinois) Memorial Hospital as one of the defendants (*Darling v Charleston Memorial Hospital*, 33 Ill 2d 236 [1965]). In the course of the litigation he persuaded the court that the hospital was independently liable and responsible for its actions. The facts are simple: Darling fractured his tibia and fibula and was taken to the hospital's emergency department. The general practitioner on call applied a cast and admitted Darling to the hospital. Thereafter Darling complained continually about pain. One day after admission, the doctor notched the cast because the toes had become swollen and dark. The toes then became cold and insensitive, and 2 days later the doctor split the cast. Ten days later Darling was transferred to another hospital and to the care of an orthopedic surgeon who amputated the leg 8 inches below the knee. The general practitioner settled out of court, but the hospital chose to defend, probably because of the traditional immunity of hospitals to malpractice actions.

> *In fact, however, the plaintiff made no contention that Dr. Alexander was the hospital's agent. Instead the plaintiff contended and the court held that* the hospital itself had breeched duties it owed the patient directly. *It was not responsible for the physician's failure, but for its own.*[4] (Emphasis supplied.)

The hospital argued that it had followed due care for hospitals in the community; it claimed that it had done all that was usual and customary and that it had not deviated from the norm of the standard of care for hospital practice. The plaintiff's lawyer introduced the bylaws of the hospital, bylaws that permitted hospital administration to require consultation. The Illinois Supreme Court thought them helpful:

> *In the present case, the regulations, standards and bylaws which the plaintiff introduced into evidence, performed much the same function as did evidence of custom. This evidence aided the jury in deciding what was feasible and what the defendant knew or should have known. (Darling v Charleston Memorial Hospital, p 332)*
>
> *Using this new measure of the hospital's duty, the Appellate Court found that the hospital was negligent (1) in failing to use reasonable care to see that only persons duly qualified to perform orthopedic surgery were allowed to do so; (2) in failing to require consultation with members of the hospital staff skilled in the techniques involved; and (3) in failing to have a sufficient number of nurses for bedside care capable of recognizing and reporting the progressive gangrenous condition of plaintiff's right leg.*[4]

The Illinois Supreme Court agreed, and a precedent was set. The case acknowledges reality in that the hospital does provide more than four walls within which medicine is practiced. The hospital with its personnel and equipment affects every aspect of the physician's practice. The Darling case left no doubt that the hospital is independently liable for the totality of the practice of medicine occurring within its walls. It is important then that hospitals follow their bylaws and that surgeons familiarize themselves with these hospital responsibilities.

Embryonal Remnants in Inguinal Hernia Sacs

Inguinal herniorrhaphy is the most common general surgical procedure performed on neonates and young pediatric patients. The vas deferens and epididymis are vulnerable to damage, including transection during inguinal exploration or hernia repair. Glandular or tubular epithelial-lined structures are sometimes found on pathologic examination of hernia sac tissue. Significant legal implications arise when embryonal remnants are mistakenly identified as true vas deferens or epididymis.[5]

This problem of misidentified true vas deferens or epididymis is sometimes magnified by time pressures imposed by legal requirements to report possible medical complications quickly. The law of the state of New York requires that significant complications be reported by telephone within 24 hours, followed by a full written report within 5 days. The report must include the names of the alleged involved physicians.

The case that follows illustrates the medicolegal consequences that can occur after the mandated immediate nonsubstantiated report of complications. The case involved an alleged bilateral vas deferens in-

jury during a bilateral inguinal herniorrhaphy in a 7-month-old boy. Review of the surgical pathologic specimen showed that both hernial sacs did indeed contain segments of vas deferens structures. These, based on the findings at reexploration, were consistent with duplication or embryonic remnants of the vas deferens. The vas deferens was found to be normal and uninjured bilaterally. The legal ramifications remain unclear. Since there is no clearcut method to retract the allegation, the physician's profile may be permanently damaged.[6]

PHYSICIAN–PATIENT PRIVILEGE

The law in considering what may or may not become evidence admissible at trial has carved out a series of what it calls privileges: attorney–client, priest–penitent, physician–patient. The privilege means that the attorney, priest, or physician may not be required to reveal, at any stage of the legal proceedings, information imported in confidence while the formal relationship exists and about matters germane to the relationship. The privilege belongs to the client, penitent, or patient and can be waived. In the case of the physician–patient relationship the release or waiver occurs when the patient signs a written release (to a stated individual) of information contained in the hospital record. Information obtained during the relationship should be segregated, kept confidential, and released only to authorized authorities. Although the law labels them "eavesdroppers," the privilege extends to nurses, orderlies, and receptionists. Patients can expect their confidences to be honored by all health care workers assisting the physician. Apart from waiver a doctor's records may be subpoenaed; the document should be kept on file after it is honored. When statutes mandate reporting by physicians, the privilege is overridden by the statute. The laws typically require reporting in instances of child abuse, infectious disease, and evidence of trauma.

A Utah Supreme Court case (*Berry v Moench*, 331 P2d 814 [1958]) involved the factual situation of a psychiatrist releasing confidential information to the parents of the patient's fiance after the parents sought to learn the psychiatrist's impression of the man. The physician responded with a letter derogatory toward the patient. The patient sued for libel and slander, and the court discussed the nature of the privilege:

> *. . . it is obligatory upon the doctor not to reveal information obtained in confidence or treatment of his patient. It is our opinion that if the doctor violated that confidence and published derogatory matter concerning his patient, an action would be for an injury suffered. (Berry v Moench, p 817)*

Privileged information about a patient cannot be made public. However, during conversations with his or her attorney, a defendant-physician has the right to reveal previously privileged information about the plaintiff. Previously privileged information can also be revealed during depositions and trials. In addition to revealing previously known information, the physician being sued has the right to conduct investigations to learn of the patient's true degree of damages or disability. For example, in *Adlerstein v South Nassau Communities Hospital* (Supp 439 NY S2d 605), the patient claimed that he had been rendered sterile by the malpractice of the defendant-physicians. The Court of Nassau County ruled that by bringing a personal injury action (lawsuit), the patient put his physical condition in controversy and must therefore submit to physical examination. He also waives physician–patient privilege.

In this ruling the court judged that the taking of roentgenograms would be permitted, although a myelogram or cystoscopic examination would be too invasive or dangerous to demand. Although the taking of semen analysis may be embarrassing or even humiliating, the court ruled it could be ordered in the case of a claim of infertility.

The court ruled it reasonable that the patient submit to (1) a physical examination, (2) history-taking, (3) semen analysis, and (4) blood studies given by a physician of the defendants' choice.

THE PHYSICIAN AS WITNESS

Physicians are with increasing frequency being called into the courtroom to offer professional testimony. Sometimes the appearance is voluntary or paid for by fee; other times it is compelled by subpoena. Most of the time the appearance is dreaded, but it need not be the harrowing experience that some physicians have suffered and most expect. Preparation is the key, preparation to the point of rehearsal. The attorney should have a list of questions that he or she intends to ask, and the attorney should be able to anticipate most of the questions that the witness will be asked on cross-examination. A rehearsal should be held a few days before trial.

At trial, the physician is well advised to avoid the role of advocate. No sides should be taken, and in no event should testimony be slanted. Testimony is most effective when it is impartial medical truth; such testimony also happens to be less susceptible to attack. Attack will surely come during cross-examination, and it will come from every angle. Answers to cross-examination should be medical truth, and the witness who wavers from an already recorded answer may find himself or herself skewered. If the physician

keeps in mind that a few points will be scored, and if the physician avoids arguing and display of anger or irritation, the experience need not be terrible. If it is thought of as an intellectual exercise with a stranger, it can even be educational. There is no substitution, however, for preparation. It should be insisted on.

CONCLUSIONS— A STATUTORY EXAMINATION

Workers' compensation is the one area in which the paths of law and medicine most frequently cross for the hernia surgeon. It is a source of great frustration to both the patient seeking compensation and the physician, unless each is well aware of the specific provisions concerning the compensable hernia.

Statutory Language

The statutory language used by various workers' compensation statutes is relatively consistent in requirements of the conditions, origin, and reporting of various illnesses and injuries deemed compensable. The laws concerning job-related hernias are an exception. Hernia statutes are much more specific as to the conditions that constitute a compensable rupture. Historically they have been made specific to protect the employer from compensating for hernias incurred by employees that in fact did not arise out of their employment. It is difficult to file a fraudulent claim for a broken arm because of the origin and nature of the injury. The nature of a hernia makes it relatively simple to abuse the standard requirements of most workers' compensation statutes. Thus it was the exceptional nature of the injury that spawned the special provisions that now are in effect.

The specific requirements for a compensable hernia vary from state to state, but most states (including Illinois) adhere to the following conditions:[7]

1. *That there be an accident arising out of and in the course of employment resulting in a hernia*
2. *That the hernia appear suddenly or immediately*
3. *That the hernia be accompanied by pain*
4. *That the hernia did not exist before the accident or event*
5. *That proper notice was given within a specified time (In Illinois the employer must be notified of the occurrence of a hernia within 15 days of the event.)*
6. *That resort to a physician takes place within*

the specified period after the incident resulting in the hernia

7. That there was immediate cessation from
work

Many believe that the ironic outcome of such statutorial provisions is that they, in fact, foster the
fraudulent claims that they were designed to prevent.
Dishonest workers, they say, will avail themselves of
these compensation requirements and follow them to
the letter. Honest workers will quite often fail to follow the provisions either through ignorance or diligence, not letting a slight abdominal pain or discomfort keep them from doing their jobs. Two examples
taken from the *Medical Journal of Australia* illustrate
the point:

> *The first man has had a small or medium-sized hernia for
> some years. He decides that he will have it operated upon at
> the insurer's expense. In the presence of witnesses, he com-
> plains of some or all of the symptoms stated in the classical
> description, and fulfills the legal obligations of reporting it.
> This patient would be accepted as a liability, yet he is dis-
> honest.*
>
> *The second man does heavy work, and accidentally feels
> a lump in the groin. It is not causing any disability, but it
> is almost certain that he acquired it during the course of his
> work, yet he does not know how, when, or where. He is hon-
> est and says he does not know when or where the hernia oc-
> curred; he is denied compensation.*[8]

Of the many parties involved in a compensation
claim for a hernia, the employee's physician has the
greatest opportunity to differentiate between the
valid and the fraudulent claim, because he or she is
the one who knows both the medical history and condition of the worker as well as the story of how the
hernia initially occurred. Following the statutory provisions alone is often an inadequate method of assessment. In fact, a second caveat needs to be registered
for the language of the statute: look at the words with
which one is dealing. What conditions constitute an
accident? What length of time corresponds to "immediately"? Is minor discomfort sufficient to describe
"pain," or must the sensation be incapacitating? Finally, is it reasonable from a medical standpoint to ask
that a physician discern the age of a hernia within a
month or even 2 weeks? These are important questions because the outcome of several cases has turned
on the definitions assigned to these words. It would
behoove the physician to become familiar with the
statutory definitions of individual states and their judicial interpretation in order that the system function
smoothly and efficiently.

Whether or not an employee has suffered an accident within the provisions of the compensation law

has been called a mixed question of law and fact that
is to be answered by the conditions of the individual
case (*Derby v Swift and Co.* 188 Va 336 [1948], p 344).
However, the generally accepted definition of a compensable accident is as follows:

> *An event happening without any human agency, or, if
> through human agency, an event which, under the circum-
> stances, is unusual and not expected by the person to whom
> it happens. Where the effect was not the natural and prob-
> able consequence of the means employed, and was not in-
> tended or designed, the injury resulting was produced by
> accidental means. (Derby v Swift and Co., p 336) (See
> also Williams v Industrial Commission, 68 Ariz. 147
> [1949]).*

Even with this fairly definitive statement of what
constitutes the event, states still differ as to the "accidental" conditions required for compensation. The
key question is, "Must a hernia arise out of an accident
in order to be compensable, or is a hernia that is incurred in the normal duties of employment sufficient
for compensability?" The question arises not from disagreement over the definition of an accident but
rather over the section of that definition that is to be
given the greatest emphasis.

States that have a propensity for strict statutorial
construction rely on the definitional phrase, "The
event was not the natural consequence of means employed." In other words, an accident causing a hernia
in an employee need be an extraordinary occurrence—the employee slipped, had a collision, fell—to
be compensable. States whose legislators are not strict
constructionalists prefer to rely on the phrase, "an
event not expected by the person to whom it happens." The injury need only be unexpected to be compensable; no occurrence outside the realm of normal
employee duties is needed for recovery.

A good example of a case of strict construction is
Allen v Wolverine Express, Inc. In this case the employee
suffered a hernia while engaged in his normal duties,
those of a truck operator. The man was originally
awarded compensation by the Michigan Department
of Labor and Industry. On appeal by the employer,
the Michigan Supreme Court reversed the decision,
stating that the hernia did not result from a "fortui-
tous happening" (*Allen v Wolverine Express, Inc.,* 279
Mich 621 [1937] p 623; see also *Hooks v City of Wyan-
dotte* 278 Mich 232 [1936], and *Williams v National
Cash Register Co.* 272 Mich 553 [1935]).

Contrasted to this case is a South Dakota ruling,
Johnson v La Bolt Oil Co., in which the employee also
sustained a hernia during the performance of his regular duties. The court ruled in favor of the employee,
stating that:

We are of the opinion that to constitute an injury "by accident," it is sufficient that the injury itself is unexpected, and that it is not necessary that the cause of the injury should be untoward or unexpected, occurring without design. (Johnson v La Bolt Oil Co., 62 SD, 391 [1934], p 395) (See also Hardware Mutual Casualty Co. v Sprayberry, 195 Ga 393 [1943], and Derby v Swift and Co., 188 Va 336 [1948].)

Interstate disagreements also occur in the area of statutorial time requirements concerning hernia. For instance, what length of time is allowed between the occurrence of an accident and the subsequent discovery of a hernia as described by the phrase, "The hernia must immediately be preceded by trauma arising out of the course of employment" (Ill Rev Stat ch 48 138.8)? The Colorado Supreme Court has held

. . . immediately means within a reasonable time, without unnecessary delay. It has been held that the word "immediately" is not synonymous with "instantly" and "without delay." (Central Surety and Insurance Corporation v Industrial Commission, 84 Colo 481 [1928], pp 491, 492)

In the same case the court ruled that a span of some 3 days between the alleged accident and the diagnosis of hernia was a sufficiently short time to satisfy the statute's language. The Illinois Supreme Court, however, denied recovery to an employee who incurred pain and in whom strangulated hernia was diagnosed less than 12 hours after the incident that supposedly caused the injury. The court stated:

This incident occurred shortly before noon on Saturday. . . . The appearance of the hernia at midnight was accompanied by pain, but it is clear that within the contemplation of the statute it was not immediately preceded by trauma arising out of and in the course of his employment. (Mirific Products Co. v Industrial Commission, 356 Ill 645 [1934])

Medical Evidence

In addition to the difficulties of statutory language there is a second area in which a physician and an employee-patient often find problems. It involves the realm of medical evidence, and the trouble stems from the fact that several stipulations of workers' compensation law dealing with hernia are arguably not realistic in light of the medical facts. The first of these inaccurate provisions deals with the presence of pain with the occurrence of a hernia. It will be remembered that the statutes generally require that in order to be compensable, a hernia must be accompanied by pain and the pain and injury must be such as to cause immediate cessation of work. Hernias that oc-

cur this suddenly and completely tend to be the exception rather than the rule. Most hernias cause a degree of discomfort, if any sensation at all.

A second provision that affects the physician and surgeon more directly involves the requirement that the hernia did not exist before the accident or event. The requirement necessitates that the physician determine the length of time the hernia has been present. The usual scenario begins with a worker going to a physician and complaining of abdominal pain or a lump that has recently been discovered. The patient states that a week or so ago he had engaged in some extremely heavy work at his job. An examination is made, the presence of a hernia is diagnosed, and an operation is performed. After the operation the physician is approached by the employer or an insurance carrier wanting to know if the age of the hernia was such that it could not have existed before the date of the employee's accident. A definitive answer is not always forthcoming. It may be possible in some cases to identify an extremely long-standing hernia by the presence of a thickened sac adherent to the surrounding tissues. If such conditions are not present, then the age of the hernia may be anywhere between a week and several months.

If a worker has what may be termed a congenital weakness or predisposition to a hernia, the condition in itself will not cause denial of compensation if that worker should incur a hernia during employment. However, if an employee does have a hernia existing before any accident, and then the hernia is aggravated or strangulated through an incident of employment, no compensation will be made (*Cuneo Press Co. v. Industrial Commission* 341 Ill 569 [1930]; see also the work of Ludes and Gilbert[9]). Thus it is advised, for the patient's sake, that careful records be kept in this area for those patients engaged in physically demanding occupations. Workers who incur non–work-related hernias should be encouraged to have them repaired while the expense would be minimal, rather than risk job-related aggravation that would be much costlier in terms of health and money yet not be compensable.

It is obvious that the provisions and language of the statutes are not perfect. But that does not change the fact that it is still the law as it now stands. For physicians or surgeons who deal with the diagnosis and correction of hernia it is only a matter of time before they are involved in some facet of the legalities concerning compensable hernia, whether through insurance questionnaires, depositions, or even in court itself. The most efficient manner for serving the patient's best interests while concomitantly reducing the time and inconvenience incurred by the physician is for the physician to become familiar with statutory provisions concerning compensable hernia. Surgeons should learn what legal requirements need to be fulfilled and discern which provisions are feasible in light of medical fact and which are not. The questions that the physicians face in court mainly concern the areas covered in this section: the traumatic nature of the hernia, the existence of a previous hernia in the patient, and the age of the given hernia. If it is not possible to give a definitive answer, the surgeon should say so but should be prepared to explain why such an answer cannot be given. Such knowledge and preparation alleviate many of the legal difficulties encountered by the physician and ensure more complete and justifiable handling of the patient's case.

REFERENCES

1. American Medical Association. The best of law and medicine, 70/73: a collection of 154 of the 161 articles published in the Law and Medicine section of JAMA from July 6, 1970–July 30, 1973. Chicago, American Medical Association, 1974:1.
2. Holder AR, ed. Medical malpractice law. New York, John Wiley & Sons, 1975.
3. Frew S, Roush W, LaGreca K. COBRA: implications for emergency medicine. Ann Emerg Med 1988; 17:835.
4. Rapp J. Darling and its progeny: a radical approach toward hospital liability. Ill Bar J 1972;60(July):883.
5. Popek EJ. Embryonal remnants in inguinal hernia sacs. Hum Pathol 1990;21:339.
6. Tolete-Velcek F, Leddomado E, Hansbrough F, Thelmo WL. Alleged resection of the vas deferens: medicolegal implications. J Pediatr Surg 1988;23(1 pt 2):21.
7. Blair EH, ed. Reference guide to workmen's compensation, section 7. St. Louis, Thomas Law Book Co., 1974:1.
8. Turnbull H. Inguinal hernia: a compensation problem. Med J Aust 1968;1:190.
9. Ludes FJ, Gilbert HJ, eds. Corpus juris secundum. Workman's compensation section 555 (13). New York, American Law Book Co., 1958.

Editors' Comment

This chapter is an overview of the medicolegal aspects of surgical practice and of the relationships between physicians and their patients. Whereas the discussion is focused on hernia through the choice of examples and recent legal cases, the main thrust of the discussion applies broadly. This chapter is thus a useful review for all practicing surgeons, particularly in the current climate of medical liability.

In his editorial comment on this chapter published in the second and third editions of *Hernia*, Nyhus highlighted the historical perspective of A.H. Iason relative to industrial liability and workers' compensation as found in the first edition. Because all of this material is still pertinent, Iason's review has been added to this Comment. In essence, the position today under workers' compensation regarding inguinal hernias is that unless the hernia has been detected during a preemployment physical, the appearance of a hernia in an employed person is presumed to be job related. Although all of us recognize that this interpretation applied in the arbitration of workers' compensation claims results in overattribution to the job of the genesis of a hernia, the presumption is likely to remain in the absence of proof that the hernia had some other cause.

Following are the salient historical facts in the worldwide recognition of the liability of employers to provide compensation for industrial accidents.

The first treatise on the subject of occupational diseases was Bernadino Ramazzini's *De Morbis Artificum Diatriba*, Padua, 1700. On November 3, 1838, Prussia took a revolutionary step—the advocacy of an employer's liability act. It was applicable only to railroad workers. In the following year, statutes were passed compelling certain classes of employers to contribute to a sickness fund.

In Europe the industrial revolution, with its consequent economic ills, brought about the first humanitarian factory legislation. The peerage became aware of the beerage. In Ruskin's phrase—concerning Dickens's *Hard Times*—it was "sullen socialism." The legislation was supplemented later by more specific regulations of the general conditions of labor. The actual impetus was given by the English Reform Acts of 1846.

The economic theory—today a truism—that served as a basis for workers' compensation laws was the doctrine of "occupational risks," which held that the risk of economic loss to employer and employee through personal injury to the latter in the course of production should be carried by industry itself. In Europe, generally, before the acceptance of the newfangled doctrine of occupational risks and the consequent adoption of accident compensation, legislative provisions of rights and remedies for personal injury in industry were largely governed by the Code of Napoleon. In the British Empire, the English Common Law prevailed.

Compensation for industrial injuries under the Code of Napoleon was based on the question of fault. An employee could not recover against a negligent employer, nor could a worker recover if the accident was the result of what was (and is) known as the ordinary trade risk. Under the English Common Law, the employer's whole duty to an employee consisted in the use of "reasonable" care for the mere safety of the worker. If the worker's injury was due entirely to the fault or negligence of the employer, compensation was recoverable if the disabled person could prove that damages actually had been sustained by reason of such injury.

There was a widespread movement against compensation legislation when it was first advocated in Europe; such a revolutionary step, it was contended, would be disastrous for industry. The compensation idea, therefore, was first carried out purely on experimental bases. The large-scale industries—mining, navigation, railway transportation—obviously carried high trade risks, and it was feared that the first applications of the enforced compensation laws would work an economic debacle. With the development of large-scale industries and more frequent use of power machinery, together with the expansion of industrial establishments, there was an obvious increase in the trade risks.

In the smaller industries a simple system and scale of compensation for personal injuries prevailed the world over. It was based on the principle that an employee injured in industry should be compensated by the person, or persons, directly responsible for the accident. The Civil Code in continental Europe generally provided legal relief for the worker. It was more readily obtainable than under the English Common Law, but in each case the person liable was supposed to have committed some fault. The plaintiff was obliged to begin suit and to prove some fault or negligence on the part of the employer according to the rules of evidence prevailing in the courts of each country.

The workers' compensation law was introduced in the Reichstag (Germany, 1881) but failed of adoption. Soon thereafter came the famous message to that body by Emperor William I, in which he recommended legislation to compel employers in certain industries to compensate injured workers without regard to the cause of the injury. The royal benefactor recommended the enactment of a bill, not only for the insurance of workers against industrial accidents, but also for industrial sick relief, invalidity, and old-age insurance. The sickness law was enacted by Germany in answer to this imperial message in 1883, the accident compensation law in 1884, and old-age and invalidity insurance laws in 1889.

The principle of compulsory compensation was first recognized in Germany, but the idea of compensation in relation to social insurance was actually in vogue before that time. (It really dates back to the early centuries—see the Kuttenberg Mining Ordi-

nance, enacted in Bohemia, between 1300 and 1310.) With the rise of the wage-earning class there came into being, established by that class (as were economic ameliorative measures generally), different forms of mutual aid.

The provisions of the early laws were, of course, hardly liberal. However, as time went on the undeniable economic value of the compensation principle became obvious to all diehards, and the provisions of the earlier laws were soon extended and broadened. Nowhere, to date, has an attempt been made to curtail in any manner the benefits to be derived from compensation legislation.

In England, the Employers' Liability Act was introduced and passed in 1880. The injured servant still had to prove fault or negligence on the part of the master and had to deal with the insurance companies that the liability acts brought into existence. However, most accidents remained uncompensated. The protection of the Common Law was considerably reduced by judicial decisions that placed in the hands of employers a strong weapon—the defense of "common employment." Lord Shaftesbury and other Tories in the House of Lords introduced tentative measures for the protection of and compensation to employees, which later were transformed into the Employer's Liability Act of 1880. This act was introduced by Mr. Gladstone. The Workmen's Compensation Act of 1897 came into force July 1, 1898.

The English courts, before compensation days, held that traumatic hernia, for example, could occur only from direct violence, resulting in a definite tearing, or rupture, of the abdominal wall. All other hernias were considered to be caused by congenital defects. Few claims were therefore made for traumatic hernia.

The United States was the last of the great industrial nations to evince an interest in social legislation, particularly as it applied to workers' injuries. The compensation movement was started in this country a full decade after the first British laws of 1897. After 1911 there was rapid progress, when nine states enacted compensation laws. By 1920, 41 states, as well as the federal government, had substituted compensation for the old liability law. By 1934 three more states and the four territories had accepted compensation, leaving only Florida, South Carolina, Mississippi, and Arkansas as adherents to the archaic liability system. By 1934 every state except Alabama required employers either to insure compensation risks or to give proof of ability to meet them. Even poor czarist Russia in 1903 had accepted the principle of industrial responsibility for industrial injuries long before it was seriously debated in American legislatures.

In the United States the principle of compensation insurance was first recognized by Maryland when provision was made for injured miners. The first constitutional law was enacted in the state of Washington, and in quick succession each state applied various methods in the adjustment of workers' claims. The first laws in the United States—in 1908—covered only workers under federal jurisdiction. In 1911, 10 American states legalized definite and certain compensation for industrial injuries. By 1916, 31 states had introduced compensation insurance, and a few years later all but 4 states had enacted legislation along compensation lines. Today all states have workers' compensation laws.

R.E.C. and L.M.N.

Hernia, Fourth Edition, edited
by Lloyd M. Nyhus and Robert E. Condon.
J.B. Lippincott Company, Philadelphia © 1995.

Supplementary Reading

Because we hope that this monograph will be used for reference as well as for study, the editors append a list of books and theses, and a few journal articles, pertaining to hernia. This list supplements the references, chiefly to journals, that appear at the ends of the chapters of this book. It is, of course, impossible to include all works on the subject. Seeking a criterion of selection that would produce a practical list, we decided to limit it to those works that are, with a few exceptions, in our combined personal libraries, since we believe they are the best on the various matters they deal with and are available in most medical libraries.

Richter AG. Abhandlung von den Brchen. Linz, Frattner, 1783.

In this classic first edition, Richter describes the partial enterocele that maintains the eponym Richter hernia.

Richter AG. Traité des Hernies, ed 2, vols I and II. Cologne, Edenkoven & Thiriart, 1798.

This two-volume French edition of his classic (Garrison No. 3146) is comprehensive. The first volume primarily deals with groin hernia and its major complications (ie, strangulation, gangrene, and fistula). The scope of volume II is broad and includes sections on perineal, vaginal, diaphragmatic, sacral, and other hernias.

August Gottlieb Richter (1742–1812), Doctor in Philosophy and in Medicine; Counselor and Physician of His Majesty the King of England; Professor of the Medical and Surgical Clinic at the University of Göttingen; President of the College of Surgeons of the same city; Physician for the Principauté of Göttingen; Member of the Academies of Science of Göttingen and Stockholm, of the Society for Physicians of Copenhagen, and of the College of Physicians of Edinburgh.

Scarpa A. Traité Pratique des Hernies ou Mémoires Anatomiques et Chirurgicaux sur ce Maladies. Paris, Gabon, 1812.

Antoine Scarpa (1747–1832), Surgeon Consultant to the Emperor and King; Professor of Clinical Surgery, Venice, Italy.

Hesselbach FC. Neueste Anatomisch-Pathologische Untersuchungen über den Ursprung und das Fortschreiten der Leistenund Schenkelbrüche. Würz-burg, Stahel, 1814. (Courtesy of Dr. Clarence J. Berne, Los Angeles)

The clarity of the illustrations is remarkable. The structures so frequently mentioned in eponymic terms relating to Hesselbach are well demonstrated.

Franz Caspar Hesselbach (1759–1816), Prosector in the Anatomical Theater of Würzburg; Member of the Physical-Medicine Society of Erlangen.

Cloquet J. Recherches Anatomiques sur les Hernies de l'Abdomen. Paris, Méquignon-Marvis, 1817.

Cloquet J. Recherches sur les Causes et l'Anatomie des Hernies Abdominales. Paris, Méquignon-Marvis, 1819.

These two volumes are bound together. The first section deals with normal anatomy, and the second section deals with the anatomy of groin hernias.

Jules Germain Cloquet (1790–1883), Doctor of Medicine; Prosector of the Faculty of Medicine of Paris; Special Professor of Anatomy and Surgery; Ex-surgeon Interne of the Civil Hospitals of Paris; Private Professor of Anatomy and Surgery; Member of the Society for Medical Education; Corresponding Member of the Academy of Natural Sciences of Philadelphia.

Lawrence W. A Treatise on Ruptures, ed 5. Philadelphia, Lea & Blanchard, 1843.

This monograph is a particularly good source for early references to Richter, Scarpa, Cloquet, Hesselbach, Petit, and Potts.

William Lawrence, FRS (1783–1867), Surgeon Extraordinary to the Queen; Surgeon to St. Bartholomew's Hospital and Lecturer on Surgery at the Hospital.

Cooper A. The Anatomy and Surgical Treatment of Abdominal Hernia. Philadelphia, Lea & Blanchard, 1844.

This American edition was taken from Cooper's second London edition. A publisher's note in a preface to the American edition, "Though the work of Sir Astley Cooper upon Hernia has been long before the public, and the importance of his contributions to Surgery universally acknowledged, yet its inconvenient size, that of a very large folio, and its great cost, have almost precluded the practitioners of the United States from having access to it; and were its possession desired, the wish could not now be gratified, as no complete copy of the work can at this period be purchased in London."

This monograph primarily relates to groin anatomy and hernias; however, other forms of abdominal hernia are mentioned briefly.

Sir Astley Paston Cooper, BART, FRS (1768–1841), Surgeon to the King and Consulting Surgeon to Guy's Hospital, London.

Teale TP. A Practical Treatise on Abdominal Hernia. London, Longman, Brown, Green & Longmans, 1846.

A presentation of concepts standard for the time.

Thomas Pridgin Teale, FRS (1801–1868), Fellow of the Royal College of Surgeons and Surgeon to the Leeds General Infirmary.

Dowell G. A Treatise on Hernia: With a New Process for Its Radical Cure, and Original Contributions to Operative Surgery, and New Surgical Instruments. Philadelphia, DG Brinton, 1876.

The "wound man" was a familiar figure in the medical literature of the middle ages. Certain illustrations in this book (p 49) are reminiscent of the wound man.

Greensville Dowell, MD (1822–1881), Professor of Surgery in Texas Medical College; late Professor of Surgery in Galveston Medical College; formerly Professor of Anatomy in Galveston Medical College; Surgeon to the Medical College Hospital; Honorary Member of Boston Gynecological Society.

Warren JH. A Practical Treatise on Hernia, ed 2. Boston, James R. Osgood & Co; London, Sampson Low, Marston, Searle, & Rivington, 1882.

Although Warren (a friend of Dr. Brown-Séquard) visited in France, the French concept of the "bandellette iliopubienne" is not mentioned in his monograph.

Joseph H. Warren, MD (1831–1891), Member American Medical Association, British Medical Association, and Massachusetts Medical Society; formerly Surgeon and Medical Director USA.

Marcy HO. The Anatomy and Surgical Treatment of Hernia. New York, D. Appleton & Co, 1892.

This is a monograph of 421 pages. Marcy borrowed freely from the old masters in production of the illustrations (Cooper, Langenbeck, and Scarpa). The text is limited to the discussion of groin hernias.

Henry Orlando Marcy, MD, LLD (1837–1924), President of the American Medical Association; Surgeon to the Hospital for Women, Cambridge, Massachusetts; Fellow of the Boston Gynecological Society; Corresponding Member of the Medico-Chirurgical Society of Bologna, Italy.

Macready JFCH. Treatise on Ruptures. Philadelphia, P. Blakiston, Son & Co, 1893.

A standard monograph on the subject. A rather extensive section on trusses is presented. A new method for strengthening the internal ring is of interest. He credits Niehans (Zesas: Zentralbl Chir, 1888) as follows: "When the inner ring had been sutured, a large layer of the periosteum from a dog's tibia was placed over the area and fixed by stitches. After recovery, a firm, tense tissue was felt to occupy the region of the inner ring which did not yield any impulse on cough."

Jonathan FCH Macready, FRCS (1850–1907) Surgeon to the Great Northern Central Hospital; to the City of London Hospital for Diseases of the Chest, Victoria Park; to the Cheyne Hospital for Sick and Incurable Children; to the City of London Truss Society; and Surgeon in London to the Merchant Taylors Company's Convalescent Homes at Bognor.

Eccles WM. Hernia: Its Etiology, Symptoms and Treatment. New York, William Wood & Co, 1900.

A large portion of this text relates to the use of the truss.

William McAdam Eccles, MS, FRCS (1867–1946), Assistant Surgeon, West London Hospital and City of London Truss Society; Examiner in Anatomy to the Society of Apothecaries; and Late Demonstrator of Operative Surgery and Senior Assistant Demonstrator of Anatomy, St. Bartholomew's Hospital.

De Garmo WB. Abdominal Hernia: Its Diagnosis and Treatment. Philadelphia, JB Lippincott, 1907.

This text is particularly well illustrated. A section on the treatment of hernia by gymnastics is of interest.

William Burton De Garmo, MD (1849–1936), Professor Special Surgery (Hernia), New York Post-Graduate Medical School and Hospital; Fellow of the New York Academy of Medicine; Member of the American Medical Association and New York State and County Medical Societies; Honorary Member of the Medical Society of Virginia.

Ferguson AH. The Technic of Modern Operations for Hernia. Chicago, Cleveland Press, 1907.

As indicated in the preface, this book presents the surgical phase of the subject. All discussions of etiology, symptoms, diagnosis, prognosis, and treatment other than surgical were omitted. Although the Ferguson operation is given in detail, other types of repair are also discussed.

Alexander Hugh Ferguson, MB, MD, CM, FTMS (1853–1912), Commander of the Order of Christ of Portugal; Professor of Clinical Surgery, Medical Department of the University of Illinois; Professor of Surgery at the Chicago Post Graduate Medical School; President of the Chicago Hospital; Surgeon to the Chicago and Post Graduate Hospitals; Fellow of the International Surgical Association, American Surgical Association, Chicago Surgical Society.

Murray RW. Hernia: Its Cause and Treatment. London, JA Churchill, 1908.

A short text of only 99 pages.

Robert William Murray, FRCS (1860–1940), Surgeon, David Lewis Northern Hospital, Liverpool; Late Surgeon, Liverpool Infirmary for Children.

Gallaudet BB. A Description of the Planes of Fascia of the Human Body, with Special Reference to the Fascia of the Abdomen, Pelvis and Perineum. New York, Columbia University Press, 1931.

B.B. Gallaudet, Department of Anatomy, College of Physicians and Surgeons, Columbia University.

Rice CO. Injection Treatment of Hernia. Philadelphia, FA Davis, 1937.

A comprehensive review of this technique. A 97.6% cure rate was reported in a selected series of 379 patients treated under supervision of the author.

Carl O. Rice, MD, PhD, FACS (1898–1985), Instructor in Surgery, University of Minnesota School of Medicine; Surgeon in Charge of the Surgical Out-Patient Department of the Minneapolis General Hospital; Adjunct to the Surgical Staff of the Minneapolis General Hospital; Surgeon to Asbury Hospital, Deaconess Hospital and Swedish Hospital, Minneapolis; Member of the Minneapolis Surgical Society, American Medical Association, Minnesota State Medical Society, Minnesota Pathological Society.

Schmieden V. Die Operationen bei Unterleibsbrüchen. Barth, von Johann Ambrosius, 1939.

Victor Schmieden, MD (1874–1945) Professor of Surgery, Frankfurt.

Iason AH. Hernia. Philadelphia, Blakiston, 1941.

This comprehensive text is divided into three sections: historical evolution of hernia surgery and technical and medicolegal aspects. An excellent author index is included.

Alfred H. Iason, MD (1891–1974), Consulting Surgeon, Long Beach Hospital; Director of Surgery, Brooklyn Hospital for the Aged; Surgeon, Manhattan General, Madison-Park, Hospitals; Director of Surgery, Queens Memorial Hospital; Attending Surgeon, Trinity Hospital; Instructor in Anatomy, New York Medical College.

Mair B. The Surgery of Abdominal Hernia. Baltimore, Williams & Wilkins, 1948.

This a concise presentation of many of the modern views of the hernia problem. The monograph includes reference to most types of hernias, including diaphragmatic.

George B. Mair, MD, FRFPSG, FRCSE (1914–) Surgeon, Law Junction Hospital, Lanarkshire; formerly First Assistant, Professional Unit of Surgery, University of Durham.

Prat D. Sobre la Anatomia del Canal Inguinal y Tratamiento de la Hernia Inguinal. Bol Soc Cir Uruguay 1948;19:218.

D. Prat, MD, Professor of Surgery, Montevideo, Uruguay.

Surraco LA. Anatomia del Canal Inguinal. Bol Soc Cir Uruguay 1948;19:121.

Luis A. Surraco, MD (1884–1970), Professor of Urology on the Faculty of Medicine, Montevideo, Uruguay.

Watson LF. Hernia—Anatomy, Etiology, Symptoms, Diagnosis, Differential Diagnosis, Prognosis, and Treatment, ed 3. St. Louis, CV Mosby, 1948.

This is one of the most quoted source books on the subject in the modern literature.

Leigh F. Watson, MD, FICS (1884–1963), Certified by the International Board of Surgery; formerly Associate in Surgery, Rush Medical College, Chicago; formerly Assistant Professor of Surgery, University of Oklahoma Medical School, Oklahoma City.

Iason AH. Synopsis of Hernia. New York, Grune & Stratton, 1949.

In the preface to this volume the author indicates that this is a condensation of his 1941 book. New material has been added.

Vogeler K. Chirurgie der Hernien. Berlin, Walter de Gruyter, & Co, 1951.

Karl Vogeler, Head of Surgery at the Krankenhaus in Stettin; Professor of Surgery at the University of Berlin.

McVay CB. Hernia: The Pathologic Anatomy of the More Common Hernias and Their Anatomic Repair. Springfield, IL, Charles C Thomas, 1954.

Although only 40 pages in length this monograph is filled with accurate information presented in a concise yet inclusive manner.

Chester B. McVay, MD, PhD (1911–1987), Clinical Professor of Surgery and Associate Professor of Anatomy, The University of South Dakota School of Medical Sciences; Surgeon, The Yankton Clinic, South Dakota.

Fruchaud H. Anatomie Chirurgicale des Hernies de l'Aine. Paris, G. Doin & Cie, 1956.

Fruchaud H. Traitement Chirurgical des Hernies de l'Aine chez l'Adulte. Paris, G Doin & Cie, 1956.

These two monographs are beautifully illustrated. Everyone interested in this subject should review these fine works.

Henri Fruchaud, Professor of Clinical Surgery, School of Medicine, Angers; Surgeon to the French Forces of Liberation; Surgeon to the Hospital Saint-Louis d'Alep.

Ogilvie H. Hernia. London, Edward Arnold, 1959.

This book was written for two reasons, according to the author's preface. He desired to assemble a number of his personal contributions into one package, and further he wished to present a review of hernia surgery that was "personal and dogmatic rather than transcriptive and obsequious." Sir Heneage Ogilvie has achieved these goals. This monograph is written in the fine British tradition of excellence.

Sir Heneage Ogilvie, KBE, MA, MCh, MD, FRCS (1887–1971), Consulting Surgeon, Guy's Hospital.

Ravitch MM, Hitzrot JM. The Operations for Inguinal Hernia. St. Louis, CV Mosby, 1960.

This book of 64 pages presents succinctly the lives of Bassini, Halsted, Andrews, Ferguson, and Lotheissen as they relate to the subject.

Mark M. Ravitch, MD (1910–1989), Professor of Surgery, University of Pittsburgh; Surgeon-in-Chief, Montefiore Hospital, Pittsburgh.

James M. Hitzrot II, MD (1929–   ), Orthopedic Surgeon, The Johns Hopkins Hospital.

Koontz AR. Hernia. New York, Appleton-Century-Crofts, 1963.

This book embodies many of the author's personal concepts as developed through his years of intense study on this subject.

Amos R. Koontz, MD, DSc, FACS (1890–1965), Surgeon to The Johns Hopkins Hospital; Consultant in Surgery to the Surgeon General of the United States Army; Emeritus Assistant Professor of Surgery, The Johns Hopkins University School of Medicine.

Nyhus LM, Harkins HN. Hernia. Philadelphia, JB Lippincott, 1964.

Lloyd M. Nyhus, MD (1923–   ), then Professor of Surgery, University of Washington School of Medicine, Seattle.

Henry N. Harkins, MD (1905–1967), Professor and Chairman, Department of Surgery, University of Washington School of Medicine, Seattle.

Calman CH. Atlas of Hernia Repair. St. Louis, CV Mosby, 1966.

Carl H. Calman, MD, FACS (1925–   ), Clearwater, Florida; formerly Assistant in Clinical Surgery, Washington University School of Medicine.

McVay CB, Read RC, Ravitch MM. Inguinal hernia. Curr Probl Surg, October 1967;4:1.

Raymond C. Read, MD, FACS (1924–   ), Professor of Surgery, Department of Surgery, University of Arkansas for Medical Sciences; Chief, Surgical Service, Veterans Administration Hospital, Little Rock, Arkansas.

Pinotti HW. Megaesôfago, Motildade do Esôfago e Teste de Refluxo Ácido, Antes e Após Dilatacão Forcada da Cárdia. Tese para concurso de docênia-livre de Clínica Cirúrgica de Faculdade de Medicina da Universidade de São Paulo, Brazil, 1967.

Henrique W. Pinotti, M.D. Department of Clinical Surgery, Faculty of Medicine of the University of São Paulo.

Zimmerman LM, Anson BJ. Anatomy and Surgery of Hernia. Baltimore, Williams & Wilkins, 1967.

A widely read and respected book.

Leo M. Zimmerman, MD (1898–1980), Professor of Surgery, Chicago Medical School; formerly Attending Surgeon, Michael Reese, Cook County, and Chicago Memorial Hospitals.

Barry J. Anson, PhD, Med Sc (1894–1974), Professor of Anatomy, Northwestern University Medical School; Member of Attending Staff, Passavant Memorial Hospital.

Johnson HD. The Cardia and Hiatus Hernia. Springfield, IL, Charles C Thomas, 1968.

H. Daintree Johnson, MD, M Chir (Canta.), FRCS, Honorary Consultant Surgeon, the Royal Free Hospital, London; Senior Lecturer in Surgery, the Royal Postgraduate Medical School, London; lately Member of the Court of Examiners, Royal College of Surgeons of England; Examiner in Surgery to London University.

Ravitch MM. Repair of Hernias. Chicago, Year Book Medical Publishers, 1969.

Gaster J. Hernia: One Day Repair. Darien, CT, Hafner Publishing, 1970.

Joseph Gaster, MD (1911–   ), formerly Assistant Clinical Professor of Surgery at College of Medical Evangelists (now Loma Linda University); former Attending Surgeon, Los Angeles County General Hospital.

Lichtenstein IL. Hernia Repair Without Disability: A Surgical Atlas Illustrating the Anatomy, Technique, and Physiologic Rationale of the "One Day" Hernia. St. Louis, CV Mosby, 1970; 2nd edition, 1986.

Irving L. Lichtenstein, MD (1920–   ), Fellow, American College of Surgeons and Pan American Medical Association.

Weinberg SR, Kovetz A, Lazarus SM. Simultaneous Prostatectomy and Inguinal Herniorrhaphy. Springfield, IL, Charles C Thomas, 1971.

Sidney R. Weinberg, MD, FACS (1912–   ), Clinical Professor of Urology, Downstate Medical Center of New York; Chief Division of Urology, The Jewish Hospital and Medical Center of Brooklyn; Attending Urologist, Long Island College Hospital, Columbus Hospital, Kings County Hospital; Consulting Urologist, Peninsula General Hospital and Samaritan Hospital.

Albert Kovetz, MD (1938–   ), Major, US Air Force; formerly Chief Resident in Urology, The Jewish Hospital and Medical Center of Brooklyn.

Stephen M. Lazarus, MD (1938–   ), Assistant Attending in Urology, The Jewish Hospital and Medical Center of Brooklyn, Greenpoint Hospital, Long Island College Hospital, Columbus Hospital.

Zimmerman LM (ed). Symposium on Surgery of Hernia. Surg Clin North Am 1971;51:1249.

Maurer H-J, Otto W. Die Hiatushernie. Berlin, Walter de Gruyter, 1972.

Hans-Joachim Mauer, Professor of Radiology, Tromsö Norway.

Wilhelm Otto, MD, Bonn, Germany.

Skinner DB, Belsey RHR, Hendrix TR, Zuidema GD (eds). Gastroesophageal Reflux and Hiatal Hernia. Boston, Little, Brown & Co, 1972.

David B. Skinner, MD (1935–), Dallas B. Phemister Professor and Chairman, Department of Surgery, The Pritzker School of Medicine, The University of Chicago Hospital; Surgeon, The University of Chicago Hospital.

Ronald H.R. Belsey, MS, FRCS (1910–), Senior Cardiothoracic Consultant, South West Region; Surgeon-in-Charge, Department of Thoracic Surgery, Frenchay Hospital, Bristol, England.

Thomas R. Hendrix, MD (1920–), Professor of Medicine and Chief, Division of Gastroenterology, The Johns Hopkins University School of Medicine; Physician, Johns Hopkins Hospital.

George Dale Zuidema, MD (1928–), Warfield M. Firor Professor of Surgery and Director, Department of Surgery, The Johns Hopkins University School of Medicine; Surgeon-in-Chief, The Johns Hopkins Hospital.

Smith RA, Smith RE. Surgery of the Oesophagus. The Coventry Conference. New York, Appleton-Century-Crofts, 1972.

R. Abbey Smith, ChM, FRCS, FRCSE, Consultant Thoracic Surgeon, South Worchestershire, South Warwickshire, Coventry and Burton Hospital Groups.

R.E. Smith, MA, MB, BCh, FRCP, Area Director of Postgraduate Medical Education, Warwickshire.

Van Ackeren H. Chirurgie der Bruche des Erwachsenen. In Baumgartl F, Kremer K, Schreiber HW: Spezielle Chirurgie fr die Praxis, Band II, Teil 3. Stuttgart, Georg Thieme, 1972.

Herman Van Ackeren, MD, Department of Surgery, Marienkrankenhaus, Hamburg, Germany.

Sorensen HR, Jepsen O, Pedersen SA (eds). The Function of the Esophagus. Proceedings of a European Symposium, Odense University, October 16–18, 1972. Odense, Denmark, Andelsbogtrykkeriet, 1973.

H. Rahbek Sorensen, MD, Professor, Odense University Hospital.

O. Jepsen, MD, Professor, Odense University Hospital.

S.A. Pederson, MD, Research Fellow, Odense University Hospital.

Corral EV. Estudio de la Utilizacion del Tracto Iliopubiano en la Reparacion de Hernias Inguinales con Abordaje por via Preperitoneal: Revision De 76 Casos. Tesis, Universidad Autonoma de Chihuahua Escuela de Medicina, Chihuahua, Mexico, 1974.

Elias Valenzuela Corral, MD, University of Chihuahua.

Petit J. Methode Originale de Traitement des Hernies de l'Aine et de Leurs Recidives: L'Interposition sans Fixation d'une Prothese en Tulle de Dacron par Voie Indirecte: A Propos de 168 Observations. Thèse pour le doctorat en médecine, Paris, Universite D'Amiens, 1974.

Jacques Petit, MD, Department of Medicine and Pharmacy, University of Amiens.

Ghahremani GG, Meyers MA. Internal abdominal hernias. Curr Probl Radiol 1975;5:1.

Gary G. Ghahremani, MD, Professor of Radiology, Chairman, Department of Diagnostic Radiology, Evanston Hospital, Evanston, Illinois.

Morton A. Meyers, MD, Professor of Radiology, Cornell University Medical College—New York Hospital, New York, New York.

Kimberly RC. Problems of Recurrent Hernia. Springfield, IL, Charles C Thomas, 1975.

Robert C. Kimberly, MD (1909–), Instructor Emeritus, The Johns Hopkins University School of Medicine.

Sanabia Vadez J. Estudio Anatomo-clinico de la Utilizacion de la Fascia Transversalis en el Tratamienta Quirurgico de las Hernias de la Region Inguinal. Doctoral Thesis, University of Madrid, 1975.

J. Sanabia Vadez, MD, Attending Surgeon, Hospital Provinciale, Madrid.

Cordiano C, Querici Della Rovere G. L'Incontinenza Cardiale: Fisiopatologia—Clinica—Terapia. Padova, Piccin Editore. 1976.

C. Cordiano, MD, Institute of Surgical Pathology of the University of Padova, Seat of Verona.

G. Querci Della Rovere, MD, Institute of Surgical Pathology of the University of Padua, Seat of Verona.

Gahagan T, Lam CR. Esophageal Hiatus Hernia—Rationale and Results of Anatomic Repair. Springfield, IL, Charles C Thomas, 1976.

Thomas Gahagan, MD (1926–1967), late Associate Surgeon, Division of Thoracic Surgery Henry Ford Hospital, Detroit.

Conrad R. Lam, MD (1905–1990), Consultant in Thoracic Surgery, Henry Ford Hospital, Detroit.

Murakami J. An Atlas of Groin Hernia Repairs Without Recurrences and Complications. Tokyo, Maruzen, 1977. In Japanese.

Jiro Murakami, MD, Head, Department of Surgery, Murakami Memorial Hospital, Gifu, Japan.

Nyhus LM, Condon RE. Hernia, ed. 2. Philadelphia, JB Lippincott, 1978.

Lloyd M. Nyhus, MD (1923–), then Professor and Head, Department of Surgery, the Abraham Lincoln School of Medicine, University of Illinois at the Medical Center, Chicago.

Robert E. Condon, MD (1929–), Professor and Vice-Chairman, Division of Surgery, The Medical College of Wisconsin, Milwaukee.

Moftah A. A Study of Factors Concerned with Herniation Through the Anterior Abdominal Wall Aponeurosis. Thesis in partial fulfillment of the requirements for the degree of doctor of medicine, Faculty of Medicine, Cairo University, 1978.

This work was performed in the surgical unit of Professor Omar M. Askar, Faculty of Medicine, Cairo University.

Ponka JL. Hernias of the Abdominal Wall. Philadelphia, WB Saunders, 1980.

Joseph L. Ponka, MD (1913–1993), Senior Staff Surgeon, Henry Ford Hospital, Detroit, Clinical Professor of Surgery, University of Michigan Medical School, Ann Arbor.

Grosfeld JL, Weber TR. Congenital abdominal wall defects: Gastroschisis and omphalocele. Curr Probl Surg 1982;19:159.

Warlaumont C. Les Hernies de l'Aine: Place des Prosthèses en Tulle de Dacron dans leur Traitement. Thèse pour le Doctorat en Médecine, 6 July 1982. Le Clinique Chirurgale du Centre Hospitalier Universitaire d'Amiens.

This work was performed in the clinic of Professor R. Stoppa, University of Amiens.

Chevrel JP. GREPA (Group de Recherche et d'Etude de la Paroi Abdominale), 1982.

This group of surgeons from France publishes a series of monographs dedicated to the subject of hernia. Communications with the GREPA may be made through the following address: Hôpital Avicenne, 125, Route de Stalingrad, F-93009, Bobigny, France.

Houdard CL, Stoppa R. Le Traitement Chirurgical des Hernies de l'Aine. Paris, Masson, 1984.

C.L. Houdard, MD, Professor of Surgery, and surgeon to the Hospitals of Paris, France.

R. Stoppa, MD, Professor, Faculty of Medicine and surgeon to the Hospitals, Amiens, France.

Excellent views of the placement of the giant prosthetic reenforcement of the visceral sac.

Lex A, Valtorta A. Hérnia: Aspecto Clínico e Cirúrgico. São Paulo, Panamed, 1984.

Ary Lex, MD, Executive Director, Central Institute and Hospital of the Clinics, São Paulo, Brazil.

Anacleto Valtorta, MD, Chief of Medicine and Hygiene, Hospital of the Clinics, São Paulo, Brazil.

Nyhus LM (ed). Symposium on hernias. Surg Clin North Am 1984;64:1.

Chevrel JP (ed.-in-chief): Chirurgie des Parois de l'Abdomen. Heidelberg, Springer-Verlag, 1985. In French, English translation: Surgery of the Abdominal Wall, 1985.

Jean Paul Chevrel, MD, Service de Chirurgie Générale et Digestive, Hôpital Avicenne, 125 Route de Stalingrad, F-93009, Bobigny, France. Prof. Chevrel and his colleagues from GREPA (M. Caix, G.

Champault, J. Hureau, S. Juskiewenski, D. Marchac, J.P.H. Neidhardt, J. Rives, and R. Stoppa) have published this exceptionally fine summary of the modern French approach to hernial problems. An English edition was published by Springer-Verlag in 1986.

Louis D. Les Eventrations Post-operatoires. Thèse pour le Doctorat en Médecine, Faculte de Médecine d'Amiens, April 18, 1985.

Didier Louis performed these studies in the surgical clinic of Professor R. Stoppa.

Ellis H, Bucknall TE, Cox PJ. Abdominal incisions and their closure. Curr Probl Surg 1985;22:1.

Harold Ellis, DM, MCh, FRCS, Professor of Surgery, University of London, England.

Timothy Bucknall, MS, FRCS, Senior Surgical Registrar, Westminster Hospital, London.

Peter J. Cox, BSc, FRCS, Senior Surgical Registrar, Westminster Hospital, London.

Bernard F. Cure des Hernies Inguinales Selon la Technique de Shouldice: Notre Experience sur 329 Cas de 1980 à 1984. Thèse pour le Doctorat d'Etat en Médecine, Facultes de Médecine, Université Paul Sabatier and Hôpital de Toulouse, France, October 1985.

This thesis was sent to Dr. Nyhus by F. Lazorthes, Toulouse, France.

Smedberg SGG. Herniography and Hernial Surgery. Doctoral dissertation, Bulletin no. 59, Department of Surgery, Lund University, Lund, Sweden, May 1986.

S.G.G. Smedberg has worked in close collaboration with Professors Albert E.A. Broomé and Åke Gullmo of the Central Hospital, Helsingborg, Sweden.

Terranova O, Martella B, Battocchio F. La Chirurgia dell'Ernia Inguinale. Congresso Internazionale in Onore di Edoardo Bassini, Atti del Congresso. Divisione di Chirurgia Geriatrica, Ospedale di Padova, Italy, 1986.

This is a collection of extended abstracts of papers presented to an international congress held November 28–29, 1986, at the University of Padua, Italy, to honor the memory of Edoardo Bassini. In developing this celebration, Professors Alberto Peracchia and O. Terranova and their colleagues performed a service to the history of hernial surgery.

Ellis FH Jr. Hiatus hernia. Clin Symp 1986;31:1.

F. Henry Ellis, Jr., MD, PhD (1920–   ), Head, Section of Thoracic and Cardiovascular Surgery, Lahey Clinic Medical Center, Burlington, Massachusetts.

Jamieson GG, Duranceau A. Gastroesophageal Reflux. Philadelphia, WB Saunders, 1988.

Glyn G. Jamieson, MS, FRACS, FACS, Dorothy Mortlock Professor of Surgery, Chairman, Department of Surgery, University of Adelaide and Royal Adelaide Hospital, Adelaide, Australia.

André Duranceau, MD, FRCS(C), FACS, Professor of Surgery, Université de Montréal, Chief, Division of Thoracic Surgery, Hôtel-Dieu de Montréal, Québec, Canada.

Devlin HB. Management of Abdominal Hernias. London, Butterworths, 1988.

H. Brendan Devlin, MA, MD, MCh (Dublin), FRCS (England), FRCS (Ireland), FACS, Consultant Surgeon, North Tees General Hospital, Stockton-on-Tees, Cleveland, England.

Hill L, Kozarek R, McCallum R, Mercer CD. The Esophagus: Medical and Surgical Management. Philadelphia, WB Saunders, 1988.

Lucius Hill, MD, FACS, Clinical Professor of Surgery, University of Washington; Surgeon, Virginia Mason and Swedish Medical Center, Seattle, Washington.

Rochard Kozarek, MD, Section of Therapeutic Endoscopy, The Mason Clinic; Associate Clinical Professor, University of Washington, Seattle, Washington.

Richard McCallum, MD, Head, Division of Gastroenterology, University of Virginia School of Medicine, Charlottesville, Virginia.

C. Dale Mercer, MD, FRCS(C), Assistant Professor of Surgery, Queen's University, Director of Surgical Esophageal Research, Queen's University, Kingston, Ontario, Canada.

Barroetaveña J, Herszage L, Barroetaveña JL, Ainstein R. Hernias de la Ingle, ed 2. Buenos Aires, El Ateneo, 1988.

The line drawings are very effective.

Barroetaveña J, Herzage L, Tibaudin H, Barroetaveña JL, Ahualli CE. Cirugia de las Eventraciones. Buenos Aires, El Ateneo, 1988.

This presentation highlights anterior abdominal wall hernias.

Jorge Barroetavena, MD, Chief of Surgical Service, Htal. Sirio-Libanes, Buenos Aires, Argentina, South America.

Radovanovic S, Radovanovic B. Abdominal Wall Hernias. Požarevac. Prosveta, 1988.

A timely survey of most hernia types.

Terranova O, Battocchio F. La Chirurgia delle Ernie della Regione Inguinale e Crurale. Padua, La Ganangola, 1988.

The Bassini, McVay, Shouldice, and Stoppa techniques are given in detail.

Madden JL. Abdominal Wall Hernias: An Atlas of Anatomy and Repair. Philadelphia. WB Saunders, 1989.

John L. Madden, MD (1912–   ), Attending Surgeon, Doctors Hospital; Clinical Professor of Surgery, New York Medical College, New York.

The drawings of the late Frank Robinson are very effective. Mr. Robinson visited the operating rooms of several contributors, thus giving his illustrations a special personal touch.

Nyhus LM, Condon RE. Hernia, ed 3. Philadelphia. JB Lippincott, 1989.

Lloyd M. Nyhus, MD, Warren H. Cole Professor and Head, Department of Surgery, University of Illinois College of Medicine at Chicago.

Robert E. Condon, MD, Ausman Foundation Professor and Chairman, Division of Surgery, the Medical College of Wisconsin, Milwaukee.

Skandalakis JE, Gray SW, Mansberger AR Jr, Colburn GL, Skandalakis LJ. Hernia: Surgical Anatomy and Technique. New York, McGraw-Hill, 1989.

John E. Skandalakis, MD, PhD, FACS, Chris Carlos Professor of Surgical Anatomy and Technique, Emory University School of Medicine, Atlanta, Georgia.

Comprehensive review.

Kogan AS, Veronski GI, Taevski BV. Pathogenetic Basis of Surgical Treatment of Groin and Femoral Hernias. Irkutsk, University of Irkutsk Press, 1990.

This work is dedicated to our anatomic and clinical studies. (The Editors)

Schumpelick V. Atlas of Hernia Surgery. Philadelphia, BC Decker, 1990.

Volker Schumpelick, Professor Dr. Med, Chairman, Department of Surgery, RWTH Aachen, Aachen, West Germany.

This is the English translation of Hernien. Stuttgart, F Enke, 1987.

Nyhus LM, Klein MS, Rogers FB. Inguinal hernia. Curr Probl Surg 1991;28:403.

A classification of hernia types is presented based on defects in the posterior inguinal wall.

Terranova O, Battocchio F, Martella B, Spirch S. Attualita' e Prospettive nella Chururgia delle Ernie e del Laparoceli. Padua, Instituto di Clinica Chirurgica I, 1991.

This is a report of the Second International Congress on hernia problems held in Padua, Italy.

Wantz GE. Atlas of Hernia Surgery. New York, Raven Press, 1991.

George E. Wantz, MD (1923–   ), Clinical Professor of Surgery, Cornell University Medical College, Attending Surgeon, The New York Hospital—Cornell Medical Center, New York.

The illustrations of Casper Henselmann are excellent.

Bulen JA, Bridgman CF. The Hernia Solution: Myths, Facts, Answers. Escondido, CA, Advanced Health Press, 1992.

James A. Bulen, MD, FACS, Chief of Surgery, Palomar Hospital, Escondido, California.

Charles F. Bridgman, PhD, former Director of the National Audiovisual Center of the National Library of Medicine, Bethesda, Maryland.

This is an authoritative guide for patients suffering from a variety of hernia problems.

Rutkow I (ed). Hernia Surgery. Surg Clin North Am 1993;73:395.

Arregui M, Nagan R. Inguinal Hernia: Advances and Controversies. Oxford. Radcliffe Press, 1994.

This represents the content of an international meeting on the subject of hernia, held in Indianapolis, Indiana, 1993.

Bendavid R. Prosthesis and Abdominal Wall Hernias. Georgetown, TX, RG Landes, 1994.

Estrada RL. Internal Intra-Abdominal Hernias. Austin, Texas, RG Landes, 1994.

Battocchio F. Testo atlante di Chirurgia Delle Ernie. Milan, Utet Periodici Scientifici, 1994.

Veleuti G, Scaramuzza P, Testa A. Le Ernie Inguinal, ed 2. Torino, Utet, 1994.

Index

Recurrent hernias (*cont.*)
preperitoneal prosthetic repair of,
165, 167–168, 169f-170f, 206–
208, 207f
prevention of, 242–244
after Shouldice repair, 223, 224t,
225t, 228–229, 233–234
Shouldice repair in, 223
sliding hernias, 305–307
tension-free repair of, 244–245
patch repair in, 245
plug repair in, 244–245, 244f-
245f
preperitoneal repair in, 245
after laparoscopic herniorrhaphy,
266t, 267, 267t
after preperitoneal prosthetic repairs,
203t, 204
rate in audit of groin hernia repair,
85t
spigelian, 390
after ventral hernia repair with
expanded PTFE patch, 332
Reduction en masse, 288–289, 289f
in inguinal hernia, 270
in interparietal hernia, 395, 396f
Reflected fibers of Colles ligament, 184
Reflected inguinal ligament, 25f, 27
Reflux, gastroesophageal, manometry
in, 550, 550f
Regional anesthesia, 218, 504–511. *See
also* Anesthesia, regional
Relaxing incision, 218–219
in anterior iliopubic tract repair, 147–
148, 148f-149f, 150
in Cooper ligament repair, 123, 126f,
128, 130
in preperitoneal approach in inguinal
hernia, 165
Respiratory system, anesthesia
affecting, 502
Respondeat superior, 585
Resuscitation
cardiopulmonary, equipment for,
505t
in strangulating hernias, 289–290
Retroanastomotic hernia
afferent loop, 476, 477f, 479f-480f
of bypassed small intestine, 482, 482f
clinical features of, 478–480
after colostomy, 481f, 481–482
efferent loop, 476, 477f-479f
after femoral-femoral bypass graft,
482–483, 483f
after gastrojejunostomy, 475–481
paratransplant, 483, 483f
prevention of, 480–481
after total gastrectomy with Roux-en-
Y reconstruction, 477f, 478
treatment of, 481

Retropubic space of Retzius, 41, 405,
405f
Retropubic vein, laparoscopic view of,
68, 68f
Retrovesical space, 405f, 408–409
boundaries in men, 408–409
boundaries in women, 409
Retzius space, 41, 405, 405f
Rhodergon velvet, 535t. *See also*
Prosthetic materials
Richter, August Gottlieb, 8
Richter hernia, 286, 311–315
clinical features and diagnosis of,
312–313
history of, 311–312
incidence and site of, 312, 313t
pathology of, 312, 312f
treatment of, 313–314
Right of abdominal domain
hernia contents affecting, 519, 519f
loss of, 275–276
and pneumoperitoneum in giant
hernias, 276, 516, 519
in ventral hernia, 323
Ripstein rectopexy in rectal prolapse,
458–460, 459f, 464
Romberg, Moritz Heinrich, 439
Rosenmüller node, 42

S

Sacral rectopexy in rectal prolapse,
458–460, 459f
Sacrosciatic hernia, 440
Scarpa, Antonio, 7–8
Scarpa fascia, 23–24, 55f
identification of, 137
Sciatic foramen
greater, 441
lesser, 441–442
Sciatic hernia, 440–448
anatomic considerations in, 440–
443
classification of, 442
comment on, 447–448
contents of sac in, 440
etiology of, 440
historical aspects of, 440
incidence of, 440
infrapiriformis, 441f-442f, 442–
443
operative treatment of, 443–447
transabdominal approach in, 444–
445, 444f-445f
transgluteal approach in, 446f,
446–447
wad technique in, 445, 447–448
subspinous, 441f-442f, 443
suprapiriformis, 441f-442f, 442
symptoms and diagnosis of, 443

Scrotum
hernias of, pneumoperitoneum in,
516
postoperative ecchymosis of, 276
Seizures from regional anesthetic
agents, 507
Semicircular line of Douglas, 238f, 382,
383f
laparoscopic view of, 65f, 68f
Semilunar line, 22, 22f, 381, 382, 383f-
384f
Sepsis
and ventral hernia development, 321
wound. *See* Wound infection
Seroma from expanded PTFE patch in
ventral hernia, 329, 334
Sex factors in obturator hernia
development, 432, 432t
Shelving border of inguinal ligament,
26, 42, 55f
Shouldice repair, 10, 217–236
calibration of internal ring in, 233
comments on, 227–229, 236
compared to Bassini repair, 217, 234–
236, 235t
complications of, 224–226, 226t
cremaster muscle resection in, 220, 230
dissection in, 220–221, 229
experience with, 229–234
general principles in, 217–219
history of, 217
local anesthesia in, 219–220, 229
postoperative period in, 223, 233
reconstruction of inguinal region in,
220f-224f, 221–223, 229f-232f,
231–233
recurrence rates in, 223, 224t, 225t,
228–229, 233–234
results of, 223–224
sedation in, 219
technical aspects of, 219–223
transversalis fascia incision in, 220–
221, 230
Shutter mechanism, inguinal, 36, 73–
74, 88, 89f
evaluation of, 119
Sigmoidectomy, abdominal, with rectal
fixation in rectal prolapse,
457–458, 458f
Silastic, 535t. *See also* Prosthetic
materials
Silk sign in inguinal hernia, 97
Silo devices
in gastroschisis closure, 354
in omphalocele closure, 344, 350
Sister Joseph nodules at umbilicus, 363
Skin
preparation for ventral hernia repair,
323
tension lines in groin, 22

Weight of patients. *See also* Obesity
 and anesthesia technique, 502
Wells rectopexy in rectal prolapse, 458–
  459, 459f, 464
White line. *See* Linea, alba
William of Salicet, 6
Women. *See* Females

Wound healing, collagen metabolism
  in, 76
Wound infection
  after inguinal hernia repair, 277
  after Shouldice repair, 225
  from expanded PTFE patch in
   ventral hernia, 329, 332, 334

and hernia development, ventral
 hernia in, 321

Z
Zimmerman repair of sliding inguinal
  hernia, 301, 306f-307f